1 MONTH OF
FREE
READING

at
www.ForgottenBooks.com

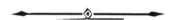

By purchasing this book you are
eligible for one month membership to
ForgottenBooks.com, giving you
unlimited access to our entire
collection of over 700,000 titles via
our web site and mobile apps.

To claim your free month visit:
www.forgottenbooks.com/free786586

ISBN 978-0-483-59311-4
PIBN 10786586

THE
DIETETIC AND HYGIENIC GAZETTE

A MONTHLY JOURNAL OF PHYSIOLOGICAL MEDICINE

VOL. XVII.   NEW YORK, JANUARY, 1901.   No. 1.

THE ESSENTIALS OF HEALTH AND LONGEVITY.

BY W. G. KEMPER, M.D.,
Manitowoc, Wis.

THE ultimate aim of the study of medicine is the prevention of disease; the bringing about of such perfection in the manner of living that but one mode of death—the gradual decay of old age—shall be probable.

It is obvious that we can make no attempt at prevention of disease unless we know the cause. In the last century an empiric flourished whose beautifully simple theory was based on his belief that all diseases were caused by buttercups. Every man, woman or child ate mutton, beef or butter, or drank milk. Cattle and sheep, with their grass, ate buttercups—consequently buttercups were the cause of all diseases. Here the one important hygienic principle was the utter destruction of this direful meadow-blossom.

Many of the theories of medicine of today are as preposterous, or as idiotic, and are built upon total error, stupidity or mere fractions of truths.

The preservation of health and the attainment of old age are of such eminent importance to mankind that, though perhaps ignorantly or heedlessly disobeying the simplest rules of hygiene, many inquirers are spending their lives in the eager search of the alchemical agent. And the heavens, the earth, the Bible, the shadowless spirit-land, even the caldrons of the votaries of the Black Prince, are explored and probed for the unattainable *Elixir Vitae*.

The more ridiculous or incomprehensible the theory of any new cult of universal health, the greater, apparently, is the following. The inanities of a mountebank who denies the existence of pain, or the realities of disease, are enthusiastically applauded by her disciples, many of whom have forfeited their physical welfare by appeasing with too liberal a hand the cravings of their too material digestive apparatus. Said a recent lecturer upon this fallacy: "Whatever may be the evidence given by the corporeal senses, we deny its reality." Here the corresponding hygienic rule is the renouncing of the corporeal senses, for they tell us falsehoods. If decayed teeth trouble you deny that they are decayed, protest against the evidence of your reason, and you may laugh at the dentist.

The ancient custom of wearing amulets to ward off disease has not yet entirely disappeared from even the most civilized communities. And the shriveled potato, to prevent rheumatism, may be found in the mysterious depths of many a pocket.

In this respect the world has made but little progress since the age of the knightly Ponce de Leon, who explored the wilderness of Florida in search of the fountain which was to restore to him his youthful ardor. Or the Flagellants, who in former centuries hoped to propitiate the Divine Being and ward off Black Death, by scourging to the blood one another's bared shoulders.

In all this rummaging for panaceas by

the world at large the very essentials of our well-being are generally overlooked or neglected—the air that we breathe, the food that is to sustain us, and the drink with which we slake our thirst. In the improper use of one or all of these lies in almost every instance the root of our afflictions. And it is a sad reflection upon our vaunted civilization that the lower the station of a race the less common is disease. Joseph L. Stickney, regarding the Basutos in Africa, writes: "They are a thriving people of great physical strength and courage; they are not yet broken by the vices and diseases that too often accompany the approach of civilization." Want compels these simple people to use that which is nearest at hand; the fresh air of the veldt and forest, the pure water of the mountain rill and unadulterated animal and vegetable food. Still lower, among the beasts in the wild state, the ravages of disease-producing germs are sought for in vain. They do not contract typhoid, cholera or malaria for the reason that the micro organisms of these afflictions do not find in their tissues the media favorable to their growth. For a similar reason the observance by successive generations of mankind of proper hygienic principles will not only overcome the inherited morbid proclivities of their forebears, but it will modify the character and virulence of pathogenic bacteria or their products, and will endow the body with a natural immunity against their evil influence; for it is necessary to infection that the tissues shall be, in some degree, disordered.

The bodily vigor is greatly augmented by the habitual respiration of pure air. An atmosphere that is charged with the exhalations of the lungs and skin is a most potent predisposing cause of disease. The oxidizing processes which effect the destruction and the elimination of effete matters from the system, and the activity of cell-growth, will be greatly weakened by even a small quantity of carbonic acid gas. Waste material, completely oxidized, will be carried off in the form of water and carbonic acid; the nitrogenous parts passing

off by the kidneys. But imperfect oxidation converts it into products closely allied to fecal excretions, with which the unrenewed air will become charged. In the midst of a close ill-ventilated atmosphere of this kind it is physiologically impossible for human beings to grow up in a sound state of body or mind. Individuals sometimes accommodate themselves to a most unwholesome atmosphere, but they will usually become victims of the first passing epidemic, to which their death will be ascribed.

The large majority of our dwellings are poorly ventilated. The absolute necessity of a constant change of air, if a perfect condition of health is desired, is but seldom considered of sufficient importance. The unwholesome emanations of the soil are not excluded. With few exceptions the bedrooms are too small and their occupants too many. They should be the largest, sunniest and most pleasant rooms in the house. They should contain plants, which exhale oxygen and absorb carbonic acid. But the fragrance of flowers in sleeping apartments is not healthful. The periodical cleansing of dwellings, by preventing the deposition of pathogenic materials, is an important factor in maintaining the purity of the air.

Breathlessness, lassitude, drowsiness, muscular inertia, anemia and neurasthenia are common results of the inhalation of air that is contaminated, or is deficient in oxygen. Individuals thus surrounded may become uncomfortably obese. The hydrocarbons, not being consumed by a sufficiency of oxygen, are deposited as fat. There is a tendency to neuralgia; aortic and pulmonary murmurs are common. All of which lead eventually to confirmed invalidism.

One of the fertile sources of infantile diseases is a poverty of wholesome air. Toward the end of the last century, in the Dublin Foundling Hospital, during a space of twenty-one years, out of 10,272 children sent to the infirmary only 45 recovered, as a result of deficient ventilation of the wards. Life spent in a pure air and deep expansion of the lungs in an atmosphere charged with health-giving oxygen will effect the perfect aeration of the blood, and will render the system tolerant to the various disease germs which are inhaled with every inspiration; and it will impart to the individual the delightful sensations of energy and vigor.

In a greater measure, perhaps, the good and bad states of the body depend on the food; but it is not always easy, with a balance in hand, to determine that which is proper for each individual. Some persons fatten on a quantity of food on which others would starve. The regimen proper for a man at leisure may be very unfit or insufficient for him that swings the sledge. The appetite would inform every person when he has eaten enough were it not for the seasonings which excite to excess. As Nature has distributed a large variety of nutritive substances a regimen conducive to health need not be uniform, but we should confine ourselves to a few dishes at a time. Desserts may be very tempting to the palate and they are not necessarily unwholesome, but as they are generally taken when hunger is satisfied they do not tend to promote good health or long life. Vinegar, mustard, pickles and other condiments, though necessary in many inactive conditions of the stomach and bowels, in health stimulate the desire for more food than the body requires.

Take simple foods, in quantities sufficient to satisfy hunger, is a dietetic rule of the first importance; and to it may be added that no meal should be taken until the previous one has been digested. Two or three repasts a day, according to the necessities of the individual, are generally sufficient. The proper mastication of food and the thorough intermixture of saliva are very necessary. The rapid feeding at lunch counters is in many cases the prime cause of poor health, needless worry, vexation and eventual breakdown in business men.

"When I see the fashionable tables covered with all the riches of the four parts of the world I think I see gout, dropsy, fevers, lethargy and the greater parts of the other diseases hidden in ambush under each plate," says Addison very truly. It cannot be denied that more sickness can be attributed to the pleasures of the table than to any other cause.

If the potency of the digestive secretions were not weakened many patho-organisms that find their way into our drinking water would be innoxious. The human body has become peculiarly susceptible to microbic invasions, and water, looked upon with suspicion as the habitat of many invisible enemies of man, is imbibed less freely than the system requires. Were it not for the continual flow of this clear product of nature through the tissues our very existence would be impossible. This constantly moving water amounts to two-thirds of our body weight, and every motion, every organic activity, every thought, requires nutritive elements which this common carrier of the organism always holds in readiness for the use and repair of every part. At the same time that it deposits constituent elements it washes from the tissues, as quickly as they are formed, the effete products and removes them through the kidneys, the skin, the bowels and the lungs and prevents their conversion into toxins of disease. The rapid removal of waste matter augments assimilation. Thus the liberal use of water acts as a tonic, improves the appetite and increases the body-weight.

Water is the supreme drink of health. Four pints at least should be daily consumed, as otherwise the effete materials cannot be removed with proper rapidity, and a coated tongue, foul breath, costiveness, tenacious secretions, fetid perspiration and a dense complexion are the results.

It is an excellent diuretic and a diaphoretic of no mean potency. A tumbler full at bed time, by aiding the rapid excretion of waste matter, will prevent that languid, weak feeling of which many well-fed people complain when they arise in the morning. A pint of water in the morning will tone up the digestive organs and stimulate the actions of the bowels; and when too liberal a diet has been indulged in the free consumption of water will prevent manifestations of the gout. It will also aid in the prevention of Bright's disease, by carrying off in greater dilution the azotic matter; care should be taken, however, that it does not contain a common adulterant, which is often contributive to the affection.

The external use of water is as salutary to the organism as the internal. "Cleanliness is akin to godliness." It opens the pores and removes all those decomposed materials that favor the reception of disease.

Some allege that exercise is a prime necessity for the maintenance of well-being; but an individual too languid to move about actively in all probability has sinned against the very hygienic rules for which I am contending, and is not in the best state of health.

Air, food and drink. This trio, rightly employed, is the catholicon, obvious and close at hand, yet unseen by many a narrow enthusiast, who, by the light of glimmering jack-o'-lanterns, is pursuing theories too ridiculous to merit the dignity of an argument. The wealth of no man is great enough to acquire it by purchase, yet it is the certain reward for the judicious practice of self-denial.

These are the elements of hygiene which are peevishly disdained by many an over-drugged and over-operated invalid, while, with astonishing faith and resolution, she is taking the prescribed doses of her last doctor's tonic. And physicians are often at fault in not considering them sufficiently in their etiological investigations. With their minds overloaded with the latest contributions of the bacteriologist they are apt to forget, or to deny the pathological influences of daily habits, temperaments and diatheses.

"Live on a shilling a day, and earn it," was the sound advice given by a great physician to a wealthy nobleman, a gourmand, who had searched the four quarters of the globe for a medicine that would drive away the pains of the gout.

Could mankind be taught and compelled to live in a manner concordant to these principles disease would, in all probability, disappear from the face of the earth; and death would supervene from a general failure of the vital powers, rather than from the abnormal action of any special organ. It would settle the vexed question of alcoholic intemperance, for I maintain that a person in absolutely perfect health will not crave or require alcohol, nor tobacco, tea, coffee or other stimulant, that in the present state of our civilization seem to be necessary.

Spartan simplicity in all that pertains to food; the respiration of air, rich in oxygen, as it is wafted from all points of the compass, and the liberal internal and external use of water, sparkling with purity, will render the body robust, the teeth sound, the joints supple, the motions free, and will give the color of health to the complexion. It will make the understanding acute, the memory happy and sleep refreshing. All the enjoyments of life will be sweetened by an ideal state of health; and, when the soft hand of the Angel of Death is laid on a gray head, dissolution will be as calm and free from pain as the going to sleep of an infant.

NON-ALCOHOLIC MEDICATION.

Mary Snoddy Whetstone, M.D.
Minneapolis, Minn.

In the tenth century of the Christian era the process of distillation was discovered by an Arabian alchemist. By it the active principal of fermented liquors was separated and drawn off.

This spirit he named *Al ghole,* the Arabian name for evil spirit. Time has revealed that the product was well named.

It was eagerly proclaimed the long-looked-for " cure-all."

" If the medical profession is responsible for the wide-spread belief that alcoholics are of service to mankind, it should not be forgotten, that it is to the members of the same profession that the world is indebted for the correction of these errors," is most truly remarked by Martha M. Allen.

We find all down through the centuries there have been physicians who doubted and opposed its claim to merit. In 1802 Dr. Beddoes of England pointed out its dangers in social and medical use.

In 1829 Dr. John Cheyne, Physician General to the forces in Ireland, said:

" The benefits which have been supposed from their general use in medicine and especially in those diseases which are vulgarly supposed to depend upon mere weakness, have invested these agents with attributes to which they have no claim, and hence as we physicians no longer employ them as we were wont to do, we ought not to rest satisfied with the mere acknowledgment of error, but we ought also to make every retribution in our power, for having so long upheld one of the most fatal delusions that ever took possession of the human mind."

Dr. Higginbotham, F.R.S., of Nottingham, Eng., the author of one of the standard medical works, and a most successful practitioner, after having used alcohol for twenty years and practiced without it for thirty years, stated in 1832: "My experience is, that acute diseases are more readily cured without it, and chronic diseases much more manageable. I have not found a single patient injured by the disuse of alcohol, of a constitution requiring it. If I ordered or allowed alcohol in any form, either as a food, or a medicine to a patient, I should certainly do it with felonious intent."

The world has had two great leaders of Scientific Temperance. The first was Dr. Benjamin W. Richardson, of England.

He was one of the most eminent physicians in the history of medicine, a great scientist, chemist and physician. No man has experimented more carefully and critically to ascertain the effects of alcohol on man, than Dr. Richardson. Through his researches the whole aspect of alcoholic medication has changed. He predicts that " the administration of alcohol will become like blood-letting, a thing of the past."

So valuable had been his researches that in 1863, the British Association for the Advancement of Science requested him to investigate certain chemical substances. He spent several years on the study of various forms of alcohol, and sent in his report.

The result of these researches were that he learned purely by experimental observation that, "in the action on the living body. alcohol deranges the constitution of the blood; unduly excites the heart and respiration; paralyzes the minute blood vessels; disturbs the regularity of nervous action; lowers the animal temperature and lessens the muscular action." So unwilling were physicians to believe these statements that his report was not accepted by the association, but was sent back for correction.

At this time Dr. Richardson was not a total abstainer, but as a result of his researches along this line he became one of the world's two great advocates for disuse of it as a beverage, and a medicine.

For the purpose of demonstrating that alcoholic medication was unnecesary as a medicine, Dr. Richardson caused the use of alcohol to be discontinued in some of the leading hospitals of London and published the results. When the brewers, who were large contributors to those hospitals, learned of this they threatened to withdraw their support, if its use was not resumed. So the administration declined to allow the experiment to be continued.

This led to the founding of the National Temperance Hospital in London in 1876.

Our other great leader and champion of Scientific Temperance is Dr. Nathan S. Davis, of Chicago, a physician of great eminence and ability. He was the founder of the American Medical Association, and author of the code of ethics which governs that body, and is a man that all physicians " delight to do honor.' He was instrumental in establishing Mercy Hospital, the first in Chicago, and was connected with it for thirty years, and during that time no alcohol was administered in its wards.

He has been a tower of strength to the National Department of Scientific Temperance, and Non-Alcoholic Medication and in the founding of the W. C. T. U. Temperance Hospital in Chicago. After a series of experiments extending through several years he reported the results in a paper read before the American Medical Association in 1851. They showed that alcohol, instead of increasing animal heat and improving nutrition and strength, it produced reduction of temperature and strength. That the effects of alcohol are simply those of an *anæsthetic* and organic sedative. Like ether and chloroform, its presence diminishes the sensibility of the nervous system and brain, thereby rendering the individual less conscious of all outward and exterior impressions. It has long been one of the paradoxes of human action, that the same individual would resort to the same alcoholic drinks to warm him in winter, protect him from the heat in summer, to strengthen when weak and weary, and soothe and cheer when afflicted in body or mind. With the fact now before us, the explanation is evident.

The alcohol does not relieve the individual from cold by increasing his temperature; nor from heat by cooling him; nor from weakness and exhaustion by nourishing his tissues; nor yet from affliction by increasing nerve power, but simply by diminishing the sensibility of his nerve structures, and thereby lessening his consciousness of impressions, whether from heat, or cold, or weariness, or pain, but has diminished his consciousness of their existance, and thereby impaired his judgment concerning the degree of their action on him.

These teachings were so contrary to the then accepted opinions of alcohol that it is stated that the paper was pigeonholed and never went to the committee on publication, as was usually done with all transactions of the society. However, it was subsequently published in the *Northwestern Medical Journal*. Dr. Davis was one of the founders of the Chicago Medical College, where he lectured for many years and faithfully taught non-alcoholic medication.

In one of his lectures given before a class of students, he said: " The supposed benefits of this class of agents in medicine, are as illusory as they are in general society.

During the last forty-five years I have prescribed for internal use *no* forms of either fermented or distilled liquors in the treatment of either acute or chronic diseases, simply because I had previously proved to my own satisfaction that their effects were a positive hindrance to the recovery of my patient. During all those years I have embraced every opportunity presented by consultation with other practitioners, to study the chemical results obtained by them, and I am certain that there is no disease that cannot be treated more successfully without alcoholic liquors than with."

It was when I was a medical student that I got an arrest of thought on the use of alcohol as a medicine. For some unknown reason to us, the leading professors were led to speak on the subject and discusses it. Except Dr. Palmer, the dean, not one was a temperance man. Yet the burden ot their testimony was, that it was harmful. One who had once been a slave to alcohol, closed his remarks by saying: " If it had never been known as a remedy, the world would be better off, for it had done more harm than good." In a paper read by Dr. Charles T. Davis, before the National Temperance Convention, speaking of the success which has attended the treatment of surgical and medical cases without alcoholic or fermented drinks in the National Temperance Hospital of Chicago, said:

" The lesson already taught has been sufficiently convincing to impress the most skeptical that alcohol is not only unnecessary as an active medical agent, but that in a majority of cases it is an actual hindrance to the recovery of the patient. Slowly but surely every year this great truth is being impressed on the minds of the medical profession." Many cases of prolonged illness or unexpected death, diagnosed as heart-failure should be attributed to alcohol poisoning. A Skilled physician was called in council to see a patient in a comatose condition. After examining the patient and medicines administered, they stepped into an adjoining room, when the consulting physician remarked: "I think some of the coma is due to the repeated doses of brandy given, and if that is discontinued, it will disappear." The suggestion was acted upon, the coma disappeared, and the patient recovered.

Many English physicians are trying to dispense with the use of alcohol in medicines. In St. George's Infirmary, London, where beer was discontinued in the treatment of transient cases, they were ready for dismissal much sooner than before. Thirty old women had been bed-ridden from one to seventeen years, being daily supplied with brandy or beer. When this was discontinued they all improved, so as to be able to leave their beds, and some went to work.

The use of beer by nursing mothers is not uncommon in some localities. Dr. Edmonds, of London, who has given much study to the effects of spiritous liquors during the period of lactation, says:

"Ladies, bear in mind, when you are told to take wine, beer, or brandy, that you are merely distilling that same spirit in your child's frame, out of blood that has been alcoholized."

It is only physicians who have the courage of their convictions, and great independence of character, who will dare to act contrary to the prejudices of the people. Dr. Richardson's prediction is our hope. "When people cease to believe in alcoholic remedies, physicians will no longer prescribe them. But when the majority desire the 'physician's prescription,' as a cover for indulgence, there will always be found physicians willing to give such prescriptions."

Again you may be told that you or your loved one "will die without it," or if you persist, the physician may refuse to assume the responsibility of your case. In the light of the above opinions, have courage to stand firm, and send for another physician if necessary. When dismissal stares a physician in the face, it stimulates his brain to find a substitute for alcohol, in his materia medica.

When a young physician I heard Mrs. Mary C. Nind relate an incident which greatly strengthened my non-alcoholic principles.

"During the session of the Woman's National Temperance League in London in 1876 there was present Mrs. Johnston, of Brooklyn, N. Y., who gave the following experience: 'I was the subject of sinking spells and lost consciousness. My physician prescribed wine at my meals and brandy when I had one of the attacks. At the time of the Woman's Crusade, I was strongly drawn to join their ranks, but thought, how can I work while using the liquors medically. I thought and prayed, and at last resolved to abandon all, and trust God for the results and enter the crusade. I did so. Soon after, while out on the work I had one of my attacks. A physician was summoned. He called for some of the best brandy. I was not so far gone that I could not protest and said "not a drop." "This is no time to be airing your temperance principles, it is brandy or death." "Death it is, then," I said, and added, "send for other remedy in his medical case, and I re-another physician." Then he found an-covered gradually. My heart trouble left me, and I have not had a serious attack for years.'"

Many physicians are prescribing alcoholics as a matter of routine. A physician giving directions to a nurse said: "If the patient's heart becomes weak, you might give a little brandy or whiskey." Seeing reluctance expressed upon the nurse's countenance, he added hastily: "Or strong coffee will do just as well." The nurse in relating this to Martha M. Allen said: "Why could he not have ordered coffee in the first place if he thought it equally good?"

Very few people seem to think of the danger lurking in the various cough mixtures, soothing syrups, and other proprietary medicines given to children and others.

There is no longer any excuse for ignorance or prejudice. Mary Allen fitly remarks: "When the home medicine-chest is purged of all its deceitful and dangerous drugs, and the family physician is requested to not administer alcohclics, there will be fewer premature deaths, and fewer lost souls to be accounted for in the day of judgment."

The use of proprietary medicines should be discontinued because of the large amount of alcohol in most of them.

Fancy good people taking Best's Tonic with 7.6 per cent. alcohol, Paine's Celery Compound containing 21 per cent., or Warner's Safe Tonic with 37.5 per cent., or Beef, Wine and Iron, whose proprietors are more honest in that story, make no pretention to hide the serpent which it contains.

I know of one man who became a drunkard from taking Ayer's Sarsaparilla, and another man had delirium tremens from taking Jamaica ginger, which is nearly pure alcohol. All coco wines and all liquid malt extracts contain alcohol except those put up in thick syrups.

My message would be incomplete if I rested without giving something better to use in the place of alcohol.

The physician has a number of remedies at his command, but for home use there are some remedies that may be found in almost any house. First is *hot water*. As an internal and external remedy its value is incalculable. A cup of hot water sipped is a most excellent stimulant. Headaches, which so often are the result of the retention of impure matter in the system, will usually be cured by drinking freely of hot water at frequent intervals and omitting the next meal.

A half teaspoonful of pulverized ginger in a cup of hot water, or hot peppermint water, is a good stimulant.

For a weak heart or a condition of shock from any cause, there is no restorative so good as applications of hot-water bottles about the heart and extremeties.

Carbonate of ammonia is one of the best remedies for strengthening the circulation, and leaves no depression behind it, and is better than alcohol in any form. Five grains in a little water is an ordinary dose.

If not at hand you may give five drops of aqua ammonia in a little water, or ten to sixty drops of aromatic spirits of ammonia, in a wineglassful of water, or two to five grains of camphor in sugar or a capsule. For poison of snake bites, put some turpentine in a wide-mouthed bottle and place the mouth of the bottle directly over the bite so no air can enter, or ammonia water may be applied the same way. A strong solution of soda may be applied and taken internally.

Another dangerous use of alcohol is in the bath. Very recently I was one of a group who entered into a discussion on the use of alcohol as a medicine. All appearing to be convinced that it was harmful and unnecessary as a medicine, one remarked: "Well, there is no harm in using it in a bath." I answered him by citing the case of a child that had a slight cold, which to relieve its mother gave an alcohol bath. After a little time had elapsed the child manifested alarming symptoms, from which the mother was unable to arouse it. At this stage I was hastily summoned, and found the child had been intoxicated by the alcohol bath. In general a plain water bath meets every indication. If there is an irritation of the skin, a little soda of ammonia or borax dissolved in the water is soothing. If there is excessive perspiration add a little vinegar or juice of a lemon to the water.

Instead of using alcohol to prevent bedsores use a teaspoonful of alum or sulphate of zinc in a pint of water to bathe the portion of the skin subjected to pressure.

For chills the best all-around safe remedy is warmth and rest. For "fainting attacks" lay the patient flat on the back without a pillow, give plenty of fresh air and remove all obstruction to circulation.

For nervous exhaustion the Edinburg Royal Hosp. no longer prescribes stimulants, but food exclusively of milk and eggs in the form of custard sweet or salt. When women learn how to prepare wholesome food for their families there will be little, if any, nervous prostration and less use for a doctor.

But what shall we do for the one who has tarried too long at the wine cup and felt the "sting of the serpent"? Dr. Andrew Clark.

of Nottingham, advises: "That when the intense desire for drink is present it will usually be found that the stomach is out of order. If one-half teaspoonful of pulverized ipecac is taken so as to produce full vomiting the desire for stimulants is immediately removed." Instead of sending one of these unfortunates to an expensive "cure," try the ipecac. Much might be written of the danger of awakening an inherited appetite for alcoholics by administering it as a medicine did time and space permit.

God's word and medical science are agreed that alcohol, whether as a beverage or as a medicine, "is a mocker, whosoever is deceived thereby is not wise."

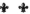

THE PHYSICAL BASIS OF MIND.*

By Brooks F. Beebe, M.D.

ONE year ago, in my opening remarks to you, I insisted upon your appreciation of the truism that *knowledge, to be of the greatest value, must be practical.* You will recall that our worthy Dean in his opening remarks a few days since called your attention to the same, or similar, idea, viz., that "you are to remember that the great aim in the study of medicine is the cure of the sick, the alleviation of suffering, the prevention of disease, etc.," which may properly be called the practical application of our science.

Another thought of greatest import is that *the central idea of all science, its object and end, is the regulation of human conduct.* Every science that the world studies and all knowledge has for its chief purpose right action, and knowledge is defined as "the consciousness of our relations to the external world, ourselves being a part of that world." The foundation of this knowledge comes to us, as you know, through impressions made upon our nervous system and that of others. "Experi-

* An abstract of a lecture delivered to the class in Mental Diseases, at the Medical College of Ohio, October 11, 1900 —Lancet and Clinic.

ence is therefore the source of all knowledge."

If, at birth, we were deprived of our five special senses, or so placed that they could not be used, we would remain as we were born—idiots. The merest tyro in philology knows that the word "education" means to bring out, to lead forth or form, not to cram into. The well-educated person, therefore, is one from whose brain he is able to lead forth ideas for the purpose of regulating his conduct or that of others. As President Jordan, of the Leland Stanford University, says: "Science is the gathered wisdom of the race. It is the flower of the altruism of the ages, by which nothing that lives 'liveth to itself alone.' "

Psychiatry, that branch of medicine which treats of the cure of mental diseases, is perhaps the broadest field of our science. It commands the respect and special attention of the most enlightened of the entire world. The word psychiatry comes from the Greek *psuche*—breath; psucho—to blow—though, very unfortunately, it has crept into meaning, soul. Psuche—breath—has direct reference to breathing as significant of life, a living, moving being or organism.

Our knowledge of mental diseases has become so greatly extended in recent years by pathological facts (the same being also true of every branch of medicine) and by experimental physiology that it is with difficulty we are enabled to recognize in the psychology of to-day that of former times. The study of mental diseases has entered a new era; it has become compulsory in most medical colleges.

Insanity and other diseases of the nervous system are on the increase, to the causes of which I will call your attention later; but in the very beginning I wish seriously to impress you with this fact, that *few diseases are more susceptible to cure when taken in the early stage.* It is just as easy to do great things as small, if one only knows how. For instance, until very recently it was considered an impossible thing to *see* internal parts of the body. The X-rays make that now very simple.

"Mind is recognized universally and instinctively as the greatest thing in man;" but do not forget that mind, to be sound, must be in a sound body—"*Mens sana in corpore sano.*" Every form of deterioration of the nervous system shows itself in lessened power. As a result of bad heredity, insufficient or improper education, pernicious environment, precocious activity, bad habits, disease, etc., there is a lessened power to know and to choose the proper thing, and a wrong choice leads to failure, to degeneration, to death. So that the physician becomes a high priest —nay, the highest priest, in the estimation of many—in the production of happiness and good to the world.

To some extent the subject of mental diseases is not an easy one to teach.

I cannot say that knowledge of mental diseases is more important than that of physical diagnosis, but, on the contrary, if only the diseases of purely psychic nature are considered, pure insanities being but few in number as compared with all the diseases that a physician treats, I should not hesitate to say that general physical diagnosis is by far the more important study, since it is necessarily called into practice, in general or special work, every day of our professional career. But you must remember, however, that a thorough knowledge of mental diseases demands a thorough knowledge not only of the entire nervous system, but an appreciation of the intimacy existing between all diseases of the body.

Medicine is entirely too great a thing for any one mind to become thoroughly proficient in all departments, and he who undertakes to practice all does so at the expense of his patient's good and his own honor and integrity. You must remember that the human house not only has many rooms or compartments, but that all of them are very intimately associated, bound together by means of the wonderful nervous system, so that we can say of man "*E pluribus unum,*" or one in many.

Many years ago Pope, in writing his "Essay on Man," said:

"Know then *thyself, presume* not God to Scan;
The proper study of mankind is Man."

He did not mean, of course, that every one should become a physician, but I take it that he had reference to the great importance that attaches to man's moral and social nature, *which is necessarily based upon his mental constitution, and that in its turn upon the physical structure of his nervous system.* And by way of parenthesis I will add that long before you have arrived at a complete and satisfactory knowledge of mental philosophy you will find your study widening out, necessarily, into the whole subject of general philosophy, or "the why and wherefore of everything."

Now, since we think, man is by far the most important creation, on earth, that his brain is the most highly organized matter known to science, and that psychic phenomena are the highest and grandest that his wonderful nervous system can produce, you can easily surmise what I think of the study of mind. If man is "the crowning glory of creation," certainly mind is the most brilliant of the jewels in that diadem, that, like a great beacon-light, casts its rays of intelligence to the entire world.

What is mind? We all agree that we must know something of the anatomy and physiology of the heart and stomach and other organs ere we can appreciate what is meant by diseases of them. So we must have a clear understanding of what mind is before we can derive much benefit from a study of mental diseases. You need not go to the dictionary for a definition. It is not there.

In the first place, mind is not an entity, not an integral part of man, like hand or heart or brain. It is a form of force, or rather an exhibition of force. Let us suppose that nerve force is identical with electricity, for which idea there are good reasons, both *pro* and *con.* As we know, it is generated by a part of the nervous system, viz., the little "neurine batteries" or cells of grey matter. That electricity would produce certain phenomena, would it not, like any other form? Besides, you must remember that it is from the particular collection or *group of phenomena* that we are enabled to give a name to particular forms of force. In this manner we investigate heat, light, electricity, motion, animal magnetism *and life itself.* We only recognize each form of force by *what it does,* by the *phenomena* which force or energy chooses to produce in a particular kind of matter for the time being. Mind, therefore, we say, is not an entity, but *an exhibition of force resulting from the collective functions of grey nerve tissue,* not only of the brain, but the entire nervous system. Then let us study it just as we study heat, light, electricity, etc., *from its own group of phenomena*—learn something of the laws conconcerning it and make the practical applitions as circumstances will permit us.

As a result of the very great progress made in the science during recent years the word psychology, defined as "the science of the soul," becomes almost a misnomer. Like many other terms, however, we hold on to it, though it is somewhat misleading. Remember, that when I use the word psychology or any of kindred derivation I have reference to *mind,* and not to *soul.* If there is a soul—that immaterial something or nothing, according to one's religious belief —it is necessarily metaphysical, *i. e.,* beyond the physical, and is therefore not susceptible of demonstration.

" Tell me not in mournful numbers
 Life is but an empty dream.
 Life is *real,* life is *earnest,*
 Dust thou art, to dust returneth."

Let us take a look at a little of this dust and see if we cannot discover something of real beauty and practical value within it. No longer does the ancient fairy tale that Adam and Eve were created adults have a hearing in our midst. This crude idea of the origin of man no longer is believed. Genesis is considered legendary by the theologians themselves. Fancy, if you can, the Almighty One stooping to earth, gathering up a handful of dust, moistening it in some way, fashioning it into a human form as a child would a mud baby, puffing into it the so-called spirit of life and then have a living, moving thinking being. What a ridiculous conception of the most wonderful and beautiful of all creation! What an unfortunate understanding of the mighty and magnificent laws that called us into existence and controls every atom of our being!

Just for a moment, what are some of the physiological facts or truths relative to the new-born babe? While *in utero* the child breathes through the blood that is common to mother and child. The tissues of the child are fed just as the tissues of the mother, and from the same blood. Its tissues take up O and give off CO_2 continuously.

At birth the cord is severed and there is instantly an interruption of blood circulation from mother to child. The child dies if it is not supplied with oxygen from another source. How? *What sets the machinery in motion?* At birth there immediately begins to take place an accumulation of CO_2 in the system, just as it does in you and me when we hold our breath for a short time; and it is only for the short time that we can hold our breath, as the act is mostly involuntarily in the adult, and entirely so in the newly-born. The accumulated CO_2 acts upon the respiratory center in the floor of the fourth ventricle; afferent nerve impulses are sent out to the so-called respiratory muscles; they lift up and dilate the chest, the air rushes in "of its own accord," and thus has breathing been established. A new physical being has come into existence, *has begun to psucho,* to breathe, to blow, and *every step* that it has taken has been fully accounted for by natural laws.

If life is worth living at all (and doubtless most of you will agree with me that it is), it certainly is worth living well; and to live it well, to accomplish the most good possible and secure the greatest amount of happiness, we must acquaint ourselves with the laws that control us. No one doubts that we are under the domain of natural laws, that *there is some power superior to man*. We must know these laws in order to use them to our best advantage, *i. e.*, to enable us to put ourselves in accord with the inevitable and not butt our puny brains against the stone wall of cruel fate.

The population of the United States is about 76,000,000 of people. *Ten times that number*, or 760,000,000, is the estimated number of gray nerve cells in the average human brain. The consensus of opinion of 76,000,000 people is an enormous force or influence. The aggregate function of 760,000,000 brain cells is also an enormous force or influence. Each cell, like each person, has its own individual characteristics and functions. Each cell has the properties of irritibility, or sensation, motion, respiration, assimilation, secretion, reproduction, etc. They all are "endowed by nature with certain inalienable rights of life, liberty and the pursuit of happiness." *Look at each cell as a person.*

The consensus of opinion of these myriads of cells is, in fact, the mind of the man, *i. e.*, the result of the totality of their function.

Think of it—700,000,000 of these cells! I apprehend that the number is almost too large for one's thorough comprehension.

We say it is about 95,000,000 miles from earth to our sun, and, of course, the same distance to "the other side" of our system, or say 190,000,000 miles as a diameter across our system. Beyond our system is another system, beyond that another, beyond that another, then another, and another, and on and on forever. *Space has no end and no beginning. So of time. It never had a beginning and will never have an end.*

What does one million mean? It will take a bank clerk a full month of thirty days, working ten hours a day, to count one million pennies, counting them one by one. Seven hundred millions of grey cells in one human brain! What an amount of energy should be generated and liberated from a properly developed brain!—*a little round world of energy.*

But what is energy or force? Energy is defined as "that power of influence, *inherited in matter*, which is capable of initiating motion or of stopping it." In the word energy, therefore, is conveyed the idea of activity, whereas with the word force is connected the idea of capability—the words changing with the ideas.

As a basis, therefore, for our study of mental diseases, as, in fact, for the consideration of any disease, we must "begin at the bottom" and try to understand something of the fundamental facts concerning the matter composing brain tissue, and then its physiology and pathology.

We are told that "all phenomena pertain to matter and are the *appreciable expression* of the force residing therein;" that "all particles or atoms of matter are under chemical and physical law; that physiology is but the chemistry and physics of living bodies; that there are many forms of force, or rather many groups of expressions of force, and that to these groups we assign different names, as heat, light, etc., including life, and mental force; that each is convertible into the others—correlation of force, as it is called—and that nothing is lost—conservation of force; that the great progress in science in the last fifty or seventy-five years, equal to that of the three hundred years immediately prior, and that again to *all* that preceded it, is a result of the recognition of the laws of correlation and conservation of force; that "life is a complex term including all the phenomena of living beings;" or that "life is a mode of motion, or, again, an exhibition of force; that we consider energy either as potential, latent: or as kinetic, active.

Whence the source of all energy? We are able to trace it back to the sun, but "thus far shalt thou go and no farther."

We say that a body, if left to itself, will fall to the earth in obedience to the law of gravitation. But when we are asked *why* matter is endowed with this property of attraction we can only fold our arms and say we do not know. We think it a very important discovery, however, to become conscious of this great law of gravitation, by means of which the systems of planets are kept in their places. And the same we can say of any other of the many laws of nature.

Vegetable seeds, for instance, placed in the ground, given a sufficient amount of sunlight and moisture, will germinate and develop into plants which have the power of chemically uniting elementary matters to form starch. This is a very simple organic compound, and is produced in this way. Vegetable life gives off or exhales oxygen and absorbs carbonic acid gas, which is just the reverse of animal respiration.

Thus there is built up the plant, the tree, great primeval forests, some of which ages ago were sufficiently submerged and compressed to become that valuable latent form of force called coal. Or, again, the starch and sugar may be converted to animal tissues. Thus food is another form of latent energy which, when converted to nerve tissue, may produce the phenomena we are to consider. Coal is, therefore, but pent-up sun-rays, a latent or potential form of energy that we see easily converted to heat, motion, magnetism, light, and electricity. And the animal kingdom is but another form of pent-up sun-rays.

So much then of *how* we came into existence; the *why* will probably never be known.

And now let us consider more specifically the mental phenomena, which collectively we have called mind, then their laws and applications. But first, what is a phenomenon? We do not *see* energy, we only know of its existence by what it does. For example, in a thunderstorm we observe a streak of light coming down from the clouds, *caused* by electricity. We do not see the electricity; we only appreciate what it does—in other words, the phenomena. And we know of the existence of any form of force *only* by what it does, or by its phenomena. Therefore a phenomenon is defined as "the *change* that takes place in the *condition* of any body," or, as I have already said, the "appreciable expression" of some form of force.

DIETS FOR EVERY DAY USE.

By J. Warren Achorn, M.D.
Boston.

If water were the only food required, every one's physical condition, other things being equal, should be as good as every other one's.

What is the difference, then, between water and what this and that one eats or drinks that makes this one neuralgic and that one anaemic, this one rheumatic and that one plethoric, this one fat and that one lean? It is either faulty food, lack of oxidization or failure to eliminate. Impaired health waits on all three.

We are prone to eat and drink the things that hurt us most, and this is as true of pie and pickles as it is of alcohol and tobacco.

The ability to let alone food known to disagree is an exhibition of control seldom seen except at state dinners.

A knowledge of what to eat and what not to should be in the possession of every one.

Our food should be fitted to us with as much care as our clothes and changed to satisfy diseased conditions whether functional or organic, or to meet the needs of bodily change incident to advancing years. We love the thing that hurts us simply because we were not taught the right thing in the beginning. Parents too often allow a child what he likes rather than what he should have. What one can eat with impunity at twenty is not necessarily the food that fits best at forty.

Then, too, the question of *when* to drink is important, aside from the drink itself. The fact that it is as much a question of *time* as quantity is not generally appreciated.

Temperament, environment, work, dress, inheritances, habits of mind and body have to do with it all, but all these conditions can be modified. Minds can be taught with patience to think in new channels; the owner of a body can be taught to keep it in repair, or in the best mental and physical state possible under the circumstances.

If a person's nutrition and strength are maintained and all the eliminative functions are working properly (the blood and urine being normal and the lung capacity and weight proportionate to the height) his food and drink for the time are approximately what they should be and his occupation and habits such as his physique can endure. Here the "physiological balance" exists or has been found; yet the disease for which he is undergoing treatment, may persist or has not been wholly relieved by regulating the foods. Cause for this persistence is probably due to some *one* food, or foods, eaten in too great quantity or too continuously, or in insufficient quantity, or to too much liquid *at meals,* or to some mental or physical *habit,* that must be sought out and overcome.

These diet lists will be found good working formulas, right in principle, but it is not expected they will act perfectly with all.

By careful attention, however, to the Notes regulating each and to individual requirements, it is hoped they can be made to relieve with fair certainty the abnormal states for which each is intended, whether due to improper foods, failure of elimination or bad habits.

GENERAL RULES.

One should be temperate in the adoption and use of foods named in the diet selected. Change in any one particular is change enough for that day.

It is too much to expect that regulation of the food will promptly revolutionize the habits of a life time.

These diets must be carefully and intelligently followed, if the results claimed for them and expected are to be realized.

No attempt has been made to furnish an elaborate bill of fare.

Health and good digestion are the first considerations sought.

Food known to disagree should be avoided. It may agree later on.

Eating too continuously of one food to the exclusion of others of the same class should be avoided.

Meats should be stewed, roasted or broiled. Fish should be boiled, broiled or baked.

Fried food in any form, especially fried fat, is indigestible.

The best time to drink water or other liquids in amount, is the same in every case —on rising, an hour and a half before meals and half an hour before retiring.

Not more than two glasses should be taken at any meal and but one when soup is indulged in. Drink slowly.

Water should be taken at the close of a meal, milk during the meal: sip after swallowing food. The mouth should be rinsed after drinking milk.

Only liquids should be taken between meals, unless fruit or other food is required for constipation or nourishment.

Constipation must be avoided: it is intimately related to all chronic disorders for which regulation of the foods is indicated.

Properly the heartiest meal should be eight hours away from sleep. If one is at work, however, and a heavy lunch causes indigestion or drowsiness this rule should not be followed. Insomnia, on the other hand, with many, is nature's signal for a light supper.

HEIGHT, WEIGHT AND LUNG CAPACITY.

MEN.

Height		Weight.	Lung capacity based on the height.	Lung capacity based on the weight.
Feet.	Inches.	Pounds.	Cubic inches.	Cubic inches.
5	1	120	183	216
5	5	125	186	225
5	3	130	189	234
5	4	135	192	253
5	5	141	195	253
5	6	145	198	261
5	7	150	201	270
5	8	154	204	277
5	9	159	207	286
5	10	164	210	295
5	11	169	213	304
6	0	175	216	315
6	1	181	219	325
6	2	188	222	338

WOMEN.

Height		Weight.	Lung capacity based on the height.	Lung capacity based on the weight.
Feet.	Inches.	Pounds.	Cubic inches.	Cubic inches.
4	10	108	116	194
4	11	112	118	201
5	0	114	120	205
5	1	118	112	212
5	2	123	124	221
5	3	126	126	226
5	4	129	128	232
5	5	133	130	239
5	6	137	132	246
5	7	142	134	255
5	8	146	136	262
5	9	150	138	270
5	10	154	140	277
5	11	158	142	284

Figures for the height and weight mentioned here are taken from the records of the Metropolitan Life Insurance Co.

The lung capacity based on the *height* for men, is in the ratio of 3 to 1—for every inch of height there should be three cubic inches of lung capacity. For women the ratio is 2 to 1.

The lung capacity based on the *weight* is derived from multiplying the weight by 1.8.

The thoracic perimeter should not be less than half the height; this is found by dividing full inspiration and expiration added, by 2.

"Milk and grains, grains and eggs, grains and vegetables or meats, grains and fruits" are compatible.

"Fruit and vegetables, milk and vegetables, milk and meats, or fats cooked with grains" are incompatible.

DIET IN CONSTIPATION.

(Copyright.)

Take a glass of hot or cold water on rising, salted to taste or flavored with lemon juice, cloves or unfermented grape juice. Orange juice, grape-fruit juice.

BREAKFAST: *Cereals*—Corn meal mush, oat meal mush, thoroughly cooked, with cream and a dash of sugar; rye mush with clear honey or New Orleans' syrup; cracked wheat, coarse hominy.

Meats—(red) Rump steak, round steak, sirloin; mutton chops, lamb chops; thin bacon with dry toast. Pepper and salt, Chutney or Worcestershire sauce.

Fish—(oily) Salmon, mackerel, blue fish, sword fish, eels, boiled or baked; (fine fibred) cod, haddock, halibut; trout or other lake or brook fish, boiled or broiled.

Eggs—Soft boiled. poached or raw, twice a week.

Breads—Cestus gluten and bran bread, corn bread; whole wheat, rye, graham and brown bread. Butter, clear honey, orange marmalade.

Fruits—Stewed prunes, stewed figs; fresh stewed fruit. raw ripe fruit. Apples, apricots, gooseberries, blackberries, strawberries, huckleberries, blueberries. Melons.

Drinks—Clear coffee, cold water. Vigor chocolate.

A. M. BETWEEN MEALS: Cold water, root beer, sweet cider, buttermilk. French prepared prunes, Turkey figs, dates.

LUNCH: *Meats*—(red) Roast beef, roast lamb, roast mutton; (white) stewed or roasted chicken, turkey, capon, duck or goose; quail, partridge or other game birds.

Any *fish* mentioned. Sardines in oil.

Any *vegetable* mentioned.

Any *bread* mentioned.

Any *fruit* mentioned.

Any *drink* mentioned. Unfermented grape juice. Milk.

Any *dessert* mentioned, if desired. Nuts, with crackers or fruit.

P. M. BETWEEN MEALS: Same as A. M.

DINNER: *Soups*—Vegetable, oat meal or cracked wheat soups. Veal, lamb or mutton broths, chicken broth, with cestus bisbak or pearl braley or okra. *Croutons.*

Any *fresh fish* mentioned. Oysters raw with horseradish.

Any *meat* mentioned.

Vegetables—Green corn, boiled onions, spinach, cauliflower, tomatoes, asparagus, celery; Brussles sprouts, radishes. sauer-kraut and cabbage. Carrots. turnips. haricots, parsnips, green beans. green peas. beet tops.

Salads—with vinegar and oil—Lettuce, dandelion, beet, cucumbers, Bermuda onions, coldslaw.

Macaroni with fruit jelly or syrup.

Any *bread* mentioned.

Any *fruit* mentioned. Fresh pears, plums, peaches or cherries, stewed or raw. Grapes.

Any *drink* mentioned. Lemonade, beer, ale. Weak tea, tablespoonful to a pint.

Desserts—Fig pudding, prune pudding, apple charlotte, apple tapioca pudding, tamarind sauce, rhubarb sauce; graham crackers, oat meal crackers; cottage cheese, fruit jam, fruit jellies; raisins, ice cream, ices. Ginger bread.

9 P. M. Buttermilk, cider, water, figs.

NOTES.

Cold water is to be preferred to hot; hot water may be used morning and evening by the anemic, in cold weather.

Coffee should be drunk not too hot; black coffee and lemon juice, on rising, has a laxative effect with many.

Only fresh foods should be eaten.

Sugar and other sweets should be eaten sparingly.

Gross eating tends to constipate; especially if the digestion is weak.

A breakfast of oat meal and cream, or rye mush and syrup, has a decidedly laxative effect. If cream disagrees, malted milk, unfermented grape-juice or prune-juice may be substituted.

Stewed fruits should be one of the regular dishes; morning and evening, if vegetables are not eaten instead. Dried plums and prunes should be minced before boiling. Dried or canned peaches tend to constipate. Bananas tend to constipate.

Fruit between meals is more laxative in action than when taken at meal time.

Tomatoes at breakfast help constipation; better eaten raw.

Avoid fruits between meals if fruit with meals is effectual. Fruit and vegetables at the same meal are objectionable, if digestion fails. Cabbage causes flatulency.

Apples at the close of every meal with many, are especially good for constipation.

If the digestion is imperfect cooked fruit is the better.

Use saccharine in place of sugar on cooked fruit.

If dyspeptic or gouty, a dash of rum or sherry may be used to flavor grape fruit, in place of sugar.

Sweets and starchy foods do not often go well together.

Sweetened coffee with starchy food is apt to produce flatulency.

Avoid eggs if the tongue is furred, if there is nausea, flatulency or loss of appetite.

Red meat tends to constipate some people and not others.

White bread tends to constipate some people and not others.

All breads must be eaten cold and in strict moderation.

All soups must be thin; soups tend to constipate dyspeptic patients.

Soups or purees should be served with grains or croutons.

The constipating effect of milk may be overcome by adding a tablespoonful of sugar of milk to each glass.

Milk and meat at the same meal are incompatible.

Root beer should contain either sarsaparilla or sassafras.

A little water poured on a tablespoonful of linseed (let stand for an hour) and drunk just before a meal, is laxative in action.

Walnuts, filberts or pecans, for lunch with fruit do not constipate; masticate thoroughly.

If fleshy, avoid corn-meal mush, oat meal, corn bread, oily fish, figs, dates, sweets, soups, beer and ale.

If rheumatic avoid the free use of tomatoes, asparagus, rhubarb, onions, spinach, soups, beer, ale and sweets.

Constipation, generally speaking, is nothing but a *bad* habit. By the persistent use of proper foods, the maintenance of regular habits and some form of treatment or exercise, the majority of cases due to faulty foods can be relieved.

ANNOUNCEMENT.

KNOWING Dr. J. Warren Achorn to be greatly interested in diet in disease we have made an arrangement with him to write a series of "Diet Lists" for certain abnormal conditions, to be published in the GAZETTE, one in every issue, during 1901. In this number of the GAZETTE we publish his diet list in constipation. For February the one for indigestion or dyspepsia will be given. We will announce in each succeeding issue of the GAZETTE the diet list which will be published in the next following number.

Department of Physiological Chemistry.

WITH SPECIAL REFERENCE TO DIETETICS AND NUTRITION IN GENERAL.

FEEDING IN TYPHOID FEVER.

ACCORDING to F. L. Keays (*Medical Record*) the routine diet in vogue at the New York Hospital throughout the active stage of typhoid fever is milk, fifty to seventy ounces being given in twenty-four hours. It is customary to keep a daily record of the amount of milk taken, so that it will not fall below what is necessary. When plain milk is not acceptable to the patient it is varied in different ways; a little brandy or a few spoonfuls of coffee or some malted milk is added; koumyss or matzoon is substituted for milk from time to time for variety. Patients who complain of hunger are given broth or beef juice. As soon as the temperature reaches normal, more active feeding is begun. The patient is given a lamb chop, or an egg boiled for twenty minutes, and finely chopped, or scraped-beef sandwiches. Proper mastication of the food is urged. Each day, as the food agrees, new articles of diet are added to the list, or those already given are increased in amount. Baked custard, bread, milk toast, and finally chicken, raw oysters, baked apple, baked potato, rice, hominy, and green vegetables are allowed, the milk all the time being cut down. The patient is kept upon this food while in the hospital and is told to continue it for several weeks after leaving.

OLIVE OIL IN GASTRIC AFFECTIONS.

THE *Medical Times* says that at the International Medical Congress Dr. Cohnheim, of Berlin, detailed his experience with large doses of olive oil in cases of severe gastric distress. In his first case the young man had suffered from an injury in the gastric region, and it seemed probable that a traumatic ulcer had resulted. The pain on eating was so great as to make the patient avoid food. A wineglass of olive oil taken before meals gave complete relief. The same remedy was tried in other cases in which stomach discomfort was a prominent symptom. Even in cases of gastric cancer relief was afforded to many symptoms. In cases of pyloric stenosis most satisfactory results were secured as far as the alleviation of symptoms was concerned. Besides, the dilatation of the stomach that existed began to diminish, and eventually in some cases disappeared completely. Cohnheim has treated twelve cases of gastric catarrh by this method with uniformly good results whenever the patients bore the oil well. In one or two cases this method of treatment was tried as an absolutely last resort before operation, and it proved successful. Patients who had lost so much in weight as to appear almost cachectic began immediately to gain in weight, and within a couple of months gained from fifteen to thirty pounds.

Professor Mathieu, of Paris, said that in certain of the country parts both of Germany and France olive oil is used as a family remedy for all stomach pains. It is most effective and has a high reputation. In his practice at the Hôpital Andral, Dr. Mathieu has often used this remedy and knows how efficient it is where less simple remedies have failed. He recommends it with confidence despite its utter empiricism and lack of claim to any scientific basis.

THE SOURCE OF OXALIC ACID IN THE URINE.

THE question as to the source of the oxalic acid found in the urine has not yet been satisfactorily solved. According to Lommel (*Deutsches Archiv für klinische Medicin*) the oxalic acid excreted by the kidneys seems to be derived only in small part from that introduced into the organism by the food. More than one hundred analyses made by this investigator under varying conditions of diet failed to show that the amount of oxalic acid excreted was greater after a mixed or a vegetable diet than after a diet free from this salt, *i. e.*, one that consisted chiefly of meat and bread. By far the greatest part of it is formed in the body itself, for even during absolute abstinence from foods containing oxalic acid this substance appears in the urine in considerable quantity—about 30 milligrams per day.

When oxalic acid has been ingested in large quantities with the food, only a small fraction appears in the urine and feces. Lommel believes it to be highly probable that the salt is for the most part decomposed during its passage through the organism, it being possible that a certain proportion is destroyed on reaching the intestine. The excretion of oxalic acid bears no direct relation to the disintegration of albumin; the introduction of food rich in nuclein, however, causes, besides an increase of uric acid, a heightened excretion also of oxalic acid. Food containing much gelatin increases likewise the output of this salt.

THE DISADVANTAGES OF RAW-MILK FEEDING.

THE objection to the raw-milk feeding of infants is based, according to Louis Fischer (*Medical Record*), upon the contamination of milk with various pathogenic bacteria. Such risk, however, is reduced to a minimum when all the principles of modern hygienic measures are rigidly enforced. It is a well-known fact that the prolonged use of sterilized or boiled milk will produce scurvy, and when scurvy exists both sterilized and boiled milk must be discontinued to give place to fresh raw milk. Does it not seem more plausible in the face of such clinical experience to commence feeding at once with raw milk rather than risk the development of scurvy and be compelled to discontinue all other forms of feeding excepting raw foods? There is a certain deadness, or, to put it differently, absence of freshness in milk that is boiled or sterilized. It seems to be the lack of this same element of freshness which in the absence of fresh meat and green vegetables will produce scurvy in the adult. Speaking of the development of scurvy in children fed on sterilized or boiled milk, Rundlett says that changes take place not in the albumin, fat, or sugar; but in the albuminate of iron, phosphorus, and possibly in the fluorin, vital changes takes place. The albuminoids are certainly in milk, derived as it is from tissues that contain them and are present in a vitalized form as proteids.

On boiling the change that takes place is due simply to the coagulation of the globulin or proteid molecule, which splits away from the inorganic molecule, and thus renders it as to the iron and fluorin unabsorbable, and as to the phosphatic molecule unassimilable. This is the change that is so vital, and it is this only which takes place when milk is boiled. It is evident that children require phosphatic and ferric proteids in a living form, which are contained only in raw milk.

Cheadle says that phosphate of lime is necessary to every tissue. No cell growth can go on without earthy phosphates; even the lowest form of life, such as fungi and bacteria, cannot grow if deprived of them. These salts of lime and magnesia are especially called for in the development of the bony structures.

FOOD IN TUBERCULOSIS.

IN his recent work on *"Treatment in Practical Medicine,"* Mitchell Bruce says anent this subject: When anorexia, discomfort, vomiting and the other evidences of indigestion, such as depression, languor, headache, constipation and turbid urine, make their appearance in phthisis, they are too often directly referred to the tuberculosis or to the fever. The patient is ordered milk, essences and every description of patented and advertised foods and "wines"; oil, tonics, malt, and the latest specific for tuberculosis are given even more freely than before. The exercise of a little common sense ought to have prevented all this. The first step to take in such a case is to prescribe a mercurial purge, followed by a saline. The second step is to order a diet of light solids, and specially to supervise the breakfast and supper menus, and to cut off stimulants and all manufactured materials, excepting a good peptonized cereal food at the evening meal. Thirdly, the times and manner of taking food must be revised. Excessive frequency and excessive amount must be temporarily avoided. If sickness be prominent and persistent, bodily rest is indicated, and the patient should lie down for half an hour before his mid-day meal and for at least two hours after it. Sometimes, indeed, obstinate cough and vomiting have to be met by confining the patient to a couch and bringing him his meals, which he takes in the reclining posture. Counter irritation is often successful in the distressing cases; feeding provokes paroxysmal cough, ending in vomiting and loss of the entire meal. A fly blister to the epigastrium, application to the pharynx or larynx, and iodin paint over a large secreting cavity are different measures called for by different conditions. The best internal remedy is a combination of sodium bicarbonate, sal volatile, diluted prussic acid, and diluted infusion of a vegetable bitter stomachic, given shortly before meals to relieve the mucous catarrh of the stomach and to promote the appetite and secretion of gastric juice. *Night* feeding in active phthisis is indicated by several conditions: That the night is too long for a patient with advancing tuberculosis to go unfed, patients with pneumonia being fed every two hours; and that broken sleep produces restlessness, increase of cough, sweats and exhaustion.

THE INFLUENCE OF FOOD UPON MILK SECRETION.

TEMESVARY, according to an abstract in the *Medical Age* from the *Centralblatt für Gynaekologie,* has recently studied the influence exerted by food upon the secretion of milk. His experiments extended upon 216 wet-nurses, who within from one to two weeks after labor were fed—for periods of four days at a time—according to the following rotation of diet: (1) Ordinary (mixed) diet; (2) milk diet; (3) preponderance of vegetable diet; (4) preponderance of animal diet; (5) rich mixed diet; (6) ordinary diet, with addition of from one and a half to two pints of beer per diem. This led to the following general conclusions: The largest amount of milk secretion occurred under a rich mixed diet, which also insured the largest absolute amount of cream. The next largest amount of fat followed upon the administration of ordinary diet, while preponderating vegetable and essentially animal diet produced the smallest amount of fatty constituents. According to Temesvary a rich mixed diet insures the most compact and best milk, vegetable diet producing the most watery secretion. The addition of beer to ordinary diet diminishes the amount of milk secreted, but noticeably increases the proportion of fatty constituents.

As to the mediate influence of maternal diet upon infants, Temesvary has noticed with all methods an equal absence of gastro-intestinal disturbance, except with the vegetarian diet, which increases the tendency to digestive complications.

Concerning the increase in weight, animal

diet, beer diet, and rich mixed diet afforded the most favorable results; next came the ordinary (milk) diet, and lastly vegetable diet.

Temesvary concludes that the composition of the mother's dietary has a considerable influence upon the secretion of milk, the most important factor, however, being of a quantitative nature. If the amount of food prove insufficient, the secretion will be scant both in quantity and fatty constituents; if abundant and highly nutritive, the milk is larger in amount and richer in fats, ordinary mixed diet occupying the middle ground.

THE ROLE OF THE SPLEEN IN THE PANCREATIC DIGESTION OF PROTEIDS.

In a recent number of the *Lancet*, Henry F. Bellamy gives a detailed account of the experiments that have been performed by Schiff and Herzen, in order to show the important rôle played by the spleen in the production of pancreatic ferments. The experiments of Schiff date back as far as 1868. They were undertaken as a result of the observations made by a number of physiologists that, at a certain period after the commencement of digestion—about five hours—the spleen became congested, and increased considerably in weight. Various experiments were performed, all of which seemed to prove that dogs, whose spleen had been extirpated, or whose splenic vessels had been ligated, were unable to procure an active pancreatic fluid. Later, the discovery of zymogen by Heidenhain and the fact that this substance could be converted into trypsin by the action of oxygen, seemed to disconcert the apparently obvious results of Schiff's work, but Herzen suggested that possibly the spleen secreted a substance which was poured into the general circulation, and, coming in contact with the zymogen, converted it into trypsin. He, therefore, believed that it should be possible to obtain this tryptogentic substance from the

spleen itself at the period of its greatest congestion. He found that by mixing a pancreatic infusion and infusion of congested spleen together an actively digesting solution was produced that would dissolve fibrin and albumin; whereas the pancreatic infusion mixed with extract of anemic spleen was without effect. It having been suggested by Heidenhain that this was probably merely due to the excess of oxygenated blood in the splenic extract, a series of experiments was undertaken with extract of anemic spleen mixed with arterial blood; they were, however, inefficient. It seems, therefore, conclusively proved that the spleen, during its period of turgescence, does secrete some substance which acts upon zymogen and converts it into trypsin, and that this substance has a specific and peculiar action. It is possible that the zymogen excreted by the pancreas before the splenic ferment is elaborated is gradually converted into trypsin by oxidation in the intestinal tract. In splenectomized animals proteid digestion appears to be accomplished chiefly in the stomach.

THE ARMY RATION IN THE TROPICS.

In a paper published in the *Philadelphia Medical Journal* and entitled "A Tropical Ration," J. R. Kean, Major and Surgeon, U. S. Vols., discusses the proper dietary in the tropics and its essential differences from that of temperate climates. He writes in part:

The diet of the average American at home contains 125 grams of proteid, whereas only 40 to 50 grams are necessary (with abundance of carbohydrates) to preserve the nitrogen-equilibrium and prevent tissue-waste. It seems that such a proteid excess (luxus consumption) is less desirable and less harmless in the tropics. That this is true is shown by the fact that in India and other European tropical colonies as soon as the wealthier natives begin to adopt European modes of life they at once lose their relative immunity to dysentery, liver-abscess, jaundice and like intestinal disorders which are the scourges of the European immigrant. It is a matter of common experience that in hot weather a diminished desire for meat on the part of most people is observed, and especially the kind of meat chiefly eaten by the American soldier—roast (baked) beef with rich gravy, and bacon. At the same time comes a longing for fresh vegetables and fruits. The appetite is lessened by long-continued heat and is more capricious. It craves variety, especially in vegetables and fruits, and a restricted and monotonous diet becomes distasteful and repulsive. Under these circumstances strength once lost is regained slowly, if at all, and convalescents do not entirely recover without a change of scene, which means, among other things, a change of diet. The importance of variety in the ration, and especially in the vegetable component, is, in the tropics, I believe, a matter the great importance of which has been overlooked.

"On one point, and only one, I believe, in the whole subject of tropical dietetics are all observers agreed, and that is as to the disastrous effects of alcoholic excess in the tropics, though as regards to what constitutes excess there is not quite so much unanimity. Now alcohol is the instinctive resort of the bored mind, and the dulled appetite, the refuge from monotony of occupation and monotony of food. The responsibility for much of the drunkenness in the army must be divided between the commanding officer who does not vary his drills and exercises and the captain who puts every day before his men the never-varying dinner of roast beef and potatoes."

THE PREPARATION OF UNFERMENTED GRAPE JUICE.

A CALIFORNIA Experiment Station bulletin states that unfermented grape juice has been used for ages, but that generally the use has been restricted to the immediate vicinity of vineyards, because the product spoils quickly unless preserved. Modern improvements in methods of preserving have resulted in greatly extending the use of grape juice. However, the methods of preservation employed have not been uniformly successful, or have frequently resulted in products injurious to health. Heretofore the expense of proper preservation has been so great as to restrict the use of this beverage almost exclusively to medicinal purposes, the price being too high for the regular consumer. The bulletin of the California Station referred to discusses the qualities of pure normal unfermented grape juice, and explains how it may be successfully and economically prepared. Analyses are reported which show that the normal juice or must of grapes contains no alcohol, glycerin, etc., which are the principal constituents of wine, but that its main constituent is grape sugar (generally 20-24 per cent.), with some acids (mainly tartaric acid), mineral matter, and nitrogenous compounds (protein). There are all substances of nutritive or therapeutic value, and pure grape juice should contain no others. Unfortunately, analysis has shown that many of the so-called "grape juices" found in the market are not pure, but frequently contain considerable amounts of alcohol, besides injurious preservative materials.

The spoiling of grape juice is due to the action of micro-organisms which, even with the greatest care and cleanliness, get into it and there find conditions specially favorable to their growth and activity. One of the first and main results of the activity of the organisms usually present is the formation of alcohol from the sugar present. The main object of all processes of preservation is, therefore, to permanently prevent fermentation and at the same time keep the juice clear and attractive in appearance.

To attain the first object there are two general groups of methods, which may be called, respectively, chemical and physical. All the chemical methods consist in the addition of germ poison or antiseptics, which either kill the microscopic organisms of fermentation or permanently prevent their growth and increase. Of these substances the principal used are salicylic, sulphurous, boracic acids, saccharin, and, of late, formalin. Many patent preservatives are found on the market, but they nearly all contain one or more of these substances as their active principle. They are all injurious to digestion and in other ways; and it may be said in general that any substance which prevents fermentation will also interfere with digestion, and is therefore to be avoided.

The physical methods work in one of two ways; they remove the germs by some mechanical means, such as a filter or a centrifugal apparatus, or they destroy them by heat, cold, electricity, etc. The physical methods, especially those which depend upon heating the liquid to a sufficiently high temperature to kill all organisms present, are considered safest and most practical.

FORMALDEHYDE IN MILK.

THERE seems to be no subject in pediatrics, says the *Chicago Clinic*, and especially in the very important division of infant dietetics, which is so generally conceded or accepted as to have no voices rising in opposition. If one thing seemed to be absolutely settled, beyond all doubt or peradventure, it was that the introduction of toxic substances into milk for the purpose of preservation is to be utterly condemned and prevented by the most vigorous action of municipal and State authorities. Moechel and Froehling, of Kansas City, however, have put themselves on record as advocating "a proper percentage of formaldehyde should be allowed to be a benefit rather than a deleterious in milk," and that it is much better than sterilization. which is known to alter the food value of

the milk. However extreme the opinion of medical men may be against sterilization we do not believe that many will be ready to accept the introduction of a rank poison as a germicide in milk intended for artificial infant feeding. The physicians above quoted maintain that: (1) Formaldehyde does not interfere with the human gastric, intestinal or ptyalin disgestion; (2) that infants which did not prosper with various kinds of infant foods or milk at once changed for the better when given milk containing formaldehyde.

It seems hardly necessary to voice a protest against the advocacy by a physician of a practice against which cities and their medical boards are waging a bitter and expensive war, on the ground that such practice is prejudicial to life and health. Such an opinion cannot be taken except as a certain license to unscrupulous milk dealers in their pernicious practices.

Halliburton (*British Medical Journal*) said that an antiseptic is inimical to the life of the organisms that cause putrefaction; it cannot therefore be harmless to the vital functions of higher animals. Formaldehyde, he says, makes gastric digestion almost impossible and effects pancreatic digestion even more readily. Arnett (*Lancet*) says that the use of formaldehyde in milk or other food is invariably injurious, especially to infants, and he contends that the use of preservatives in milk is largely responsible for the great infant mortality in our large cities.

Certain it is that the introduction of toxic substances into food for those of even the best health is injurious; such preservatives when given to a sickly infant must be markedly deleterious, and in this day, when milk can be secured pure and free from injurious bacterial action, without any artificial means of preservation, the use of formaldehyde is never justifiable and is mentioned only to be condemned in the strongest terms.

THE NUTRITIVE VALUE OF LEGUMES.

In Farmers' Bulletin No. 121, published under the auspices of the U. S. Department of Agriculture, Mary Hinman Abel writes concerning the nutritive value of legumes as follows:

The different kind of legumes are so similar in their general character, nutritive constituents, and digestibility that in these regards they may be treated together. Even in an immature state, as green peas and beans, they are, as regards composition, equal or superior in nutritive value to other green vegetables, and the ripened seed shows by analysis a very remarkable contrast to most of the matured vegetable foods, as the potato and other tubers, and even to the best cereals, as wheat. This superiority lies in the large amount of nitrogen in the form of protein that they contain. Another characteristic of the legumes brought out by analysis is the large percentage of mineral matter in them, the excess being chiefly in lime and potassium salts. In some instances they contain a large amount of fat; for instance, 17 per cent. in the soy bean and 50 per cent. in the peanut.

Fresh string beans, sugar peas and shelled peas, like other fresh, succulent vegetables, contain considerable water, which, with the materials dissolved in it, forms the plant juice. They somewhat resemble cabbage in percentage composition. Fresh shelled beans, peas, and cow-peas contain a fairly large amount of protein or nitrogenous material, the nutrient which serves to build and repair body tissue as well as to furnish energy. They also contain considerable carbohydrates and small amounts of fat, both these classes of nutrients serving to supply the body with energy. The amount of ash or mineral matter in the legumes varies in amount. It doubtless serves the same purpose in the body as mineral matter found in other food materials. The canned legumes, which are simply cooked foods sterilized and kept in such a way that they cannot ferment. resemble in composition the same materials uncooked. The dried legumes contain some water, though to the eye they seem to be perfectly dry. They contain a high percentage of protein, in this respect surpassing the other seeds commonly used as food, such as wheat. They approach animal foods as regards protein and total nutritive value, most of the legumes containing carbohydrates in place of the fat found in animal foods. Fats and carbohydrates, however, serve the same purpose in the body, although the fats yield two and one-fourth times as much energy per pound as carbohydrates.

Vegetable foods are nearly all rich in starch and other carbohydrates which supply an abundance of carbon to the system; but they contain, in general, comparatively little nitrogen, an element that is of first importance in a dietary. Therefore, the very large percentage of this constituent found in the legumes constitutes for us their special interest, and the true nature of the compounds in which this nitrogen exists is also of the utmost importance.

Most of the nitrogen found in the pea, bean and lentil is in a form very useful as food. It is called by Liebig "plant casein," on account of its general resemblance to the casein of milk. Although its action as a food is similar to that of the nitrogenous matter of other vegetables, it is markedly different in some of its characteristics from, for instance, the gluten of grains. Pea and bean flour will not form a dough with water and cannot be utilized for making porous bread.

WHAT IS YEAST?

Yeast is the scum which rises when farinaceous and vegetable substances are in a state of fermentation with water, says a writer in *Food and Cookery*. It is also called "barm." It is used or added to substances intended to ferment in order to hasten the process of fermentation.

Scientifically speaking. yeast is a minute fungus of the genus Saccharomyces. A single plant is a round or oval one-celled, microscopic body, which reproduces in two ways—either by sending out buds which break off as new plants, or by forming spores which will grow into new plants under favorable conditions. It grows only in the presence of moisture, heat and nutritive material. If the moisture is not abundant the surrounding substances absorb that which already exists in the yeast-cells, and so prevent them from performing their functions. Yeast develops best at a temperature of 77°-95° F. (25°-35° C.). It is also believed that some nitrogen is necessary for the best development of yeast, and that such development is most complete in the presence of free oxygen; but why these things are so is not yet clearly understood.

If a dish of malt extract, originally free from yeast, be exposed to the air, alcoholic fermentation, such as could be produced only by yeast, will soon set in. Such yeast is known as "wild yeast," and all yeasts have been cultivated from it. The oldest method of growing yeast is, perhaps, that used by the Egyptians. A little wild yeast was obtained and set in dough, a portion of which was saved from the baking; there it went on developing as long as materials held out, and thus the bit of dough, or "leaven," contained so much yeast that a little of it would leaven the whole loaf.

A microscopical examination was recently made of some bread over 4,400 years old, found in Egypt with other remains of a long-vanished people. It was made of ground barley, and the yeast-cells were plainly visible. A similar process of raising bread with "leaven" is still carried on in some regions of Europe. The "wet" or "potato yeast," so common before the days of patent yeast, was made by a similar method. Wild yeast was cultivated in a decoction of hops, or potato and water, and some of the material thus obtained was mixed with the dough. The "barms" so much used in Scotland are made by letting yeast grow in malt extract of flower. Brewers' and distillers' yeasts are taken from the vats in which malt extract has been fermenting. Compressed yeasts are made by growing yeast-plants in some sweet liquid, then drying the material to check their growth, and pressing it; sometimes a little starch is added to make the little cakes keep their shape. The strength of any yeast depends on the care with which it is made and preserved. Ordinary brewers' yeasts are likely to be full of the bacteria which set up lactic or other fermentations in the bread, and give it a disagreeable taste and odor. They are very susceptible to changes in the weather, and cannot be always relied on. Compressed yeasts, if carefully made, are more uniform in strength and composition. Usually a few of the microscopic plants or bacteria other than yeast are allowed to remain, as the slight acid taste they give to the bread is considered an advantage.

Dough made with a proportion of yeast, say one ounce of compressed yeast to six pounds of flour and allowed to stand, becomes what is technically termed a *sponge.* When this dough is baken it develops carbonic acid gas, which necessarily makes the bread lighter than it would otherwise be; it also removes some of its saccharine matter. The consumption of yeast in Great Britain is so great, that in addition to the great quantity supplied by English brewers. enormous quantities are daily imported from France, Holland, Belgium, and Germany.

THE ADVANTAGES OF A MIXED DIET.

A MIXED diet, says Dr. Cosgrave in the *Hospital Nursing Mirror*, is best, as there no article of diet—except milk—which has the different elements in proper proportion, and although milk will do during the enforced rest of illness, a more solid diet is necessary for those going about and doing work.

Each person requires daily about 300 grains of nitrogen and 4,000 grains of carbon. A pound of lean meat contains the right quantity of nitrogen, but four pounds would have to be eaten to get enough carbon; so four pounds of potatoes contain the right amount of carbon, but twenty pounds would have to be eaten to get the required nitrogen. By using a mixed diet of meat and potatoes, about three-quarters of a pound of meat and three pounds of potatoes give the required amounts.

Experience has led to the use of all these classes of foods at the chief meals. Thus a breakfast of tea, bread and butter and fried bacon, or a boiled egg, has all classes represented, as has also a dinner of water, meat (fat and lean) and potatoes.

The recognition of this necessity is also shown by the way in which certain articles of food are commonly combined; thus, chicken, the flesh of which is nearly free from fat, is usually taken with bacon, bread sauce adding a carbohydrate. Bacon also goes with rabbit, and with cabbage and potatoes; indeed, the large proportion of fat in bacon makes it a useful addition to many other foods. Again, boiled dumplings and Yorkshire pudding are frequently served with meat. Irish stew is another good example of a dish which includes all classes of food. Curried chicken and curried lentils represent the combination of carbohydrates with animal and vegetable proteids.

The most common defects in diet are:

1. Deficient nitrogenous foods (proteids). This results partly from the dearness of meat, which is the usual source of our nitrogen, and partly from not using the cheaper vegetable sources. The ease with which bread and tea can be got ready is another cause.

2. Want of fresh vegetables. Many people think they cannot digest vegetables and so avoid them; this is a frequent cause of ill health.

3. Want of salts. This occurs chiefly in those who do not take fresh meat and vegetables. White bread, for example, is wanting in phosphites, but these can be obtained from eggs, milk, meat, etc. For this condition fresh meat, fresh vegetables, raw or stewed fruits, rhubarb, oranges, lemons, ets., should be taken. The free use of vegetable soup is highly desirable.

4. Want of fat. This is most frequent in children and in delicate adults. Bacon, butter, cream and suet puddings can often be taken when fat in other forms is rejected.

A few examples of food values may be given:

Eggs are equal in food value to the same weight of butchers' meat. The yolk is the richest part, as it contains more of the fat; it gives nearly six times as much force to the body as does an equal weight of the white.

Rice, which is the main food of one-third of the human race, contains only one part of flesh-formers to ten of heat-givers, and so has too little nitrogen to be in itself a perfect food. Taken with milk, or with eggs, etc., as in curry, this deficiency is made up. It is best steamed till tender, as boiling removes much of its nitrogen and mineral matters, neither of which it can afford to lose.

Oatmeal has one part of flesh-formers to about five of heat-givers, but is wanting in fat and is therefore best taken with milk.

Many experiments have been made to determine the time required for the digestion of food; the following table illustrates the range of time:

	Hours.
Tripe	1
Chicken	2¾
Non-oily fish	3
Roast beef	3
Roast mutton	3¼
Roast veal	4
Roast pork	5

ABSINTHE AND ITS EFFECT.

DURING the Algerian war, which lasted from 1844 to 1847, says a writer in *Health*, the French army were more in danger from African fevers than from their Algerian enemies. Several things were tried as antidotes or preventives by the skilful army physicians. Finally absinthe was hit on as the most effective febrifuge.

The soldiers were ordered to mix it in small quantities three times a day with the ordinary French wine. The luckless happy-go-lucky privates grew to like their medicine, which at first they swore at bitterly for spoiling with its bitterness that beautiful purple vinegar they fondly fancy is wine. But when absinthe alone began to usurp the time-honored place of claret in the affections of the French army the evil became an unmixed one.

Absinthe straight as a beverage is an entirely different thing from absinthe mixed as a medicine or an occasional tonic. The victorious army on their triumphant return to Paris brought the habit with it. It is now so widespread through all classes of Parisian society—and Paris gives the cue to France—that French men of science and publicists regard the custom of absinthe tippling as a vast national evil.

The consequence of the use—and use of this drug ripens to abuse, even with men of unusual will power—has been in France disastrous to a dreadful degree. Many men of remarkable brilliancy have offered up their brains and their lives on the livid altar of absinthe. Baudelaire, who translated all of Poe's works into French, had a terribly grotesque passion for the pleasant green poison. In one of his mad freaks this minor French poet actually painted his hair the same tint as the beverage that corroded his brain, possibly from an odd fancy to have the outside of his head correspond with or match the inside.

Alfred de Musset, who was the French Byron *plus* a tenderer, naiver touch, also fell a victim to the drug after George Sand gave the final smash to his fragmentary heart. A frightful historic pun occurred in this connection. Towards the end, when the great poet, growing more morose every day, hid from his old companions and was missing from his favorite haunts, one man, not aware of his infirmity, exclaimed: "Why is it that our dear de Musset absents

himself from us nowadays?" And a grim wit lispingly answered: "For a woman'th reathon, my friend; he abthinth himthelf jutht becauthe he abthinth himthelf." *Il s'absente parcequ'il s'absinthe.*

Paul Verlaine, a French literateur, is another absinthe fiend, and Guy de Maupassant is reported to have burned his brains away with the same emeraldine flames. The brain disease caused by this drug is considered almost incurable. Far worse than alcohol or opium, it can only be compared to cocain for the fellness of its clutch on poor humanity.

What, then, is this dreadful drink composed of, and how is it made? The answer is easy enough, though the process, to ensure perfection in the evil, is not so. Absinthe may be technically described as a redistillation of alcoholic spirits (made originally from various things, potatoes, for instance), in which, to give it the final character), absinthium with other aromatic herbs and bitter roots are macerated. The chief ingredient is the tops and leaves of the herb *Artemisia Absinthium*, or wormwood, which grows from two to four feet in great profusion under cultivation, and which contains a volatile oil, absinthol, and a yellow, crystalline, resinous compound, called absinthin, which is the bitter principle. The alcohol with which this and the essentials of other aromatic plants are mixed holds these volatile oils in solution.

It is the precipitation of these oils in water that causes the rich clouding of your glass when the absinthe is poured on the cracked ice; double emblems of warnings of the clouding and the crackling of your brain if you take to it steadily. Thus every drink of the opaline liquid is an object lesson in chemistry that carries its own moral.

The continued use of absinthe gives rise to epileptic symptoms as an external expression of the profound disturbance of the brain and nerves. One large dose of the essence of the wormwood, indeed, has been noted as causing almost instantly epileptiform convulsions in animals.

But the drug it not without its uses from

a broad point of view. As the name implies, it is an anthelmintic, or a pretty safe cure for certain kinds of animal life that sometimes infest the intestines of men. This peculiar property was well known to the Greeks, who had a wine infused with wormwood called absinthites.

In some parts of Germany wormwood is used in lieu of hops for brewing of certain brands of beer, and it unquestionably has valuable tonic properties. Absinthe is made almost everywhere.

The first effects of it are a profound serenity of temper and a slight heightening of the mental powers, coupled with bodily inertia. This is the general rule, but, as a famous physician once remarked of a dreadful disorder in his lecture room, "Gentlemen, the chief glory of the beautiful disease I am now explaining is the remarkable variety of its manifestations."

OYSTERS AND DISEASE.

WITH the advance in our knowledge of the subtle and unexpected ways in which disease may be transmitted, says an editorial in the *Boston Medical and Surgical Journal*, suspicion has from time to time, and not unjustifiably, fallen upon the oyster. It has been easy for a somewhat vivid imagination to picture the contamination to which oyster beds may be exposed, and to conceive of the possible multiplication of pathogenic bacteria or other agents inimical to health within their shells. Admitting these facts, it is a short step to imagine the effect upon man of eating such oysters and to add another terror to the constantly increasing number with which we are surrounded. Fortunately in this, as in many other matters, an appeal to experiment does much to clear the way for a calmer and more rational interpretation of the facts. This service has lately been rendered by an exhaustive and painstaking study on the general subject of oysters and disease undertaken by Professor W. A. Herdman, of Liverpool, and Professor Rubert Boyce, also

of Liverpool, and both of University College. Their work is published in full, with plates, in the second volume of the Thompson Yates Laboratories Report, and well repays a careful perusal. The conclusions of these investigations are of moment, and should be generally known both by the raisers and consumers of shellfish. In general their experiments, in common with those of others, go to show that oysters and other shellfish used as food must from their nature and the circumstances of their cultivation and sale be regarded as liable to contamination from pathogenic and other organisms of their products. Recognizing this fact, the following statement made by the writers is sufficiently self-evident: "Shellfish must not be taken as food from grounds where there is any possibility of sewage contamination; after removal from the sea, while in transit, in store or in market, they should be carefully protected from any possibility of insanitary environment; they should not be kept longer than is absolutely necessary in shops, cellars, etc., in towns where, even if not running the risk of fresh contamination, they are under conditions favorable to the reduction of their vitality, and the growth of their bacterial contents—the fresher they are from the sea the more healthy they are likely to be; finally, only absolutely fresh shellfish should be eaten uncooked, and those that are cooked must be *sufficiently cooked*, raised to boiling point and kept there at least ten minutes."

Among the details of their experiments several matters of great interest were brought out. The vexed question of "greening" in oysters was one. The investigation showed that there are several perfectly distinct varieties of greenness, some being entirely healthy, and others indicating an excess of copper; in certain American oysters, for example, it was distinctly proved that their green color was due to copper, and also that the copper is situated in the blood cells, or leucocytes, which are much increased in number. This condition they call a green leucocytosis. On the other hand experiments in feeding oysters with no clear evidence of any absorption of the metals accompanied by greening.

The investigations on the presence of typhoid bacilli in oysters is also of much importance. They did not find the bacillus in any oysters obtained from the sea or from markets, but were able experimentally to inoculate oysters with typhoid and recover the organism from their bodies up to the tenth day. It appears, however, that the bacilli do not increase in the body or tissues, and probably die in the intestine. Sea water was found inimical to the growth of the bacilli and the washing of infected oysters in a stream of clear sea water led to a great diminution or, in some cases, a total disappearance of the bacilli in from one to seven days. The colon group of bacilli is frequently found in shellfish, but probably not in those living in pure sea water. It is unsafe, however, to infer from this that the presence of colon bacilli invariably indicates sewage contamination. Further investigation on this point is desirable. The writers inform us with reference to their negative results regarding typhoid that their samples of oysters were in no case, so far as they were aware, derived from a bed known or suspected of contamination with typhoid.

As a result of their investigations they feel amply justified in sounding a warning note regarding the raising and selling of oysters. They urge the greatest possible care in the prevention of contamination, and for the regular inspection of the grounds by qualified persons. Foreign oysters should be as carefully inspected as those raised at home, and a systematic quarantine established.

The report is, in a general way, reassuring, and yet, throughout, it recognizes a real danger, provided the utmost precaution be not taken to guard the oyster beds as we would any other source of food supply. It is well that we should be fully aware of all the facts and insist upon the legal enforcement of close inspection. When this is done we may, no doubt, still enjoy our oysters, with the practical assurance of their harmlessness.

ON SOME NON-ALCOHOLIC BEVERAGES.

Dr. E. MacDowell Cosgrave, in a lecture on the subject of beverages, published in *The Hospital Nursing Mirror*, says in part:

One group of beverages in common use contains tea, coffee, and cocoa. These are non-alcoholic, and are stimulant and restorative. They are generally taken hot; this adds to their restorative effect. Although from the milk and sugar they contain they have some food value, generally these additions are only sufficient to give flavor. As they are all made with boiling water, they are safe drinks when the water supply is contaminated.

Tea.—The ordinary black tea is made from leaves which, after picking, are left in heaps until a process of fermentation has taken place.

Tea is made by infusing the leaves by pouring boiling water upon them. The kettle should be filled with fresh cold water, and, as soon as the water boils, it should be poured over the leaves, previously placed in a scalded-out teapot. Water that has been boiled for any length of time has its air expelled, and does not make good tea.

Tea should not be allowed to "draw" too long. At the end of five minutes or so it it will have exhausted the good of the leaves. If tea has to be kept for a latecomer it should not be allowed to stand on the leaves, but should be poured into another teapot or heated jug. Tea during "drawing" should not be placed on the hob, but under a cosy.

The restorative effect of tea is partly caused by the thein, which is practically identical with the caffein of coffee, and partly by the warmth of the fluid. Tea contains tannin, which is commonly blamed as a cause of dyspepsia, and various devices have been adopted to exclude it; but it is harmless, and properly made tea is unlikely to do harm unless it is taken without food, when it provokes the stomach to secrete gastric juice, although there is nothing to be digested; or when it is taken very hot after a meat meal, and then it is not the tea which does harm, but the hot fluid, which kills the pepsin necessary for the digestion of meat. In some cases where dyspepsia already exists, tea-drinking does harm, as the large amount of hot fluid relaxes the already distended stomach and leaves room for flatulence to collect.

Nervousness sometimes follows tea-drinking, but only in cases where it is drunk to force the brain to work beyond its natural powers, and without proper food being taken; as a result the nervous system becomes overstrained.

Coffee.—The best coffee is made from "berries" that have been freshly roasted and ground. To get the strength it needs boiling, but this dissipates the aroma; the best compromise is to make an infusion, pour it off into a heated jug, then to boil the grounds and add this decoction to the infusion previously made. It should be made very strong, so as to bear diluting with plenty of hot milk without tasting weak; this makes coffee a useful beverage for those who cannot take solid food. It is a strong heart-stimulant, and invigorates without subsequent collapse.

Coffee is often adulterated. A simple test is to throw a little into a wine glass of water; if it is pure, it will float and will hardly tinge the water; if, however, chicory or dandelion are present they will sink and color the water red. Many people like the addition of a little chicory.

Cocoa.—This is a milder and less stimulating beverage than either tea or coffee, and contains more food; unfortunately it is less refreshing. The seeds broken up are called cocoa nibs; after prolonged boiling and removal of the floating cocoa-butter, they yield a good beverage.

Prepared cocoas are often used; they contain less cocoa-butter, and are more quickly prepared than the nibs. In some (wrongly called "soluble") the cocoa is ground up with starch; with boiling water the starch forms a mucilage in which the fine particles of cocoa remain suspended.

Chocolate is cocoa ground up with sugar and flavored with vanilla; it generally contains a little starch. Van Houten's cocoa is prepared from the nibs, some of the fat being removed; as it does not contain starch, it forms a thin drink.

All preparations which have drugs, such as kola, added, should be avoided.

Artificial mineral waters have as their basis water surcharged with carbonic acid gas. Soda water, potash water, and lithia water have those salts added, but not in the "lowering" amount often ascribed to them. Indeed, such mineral waters are practically no more lowering than an equal quantity of plain water.

Lemonade and ginger-ale contain in addition to the flavoring agents a considerable amount of sugar, and so are not such refreshing drinks; it is the sugar that causes the lasting froth. Ginger-ale is a pleasant adjunct to a convalescent's meals; if too hot, it may be diluted with an equal quantity of soda water.

Home-made lemonade, made by pouring boiling water on a cut-up lemon (the white rind being removed) and a little sugar, forms a refreshing acid drink.

Of the natural mineral waters, Apollinaris is the best as a beverage, and should always be used abroad if the water supply is doubtful. It is a very pure water, and every precaution is taken in washing and filling the bottles so that it may not be contaminated.

SCIENTIFIC DIETETICS.

WHEN we order this thing and that thing for a sick person to eat, says Dr. John Janvier Black in his recently published book, *"Forty Years in the Medical Profession,"* do we do it thinkingly or unthinkingly? Surely, we should think in carbon and hydrogen, oxygen and nitrogen. Given a patient with contracted kidneys and hypertrophy of the left ventricle, and other ills perchance following in the wake of these, of what use is medicine, of what use are pills and powders, if we allow such a patient to stuff himself with an excess of nitrogenous food?

When we order our pills and potions and powders in such a case, let us think in carbon and hydrogen and oxygen and nitrogen, and see to it that we do not increase his blood-pressure by food whilst we are endeavoring to control it by drugs. In such a case, if I must abandon one course of treatment and keep only to the other, give me diet; "throw physic to the dogs."

Another practical point in dietetics is—study the individual. It is very true that what will nourish one man will poison another, and further, what will be proper for a well man may kill a sick man. Some individuals can live on milk alone when they try; with others it is impossible. Many a man can eat mutton and grow fat on it, so he can eat eggs and thrive; to others, again, these are poison. Such are mere idiosyncrasies, and it is well to remember them. I believe the principles of diet and nutrition, the effects of alcohol and tobacco and such, should be taught to some extent in the schools; not fanatically, but reasonably. Some general knowledge on this score would add much to the general health of a people and be of assistance to physicians in treating the average man. There is a diet for the young, for the man of middle age and for the aged person. We commence with milk, with the complete food, the balanced ration. We go through all the luxuries of a lifetime, and as we approach toothless old age we come back again to childhood and to childhood's ration—milk, and in extreme old age the nearer we adhere to the simple milk diet the better and happier we are, and the longer and more satisfactorily we live. My observation and experience lead me to believe, as intelligent persons grow to middle age and beyond, they, as a rule, become careful as to diet.

There is, no doubt, much suffering from improper diet, and bad cooking is responsible for many ills, and doubtless many deaths. A little observation of the inner life of the poor will cause one to realize in a high degree the utter discomfort and utter misery, even unto death, which come to those untutored and unskilled in providing, in choosing and in preparing properly for the table even the simplest of foods. Education, supervision, the evolution to a higher plane of living for these people is the only corrective for such pitiable ignorance and carelessness. These people need supervision, they need instruction. The principles of cooking practically taught in schools would help out in this work. Call it paternalism if you will, but as we grow wiser in government such matters must come up and be taken up before we reach the highest civilization.

The simplest chemical classification is Liebig's nitrogenous and non-nitrogenous. The nitrogenous group are tissue-builders or flesh-formers; the non-nitrogenous group furnish the body with the fuel and keep up the animal heat, and are the force-producers. The tissue-builders also produce some force and heat. There is some nitrogen in vegetables, though not a great deal. The outside coverings of the starch granules contain some nitrogen, for example. Nitrogenous foods also are not absolutely nitrogenous, as they contain some fat and glycogen. The uses of food are to serve the body with materials for growth and renewal, and with power, much as fuel does for the steam engine. The consumption of fuel furnishes the power. The starches and sugars furnish much of the power to man. The original force is in the heat of the sun; this is stored by the plants in the latent form of chemical compounds, as Professor Thompson says. The main force of power is oxydation, chiefly of carbon. Wherever it goes, or any waste product goes, it is not destroyed, it only changes its form; you cannot destroy matter. Take urea; it is matter merely of our food in a changed form, something like ashes from coal. The urea and other débris, if not gotten out of the body, blocks the system and prevents the normal processes of oxydation, which must go on properly to give one good health.

Water is to be looked upon as a food, composing as it does seventeen per cent. of the weight of the body, and much of it passes through the body unchanged. Withhold it, and life is impossible. I am sure, as a remedy, it is not half appreciated. Many persons do not drink water enough, and suffer accordingly, whether sick or well. Others, again, may take too much, and it is the duty of the physician to study each case and set his patient right on so important a matter. Of course, much of the water we take goes in as part of our food, and this fifty to sixty per cent of water in our solid foods must be taken into account.

Thompson, quoting from Von Pettenkofer and Voit, shows that during the performance of hard labor the consumption of albumin remains practically the same as during rest, whereas three and one-half times as much fat is consumed, and the amount of carbohydrates is the same, hence for hard laborers give plenty of fat pork, butter, oil and such. A workingman will take from fifty to seventy-five ounces of solid food in twenty-four hours, and about the same amount of water by weight. The ration should contain one part of nitrogenous food to three and one-half parts of non-nitrogenous food. The average albuminous food gives about sixteen per cent of nitrogen. Cow's milk and wheat flour approach nearest to a balanced ration of all food as to their nitrogenous and non-nitrogenous proportions. In cow's milk the proportion is one to three, and in wheat flour one to four and one-half.

These are matters of great practical importance, and all physicians should be more or less familiar with them. The destruction of the carbohydrates in the body is very complete when eaten in excess, and they do not produce fat like fatty foods taken in excess. This is an important practical point. The carbohydrates are more or less fattening when eaten with albumin and fats, because they check the consumption of albu-

min and fats and leave more of them to be converted into tissue fats. Eaten alone they are not so fattening; for example, the Chinaman, living mostly on rice, is not usually overfat. Another practical point: When you have children growing rapidly and using their force in the ceaseless activity of the young, see that they get sufficient of proteids in their daily ration. The food of certain articles of diet is most important to the physician, whether to make up a ration for the soldier, for the laborer, the professional man, or women or children, or, more than all, of the sick entrusted to his care. Of albuminous matters used as food, one-third of it is excreted as urea. This is important to remember when the kidneys are diseased and cannot get rid of this urea, although as before said, some are beginning to deny that urea unexcreted is the great offender it has heretofore been given credit for.

Probably most persons over thirty-five years of age consume too much nitrogenous food, especially those who inherit gout. These gouty, bilious people are usually the strong and healthy, and, as a rule, have ravenous appetites; they live to eat, rather than eat to live. They often incline to be good drinkers of wines, spirits and malt liquors, but, as a rule, much to their disadvantage, are light water-drinkers. If they drink more water the ill effects of a vicious metabolism, of vicious tissue change in nutrition and secretion, would be carried out of the system more generally in the various secretions and excretions. It is surprising to see how soon one who has been a free meat-eater can come down to almost a non-nitrogenous diet and enjoy life and feel lighter and better and more contented in every way, provided the excess of nitrogen he had been taking was doing him harm. One must know something of the chemical composition of foods to lay out such a diet, for it will not do to tell a patient to live on milk and eggs and fish and all manner of vegetables, and to avoid only red meats and the black meat of poultry, etc.

The average fish diet is surely not the

light diet we unthinkingly are apt to take it to be; nevertheless fish is a safer and lighter diet than red meats and such, even if we take the stronger fish like cod. Fish diet does not load the blood with as much waste as the heavy meats do, requiring the getting of more oxygen by exercise to eliminate them from the system. Thus fish diet does not render the overfed man dull, like heavy meats, nor is there any truth in the common belief that fish diet is the best brain-food from the excess of phosphorus it contains.

Eggs are most completely digested, and hence are very nutritious as to their weight, and make a well-balanced ration with carbohydrates alone. The yolk is rich in fats, containing olein, palmitin, yellow pigment and lecithin. It also contains grape-sugar in very small amount, phosphates, iron compounds and sulphur.

Notwithstanding the general belief to the contrary, experiment shows five minutes' actual boiling to be the proper time to boil 167°. A coddled egg is never boiled, for then the heat must reach 212°. At fifteen cents per dozen, hens' eggs are cheap food. At thirty cents per dozen they are expensive food.

Physicians should be able to instruct the families they attend as to their food supply and the nutrients required by different families to keep them in good strength and good health. A family where most of the members are laboring men and women surely requires a different food supply from the family of men and women living a quiet life of ease and comfort. Practically no thought is taken of this either by families or physicians. I am sure, as society goes on to the evolution of a higher civilization, it will be the duty and the every-day work of the family physician to take charge of such matters in the families they attend, and thus lead to a more general rational living, and to better, happier and healthier lives for the individual.

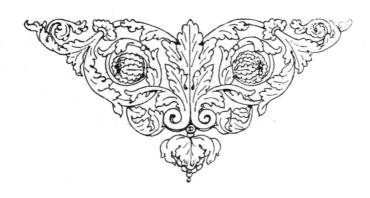

Department of Hygiene.

WITH SPECIAL REFERENCE TO STATE AND PREVENTIVE MEDICINE.

--- --- --- --- -

THE OUNCE OF PREVENTION.

LOOKING over the Progress of Medicine, so frequently alluded to in current medical literature, the one word which epitomizes the changes of the past quarter of a century is *Prophylaxis*. The study of how to cure has merged into that of how to prevent disease. Science reiterates and emphasizes the new rallying cry, "An Ounce of Prevention is worth a Cartload of Cure!"

Cures are undoubtedly more prevalent than in the days of our ancestors, but it is chiefly because preventives have multiplied a hundred fold.

Among the effective prophylactics none occupy so wide a range as the oxygen group. Suboxidation complicates and retards the treatment of all modern diseases. Whatever will give us air, or its vital element—oxygen—will modify disease and facilitate its treatment, by whatever name it may be called. We are learning to breathe a little better than we did, and we ventilate our dwellings a little better. The improvements in this respect are adding to the span of life and to the sum of human enjoyment. But there is still a prevalent degree of oxygen famine. The bicycle, golf, football, tennis, rowing, sea voyages and mountain climbing are all on the right track, but there are millions who are wholly deprived of these privileges. The searchlights in materia medica are all hunting for economic and safe methods of relieving the universal famine. The "Tonics" are valuable to just the extent that they either supply or induce *an increased absorption of oxygen*, or as they act as *oxygen carriers*. Patients do not assimilate appreciable quantities of iron, but it is often an excellent tonic, because it is one of the best oxygen carriers. Most of the reputed tonics act thus vicarously, by either inducing, supplying or conveying an increment of oxygen. The reason why so much "tonic" treatment disappoints the physician and his patient is because the needed increase in the vital element is not supplied.

We speak of this element as a physiologic agent. Indirectly it is probably the most universally invoked of all our adjuvants in the treatment of chronic ailments. Patients are sent in all directions in search of it, across the seas, up the heights, and to "salubrious" retreats, where a more uniform or congenial temperature invites to out-door living and out-door sports, or where some more or less harmless spring waters generally get all the credit for any good results that follow.

How to make this element more freely accessible to the millions who cannot afford to sail the seas, climb the mountains or tarry at the watering places becomes an important and decidedly democratic desideratum and a problem for the physiologist of the future to study.

As a medicinal agent oxygen has had its ups and downs. Quack chemists have made it, quack medicine men have advertised it under various delusive names and quack doctors have used it for all sorts of purposes, legitimate and illegitimate. Some good men in the profession, who ought not to be so easily diverted, have almost entirely avoided it on account of this mixed history. They should remember that such has been the story of nearly all the meritorious laboratory products. Priestly and Lavoisier were accounted quack scientists when they announced the isolation of oxygen; yet oxygen asserted itself and still asserts itself as the most universal and most potent of all the chemic elements. Without it neither sounding brass nor tinkling cymbal could either sound or tinkle. It is and ever has been, as it will ever be, a *sine qua non* of all chemical and vital affinities—the sole condition of life itself. An inadequte supply of it to the vital economy means degeneration and disease. Whatever learned phrases we invent to describe the condition, in the end most mortals are asphyxiated. Not in a crude way, like beautiful Desdemona, but by the refined processes so prevalent in civilized society.

Spurgeon's now much-quoted Jeremiad against Debt, Dirt and the Devil may sound a trifle blunt, coming from a reverend source, but it is a valuable object lesson for the medical profession.

Debt is a monster millstone about the neck of many a struggling mortal, and is answerable for much of the current mental, moral and marital misery and for social crimes innumerable.

Dirt is the omnipresent and incessant foe to human life, happiness and longevity. Against it Lieutenant General Cleanliness and Admiral Antisepsis led the reorganized and newly-weaponed Army and Navy of attack and invasion.

The *Devil* is not now quite so necessary to theologians as he once was, but he still heads the wavering and decimated hosts of the mythologians. Instead of a distinct entity he is now held to be a symbolic embodiment of the whole D family, *Debt, Dirt, Divorces, Darkness* and *Death.*

To his list of antidotes and antagonists—Hard Work, Honesty, Soap and Scrub Brushes the great preacher might have appropriately added that Mauser-Maxim-Machine-gun-Lyddite of modern ammunition—Oxygen. This is the explosive which can reach the enemy, even behind his most effective breastworks, and in lurking ambush! This element is always to be had for the asking, is prepared by Nature, who is an honest expert and is an always loaded magazine rifle. It can be safely and successfully sent on reconnoisances into the most intricate passes. It protects its own sharpshooters from harm and is a faithful ally in the effort to locate and dislodge the germ enemy, whole platoons of which it eventually annihilates if it be persistently invoked. The treatment of wasting diseases, and especially of consumption, has finally settled down to the constant and unrestricted use of fresh air. All the other vaunted specifics have proved delusive and are being quietly discarded. Climate (oxygen) and hygiene now hold the boards.

❧ ❧

HALF TRUTHS AND HUMDRUM IN THE FIELD OF HYGIENE.

THE world is full of "cranks," the term generally being applied in a more or less deprecatory if not sometimes despicable sense. Many people look upon "cranks" as the direct or indirect cause of most of the social troubles of the day and age. To such people a "crank" is a criminal by implication, if not in fact.

This is an unwarranted and perhaps often unconscious misconception of the character and of the facts in the case. In the mechanical world the crank is a most essential factor, the very keynote to power. In its crude form power is merely pressure in one direction, and therefore unavailable for human processes. The crank transforms this into rotary motion and thus makes locomotion and every form of machinery possible. Without the interposition of the crank to turn their energy into useful work the steam engine and the dynamo would be no more than curiosities and playthings.

The social, sanitary and "moral" crank is quite as essential in the general makeup of human society. Each has his specific and usually legitimate mission. That portion of society coming in immediate contact with him is compelled to make due allowance for the one-sidedness of his particular fad; but in the grand whole he has no occasion to apologize for living, or for his presence in any particular community.

Premising our remarks by this general disclaimer of prejudice against the genus "crank," our immediate business is with "hygienic" cranks. They form a numerous family, are as dissimilar as if each included a distinct family of his own, and are annually multiplying. One has never looked beyond the bathtub, and so is a hydropathist, or a "hydriatist," a term dragooned into use since the Century Dictionary was compiled. He swears by Priessnitz, Shaw and Trall, or else he never heard of these pioneers, and imagines himself a discoverer! He baptizes his patients, right and left, early and late, soaks, showers, steams and sponges them, squirts water over, under and through them, or pumps them full and parboils them alternately and at regular intervals.

Shoulder to shoulder with this modern reminiscence of Neptune and the Sea-nymphs stands the Diet crank. His name is legion, but each one is a man of a single fad. The latter varies from train oil emulsion and terrapin-on-toast to unleavened bran mash, and from the cannibalism of raw meat to roasted potatoes, rice croquets and raw wheat. One is morally certain that the unpardonable dietetic sin consists in partaking of more than one meal in twenty-four hours; and the next one recommends feeding every two hours during the day, regretting that the night cannot be broken up into lunch hours with omelets and oysters, broiled steaks and lobster salads galore. One is convinced that mastication is the keynote to the Millennium; another that water drinking will ward off the ingestive sins of the world; another sounds the praises of a milk diet, and the next denounces the products of the dairy as the most prolific source of tuberculosis.

Thus the masquerade goes on, no two advocates in agreement, but each confident he is the trusted custodian of a saving grace.

Near of kin are the exercise cranks. According to these you have but to become a Sandow, a football captain or a golf champion to mock at the health teachers and outlive the centenarian.

The latest fanatic in this line hails from Chicago, and proves beyond a peradventure, by at least three or four examples and numerous inferences, that after reaching thirty-five no man or woman should take any exercise whatever! He insists with apparent seriousness, that, in effect, every muscular movement indulged after reaching that age is a physical injury and a menace to longevity!

The next specimen of the genus worships Psyche. Everything is mind, soul, suggestion. Think a thing and you are that thing. There is no such thing as feeling. Toothache is a groveling delusion, and a broken leg a figment of the imagination. This too, too solid earth is a physical fraud, a phantom of a sinful and unbelieving brain. God is, and Mother Eddy is, and that is all that is necessary.

Finally, the humdrum hygienists are a host. They have been telling the same story, reciting old saws and see-saws about orthodoxy in diet, "taking cold," regular exercise and systematic coddling for the last four generations. All their philosophy consists of folklore that was old when Moses made love to Zipporah in the Kenite Oasis. A new idea would endanger their reason; so they are satisfied with the old, which they con, over and over, year in and out, like poll-parrots, or flesh-and-blood phonographs that can be rewound to the end of time, but who remain unconscious of their own stupidity and proud of their accumulations of dry-as-dust platitudes.

❧　❧

GOETHE'S HYGIENE.

THE fame of Goethe, the great age to which he lived, and his reputation as a model of physical as well as mental manhood give a special interest to Dr. Bode's article on "Goethe's Hygiene" in the *Hygienische Rundschau*, No. 15, which is commented upon in *Janus* for November. Though justly considered one of fortune's greatest favorites, Goethe owed physically less to nature than is generally supposed. "He suffered much in lungs, heart and kidneys, his digestive organs troubled him greatly, gout gave him bad hours, besides which came external evils or ulcerations on cheeks, eyes, feet, etc." He had serious hæmoptysis in his 18th year, and was "given up" several times, 1767, 1768, 1817, 1823. In 1788 Schiller found him looking much older than his years. His sentiveness was sometimes a burden to him. He loved warmth and light and hated the winter He was upset by some decayed apples in Schiller's desk, which did not affect the weaker poet. Neither tea nor coffee agreed with him, and his temperament varied with the barometer.

All these disadvantages, however, were outweighed by an excellent appetite and power of sleeping, and a deliberate care for his health, the absence of which he blamed in Schiller. He thought much of the power of will in warding off infection and maintaining strength and vigor and he used it to convert his naturally passionate and excitable temperament into the Olympian serenity which characterized his later years. Equally important was his love of fresh air and exercise. He introduced river bathing at Weimar, and converted the local physicians to his views. Walking and riding were his favorite exercises and he was among the first to practice mountaineering as a sport. His teeth were perfect to his 83d year, and he could boast that he had never suffered from tooth or headache. He was fond of fruit and drank wine to the extent of a bottle, or a bottle and a half, daily. Tobacco he abominated. With regard to medicine, he held the curious view that, though physicians might maintain or restore health, they could not prolong life. "We live so long as God has ordained, but it is a great difference whether we live like poor dogs, or are well and vigorous, and here a clever physician can do much." Of his own medical adviser, he said in 1827. "That I am still so well is owing to Vogel," and a year later, "Vogel is a born doctor and one of the most genial of men"; while the latter said of the poet, "Goethe had a singularly high opinion of genuine disciples of healing art, and was a grateful and compliant patient."

SANITATION IN THE FIGHT AGAINST CONSUMPTION.

EVERY well informed and reflecting physician knows, says the *N. Y. Med. Journ.*, that it will not do to concentrate our efforts in any particular direction to the exclusion of other points. The segregation and enlightened treatment of persons actually affected with tuberculous disease, as well as measures for destroying or sterilizing their sputa, are indispensable, but one great element in any successful strife against the spread of the disease lies in strengthening the resistive powers of persons who have not yet been attacked, and chiefly by improving the homes of the poor and their modes of life. This was very effectively pointed out by Dr. Beverley Robinson, of New York, in the January number of the *St. Louis Courier of Medicine*.

If we admit, says Dr. Robinson, that without the bacillus there is no tuberculous disease, yet, even with the bacillus, there must be the soil ready or prepared for its growth and development, with all its evil consequences. In a healthy individual, he thinks, it is more than probable that the bacillus will prove innocuous. for it will meet with a barren soil and, taking no root, will breed no disease; susceptibility, hereditary or acquired, must exist, or the microbe's attack is ineffective—literally, it does little or no harm to persons who are in perfect health. On this point, we think, the profession is quite in accord with Dr. Robinson; indeed, the opinion he expresses seems an almost unavoidable inference from the observation that so many escape the disease throughout a long life, although practically exposed to it well-nigh continually.

Dr. Robinson would have legislation enforcing an adequate supply of pure air in the tenement-houses, with the free penetration of sunlight and cleanliness made obligatory. Perhaps it is not practicable for legislation to do more in these directions than to enforce a certain minimum of requirements; but, seeing what reforms have already been brought about in the sanitary surroundings of the poor, mainly as the result of medical teaching, we may confidently hope for a speedy and ample extension of these improvements—with legislation if necessary, but independently of it by preference.

ADVANTAGES AND LIMITATIONS OF STERILIZING AND PASTEURIZING MILK.

MILK, said Dr. Blackader, of Montreal, in a paper read before a recent meeting of the New York Academy of Medicine, obtained under unfavorable conditions and kept at a rather high temperature contained many bacteria, and in addition, their spores and toxins. According to our present knowledge, all forms of bacteria were undesirable in an infant's food. It had been shown that 99.8 per cent. of the bacteria could be destroyed by pasteurization. The older the milk was the more difficult it was to pasteurize it. Pasteurization at 70° C. destroyed the vast majority of the forms liable to produce extensive and rapid change in the quality of the milk. It was necessary in most instances to maintain the pasteurized milk at a low temperature in order to preserve it from further change.

However, the same could be said of milk heated to 100° C. Milk exposed to 60° C. or 140° F. had ninety-six to ninety-nine per cent. of its bacteria destroyed. Russell had found that when milk was heated in tubes to 140° F. tubercle bacilli were not entirely killed because the little pellicle which formed on the surface of the milk protected the bacilli to some extent. If this pellicle was broken up complete destruction of the tubercle bacilli was assured. Milk raised to 100° C. was markedly altered in taste, smell, and chemical composition. The albumin and globulin were coagulated, the lecithin and nuclein were destroyed, and the organic phosphates converted to some extent into the inorganic phosphates. For the coagulation of milk in the stomach calcium must be present in a more or less free form. It was probable that the preliminary curdling of milk was an aid to digestion. It was also probable that in milk heated in this way certain useful ferments were destroyed. As long as milk could be rendered practically sterile at comparatively low temperatures it seemed useless and even deleterious to subject the milk to a higher temperature. It was generally stated that milk was pasteurized at 157° F.

EXAMINATION OF DRINKING WATER IN ILLINOIS.

DURING the last few years, according to *Science*, several thousand samples of drinking water from various ordinary housewells throughout the State have been sent to the State University of Illinois for analysis and report as to quality. By far the greater proportion of these water samples have proved, upon analysis, to be contaminated with drainage from refuse animal matters, and consequently have been regarded with grave suspicion, or have been pronounced unwholesome for use as drink. The present prevalence of typhoid fever in a number of places in the State makes it desirable that the public should remember that the State has made provision for the examination of all suspected waters. It is not practicable to isolate actually the typhoid-fever germs or to prove directly their absence from waters submitted for analysis; this for the reason that the work entails more labor and time than are made available by the means which the State provides. However, the chemical examination is sufficient ordinarily to show whether the water is contaminated with house drainage or drainage from refuse animal matters or whether it is free from such contamination. Any citizen of the State may have examinations made of the drinking water in which he is interested, free of charge, by applying to the Department of Chemistry of the State University.

It would, no doubt, be advisable if this practice were general throughout the various States. It is altogether probable that by such means, carefully carried out, a considerable protection against epidemic disease might be secured.

THE USE OF TOBACCO ON ACTIVE SERVICE.

In the face of all that has been said, and apparently proven, against the use of alcohol and tobacco, we occasionally meet with some one who advocates the use of one or the other or both, under certain conditions. The London *Lancet* says that the war in South Africa has taught many things of greater and of less importance. Perhaps nothing that it has demonstrated has been more marked than the important part which tobacco plays in the soldier's existence. Whether this is to be reckoned as a great fact or a small one there can be no doubt about the truth of it. Yet the Duke of Wellington's armies had no tobacco worth speaking of. If they did not forbid its use, at any rate the Iron Duke's officers were directed to advise their men strongly against it. What a curious contrast with the campaigning in South Africa, where marches and privations as long and as stern as any suffered by our great-grandfathers were borne by the volunteers and soldiers of to-day with a grumble only when their "smokes" failed them. We have it from many who took part in the forced marches leading to Paardeberg, to Bloemfontein, to Pretoria, and beyond, that rations were but two or three biscuits a day the only real physical content of each twenty-four hours came with the pipe smoked by the smouldering embers of a camp fire. This pipe eased the way to sleep that might otherwise have lingered, delayed by the sheer bodily fatigue and mental restlessness caused by prolonged and monotonous exertion. It is difficult, then, to believe that tobacco is anything but a real help to men who are suffering long labors and receiving little food, and probably the way in which it helps is by quieting cerebration—for no one doubts its sedative qualities—and thus allowing more easily sleep, which is so all-important when semi-starvation has to be endured. The cases of acute mental derangement in the course of campaigns such as the present are many. There have, indeed, been many in South Africa. It would be most profitable and interesting could medical officers have taken special note of the capacity for sleep previously evidenced by those who broke down, and also of their indulgence or non-indulgence in tobacco. We are inclined to believe that, used with due moderation, tobacco is of value second only to food itself when long privations and exertions are to be endured. Two features are to be noted with regard to the smoking practiced on active service. It is almost entirely in the open air, and it is largely on an empty stomach. The former is always an advantage; the latter we generally reckon a most unfavorable condition. Shall we see in the near future patients with tobacco amblyopia or smoker's heart acquired while the trusting friend of tobacco thought that he was enjoying unharmed the well-earned solace of a hard day's march? We believe not, and that the open air will have saved what might have been the untoward results of smoking when unfed.

THE REVIVAL OF CARBOLIC ACID.

CARBOLIC acid is a misnomer, as the substance so-called is not an acid. Its proper name, phenol, seems a long way from general adoption, and perhaps it is not well to urge the change, as the results might be serious, due to a misapprehension of the less frequently employed term. Carbolic acid has had a singular history. In the seventies it was regarded as the first of antiseptics. Later its poisonous properties were recognized and it fell into disuse, and other more powerful and less dangerous antiseptics came into vogue. The symptoms of poisoning by carbolic acid, the nephritis with its albuminuria and smoky urine, are so well known that they need no description. The occasional occurrence of such severe complications led to a reduction in the strength of carbolized solutions used in surgery until their antiseptic value was practically *nil*. At the same time their poisonous properties were not very greatly lessened. Of late attention has been directed to the frequency with which carbolic acid causes gangrene, particularly of the fingers and toes. This effect is produced when very dilute solutions are employed, if they are kept in contact with the parts for several days. The observation of Palmer, that alcohol was a perfect antidote for strong carbolic acid bids fair to give the drug a range of usefulness that it has never before had. It is apparent that it is the amount of carbolic acid which is absorbed that causes its poisonous properties. A dilute solution having little or no effect in occluding the vessels is very readily taken up. Strong carbolic acid, on the contrary, seals the vessels and prevents absorption. By the term "cure" or strong carbolic acid is meant the liquefied crystals, the solution containing about 95 per cent. of the acid. Experience has proven that this may be applied to an excoriated or ulcerating surface almost with impunity, so far as the absorption is concerned. The depth to which the caustic may extend is variable. Before the neutralizing effect of alcohol was known the strong acid was rarely used, as it was impossible to know how deep it might go. Now a strong acid may be applied and left for one or two minutes, or even longer if it seems desirable, and its action can be immediately suspended by the application of alcohol.

This application of the strong acid seems to be the best method of treating a suppurating focus. An abscess may be washed with it, destroying the pyogenic membrane, a single application making the cavity aseptic. This followed by alcohol would limit the further action of the drug; the same is true regarding ulcers, sloughs, and necrotic areas. The brilliant results that have been achieved by Phelps in treating deep suppurations about the hip, and suppuration of the middle ear, bid fair to make this one of the most important surgical means of dealing with suppuration.—*Medicine.*

PHYSIOLOGICAL EXPERIMENTA-TION OF ANIMALS.

AFTER recounting the difficulties which legislation had placed upon the scientific research of the physiologists in England, in an address before the students of the Denver College of Medicine, *Colorado Medical Journal,* Sir Edward Foster said:

"I suppose you don't experience the sort of thing here, but in the rest of the world we are stimulated by difficulties; and I think there can be no doubt that the fact we have to fight against difficulties in the progress of physiological inquiry occasioned by the Act has really stirred us up to more active and more earnest inquiry than if the Act had not passed; but if the question comes before you, don't you be too much influenced by the beneficial effects of difficulties. (Laughter.) Resist, as I have said to everyone in America, resist interference with your inquiries. I heard the Lord Chief Justice of England, when this matter was being discussed in the House of Lords, I heard him say, 'You must remember, my lords, that this is essentially a penal act.' I, a professional physiologist, sat in the gallery of the House of Lords and heard the highest legal authority state that the legislature were about to treat me as a felon. They were about to bring into action what he called a penal act. Don't you allow yourselves for a minute to get crippled by all these special certificates.

"Indeed, no legislation at all is necessary. I speak not for myself; I speak for all my brethren. We are not cruel. We never cause pain if we can possibly help it, and the whole progress of physiology is dependent upon the experiments upon living animals. The other people may say what they like, but if you read the whole story of physiology you will see that every step has been based upon an experiment on living animals. I have just come from delivering a course of lectures in San Francisco on the history of physiology. I always knew that our science was based on experiments, but I never knew it as I know it now when I have had to read carefully the old authorities and trace out all their work. Every one who has made an advance has made it by experiment on living animals. And in the old time, for instance in the seventeenth century, in the '60's or '70's of the seventeenth century, just following Harvey, there was a man. Richard Lower, who did very great work on the circulation, on respiration and other parts of physiology, and so far as I can make out from reading his works he must in the quiet retreat of Oxford have performed just as many experiments, indeed, I believe on the whole he performed in the same time more experiments than Claude Bernard; and Harvey himself, in his great work on the heart, says not only once, not twice, but several times, that he came to the truth first of all by observing certain facts in the animals and then testing those facts by repeated experiments on living animals. And it is a duty of the whole medical profession to see that the physiologist is not hampered in his important inquiries by any misdirected legislation."

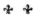

INFECTION INCREASED BY THE USE OF ALCOHOL.

WHILE direct experimentation upon man for the purpose of determining whether or not the use of alcohol renders him more susceptible to infection, has not been undertaken, but says *Mod. Med.* every physician is fully cognizant of the fact that when an alcoholic habitué becomes diseased, his chances for recovery are much less than those of the total abstainer. The inebriate who contracts pneumonia—a disease to which on account of his indulgence in alcoholic beverages he is prone—stands a very poor chance of recovery. The surgeon also recognizes the inability of wounded tissues of the drunkard successfully to combat infection and to heal by first intention. Because of these conditions the surgeon frequently hesitates to operate upon such an individual.

While these facts have been familiar for years, very little has been done to determine the real cause which in such cases renders the vital principle of the body unable to cope successfully with disease-producing agencies.

Some years ago Dr. Abbott carried on a number of experiments which had a practical bearing upon this subject. His experiments consisted in feeding rabbits upon alcohol, and later inoculating them with some pathogenic micro-organism. The result showed that in every case, control animals were much less susceptible to infection than the animals which had been fed upon alcohol, thus clearly demonstrating that alcohol greatly decreases the ability of the animal body to resist disease.

Dr. Laitinen (*Zeitsch. f. Hyg. und Infect.*, July 19, 1900; *Br. Med. Jour.*, September 23) recently conducted a number of experiments similar to those of Dr. Abbott. In these experiments Dr. Laitinen used 342 animals—dogs. rabbits, guinea pigs, fowls, and pigeons. The animals were inoculated with anthrax tubercle. and diphtheria bacilli. These were chosen as types of acute infection. chronic infection, and pure intoxication. A twenty-five-per-cent. solution of ethylic alcohol in water was used in most cases. When employed in greater strength, the alimentary mucous membrane of birds became inflamed. In a few cases dogs were given fifty-per-cent. solutions of alcohol.

The alcohol was administered either by an esophageal catheter, or by dropping it into the mouth by means of a pipette. The dose was graduated according to the weight of the animal, being from one and one-half c.cm. in the pigeon to sixty c.cm. in some of the dogs. It was administered in a variety of ways and for varying times; sometimes in single large doses, at others in gradually increasing doses for months at a time, in order to produce here an acute and there a chronic poisoning. In all cases Dr. Laitinen found that without exception the effect of the administration of alcohol, in any form whatever, was to render the animal distinctly, sometimes markedly, more susceptible to infection than were the controls.

Such convincing proof of the devitalizing nature of alcohol should certainly carry a great deal of weight with it, especially when obtained by such eminent investigators. This, coupled with the practical experience of the physician in dealing with patients who have been in the habit of using alcoholics, should be a warning against the administration of alcohol in any form; for the object to be sought in the treatment of disease is to increase the vital activities of the tissues, and thus render them more resistant to infection.

The administration of alcohol for the purpose of increasing bodily resistance is certainly in nowise a rational or scientific procedure, and its use is certainly not upheld by men who have carefully studied its therapeutic properties.

THE ORIGIN OF DISEASE.

WHILE the writer of the following paper may be a little over sanguine in his views, what he says is nevertheless full of good sense: "Reading in a medical journal an article on the etiology of epilepsy," says this writer in London *Health*, "suggests the important subject of the origin of disease as a topic for careful consideration. Whatever science achieved in this study of causation, by its researches with the microscope, and by chemical analysis, it has only made more apparent the fact that human beings are largely responsible for their own ills.

"A knowledge of how to recognize and get rid of disease, in its beginnings, is now needed, so that suffering may be lessened and life be saved.

"Whenever, in my study of disease, I trace back the history of any case, I find certain conditions present at the beginning, and these are the same in 90 per cent. of all diseases. They arise from external causes, and affect the body, first, at its surface, the skin, rendering it inactive for a shorter or longer time, with consequent disturbance in all the vital processes, depleting the body of alkalies, by eliminating them as alkaline carbonates. Chemically, skin inaction is a self-poisoning process; for the skin is an all-important organ, for elimination of waste products, and any condition that interferes with this function causes one or more of the other organs to take up the work vicariously, and overwork or disease of that organ results.

"An inactive skin may be the result of some mental state, as grief, fear, anger, care: or it may be caused by a nervous shock, by over brain work, or may arise from exposure to dampness, cold, or heat, or from tight clothing, etc.

"As a consequence of these disturbing causes there is contraction at the surface of capillaries and pores, retention of carbonic acid and other waste products of the body, with arterial tension, that makes the heart work at a disadvantage.

"I believe that an inactive skin is the origin of functional derangements, and also of the occlusions of tissues that give rise to aneurisms, acute mania, coma, sunstroke, apoplexy, cholera infantum, tumors, cancer, rheumatism, dyspepsia, eczema, fevers, paralysis, kidney, and other organic diseases; and that this abnormal condition of the skin holds persons in the constitutionally debilitated state (by the same self-poisoning process), that manifests itself in the many nervous affections that are presenting new complications for study each year.

"To help bring about better health conditions, several important suggestions are presented. Such as the diffusion of practical knowledge that will enable people to help themselves, by attention to hygienic methods of living, so that, if they are in a malarial region, for example, they may keep themselves proof againt all miasma.

"Line upon line and precept upon precept," being required by each generation. Restoration to a normal condition is possible at the beginning of each disturbance of function in the body, and this can be understood and attended to by all intelligent persons.

" Retrocession of an exanthema is liable to prove fatal, and death ensues in a few minutes if the skin is wholly occluded. Any partial occlusion or inaction causes a relative amount of disturbance in the vital, chemical changes, which, when they are held at their normal balance, maintain the body in health.

"Any deviation from this balance in the growth and repair of tissue, and the elimination of waste matter, causes the individual to become susceptible to disease. Take a case of pneumonia. The first stage of chill causes a contraction of the skin, with occlusion of pores and capillaries, and retention of waste matter that must be got rid of by some other eliminating organ, or remain in the body and chemically deteriorate, thus furnishing a fertile growth of bacteria and other low forms that flourish under such circumstances. This contraction at the surface of the body congests the lungs, that is, over-crowds them with blood driven from the skin by the effect of the chill, and the heart works at a greater speed and under difficulties that cause overstrain.

"Remove the pressure (arterial tension), by restoring the skin to its normal action, and amelioration of the whole condition begins at once. Kidney diseases (when not produced by drugs) result from the functional derangement of the skin, causing vicarious elimination of waste products, and overwork and disease of the kidneys ensues. Restore and hold the skin to its normal work, and the kidneys are relieved and restored to a healthy state.

"Rheumatism originates in 'a chill,' or exposure to cold, or dampness, and the same skin inaction and self-poisoning processes result as in other diseases.

" Consumption begins in a series of 'colds,' which means lack of vital action at the surface of the body, and the consequent overwork and disease of lungs and other organs.

Illustrations can be multiplied, but they all show a similarity of conditions in the earlier stages of disease, and the need of checking these in their incipiency, so as to stop further retrograde processes.

"How best to restore the skin to its normal activity, where functional disturbance has arisen, is a question of vital importance, for on reading medical journals, I find records of various combinations of therapeutic treatment, but no recognition of the need of such adjuvants and hygienic means as will restore and hold the skin to its best functional activity. Bathing, the inducing of profuse sweating, and friction, are the usual methods of bringing about a skin reaction.

"Bathing is often done improperly causing a great loss of vitality and strength, instead of benefit.

"Profuse sweating is also a depleting process, but shows a tendency in the system to reaction at the surface that ought to be made available at less expense to the patient. By friction of the skin, properly applied, the reaction can be best brought about. To do this it is necessary to stimulate the whole surface of the body by rubbing, in harmony, with the circulation.

"Most persons will rub 'down,' or in any direction, no matter what, so long as it is vigorous, without any practical knowledge or attention to the needs of the case, or to the physiological processes, which should be helped, not hindered, by artificial means.

"Slow, firm movement, causing pressure in the direction of the venous circulation, will restore the skin to its vital activity best. This can be done by the hand; but by application of a properly-constructed flesh-brush, which will help restore the skin to its action, and also restore the electrical conditions of the body to a normal balance, the whole system is regulated, and disease abated.

"Having carefully tested this method during a period of ten years, I have been able to rapidly restore persons from both acute and chronic diseases."

INDIVIDUAL RESISTANCE IN DISEASE.

VARIATIONS in severity of symptoms depend on the varying violence of the attack and 'the varying capacity of resistance. Dr. Durham dismisses the former on account of "our scanty knowledge of the laws which govern the variations of the parasite." This well-founded admission reveals a gap says *The Contemporary Review* in the very foundations of bacteriology, sufficient to render the entire edifice of doubtful stability; but let that pass. More is known about the effect of resisting power in individuals. It may be due to specific immunity acquired by a previous attack or transmitted from a parent, or it may consist in a natural refractoriness. Several classes of persons may be distinguished, all capable of harboring specific organisms without showing any recognizable signs of it. One very important class is formed by those who have had an attack and recovered, but in whom the specific micro-organisms remain for an indefinite time. Dr. Durham mentions diphtheria, enteric fever, and plague. The bacilli of all these diseases have been found in patients weeks and months after their apparent complete recovery. Dr. Klein has recorded the same thing of scarlet fever. This is in keeping with a pretty common occurrence. A child has diphtheria or scarlet fever and is sent to the hospital. In due course it is sent home quite well, but at once, or perhaps after a time, other children in the same house take the disease. Then there is an outcry about "premature discharge." The same thing happens in private houses. One person suffers from some infectious illness, and is shut off from the other inmates, who remain quite well. The patient recovers and returns to ordinary life, and presently some one else takes the disease.

A second class consists of those who, having never had a previous attack, are exposed to infection and take it, but in so slight a form as to escape notice. The most familiar examples of this are furnished by dipththeria and plague. The most trifling of sore throats and a slightly enlarged gland may represent these formidable diseases, respectively. A third class—or perhaps it is only a difference of degree—is formed by those in whom the infective agent lodges, but remains wholly inactive. Here again, diphtheria, which has been more carefully studied in this connection than any other disease, furnishes examples. Virulent cultures of diphtheritic bacilli have been obtained from healthy children.

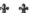

FEEDING IN TYPHOID FEVER.

THE effects of a more generous diet on the treatment of typhoid fever than is the usual practice are discussed by Dr. G. W. Moorehouse in the *Boston Med. and Surg. Journal*, Nov. 15th, 1900, and reviewed in the *Med. News*. In a study of a series of 150 cases of which Dr. Moorehouse reports 117, the average time the patients were kept on a milk diet was ten days. As soon as the appetite began to return to any patient soft typhoid diet was at once ordered without direct reference to the temperature. The appetite and not the temperature was the guide to the continuance and increase of the diet once begun. The typhoid diets adopted by the writer are: (1) Milk diet, eight ounces every two hours, subject to special directions as to night feedings; (2) liquid typhoid diet, consisting of milk, milk with tea or coffee, albumin-water, beef-tea, malted milk, chicken-broth and barley-water, beef-juice and barley-water; broths, milk whey, junket, strained soups or gruels may also be given; (3) soft typhoid diet, to be added to the milk or liquid diet (a) ice cream, well cooked (boiled) rice, broths thickened with it; (b) soft boiled or poached egg on soft toast, blanc-mange and milk puddings, calf's foot and other gelatin jellies; (c) gruels, crackers or bread softened in milk or broths, macaroni, finely-minced or scraped meats; the increase in diet to be very gradual, one addition only each day; (4) typhoid convalescent diet, to be added to anything above, the soft parts of oysters, a sweetbread, chop, cutlet, squab, game (small), chicken, fish, steak, rare roast beef; a mealy baked potato may also be given with any of the meats; (5) full typhoid diet, 6 A.M., milk; 8 A.M., a cereal with cream and a little sugar, milk with tea or coffee, egg on toast, bread or toast with butter; 10 A.M., bread and butter, with gruel or milk, or broth with egg; 11.30 A.M., soup, meat or fish (anything mentioned above), ice cream, blanc-mange, or milk pudding; 2 to 3 P.M., like 10 A.M.; 4 to 4.30 P. M., creamed chicken or a bit of cold chicken or roast beef, bread, and milk flavored with tea or coffee; 6 P.M., cocoa, gruel or broth; at night, milk two to four times. Any change from a less to a more generous diet should always be gradual. The mortality in the 150 cases, thus fed, was 8.67 per cent. There were relapse-like rises of temperature in 30 of the 117 cases. In nine cases this relapse occurred before, and in 21 after, a more generous diet was begun. The writer believes this high proportion (18 per cent.) of relapse to be due to the fact that he has doubtless included among the cases of relapse many which would not be so classified by others. The temperature charts show very clearly that the increased feeding does not interrupt the deferescence. The important features in these diet lists are (1) the article permitted, and (2) the directions for the increase in diet, insuring the gradualness of any increase from a less to a more generous diet level. The new level was in the average case in about four or five days. Moorehouse says that patients fed generously begin to put on flesh at once, and show a continuous gain in strength and spirits as well as in flesh. He thinks that liberal feeding is a distinct advantage as regards prompt recovery of normal condition.

✠ ✠

THE DIETETIC AND MEDICINAL TREATMENT OF DIABETES MELLITUS.

By R. B. Glass, M.D.

(Extract from Clinical Report.)

The more prominent symptoms in diabetes mellitus, viz.: thirst, inordinate appetite, copious diuresis and emaciation, are unquestionably dependent upon the amount of glucose in the blood and tissues. Our first duty is to combat all disorders of skin, stomach, bowels, and internal organs. Regulation of habits of life, correct diet and proper clothing are valuable means toward perfect recovery. Withdraw from the diet as completely as possible (but not too suddenly) all sugar-producing articles—the most important being potatoes and bread.

Admissible foods are cheese, eggs, poultry, game, oil, fats, butter, pure cream and fish. Green vegetables such as spinach, lettuce with plenty of oil and mustard, onions, water cress, cabbage and celery. Soups prepared from meat or the above vegetables are greatly relished. Tea or coffee without milk or sugar. The vegetable kingdom abounds in articles containing a large percentage of sugar, and these must be rigidly excluded.

The non-admissible foods are liver, honey, milk, beans, peas, parsnips, turnips, potatoes, carrots; sago, rice, macaroni, vermicelli, tapioca. Avoid sweet fruits, such as oranges, pears, apples, plums, currants, gooseberries.

As to the medicinal treatment, I have found nothing which in therapeutic force equals arsenauro. The results as described in the following case are practically identical with those secured in several others which recently came under my care.

Miss H., clerk in confectionery, ate much candy, noticed constant thirst, drank water frequently, ravenous appetite, voided urine to the amount of nine pints in twenty-four hours. Thought she had a tape-worm, her appetite being insatiable. Polyuria and an eczema of the genitals prompted her to consult me. Examination revealed spongy gums, carious teeth, eczema of the genitals with distressing pruritus, very weak heart, breath sweetish, swelling about both ankles. Specific gravity of urine was 1.049, sugar 12 per cent., albumin a trace; placed her upon a diet of fresh meat, eggs, sardines, cheese, peanuts, tea and coffee; ordered a warm bath every evening, the alimentary tract flushed with a saline once weekly. She followed instructions implicitly. Arsenauro was given, ten-drop doses in a full goblet of water, t. i. d. the first day, twelve drops four times a day the second day, thirteen drops four times third day, fifteen drops four times fourth day, eighteen drops four times fifth day, twenty drops three times sixth day. Urine was then examined; great improvement, quantity reduced to fifty-two ounces, specific gravity 1.030, patient had gained three pounds in a week. For two days I continued the same dose of arsenauro, patient's condition remaining stationary. I then increased the dose to twenty-two drops in a full goblet of water t. i. d. As she was slightly constipated, I ordered a saline to again flush out the alimentary tract (as I consider this most important in all cases). Arsenauro was gradually increased until forty-eight drops were taken t. i. d., when physiological effects showed. The quantity was reduced to forty-five drops t. i. d. and continued for ten days (the

patient feeling most comfortable). I found that rapid amendment had set in, pruritus gone, eczema had almost disappeared, swelling about the ankles gone, quantity of urine reduced to almost normal, with a trace of sugar. The restricted diet was continued three weeks longer—the sugar had then entirely disappeared, the patient had reached her original weight and felt perfectly well.

There are certain important facts to bear in mind in the treatment of diabetes mellitus with arsenauro or mercauro.

First.—Administer a saline and flush out the alimentary tract. For this purpose two teaspoonfuls of Carlsbad sprudel salt should be dissolved in one pint of hot water and the patient should be directed to take this quantity in three portions at least one hour before breakfast.

Second.—See that the digestive organs are in good condition. I usually follow the saline with 3 grs. of caroid and 3 grs. of bicarb. soda in powder, to be taken just after meals for four or five days.

Third.—Now begin the use of arsenauro or mercauro. If the case in hand be complicated with Bright's disease, then mercauro should be given preference.

Uncomplicated diabetes demands arsenauro.

Method of Administration.—Commence with a small dose, say five drops in one-half goblet of water after each meal. Day by day increase the dose in drops until the patient gives evidence of physiological saturation. This will be observed when under the lids puff or there are loose, griping evacuations. Some patients will show this early, at eight or ten drops; others will not manifest this intolerance before reaching sixty or eighty drops, but each case is a law unto itself, and it is imperative that this point of saturation be reached in each individual.

When these untoward manifestations are apparent, the solution should not be increased, but the quantity lessened a few drops to a dosage which does not produce these symptoms, the patient being continued on this lessened dose (which does not irritate) for eight or ten weeks, before permanent results are to be expected.. It is well to keep the patient on the solution long after the disappearance of all sugar. No affection carries in its train more debility and discomfort than diabetes. Persons experience a degree of debility known scarcely to any other form of malnutrition.

It may be said that arsenauro and mercauro have the power to cure diabetes mellitus by quieting the irritation of the vaso motor centers whence the glycosuria and other symptoms of diabetes emanate.

Arsenauro and mercauro are powerful blood makers and blood builders and exercise their specific influence by virtue of their nutritive effect upon the nerve centers.

Malnutrition and its accompanying debility, whenever met, are positive indications for these tonic alteratives; and for the ill nourished and anemic child with a weakly constitution, arsenauro and mercauro produce astonishing results.

A strict adherence to a proper dietary is absolutely necessary.

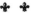

INFLUENCE OF LIGHT ON THE SKIN.

THE influence of sunlight on the appearance of the skin can hardly be overrated, says *The Family Doctor*. Recent experiments with the electric light, which of all artificial illumination most nearly resembles sunlight, have shown how important a part light plays in promoting growth. It has long been known that plants deprived entirely of light soon droop. Some time ago the beneficial action of light was forcibly illustrated. At the close of a public lecture it was found that some buds which had remained on the table had actually blown under the influence of the electric light, while others which had been kept in the dark had made no progress whatever. Animals, too, are well known to have similar susceptibilities, and it is certain that much of the pallor observable in the faces

of those whose lives are passed in our gloomy courts and alleys and underground work-shops is due to insufficiency of light. No wonder that children reared in badly lighted nurseries, and æsthetic people who delight in small windows, with colored glass still further to dim the entering light, should pay the inevitable penalty in pale face and impaired health. Certain skins are very susceptible to the direct action of the sun's rays. Freckles or small spots of discoloration are due entirely to an exceptional formation of pigment in the favoring light of the sun, and sometimes fade as rapidly as they come. The heat rays of the sun act in just the same manner as a fire or mustard plaster, causing general pigmentation or sunburn. Absence of light is said to stimulate the cells in which pigment exists, causing them to contract and so hide the pigment; hence the surface becomes lighter in color, returning to a darker tint again on the reaction of light.

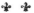

THE HYGIENE OF MANIA.

DR. ANTOIMIE, director of the Insane Hospital of Voghera, recently made an interesting address on the hygiene of mania before the Italian Society of Hygiene. The able chairman of the conference observed that the progress of civilization, the incessant intellectual work, the sharp struggle for existence, and poverty, have for the last twenty years doubled the number of insane people in Italy, which is very nearly 33,000. He went on to speak of the active means that they might take concerning the mania either of persons under treatment or persons who have already been treated, and again persons who might require treatment in the future. For the first mentioned, a vigilant and intelligent care is necessary, in the choice of the duty (or work), which they wish to assign to them in (the) society, so that they be not constrained to fight a battle superior to their physical and mental forces. For the second, it is desirable that the work of the patrons of the discharged patients should not be limited only to pecuniary help, but should surround them by a moral guardianship.

For the third, it would be useful to give to the insane hospitals more room for workshops, thus taking away the appearance of prisons, of great barracks, of cemeteries of the reason.

Dr. Antoimie talked at length of malnutrition as an important cause of mania, and he concludes by saying that he has not finished the argument, but only to give some advice in view of the benefits that can be drawn from a better-understood hygiene in the treatment of mania.—*Exchange.*

THE ELEVATOR DISEASE.

THE *London News* is responsible for the following warning, says the Boston *Med. and Surg. Journal,* which we believe may have an element of truth: "It looks as though people with weak hearts had, after all, better climb ten flights of stairs than effect the ascent by means of the lift. This convenient institution is becoming ubiquitous. We soar up to the topmost story of the sky-scraping flat, we descend through geological strata to the twopenny tube by its assistance. We thought we were thereby saving our vital energies and lengthening our lives. The doctors seem to hold another opinion. Lift attendants have died sudden deaths; people with weak 'hearts have noticed ominous sensations when in the elevator. We are told the sudden transition from the heavier air at the foot to the lighter air at the top is extremely trying to the constitution. Even millionaires and bishops and aldermen are now voluntarily tramping up stairs and avoiding the swifter but insidious route. In fact, a new disease has swung into our ken, 'liftman's heart.' We had all of us been risking this malady without knowing it. It is true

most people have experienced the singular sensation of internal collapse when the lift floor sinks beneath the feet, but none of us suspected the results might be so serious. Every new notion for health and comfort seems to bring its particular Nemesis."

STAMPING OUT MALARIA IN ITALY.

PROFESSOR GRASSI, to whom the credit of demonstrating the mosquito conveyance of malaria is largely due, says the *Med. Press and Circular,* has undertaken the task of stamping out the disease in the south of Italy. He proposes commencing operations on the Mediterranean side of the peninsula below Naples, over an area which covers about 30,000 square miles, with a population estimated at close upon two and a half millons. His scheme comprises the rendering mosquito-proof of all houses by means of wire gauze, and the withdrawal of their owners within the protected houses between sunset and sunrise, not a very easy thing to enforce, by the way. Those already suffering from the disease will be supplied gratuitously with quinine, and some idea of the magnitude of the undertaking may be gathered from the statement that the cost of the necessary quinine will exceed £20,000 annually. The firm of Bisleri, of Milan, have generously offered to provide this enormous amount free of cost should the enterprise prove a failure. The rules of hygiene are to be enforced where necessary by the aid of the military, but, interesting as is the experiment, we must confess to scant confidence in methods which have to be enforced at the bayonet's point. To educate this large population to the necessity for these drastic measures, on the other hand, is indeed a task from which the boldest might well shrink; moreover, years would be required before any method of instructing this ignorant populace could produce any tangible effect.

EXTEMPORANEOUS METHODS OF WATER PURIFICATION.

SURGEON-MAJOR SCHUCKING of the Austrian army is of the opinion that of the various methods of purification there are only two that can be taken into account for the use of troops in the field: (1) filtration; (2) purification by the addition of chemical agents. Among filters aiming at the sterilization as well as the clarification of water, the Berkefeld-Nordtrueyer alone is so constructed as to meet the exigencies of war. But although well adapted for use in field stations, it can only be carried in baggage wagons. Portable filters only clarify muddy water. The use of them therefore requires to be supplemented by some means of destroying micro-organisms. After extensive experiments and researches (Traube, Lode, Kratschmer, Vogel) such a means has been found in hypochloride of chlorine. This chemical agency certainly kills all bacilli in thirty minutes.—*British Medical Journal.*

CANNOT ENFORCE PURE BUTTER LAW.

THE State Board of Health of Missouri has decided to withdraw its butter inspector from St. Louis, and to make no further attempts to secure the enforcement of the pure butter law in that city as long as the bench of the Court of Criminal Correction is occupied by Judge Clark. The sale of oleomargarine as butter will then be practically unrestricted. The law prohibits the coloring of any substance desired to be used as a substitute for butter, and also the manufacture, sale, or keeping for sale, of any such substance. It does not place any restrictions on the manufacture or sale of oleomargarine, or butterine, if sold on its merits, and not as an imitation of butter.

DISINFECTION OF THE HANDS BY MEANS OF ESSENCES.

EUGENIO CALVELLO draws the following conclusions from a series of experiments: 1. That washing with soap and water and alcohol does not make the hands aseptic, although it does diminish the number of germs to a great extent. 2. That the methods of Fürbringer and Ahlfeld do not result in complete disinfection. 3. That seven to eight per cent. solutions of essence of cinnamon, eleven per cent. of essence of thyme, and seventeen per cent. of essence of geranium act precisely as do solutions of bichloride used according to Fürbringer's method, and should be given the preference in modern surgery, because they do not cause the alterations that bichloride does. 4. Nine-per-cent. solutions of essence of cinnamon, eleven and twelve per cent. of essence of thyme, and eighteen per cent. of essence of geranium assure complete disinfection of the hands. 5. The essence of patchouli has no antiseptic powers.—*Giornale Internazionale delle Scienze Mediche,* September 15, 1900.

HYDROGEN DIOXID AS A LOCAL ANÆSTHETIC.

INJECTED under the epidermis hydrogen dioxid produces immediate and complete anæsthesia of the whole skin. Dr. H. E. Kendall in the *Medical Record* says: "I have used it for over a year in opening abscesses, cutting off redundant tissue in ingrowing toe nails, opening the pleural cavity, and in one case the abdominal cavity. I do not think any absorption takes place, as the intercellular inflation from the gas generated seems to produce such pressure that the skin cuts like frozen tissue."

Department of Physical Education.

WITH SPECIAL REGARD TO THE SYMMETRICAL DEVELOPMENT OF THE BODY.

PHYSICAL TRAINING THE FUNDAMENTAL PART OF UNIVERSAL EDUCATION.

OUR knowledge of how to educate children is undergoing a very great change. The importance of physical training as a part of the scheme of universal education is now recognized by our leading institutions of learning but its full import does not seem to be grasped by the average school teacher or the masses.

Mr. W. W. Hastings in an address says:

"The problem of the age is life, development, conservation of energy.

"That which has absorbed the maximum of our attention as educators, is intellectual development; the result passes for education. The more advanced method by which this much coveted end is being hastened to-day is by the conservation of energy, by the study of economy in the use of the student's time, by teaching him only those things for which he finds an application, by making his path easy. It is not entirely clear but that for the development of individuality of students, too much thinking is done for them. The saving salt to their originality is the inculcation of this practical utilitarian point of view. But the latter has not seemed adequate for the desired end. The independent thinking of a few decades ago, which almost single handed forged its way through all difficulties is responsible for the independent vigorous minds of to-day.

"Economy of expenditure means conservation of energy, but the latter does not necessarily mean true development. A man may by skillful manipulation of his affairs avoid bankruptcy, and yet be gasping for life in a business way. A man may by attention to diet, sleep and other physical hab-

its prolong his existence indefinitely, and all the time be tottering upon the brink of the grave, but this is not *living*. Economy is good, expenditure is better. The vigorous use of his faculties makes the man. That education which does not include the cultivation of vigorous, healthy, normal thinking, is no education. The law of the universe that each form of life prepares the way for something higher, culminates in man himself. The physical exists for the mental, the mental for the spiritual. Brain requires to be fed with rich red blood, the spiritual life demands a clearness of vision to see God.

"Whenever a man ceases to be dependent upon a brain to do his thinking, then will energetic thought cease to be dependent upon physical energy. The teacher who attempts the development of the life of an individual without measuring his physical vitality, is as wise as the builder who attempts to bridge the Niagara without a knowledge of the strength of materials.

"The period at which in a peculiar sense rich full life is made, is that of childhood when public school teachers have the responsibility. It is the period of ceaseless activity, of inquisitiveness and acquisitiveness, of latent power, of growth of development. The ultimatum of our endeavor is not head cramming with book learning, but the formation of character. In the final analysis force of character depends upon the sustaining power of a strong physique. There are no doubt many practical and historical exceptions, but health of mind and clearness of mental vision are not the natural products of a diseased body or of weakness and atrophy, any more than a morbid diseased imagination, a weak memory and a variable judgment are the fruit of a healthy organism. The severe concentration of our modern thinking is making "little old men and women" of our boys and girls, is sapping vitality during the period in which it should be stored. The thoughtful teacher is beginning to recognize that health and development, not book learning are his first care; that individuals not things are to be taught; that thinking not knowledge is power. He wants a working basis for the production of physical and intellectual power.

"Upon the collection of a large number of physical measurements very accurate standards of normal development may be obtained. According to the generalizing method the mean development of each sex and age is regarded as the type or norm for that sex and age. The first thing to know then is whether and how much a child varies from the normal of his sex and age, and what kind of exercise will correct his peculiar defects."

ATHLETICS AND PRACTICAL PHYSIOLOGY IN MEDICAL SCHOOLS.

Dr. Bayard Holmes (*The Plexus*, October) says: "Medical schools are now provided with lecture rooms, laboratories, libraries, and clinical conveniences, but with hardly an exception they are destitute of gymnasia, athletic fields, and lavatories. Before our education reaches that efficiency which the subject demands, these equipments must be added, and probably at the same time the feeding and social necessaries of the student will be improved and provided for, either from the student initiative or by the co-operation of the college and student."

SLEEPING POSTURE.

The question frequently is asked, "What is the proper or best position during sleep?" We answer, "If healthy and natural, the most comfortable position for you is the one to choose." If you have an abnormal stomach and eat unwisely, it will be unsafe to lie upon your back, because the full stomach will press heavily upon the largest artery and most important nerve plexus in the body and perhaps cause serious results.

But if you are in normal health and temperate, I consider it preferable to lie on the back much of the time during sleep, for the following reasons:

1. In this position one can lie more thoroughly relaxed than in any other.

2. All of the trunk organs are in good position with relation to each other and to gravity.

3. The circulation is more free and regular.

4. If the room is properly ventilated the poisonous expired air will be readily removed at each breath and replaced with fresh air. While if lying on the side one is likely to breath more or less vitiated air.

Women are sometimes advised for plevic troubles to "sleep on the stomach." This is a good position to relieve uterine displacements, particularly if the hips be elevated, but I should not advise any one to sleep long that way because one is almost certain to get the arms and the neck in a cramped position, thus breaking the harmony of circulation. Besides, it is well nigh impossible to keep the lungs plentifully supplied with fresh air with the face so close to the pillow as it must be in this position.

It is commonly supposed that the heart's action is better when one lies on the right side than on the left. It is certainly safer for the gormand to sleep on his right side, because the stomach will then give the heart more freedom. Even a light eater may have his stomach so distended with gas as to cause palpitation of the heart when he lies on his left side. But one with a natural stomach need not trouble about his heart, no matter what position he assumes.

Watch a healthy baby asleep; note how it lies heavily on its back with arms and legs outstretched resting on the bed. Occasionally it turns on the right or left side, still keeping the limbs as fully relaxed as the body. Verily we must "become as little children if we would enter the kingdom of health."

It is not so much the posture during sleep which counts for health as it is the perfect relaxation of nerves and muscles and the deep rhythmical breathing of pure air.

My advice is: Be kind to your stomach, open wide your windows, use a very small pillow, relax completely, lie on your back and take wide breaths as you fall asleep, then let Nature take care of your sleeping posture and you will waken as fresh as the glad new day.—*Mrs. E. L. Sessions.*

MASSAGE IN JAPAN.

"As every one knows," writes Dr. X. C. Wood in the *Philadelphia Medical Journal,* "massage has been largely practised in Japan almost from time immemorial. In a recent tour through that country one of the most interesting and curious sights that I witnessed was a little 'tot' between five and seven years old, with the utmost seriousness and earnestness, and with a marked degree of skill, standing and massaging the age-stricken trapezius and other muscles of the shoulders of an old grandfather or grandmother squatting before him. The common belief that the blind have in Japan a monopoly of the practice of massage appears to be only so far correct that probably 90 per cent. of the practitioners of the art are blind persons, who wander about the streets blowing a peculiar double whistle whose two weird notes may be heard at almost any hour of the day or night, pleading for work and sustenance.

"In order to make out the differences between the art as practiced by the Japanese

and the Europeans, I ordered a masseur in Yokohama, Tokyo, Kioto, Mianoshita, Nikko and one or two other places. As was perchance naturally to be expected, Yokohama being simply a foreign excrescence on the Japanese body corporate, the masseur in that city was not blind and seemed simply to be badly trained in the European methods. I could not make out any difference between him and a second-class American masseur.

"Kioto is the center of all that pertains to Japanese religion, art or customs, having been the capital of old Japan, and being still the culture capital of the country. The masseur I saw there possessed great skill; his methods, however, did not differ very greatly from those to which we are accustomed, except in one motion, which seems to me the most efficient I had ever had practiced on me, for the purpose of deep kneading between groups of muscles or of muscles situated much below the surface. The motions were so quick that in the absence of ability to talk with the practitioner it was a little difficult to perceive exactly how they were made, but I finally made out that the procedure might be termed a rolling use of the different joints of the fingers; first, the tip; then the distal intraphalangeal articulation; then the next joint; and then the knuckles applied one after another with great rapidity and force; the maximum of the force sometimes being reached with the second intraphalangeal joint, the knuckles only pressing lightly; in other cases the knuckles themselves giving the main blow. It was apparently when it was desired to penetrate deeply between two closely placed muscle groups that the maximum force was applied with the second intraphalangeal joint.

"One or two somewhat curious differences between the Japanese customs and our own were noticeable. In one of the places a woman, old, blind and ugly, was sent to do the work. The length of the séances seemed to be arranged according to the desire or the ability of the person operated upon to pay, and were remarkably cheap, even when the foreign price was demanded. Thus, asking the charge at one of the hotels, before engaging an operator, I was told 'Thirty sen,' that is, fifteen cents an hour. On expressing surprise, saying I had always paid forty sen, the man replied, 'Oh, yes, that is the price for the foreigner.' Not considering myself seriously cheated I paid the forty sen, or twenty cents, for an hour of labor sufficiently hard to make the operator sweat freely."

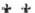

MOUTH-BREATHING AND ITS RE-LATION TO DISEASES OF THE THROAT, NOSE AND AC-CESSORY CAVITIES.

MOUTH-BREATHING, says Mayo Collier, *N. Y. Medical Journal,* is evidence that the physiological function of the nose—the warming, the moistening and the filtering of the air—are more or less in abeyance, and so lost to the respiratory function; and deficient nasal respiration means nasal obstruction in its wider sense. Long-continued mouth-breathing, even when the nose is healthy, begets more or less complete atrophy of the muscles and tissues of the external nose with collapse of the alæ, and gives a sharp and pointed expression to the features. So that mouth-breathing, if persisted in even in the hypothetical condition of a healthy and patent nose, would ultimately induce anterior nasal obstruction from atrophy following disuse of the nose valve. This would be followed by swelling of the lining membrane of the nose and accessory cavities from vascular dilatation, which again would lessen the capacity of the nasal respiratory tract and tend to set up nasal obstruction. A vicious circle is thus set up. Obstruction to nasal respiration may set up a rarefaction of the air contained in the frontal, ethmoidal, sphenoidal, or maxillary sinuses, and cause congestion of the lining membrane and a possible outpour of fluid and blockage of the natural vent, even though there is no previous disease or ca-

tarrh present. So that in diseased conditions of these sinuses the first step in treatment is to see that there is a free inlet of air to the respiratory passages; this holds good in both the chronic and acute cases. Politzeration is of little value; a permanent and continuous air supply must be established. The association of mouth-breathing with high palate, a symmetrical upper jaw, prominent nose, open mouth, and thin, flattened face is a constant one. A small increase in pressure from without, constantly applied to the walls of the nasal box, pushes up the palate, disarranges the mandibular arch, and causes general atrophy and an undeveloped condition of the whole upper jaw. If such cases are taken in an early stage and the nasal respiration restored the constant stream of air passing through the nose moulds and expands the upper maxilla, and, in time, the greater part of the deformity will disappear. Further, the anæmia, loss of weight, and listlessness, of children with post-nasal growths, is probably due to the want of proper oxidation at night. Remedy this and their return to health is usually prompt.

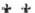

THE EFFECT OF MODERN EDUCA-TION UPON CHILDREN.

THE stress of modern education has enormously taxed the brains of children by the multiplicity of studies. Children cannot assimilate the ideas in widely differing department of knowledge at one and the same time. The effort to do so deranges in many instances the entire nervous system of the child. The so-called nervous child is not only not normal, but may be the victim of the education methods of the present day. The examination system is often a horror to such a child, as the writer knows from his own experience. The studies required of a growing child should never be allowed to disturb the health or interfere with proper rest and exercise. The modern city child seems to be unable to endure the burdens of civilized life as easily as did the children of the past, who were brought up in the country and spent the greater part of the time in the fresh open air. Whether our fathers were more hardy and robust as children than the progeny of the present generation may be an open question, but certainly the conditions of civilized life have so completely changed that at the present day mental and physical education possess equal importance for the growing child. The mind of the child to-day is too often developed at the expense of its vitality and health.—*W. M. D'Aubigné Cahart, M.D.*

ACOUSTIC EXERCISES FOR DEAF-MUTES.

ACCORDING to the *Journal of Laryngology* for October, says the Charlotte *Med. Journal*, V. Urbantsclistch emphasizes the importance of acoustic exercises in all cases for developing the sense of hearing. He then treats of methodical acoustic exercises for deaf mutes. He answers several important questions bearing on this subject.

What cases are suitable for acoustic exercises? The exercises are always at first experimental, because the result cannot be foretold in any individual case. Success has been achieved even in deafness due to cerebrospinal meningitis. The author is quite opposed to Bezold's view that all who cannot hear tuning-forks a[1] to b[2] should be passed over, for even in such cases he has had good results.

How long should the exercise be continued? The more difficulty there is in arousing perception of sound, the more are special exercises required, whereas these may be limited or omitted whenever ordinary sounds are perceived or the deaf-mute can hear his own voice.

What are the results of acoustic exercises? The result of the exercises will vary with the nature and duration of the daily practice: with the amount of hearing-power already present, and with its ca-

pacity for development; with the intellectual condition of the patient, and with his interest in the exercises. In some cases in which hearing-power is apparently absolutely wanting, a trace of hearing may be awakened which is capable of further development. As a general rule acoustic exercises raise the hearing-power, thus a mere trace of hearing becomes a hearing of tones, this again a hearing of vowels, words and sentences. The capacity for development of each individual case cannot, however, be estimated; it varies even in a right and a left ear which at the start were functionally equal.

What is the practical worth of acoustic exercises? These exercises have a favorable influence on speech, on its hardness and its modulation, and also on the possibility of learning a dialect. As his hearing-power improves social intercourse becomes easier for the deaf-mute, and at the same time the difficulty of earning his living diminishes.

THE TRAINING OF SIGHT.

LORD WOLSELEY having lately remarked upon the good sight of the Boers as one cause at least of their good shooting, and having ascribed this good sight to its constant exercise in the open air, Mr. Brudenell Carter has pointed out that it is not merely a question of open air but of the training of the sight upon things that are far off and difficult to see. The defective vision possessed by so many children who have been brought up in towns is not caused by errors of refraction alone, common as these are, but by an actual deficiency in acuteness of vision, a lack of development in the nervous structures involved in the act of seeing. "Vision," he says, "like every other nerve function, must be cultivated for the attainment of a high degree of excellence. The visual power of London children is not cultivated by their environment. They see the other side of the street in which they live, and the carts and omnibuses of the thoroughfares. They scarcely ever have the visual attention directed strongly to any object which it is difficult to see or which subtends a visual angle approaching the limits of visibility; and hence the seeing function is never exerted, or at least is not habitually exerted to anything like what should be the extent of its powers. With a country child the case is widely different." Mr. Brudenell Carter would like to see a place given to excellence of vision among the various physical qualifications which are habitually tested by competition and for which prizes are awarded, and he urges the desirability of volunteers taking up the exercise and training of the sight. "It is at least certain that our riflemen would not shoot worse for having learned to see better."—*The Hospital.*

THE HUMAN EYE AND HOW TO CARE FOR IT.

DR. REIK, writing in the *Cosmopolitan* for September, says that the excessive use of alcohol and tobacco effects the eyes very seriously and that for some people tobacco is a poison and produces a lesion in the nerve of the eye leading to blindness. The most important thing of all, however, in order to take care of the sight is to get sufficient light to work and read by. The most desirable location of a light to read by is from above, behind, and to the left of the body. Of artificial lights the incandescent electric is the best, though the use of incandescent mantles has much improved gaslight. Where coal oil is the only illumniant the so-called student lamps make a very satisfactory light.

THE FIRE THAT KINDLES POWER.

No matter how skilfully constructed or how powerful the locomotive may be, unless the water used to run it is boiling the train will not move an inch. What the boiling water is to a locomotive, enthusiasm is to a man. No matter how great his ability or diversified his talents, unless he is filled with that enthusiasm which generates energy, great motive power, as the boiling water generates the steam which propels the train, he will never accomplish anything noteworthy. Every successful person, whatever his profession or occupation, is filled with this stimulating force. It is this which enables him to overleap obstacles, to spurn hardship and privation, to dare any dangers in order to reach his goal.

You cannot hope to accomplish much in the world without that compelling enthusiasm which stirs your whole being into action. You cannot have this soul-energy unless you are in your right place, unless you are in love with your employment. Your work must be to you what his violin was to the great master, Ole Bull. The famous violinist had an almost idolatrous affection for his instrument. He used to talk to it, pet it, caress it and then breathe his very soul into it. The violin responded to his caress, and with it the great artist swayed multitudes as forests are swayed by the tempest.

To be filled with the enthusiasm that wins, your work must be to you your life, your all.

In one of the art galleries in Paris stands a beautiful statue in the modeling of which the sculptor sacrificed his life. He was so poor that he lived and worked in a small garret. One night, when the clay model of his beautiful conception was almost completed, a heavy frost fell upon the city. The sculptor, shivering in his garret, knew that if the water in the interstices of the clay should freeze, the lines of beauty would be distorted and his model ruined. Forgetting cold, hunger, everything but the conception which he had called into being, he got up and wrapped his bedclothes around the lifeless clay. In the morning the sculptor was found dead, but his model lived and other hands molded it in marble.

This was carrying enthusiasm to extremes, but it is an example of the indomitable power, heroism, which enthusiasm generates.

This immortal fire kindles sleeping powers, stimulates latent energies and arouses resources undreamed of before. It multiplies ability and often takes the place of talent.—*Success.*

THE COOK AND THE DOCTOR.

MR. C. CHAMPEAUX, who writes for the *Caterer Monthly,* seems to think that the cook should have as marked distinction, or title, as the pharmacist or even the doctor. He says:

"The foundation of all health is good digestion, and this foundation is conditional on the knowledge of the person who prepares the food for the family or individual. There are thousands of different kinds of foods and hundreds of different ways of preparing them, the difference between these ways often meaning the difference between health and disease. Is it not, therefore, the expert knowledge that chooses and discriminates, worthy the name of a science, and, further, worthy the respect accorded to other recognized sciences?

"What knowledge is required to be a pharmacist? The Codex—the drug code, sanctioned by legislation. The cook does not learn the culinary science so easily as the pharmacist learns the Codex. The culinary science requires more instruction and practice than that of pharmacy, because the cook, besides being precise, has to create pleasure; he must soothe the palate and please the eye, as well as build up the body.

"If Dame Cookery had had a Hippocrates to develop it in Greek of a Celsus to profess it in Latin; if to learn to cook it were necessary to know Greek and Latin, the cook, having become a doctor by the accessory sciences and a pedant by profession, would be looked upon everywhere as at least the equal to the pharmacist, and would write after his name the initials of his degree in the university of his calling.

"To understand the art of cooking is, for instance, to understand fermentation also. There is no healthy digestion without proper fermentation, so a chef must understand how to combine his dishes in order to awake and sustain the appetite and protect the digestion of his patron by a happy choice of agreeable condiments that will combine the saccharifiable and saccharifying principles.

"If the cook wants to make, say, a sauce chasseur, he will use salad oil to fry his eschalottes in, and will skim that oil off before sending his sauce to table; if a sauce piquante is required he will use vinegar with his eschalottes and then reduce it by evaporation; if some one asks for a Bordelaise sauce he will add some claret and then reduce by evaporation. If he makes paysanne or any other vegetable clear soup, he will put a piece of clarified fresh butter in a thoroughly clean pan, season his cut vegetables and add them to the butter, and instead of evaporation, it will be extraction of liquids. By covering his pan hermetically and putting it on a slow fire, he will extract the juice of the vegetables, and in their own juice they will cook and become tender; then he will add to them a good consommé, and as it simmers skim off the butter and finally produce a soup that will fortify the digestive organs of anyone. This I call chemistry."

IS IT TRUE THAT THE SPAN OF LIFE IS LENGTHENING?

FROM statistics and the result of certain changes in the methods of living, we can safely affirm that the span of life is steadily lengthening, says the *Royal Magazine,* of England. Three thousand years before the Christian era the average duration of life was said to be three score years and ten; this would make middle age come at thirty-five. Dante considered that year the middle of life's arch, and Montaigne, speaking for himself at the same period of life, considered his real work practically ended, and proved that he thought he was growing old by falling into the reminiscent age.

At the present time fifty years is considered as middle age. In the days of the Revolutionary War prominent men at that time were looked upon as old at fifty years. We are justified in supposing that the span of human life will be prolonged in the future because the possibility of living to an older age has been demonstrated by the great advances made in medicine and hygiene during the past ten years.

We have attained a vast amount of knowledge as to the causes of disease, and new remedies for their successful treatment have been discovered. We have no new diseases, at least, of any serious character, and we are better able to treat the old ones, which, like old foes, appear to us with new faces.

One of the most interesting and trustworthy statements in respect to old age is the report of the habits of centenarians, made some years ago by a commission appointed by the British Medical Association. Without going into particulars of the different cases it is valuable to note, generally, the result of this investigation.

It seems that most of these old people were small or medium of stature and of spare habit of body; the voice was rarely feeble; most of them had lost their teeth, but nearly all enjoyed good digestion; one old man of ninety-eight, a clergyman, placing his hand on the organ in question, and saying that he never knew what it was to have a stomach. Nearly all of them had enjoyed uninterrupted good health, and many had never known what it was to be sick.

They were all very moderate in eating, most of them using little animal food. Few indulged at all in intoxicating drinks, and those only in notable moderation. They took considerable outdoor exercise, and nearly all possessed the good-natured, placid disposition.—*New York Herald.*

THE CURABILITY OF INEBRIETY BY MEDICAL TREATMENT.

T. D. CROTHERS believes that when inebriety shall be more generally studied and treated as a disease by the profession, a degree of curability will be obtained far beyond any present expectation. The continued or occasional excessive use of spirits to intoxication is not the disease, but is a symptom of some central irritation and exhaustion; also of poisoning and starvation. Many of these cases are self-limited, and follow a certain course, dying away after a time. The subsidence of the drink symptom by the removal of the exciting causes and building up the system to greater vigor and health is the only rational treatment. The highest medical judgment will be needed to determine the exact condition in each case, and the possible range of remedies required—not any one drug or combination of drugs, not so-called moral remedies, not appeals to the will power, but a clear, broad, scientific application of every rational means and measure demanded.—*St. Louis Medical Review,* October 13, 1900.

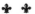

TREATMENT OF ACUTE ALCOHOLISM.

THE expectant plan is the most rational. Opiates are dangerous, because they additionally derange digestion, and, acting as powerful cardiac sedatives, tend to paralyze the heart, and, finally, because they check elimination, interfere with the normal secretions and digestion. Sleep is never to be attained at risk of hazard to the patient, but, is to be expected as one of the harbingers of a convalescence not to be enforced. In acute alcoholism, as in many other acute diseases, the vis medicatrix is fully adequate in most cases to produce the happiest results.—DR. J. K. BAUDUY, *St. Louis Medical Review,* December 1st.

EXCLUSIVE SOUP DIET AND RECTAL IRRIGATIONS IN TYPHOID FEVER.

BASING his statements upon a personal experience of one hundred and fifty-three cases in private and hospital practice during the last ten years, A. Siebert gives the following as the results of this mode of treatment: 1. Delirium, headache, insomnia, nausea, vomiting and tympanites usually disappeared within forty-eight hours of treatment. 2. Tympanites, nausea, and vomiting never developed in any patient, even when complicating pneumonia was present. 3. The fur on the tongue disappeared within a few days. 4. Appetite came frequently on the fourth day of treatment, even when the thermometer registered 102° to 103° F.. 5. Even excessive diarrhœa (fifteen to twenty five daily stools) disappeared invariably within the first week of treatment. 6. In all uncomplicated cases the temperature began to decline within twenty-four to forty-eight hours after the beginning of treatment and invariably would reach the normal figure within ten to twelve days. 7. In cases complicated by pneumonia, nephritis, or phlebitis when treatment began, the temperature usually remained in accord with the inflammatory conditions found until these also disappeared; while the cerebral, gastric, and intestinal disturbances usually subsided as rapidly as in the uncomplicated cases, excepting anorexia. 8. Complications, when not present at the start, were very rare and then usually developed within the first two days. 9. Intestinal hemorrhage was noticed in three cases, none ending fatally. Perforation did not occur. Five feedings were given during the day. After an initial purge the patients seemed to do as well for forty-eight hours on cold water alone as on any kind of food. Then soups were given made of barley, oatmeal, rice, and peas, strained and well salted and peppered. Two days later lentil soup and the yolk of a fresh egg were added to the oatmeal, rice, and barley soups. An adult was allowed half a pint of two kinds of soup alternating, every three hours. Five to fifteen drops of dilute hydrochloric acid were given before each meal unless hyperacidity prevailed, but no other medicine. Cold water was allowed ad libitum.—*Northwestern Lancet,* October 1, 1900.

A HARVARD STUDENT'S DIET.

IN commenting on the diet of a student in Harvard College, the *N. Y. Sun* has this to say:

"Several theoretical and practical diet reformers and economists, vegetarian, antivegetarian and eclectic, have propounded cheap and not always filling bills of fare, by the practice of which health and wealth may be saved. It is as clear as mud that good buyers, frugal cooks and judicious feeders may live on a few cents a meal and families, large, small and medium, on $1.50 or $2 a week. Excellent examples of household economy are set before the country. If they were followed there would be a great increase of accumulation and the interest rate would go down. But we fear that they are not followed. Perhaps the statistics of the next-to-nothing dieters are ungenerously distrusted. Perhaps the lust of gain is less strong than Bishop Potter imagines. At any rate the butchers keep on carving meat for others and fortunes for themselves and the procession of grocers and bakers at the receiving teller's window is not diminishing.

"Still, let us not be weary in well-doing and let us applaud those who are willing to mortify the flesh and fatten the bank account. The proselyting missionary of thin living might become wearisome, but he who lives thinly for himself alone and unsustained by the name of science or the hope of making the rest of the human race sit down at his modest ordinary, is a rare and independent spirit, worth knowing. Such a one is a certain member of the present senior class of Harvard College. His name is given. not with entire correctness, by the *Boston Advertiser*, but is here omitted. The young man is not dieting for the sake of fame. "He went to Harvard to conquer obstacles," says the *Advertiser*, "and has already earned a scholarship for his first rate work last year." He boards at Randall Hall, where some 1,000 students have their commons. He lived last year and is living this year on this meal taken three times a day:

2 Baked Potatoes............... 4 cents
Bread .... 1 "
Hot Water.................... 0 "
                                —
    Total .... 5 "

"Evidently this young man bothers himself very little with the researches of Prof. Atwater on the value of food save in cents. His problem is to sustain life sufficiently and cheaply, and he finds that six baked potatoes and three portions of bread fill the bill and *him*. The hot water may be regarded as free medicine or free luxury.

The monotony of such meals is probably much less than it seems. The wearied frequenter of restaurants usually finds himself ordering about the same breakfast, luncheon and dinner day after day. To be sure his breakfast, and his luncheon and his dinner, will be three different meals in substance as well as in name, but in vain do most of the fish of the sea and the fowls of the air appeal to him. In that great ocean of a bill of fare he has his three regular routes. Reduce them to one and you have the simple system of what the Boston Town Clerk called "the pore scolers of Hervert College." The simplicity of the baked-potato-bread-and-hot-water proposition is a merit. The amount of nervous tension and wear made necessary by the study of bills of fare, the amount of heat, ill temper and disappointment caused by the daily attempts to make new ventures and experiments is appalling. In the strict sense, the Randall Hall five-cent meal is not scientific. In a higher and better sense it is philosophic. It avoids friction. It is a certainty and a relief. The machine must be kept up. This will keep it

up and keep it up well. The young man in question "appears as powerful to-day as when on the football field on the Pacific Coast." He is not trying to force his method of stoking upon anybody else. But it is good enough for him and costs only $1.05 a week.

"It is rather strange that nobody, so far as we remember, has imitated Dr. Dio Lewis's experiment of living for a time upon baked beans. The Harvard philosopher who will try that can live easily and abundantly for a good deal less than a dollar a week. Cambridge is near the heart of the Great Bean District and should be true to the transcendental staple. It is true that Cicero somewhere explains the aversion of the Pythagoreans to beans on the ground that beans produce "an inflation of the stomach which makes against the tranquility of the mind seeking for truth;" but who seek truth more earnestly than the Bostonians? They may not find it, but they find the beans and they can 'find themselves' cheaply by means of beans. Baked potatoes, bread and hot water are an excellent good meal, but in beans is a mystical virtue."

DIE RICH, DIE DISGRACED.

"THE day is not far distant when the man who dies leaving behind him millions of available wealth, which was free for him to administer during life, will pass away 'unwept, unhonored and unsung,' no matter to what uses he leaves the dross which he cannot take with him. Of such as these the public verdict will then be: 'The man who dies thus rich dies disgraced.'

"The result of my own study of the question, 'What is the best gift that can be given to a community?' is that a free library occupies the first place, provided the community will accept and maintain it as a public institution, as much a part of the city property as its public schools, and, indeed, an adjunct to these. It is no doubt possible that my own personal experience may have led me to value a free library beyond all other forms of beneficence. When I was a working boy in Pittsburg Colonel Anderson of Allegheny—a name I can never speak without feelings of devotional gratitude—opened his little library of 400 books to boys. Every Saturday afternoon he was in attendance at his house to exchange books. No one but he who has felt it can ever know the intense longing with which the arrival of Saturday was awaited that a new book might be had."—*Carnegie.*

APHORISMS FOR CHILDREN.

1. ANIMAL food once a day and in small quantities, if the teeth can masticate, is necessary to a rapidly growing child.

2. Avoid a too nourishing diet in a violent-tempered child.

3. Avoid seasoned dishes and salt meats, pastry, uncooked vegetables, unripe food, wine and rich cake.

4. Never tempt the appetite when disinclined.

5. Insist on thorough chewing; a child who eats too fast eats too much.

6. Vary the food from day to day but avoid variety at one meal.

7. Take care that the child's food is well cooked.

8. Wine, beer and confections should never be given to a young child.

9. Give no food between meals; the stomach requires rest, like any other organ than anything else.

10. Remember that over-feeding and the use of improper food kill more children of the body.

11. Give no laudanum, no paregoric, no soothing syrup, no teas.

12. Remember that the summer complaint comes chiefly from over-feeding, and the use of improper food, but never from teething.

13. When children vomit and purge, give them nothing to eat for four or five hours.

14. Do not bring a child under three years of age to your table to eat.

SANGUIFERRIN IN THE TREATMENT OF ANEMIA.

ALLOW me to report the following: A most unusual and remarkable progress in the case of anemia, caused by long-continued opium poisoning. Early in May was called to see Mrs. B., age 48, who was suffering from chronic opiumism. Under my special treatment she improved unusually slow. I found she had atrophy of the liver and paralysis of the ascending colin. A careful microscopical analysis of the blood showed the red corpuscles reduced to 2,862,000, and some were much distorted and undersized. Specific gravity, 1038; hæmoglobin, 40 per cent. Repeated weekly analysis marked only a very slow progress, and I was much worried. She had not been out of home for two years, and while I mastered her case, so far as opium was concerned, she was no better physically. Her weight at the time she became my patient was 90 pounds, and she gained only two pounds the first month. On June 1st I was induced to use Sanguiferrin. She improved from the start, and at the end of two weeks was eating fairly. The red corpuscles numbered 3,195,020; specific gravity, 1040; hæmoglobin, 40 per cent. She left for New Orleans August 1st, weighing 129 pounds and her blood in the following condition: Specific gravity, 1057; hæmoglobin, 75 per cent.; red corpuscles, 4,299,000. She eats well, sleeps well and enjoys life.

Case 2. Mrs. S., age 31, suffering from dysmenorrhea from puberty, married eight years, never was pregnant. After two months under Sanguiferrin finds herself relieved of her suffering and pregnant.

DR. OZIUS PAQUIN.

EDITH—Uncle George, is it a painful operation when a man has his leg pulled? And do they take anything?

Uncle George—Gas is usually administered, I believe.—*Boston Transcript.*

THE PREDATORY MOSQUITO.

EVERY physician who "keeps tab" on the advances and discoveries of medical science is now aware that there are two kinds of mosquitoes—the good and the bad. We presume, however, that some one will dispute this statement and say of this insect as the average army officer says of the Indian, "There's no good mosquito but a dead mosquito." It's true that they all sting, but some of them add insult to injury by injecting the malarial virus into her unsuspecting victim. We say *her,* because we believe the male mosquito is a better behaved insect than his spouse and does not "present his little bill" at inconvenient times.

These few remarks are but prefatory to the announcement that the Palisade Mfg. Co. has prepared and is now mailing to physicians an illustrated folder, showing in sepia the distinctive differences between Culex (the non-malarial) and Anopheles (the malarial) mosquito, with instructions as to how to detect the good insect from the bad. A copy will be mailed to any physician who has not as yet received one.

✠ ✠

"WHAT is an anecdote, Johnny?" asked his teacher. "A short, funny tale," answered the little fellow. "That's right," said the teacher. "Now, Johnny, you may write a sentence on the blackboard containing the word." Johnny hesitated a moment and then wrote this: "A rabbit has four legs and one anecdote."—*San Francisco News Letter.*

✠ ✠

A COMMENDATION.

HAVE given Dad's Quinine Pills a thorough trial and find they act entirely as represented. I cheerfully recommend them to the profession.

GEO. W. EWING, M.D.
Middleton, Mass.

NEW CURE FOR ASTIGMATISM.

AN English popular journal is responsible for the following gem: "In the public schools of some cities measures are taken, by presumably competent officials, to test the children's eyesight upon the assumption —often too well founded—that the parents are not sufficiently watchful in that important particular. A little boy came home one day, soon after the term had commenced, with the following note signed by the principal: 'Mr. Green: Dear Sir—It becomes my duty to inform you that your son shows decided indications of astigmatism, and his case is one that should be attended to without delay.' The father sent this answer the next day: 'Mr. Kershaw: Dear Sir—Whip it out of him. Yours truly, John Green.'"

MASSAGE as a separate and independent study is the latest novelty at the Berlin University. Two courses of massage—one of six months' duration for students and one of one month for doctors—will be held under Professor Zabludowski's direction at the new University institute for massage and Swedish gymnastics.

✠ ✠

WORTHY OF HIS HIRE.

A STRANGER got off the car, and, accosting a newsboy asked him to direct him to the nearest bank.

"This way," said the newsie, and, turning the corner, pointed to a sky-scraper just across the street.

"Thank you, and what do I owe you?" said the gentleman pulling a penny out of his pocket.

"A quarter, please."

"A quarter! Isn't that pretty high for directing a man to the bank?"

"You'll find, sir," said the youngster, "that bank directors are paid high in Chicago."—*Chicago Tribune.*

Department of Notes and Queries.

FREEDOM OF DISCUSSION BETWEEN EDITOR AND READER.

THIS Department is designed to furnish a frank, cordial and thorough interchange of ideas between Editor and Reader.

To avoid the conventional pitfall into which so many of these Departments drift, patrons who desire to avail themselves of its privileges are requested to scrupulously refrain from personalities, to make their inquiries and responses brief, to the point, and of general interest. By strict observance of these rules the Department can be made of immense practical value to all our readers.

Query 63. Is there any preparation, any course of diet or any mode of living that will aid one in getting rid of the tobacco habit?
W. W. P., Tenn.

Answer.—There are numerous substitutes and antidotes advertised to cure the appetite for tobacco; but so far as we know none has been found that in any degree satisfies the habitué unless it contains a considerable percentage of very rank tobacco, which of course makes it a cruel delusion and worse than worthless.

The most essential factor in the cure of the habit is *will power* and a fixed determination to break off at any cost.

It usually requires three months for the system to adapt itself to the deprivation and to eliminate the taint of the weed from the tissues. If the victim will set his face as a flint and bear the tortures of unsatisfied craving for the necessary length of time, he can surely come off victorious. If he occasionally yields to temptation during this term it will take much longer.

If chewing is the habit various substitutes of a harmless nature, to take the attention, will be found of service, one of the best being *calamus*, or sweet flag root. It is tonic and stomachic, has a pungent taste and is harmless. Cloves, cassia buds, cinnamon, licorice root, lemon drops, and, poorest of all, chewing gum, have been used.

If smoking is the vice cubeb cigarettes in moderation may be indulged when the craving is likely to get the upper hand of the would-be reformer. In either case total abstinence from tobacco is absolutely essential. No man ever stops who undertakes to do so gradually.

Various hygienic resources may be invoked, and will be of material assistance. To favor elimination of the nicotine and soothe the nervous system a semi-weekly Turkish bath is one of the best. In the absence of facilities for this the full hot bath followed by a cold plunge, shower or sponging and vigorous friction will furnish a fair substitute. For those who react well a momentary cold bath and prompt rubbing, on alternate mornings, is advisable. The diet should be thoroughly nutritious, and it will be well to have the patient take a cup of hot bouillon or beef extract between meals and at bedtime. The latter may be resorted to whenever the nervous system is greatly depressed for lack of its accustomed stimulo-narcotic.

In the way of medicine, about the only rational and harmless class of drugs is found among the genuine nerve tonics. One of the best of these in our hands has been Horsfords acid phosphate, to which has been added tincture of nux vomica and capsicum, a teaspoonful of each to the ounce of phosphate. The dose of this mixture is one-half to one teaspoonful in a glass of water, three or four times a day. It should never be taken clear.

Valuable auxiliaries are found in plenty of outdoor air, moderate exercise, lively social surroundings and interesting occupation.

Query 64. Is rope-climbing too violent for a boy of twelve?
W. W. P., Tenn.

Answer.—Not if indulged in moderation at the outset, that is, without "violent" effort.

Query 65. Can you suggest the best means of developing the body?
W. W. P., Tenn.

Answer.—If children are clad in clothing that does not impede their limbs or interfere with bodily movements, and are taught to avoid cramping, unnatural and hurtful positions and attitudes, their natural spirits, physical restlessness and ambition will generally prompt a sufficient degree and variety of movements to bring all the muscles of the body into healthful play. There are exceptions in which it is necessary to adopt some system of training in order to ensure a harmonious development. A description of any such system would be out of place in this department, since it would require a small volume to compass it. Our Department of Physical Education will give you many apt suggestions from month to month.

The market is well supplied with compendiums on this subject, and it would be well to have one at hand for reference. We would at the same time caution you not to carry any "system" to extremes. The "Professors" of physical culture and health exercises sometimes overdo the matter by advising too much "system." Children's muscles as well as their minds can be seriously injured by being over-urged—too rapidly developed.

Query 66. What remedy would you suggest for cold feet?   W. W. P., Tenn.

Answer.—To advise intelligently in this case or any other case it is necessary to know the cause of the condition. The radical and sometimes the only cure for physical ailments is the discovery and removal of their cause. Having no clue to the cause in this instance we can only advise in a general way.

In all cases cold feet are a serious annoyance and source of suffering. In many cases they constitute a perpetual menace to health. The condition is often a symptom of some form of disease or constitutional debility. In certain cases it seems to be a bodily habit or idiosyncrasy. People afflicted in this way do not notice that their feet are cold, because they are never warm. Such a condition cannot fail in time, to tell on the health. It consists essentially in an imperfect or uneven circulation of the blood. Whatever will aid in correcting this deficiency or habit will merit the name of "cure." The necessary auxiliaries may include all the hygienic agencies at command—nourishing diet, rational exercise, fresh air and sanitary surroundings. Among the special exercises may be mentioned walking, the most valuable and universally available of all forms of exercise, jumping, kicking, stamping, swinging the legs, bicycle riding, and especially slapping the soles of the feet vigorously with an old slipper or an appropriate paddle. The latter is perhaps more thorough and lasting in its effects than some of the others, but it will not take the place of exercise.

For people who cannot take adequate exercise a very hot footbath for ten minutes, followed by a cold dash, should be frequently indulged, especially before retiring. One should never attempt to sleep with cold feet. Better go to bed with a hot footstone, a hot water bag or a heated brick than to brave the nightmare of cold feet.

Query 67. Do you consider cod liver oil a food proper, and as such is it possessed of any marked superiority over other fats and oils? Or does its reputation depend upon medicinal constituents contained in it? I have used it in my practice for many years without any satisfactory understanding of its action. I have met with numerous failures in its use, have many times been obliged to forego its exhibition on account of its un-

palatability. or the strong prejudice of patients against its taste or smell, or both, and have sometimes wondered whether its lack of uniformity in action does not prove that its virtues have been exaggerated, and whether it has any genuine value beyond the quantity of oil it contributes.

A journal that begins its name with DIETETIC ought to have definite ideas as to the real value of this long-used and universally lauded article of—which is it, diet or treatment?—and what preparation of it do you recommend? Is "Hydroleine" a reliable form of cod liver oil?
                                          J. M. C., Colorado.

Answer.—In the first place cod liver oil is an animal oil. For this reason it may be assumed that it is more assimilable than oils of vegetable origin. This assumption is, however, disputed. But the advocates of its use, representing the vast majority of the medical profession, do not by any means rely upon its virtues merely as an oil, since, as such, it is probably not much more valuable in the human economy than olive or cocoanut oils, beef marrow or mutton fat.

Fat in some form is an essential constituent of every wholesome dietary. It is an unorganized tissue, but it is prerequisite to every phase of vital transformation. Every new blood globule must have its filmy envelope of fat. It is also the fuel of the system, affording more than twice as much heat as the same quantity of the proteids. or cane sugar, or than the mixed proteids and carbo-hydrates.

Those who make frequent autopsies are constantly surprised at the quantity and general distribution of adipose tissue found in subjects who in life passed for decidedly lean persons. It is the harmonious distribution of fatty tissue that gives to youth and adolescence, to blooming maiden and blossoming bride those symmetrically rounded outines that clothe the unattractive scaffolding and hide the coming wrinkles, and therefore fat is the principal source of physical beauty. The belle who is the center of admiration when in the flush of health dreads to expose her haggard outlines after a run of typhoid, and the waning prima donna or theatrical star resorts to every known artifice to hide the fact that time and dissipation have begun to make sad inroads on her artistic outlines. They are burning up their adipose tissue, their "plumpness" and "freshness" on the altar of their art, or of their folly.

While the use of fats. and especially of cod liver oil, has been urged in wasting diseases and diseases characterized by innutrition or malnutrition since time immemorial, few have stopped to inquire just how they act, what specific function they fulfill, and to what limitations they are subject.

A patient suffering from any form of wasting disease first consumes his stored-up supply of fats. When this supply is exhausted, if fresh material is not adequately supplied, or if the supply be in a form not readily assimilable, the organized tissues are sacrificed, and the system begins to consume itself to meet the vital demand. This satisfactorily explains the necessity for a due proportion of fats in all dietaries.

In all wasting diseases there is a tendency to retrograde metabolism. It is found that even an excess of fats, if supplied to these cases in strictly a dietetic form does not generally arrest this tendency toward degenerative metamorphosis. Empirical observation during several generations past seems to have established the fact that cod liver oil acts in a double capacity. It supplies the required fat food, and it checks the degenerative tendency. On just what principle or constituent of the oil this result depends has not been satisfactorily determined.

Admitting that the article in question has specific virtues it follows that all the conditions connected with its administration to invalids must be as nearly perfect as possible, otherwise the results cannot be expected to be uniform. Much of the oil in the market, regardless of its lying labels, is either semi-rancid or largely adulterated. The fresh oil derived from healthy livers before putrefactive changes have set in should give uniform results, when exhibited to subjects presenting similar conditions. But human stomachs are very whimsical, and the stomach of an invalid is always lacking in normal digestive ability. It is also true that in its concentrated and unmodified condition this oil is disagreeable to most palates and intolerable to many stomachs. Hence the numerous "emulsions" and "creams" vaunted in the market. Some of these contain little or no cod liver oil, but are made up of vegetable oils emulsified with cheap gums, gelatin or what not, and flavored to cheat the palate. Such preparations have little or no value—some of them are villainous—and they have no doubt had the effect to discredit genuine and worthy products. What is required is minute mechanical subdivision and some degree of predigestion. All the leading manufacturers of emulsions claim to have accomplished these two objects, each in his own way. The first is usually accomplished by mechanical agitation with some form of alkali, and the latter by the introduction of pancreatin. If either process is imperfectly performed the results are unreliable and unsatisfactory, even when all possible honesty is practised and genuine cod liver oil only is used. It is hardly to be wondered at that results are not uniform, since so few preparations in the market are based upon all these essential conditions. If the oil at the outset be tainted, if the emusification be imperfectly performed, or if the pancreatin used be inert and the mechanical manipulation carelessly attended to, the product is comparatively worthless and disappointment will inevitably follow its use.

As an exponent of Dietetics the GAZETTE has "definite ideas" on this subject. We do not agree with the medical pessimists or nihilists who assert that cod liver oil is of no more value than lard, cotton-seed or peanut oil. We do not consider it judicious to set aside the accumulated evidence of several generations of observers as to the efficiency of cod liver oil, aside from its nutritive properties. *It is unquestionably both a food and a treatment.*

As to recommending particular preparations we are not inclined to discriminate against any manufacturer who observes the essential requisites we have named, viz.: *purity and absolute freshness of the oil used, minute subdivision by means of emulsification,*—milk being a good model,—and *pre-digestion by means of fresh and active pancreatin and an unobjectionable alkali.*

We have used the oil unmodified, but have found it not well tolerated *except by those who did not need it.* We have used nearly all the different preparations now in the market, and among our preferences is the Hydroleine of which you inquire. Hydroleine is one of the oldest of the many candidates; it has been before the profession for years, is scientifically prepared, uniform in quality, does not offend the palate, is a beautiful emulsion, and carefully pancreatized. It responds to all the most critical tests of a perfect product, and none of its competitors seem to have improved upon the process used in its preparation.

THE DELICATE NUTRITION SNAIL.

SNAILS are not only regarded as a great delicacy in Paris, but are reckoned as very nutritious. Hygienists say that they contain 17 per cent. of nitrogenous matter, and that they are equal to oysters in nutritive properties. Nearly one hundred thousand pounds of snails are sold daily in the Paris markets. They are carefully reared for the purpose in extensive snail gardens in the provinces, and fed on aromatic herbs to make their flavor finer. One snaillery in Dijon is said to bring in to its proprietor seven thousand francs a year. Many Swiss cantons also contain large snail gardens, where they are grown with much pains. They are regarded as great delicacies.

THE CHACMA BABOON.

Two officers escaping from Pretoria were about to cross a river, when they saw on the opposite bank a troop of these baboons coming down to drink. They were so sensible of the danger of irritating these beasts, or of making the troop utter their barks and yelps of alarm, that they remained for two hours up to their necks in water until the troop retired. Some surprise was expressed that the officers should pay regard to "a troop of monkeys." Any one who shares this feeling may see at the Zoo, probably for the first time in fifteen years, a full-grown male Chacma. A soldier writing home from the front described a locust as "something between a bird and a fly." This baboon is "something between a monkey and a boar." Its head, shoulders, tusks, and muscles show immense strength, and its size is greater than the measurements given in a recent work on South African mammals. It is 3 feet 8 inches long from the nose to the end of the body, and when it stands upright its head is 4 feet 4 inches from the ground. The baboons have maintained their place in South Africa against all enemies, including man, and are likely to do so for some years to come.—*Spectator.*

To be a good cook means the knowledge of all fruits, herbs, balms and spices, and of all that is healing and sweet in fields and groves, and savory in meats. It means carefulness, inventiveness, watchfulness, willingness and readiness of appliance. It means the economy of our great-grandmothers, and the science of modern chemists. It means much tasting and no wasting. It means English thoroughness, French art and Arabian hospitality. It means, in fine, that you are to be perfectly and always ladies (loaf-givers) and are to see that everybody has something nice to eat.—*John Ruskin.*

CATFISH "SALMON."

A PETITION was presented October 8, ult., to the police jury of Concordia Parish, La., for seining privileges, brought to light by the fact that thousands of tons of spoonbill catfish are caught in the waters of that parish every year, canned and chemically treated, shipped East, and sold in the market as salmon. The petition made known this fact, and further showed that the desire of the petitioner was to continue the practice of converting catfish into salmon on a grand scale. He wants to erect a large factory for this purpose.

This industry has been prospering for years in a quiet way, though the attention of the Government was once called to it, and an investigation was made. So perfect is the imitation that it can only be detected by the small pieces of blue skin that get into the cans through the carelessness of the packers.

VERY OLD PEOPLE.

MORE people over one hundred years old are found in mild climates than in the higher latitudes. According to the last census of the German empire, of a population of 55,000,000 only 78 have passed the hundredth year. France, with a population of 40,000,000, has 213 centenarians. In England there are 146; in Ireland, 578; and in Scotland, 46. Sweden has 10, and Norway, 23; Belgium, 5; Denmark, 2; Switzerland, none. Spain, with a population of 18,000,000, has 401 persons over one hundred years of age. Of the 2,250,000 inhabitants of Servia, 575 have passed the century mark. It is said that the oldest person living is Bruno Cotrim, born in Africa, and now living in Rio de Janeiro. He is 150 years old. A coachman in Moscow has lived for 140 years.—*Indian Medical Record.*

THE
DIETETIC AND HYGIENIC GAZETTE
A MONTHLY JOURNAL of PHYSIOLOGICAL MEDICINE

| VOL. XVII. | NEW YORK, FEBRUARY, 1901. | No. 2. |

THE NEWLY DISCOVERED ELEMENTARY GASES OF OUR ATMOSPHERE.

By THEODORE W. SCHAEFER, M.D.,
Kansas City, Mo.

IN ancient times the air, like fire and water, was regarded as a simple substance, but the investigations of Rutherford (1772), Priestly (1774), Scheele (1775) and Lavoisier (1774-1787) have shown that the atmosphere contains two gases, oxygen and nitrogen, the former possessing the power of supporting combustion and respiration, whilst the latter was shown to be incapable of sustaining animal and plant life.

Previous to the discovery of the composition of the atmosphere the presence of carbon dioxide was demonstrated in the air as far back as in 1764, by Macbride, from the observation that quicklime, after long exposure to the air, acquired the property of effervescing with acids.

Until very recently (1894) we considered the atmosphere, besides its constituents oxygen, nitrogen, carbon dioxide and aqueous vapor, as a kind of *terra incognita,* so to speak, because from the very nature of things the gases of the air are less easily approached by the aid of our senses than the other terrestial substances. It is for this reason that our knowledge of the composition of the air has not been enriched for over a century and we simply rested content with the knowledge that it contained only oxygen and nitrogen as its chief constituents.

A suspicion has always existed that the nitrogen found in the atmosphere may be a compound body. Even Cavendish (1784), when experimenting with air which he had confined in a tube over an alkaline solution, to which oxygen was gradually supplied and through which he passed a series of electric sparks, noticed that invariably a small residue of gas escaped conversion into oxides of nitrogen and consequent absorption by the alkali, and found the nitrogen residue eventually reduced to about 0.8 per cent. This residue, strange to say, was unaccounted for and not investigated until the year 1894, when Lord Rayleigh made the discovery that atmospheric nitrogen is specifically heavier than nitrogen obtained from other sources. The subject was further investigated in the following year—1895—by Professor Ramsay and Lord Rayleigh by the old method of Cavendish just mentioned, as well as by the newer one of making atmospheric nitrogen combine with magnesium at a red heat. They found that the unabsorbable residue possessed a spectrum hitherto unknown and a density of 20. They named this new gas "argon," or inactive, having scarcely any affinity for other elements. It is present in atmospheric air to the extent of about one per cent. Continuing his researches in the same year Ramsay, in search for argon, discovered another gas in the mineral cleveite, possessing a spectrum (a bright yellow line near that of sodium), which had been previously discovered in the year 1868, in the chromosphere of the sun by Jannsen, of Paris, and named "helium" by Frankland and Lockyer. Helium is a constituent of atmospheric air and has a density of 2 and, like argon, is chemically inert. Subsequent liquefaction of crude argon by means of liquid air, prepared by a process invented simultaneously by Linde and Hampton, gave a residue which was named by Ramsay and Travers "krypton," meaning hidden; traces only being present. Ramsay and Travers have since announced the presence of additional elements in liquid argon, which they have named "neon," "metargon" and "xenon."

The atomic weight of helium is 4; neon, 20; argon, 40; krypton, 82, and xenon 128. These atomic weights for the newly discovered gases are not reconcilable with Mendelieff's periodical table and so an extra group had to be constructed for them. They all agree in being mono-atomic, *i.e.*, their molecules consist of single atoms, and they have no tendency to form compounds, that is to say, they possess no valence.

Until very recently we considered the composition of the air as very simple; it now appears marvelously complex, containing oxygen, nitrogen, carbon dioxide, aqueous vapor, ammonia, hydrogen, hydrocarbons, argon, metargon, helium, krypton, neon, xenon and, within the last two years, "coronium" has been added, and others seem likely to follow—surely we are getting a long, long way from simplicity, says Dr. W. A. Jones.

The discovery of coronium recalls some very interesting speculations. It is generally recognized that heat, if sufficiently great, has the power to decompose compounds, *e.g.*, water is decomposed into hydrogen and oxygen at the temperature of molten platinum. This being the case, we would look for the most elemental substances, or *the* elemental substance, where the heat is greatest, as in the sun. During the eclipse which passed over the western part of the United States in 1869 the spectrum of the corona, the halo which surrounds the sun when in eclipse, was first accurately studied. A characteristic and bright line was observed in the green portion of the spectrum, and, as it could not be identified with any terrestial element, it was named "coronium." Prof. Nasini now feels sure that he has discovered the same substance in the gases issuing from certain Italian volcanoes—quite the natural place to look for it. The most striking property of coronium is its specific gravity, seemingly much less dense than hydrogen—the lightest substance known. The researches of Gruenewald made it appear probable that helium and coronium are compounds of hydrogen. Both these are now known, and it seems more puzzling than ever.

About five months ago Prof. Armand Gautier completed his researches, proving the constant presence of two volumes of hydrogen in every 10,000 volumes of air, putting the amount of helium, not yet accurately determined, at half that of hydrogen.

The theory of the constitution of mixed gases of Dalton supposes that the oxygen and nitrogen of air form independent atmospheres, the one gas not pressing upon or interfering with another. If each of these atmospheres were of uniform density, their heights would obviously be inversely as the densities of the two gases. (Graham's Elements of Inorganic Chemistry, 1858, page 251.) According to Laplace, the pressure of each atmosphere diminishes in logarithmic proportion to its density. The formula used for such calculation is well known, being in general use for the determination of heights by the barometer.

According to Dr. Gustavus Hinrichs the atmosphere of our globe consists of five well-defined strata or separate atmospheres:

1. *The lowest atmosphere,* containing the aqueous vapor and clouds—the real "atmosphere"—and, also, carbon dioxide gas. The height of this layer is 2 myriameters, or 12 miles.

2. *The oxygen atmosphere* reaches to about 5 myriameters, or 30 miles, where the amount of oxygen becomes less than 10 per cent. in volume.

3. *The nitrogen here forms 86 per cent. by volume* of *the air,* and gradually dimin-

ishes to 4 per cent. at the height of 10 myriameters, or 60 miles.

4. *The helium atmosphere* here shows the largest per cent., namely 16. It gradually gives way to

5. *Hydrogen*, which at the height of 17 myriameters, or about 100 miles, already constitutes 90 per cent. by volume of the air, and finally is the only gas present in the upper layers of our atmosphere.

Meteorites are known to contain hydrogen and helium, occluded in the iron; these gases may have been taken up while traversing the upper layers of the atmosphere. The auroral beams are seen in those parts of our atmosphere where helium prevails, while lower forms of the aurora are indicative of the krypton in the lower strata.

We know practically nothing of the physiological importance of the newer constituents of the atmosphere.

PRACTICAL POINTS ON FEEDING THE SICK.

IN an address on the above subject before the Rocky Mountain Inter-State Medical Association Dr. E. A. Irwin in part said:

" Recent studies and experiments by various authorities have shown that very frequently the malnutrition, anæmie and other complications following the acute, continuous fevers have been due to the practice of restricting the diet too much. This is especially so in typhoid fever, in which disease many writers, during the past two years, have advised a much more liberal feeding than usually practised.

"Milk, broths and beef tea, all in too small quantities, have for years been the routine diet for typhoid. Often the milk has been the least digestible and the beef teas unpalatable. The more liberal diets recommended even during the height of the fever have included solids, such as meat, sweetbreads, toast, eggs and some vegetables, together with milk, peptonized milk, buttermilk, custards, ice cream, etc., and an abundance of cold water.

the duration of the disease, they were ali-

" Dr. Bushuyers, a Russian army surgeon (quoted in *Progressive Medicine,* March, 1899) experimented on about ninety cases of typhoid among soldiers with a liberal solid diet, with an equal number at the same time on the old regimen. He concludes that, perforation, hemorrhage and relapse are not increased, even being less among his cases with liberal feeding, while there was less tympanites and gastric distress, strength was preserved, convalescence shortened, nervous symptoms, sordes and dry mouth less troublesome.

" Marsden (3), (*London Lancet,* Jan. 13, 1900) experimented on 200 cases, with a similar result. He noted that fish seemed to increase the diarrhoea. Marsden's cases showed 13.5 per cent. of true relapse, 27 cases, which is too high. His dietary consisted of milk, peptonized milk, bread and milk, fish, potatoes, chicken, bread and butter and minced meats, according to the condition of the digestion and appetite. He noted as a result a lessened tendency to post-typhoid complications, such as anemia, abscess, gangrene and asthenic conditions.

" My own experience has been limited to twenty cases. These being in the Cook County Hospital, there was not much variety to the diet. Meat and eggs were our only serviceable solids.

" In most cases on admission I found not even milk was tolerated. It seemed to increase the gastric distress and tympanites and showed undigested curds in the stools. This was remedied by giving the milk partially peptonized, or in a few cases completely peptonized for a few days. With this the gastric disturbance ceased quickly in all but one case (in which nausea, pain and vomiting persisted for three weeks), and the tympanites lessened in all cases immediately, disappearing completely in most of them.

" The patients took from three to five pints of partially peptonized milk daily.

" As soon as they showed an appetite, which usually occurred on the third or fourth day after admission, irrespective of lowed dry toast and soft poached or boiled egg, etc.

"In no case where given was there any sign of the toast and egg not being digested, tympanites was not increased, nor did undigested particles appear in stool.

"Vegetables and meats were not allowed early, because of the poor character or bad preparation of those obtainable at the county hospital. In all these cases convalescence was early and rapid, emaciation never marked, mental torpor absent entirely, while nervousness, neuritic symptoms and delirium were slight.

"There were no relapses. One death—a peculiar typhoid—which continued for seven weeks with low morning and high evening temperature.

"These 20 cases contrasted markedly to 25 cases I had one year before, in which the diet was not so carefully attended to. Milk was the chief diet, and it was not always good; it was seldom modified, and was given in insufficient quantities. Soft milk toast was allowed only after normal temperature had been maintained for two days, and was stopped if the temperature rose again. These cases all had marked tympanites, great emaciation and exhaustion, and their convalescence was 50 per cent. longer than among the twenty.

"It is not a question of liquid or solid food, but one of digestibility. Other things being equal, liquids are more easily digested in fevers than solids, because they supply the water which is deficient in the secretions.

"It is necessary then to secure a diet that is easily and completely digested and assimilated and to give it all that the system needs for nourishment. A healthy adult requires, according to Kirke's physiology, 120 grams of proteid, which is represented by about two quarts of cow's milk, but during the fatigue of fever twice as much nitrogen is eliminated by the urine as in health, hence more proteid or carbohydrate is required to make good the waste, and on our ability to supply this, by feeding, will depend the emaciation and other results of malnutrition in our patient.

"The same considerations hold in the other acute fevers, as pneumonia, scarlet fever and influenza. In these the gastric disturbance is especially marked at the onset, but passes off early, when the patient should be fed to the limit of his digestive capacity, because of the great tissue destruction and elimination of nitrogen in those diseases. The importance of this matter is evident, but it is easily neglected or overlooked.

"Early in the disease milk, prepared to suit the case, is usually the best diet. It may be given fresh, or with the addition of lime water or soda, or partially or completely peptonized; also the beef juices, broths, etc., may be given and later the easily digested solids or semi-solids, looking to the digestibility rather than solidity of the material. Proteids are, as a rule, more easily digested during fevers than starches or carbohyrates.

"Custards and ice creams are good and are usually relished by the patient. Eggs, soft poached or boiled, or the yolk of hard-boiled eggs; rare broiled steaks, sweetbreads, calves brains, etc., roasts. Toast, if well dried, then quickly browned, is good and is better digested if given dry. The patient enjoys the performance of the chewing, etc."

In the discussion which followed, Dr. Hershey said:

"There is one thing I would like to call attention to which Dr. Irwin has left out, and that is the feeding of albuminated water in the diarrhoea which so often complicate low forms of fever. I have never yet seen a stomach so irritable that could not take albuminated water, nor have I ever seen a diarrhea, it matters not how long standing, that plain, simple albuminated water will not cure. The white of one egg beaten thoroughly, just the same as they prepare frosting for a cake, then beat it into a glass of cold water, is the remedy by which I control diarrhoeas of months' standing. I never had a case of typhoid fever with a diarrhoea complication that I did not put the patient upon the treatment at once."

THE THERAPEUTICAL DRINKING OF HOT WATER—ITS USE AND ORIGIN.*

BY EPHRAIM CUTTER, M.D., LL.D., OF NEW YORK CITY.

I. ITS USE.

1. *The Water Must be Hot, not Cold or Lukewarm.*—This is to excite downward peristalsis of the alimentary canal. Cold water depresses, as it uses animal heat to bring it up to the temperature of the economy and there is a loss of nerve force in this proceeding.

Lukewarm water excites upward peristalsis or vomiting, as is well known. By hot water is meant a temperature of 110 to 150 degrees Fahr., such as is commonly liked in the use of tea and coffee. In cases of diarrhea the hotter the better. In cases of hemorrhage the temperature should be at blood heat. Ice water is disallowed in all cases, sick or well.

2. *Quatity of Hot Water at a Draught.*—The urine of a healthy babe suckling a healthy mother (the best standard of health) stands at a specific gravity, varying from 1015 to 1020. The urine of a patient should be made to conform to this standard and the daily use of the urinometer tells whether the patient drinks enough or too much hot water. For example if the specific gravity of the urine stands at 1030 more hot water should be drank, unless there is a loss by sweating. On the other hand, should the specific gravity fall to 1010, less hot water should be drank. The quantity of hot water varies usually from one-half to one pint or one and a half pints at one time drinking.

The urine to be tested should be the " urina sanguinis," or that voided just after rising from bed in the morning, before any meals or drinks are taken.

The quantity of urine voided in 24 hours should measure from forty-eight to sixty-four ounces. The amount, will, of course, vary somewhat with temperature of the

atmosphere, exercise, sweating, etc. The urinometer will detect at once whether the proper amount of hot water has been drank, no matter whether the patient is present or absent. Another test is that of odor. The urine should be devoid of the rank " urinus " smell, so well known, but indescribable.

3. *Times of Taking Hot Water.*—One hour before each meal, and half an hour before retiring to bed, thus allowing the hot water time enough to get out of the stomach before the food enters or sleep comes, and avoids vomiting. Four times a day gives an amount of hot water sufficient to bring the urine to the right specific gravity, quantity, color, odor, and freedom from deposit on cooling. If the patient leaves out one dose of hot water during an astronomical day, the omission will show in the increased specific gravity as indicated by the urinometer, in the color, etc. Should the patient be thirsty between meals eight ounces of hot water can be taken any time between two hours after a meal and one hour before the next meal. This is to avoid diluting the food in the stomach with water.

4. *Mode of Taking the Hot Water.*—In drinking the hot water it should be sipped and not drank so fast as to distend the stomach and make it feel uncomfortable. It is most comfortably taken by sipping from a saucer.

5. *The Length of Time to Continue the Use of Hot Water.*—Six (6) months is generally required to wash out the liver and intestines thoroughly.

As it promotes health the procedure may be practiced by well people throughout life and the benefits of "cleanliness inside" be enjoyed. The drag and friction on human existence, from the effects of fermentation, foulness and indigestible food, when removed, give life a wonderful elasticity and buoyancy, somewhat like that of the babe before alluded to.

6. *Additions to Hot Water.*—To make it palatable, in case it is desired, and medicate the hot water, aromatic spirits of ammonia, clover tea blossoms, ginger, lemon juice,

sage, salt and sulphate of magnesia are sometimes added. Where there is intense thirst and dryness, a pinch of chloride of lime or nitrate of potash may be added to allay thirst and leave a moistened film over the parched and dry mucous membrane surfaces. When there is diarrhea, cinnamon, ginger and pepper may be boiled in the water and the quantity drank, lessened. For constipation a teaspoonful of sulphate of magnesia or one-half teaspoonful of taraxacum may be used in the hot water.

7. *Amount of Liquid to be Drank at a Meal.*— Not more than eight ounces. This is in order not to unduly dilute the gastric juice or wash it out prematurely and thus interfere with the digestive processes.

8. *The Effects of Drinking Hot Water are the Improved Feelings of the Patients.* —The feces become black with bile washed down its normal channel. This blackness of feces lasts for more than six months, but the intolerable fetid odor of ordinary feces is abated and the smell approximates the odor of the feces of healthy infants suckling healthy breasts; and this shows that the ordinary nuisance of fetid feces is due to a want of washing out and cleansing the alimentary canal from its fermenting contents. The urine is clear as champagne, free from deposit on cooling, or odor, 1015 to 1020 specific gravity, like infants' urine. The sweat starts freely after drinking, giving a true bath from center of body to periphery. The skin becomes healthy in feel and looks. The digestion is correspondingly improved, and with improvement comes a better working of the machine. All thirst and dry mucous membranes disappear in a few days, and a moist condition of the mucous membrane and skin takes place. Ice water in hot weather is not craved for, and those who have drank ice water freely are cured of the propensity. Inebriety has also a strong foe in the use of hot water.

9. *Summary of General Conditions on the Therapeutical Drinking of Hot water.*— (*a*) Foundation for all treatment of chronic diseases.

(*b*) Excites downward peristalsis.

(*c*) Relieves spasm or colic of the bowels by applying the relaxing influences inside the alimentary canal, just as heat applied outside the abdomen relieves.

(*d*) Dilutes the ropy secretions of the whole body and renders them less adhesive, sticky and tenacious.

(*e*) Inside bath.

(*f*) Dissolves the abnormal crystalline substances that may be in the blood and urine.

(*g*) Necessary to have the hot water out of the stomach before meals.

(*h*) Use is to wash down the bile, slime, yeast and waste, and have stomach fresh and clean for eating.

(*i*) Promotes elimination everywhere.

(*j*) If objection is made, it must be remembered that we are seventy-five per cent. water.

(*k*) The gas sometimes eructated after drinking hot water is not produced by the hot water, but was present before and the contractions of peristalsis eject it, or, sometimes, it is that air is swallowed in sipping, as horses suck air. The amount of gas contained in the alimentary canal is larger than most are aware of.

(*l*) Some physicians have advised against hot water, on the ground that it would burn the coating of the stomach. If this is so then a denudation of the lining of the stomach continuously for forty years is compatible to a state of otherwise perfect health, with no sign of illness for that period of time, and is also compatible with the numerous cases that have occurred under the use of hot water as a foundation for treatment during the past forty years. Again, the same physicians drink tea and coffee at the same temperature, and this act belies their warning and shows their inconsistency and want of consideration before speaking.

II. ORIGIN.

This communication is amended and republished by request. Its first publication was in 1883. Since then further knowledge has been brought to light as to this practice which may well be noted here, with that, which obtained in 1883. The therapeutical drinking of hot water by the sick and apparently well has become so common that any matters of history connected with same are of interest.

Alain Rene Le Sage, 1668-1747 A. D., in his novel of "Gil Blas," presents the character of Dr. Sangrado bleeding and giving hot water to his patients.

Smith, "Traité de Vertus Medicinalis de l'Eau commune," a Paris, 1716, is an author that needs consulting for priority; have not been able to get the volume though have sent to Europe for it.

Several hundred years ago hot water was used in Europe in the treatment of specific blood poisons.

Gustavus L. Simmons, M.D., formerly president California State Medical Society, my class-mate Harvard Medical School, lately visited me in full health and vigor; he stated that while a medic (1855-1856) he found that large quantities of hot water were drank at water cures to such good advantage that he had followed the practice ever since.

A lady now living recently told me that once visiting my mother in 1838, she found her drinking a large cup of hot water before her meals, because of indigestion.

Dr. James H. Salisbury concluded in 1858 experiments on feeding men singly on different articles of food, and at this time apparently discovered that the drinking of hot water before meals would relieve the distressing effects of indigestion, etc. To him has been largely given the credit of being the discoverer of this practice; yet "there is nothing new under the sun," and I have no doubt that further and more complete evidence may be obtained as to the history of this practice. These are days when the people are getting back to Nature's methods; the physicians of several centuries ago were wiser in some matters than we have been with all our advances in pathology. Hence, if any one can throw further light on the history of this simple,

natural, cheap and effective means of relief, let him do it.

120 Broadway, Equitable Building,
New York, Jan. 17, 1901.

WATER.

SINCE the days of Hippocrates and Galen, says Dr. C. T. Dremsen in an address before the Tri-State Medical Association, water and diet are the only two remedies which have survived. I know of no remedial agent to-day, he adds, more flexible in character and covering a wider range of possibilities and usefulness than water.

If the physiologic and therapeutic action of water were better understood by the profession at large, he continues, I am certain that many diseases would be prevented and that others, considered incurable, would be markedly benefited if not entirely relieved.

" So simple a thing as water drinking is not methodically taught in any of our schools in this country to-day so far as I have been informed. Observation has taught me during the past few years, dealing largely during that time with patients of other physicians scattered throughout the country, that this is a most sadly neglected subject, hence it is for that reason I select this subject upon which to address you this evening.

" From what I have been able to ascertain, it is my belief that not six per cent. of our population drink a sufficient quantity of water to carry on physiologic secretion and excretion; and that is not all, less than two per cent. drink water as it should be drunk. When we realize fully that water is the only natural solvent and eliminator, and that the human system might quite properly be likened to the waterworks and sewerage system of a great city, we can begin to comprehend what prolonged deficiency might be.

" Physiology has told us much, but we have fallen asleep, and the good ship health, laden with precious fruit, noiselessly puts to sea and leaves us dreaming. The fault lies with us, we medical men; we do not endeavor to impress, either upon our patients or the public, the importance which the subject demands. Man is given to think that he should satisfy hunger by food and likewise thirst with water, and so he does in his natural state, but we forget that environment is a strong and powerful agent, and sometimes makes habit—and habit changes man's desires, and with this comes unnatural man.

"I will illustrate: Follow the little one at the age of three during the livelong day, and observe the many interruptions of mother or nurse by the cry for water. All day long the young animal drinks and drinks and drinks, seeming never to be satisfied; follow him at the age of eight to the school—there see what happens. If he wants water during the study hour, and wants it often, he is usually requested by his teacher not to want it quite so often, and if he does, in all probability he will incur the teacher's displeasure, if not absolute disfavor. So he goes through his school life, actually taught as it were, to curb this most natural and healthful desire. The same individual, when adult life is reached, becomes a banker or a clerk, we will say, and after the morning meal he goes hurriedly to his place of business (and in this day and age everything has a tendency to business, not even have any of the professions escaped), and there he sits and drills as hard, if not harder, than any day laborer on the streets, and if thirst should come he pushes it aside and continues in the mad rush of competition until the business hour is closed. Thus nature is thwarted in her every effort to keep him well and strong. As time goes on he develops one of the many so-called chronic diseases; it may be rheumatism or it may be gout; if he is a clerk, then it is rheumatism; if a banker, then gout; nevertheless, it has for its origin the same cause and the same results: faulty digestion, faulty assimilation, and faulty elimination, followed by faulty organization. Great harm has come to hydrotheraphy through

charlatans, but not an inconsiderable amount has resulted, I regret to say, by well-meaning and reputable members of our own profession. It was but a few years ago, at one of our national medical association meetings that a member of the association, an ex-president of the same and professor in one of our schools of medicine to-day, read a paper on this subject. He was an enthusiast, and advised the drinking of large quantities of water at any and all times; in fact he even urged the drinking of large quantities of water during meals. He had forgotten that physiology teaches (if it teaches anything at all) that the saliva plays one of the chief rôles in the digestion of the starchy foods, and that large quantities of water taken during meals would not only dilute the gastric juices, but also encourage the bolting of food. Every one knows, or should know at least, that water should never be taken nearer to the meal hour than thirty minutes. I make it a rule to tell all my patients to wait at least one-half hour after having drunk water, before taking their meals. Furthermore, I direct them that during their meals it is best not to drink more than one cupful of fluid, and even then that is best drunk after the meal is finished. Again I tell them to wait at least an hour and a half or more after eating before water drinking is resumed; at the expiration of that time I advise them to drink freely every few minutes until four to six glassfuls have been drunk, repeating this after each meal, except the evening meal, from one to two glassfuls being quite sufficient at that time, for the reason, if more is drunk diuresis will interfere with sleep.

"Much harm comes from drinking water too hot or too cold. In nearly all healthful localities there are usually to be found springs the temperature of which ranges from about 54° to 60° F. This is man's natural drink, and any deviation from such, if long persisted in, cannot fail to work great injury. Three pints of cold water drunk within thirty minutes, at a temperature of 45 degrees, has had the effect upon me of lowering the pulse from 80 to 50 beats per minute, and the same amount of warm water taken in the same way has increased it to as high as 97. I point this out to show the very powerful influence that this agent has in regulating heart action.

"The taking of water internally is not alone useful as a solvent and eliminator in the processes of life and death, but maintains that degree of tension in the tissues which is absolutely necessary for the circulation of the lymph stream. The effect of cold water will not only lessen the frequency of the pulse but improves its quality and arterial tone, whilst warm water, on the contrary, produces relaxation and increased pulse rate. This influence is undoubtedly brought about through the vasomotor nervous system. If hot water is used by enteroclysis there is not a drug in the whole pharmacopœia which is a safer and quicker diuretic. If you doubt this, first irrigate the colon with large quantities of hot water, and after it has been ejected fully, inject again with about one pint or less of water at a temperature of 115° to 120° F., and observe the result. Complete absorption takes place in about twenty minutes and urination is freely induced. Irrigation given in this way provokes diuresis in two ways—by the stimulating effect of heat on the circulation, kidneys, and by direct absorption. In case of shock from all causes and profound toxemia, malarial or otherwise, how indispensable this agent should prove to be when coupled with other well-known measures. These are only a few hints, but sufficiently suggestive."

HOW NORMAL BODY TEMPERATURE IS MAINTAINED IN COLD WEATHER.

In a recent number of *Good Health* Dr. C. E. Stewart says: "The marvelous ease and efficiency with which the human body, when exposed to extremes of heat or cold maintains a normal temperature and at the same time replaces the waste which must necessarily result from this ceaseless activity, affords a fascinating and highly instructive subject for study.

Whether exposed to a temperature of 100° F. above, or 20° F. below zero, the body maintains a normal temperature of 98.6° F. What enables it to do this? Before discussing this, let us refresh our memories with the fact that it is the food which we consume daily that furnishes the heat and replaces the waste occasioned by the various activities constantly going on within the organism. While the heat produced in the human body, like the heat produced from burning wood or coal, is a result of oxidation, its production and dissipation are controlled by what is known as the "heat mechanism." This heat mechanism consists of two parts, one having for its function heat production, the other heat dissipation. In order that an equilibrium be maintained, there must be a very intimate relationship between heat production and heat dissipation. This relationship is under the control of the nervous system, and is known as heat regulation.

The mechanism having control of the production of heat consists of heat-generating tissues, which are to be found in every part of the body, in fact, wherever there is vital activity going on, and heat-generating nerves and centers. The nerves are found supplying the various muscles of the body, while the nerve centers are located in the brain and spinal cord. There are three classes of nerve centers concerned in the heat mechanism, one class, when stimulated, giving rise to an increased production of heat, and another class, when stimulated, causing a diminished production. These are associated with and control a third class known as general or automatic heat-producing centers. The heat-producing and diminishing centers are located in the brain, while the general or automatic centers are in the spinal cord.

That part of the heat mechanism which has to do with the dissipation of heat, while to a certain extent under control of the nervous system, and in a measure subservient to the heat-generating process, is chiefly affected by means of the skin and lungs, and other processes through which heat is lost from the body. Nearly all of the heat dissipated by the body is lost through the medium of the skin, by the conduction and evaporation of water from the skin and lungs, and in warming drink, food, and inspired air. Anything modifying these different processes will affect heat dissipation.

So long as heat dissipation keeps pace with heat generation, and *vice versa,* a normal, equable temperature will be maintained, and in order that such be the case, it is necessary that some mechanism have a governing influence over them. Such a mechanism exists. It is known as the heat-regulating mechanism, and is found in the skin. Both heat-generating and heat-dissipating processes are readily influenced by impulses generated in the nervous mechanism of the skin. To illustrate this point we call the reader's attention to a fact familiar to all, *i.e.,* when cold is brought in contact with the skin the latter becomes pale as a result of the contraction of the small blood-vessels; the quantity of the blood is thus lessened, and the temperature lowered; less sweat is secreted, and the skin is made a poorer conductor, all of which diminishes the amount of heat lost by radiation and conduction. While the body makes every effort to conserve its heat and maintain an equable temperature, external cold, even when applied for only a short time, abstracts more heat than is conserved by the process just described, and were it not for the fact that cold, in whatever form it may be applied, starts impulses in the skin which excite the heat-generating tissues so that there is an increased production of heat, we should be in danger of losing our lives long before the theremometer reached zero.

The shivering dog illustrates the point very clearly. While the dog's master is building a fire to keep himself warm the dog curls himself up on the ground and begins to shiver vigorously; this is his method of keeping warm. The cold coming in contact with his skin has sent impulses to the heat-accelerating centers in the brain, these in turn having conveyed impulses to the general or automatic centers located in the spinal cord, which have control over the heat-producing tissues. The muscles, being the chief source of heat production—producing more than one-half of the heat in the body—at once set to work to contract involuntarily, causing the phenomenon of shivering and a consequent increase of heat, with the result that the dog's body is soon warmed.

While the body is capable of adjusting itself to a considerable variation of extremes with reference to heat and cold, reason tells us that we must assist these natural processes to a certain extent. During the hot months of summer and in hot climates the character of food and the kind of clothing are different from those used during the winter or in cold climates. With reference to clothing and food we quote from "Landois and Stirling's Physiology" as follows: "Warm clothing is the equivalent of food. As clothes are intended to keep in the heat of the body, and heat is produced by the combustion and oxidation of the food, we may say the body takes in heat directly in food, while clothing prevents it from giving off too much heat."

"Variations in the temperature of the surroundings affect the appetite for food; in winter, and in cold regions, the sensation of hunger and the appetite for fats or such substances as yield much heat when they are oxidized are increased; in summer and in hot climates they are diminished. Thus the mean temperature of the surroundings, to a certain extent, determines the amount of heat-producing substances to be taken in the food."

From the foregoing it will be seen that as cold weather approaches there must necessarily be a change in the quantity and also to a certain extent in the character of the food taken. The increased oxidation resulting from the impulses originating in the skin as a result of the cold cannot take place unless an increased amount of fuel, in the form of food, be taken. The food substances which supply energy to the body are classified as carbohydrates, which include starches and sugars; nitrogenous, which include albumins of various sorts found in eggs, meats, etc., gluten of wheat, casein of milk, peas, beans, and lentils; and fats, which are found very widely distributed in both the vegetable and animal kingdoms.

The amount of heat produced by the oxidation of the various food substances is estimated in calories, the calorie being the unit of heat, and representing the amount of heat required to raise one gram of water one degree centigrade. By burning the various food substances it has been determined that one gram of nitrogenous food yields 5,778 calories, one gram of carbohydrate yields 4,116 calories, and one gram of fat yields 9,312 calories. During the oxidation or burning of these various food substances carbonic acid gas, urea, and water are given off in the form of waste products, which are excreted from the body by the skin, lungs and kidneys.

It has been estimated that it requires about two and one-half million calories of heat to meet the demands of the human organism during each twenty-four hours. The amount of heat can be obtained from the food substances just mentioned, which are found to meet the demands of the body best in proportions of 120 grams of nitrogenous food, 90 grams of fat and 330 grams of carbohydrates. The nitrogenous food goes to build up muscles substance and furnish heat and energy; carbohydrates and fats go to form fat and to supply heat and other forms of energy.

During the winter season in cold latitudes the amount and proportions of the food substances must necessarily be changed in order to meet the requirements of the system. Man, as a rule, is more active during cold weather than during the heated season, this fact at once making it apparent that an increased amount of energy and heat-producing food will be necessary. This is best supplied by carbohydrate and fatty foods.

On the other hand, the decreased external temperature calls for foods rich in material which will supply heat. Fats and nitrogenous foods are best suited for this purpose. Fats are especially indicated in cases where an increased production of heat is required. This fact is well understood by the inhabitants of the Arctic regions, who, while not necessarily requiring a large amount of energy-producing food, do require an abundance of heat-generating material; this they obtain from the fat of the various animals native to their locality. In this latitude a mixed diet best meets the demands of the system at all seasons of the year.

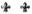

TO CURE NAUSEA.

A PHYSICIAN advances the theory that the distressing sensation of nausea has its seat in the brain and not in the stomach, and that relief may be obtained by cooling the base of the brain. He claims to have tested this often and thoroughly in the case of sick headache, bilious colic, cholera morbus, and other ills in which nausea is a distressing symptom, without a single failure; also, that he once relieved the nausea resulting from cancer of the stomach by the application of ice to the back of the neck and occipital bone. The ice is to be broken and the bits placed between the folds of a towel. Relief may be obtained by holding the head over a sink, or tub, and pouring a small stream of water on the neck. This is worth remembering, as a relief for sick headache, to which so many are subject.—*Exchange.*

MORE doctors, it is claimed, are kept busy in Australia than in any other country on the planet; at the same time, Australia consumes more animal food than any other country.

HEALTH, A BIRTHRIGHT, AND HOW TO MAINTAIN IT.

BY ALEXANDER WILDER, M.D.

WHEN after his death a sale was made of the effects of Boerhaave at Leiden, a book was offered as containing in it a synopsis of his medical learning. The eager purchaser found in it simply these words: "Keep the head cool, the feet warm, the body open, the digestion regular, and a fig for doctors."

John Abernethy was as terse as well as curt in his utterances. He regarded imperfect digestion as the cause of the numerous complaints, and advised his patients accordingly. A visitor with facial neuralgia or tic douleureux received this counsel: "This disease comes from a cold and bad digestion; remove one of the parents and you will have no propagation."

Nevertheless maxims like these, the outcomes of lifetimes of experience and observation, seldom attract much attention. Yet health is the birthright of every human being. It is contagious from one to another as no disease or epidemic ever was. But for the zealous efforts to subvert it, to create and disseminate disease, health would be universal and there would be neither pestilence nor contagion. We have epidemics and blighting diseases simply because niduses are provided for them, and because they are propagated. The maintaining of health is the first duty. We cannot dispense charity when we are poor and destitute ourselves, and we cannot render and reciprocate the good offices which are due between each individual and his neighbor, except we are in proper health and condition. Health is the inheritance of each, and the art of its preservation is the chief knowledge which should be inculcated in everywhere. Every one, professional or homes, taught in schools, and made familiar laic, adult or child, male or female, should learn it thoroughly.

Diet and hygiene belong, therefore, at the very foundation of all that we ought to learn. With these well learned and observed, it would be almost impossible to contract disease. We would then fulfil the prediction of the Hebrew prophet: "There shall be no more thence an infant of days nor an old man that hath not filled his days, for the child dying shall be a hundred years old."

The source of our many bodily woes is found in the digestive system. The food too frequently is not properly digested and assimilated that it may meet the needs of the body; and in turn the waste material of the body is not duly separated from it and eliminated. It is to this slackness of the secerment and excretory functions that the tendency to putrid, exanthematous and febrile diseases exists. Some external cause may develop them in particular forms, but they, all alike, whatever they may be named, whether the rheumatisms and pneumonias, the influenzas, the scarlet fever or typhoid, smallpox, measles or diphtheria, originate from a common cause. The body has been made unhealthy first or there would be none of them. A healthy person never contracts disease.

The body is nourished, built up and kept in repair by the proteids and albumen products which are derived from the food that is eaten. On the other hand it is kept in health by the regular eliminating of the morbid, effete and waste products which are formed in every region of the corporeal structure. As fast as the various proteid substances are fully assimilated to the organism and are duly employed in its offices, they become such dead and waste material. Chemically they have from albuminates been transformed into urates and compounds of that analogy. It is the office of the liver, kidneys and the various emunctories of the body to hurry them out. If they remain unremoved they disorder the body and render it a prey to every morbific activity.

The diseases incident to autumn and winter, whether rheumatisms, pneumonias, influenzas, scarlet fever, measles, smallpox, diphtheria, etc., are all outcomes of the uric acid diathesis.

If the morbid accumulations should be re-moved, the inside of the person thus cleansed as well as the outside, none of these diseases would exist. There is no other mode of prevention to be depended upon. No epidemic can be arrested, no disease averted by any makeshift, except the clean-sing process. It is not drugging that is required so much as it is a proper purgation and renovation.

Nevertheless I confess that I have not learned to dispense with medicines. I re-fused them when a child and sought to learn how to keep from wanting them in after life. I believe that there is a more ex-cellent way, but I have not found it. Yet there is much in dieting aright to cure as well as avert disease. For example, vegetable acids will enable the body to expel its morbid uric acid substances. Thus, lemon juice, which is so effective to avert and cure scurvy, is equally so for measles and smallpox. This was demonstrated conclusively twenty years ago by a physi-cian in Ironton, Ohio, in his own person and practice.

The same thing may be said of cream of tartar, which is an acid salt from grapes. The free use of it will eliminate uric acid accumulations from the body and so cure and prevent the diseases which they oc-casion.

A physician in Atchison City, the health officer, imputes similar benefits to the vin-egar of cider. He arrested a smallpox epi-demic with it, and found it a remedy as well as a preventive. He prescribed a dose of two table-spoonfuls in water four times a day.

It is very probable that these vegetable acids are dietetic rather than what are termed medicinal. Their principal merit is that they minister to health and enable in-dividuals to take care of themselves. Yet it will be perceived that there is a rational principle involved in their use, and this is sufficient for rational and intelligent persons.

Yet in most of these advanced questions I am a student endeavoring to learn, rather than a master ready to teach. I have sought to know what is wholesome and true, and to conform to it as well as I am able. The matter of dietetic reform has always at-tracted me, and I prize hygienic treatment far beyond medication. I do not profess to have attained very far; I never claim to be in a place because I see it at a distance ahead. But there is a way for the true and the sincere, and in that I would walk.

DIETS FOR EVERY DAY USE.

By J. WARREN ACHORN, M.D.
Boston.

GENERAL RULES.

ONE should be temperate in the adoption and use of foods named in the diet selected. Change in any one particular is change enough for that day.

It is too much to expect that regulation of the food will promptly revolutionize the habits of a life time.

These diets must be carefully and intelli-gently followed, if the results claimed for them and expected are to be realized.

No attempt has been made to furnish an elaborate bill of fare.

Health and good digestion are the first considerations sought.

Food known to disagree should be avoid-ed. It may agree later on.

Eating too continuously of one food to the exclusion of others of the same class should be avoided.

Meats should be stewed, roasted or broiled. Fish should be boiled, broiled or baked.

Fried food in any form, especially fried fat, is indigestible.

The best time to drink water or other liquids in amount, is the same in every case —on rising, an hour and a half before meals and half an hour before retiring.

Not more than two glasses should be taken at any meal and but one when soup is indulged in. Drink slowly.

Water should be taken at the close of a

meal, milk during the meal: sip after swallowing food. The mouth should be rinsed after drinking milk.

Only liquids should be taken between meals, unless fruit or other food is required for constipation or nourishment.

Constipation must be avoided: it is intimately related to all chronic disorders for which regulation of the foods is indicated.

Properly the heartiest meal should be eight hours away from sleep. If one is at work, however, this rule should not be too strictly adhered to.

DIET IN DYSPEPSIA.

(*Copyright.*)

Drink a glass of hot or cold water on rising, salted or flavored to taste; or of beef juice cold, or of hot beef tea; or of hot milk and German Seltzer (half and half), if faint or in need of nourishment.

BREAKFAST: *Cereals*—Rolled rye, rice, fine hominy, farina, wheaten grits, shredded wheat, Ralston's Breakfast Food, Malted Breakfast Food; rye mush, oatmeal. Eat with cream and sugar or with milk and a dash of sugar, with milk alone or with salt or butter.

Meats—(red) Rump, round, or sirloin steak; scraped meat-ball; mutton chops; thin bacon with dry toast; broiled tripe. Pepper, salt.

Fish—Weakfish, whitefish, smelt, cod, the *lean* of shad or bluefish, "tinker" mackerel, perch, pickerel, trout, bass.

Eggs—Raw, soft boiled, poached; eat with stale bread or Cestus Phosphated Crackers.

Breads—Gluten bread, whole wheat, rye bread, hoe-cake; unsweetened rusks, zwieback, soda crackers. Butter (spread thin), clear honey, on dry bread; prune marmalade.

Fruits—Stewed prunes (minced), baked or stewed apples, peaches, orange juice, pineapple juice, melons.

Drinks—Clear coffee, cereal coffee, Phillips' Digestible Cocoa, hot milk taken during the meal, hot or cold water taken at the close of any meal, beef tea, weak tea.

A. M. BETWEEN MEALS: A glass of milk

NOTES.

Six grains of salt and six of soda added to a glass of hot water make a desirable morning drink. Lemon juice or a little weak tea also make an agreeable flavoring.

Coffee, if it tends to disagree, should not be taken with any meal where cream is used.

Sugar in any appreciable quantity is apt to cause fermentation.

Sacchrine tabloids are a substitute for sugar; they do not cause fermentation.

Oatmeal and rye were better eaten without sugar. Oatmeal is less irritating if strained.

Liquid with meals produces "dyspepsia of liquids." Ice water aggravates dyspepsia.

The gastric juice loses its antiseptic action if diluted, and its digestive power also.

Strong tea precipitates pepsin and hardens the fibers of red meat. Tea goes best with eggs or fish.

If there is morning nausea, eggs are contra-indicated; the whites, however, may be eaten at any time.

Some form of toast for breakfast is to be preferred to eggs or meat.

Arrow-root cooked with milk is very soothing to an irritated stomach.

Milk usually agrees better if cut with lime-water or Vichy.

All bread should be at least one day old; it digests better if toasted and re-dried in the oven. Buttered toast is an indigestible article of food.

Potatoes go best with the morning meal, baked, with the jacket on; do not mash.

Meat and milk at the same meal are incompatible; they are the same thing.

Mutton digests easier than beef, and the breast of chicken or turkey easier than either.

Boiled meat or fish breaks up easier—is softer than when roasted or broiled.

Ham boiled until it is tender as chicken, cut thin and served cold, is allowable.

Hot fat is more indigestible than cold. Butter, olive oil, Terraline and Vigor Chocolate are fats that usually disturb dyspeptic stomachs; fats that do should be avoided.

"The longer food remains in the mouth the less time it will spend in the stomach."

Raw ripe fruit sets well on many a weak stomach. Unripe fruit, or over ripe fruit are both to be avoided; the former irritates, while the latter decomposes, and causes diarrhea.

The skins and seeds of fruit or vegetables are indigestible, so are skins of fowls or fish.

Do not eat fruit and vegetables at the same meal, the time of their digestion is *different;* the same rule applies to proteids and farinaceous foods; one or the other should greatly predominate.

If vegetables cannot be eaten on account of flatulency, indigestion, etc., purées of tomatoes, asparagus, potatoes and fresh peas in small quantity may be tried—or of sweet corn and celery.

All soups or purées must be thin and eaten in small quantities. Bean and pea soup were better made of bean or pea *flour.*

Not more than two vegetables should be eaten at a meal.

A weak digestion does better work on three foods than it does on six.

A teaspoonful of old brandy or whiskey taken at meal time helps the digestion of old people.

or water, hot or cold; raw egg in Madeira wine or milk; *whipped egg*, flavored with Medford rum; hot beef tea; beef juice, warm or cold.

LUNCH: *Meats*—(red) Meat juice, stewed beef, venison, sweet-breads, ham, scraped raw ham (white); stewed or roasted chicken, turkey, capon, squab, quail, wood-cock, plover, and prairie chicken.

Any *fish* mentioned.

Any *vegetable* mentioned.

Any *bread* mentioned. Phosphated crackers with plenty of butter, Somatose biscuit. Bent's Water Crackers.

Any *fruit* mentioned. Bananas,— the ripe fruit, baked.

Drinks—Weak tea (one-half ounce to the pint), weak cocoa, butter-milk, unfermented grape juice, water.

Desserts—Any mentioned, if desired.

P. M. BETWEEN MEALS: Same as A. M.

DINNER: *Soups*—Oyster, beef, or mutton soup, bouillon; add tapioca, vermicelli, Cestus bisbak, or barley. Hominy, bean, pea, and tomato soup. Serve with *croutons*.

Any *fish* mentioned. Oysters stewed (the soft parts), with horse-radish, lemon juice or pepper and salt; little-neck clams.

Any *meat* mentioned.

Vegetables—Mealy, well-baked potatoes, with butter or platter gravy; rice in place of potato, raw tomatoes, peeled and sliced; very young Lima beans, new string beans, thoroughly boiled onions, new peas, asparagus tips, stewed celery, plain lettuce, French peas, French string beans; Macaroni, plain or served with tomato.

Any *bread* mentioned. Soup sticks.

Any *fruit* mentioned.

Any *drink* mentioned. Water, milk, Vigor chocolate, China tea.

Desserts—Gelatin creams, b l a n c mange, sponge cake, floating island, rennet custard, whites of eggs custard; rice, tapioca, milk, and farina pudding; baked or stewed pears; apple sauce, not too sweet; ice cream, eaten slowly.

9 P. M.: Hot water, hot milk, adding a tablespoonful of Medford Rum; beef juice. Basbak in milk.

If the digestion is very weak, flatulent, etc., both fruit and vegetables will have to be tabooed.

If there is flatulency and fermentation, all food should be as *sterile* as possible and eaten dry, that it may be thoroughly masticated.

Raw vegetables as a rule do not irritate the stomach; they cause flatulency, however.

If digestion is slow, four hours or more must elapse before food is taken again; in this event it may be found necessary to eat four meals a day. If the stomach is dilated and digestion very slow, two meals a day only, may be tried.

Food that makes the mouth water stimulates digestion; food that causes disgust aggravates dyspepsia by stopping secretion.

Every attack of indigestion causes a relapse and it takes time to recover from indiscretions of this sort. "Eat with strict regularity."

Half an hour's rest before meals is indicated if tired, especially before supper, while sleep after meals is not advisable.

Exercise may begin an hour after meals, and stop half an hour before. When resting one should lie flat and *stop thinking*.

Mental work immediately after a meal is apt to retard digestion. Hurry and worry at meals cause dyspepsia.

Dyspepsia is often due to decayed teeth, unclean mouth, post nasal catarrh, unclean cooking utensils and tobacco.

A dyspeptic should keep warm, especially in the back and over the abdomen.

Exposure to cold by affecting the circulation disturbs the stomach.

Avoid constipation by the persistent use of laxative food—oatmeal, rye mush; whole wheat, gluten bread; baked apples, stewed prunes, raw tomatoes; lettuce with oil; grape juice, butter-milk; Vigor Chocolate, water.

Oil between meals, or on retiring, if starches and sweets are withheld, relieves constipation by giving a lazy liver something to do. One of the common causes of constipation is atony of the big intestine. Scybalæ evidence this. Oil frequently relieves this condition, also.

If wakeful, or awake and faint at night, Medford rum in milk or water may be used. Eat a cracker at the same time.

EXTRACT FROM PREAMBLE, (See issue of January *Gazette*.)

"If a person's nutrition and strength are maintained, and all the eliminative functions are working properly (the blood and urine being normal and the lung capacity and weight proportionate to the height) his food and drink for the time are approximately what they should be and his occupation and habits such as his physique can endure. Here the "physiological balance" exists or has been found; yet the disease for which he is undergoing treatment, may persist or has not been wholly relieved by regulating the foods. Cause for this persistence is probably due to some *one* food, or foods, among those allowed, eaten in too great quanity or too continuously, or in insufficient quantity, or too much liquid *at meals*, or to some mental or physical *habit* that must be sought out and overcome."

Note—"Milk and grains, grains and eggs, grains and vegetables or meats, grains and fruits" are compatible. "Fruit and vegetables, milk and vegetables, milk and meats, or fats cooked with grains" are incompatible.

DIETETIC TREATMENT OF DIA-
BETES.

Dr. N. S. Davis, Jr., emphasizes the point that a strict diabetic diet, that is, one containing no carbohydrates, should not be adopted too suddenly. Not infrequently coma has been precipitated, he says, by too sudden and great a change. Indigestion may be produced in other cases. From the beginning all sugar should be forbidden, but the starchy foods should be diminished day by day during the first week of treatment, so that all will be excluded at the end of that time.

Gerhardt's test with perchloride of iron should be constantly made. If the reaction is positive or if acetone or diacetic acid is demonstrated, lessen the albuminoids and increase the carbohydrates in the diet. (Ebstein's Rule.)

When by suitable treatment of a moderately severe, or severe case, the sugar is reduced to 500 grains daily, the case may be regarded as well controlled.

Another point is, that excellent results can often be obtained by intermittently restricting the diet closely. From two to six times a year, and from two to four weeks each time, this should be done. One or two "fast days" in a week is a good practice. The following is a "strict diet" *ménu:*

Breakfast—Tea or coffee without sugar or cream; one egg and bacon, and two or three slices of nut-bread with butter.

Dinner—Bouillon or broths; beef, mutton or chicken; spinach, asparagus, or wax beans; salad of lettuce or tomatoes, with cheese; black coffee without sugar.

Supper—Tea or coffee without sugar or cream; meat, fish, or mushrooms; a salad of tomatoes, lettuce, or chicory, etc.; two or three slices of nut-bread.

DIET IN TREATMENT OF SCIATICA.

The diet is a matter which does not receive the attention its importance demands, says Dr. A. P. Williamson. Care in this direction is always fully repaid by the good effects produced. The food should be liquid and very nourishing. It is best given in small quantities and at frequent intervals. Pain is said to be the cry of the tissues for nourishment, and if its severity is a criterion of the quantity of food needed there can be little danger of overfeeding. Milk, with salt to aid its digestibility, especially when given hot, is the very best food to be found. Home-made broths come next, and then preparations of blood, such as bovinine. The patient's palate may be consulted, but care is to be taken to avoid beef and uric-acid-forming foods in general. In this connection it cannot be too frequently repeated that in all diseases of the rheumatic or gouty diathesis large quantities of hot water should always be given the patient, say from two to four quarts every twenty-four hours. The rectum should be flushed every day, or every other day, with large quantities of water, as hot as can be comfortably borne.

Dr. J. Warren Achorn's diet list in Biliousness will be published in the March Gazette.

Department of Physiological Chemistry.

WITH SPECIAL REFERENCE TO DIETETICS AND NUTRITION IN GENERAL.

THE PHYSIOLOGY OF BODY COVERINGS.

A POPULAR author speaks of the "fatal invention of clothes," implying that the human race would be better off if the habit and fashion of wearing apparel had never overtaken the race. Like other extreme views, it is an over-statement of the case. The original man was, no doubt, hirsute; in other words, he was clothed without the aid of a tailor, shedding and renewing his glove-fitting suit in the spring and fall, with the horse and dog. Animals indulge their distinct summer and winter suits, thus equalizing the conduction or radiation of heat to comport with the surrounding temperature. Animals inhabiting cold climates are protected to a certain extent by a thick layer of fat under the skin. The fat prevents the too rapid waste of heat by conduction and radiation, and this conserves body warmth.

The aboriginal man inhabiting temperate and cold climates supplemented this internal or subjective power of resistence by artificial coverings of the furs and skins of wild beasts, or of bark mattings, the evolution of which has developed all our thousands of varieties of textile fabrics.

Many things affect the rate at which the body evolves and surrenders heat. First, its pose or position has much to do with the question. The overheated fowl spreads its wings, plumes its feathers, admits the air, and thus hastens the dispersion of heat. Some animals erect their hair, or throw themselves into the water, after which evaporation rapidly lowers the temperature.

Drawing the parts of the body together, that is, by approximating the head and limbs, tends to retain body-warmth. The rabbit in winter sits closely crouched behind a tuft of grass or a clump of bushes to econ-omize heat. Experiments show that if a rabbit be exposed to cold with his limbs extended, his internal temperature will rapidly fall several degrees. Children insufficiently covered instinctively "curl up" in bed. It was a mistake when our Spartan mothers told us we would be warmer if we would "straighten down like little men."

The heat of the body is not, however, derived from clothing. It is the oxidation and conversion of food that evolves animal heat. Clothing merely interferes with its loss or dispersion. In cold climates what we term "warm clothing" is in a sense the equivalent of food.

In estimating the value and influence of clothing it has been customary for physiologists to attach too much importance to the single item of its *capacity* for *conducting heat.* It has been almost universally assumed that in winter those substances or materials which are poorest conductors are best to be used as material for clothing, and that in summer the conditions are reversed when good conductors are best. Accepting this theory, it is not difficult to decide what materials are best for winter and what for summer apparel. But more comprehensive inquiry establishes the fact that other considerations must be taken into account. Several of these may be grouped as follows:

1. *Capacity for radiation.* Coarse materials radiate heat more rapidly than fine. But it is a popular fallacy that *color* affects the rapidity of radiation.

1. *The relation of the fabric to the sun's rays.* Dark colors absorb more heat from the sun's rays than light colors.

3. *The hygroscopic properties* of a material bear an important ratio by determin-

ing what proportion of moisture from the skin it can take up and carry off by evaporation. The same weight of wool takes up twice as much as linen; but flannel next the skin is not so easily moistened as linen, nor does it favor such rapid evaporation. Thus the non-conducting properties of wool are not the only ones to be considered.

4. *Permeability to air* is an important factor; in fact, more important than physiologists have been in the habit of conceding. Permeability favors conduction and, *prima facie*, lessens heat-conserving capacity. But contact of air with the integument induces more thorough oxidation of the blood and better elimination of toxic refuse; hence, it increases heat-production and indirectly diminishes heat-loss. If the sole object of nutrition were the production of heat and the chief object of clothing to prevent heat-loss, the subject of best materials for clothing would be very much simplified. But this is not the case.

In a future number of the GAZETTE we will take up the subject of clothing and discuss it further.

THE AVAILABILITY OF THE DIFFERENT CLASSES OF NUTRIENTS IN FOOD OF MIXED DIET.*

THE value of food for nutriment depends not only upon the total amounts of nutrients, but also upon the amounts which the body can make available for its support. The proportions of the different nutrients which the body can digest and utilize from different food materials are learned by digestion experiments. Such experiments involve the accurate measurement of the amounts of the different kinds of nutrients consumed in the food during a given period and the corresponding amounts excerted in the feces. This last material is made up of the undigested residue of the food, and of the so-called metabolic products. The latter consists mainly of residues of the digestive

* From the report of the Storrs Experiment Station, 1899.

juices. Later research has shown that in man the actual amount of undigested nutrients makes up relatively a much smaller portion of the intestinal excretion than was formerly supposed. Indeed some investigators are inclined to take the ground that the nutrients in ordinary food materials, properly prepared, are almost wholly digested by persons in health, and that the solid excreta are almost entirely made up of the so-called metabolic products and residues from the alimentary canal. While the feces do not give an exact measure of either the actual amount of the different nutrients which remain undigested in their passage through the alimentary canal or of the amounts of digestive juices used for the digestion, they do give us a measure of the availability of the food for use in the body. If the same quantities of two different food materials require the same amounts of digestive juices to prepare them for absorption, but the first is more completely digested, *i.e.*, leaves less undigested residue than the second, the first is more available. So, likewise, if both are equally digestible, but the former requires more of the digestive juices to digest it, it may be regarded as really supplying a less amount of available material to the body.

The experimental data as to the digestibility of different kinds of nutrients in different classes of food materials are as yet limited. There are on record a considerable number of digestion experiments with men. In some of these single food materials were used. In others an ordinary mixed diet of more or less varied character was employed. The experiments with single food materials or with very simple mixed diet give data for estimating the coefficients of availability of the nutrients of individual food materials. From such data we have prepared tentative coefficients for the availability of the nutrients of a number of the more common kinds of food materials such as meats, milk, wheat, bread, potatoes, etc. It is, however, a question whether these coefficients could be correctly applied to the same food materials when they are eaten in the usual way as components of an ordinary mixed diet. Fortunately we have a means for obtaining a reasonably definite idea as to their accuracy under the latter conditions. There are now on record the results of about 100 American digestion experiments with men on mixed diet. Most of these were conducted by Prof. C. E. Wait at the University of Tennessee, Knoxville, and by the writers and associates. In these experiments 13 persons have served as subjects. The diet in each case was simple and made up of common food materials, and was entirely normal in amount, proportions of ingredients, and method of cooking. In each experiment the ingredients of the feces were compared with the total amounts of nutrients in the food. The coefficients of availability thus obtained apply, therefore, to the total food eaten and not to the individual food materials. Now if the coefficients of availability which were assumed for the different kinds of food materials, as above described, represents the actual availability of the same materials when they are eaten in mixed diet, then by applying them to the materials consumed in these experiments we should get estimated results which would agree with those found by experiment. We may, therefore, use the agreement or disagreement of the estimated availability of the total nutrients of the diet used in these experiments with the results actually found as a measure of the correctness of the assumed coefficients of availability. This has actually been done. Using the coefficients as first assumed there was some discrepancy between the computed and experimental results. The coefficients were slightly altered, the change being such as seemed to us most probably correct, and the computations were repeated. In this way coefficients were found which brought results agreeing very closely with those of actual experiments.

In selecting coefficients for availability, food materials were divided into the following groups: (1) Animal food materials, as meats, fish, milk, etc. (2) Cereals, such as wheat flour, corn (maize) meal, etc. (3) Sugars and starches. (4) Vegetables, as potatoes, cabbage, turnips, etc. (5) Fruits.

The coefficients of availability assumed are shown in the following table:

Coefficients of availability of nutrients of different groups of food materials and of total nutrients of mixed diet.

	Protein.	Fat.	Carbohydrates.
	%	%	%
Animal foods, - - -	97	95	98
Cereals, - - -	85	90	98
Legumes, dried, - - -	78	90	97
Sugars and starches, - -	—	—	98
Vegetables, - - -	83	90	95
Fruits, - - -	85	90	90
Vegetable foods, - - -	84	90	97
Total food, - - -	92	95	97

In applying the assumed factors for availability (coefficients of availability) to the results of actual digestion experiments with men upon mixed diet the method employed was, in brief, as follows: The amount of available protein, for example, was calculated upon the assumption that 97 per cent. of the protein in animal food, 85 per cent. of that in cereal food, 78 per cent. of that in the dried legumes, 83 per cent. of that in vegetables and 85 per cent. of that in fruits can be utilized by the body. The sum of the amounts of protein thus computed as available in the different groups divided by the total amount of protein in the food eaten gives the calculated coefficient of availability. The computed coefficients of availability for the fats and carbohydrates were obtained in a similar manner.

The average variations between the coefficients as found and as calculated are inconsiderable. In some individual experiments they reached 5 per cent. for one or more nutrients. In some cases the calculated values were larger, in others they were smaller than those found by experiment. These variations in individual experiments are not at all surprising. Different specimens of the same food material may differ in availability with differences in composition and method of cooking, just as different persons may vary in their capacity to digest the food. But these minor variations disappear in the average of a large number of experiments, as is seen in the figures for all the experiments together. In the whole 93 experiments averaged in the above table the coefficients for the availability of protein were 93.3 as found, against 93.6 as calculated; the corresponding figures for the fats were 95.0 against 94.5, and for carbohydrates 97.7 against 98.1. These agreements seem to us to be reasonably close.

CONSTIPATION.

SOME observations have recently been made, says *The Hospital*, in regard to the conditions which conduce to constipation which are certainly worthy of consideration, and all the more so since they seem to explain, to a certain extent, one of the great difficulties which always stand in the way of securing a proper action by the use of aperient drugs—namely, the tendency to constipation which so constantly follows their cathartic action. According to E. Roos, writing in the "Munchener Medicinische Wochenschrift," an important factor in the production of the normal peristaltic action of the bowels is the stimulation of their coats by the products of the normal flora which inhabit the intestinal tract. Accordingly he cultivated the coli bacillus, and enclosed the culture so obtained in gelatine capsules, which he then coated with collodion and keratin so as to ensure that they should pass through the stomach into the intestines undissolved. These capsules he then administered to several patients during five days, with the effect of relieving them for a couple of weeks of the constipation from which they had previously suffered. The same experiment performed with dead bacilli proved negative. He then used cultures of the bacillus by which lactic acid is produced. These produced increased peristaltic action and caused flatulence, but did not relieve the constipation. Yeast given in the same way, however (in capsules coated as before with keratin), produced no gastric disturbance or flatulence, but after a few days acted as an aperient.

Perhaps it has been too much taken for granted that the action of aperient medicine must, as a natural consequence, be followed by a reaction in the form of constipation. That this is a common sequence no one can doubt. Nothing, for example, can be more striking than the effect of a calomel and colocynth pill upon a patient unaccustomed to aperients, unless it be the disappointment which follows upon an early repetition of the dose. Yet, unless we are to believe that the aperient has removed some ingredient from the intestinal canal, something which usually acts as an intestinal stimulant, it is by no means easy to explain why such an effect should be produced. It is common enough to hear the matter explained on the hypothesis that it is not the mercurial, but the onflow of the bile thereby set up that causes the aperient effect. Perhaps. But bile is formed too quickly, and the charge in the intestine is too rapidly replaced to make this explanation entirely satisfactory. If, however, extending the suggestion put forward above, we are to imagine that each portion of the intestine is inhabited by its own special flora, by whose action the successive changes undergone by chyme in its passage along the canal are assisted, and by the products of whose action the intestinal peristalsis is stimulated and maintained, then it is easy enough to see that the taking of an aperient may so upset the whole fermentative economy of the digestive tract as to displace the microbic elements proper to each district, and that this may have the effect of putting a stop to normal action of the bowels until each portion of the intestinal canal has become recharged with its normal fermentative organisms. The subject is an interesting one, and evidently has an important bearing upon the question of the cause of the aperient action of certain kinds of food which seem on analysis to contain no substance of an aperient nature. Perhaps such materials merely form a proper medium for certain micro-organisms by whose products peristalsis is kept up.

THE QUESTION OF DIET IN BRIGHT'S DISEASE.

" WE have on a number of occasions called the attention of our readers," says the editor of *Therapeutic Gazette*, "to the change which is taking place in the opinion of skilled clinicians concerning the diet which should be instituted in the treatment of chronic nephritis. It will be remembered that on one occasion we pointed out that in many instances a diet of unskimmed milk is very much better for the patient than a diet of skimmed milk, although the latter is the one which is usually advised; the advantage in the unskimmed milk over that which has been skimmed depending on the fact that it contains more of the cream, and is therefore more nutritious. While it is true that some patients are not able to digest the cream, others are quite able to do so, and should not be denied the advantage to be gained by this increase of nourishment.

" Again, we quite recently called attention, editorially, to the fact that investigation failed to reveal any good reason for forbidding such patients the use of red meats and allowing them white meats; the two varieties of meat differing one from the other so slightly in their constitution that one could not be considered more harmful than the other. Our attention has been called once more to this important matter by the review of the treatment of Bright's disease which has been contributed by Prof. J. Rose Bradford, of University College, London, to the volume of 'Progressive Medicine' for December, 1900. As he well points out, the principle of the treatment of Bright's disease is chiefly to spare the kidneys as much as possible, because of the very prevalent view that owing to the damaged condition of the renal structures the excretory activity of the organ is very considerably impaired, and for this reason it has been the custom to cut down the nitrogenous ingesta as much as possible. It is on this basis that the milk diet in Bright's disease was instituted. But the matter is not as simple as it seemed at first sight, since the proteid ingesta cannot be diminished below a certain quantity, and it is well known that during starvation the execretion of nitrogen is still fairly free. If proteid food is to be strictly withheld from the patient his proteid tissues will undergo disintegration; and on the other hand, if too much proteid is given, it may be disadvantageous. It would seem probable, too, that in severe cases of nephritis there is a rapid breaking-down of proteid material, so that the patient rapidly loses strength and weight, unless he is provided with a considerable quantity of food containing albumen, and doubtless in many instances a rigid adherence to a strict milk diet actually tends to weaken the patient.

" More recent clinical observers have shown themselves to be in favor of allowing a more liberal diet, on the ground that with the improvement in general health we might expect an improvement in the condition of the kidney. Or, to express it in Bradford's words: 'The modern tendency is not to restrict the diet in cases of chronic Bright's disease to the same extent as was formerly the case.' Patients with chronic Bright's disease may pass as much as from twenty to forty grammes of dry proteid in their urine each day—an amount equivalent to that found in one to two pints of milk. Inasmuch as the minimum amount of proteid necessary for an adult is that contained in from three to four pints of milk, namely, from seventy to eighty grammes it is obvious that a milk diet may at times be insufficient. Further than this, it is perfectly possible that the administration of many pints of milk a day dilate the stomach and overload the digestion. While permitting the patient to use a liberal diet may considerably increase the amount of albumin in his urine, this should not be considered the chief gauge as to the advisability of this free feeding, but we should study the patient's general condition, and if he improves in strength and nutrition under the increased diet, it is a fair supposition that the advantages gained are of greater value than the disadvantages associated with an increased albuminuria.

" Mills has also recently written upon this subject, and expresses the belief that red meat is permissible to many of these patients once a day, and that chicken, eggs, and fish may all be used. There are two other points which it is important for us to remember in this relation. One is that alcohol should be forbidden to all these patients except in rare instances, and the other is that in acute nephritis, which is an entirely different condition from that which we have been discussing, a rigid milk diet is usually to be insisted upon.

"These remarks are still further indorsed by the paper of Robin, of Paris, recently published and quoted in the *British Medical Journal* of October 13, 1900: 'In a paper on this subject read in the Section of Therapeutics at the recent International Congress of Medicine, Robin said it is recognized that the same system of diet is not suitable for all sufferers from Bright's disease. In particular the exclusive use of milk causes in some of them an increase, at least for a time, of albumin in the urine. Further researches prosecuted for many years have convinced him that an exclusive milk diet diminishes albuminuria always less than a vegetable diet, sometimes even less than the use of meat alone. In all cases a mixed diet of milk and vegetables or of milk and meat has a better effect than the exclusive use of milk. The following is the system that he adopts for the purpose of ascertaining the regimen most suitable for each patient: He begins by giving only milk. This has the effect of first increasing the amount of albumin in the urine; then it diminishes, and remains stationary. At this stage vegetables are added to the diet. New oscillations are then produced; when these have ceased meat is cautiously allowed, whilst milk and vegetables are continued. In this way it is easy to ascertain which of the three systems of diet—milk, milk and vegetables, or milk, vegetables, and meat—brings about the most marked dimi-

nution in the amount of albumin eliminated. It is important, also, to ascertain the value of each alimentary substance in regard to the production of albuminuria. Some researches which Dr. Robin has made on this subject have led him to the following conclusions: Bread has no effect on the albumin; wine causes an increase; amongst meats, beef and veal are more to be recommended than mutton or fowl; fish should be forbidden.' "

PURPOSE OF DIETETICS.*

Is the purpose of the science of health or dietetics only to point out to man the ways. by means of which he can save his physical or bodily being from sickness and disease? How ready are we to attribute to the rationally applied exercises, which make out only one of the means of promoting bodily health, only this one effect and only this one purpose. Harvey, the discoverer of the blood circulation, already laid down the fundamental law that mental and bodily life have their origin in one and the same source, and that they are subject to the same higher laws. The muscular system as the motor part of the body, and the digestive organs as the assimilating part, necessarily belong together with the functions of the mind. Frequently the superiority of the mind reveals itself in opposition to the body, and history records men of high genius and heroic strength of character, who had a crippled body only at their command. But to draw conclusions from such cases would lead to pitiful errors. On the contrary, it appears that the organism is capable of the highest manifestation of strength only when all its parts have arrived at the highest state of development. Thus our vital energy will be able to set free its entire latent power only when body and mind have been developed in harmony. The true mental education must, therefore, always go hand in hand with the highest bodily or physical culture.

* Translated from the "Schweizer Turnzeitung" by Carl L. Schrader for Mind and Body.

All the powers within us we have to gain by means of personal efforts. Through untiring efforts we shall also be enabled to restore the physical strength, which through the intensive mental strain that characterizes our century has been lowered to such an extent. Thus the art of life calls out to man: Dare and be well, and through perseverance and strength of will you shall be victorious. Our physical strength has not decreased in the same ratio as our mental capacity has increased. Like ore in the mine it lies latent, hidden in our body, and it requires but efforts of our will to bring it forth from within. Everybody ocasionally notices in himself that his physical capacity increases to an extraordinary height when, through emulation, a certain surplus of energy is permitted to disengage itself in one's extremities, and create in them an insuppressible desire for activity. In such exalted conditions, as it were, great thoughts and bold resolutions find their origin, and the mind attempts problems from which it used to shrink before when it was in an obtunded consciousness from physical exhaustion.

Does such a general condition exist in our public life? Indeed, no, and yet it must be the desire of every true friend of humanity that such a condition be brought about. The old proverb: "Mens sana in corpore sano" (a sound mind in a sound body) is as significant to-day as it ever was, and it should be revived with greater seriousness, so as to arrest the physical diseases of our generation, the overtaxation, and fatiguing of our mental strength, and to restore the robust health and youthful freshness of our forefathers. How many people to-day are not sick who, nevertheless, cannot be called well? They lack the joyful bell-like laughter of an everlasting vitality. One is tempted to say, they live not but are only existing, they merely vegetate. How many have ever, from birth on, experienced the real joy of a perfect health. Their pleasures were only half pleasures, their ailments lasting, chronic, and constantly growing. Only by means of incessant urging and unnatural stimulants are they able to enjoy life. The result of this artificial excitation is a fatiguing reaction that follows. If such a condition is of any long duration, the innervation of the body must weaken the mind. Fatigue and total prostration alternate with sudden excitements and overstimulations. The will and the moral strength are impaired until a total passivity takes possession of the physical as well as the mental life. During such relaxing resignation we blame our ancestors and nature that they gave existence to such a weakly body. Both nature has created in us the ability to produce life anew and make it desirable. "The sick must in the main help themselves," as the eminent Dr. Duehring used to say. But very rarely does man think of his own fault and his own help. Nothing should be too much, nothing too expensive, for us to gain this most valuable treasure of health.

Who, then, is responsible for our low state of health? How apt is one to reply: It is our culture, our refinement, our civilization, which bring all this about. But there is no greater folly than to accuse culture that it permitted humanity to degenerate. The true sources of all physical evil in mankind are effeminacy and ignorance, and history gives us sufficient data to prove that the greatest and best cultured peoples were not extinct on account of their culture, but because they lost their strong, natural way of living, thereby lowering their regenerative ability, while the requirements put on the mental and bodily strength were constantly increasing. By culture we understand the result of natural and rational development of all noble human faculties to an always higher aiming power and completeness. Wherever a bodily organ is destroyed or a mental faculty is crippled and its strength ceases, there the paths of nature have been deserted and the laws of culture disobeyed. Wherever we trace normal life in nature, be it in the kingdom of plants or in that of animals, there we find this striving for perfection, for completeness. The development to higher and better forms is the principle of nature's operations in vegetable as well as in animal life. But while the animal is under the immediate constraint of instinct, impulses, and senses, man possesses self-reliance and independence; with him the moral law takes the place of nature's constraint; the simplest, most general nature purpose becomes a clearly defined and willed moral action. The primal phenomenon of the mind, then, is the production of moral strength. Therefore athletes and gladiators, the Olympic victors, and the Roman triumphators were not the ones to win places of honor in the world's history, but those intellectual heroes, who, through moral strength, won victories over external powers, albeit they appeared defeated. Their untiring obedience to the laws of the higher world filled them with enthusiasm and courage, and to bring such obedience, in the realm of our physical life, to a practical application is the purpose of dietetics. With the same sacrificing enthusiasm and the conscientious fulfilment of his duty man must strive to educate all organs of his body so as to remove all imperfections. Thus life and soul, in brotherly concord and complete harmony, must be made serviceable to the general law of nature: Through development to perfection.

WATER DRINKING.

MORE attention, perhaps, is given at present to the drinking of water for therapeutic purposes than to any drug in the materia medica. Scarcely any writer, in the treatment of disease, fails to give water a very prominent place.

"The importance of water to the vital economy must be recognized," says the editor of *Modern Medicine*, "when we remember that the living organisms which compose the human body, as well as of other animals, are submerged in water. Water drinking," he continues, "is an internal bath: it dilutes the fluids of the body in which the cells and fibers are bathed; it purifies the body by diluting the medium in which it lives. By the free use of water the movement of the mass of liquid in which the living elements of the human body perform their work, is quickened, and the stream of life runs clear and pure. It has been shown that water is absorbed from the stomach very slowly. This takes place chiefly in the intestine. Absorption is stimulated, however, by the presence of CO_2. Distilled water charged with CO_2 is the best of all drinks as a beverage for use. It is soothing to the stomach, and is rapidly absorbed; hence more readily quenches thirst. The presence of mineral salts of any kind lessens the rate of absorption.

"To the great thinning of the blood which follows copious water drinking is due the remarkably increased activity of the kidneys, skin, and bowels which it produces. Examination of the urine shows not only that the quantity is increased by water drinking, but that the urea and other solid constituents are also increased. Fleming, in experiments for the purpose of determining the physiological effects of the Turkish bath, showed that the perspiration produced in profuse sweating after copious water drinking contains a larger per cent. of chloride of sodium than does the urine. An increase in the amount of urea and other nitrogenous principles (1.55 per cent.) was also noted.

"Baron Liebig showed long ago (and his observations have been many times confirmed) that water drinking powerfully influences metabolism, increasing both assimilation and disintegration, but especially the former.

"Water is a medium by which nutritive material is conveyed to the tissues and waste matters conveyed out of the body. Thus it is evident that by increasing the amount of water introduced into the body, the movement of the vital fluids, the blood and lymph, may be accelerated almost at will. By the increase in the volume of blood, the blood pressure is raised, the heart movements become more energetic, and the functions of the glands and other forms of activity are increased. This is true of the secreting glands as well as of the kidneys and other excreting glandular organs. Increased movement of blood through the lungs secures greater absorption of oxygen by which the various metabolic and catabolic processes are facilitated; retrograde metamorphosis is more completely accomplished; uric acid, urates, oxalates, and other products of imperfect oxidation are diminished or made to disappear entirely; in short, the patient lives a more highly vitalized and functionally active life.

"The effect upon the blood of copious water drinking suggests it as a valuable measure in cases of dropsy, whether general or local in character, especially the latter. The increase in the specific gravity of the blood due to the rapid withdrawal of water by the kidneys and the skin, even to the extent of impoverishing the blood, prepares the way for the absorption of the dropsical fluid; and by a repetition of this measure from day to day, most remarkable therapeutic results may sometimes be obtained. Distilled water charged with carbonic acid gas should be employed, without the addition of sugar or any other substance, unless it be fruit juices of some sort. The dose should be from one to two pints, and should be taken preferably before breakfast or an hour or so before dinner. The writer well remembers a case with which he became acquainted while in Bellevue Hospital nearly twenty-five years ago, under the late Dr. Austin Flint. A patient under treatment for general dropsy from organic disease of the heart, which had proved so refractory to all measures which 'had been employed, including diuretics of all sorts, was finally given up as a hopeless one, and the patient was permitted to drink copiously of water, which had previously been denied or allowed only in very stinted quantities. She drank in the course of the day two or three quarts of water. As a result, profuse diuresis occurred, the dropsy disappeared, and the patient made, for the time being at least, a very good recovery, and was soon able to leave the hospital.

"Profiting by this experience, the writer has made use of this measure in many cases of dropsy, with most gratifying results, and has never found it necessary to require dropsical patients to refrain from drinking water freely. It should be taken *in large quantities and rapidly*. When practised for the purpose of carrying off the dropsical effusion, the water drinking should be confined to two periods daily, morning and evening, no fluid whatever being taken between these hours.

"When it is desired to increase the volume of the blood and to introduce permanently a larger proportion of water, the water drinking should be managed in quite a different manner. A small quantity should be taken at frequent intervals, and the amount in the course of a day may sum up to several pints; but the quantity taken at any one time should not exceed four to six ounces. This quantity may be taken every hour or hour and a half with advantage.

"When the amount of water supplied to the body is insufficient, the condition of the body becomes in some degree comparable to that of a stagnant pool; while an abundant supply of liquid so encourages its activities that it may not inaptly be compared to the flowing mountain stream.

"Water is not a mere mechanical conveyer of poisons out of and of foods in; it is a powerful vital stimulant, a divinely appointed agent which the *vis medicatrix naturæ* can use in her healing work.

"Cold water drinking is especially indicated in all the cachexias and diatheses. In rheumatism it is useful as a means of diluting the blood so that it can dissolve and carry out of the body a larger amount of uric acid and allied substances; and as a means for encouraging activity of the skin and kidneys, it is always useful in this disease.

"In obesity, water drinking is essential as a means of dissolving and carrying out of the body the large amount of broken-down material which results from the increase in tissue destruction set up by exercise, hot and cold baths, and other means employed to reduce weight. To forbid the free use of water in obesity is a grave error.

"In diabetes the free use of water is not injurious, but advantageous. The blood contains an excess of sugar. All the sugar that is not oxidized must be removed from the body by the kidneys and skin, chiefly by the former. The specific gravity of the urine in these cases is always high, indicating a similarly high specific gravity of the blood. It is evident, then, that water is needed in cases of this sort for the purpose of maintaining a proper degree of fluidity of the blood and for facilitating the removal of the unused sugar, the presence of which interferes more or less seriously with the various vital functions. While the free use of water in diabetes will of course have the effect to increase the quantity of urine daily discharged, the amount of sugar, which is a matter of most serious importance in this disease, is not increased. Indeed the amount of sugar has appeared to be somewhat decreased, doubtless as the result of the increased oxidation which takes place within the body under the influence of free water drinking.

"In fevers, water drinking is essential as a means of aiding the kidneys and the skin in the elimination of the toxins to which the rise of temperature is due, in aiding the liver in its work of destroying the fever poisons, oxidizing leucomaines, and promoting the reduction of temperature by securing an increased evaporation from the skin.

"In cases of chronic inactivity of the skin, cold-water drinking is an exceedingly valuable measure, but it must be employed with discretion, as inactivity of the skin usually means an inactive mucous membrane, so that liquids are absorbed with difficulty. In cases of chronic dilatation of the stomach, water drinking, while indicated as a means of relieving the general condition, may be inadmissible on account of the state of the stomach. In these cases water may be introduced by enema.

"Copious water drinking is one of the most effective means of relieving a common cold, by aiding in the elimination of tissue poisons, the accumulation of which gives rise to the difficulty known as 'a cold.'

"One or two glasses of cold water taken half an hour or an hour before breakfast prove in many cases an almost perfect panacea for chronic inactivity of the bowels. Hundreds of patients have been cured by this simple remedy alone.

"Chronic biliousness, which is nothing more or less than chronic toxemia resulting from the putrefaction of animal food substances in the alimentary canal, requires the free use of water. Eight or ten glasses a day would be none too much in cases of this sort.

"In cases of gall-stones and infectious jaundice, water drinking is certainly indicated. The amount taken should be ten or twelve glasses a day, if possible, so that the liver will be thoroughly flushed and the bile so diluted that it will be able to dissolve and remove any concretions which may be present. In cirrhosis of the liver arising from either indigestion or alcohol, water drinking is essential as a means of aiding the liver and the kidneys to perform the work required of them in the removal of a large quantity of alimentary poisons in addition to the toxins naturally produced within the body by the physiological processes of tissue change.

"The temperature of the water drunk should ordinarily be about 70° F. In special cases water at 60° and even 50° may be employed. Very cold water is indicated only in fevers, in constipation, and in small quantities in hypopepsia.

"The quantity of water taken must depend on the effect desired. In fevers, a good rule is to take a glass of water every hour. In hypopepsia, one-third or one-half a glassful of cold water may be taken half an hour before eating. For inactivity of the bowels, one or two glasses of cold water should be taken on retiring at night, and as much more on arising in the morning. A thirst for water is almost always an indication that it may be taken with advantage, no matter whether such use is in harmony with the established canons of hygiene or not. It is safer to trust to the natural instincts than to pin one's faith to a theory.

Almost the only decided contraindication is in connection with meals, when free water drinking prevents proper insalivation of the food.

"The purest water is universally the best. Whatever beneficial effects are obtained from water drinking must be attributed to the water itself, and not to any ingredients which it contains. Mineral waters are simply diluted drugs. The ingredients may be obtained at any drug-store, and if diluted to the same extent as that in which they are found in the so-called natural waters, the effects obtained from their use would be the same. Medical experience has shown that the best of the so-called mineral waters are those which contain the least mineral ingredients. The very best water is distilled water which has been well aërated. Water obtained from natural sources is generally more or less contaminated, that from lakes, streams, and rivers being necessarily defiled by the fish and other creatures which live in natural bodies of water, and by surface drainage, which, after every rain, washes out quantities of filth.

"Water obtained from public supplies should always be boiled; indeed, this precaution is a wise one under nearly all circumstances.

"Hard water should always be boiled for a long time to eliminate, so far as possible, the lime which it contains; but even when boiled it is by no means free from this injurious ingredient. The larger the amount of saline ingredients, the more slowly the water is absorbed. The presence of acids encourages absorption. Carbonated distilled water and diluted fruit juices without sugar are the best drinks."

ART OF THE PARIS COOK.

Since the day of Napoleon I., says R. Barnes in the *N. Y. Sun*, the Académie de Cuisine has regulated the art of the French kitchen just as the forty Immortals look af-ter the language of the French nation. The cookery academy conducts classes, has its big corps of apprentices, sits in solemn conclave, for instance, on whether wax flowers can be legitimately used in the decoration of banquet pieces, decorates its members and bestows medals and diplomas that mean everything to the ambitious and artistic French cook. One of the most important retired *chefs* of the day is president of the Académie, and it is only after years of proved superiority in the kitchen that a man can hope to be elected as an associate or a member of this grave and powerful organization.

That is one of the reasons why French cookery is kept up to its present lofty standard, and why it is taken so seriously by its pupils and master workmen. It is on the whole, a very big thing to be a first-class cook in Paris. * * *

What is sure to produce a deep impression on the American mind is the appearance and the importance of many of the officers of the Académie de Cuisine. Some of them are heads of kitchens, the savory odors of whose perfectly done game and exquisitely mixed gravies have been wafted around the world; and some of them, the most important, are independent artists, the exponents of a specialty and not officially connected with any restaurant or kitchen. Such a *chef* is only produced in Paris, and in his own profession he is an object of extreme envy and admiration. Having proved his genius, he retires and lives and works in his own kitchen—an atelier is what he calls it —a really beautiful workshop, glass-roofed, walled with tiles decorated with framed diplomas, valuable autograph letters and photographs, and furnished with the necessary utensils in ancient pewter and the sort of copper that artists prize. About the room are strange little gas ovens. * * *

To such a man as this come rising and gifted young cooks, who have already got diplomas from the academy classes and well-known restaurant *chefs*, but wish to perfect themselves in some particular branch under a recognized genius of the day. To enter one of the great man's classes it is essential to be already accomplished and, furthermore, endowed with talent and ambition; for Benjamin Constant, Gérome, or Rodin would no more think of accepting a beginner in his studio than would one of these independent *chefs*. Years of devoted labor and the consciousness of great gifts have placed him beyond the drudgery of teaching, and his income flows from his reputation.

To him the heads of restaurants appeal with liberal payments for designs for new dishes. He composes and sells exclusive recipes; he goes to *cafés* at certain hours during the day or night, and in the kitchen over his own table or stove prepares just so many portions of his special dish, and the patron of the restaurant pays him well for such services. Added to these sources of income he edits cookery books, occasionally contributes an essay to a culinary magazine, and if one is a clever cook and composes a salad, he will, for a consideration, taste, criticise and give improving suggestions.

There is one famous specialist in Paris, Gustav by name, who earns $15,000 a year by merely going the rounds of a few restaurants every evening and preparing a certain number of game dishes at each. Days in advance, a lover of good food must leave his order with the head of the restaurant for one of Gustav's famously good ducks. A date is then fixed when the gourmand can hope to enjoy the services of the gifted cook. and when the opportunity to profit by the great *chef's* art comes round an elaborate supper is the fitting environment for the faultless duck.

Down in the restaurant kitchen Gustav himself touches nothing. He merely directs, standing, like Napoleon at Austerlitz, impassively regarding the progress of the great triumph of mind over matter, and controlling the forces that transform crude fowl flesh into a dish of most exquisite savor. Often enough the evening rounds of a man of Gustav's importance include a call at a private house for the purpose of preparing one of his great dishes at a side table in the dining-room, right before the eyes of the interested guests. Of late years, having a notable cook in to do what Americans would call "stunts" at a great dinner party has been one of the most popular Parisian fashions. The *chef,* whether Gustav or another, is apt to charge about 100 francs, or as high as 200 francs (the equivalent of $40) for his services in preparing a single course for a table full of people. He brings his own utensils and possibly his own oven, one of those strange round drum-shape inventions, to set on a range or a gas frame, inside which everything can be cooked, from the most delicate little cakes to the heaviest roasts.

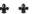

MEDICAL USES OF FRUITS.

A LONDON physician has a very interesting paper on the uses of fruits in the relief of diseased conditions of the body. To us, says *Health*, this article is worthy of careful perusal, coming as it does from one who has made the medical uses of fruits a study for nearly a generation. The physician says that he does not want it understood that edible fruits exert direct medicinal effects. They simply encourage the natural processes by which the several remedial processes which they aid are brought about.

Under the category of laxatives, oranges, figs, tamarinds, prunes, mulberries, dates, nectarines, and plums may be included. Pomegranates, cranberries, blackberries, sumac berries, dewberries, raspberries, barberries, quinces, pears, wild cherries, and medlars are astringent; grapes, peaches, strawberries, whortleberries, prickly pears, black currants, and melon seeds are diuretics; gooseberries, red and white currants, pumpkins, and melons are refrigerants; the lemons, limes, and apples are refrigerants and stomachic sedatives.

Taken in the early morning an orange acts very decidedly as a laxative, sometimes amounting to a purgative, and may generally be relied on.

Pomegranates are very astringent, and relieve relaxed throat and uvula. The bark of the root in the form of a decoction is a good anthelmintic, especialy obnoxious to tapeworm.

Figs, split open, form excellent poultices for boils and small abscesses. Strawberries and lemons, locally applied, are of some service in the removal of tartar from teeth. Apples are correctives, useful in nausea, and even seasickness and the vomiting of pregnancy. They immediately relieve the nausea due to smoking. Bitter almonds contain hydrocyanic acid, and are useful in simple cough; but they frequently produce a sort of urticaria or nettle-rash. The persimmon, or dyospyros, is palatable when ripe, but the green fruit is highly astringent, containing much tannin, and is used in diarrhea and incipient dysentery. The oil of the cocoanut has been recommended as a substitute for cod-liver oil, and is much used in Germany for phthisis. Dutch medlars are astringent, and not very palatable. Grapes and raisins are very nutritive and demulcent, and very grateful in the sick-chamber. A so-called grape has been much lauded for the treatment of congestions of the liver and stomach, enlarged spleen, scrofula, tuberculosis, etc. Nothing is allowed but water and bread and several pounds of grapes per diem. Quince seeds are demulcent and astringent; boiled in water they make an excellent soothing and sedative lotion in inflammatory diseases of the eyes and eyelids.

ELLA WHEELER WILCOX ON HAPPINESS.

ELLA WHEELER WILCOX, in a recent number of the *Chicago American*, takes up the subject of happiness and treats it in the following bright and interesting manner:

"How much happiness are you getting out of life?

"How much enjoyment of the days of each week?

"You had better pause and ask yourself this question.

"If you are merely getting through the present, with an idea of being happy in the future, I fear you are making a mistake.

"Happiness is a habit. It is influenced more or less by environment and circumstances, to be sure, and it can be shadowed temporarily by sorrow and augmented by good fortune.

"But in the main, happiness must come from within you.

"Unless you obtain some happiness every day now, you will not find it on any to-morrow.

"If you are restless, despondent, irritable and discontented, from dawn till bed-time, and wear the hours away in an impatient waiting for better times, you are forming a mental habit which will pursue you when the 'better time' comes.

"I know what I am talking about. I have seen it proved over and over again. You are building your brain cells, hour by hour, day by day, to think a certain kind of thoughts, and no change of external conditions will undo this work which you are now engaged upon.

"Of course, I am not addressing people suffering from some great loss or sorrow. Experiences of that nature must wear away; they cannot be overcome in a moment, or argued out of the heart. But they do not last—God has sent time to comfort the sorrowing.

"It is the people who are discontented with their work, and with their environment whom I address. People who are working for the future and hating the present.

"I believe in a progressive discontent. It is a means of growth. But I believe in forming a habit of being happy about something every day. While you work and strive to change your conditions, look around you and find a cause for enjoyment.

"Think of yourself as one who set forth on a journey to a desired goal. Instead of shutting your eyes and straining forward to the end, open them and take note of the blue sky, the green world, the birds, the children, and the lovers as you journey along. Be glad that you are alive; enjoy the rainstorm; take pleasure in passing a word with the friends you encounter and sit down by the roadside and converse with them now and then. Say to yourself, 'This is very cosy and cheerful. I will be happy with my friend,' and all the time rejoice that you have a goal toward which you are pressing.

"Get something out of the journey every day—some hour of · enjoyment, and even if some accident prevents you from reaching your dreamed-of destination, or delays you long, still you have some golden hours of pleasure strung upon the thread of life. And, better still, you have formed the habit of enjoyment—you have practiced being happy! And when you do reach your goal you will know how to appreciate the things you have longed for.

"Do not tell me that you have nothing to enjoy—nothing to be glad of in your present; I know better. God never made a day that did not possess some blessing in it if you look for it. Learn to be happy while you strive for things to make you happier."

THE INFLUENCE OF TEA ON DIGESTION.

DR. JAMES W. FRASER has recorded the result of an interesting series of experiments on the action or our common beverages on stomachic and intestinal digestion. The results obtained from an exhaustive series of experiments and analyses show:

"1. That it is better not to eat most albuminoid food-stuffs at the same time as infused beverages are taken, for it has been shown that their digestion will, in most cases. be retarded, though there are possible exceptions. Absorption may be rendered more rapid, but there is a loss of nutritive substance. On the other hand, digestion of starchy food appears to be assisted by tea and coffee; and gluten, the albuminoid of

flour, has been seen to be the principle least retarded in digestion by tea. From this it appears that bread is the natural accompaniment of tea, when used as a beverage at a meal. 2. That eggs are the best form of animal food to be taken along with infused beverages, and apparently they are best lightly boiled if tea, and hard boiled if coffee or cocoa, is the beverage. 3. That the casein of the milk and cream taken with the beverage is probably absorbed in a large degree from the stomach. That the butter used with bread undergoes digestion more slowly in the presence of tea, but more quickly in the presence of coffee or cocoa; that is, if the fats of butter are influenced in a similar way to oleine."

FOOD VALUE OF FRUITS.

IN recent years the growing of fruits has assumed great commercial importance in many regions of the United States, says C. F. Langworth, Ph.D., in *Sanitary Home*. especially in the south and on the Pacific Coast. The amount of fruit has undoubtedly increased with the greater production and facilities for shipping and marketing.

Many stations have reported analyses of fruits and made extended studies of the different methods of growing fruit trees, their soil requirements, enemies, etc.

The stone fruits constitute an important group, and have been studied for a number of years by the California and Oregon Stations. Fresh peaches, apricots, cherries, prunes and plums are general favorites, while enormous quantities of these fruits are canned, dried or preserved in some way. It is interesting to compare the composition of these fruits, fresh and dried, with each other and with some of the staple articles of diet.

It must not be forgotten, however, that fruits are valuable for other reasons than the nutrients which they furnish. They contain acids and other bodies which are believed by physiologists to have a beneficial effect on the system and, doubtless, very often stimulate the appetite for other food. They are also useful in counteracting a tendency to constipation. Another point—and one entirely apart from food value—should not be overlooked. That is, fruits add very materially to the attractiveness of the diet. It is not easy to estimate their value from this standpoint, since often the appearance of food has a value which cannot be measured in dollars and cents.

ACIDITY OF THE MOUTH DURING SLEEP.

THE dentists tell us that an acid condition of the fluids of the mouth plays an important part in the etiology of dental caries: also that the causes of that affection are particularly active during the hours of sleep, when saliva stagnates, so to speak, instead of being subjected to the agitation and renewal incident to the chewing and other movements that to some extent are almost continuous except during sleep. However carefully we may cleanse the teeth and rinse them with antiseptic solutions on going to bed, therefore, we are guarding but temporarily against decay, it gains on us while we are asleep. Possibly those who suffer with insomnia may snatch a crumb of comfort from this reflection, but we fear there is in it no consolation for the mouth-breathers, for the desiccation of the mouth which takes place in them during sleep, while enough to give rise to considerable discomfort on their waking, is quite insufficient to hamper pathogenic bacteria in their work of destruction.—*New York Medical Journal.*

VEGETABLE DIET.

PERHAPS no stronger argument could be advanced in favor of a vegetable diet than the enormous bulk, strength and endurance of the Japanese wrestlers. Imagine a set of men, the tallest not more than five and a half feet high, with weight ranging from 200 to 300 pounds, chest girth varying from 44 to 58 inches, and lung capacity reaching as high as 6,000 cubic centimeters! Yet the staple food of these men is rice, with a little fish; but, withal, they can hold their own against the picked men of any of the flesh-eating peoples, both for strength and endurance. The writer has frequently seen the coolies handling cargo on the Bund in Yokohama, working ceaselessly from 6 A.M. until 6 P.M., and at midday has seen them produce their simple meal of a few ounces of rice and fish, packed in a tiny piece of matting, eat it with the utmost gusto, and then resume their labors, like giants, refreshed. Meat is certainly not indispensable to produce and maintain brawn and muscle, as witness the splendid physique and staying qualities of the Scotch and Irish peasantry, whose principal articles of diet are oatmeal and potatoes!

"NOISELESS MILK."

A DAIRYMAN whose dairy was near Indianapolis, says *Southern California Practitioner,* was taken sick and went to the Hoosier capital for treatment, and, while there, lying in bed convalescing, he was greatly annoyed by being awakened at an unearthly hour each morning by the man delivering milk. This caused him to improve his convalescing hours by developing a scheme to furnish noiseless milk. As soon as he got well he had all of his milkmen shod with rubber-heeled and rubber-soled shoes, and rubber tires put on all of his wagons. He presented each one of his customers a rubber mat upon which to set the milk can by the door, so that there was no noise from that, and he had his horses all shod with rubber shoes, and then began to exploit his noiseless milk. The result has been immense. His business has quadrupled and his noiseless milk has gained great popularity.

There is a lesson in the above instance that I believe will be of great benefit. Let us all endeavor to reduce the noises of our cities. The rubber-tired vehicles have reduced greatly the noises on our streets. Many people are learning the personal advantage of wearing rubber-heeled shoes; this is materially lessening the street din. One physician in Los Angeles told us that his buggy with the rubber tires would last four times as long as one with metal tires. We do not doubt this, and on the same principle we believe that the man or woman who wears rubber-heeled shoes will be protected and life will be prolonged, as is the life of the buggy with the rubber tires. The cement and stone walks of our city are not the walks that nature made for us. They are hard and unyielding, and every step is a shock to the human system, but with the rubber heels this unnatural inelasticity of the city sidewalk is counterbalanced and the person steps lightly and briskly along, feeling that it is a real joy to be alive. We believe that there is nothing more important for the American people than to overcome their general nervous condition, and the use of rubber heels is an important step in that direction.

VALUE OF MEAT IN THE PREVENTION AND TREATMENT OF PULMONARY TUBERCULOSIS.

F. Parkes Weber directs attention to the infrequency with which tuberculosis and gouty diseases are found in the same individual, and suggests that there may be some substance circulating in the blood of gouty subjects, in minute quantities, yet sufficient to have an antagonistic action toward the growth of tubercle, and that this is likewise the case in persons taking an unusual amount of food. In accordance with this view he advocates the use of a preponderatingly proteid rather than carbohydrate diet in tuberculous individuals, laying stress on the necessity for seconding the treatment by abundant out-door exercise.

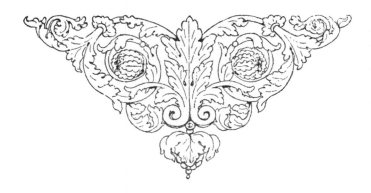

Department of Hygiene.

WITH SPECIAL REFERENCE TO STATE AND PREVENTIVE MEDICINE.

DOCTORS, DRUGGISTS AND DOMESTIC MEDICINE.

THE people of average, and especially those of more than average, intelligence in every community are, every year, becoming better informed in relation to the laws of health and the nature of the commoner forms of disease. As a result they may not be less respectful to real medical talent, but they are becoming critical of the practical results of prevailing medical practice, and are demanding reasons for much that was formerly accepted without question. Physiology, hygiene and sanitation, such as it is, is being taught in all the schools; hundreds of laymen have become regular subscribers to medical journals, and these, in turn, are gradually introducing more or less matter that is adapted to lay reading; in addition to which scores of "health" journals address themselves wholly to the laity. It is becoming a common thing for families to own and use a fever thermometer and a well-stocked medicine cabinet. To such an extent has this business increased within a decade that the great army of medical practitioners begin to sorely feel the inroads that are being made in their incomes. In a large majority of the minor complaints the people treat themselves, and they do not hesitate to assert that they are quite as successful as the average practitioner. Nor is this to be wondered at when we realize that all the quacks, and their name is legion, and, more's the shame, many of the reputable members of an honorable profession secretly resort to tricks and dishonorable methods to increase their fame and their incomes.

To this cause is attributable the immense increase in the number of proprietary medicines and secret nostrums, and the almost incredible amount of capital now represented in the manufacture of these seductive preparations.

Philanthropists deplore the condition, and medical men predict the direct results in the near future, but neither of them propose a practical remedy. There is no question but that thousands of sudden deaths occur every year that are directly attributable to this growing habit of self-medication chiefly by means of some of the loudly-extolled and plausibly advertised "cures." Since quick results are insisted upon the promulgators of these panaceas aim at this effect regardless of subsequent injury to the insistent recipients, however serious this may prove to be.

A careful analysis of the more popular of the secret nostrums now in use shows them to be based on sedation or stimulation. Bromide or chloral, juice of the poppy or product for tar, the endless changes are constantly rung on possible combinations of these universal sources of narcotism, and on the thousand and one forms of the spirit of wine or the spirit of corn. The one obtunds the sensations and lulls the patient to ease, which is easily and ignorantly mistaken for betterment. The other prods the flagging forces to a semblance of new life, for both of which effects deluded mortals are willing to pay twice, once in the cost of the panaceas and once in the ultimate loss of vital force. Faith in the false inspiration of the still and in the "curative" power of drugs is strictly in proportion to the prevailing ignorance and superstition. Competent and candid medical students have finally admitted that the province of the physician is to provide the necessary material, remove obstructions, and assist in directing natural processes, while Nature herself ultimately does all the curing. Not that this fact by any means cheapens the physician's skill; rather, it requires more acumen and better judgment than ever.

The manufacturing proprietors have taken up the question of materials, and are supplying food products of every conceivable kind, in forms adapted to every condition of the system. Their efforts are giving brilliant results, because they give jaded and ailing digestive organs that complete rest which often turns the scale. But since the arm tied up in a sling, and kept at perfect rest, eventually becomes atrophied and helpless, so, the stomach that has all its work done for it soon becomes unable to act for itself.

It is useless to shut our eyes to the existence of this evil of the domestic practice of medicine, or to the fact that it is rapidly assuming more and more extensive proportions. It is not that the people have learned too much, but that they know too little. A better knowledge of the nature of disease and the action of drugs will go far towards abolishing the practice of self-medication. The people would be more than glad of a safe guide in matters of health. They are afraid of the quacks—except the very unctious fellows who have an unsuspected gift of "od force" or hypnotism—and they are almost as much afraid of a certain class of doctors who deceive and impose upon them by insisting upon scare diagnoses and making exorbitant charges for insignificant services. The better classes, all the more intelligent, are quite willing to pay for adequate attention and honest skill, but they never feel quite sure that the doctor is not magnifying his office for the sake of his fame or his fees, in at least half the cases to which he is called. In yielding to this feeling of distrust they often make the fatal blunder of neglecting to call the doctor in cases of great gravity until it is too late, even with the aid of the best medical skill, to save them.

There is a limited circle within which the layman may treat himself and family. Beyond that circle it is neither prudent nor economical to go. Outside that limit the very best obtainable medical skill is none too good, and should be promptly invoked and implicitly obeyed. The promonitory symptoms of some of the most dangerous diseases are very obscure and insidious. To the unskilled eye and touch they mean no more than the passing symptoms of a slight cold, or the flush of an ephemeral fever. The skilled eye, ear and tactile sense of the trained physician detect the lurking danger in time to forefend it. Sometimes it is a specific poison or infection that must be counteracted; sometimes it is an explosive crisis in connection with some inherited or acquired diathesis, and again it is merely an accumulation of obstructions that need to be swept away, or it may be some special nutrient principle that the system is clamoring for.

No one will dispute the assertion that most people take too much medicine. Dosing for every trifling ailment becomes a chronic habit. Failing of relief from the use of one vaunted cureall or concoction, they try successively, perhaps, a dozen others, in the vain hope that some one of them will "hit the case."

In a measure the doctors themselves are to blame for this state of affairs. They have both talked too much and schemed too much; and in this respect there is no distinction as to schools, regulars—there never was such a thing as an "allopath," except in the lively imagination of Hahnemann and some of his early disciples—homeopaths, eclectics or what not, all have been more or less culpable. The principal sinner, however, has been the druggist. He began by prescribing over the counter; he will end by going *under* the counter! His shelves groan with their load of "patent" and proprietary remedies, and his showcases and display spaces are a-glitter with sensational advertisements. For a time he made money rapidly. To-day he has to scratch hard and twist in all directions to make the two ends of the year meet. He has robbed the practitioner, and the latter is retorting in kind; no longer submits to the wholesale duplication of his most important prescriptions, and in many cases supplies his own drugs. The manufacturing pharmacist makes it unnecessary for him to know much about pharmacy, supplies him with all needed combinations, in better shape than he could compound them himself, and the retail druggist begins to realize that he has committed business suicide. Grown desperate over his waning patronage and profits he is now trying another "dodge." Instead of selling the products of the manufacturing chemists and pharmacists, he is decrying them, and inducing his customers to purchase similar preparations put up by himself, or at least bearing his label.

This is the status at the opening of the new century. What will be the outcome of this triangular crossfire of clashing interests it is hard to predict.

A FEW REMARKS ON THE DIAGNOSIS OF REMITTENT MALARIAL AND YELLOW FEVER.

To make a differential diagnosis between malarial remittent and yellow fever is, to my judgment, one of the most perplexing questions to the medical man, not familiar with the tropical fevers of the country, for the resemblance of the symptoms of the two infectious fevers are so remarkable that one is very often driven into the dark during the first days of the appearance of the disease, and, although we consider the presence of albumin in the urine of a yellow fever patient as its most valuable diagnostic point, we do not as a rule, get this element until the third or fourth day, and there are many cases of remittent malarial fever, the urine of which at the third or fourth day, would show traces of albumin.

The early symptoms of the two diseases are remarkably alike. In both the onset may be abrupt, or it may be preceded by headache and general malaise for several days. A sudden chill at the onset is a common feature of our malarial fevers of the States, but unfortunately it is not present in every case met with in this country, and this circumstance will tend to increase our doubts as to the character of the fever.

In both there are severe pains about the body, especially the bones and joints, although we might be inclined to think that those of yellow fever are of a more excruciating nature.

The temperature in remittent fever rises rapidly to 103 F. in very mild cases, to 105 or 106 F. in the severer forms; the same may be said of the temperature in yellow fever.

The typical pulse in the latter disease is at first usually full, and slows down gradually, having no corelation with the temperature, a point which I may consider worthy of note in connection with the malarial fevers of this country.

In like manner an irritable stomach with uncontrollable vomiting exist in both diseases as well as the tendency to a jaundice condition.

In the two fevers a hemorrhagic type of the disease is found also.

All these points of similarity will naturally increase the difficulty and dangers of dealing with the two infections, for while in one quinine is indicated, in the other it would be hazardous to administer the alkaloid.

The greatest aid in the clinical differentiation between remittent and yellow malarial fever would be the appearance through the microscope of the plasmodium malariæ in the blood of a patient of the latter disease.

It seems then scarcely necessary to emphasize the increased diagnostic value of this sign, and we must, while waiting for further discoveries, rely upon the only means of observation, in order to arrive at an early conclusion.

I. P. AGOSTINI,
Act'g Asst. Surgeon U. S. Army.
San Luis, Cuba, January, 1901.

THE PHYSICIAN IN THE TWEN-
TIETH CENTURY.

UNDER the above title, among many other excellent things, Dr. Andrew H. Smith of New York, said, in a paper read before the New York Academy of Medicine: " The tendency of modern research is to give especial prominence to preventive medicine. The revelations of the microscope during the past decade have taught us many impressive and valuable lessons in the prevention of disease, while they have scarcely afforded us a single practicable suggestion as to cure.

" The triumphs of antiseptic surgery lie much more in the direction of keeping germs out of the system than of expelling them after they have effected a lodgment. And this is, beyond doubt, typical of the line in which medicine as a whole is to have its principal development in the near future. And it is this, too, which will command the attention of the laity, and win their confidence. As a consequence, instead of relying upon this or that method of cure in case they should become ill, men will prefer to put themselves under such direction as will tend to avert illness. And this will be the chief province of the family physician. To relieve suffering is a god-like office, but to prevent suffering is a higher office still. The good Samaritan rendered a service that shall be a proverb for all time, but if the traveller had journeyed from Jerusalem to Jericho in the company of a Roman soldier the tender ministry of the Samaritan would not have been required.

"Descartes has said: 'If it be possible to perfect the human race, it is in medicine that we must seek the means.' While not anticipating the perfection to which he refers, we may well believe that whatever progress is made toward it will be worked out essentially through the agency which he indicates.

" But to return from this digression, what in detail is to be the character of this improved relation between the medical prac-
titioner and the families under his charge? I can best illustrate my view of this by taking up the life of a young married pair and tracing step by step the position which their medical adviser should occupy toward them as the family life develops.

" In the first place, this medical adviser should be selected with the greatest care and with reference to his practical knowledge and sound judgment. He should not be too much their senior, for it should be no part of their plan to change without the gravest reason, and the doctor should be young enough to continue in his position, in the natural order of things, for the greater portion of their lives. They should begin by placing before him the medical history of each as completely as it can be obtained, together with all the facts they possess touching the medical history of all their ancestors. This information should constitute the beginning of a minute and careful record, to be kept by the physician and transmitted to his successor. This record should contain the results of a careful physical examination, so that the state of health of each one shall be known from the beginning. These examinations, as thorough and exhaustive as those required by the most careful life insurance companies, should be repeated at stated intervals and duly entered upon the record. It should be impossible that the first manifestation of a detectable chronic affection should be by a disastrous explosion. Sudden death from unsuspected heart or kidney disease, for example, should be relegated to traditions of the past.

" At the birth of every child every important circumstance connected with the event, as also the subsequent lactation, should go on record. The progress of dentition, the age at which the child walks and talks, the closure of the fontanelles, the particulars of vaccination—all should be entered in due order. The occurrence of one of the contagious diseases of childhood should be the subject of especial care in recording. The source of contagion, the period of incubation, the character, intensity and duration of the eruption, the complications, the treatment and the sequelæ—each should be carefully noted.

"The value of such a record would not end with the subjects of it. The next generation would profit by it perhaps as much as the present. Heredity is an influence the power of which it is difficult to estimate, for the very reason that the absence of such record as I propose prevents our tracing it backward in the family history. With such a record, however, we know from the history of the parents what to expect in the children, and the timely use of precautionary measures might avert a great deal of suffering and disease. Dr. Holmes has said that the proper time to begin the treatment of some diseases is a hundred years before the birth of the child.

"As each child grows older, nothing that can have an influence, present or prospective, upon its physical condition should escape the scrutiny of the doctor. The food given it, the clothes it wears and the habits it forms should all come under his observation. Even parental discipline should be open to his criticism, the timid and nervous child being screened from harsh rebuke, while on the other hand, the evils of good natured indulgence on the part of the parents are pointed out. They should be made to understand the supreme importance of the future health of the child, of making obedience the first habit to be acquired; and also that this can be done without the least harshness, by beginning at the first moment of intellectual consciousness.

"It will be inferred from this sketch of his duties that the family physician of the future will need to be a man of varied culture and great learning, of deep sagacity and sound judgment. He will need to know much more than how to make a diagnosis or how to write a prescription. He will have daily use for more varied knowledge than any other man in the community. His preparation will require as its foundation a thorough preliminary education in lines that will give the greatest development to the reasoning faculty, for a man cannot become a good physician by studying medicine only. He will need to be trained to view a question from all points and take account of everything that may throw a sidelight upon it. He will require a detective's quickness of perception, a lawyer's skill in weighing evidence, a business man's method and system, and a clergyman's self-abnegation. His professional training might well omit a great deal that now occupies time and yields no practical results, while it should embrace much that never yet has entered into a medical curriculum."

"LIFE CAPITAL."

In reviewing the tables of statistics in the annual report of Mr. Shirley Murphy, Medical Officer of Health to the county of London, *The Hospital,* in reference to the death-rate says: "If other things were to remain the same it is obvious that the ratio of the deaths to the population in any community ought to give a fair basis on which to judge of its healthiness and to estimate the average prospects of life offered to every infant born to it. No sooner, however, do we penetrate below the mere surface of things than we find that a multitude of circumstances besides mere healthiness influence the mortality in a district, and that the most erroneous conclusions may be arrived at by a casual comparison of crude death-rates. The point to which we would just now specially direct attention is one which is insisted on by Mr. Shirley Murphy in regard to what he speaks of as 'life capital,' namely, that death-rates tell us little unless we know the sort of people who die, and that in estimating the influence of any variation of its death-rate upon a community we must not merely count the number of the dead, but must carefully consider what prospects of life they would have had if disease or accident had not carried them off, so that we may estimate the loss of 'life capital' to the community involved by their decease. Putting the matter in that peculiarly impersonal manner which statisticians love, it is clear that a very considerable increase in the number of deaths among those whose life's work is done—say those between seventy and eighty years of age—might not only be no loss, but might even be an actual gain to a community by relieving it of the burden of supporting so many non-producers. The death of a child, however—a child which has within it a potentiality of many years of active productive life—is quite another affair; while the death of a young person who has weathered all the accidents of childhood, and is just beginning to repay the trouble spent in rearing and education, is a dead loss from an economic point of view. If, then, we are in any way to understand the bearing of any variation in the death-rate upon the prosperity of a community we must express our losses, not in numbers of deaths, but in quantity of 'life capital' destroyed.

"What Mr. Shirley Murphy has done is, first of all, to construct a 'life table' for London from the accumulated statistics collected during the ten years 1881-90. In this table the whole population is divided into twelve age-groups, and the mean future life—in other words, the prospect of life—is calculated for each age-group, and this is done for males and females separately; a matter of some importance, seeing that the females all through have a prospect of longer life than the males of the same age-group. Having, then, got his 'life table' he has sorted out all the deaths in London according to sex and age, and for each year since 1891, and applying the 'table' to each group, he has been able to show how far we are gaining or losing, improving upon or falling back from what we may call the 'standard' of 1881-90, and to express this not merely in number of lives, but in number of years of 'life capital' saved or lost in comparison with the standard.

"From this it appears that the year 1897 was the healthiest year of those under consideration, the number of lives saved, as compared with the standard, being 10,336, while the amount of years of 'life capital' saved was 367,815. Since then we have gone back considerably, the lives gained in the year 1899 being only 3,568, while the 'life capital' gained was but 264,297. Now here comes an interesting thing, and a thing which shows the importance of working out the statistics in a careful manner. At first sight a drop from ten thousand to three thousand in the number of lives gained appears a frightful fall; but on examination it appears that the year 1899 was almost as good as the year 1897, both in regard to lives saved and 'life capital' saved among people under twenty-five years of age. Almost the whole loss occurred in the older people, commencing in men at the group over thirty-five and in women at the group over forty-five.

"Now, if we turn to particular diseases, we find that the death-rates for the different years are divided into those for people below and above twenty-five years of age; but the life table has not been applied to the individual diseases. Nevertheless, we find some interesting facts. There are certain diseases in regard to which we were distinctly worse off in 1899 than in the 'standard' period; for instance, diphtheria, diarrhea, cancer, and influenza. The whole of the increased loss of life from diphtheria fell upon the young; there is no difference at all among those above twenty-five. With diarrhea, again, not only does all the increase fall upon the young, but even more, for among those above twenty-five years of age there is an actual improvement, all of which is neutralized by the increased mortality from this disease among the young. Thus we have in diphtheria and diarrhea, two diseases against which we must place a very heavy loss of 'life capital,' for they kill those who have their whole working life before them. In regard to cancer the boot is on the other leg. Both in old and young cancer has increased; but the increase is twenty-five times as great in the older group as it is in the younger, so that the drain of this disease, great as it is upon 'lives,' is not so great upon 'life capital.' "

THE GERMICIDAL AND DEODO-RANT PROPERTIES OF EUFOR-MOL.

By Thos. Maben, F.C.S., Glasgow,

Glasgow, Scotland.

A PERFECT disinfectant must possess several attributes; in particular, it must be both germicidal and deodorant, that is to say it must not only kill the bacteria that cause disease and propagate it, and in this way act the part of an antiseptic, but it should also deodorize any foul smells that may arise from decomposing or fecal matter. There are many germicides that are not deodorants, there are some deodorants that have little or no value as germicides; and there are some so-called disinfectants that are neither the one nor the other, for they do not kill bacteria nor do they deodorize, they simply create a new odor, which may or may not cover the smell it is intended to displace. If, therefore, a preparation can be brought forward that is germicidal and deodorant, and that, in addition, possesses a grateful and refreshing odor of its own, while being in the ordinary sense of the term non-poisonous, then we may claim that we have here the ideal disinfectant.

Just such a preparation is found in Euformal, a liquid composed of substances every one of which possesses, more or less, valuable antiseptic properties. The basis is a five-per-cent. solution of formic aldehyde, with which are combined eucalyptus oil, oil of wintergreen, menthol, thymol, boric acid and fluid extract of wild indigo, a combination the value of which is by no means so well known as it ought to be.

The use of formaldehyde is comparatively limited considering its value as an all-round disinfectant. It is much in demand for general hospital and sanitary purposes, but it has never taken its proper place in the sick-room for reasons presently to be explained. The virtue of formaldehyde lies in the fact that while it is a powerful germicide it has also the property of forming new chemical compounds with those gases that cause unpleasant smells; the compounds formed being perfectly inodorous. Further, this result is obtained without introducing any new odor, the substance in itself being practically without smell. This remarkable property is explained by the chemical constitution of the gas, formic aldehyde being an unsaturated compound, which greedily takes up sulphur and nitrogen, and thus destroys the unpleasant odor produced by those bodies that evolve sulphuretted hydrogen and other foul-smelling gases. It may, therefore, seem to be surprising that formaldehyde has not been accorded a prominent position as a bedside disinfectant, but the reason is not far to seek. Hitherto it has usually been recommended in the literature on the subject to use formalin or formaldehyde in the state of gas, and special apparatus is recommended for vaporizing the solution, or for subliming the tablets supplied for the purpose. It is, however, a well-known fact, and one that has been impressed on medical men by painful experience, that the vapor of formaldehyde has a decidedly irritating effect on mucous membranes, whether of the eyes, nose, or throat, and consequently its use in that form has been found to be inadmissible in the sick-room. It is true that the quantity vaporized can be limited, but no matter what the amount may be of gas that is formed the process of gaseous diffusion ensures that the air of the apartment immediately becomes uniform in composition, and thus the irritating effect of even a very small proportion of vapor is at once felt by the patient. Formaldehyde has also been recommended in throat and bronchial effections and in hay fever, but the results of its use have usually been so very unpleasant that many medical men who have tried it have been compelled to give it up altogether. It has thus fallen into disrepute in certain directions, a disrepute which is undeserved, but which, nevertheless, is not at all surprising in view of the facts just stated.

The other ingredients in Euformol all possess, in greater or less degree, antiseptic properties, and in addition most of them have fragrant odors. Euformol, therefore, not only possesses the wonderful germicidal and deodorizing properties of formaldehyde, but it naturally carries with it a refreshing and invigorating odor such as cannot be obtained from the use of that agent alone. Consequently it should prove of inestimable value, provided pracautions are taken to guard against the objections just spoken of. In order to obtain the best results in the sick-room, with no discomfort to the patient, the Euformol should be diluted with ten times its bulk of water, and the mixture sprayed by means of a fine atomizer, several times a day, for one or two minutes each time, care being taken to direct the spray away from the bed. The result will be to instantly purify the atmosphere, clearing it effectually of all germs and bad smells and replacing these by the delightfully refreshing odors of the volatile oils. In this way no unpleasant or irritating effect is experienced, while the change from a stuffy, malodorous apartment to pure, sweet, fresh air, for that is what actually takes place, is inexpressibly grateful both to the invalid and the nurse. The spray is sufficient to deodorize the atmosphere, while the liquid does not vaporize so readily as to cause any annoyance, the maximum of benefit being thus secured with no discomfort at all to any one. Used in this way, Euformol is a very inexpensive preparation, although the apparent first cost is higher than that of some much less active disinfectants.

As a deodorizer of enteric and bad-smelling feces nothing can approach Euformol in value. The best way to use it for this purpose is to pour a teaspoonful or so into the empty bed-pan and leave it there. The liquid vaporizes to a small extent, the vapor filling the pan, with the result that when the latter is used the smell, no matter how offensive, is at once completely destroyed. Euformol is also of inestimable value in the pathological laboratory, and in every case where putrid odors arise from decomposing animal or vegetable matter. Undiluted Euformol, sprayed freely over a cadaver, effectually prevents any smell arising no matter what the disease has been, and the

preparation is thus, in such cases, indispensable. As a preventive of perspiration of the feet, and as a deodorant when this condition becomes offensive, nothing better can be used. It is also invaluable for cleansing the surgeon's hands and for the disinfection of surgical instruments, for which purposes it should be used diulted with about four volumes of water, thus giving a solution containing about one per cent. of formaldehyde. Although the tendency is to slightly harden the tissues, this strength has practically no influence on the cuticle, and as the preparation is quite harmless so far as metals are concerned surgical instruments are not affected by it.

In view, therefore, of its excellencies in all these directions, and also of the fact that it is non-poisonous, we are justified in regarding Euformol as an excellent disinfectant.

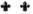

BAKING ALIVE.

"Baking alive is the latest thing in American medical science," says the London *Health*. "Three large human bakeries," continues *Health*, "are in operation in the United States, one in Chicago, Philadelphia and New York respectively, and the popularity of the new treatment is growing daily. Many doctors of note are prescribing 'baking' instead of medicine for certain forms of disease.

"The application of hot air as a therapeutic agent is an old idea. In fact, it is a very old one. All that is claimed by the modern bakers of persons is the manner in which the heat is applied, and the very high degrees which can be stood—the baking of persons up to 400° F., which is 188° above the boiling point of water, being quite possible without danger to the human system.

"When the heat is first turned on," says *Popular Science*, "the patient experiences no sensations other than mild warmth. A trained nurse is in constant attendance during the baking process, and the temperature, respiration, and so forth, are carefully watched. Up to about 150° F. little inconvenience is felt. Then the patient becomes thirsty. Sips of water are given from time to time.

"The giving of water is thought to add somewhat to the efficacy of the treatment through the gentle reaction which it induces. When 180° have been registered in the central cylinder—the degrees being indicated on a long thermometer—the patient feels thousands of tiny streams of heat impinging against his body. These streams are pouring through the perforations in the circulating jacket. The lower extremities now become somewhat numb, and the feet feel as if, to use a common expression, they had 'gone to sleep.' One seems now to be literally swimming in perspiration. This is given off from the top of the machine in the form of steam, which comes out through the funnels in a continuous stream.

"At 200° one experiences a dreamy sensation, and from this point up to 280° the baking experience is really quite pleasant. Water boils at 212° F., and yet at 280° F. a human being does not suffer the least inconvenience. It is endured for upwards of an hour. In certain cases, however, much higher temperatures are required. In some conditions from 350° to 400° F. are necessary. Heat at these high degrees is not so very pleasant. The body seems to be literally roasting. The blood at 150° seems actually to be boiling, and can be felt to be coursing through the veins at racehorse speed. The heart thumps wildly, or else seems to have disappeared altogether.

"Bags of ice are constantly applied to the head when these degrees of heat are administered. Sips of ice-water are given from time to time. A very remarkable fact in connection with the baking is that at times the temperature of one's body is actually raised five or six degrees. In cases of fever this is considered a decided advantage, as it brings on the crisis, and the reaction sets in much more rapidly than it otherwise would. After the baking the patient feels weak. He is then rubbed, and made to rest until com-

pletely restored to normal condition. A two-thirds' rest makes one feel as if he had enjoyed a pleasant, dreamless sleep. On going out into the air a species of exhilaration is experienced, and one seems better fixed for mental and physical exertion than he was before the baking.

"The principal forms of disease in which hot dry air is used are: Gout, inflammation, rheumatism, lithæmia, obesity, œdema, and all forms of pain—congestive, neuralgic, and even psychic. Some very remarkable cures have been reported among the 3000 persons who have already been baked in America. Persons have been able to walk after years of affliction with deforming rheumatism, and in certain cases chronic forms of disease have been cured."

SANITATION AND THE MOTORISTS.

Sanitation, and particularly street sanitation, is receiving a great deal of attention at this time in all the cities and large towns throughout the civilized world. "If, as we believe to be the case, the motor car has a great future before it, the whole question of the pavement of our streets," says *The Hospital*, "will have to be reconsidered. Regard for the horse has hitherto dominated the whole question of roadways. Obviously the smoother and the harder the surface of a road the less will be the power required to move wheeled vehicles upon it. But unfortunately the harder and smoother the surface of the road the more difficult it is for the horse to obtain a foothold. Hence the objections so often raised to the use of asphalt, notwithstanding that it is in itself an almost ideal material from which to construct road surfaces. It is hard, it is smooth, it is durable, it is capable of being repaired, bit by bit, without tearing up the whole roadway, and, above all, it can be kept clean. But the horses slip, and this has been a fatal obstacle. With the introduction of the motor, however, the conditions may be altered, and if we consider the immense advantages which asphalt possesses from a sanitary point of view and the economy in motive power which must result from its smoothness, we may be quite sure that in proportion as the horse becomes non-essential the use of asphalt, or some similar smooth and cleanly road surface, will come more and more into vogue in all towns where the gradients allow of its employment. It is the sanitary aspect of asphalt pavement which especially appeals to us. So far it seems to be the only form of road surface which is capable of being kept decently clean, and this is a matter of the first importance. It is not a mere question of taste and esthetics. If we are to accept the conclusions arrived at by Dr. Waldo, medical officer of health to the parish of St. George the Martyr—conclusions arrived at after very careful investigation of the facts —a very considerable proportion of the mortality from diarrhea one of the most fatal of diseases among town children, is due to the pollution of milk and other articles of food with street dust, in other words, with dried horse dung highly charged with deleterious micro-organisms. Filthy street dust we must always have with us, unless we have streets that we can wash. It is probably to the facility with which asphalt can be washed that we must look for the explanation of the largely diminished death-rates which have been noted in certain towns after the introduction of this material as a paving. It is claimed that in New York the death-rate has gone down from 38.37 per 1,000, to 1892, to 26 per 1,000 in 1896, when the cleaner streets, due to the large extension of asphalt pavement, had begun to show their influence upon the health of the population; and although we can hardly doubt that the introduction was, in this case, only one item in a general improvement in sanitary conditions, the benefits which have already resulted in London, in Paris, and in many other large towns, from the use of asphalt in courts and alleys has been such as to show how great would be the advantage of its more extended use. Not until all our streets are provided with a hard, smooth surface, which can be thoroughly cleansed, shall we even begin to see what town life might be made. It is to the motor car that we must look to bring this much-needed reform within the range of practical politics."

DIRECTIONS TO CONSUMPTIVES.

Dr. DUKEMAN states in the *Medical News* that he gives the following advice to patients suffering from pulmonary tuberculosis:

" 1. You must live in the country, and there make every effort to try to get well.

" 2. A patient who tries to get well has ten times as many chances of getting well as the one who is careless and indifferent.

" 3. You must avoid worry, anxiety, and excitement.

" 4. Be hopeful and cheerful, for your disease can be cured if you will but do your duty in strictly following the advice here given.

" 5. As a rule do not leave the house during the winter months until one hour after sunrise. Live out of doors all day. Remain indoors only on rainy and very windy days. Remain in the sunshine as much as possible, and the greater part of the time recline on a couch or in a hammock in a comfortable position. Protect your head from the sun's rays, the rest of the body lying bathed in the warm rays of the sun.

" 6. Always breathe through the nose and take your breathing exercises regularly, as I have instructed you.

" 7. Avoid dust as you would rain and dampness, and all places where the air is bad, such as theatres, concert halls, or any crowded meeting-place or lodging-houses.

" 8. Take your walking exercises regularly as prescribed, but never walk when you are tired or when you have a high fever (temperature 100° F. or over).

" 9. Dress neatly. Be clean and comfortable, but never wear a chest protector, as they are injurious; wear woolen undergarments as well as woolen socks, and thick-soled shoes to keep your feet warm and dry.

" 10. Never stay or sleep in an overheated room. In this climate, however, in the mornings and evenings during the winter months, you should have a small fire to keep your sitting-room comfortably warm, at about 65° to 68° F. Do not heat your room with an oil stove.

" 11. Never use your sleeping room as a sitting-room. Keep all the windows open in your sleeping room all day long, and one window open all night. On cold evenings close the windows a little before sundown, and then when you go to bed open one window, for you must have fresh air while you sleep. Fresh night air is as good for you while you sleep as is day air while you are awake.

" 12. Retire every night before nine o'clock. Have at least nine hours sleep; when thoroughly rested, get up any time after 7 A. M.

" 13. Never expectorate in any place where it can dry. Indoors always expectorate in a spittoon which is partially filled with water containing some anti-septic solution, such as carbolic acid (teaspoonful to pint of water) or some other antiseptic. When you cannot conveniently get to the spittoon, use your pocket-flask. Never swallow your expectoration. Never expectorate in your handkerchief, nor use the same handkerchief to wipe your nose which you have used to wipe your mouth. Always cover your mouth with your handkerchief while coughing or sneezing. Never cough while at the dining-table; by a little effort you can suppress the cough.

" 14. Never kiss any one, for your disease is infectious.

" 15. Keep your teeth clean by brushing them after each meal, and use your mouth and nose-wash night and morning, as advised.

" 16. Take a warm bath twice a week, to be followed by a rapid sponging with cooler water and a vigorous rubbing with a rough towel. If you are too weak to do the

latter, and you do not have an attendant, rub your entire body with alcohol.

" 17. Never use tobacco in any form. Never use any alcoholic beverages without the special directions of your physician.

" 18. Coax your appetite with a varied nutritious diet as per diet-list given, and eat all you possibly can. A good nutritious diet, plenty of fresh air and sunshine are the best medicines.

" 19. Should there be any intercurrent symptoms, such as indigestion, diarrhea, constipation, restless nights, increased cough, pain, blood-streaked expectoration, do not be alarmed, but notify your physician without delay.

" 20. By carefully following the above instructions, as well as the advice given you at the office, the chances of your getting well are greatly in your favor."

Dr. Dukeman has but little faith in drugs in the treatment of this disease; he has tried them all and found them wanting. His main hopes are to induce patients to go live in the country and eat plenty of easily digestible, nutritive food, especially milk, eggs and beef. One patient who ate as many as ten or twelve eggs daily for months recovered without any medicine other than a digestive mixture. He insists on patients living an easy, regular life in the open air and sunshine. In fact, if he can impress them with the absolute necessity of giving up everything else and employing themselves in taking every precaution against negligence, using every effort in trying to get well, improvement generally follows.

THE CURE OF CORNS ON THE SOLE OF THE FOOT.

ELLIS, of Gloucester, writes to the *British Medical Journal*, vol. ii, 1900, *Therapeutic Gazette*, that if the patient will give the toes free play by adopting boots and socks having a straight inside line, avoid the conventional eversion of the foot, and acquire the habit of pressing the toes against the ground in every step, the callosities will disappear. They are due to defective function of the toes. Removal may, of course, be hastened by the use of solvents, such as a mixture of salicylic acid and collodion.

Another correspondent writes that he has found that corns on the sole of the foot rarely resist the following treatment: A piece of salicylic and creosote plaster muslin, as suggested by Unna, is cut rather larger than the corn and applied to it. This is removed each or every alternate day. As much of the corn as is then removable is ground off with pumice stone, and another piece of the plaster muslin applied, and so on until tne part is normal. He uses the muslin plaster containing acid salicylic 20 per cent., creosote 40 per cent., and has found that it is more comfortable to wear if it is "backed" with one or two thicknesses of ordinary plaster. Of course a properly fitting boot with a sufficiently thick sole is a *sine qua non*.

Still another writer suggests that the best relief he found was to take a piece of moderately thick leather, circular, about two inches in diameter, and cut a small hole—size of corn—in the middle. There is no need of fastening the leather to the foot; he found it retained its position on fixing it in place after putting on the sock.

Finally the following treatment is suggested: Soak a piece of lint or cotton-wool the size of the corn with acetic acid (forming in fact a compress), to be well covered with a piece of gutta-percha sheeting; bandage lightly. Do this for three consecutive nights.

THE EFFECT OF COLD UPON THE MIND.

Extreme cold, as is well known, exerts a benumbing influence upon the mental faculties. Almost every one who has been exposed for a longer or shorter period to a very low temperature has noted a diminution in will power, and often temporary weakening of the memory. Perhaps the largest

scale upon which this action has ever been studied, says London *Health*, was during the retreat of the French from Moscow. The troops suffered extremely from hunger, fatigue and cold—from the latter, perhaps, most of all. A German physician who accompanied a detachment of his countrymen has left an interesting account of their trials during this retreat.

From an abstract of this paper by Dr. Rose in the *Medicinische Monatschrift*, we find that the earliest symptom referable to the cold was a loss of memory. This was noted in the strong as well as those who were already suffering from the effects of the hardships to which they had been exposed. With the first appearance of a moderately low temperature (about 5 degrees below zero F.) many of the soldiers were found to have forgotten the names of the most ordinary things about them, as well as those of the articles of food for which they were perishing. Many forgot their own names and those of their comrades. Others showed pronounced symptoms of mental disturbance, and not a few became incurably insane, the type of their insanity resembling very closely senile dementia. The cold was probably not alone responsible for these effects, for a zero temperature is rather stimulating than paralyzing in its action upon the well-fed and the healthy. These men were half-starved, poorly clad, worn out with long marching, many already weakened by dysentery and other diseases, and all mentally depressed, as an army in defeat always is. It needed, therefore, no very unusual degree of cold to produce the psychic effects observed under other circumstances only as a consequence of exposure to an extremely low temperature.

THE PROPHYLAXIS OF GASTRIC ULCER.

While the etiology, pathology and treatment of gastric ulcer have been the subject of extended discussion, very little has been written, says the *Medical Times,* about the prophylaxis of this affection. Ulcers with the characteristics of the conical ulcers that occur commonly in the stomach are found in but two other parts of the digestive tract, in the duodenum and in the lower end of the esophagus. As these parts, like the stomach, are frequently bathed in gastric juice, it is evident that some change in this fluid is the underlying cause of this type of ulcer. The comparative rarity of gastric ulcer shows that this change in the gastric secretion is only the predisposing cause. There must be an immediate cause for the production of the ulcer. These immediate causes can be guarded against.

There are two general conditions in which gastric ulcers are especially prone to develop—anemic and subseptic states, by which latter state is meant a condition in which, owing to the presence of a purulent focus somewhere in the body, septic material finds its way in small amounts into the circulation. It is important at such periods that patients should be warned of the danger of the development of gastric ulcer and given precise directions how to avoid the local irritation that must concur with the underlying condition for the production of the ulcer. Young anemic girls are prone to be lovers of candy and small, sharp pieces are sometimes swallowed. A taste for spices and for pickles so frequent during anemic conditions leads to the ingestion of acids and local irritants that are liable to injure the gastric mucous membrane in its state of lowered vitality. Cooks are especially apt to take superheated food, but all young women patients must be warned of the danger from this source. Seamstresses often lean for hours with some portion of a vibrating sewing-machine touching their epigastrium. Anemic governesses as school teachers lean against desks, which, when the stomach contains food, may prove a sufficient cause to locally depress the already sluggish circulation in the stomach walls. All of these patients must be told of the absolute necessity of never swallowing coarse or insufficiently masticated food.

Bread crusts should be removed or chewed very thoroughly. Raw apples and other uncooked fruit or vegetables, even celery, should be chewed very carefully before swallowing, or avoided entirely. At no time should the patient be allowed to take a large meal.

Fatal perforation in cases of latent gastric ulcer occurs particularly in patients, who, having missed a meal for some reason, eat with more than ordinary heartiness at the next one. In general, the advice should be given to eat five or six times during the day rather than to limit the eating to ordinary meal times with the danger of mechanically injuring the stomach.

⁘ ⁘

PARTHENOGENERATED MAN.— CHICAGO UNIVERSITY PROFESSOR THINKS HE IS A POSSIBILITY IN A FUTURE GENERATION.

CHICAGO, Sept. 26.—Artificial reproduction of human beings is possible, according to scientists who have followed the work of Dr. Jacques Loeb, of the University of Chicago. They are of the opinion that, theoretically, artificial parthenogenesis of human beings is as possible as the artificial reproduction of starfish and worms accomplished at Wood's Hole, Mass., by Dr. Loeb, last summer. But they say the difficulties of the method are so great that the accomplishment may have to be left to scientists of future generations. This opinion was brought to the university yesterday by Dr. Frank R. Lillie, who arrived from Wood's Hole to take up the work of the new position as associate professor of zoology. Dr. Lillie has intimate knowledge of Dr. Loeb's work. He said:

"This summer at Wood's Hole laboratory, Dr. Loeb extended his work to new groups of life. The work is artificial parthenogenesis, that is, reproduction without fertilization. Before this he had confined his work to sea urchins; this year it was extended to starfish and also to worms, an entirely different group. He developed starfish and worms from unfertilized eggs. There is no reason to doubt that the same principles apply to all of the other animals, including man. But we have not any inkling of the method of accomplishing artificial parthenogenesis of vertebrates. The discovery of such practical method may be reserved for investigators of other generations.—*New York Sun.*

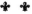

THE PRESERVATION OF THE TEETH OF SCHOOL CHILDREN.

RULES recommended by the School Children's Committee of the British Dental Association, and circulated for the information of managers and teachers of national schools in Ireland:

"Without good teeth there cannot be good mastication.

"Without thorough mastication there cannot be perfect digestion, and poor health results.

"Hence the paramount importance of sound teeth.

"Clean teeth do not decay.

"The importance of a sound first set of teeth is as great to the child as a sound second set is to the adult.

"Children should be taught to use the tooth brush early.

"Food left on the teeth ferments, and the acid formed produces decay.

"Decay leads in time to pain and the total destruction of the tooth.

"The substance of the following rules should therefore be impressed constantly upon all children:

"1. The teeth should be cleansed at least once daily.

"2. The best time to clean the teeth is after the last meal.

"3. A small tooth brush, with stiff bristles, should be used, brushing up and down and across, and inside and outside and in between the teeth.

"4. A simple tooth powder, or a little soap, and some precipitated chalk taken

upon the brush may be used if the teeth are dirty or stained.

"5. It is a good practice to rinse the mouth out after every meal.

"6. All rough usage of the teeth, such as cracking nuts, biting thread, etc., should be avoided, but the proper use of the teeth in chewing is good for them.

"When decay occurs it should be attended to long before any pain results. It is stopping of a small cavity that is of the greatest service.

"In 10,000 children's mouths examined eighty-six in every 100 required skilled operative treatment."—*Journal of the British Dental Association.*

HOW NATURE CURES.

AN eminent nerve specialist has lately explained how and why it is that tired persons find in the parks and in the country, unconsciously to themselves, the rest that restores their worn and weary nerves. The scientific theory, stated in plain language, is that a change from the office or shop or noisy street to the calmness and beauty of Nature actually switches the nerve currents to new lines of sensation, just as "central" at a telephone switchboard opens a line of communication, unseen to the caller, when the bell rings. In this entire change of thought and of sensation lies the medicine that ministers to a nerve diseased.

It seems entirely reasonable that the over-strained nerves of concentration, for example, are relaxed and therefore rested when thought is suspended or diffused in a sort of miscellaneous enjoyment of the delights of the park or the fields. The frayed nerves of worry and perplexity and annoyance must get a respite when one is listening to the song of a robin or to the soft sighing of the wind through the pine branches. To start the currents on the nerves that convey to the mind impressions of pleasure—of the calm and peace and ineffable content of nature—is "treatment" that is none the less effective because it costs nothing and you are not thinking about it.

Indeed, the nature cure is better than the faith cure in this, that you don't have to exercise your faculties or your faith to receive its benefits.

THE MORTALITY AND MORBIDITY OF PHYSICIANS.

ALFRED MOEGLICH has collected a series of statistics which give results sufficiently discouraging to the medical practitioner who aspires to reach the scriptural age of threescore and ten. Of all the professions, medicine offers its devotees the least promise of a ripe old age; the average time of death varying from fifty-two to fifty-six years, according to different authorities; while for the clergy, for example, it is ten years later. The combination of pedagogy with medicine appears to be particularly fatal, for one set of figures in which the normal death-rate is represented by 100 gives 111 as the factor for physicians, and 113.8 for medical instructors. Of the causes of death infectious diseases rank highest and, among these, typhoid fever occupies so prominent a place as almost to entitle it to characterization as an occupation disease. Tuberculosis comes next, the death-rate from this cause among physicians being almost double that of the clergy. Altogether it is rather a melancholy fact to realize that the men whose life work it is to teach others how to keep their health, or to regain it if lost, should themselves be unable to profit by their own knowledge and should be so completely at the mercy of the great bodily and mental stress to which their calling subjects them.—*Deutsche Aerzte-Zeitung,* November 15, 1900.

THE SWEAT OF PHTHISICAL PATIENTS.

DE RENZI and G. Boeri reported at the Congress on Tuberculosis recently held in Naples, that they have made researches on this subject, taking as their starting-point an investigation by Sather, in which it was shown that the sweat of phthisical patients contains tuberculin amongst the other toxic substances, and has, therefore, a curative action by eliminating notable quantities of toxins. From their own researches the authors have come to the conclusion that the sweat of consumptives differs from that of healthy persons only in being more toxic; it does not, however, produce a form of poisoning materially different. The sweat of consumptives, like that of healthy persons, produces a febrile reaction in tuberculous guinea-pigs; but if the dose injected is excessive it causes collapse and death. They hold that the febrile reaction is not attributable to tuberculin, because it is not peculiar to the sweat of tuberculous subjects, and because in a less degree it shows itself even in non-tuberculous guinea-pigs. The greater degree of pyrexia set up in diseased than in healthy guinea-pigs is to be attributed to the greater readiness with which tuberculous guinea-pigs become febrile from any cause. The pyrexia is not attributable to infection by micro-organisms in the sweat, since it persists after sterilization. It is due to the chemical principles of sweat, even that of healthy persons, as to which principles the authors at present can only say that they resist heat. Nevertheless, they believe that within certain limits the sweating of consumptives, when it is not very profuse, is more or less curative, as may be gathered from its marked toxicity. —*Lancet.*

FELKIN and Emin Pasha state that castor-oil plants about a house, and especially at the doors, are a protection against mosquitoes and malaria.

THE MEDICINAL VALUE OF HONEY.

Honey has more value as a medicinal agent than most people think. It is composed chiefly of sugar and water, but also contains volatile oils derived from the flowers, also gum and wax. Many children who will not take medicine except under great pressure, will willingly eat honey, which acts, when taken alone, as a laxative. A gargle composed of sugar and water is good for sore throats. It is also often used to disguise the taste of other medicines which are not pleasant.

THE "LAUGHING PLANT."

This plant grows in Arabia, and has been given its name, says *Health,* from the effects produced by eating its seeds. The plant is of moderate size, with bright yellow flowers, and soft, velvety seed-pods, each of which contains two or three seeds, resembling small, black beans. The natives of the district where the plant grows dry these seeds and reduce them to powder. A small dose of this powder has similar effects to those arising from the inhalation of laughing-gas. It causes the most sober person to dance, shout, and laugh with the boisterous excitement of a madman, and to rush about cutting the most ridiculous capers for about an hour. At the expiration of this time exhaustion sets in, and the excited person falls alseep, to wake after several hours with no recollection whatever of his antics.

Doctor—And you say you can't pay me?

Patient—That's right, doctor; you see, I spent all my money to buy that cook book for my wife.

"That's not right."

"Well, doctor, you shouldn't complain; if I hadn't bought the book I wouldn't have needed your services."—*Yonkers Statesman.*

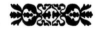

Department of Physical Education.

WITH SPECIAL REGARD TO THE SYMMETRICAL DEVELOPMENT OF THE BODY.

THE DREAD OF OLD AGE.

"I DON'T want to live to be too old," is a common remark, says Dr. C. E. Page in *Health Culture.* " The reason for this," he adds, " is that old age is apt to be associated with decrepitude, pain and all manner of physical inconveniences. But in one sense, and a very important one at that, old age is simply a question of health. A feeble and effeminate dyspeptic, often ill and likely to be snuffed out before forty, is an older man than the octogenarian who has lived in a way to keep supple, strong, free from ailments, and altogether in the swim, mentally and bodily. The latter is, so to say, eighty years young, while the other is forty years old, and really too old for anything.

" All-around physical training and rational living habits as to clothing, diet, etc., will secure to most persons a clean, sound, delightful life to the end. William Cullen Bryant probably got as much pleasure out of life as any one could desire, and his life was a most busy and useful one up to the age of eighty-four, when he died in a natural and comfortable manner, like the snuffing out of a candle. He was never ill, he enjoyed his food, exercise was a pleasure, as it is bound to be to every one of us who keeps in training, and he kept young in feeling and socially in the fashion to the last, and all this without doing penance in any shape. His habits were exceptionally wise. Here they are in brief: He rose early, took the air bath that I have practised and taught for a good many years, with light all-around exercises, free arm work, chair swinging. etc., for an hour or less; then a quick sponge bath and good towelling. A light breakfast of fruit and bread, after which a little time was spent with his stud-

ies, and then he walked to the office of the *Evening Post,* nearly three miles, and after performing his duties there walked back, " whatever be the weather or the state of the streets," to quote his own words. He used neither tea, coffee, tobacco nor spirits in any form, beyond the rarest exception of a glass of wine. In town, where he dined at six or later, he took but two meals a day. His diet was simple—fruit, vegetables, whole meal bread, with but a modicum of fish, flesh or fowl. " I abominate all drugs and narcotics," he said, " and have always avoided everything which spurs nature to exertions which it would not otherwise make. Even with my food I do not take the usual condiments, such as pepper and the like." Another characteristic of Mr. Bryant, relating to his penchant for physical training—he never took the elevator to his high-up office, but climbed the stairs as the next best thing to hill climbing."

" The entire muscular system requires exercise, and we know that a horse travels with less fatigue any given distance when he has some up and down hill work to do, than over a dead level course. The level working muscles, so to say, are resting while the uphill ones are working, and vice versa. To a person tired from over resting exercise is in the highest degree restful. The everlasting loafer and sitter has a tired feeling all the time, which can only be driven away by gradually working up in his activities. It has often been observed that the first mile in a walk is done with considerable effort, when the second is done with less, and the third with still less inconvenience, and even with ease."

In short, one of the best means of

reaching old age gracefully and happily, finally to die easily and contentedly, is to continue to exercise, within the limit of one's strength, to the end. The contrary opinion notwithstanding, man is never so old but what judicious exercise, short of fatigue, will benefit by helping to eliminate the effete, worn-out products of the body. Old people frequently hasten death by self poisoning. We remember hearing an elderly man during his last illness remark, "I would not die had I have not quit work.'"

PHYSICAL CULTURE.

However it has come about, whether through the increasing devotion to athletics or for other reasons, says the editor of the *Boston Med. and Surg. Journ.*, it is clear that physical culture in the broad sense is occupying a more and more conspicuous place in education. This must certainly be regarded as an unqualified good, and chiefly because it is based on a system which may justly lay claim to a scientific basis. Physical training is gradually but surely becoming rational; the excesses to which competitive athletic events are always likely to lead will surely be modified by a knowledge of the physiological effects of training. Both directly and indirectly the present zeal for physical culture, designed not only to make the strong stronger, but also the weak strong, is doing much toward the general development of the masses of young men and women. Institutions have, however, been slow in completely recognizing the dignity of this branch of education by establishing a definite department under the jurisdiction of a competent head. It is, therefore, of particular interest at this time that the Massachusetts Institute of Technology has taken action to install a new department devoted to physical culture. The formal announcement of this fact was made by President Pritchett at the annual dinner of the Alumni Association recently held in Boston. It was announced that the corpor-

ation had voted to give the land for the building, which is to be a memorial to the late General Walker, former president of the Institute. In this building is to be established the new department, provided the necessary endowment fund can be raised, under the charge of "a man who shall be able to do for the physical side of the students what the heads of other departments now do for the intellectual side." It is sincerely to be hoped, and there is small doubt that the hope will be realized, that this somewhat unique department of a great educational institution may be generously maintained. It will prove not only of service to the institution with which it is connected, but will undoubtedly serve as a stimulus toward the establishment of similar departments elsewhere. The time is undoubtedly ripe for just this line of work, and we are gratified to see that so worthy a memorial is to be erected to the lamented president of our most conspicuous technical school.

The tendency everywhere apparent is further shown by the recent meeting in New York of the various physical directors of the larger gymnasiums connected with our schools and colleges. The strength which comes from organization will no doubt show itself by renewed and systematic attempts toward raising the standard of this department of school and university work. The very general introduction of physical training into the public schools has already been productive of much benefit to the pupils. The idea, recently suggested for the Brookline, Mass., schools of giving special treatment to pupils of imperfect physique, is also unquestionably a step in the right direction. The whole movement toward bringing about a symmetrical physical development, beginning with the very young, is in every way commendable.

In the hands of competent men there is small danger of attaching undue importance to this fundamental branch of a child's education.

CLINICAL EXCERPT.

From the Notebook of Dr. H. B. Boice, Trenton, N. J.

Student, male, age twenty. Father living, mother dead of cancer. Subject most resembles mother. General health good; has had no serious diseases.

Injuries: Collar bone broken, sprained knee, deep cut in scalp.

He is finely built, medium height, 67.2 inches; weight, 140; skin clear; pulse 70 (strong). Upper chest expansion two and a half inches; at ninth rib, two and three-fourth inches. A year ago each of above measurements one inch less. There is marked mitral regurgitation, which did not appear a year ago. He has played football, basketball and baseball. His companions in these games speak of him as being a "stone wall" when they come up against him. In a match game of basketball, on the day before I examined him he played through the entire game "without once getting out of breath." He has never known what it was to be exhausted in any game.

It is little short of marvellous to me, knowing the conditions of extreme rib immobility and marked heart disease, that he should have not only come through the games he has in safety, but with a freedom in respiration surpassing any of his companions.

MASSAGE IN SKIN DISEASES.

Dr. Tibbles says massage in the treatment of skin diseases encourages the circulation, induces more active nutrition, and materially assists in the removal of diseased tissues, infiltrations and effusions by increasing molecular changes by means of mechanical stimulation. As usually performed, however, it is in many cases an unpleasant duty, and consequently seldom carried out so regularly or thoroughly as it ought to be. I have found that in a great many cases the massage can be sufficiently well performed by using an india-rubber roller instead of the hand, thus avoiding unpleasant contact with the skin. I have now recommended this method in skin cases for some time, and find it answers admirable. It is easy of application, and can be applied largely by the patient, though the back must be massaged by some other person. The roller I usually recommend is the ordinary roller used in photographic work, and there are others made which act equally well.

Another method of stimulating the skin in isolated patches is by the use of a blunted Volkmann's spoon or by a curette, both of which instruments I have used with benefit. This method, however, is best applied to the face and neck, and can only be performed by the surgeon. I have found it of great value in obstinate cases of acne and psoriasis and localized indurations.

A LIBERAL EDUCATION.

That man has had a liberal education who has been so trained in youth that his body is the ready servant of his will, and does with ease and pleasure all the work that, as a mechanism, it is capable of; whose intellect is a clear, cold, logic-engine, with all its parts of equal strength, and in smooth, working order, ready, like a steam engine, to be turned to any kind of work, and spin the gossamers as well as forge the anchors of the brain; whose mind is stored with the great and fundamental truths of nature and the laws of her operations; who, no stunted ascetic, is full of life and fire, but whose passions are trained to come to heel by a vigorous will, the servant of a tender conscience; who has learned to love all beauty, whether of nature or of art, to hate all vileness, and to respect others as himself.—*Huxley.*

VACATION SCHOOLS.*

THE vacation school movement originated in the desire of citizens to provide other influences than those of the streets for children living on the streets during July and August; popular observation, school reports, and statistics of juvenile arrests showing this interim in school occupation to be injurious mentally, morally, and physically. Other phases of this work are "fresh-air parties," and "country weeks," summer camps, and farms; also "summer playgrounds" that have developed into vacation schools as it became apparent that games have a strongly educative influence, and that the play spirit carried into certain forms of instruction increases the attractiveness of play-grounds.

Vacation schools (the play-ground continuing as a less highly organized and less expensive department of such schools) have within six years opened by private initiative in over twenty cities, in Newark, Philadelphia and New York being under municipal conduct—the final object of all effort elsewhere. They are for children under sixteen years of age, and continue six weeks in July and August, with only morning sessions. The attendance is voluntary; therefore, to be successful, their methods must be popular. The best results do not follow training "across the grain" after artificial methods. It is more than suspected that children in general, and the individual child, also, indicate lines of least resistance that educators should take advantage of as aids to fullest development. Play is the way of living of all young animals—their natural method of preparing for existence later. The majority of plays enjoyed by children require much hard work. Therefore the spirit of play (enjoyment), cunningly permeating vacation school curricula, secures as regular attendance and faithful work as do truant laws—work, however, of a different character.

---

* Author's abstract of paper given in the symposium on "The Medical Aspect of the Home" of the American Academy of Medicine, at its twenty-fifth annual Meeting, Atlantic City, N. J., June 2-4, 1900.

The design is to *supplement* public schools, and to give these children certain essential advantages that parents of intelligence and means supply by their own preference through home environment or travel. One chief present function of vacation schools that time is demonstrating is that of experiment stations, with a positive influence upon regular school methods and ideas. No books are used. The instruction is, briefly, according to the laboratory method.

To encourage muscular ability and accompanying executive qualities of mind (furnished by home environment one hundred years ago) manual training is prominent in the form of wood work, as carpentering, whittling, fret sawing, chip carving; or of household arts, as cooking, care of rooms and of the sick, sewing, mending, embroidery. The use of a score of different tools, of varieties of wood and other materials, is fascinating to practically all children, even when there exists a strong liking for books. Their natural creative instinct, the delight of seeing and owning the results of their labor, and enjoyment of occupations that permit free movement instead of exacting the quietness so irksome and unwholesome for them—all are utilized by the wise instructor for certain educational purposes.

Manual dexterity is as great an advantage to professional men, with its accompanying mental qualities, as is book learning to the so-called "industrial classes." Such manual training will promote home thriftiness and decencies, both within and without the house, where the ability to drive a nail and take a stitch, and the mental executive bias thus nourished in education—instead of neglected—counts for much in making homes. Such training, combined with regular school work, recognized in the schools on an equality with the latter, must encourage the hand skill our times are suffering from lack of, thus lessening the overcrowded ranks of inefficient teachers, clerks, etc., eventually giving us a higher grade of material achievement, a more comfortable living.

Of prime importance is the consideration

that there must result a higher class of citizen because of certain mental and moral qualities that manual work cultivates in children. They can only be enumerated here. They are intelligent observation, practical judgment, executive ability and habit, accuracy, perseverance, and the ambition to produce honest and creditable results. We must recognize the great social need of such qualities as these, conspicuously in the poorer homes and by "wage earners."

To city children nature study is partial compensation for the great misfortune that their childhood cannot be passed in the freedom, beauty and wholesome simplicity of country living. As the summer season dictates, this is the chief feature of vacation schools. Indoors flowers and other phenomena of the vegetable kingdom are studied from samples in the children's hands; aquaria, window boxes, pet animals, and museum specimens encourage habits of interested observation and powers of description. A school garden out of doors gives every child the supreme joy of trowelling, planting, watering, and watching developments under his own fostering care. The visiting insects and other animal life, weeds, varying conditions of soil and temperature, under educated oversight teach him the interdependence and harmony of natural laws.

This is knowledge at first hand, the most lasting kind. Acquaintance with vines, shrubs, and flowering plants for making home attractive encourages them to develop the possibilities of their own backyards and little corners of earth. School gardens in Germany, Russia, France, and Switzerland are numerous, and they are increasing in America. Educators begin to recognize not only the immediate value of this garden work for both bodies and minds; but the political and social expediency of early interesting boys and girls in productive occupation. In countries where agriculture is the basis of much of their prosperity, free schools properly should cultivate intelligent interest in this direction even in the mass of young children, with primary scientific instruction in more advanced grades,

that our public schools may recruit the farm as well as office and shop, and that the people may have at least the rudiments of a culture that nature evidently intended, but of which accidents of a short-sighted civilization threaten to deprive them.

Excursions take place every week—a very efficient drawing card utilized to its fullest pedagogic possibilities. These peripatetic schools or classes, with special instructors, visit city parks, museums, art galleries, industrial establishments, and points of local historic or scientific interest. The excursions most largely arranged for are into the country for nature study and sketching first, closing the event after lunch with free play and enjoyment. Although tens of thousands of children have been transported by boats and electric or steam cars, no accident to life or health has occurred. The numerous little groups into which the school is divided, each with a teacher, go to their several study grounds previously assigned; it may be a river path, a wood road, a field hedge or hillside, for their class work. "Bird day" is prepared for during the preceding week by handling and studying mounted specimens of birds native to that locality, learning their song and habits, and why this excursion must be in late afternoon hours and to a place of running water, trees, and underbrush. They taste the hunter's intensity of enjoyment in the stealthy approach and quiet waiting, and the child's irrepressible delight when the game is found. Sympathetic acquaintance with habits and beauties of living creatures we trust may eventually supplant the primitive slaying instinct of the race. In corresponding fashion they have "insect," "rock," "beach" and "flower" days, when the objects studied in the classroom are greeted in their habitat with the delight of welcoming old friends; or it may be a day to a well-equipped model farm.

To learn facts is not the only, nor perhaps the chief object of all this nature work. The child is inevitably forming tastes that will guide him in choice of recreations and of occupations (at least in his leisure time). That successful eight-hour-day agitation may be a benefit, it concerns us all to encourage those extra free hours being given to objects not less wholesome than the former labor. Interest in country phenomena, love of its sounds and sights, simple ability to make a yard and house attractive, cultivated in the childish brain, must often influence home-makers to choose suburban living in these days of cheap rapid transit and high city rents for cramped quarters. This movement, more fully developed in schools it is reasonable to believe will materially help to solve the tenement-house problem for many thousands and encourage the tide of population to ebb countrywards.

Art and nature study are correlated in these summer programmes. Accuracy of observation is increased by a water-color sketch. Foliage and fruit, mounted birds and butterflies, human models, and finally landscapes are given them to reproduce in color. Without seeing it, one can hardly believe how much a skillful teacher can accomplish with children from eight to fifteen years of age in brush, outline, and composition work and design, training them to see appreciatively. To cultivate memory, or imagination, and strengthen their understanding of language, a word picture may be read them for reproduction, of perhaps a moonrise on the ocean or of a harvest field; or a story is given them to illustrate. Decoration is introduced to them by applying their flower sketches to designs for book covers, wall papers, etc., or geometric figures may be used, with the final object of forming tastes. On excursions it means more than the present event to call attention to the ripples, cloud shadows and varied craft upon the water outlines against the horizon, views on roadways, and pictures made by groupings of trees and rocks, sunset glow, and noonday haze. To many children these are the only opportunities of their lives to pass a country day in the companionship of an educated, refined, and sympathetic friend. The novelty of the impression renders them most vivid and lasting. We can only mention the fact that music also is utilized for its æsthetic influences.

The advantages of outdoor gymnasia do not need demonstration. Imagine a wide-spreading American elm, with leafy shadows flitting over groups of children from hot city streets, who, under the guidance of an expert are keenly delighting in their achievements on bars, ladders and swings. This I saw in one of the very few schoolyards where the city fathers have preserved a beautiful tree. About the gymnastic games following the apparatus work I would say a word. It is almost appalling to think that the last stronghold of children—their play—is being invaded and utilized for pedagogic purposes. The truth is that play and playgrounds are being municipalized out of the world. With no opportunity but ill-smelling streets and prison-like yards, with policemen and ordinances coercing active play into chiefly a dodging out of sight and into even criminal mischief, from the repressed play hunger of growing boys and girls, it has come to pass that city children are forgetting how to play, and losing the vigor of body and character given by play. The recognition of this is behind the playground movement, and must not be forgotten as school boards take up vacation work. We believe thoughtful citizens should be jealous for preserving genuine play in vacation schools.

Gymnastic games, devised for play, for exercise, for mind and for character, have been adopted to the city conditions of small space and large numbers. Briefly characterized: they are competitive—to arouse interest and enjoyment; the competition is between groups—to encourage the spirit of coöperation as well; they require physical and mental force, and are simple to execute. If too elaborate they will not be popular. The stimulation of laughter and fun, the muscular and circulatory invigoration accompanying these active outdoor games, the onlooker must contrast with a school-room gymnastic ten (or fewer) minutes, in narrow aisles and heavy atmosphere, with formal movements. There can be no doubting which furnishes the physical and mental refreshing—the ideal of school recesses and calisthenics. The same appropriation expended for game specialists, instead of gymnastic instruction, would accomplish very much more for children *under the limitation of time and surroundings at present necessary in public schools;* besides furnishing children with plays to be used elsewhere, and, fully as important, assisting character building. Under wise control these games encourage regard for fair play and justice, powers of leadership and initiative, ideas of coöperation to win and of friendly competition, intensity of effort, agility of mind as well as of body, resourcefulness, generosity and courtesy.

Earnest students of the times have awakened to the question. How does free public education *train for self-government?* Its solution was first undertaken in certain higher (private) institutions, Amherst college among the leaders, by establishing a student governing body. This, like college gymnastics twenty years ago, was soon recognized as beginning too late to effect the best results. Primary and grammar grades are social and moral as well as intellectual seed times. In them the child, *fitting for membership in a self-governing community, is trained to obey an autocrat.* The development of reasoning powers upon questions of personal, and particularly of social conduct is wholly neglected. Yet in school government, under the supervision of scholarly minds, is the great opportunity of school systems to cultivate those ethical forces by which the career of individuals and the success of present civilization must be ultimately determined.

A few lower grade and vacation schools are experimenting to harmonize conditions of school life with democratic government—decided upon by the forefathers, and the results are encouraging. Children, proud of the responsibility of making and administering their own laws, responsive to the influences both of public opinion (in their classes) and from the principal's office, are growing into an understanding of and loyalty to social order, are developing powers of discrimination as to motives and persons,

are acquiring an inclination toward upholding community interests—all of which, starting in a play experiment, cannot fail to influence for the better the mature man and woman. They are practising a form of obedience higher than that developed by personal authority, cultivating the only spirit of obedience that should guide self-respecting members of a democracy—voluntary obedience to the right whether called for through the agency of relationship, of events, or of government.

This is the *motif* in the vacation movement—to care for less favored children during summer months, to help fill gaps in their training, and to connect certain broken currents between school and citizenship. Good teachers are needed, manifestly, to hold voluntary attendance, to give the special instruction indicated, and to conduct such experimenting efficiently.

HELEN C. PUTNAM, A.B., M.D.,
Providence, R. I.

PREVENTIVE MEDICINE.

THE results of general application of sanitary measures are that the general mortality has, during the last fifty years, been reduced one-half. The individual longevity of man has increased more than three years, that of women three and a half years. The mortality of the British troops is only two-fifths of what it was at the time of the Crimean War, among those in the East Indies one-third, and among those in the West Indies one-tenth. Dr. Parker of London has estimated that smallpox has diminished 95 per cent.; deaths from fevers generally have declined 82 per cent., deaths from typhus fever 95 per cent., deaths from enteric fever 60 per cent., deaths from scarlet fever 81 per cent., deaths from diphtheria 59 per cent., and deaths from phthisis 46 per cent. The mortality from surgical operations, has, through the teaching of Lord Lister, been reduced 20 per cent., the surgeon no longer dreading septicemia, gangrene, etc., when in former times almost every other amputation resulted in death. It is estimated that the operation for ovariotomy had added 40,000 years of useful life to women in Great Britain, with a like proportion for other countries.—Dr. William Bayard, *Montreal Medical Journal*.

SULPHUR AS A PREVENTIVE OF MOSQUITO BITES.

ONE of our readers informs us that, having seen a statement in some English medical journal to the effect that sulphur, taken internally, would protect a person against flea-bites, it occurred to him to try it as a preventive of mosquito bites. Accordingly, he began taking effervescing tablets of tartar-lithine and sulphur, four daily. He provided himself with several lively mosquitoes, and having put them into a wide-mouthed bottle, inverted the bottle and pressed its mouth upon his bare arm. The mosquitoes settled on his skin, but showed no inclination to bite him. If this gentleman's experience should be borne out by further trials, it might be well for persons who are particularly sensitive to mosquito bites to take a course of sulphur during the mosquito season, especially in view of the growing opinion that the mosquito is the common vehicle of malaria.—*N. Y. Medical Journal*.

DOCTORS AND EDITORS.

FROM the following, the origin of which, says the editor of the *Iowa Medical Journal*, is not known, it would seem that the doctor has not all the worst of it.

"The doctor from Algona said that newspapers are run for revenue only. What in thunder do doctors run for, anyway? Do they run for glory? One good healthy doctor's bill would run this office six months. An editor works a half a day for three dollars with an investment of $3,000; a doctor looks wise and works ten minutes for $200, with an investment of three cents for catnip and a pill-box that cost $1.37. A doctor goes to college two or three years, gets a diploma and a string of words the devil himself cannot pronounce, cultivates a look of gravity that he pawns off for wisdom, gets a box of pills, a cayuse and a meat saw and sticks out his shingle a full-fledged doctor. He will then doctor you until you die at a stipulated price per visit, and puts them in as thick as your pocketbook will permit. An editor never gets his education finished; he learns as long as he lives, and studies all his life. He eats bran mash and liver, he takes his pay in hay and turnips, and keeps the doctor in town by refraining from printing the truth about him. We would like to live in Algona and run a newspaper six months and see if the doctor would change his mind about our 'running a newspaper for revenue only.' If we didn't get some glory out of it we would agree to take one dose of his pills, after first saying our prayers. If the editor makes a mistake he has to apologize for it, but if the doctor makes a mistake he buries it. If we make one there is a lawsuit, tall swearing and a smell of sulphur, but if the doctor makes one there is a funeral, cut flowers and a smell of varnish. The doctor can use a word a foot long, but if the editor uses it he has to spell it. If the doctor goes to see another man's wife he will charge the man for the visit. If the editor calls on another man's wife he gets a charge of buckshot. Any medical college can make a doctor. You can't make an editor. He has to be born one. When a doctor gets drunk it is a case of 'overcome by the heat,' and if he dies it is heart-failure. When an editor gets drunk it is too much booze, and if he dies it is a case of delirium tremens.

"The editor works to keep from starving, while the doctor works to ward off the gout. The editor helps men to live better, and the doctor assists them to die easy. The doctor pulls a sick man's leg, the editor is glad if he can collect his bills at all. Revenue only? We are only living for fun and to spite the doctors."

CHOKED BY IMAGINATION.

THE fact that the throes of the imagination under great nervous excitement often produce a corresponding physical frenzy was illustrated recently in the case of a man who had gone to sleep with his artificial teeth in his mouth.

Waking suddenly with a choking sensation, he found his teeth had disappeared. He looked in the glass of water where they were usually deposited, did not see them there and realized they must be far down his throat.

Choking and struggling, he hammered on the door of a friend sleeping in the house, who, seeing his critical condition, vainly tried to draw the teeth out of the sufferer's throat. He could feel the teeth, but had not the strength to extract them. He ran for a blacksmith who lived a few doors away, but the blacksmith's hand was too big to put into the man's mouth.

A doctor had been sent for, but he was so long in coming that the victim of the accident seemed likely to die of suffocation before the physician arrived. A little girl of ten years was brought under the impression that her small hand might reach the obstacle and withdraw it, but she got frightened and began to cry.

The sufferer became black in the face, his throat swelled out, and his friends expected every moment to be his last, when finally the doctor arrived. He heard the history of the case, saw that the teeth were not in the man's jaws nor in their nightly receptacle, felt the throat and cast his eyes seriously upon the floor.

There he saw the whole set of teeth. He adjusted them in the jaws of the patient, told him to breathe freely, and every symptom of suffocation disappeared.—*Philadelphia Record.*

WENT AROUND THE SPOT.

BEFORE Bismarck reconstructed the map of Europe, and made a united Germany, says the *London King,* a dozen little principalities used to annoy travelers by stopping them at their frontiers until they had satisfied the custom house demands. A Yankee once had his carriage stopped at the frontier of a petty prince's country. The Herr Ober, controleur at the custom house, came forward and, much to his indignation, was received in a nonchalant way. The Yankee was ungentlemanly enough not to get out of his carriage or even to take off his hat. The Herr Ober sharply demanded the key of the tourist's trunks, which his subordinate began handling roughly.

"Here, hands off," shouted the Yankee. "I didn't come here from the United States of America to be controlled by you. Put those trunks back. I'll not go through you at all. I'll turn back. I'm in no hurry and don't care for losing a day. You're no country. You're only a spot. I'll go around you." And he did.

MEMBRANOUS CROUP.

THE treatment of membranous croup has not met with such striking success as to render the introduction of a new remedy undesirable. And when this remedy comes to us with a long list of successes to back up its claims they are assuredly worth investigating. We refer to the brown iodized calcium, which has proved a remarkable remedy in true membranous croup, the non-diphtheritic variety. For it has been shown that there is a membranous croup which is distinct from laryngeal diphtheria. For the former iodized calcium is presented as a specific; for the latter, true calcium sulphide is likewise advocated. Both remedies are supplied by the Abbott Alkaloidal Co.

A NOTABLE DISTINCTION.

THE current number of the *Canadian Journal of Medicine and Surgery,* which is one of the representative journals of Canada, contains an article which is, perhaps, one of the most scientific ever written upon the subject of the treatment of bronchitis. All the various methods of treating this affection are discussed in detail and their merits compared; numerous formulæ of the official drugs of the Pharmacopœa are also suggested. There is, however, but one proprietary remedy mentioned as being of sufficient value to merit distinction. This remedy is Angier's Petroleum Emulsion, and the writer states that it is of specific value in affording prompt relief from the symptoms of inflammation of the respiratory tract. Cough is promptly checked, expectoration made easy and free from effort and the sensations of irritation and inflammation in the chest are almost immediately abolished.

The writer of the above article states that these beneficial effects of Angier's Petroleum Emulsion are noted even in the chronic, obstinate forms of bronchitis, and that this remedy may be relied upon to effect a cure.

THE effect of music on the sick was discussed at length at the meeting of the International Metaphysical League recently held in New York. It was said that the therapeutic value of music has passed beyond the experimental stage and is no longer a mere theory. So many and varied are the natures of the diseases influenced beneficiently by it that it is impossible to draw the line and say that it is better for this or that disorder, for music acts directly upon the mind, and mental states are mirrored in the flesh. We do not claim music to be a cureall, but an adjunct, and as such it should have an honored place in the homes of those who would heal, in the hospitals, sanatoriums, and prisons.

EDITORS AND DOCTORS.

IT is an old story that every man thinks he can edit a newspaper more successfully than the editor, and it is false. And there is one other field of human endeavor in which every man thinks himself supreme; namely, curing rheumatism and colds. In a lively career of three months with inflammatory rheumatism I have made a collection of some 200 "sure cures" from kindly-disposed persons, who felt that I needed their services. No two agree. The only easement I have found lies in famine, and no man or set of men can have a proprietary interest in that formula. Therefore, oh, fellow sufferers, let me join the Dr. Knowalls and prescribe this "sure cure:" Quit eating, quit drinking, quit smoking, quit bathing, quit worrying; if these fail, quit breathing. Money refunded if no cure.— *N. Y. Press.*

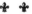

SHEEP WITH ARTIFICIAL TEETH.

A NEW SOUTH WALES correspondent of the *Liverpool Journal of Commerce* says that a pastoralist of Hargreaves, near Mudgee, has tried dentistry for sheep, with great success. He had a valuable American ram, which found great difficulty in masticating its food, owing to the loss of teeth. Artificial teeth were inserted, and the animal has since vigorously attacked its fodder. This is believed to be the first experiment of the kind in the colony.

HAGEE'S Cordial of Cod Liver Oil with Hypophosphites of Lime and Soda is the remedy for grippe. It restores health, and has the further effect of curing the disagreeable post-grippal symptoms so often seen. Thus, night-sweats, loss of weight, and the entire train of nervous symptoms, such as intestinal neuralgia, headache, brain fag, eye strain, etc., quickly yield to its action. It is pleasant to take, efficient in action, and a great builder of all the tissues.

THE TEETH OF THE NATION.

IF we were a truly military nation, we certainly should give more attention to the children's teeth than we do at the present time. A committee of the British Dental Association some time ago investigated the mouths of a large number of school children, with the result that they found that 84 per cent. of those examined had carious teeth. Of course all these 'children were not suffering from toothache. If they had been something would have been done. The mischief is that dental caries often goes on until it has ruined the tooth for all useful purposes before any serious pain is produced, and that the children of the poor, when caries has gone on to such a stage as to cause toothache, have often nothing before them but extraction. Hence many troubles, much crowding and ill-development of the permanent teeth, and much future inability to tackle "bully beef." It is in the stage before toothache that preventive measures can best be taken, and this means that the dentist must go to the schools.

A great deal is being said just now about the necessity of providing free meals for school children, and although such a proceeding spells rank socialism, so, it must be remembered, does free education. For there is something before even food, and that is teeth. It must be remembered that there is a great hereditary and instinctive tendency among all but the very lowest type of the human race which drives parents to provide their young with food. Food of a sort then the children will be sure to have. On the other hand, there is no inborn instinct which drives parents to look after their children's teeth. Yet we as a community object to nature's method of eliminating the toothless ones by starvation. So we keep these weakly ones alive sometimes in hospitals, sometimes in jails, sometimes in workhouses, but always at great expense, while the great multitude of those who are not thrown entirely upon our hands, lead a less healthy and less productive life than would be the case if they had been thrown upon

the world uneducated, perhaps, but with good teeth. That the State should take care of the children's teeth is a matter not to be lightly put aside on the plea of its socialistic tendencies. It is a matter of both military and national importance.

Whether the State might not dig even deeper to the root of the matter, destroy all feeding-bottles, and punish with fine and imprisonment all mothers who do not suckle their own infants, is a still larger question which we will leave the Socialists to discuss. —*The Hospital.*

THE GENERAL CARE OF THE SKIN, CONSIDERED FROM THE POINT OF VIEW OF PROPHYLAXIS.

THE author discusses the management of the skin and its appendages during health. One essential element in the due care of the skin is not to remove prematurely, or to too great an extent, much of the outer epidermis. The author does not approve of the indiscriminate use of soap; moderate friction is far better, and the loofah forms the best flesh brush. He is a warm advocate of cold baths, where not contraindicated by age or weakness. Hot baths should not be indulged in frequently. Distilled or rain water is by far the best for toilet purposes; hard water acts deleteriously to the skin, yet artificial additions to water for the purpose of softening it are apt to be harmful. The article closes with some general remarks on the toilet of the hair and nails. —*Dr. W. A. Jamieson, in N. Y. Medical Journal.*

THE basis of success rests in a person's power to stand alone; and no man will ever be the magnet to attract success until he can stand alone, straight and tall as a liberty pole, glorying in the position; free from fear, independent of public opinion, and daring to be himself. Here is the strength that draws still greater strength; here is that which all men adore, and before which all assumptions of greatness doff their tinsel crowns.—*Helen Wilmans.*

THE BREVITY MEDICAL CLUB.

History of the Club and Proceedings of First Meeting.

Conceived Christmas morning and born Christmas afternoon, 1900. Respiration fully established within thirty minutes. Vision and revision congenital.

Membership mentionless; officers honorless; place of meeting immaterial, but always at the office or residence of some member who invites it.

Objects: Promptness, Precision, Perspicuity, Pithiness, Pertinency, Progress.

AXIOMS: APHORISMS AND CATECHISM.

There is no fool like a long-winded fool.

A tale is well told that is told in three sentences.

The value of a book, essay, or sermon depends upon the proximity of Preface and Peroration, Introduction and Finis.

Never open your mouth or ink your pen until you have something worth saying and have hunted down the fewest and most incisive words in which to express it.

The quintessence of knowledge is in knowing when to quit.

Life is too short for gossip and chatter.

The true secret of Longevity lies in the daily practice of uncompromising Brevity.

The Telegraph has added a dozen years to every business man's life by teaching him to say in ten words all that formerly dwadled through half a page.

Not Density but Condensity.

The First Paper read before the Club and submitted to the crucial test of criticism from the club standpoint follows:

(As Thought and not Authority carries weight, no name will be attached to any paper read before the Club. This note must be considered as a standing explanation.)

THE VALUE OF OXYGEN IN CARDIAC LESIONS.

Fifteen years ago there wasn't much Oxygen in the air. (This is not a chemical postulate.)

To-day this element and various dilutions and adulterations of it are being pumped into thousands of subjects every week and almost everywhere, subjects mostly moribund, from a great variety of causes.

Subjects *in articulo mortis* from pneumonia, or uremia, are deemed especially eligible to the pumping process.

What are the facts without the fads, and what is the rational place and value of the agent in these and other analogous cases?

Is it merely another fashion like that of antipyrin, antisepsis, antitoxin, chloral, the bromides? Or has it a legitimate field and function among rational therapeutics?

Unquestioned authority asserts that the only genuine muscle tonic is pure Oxygen. The heart is a muscle, the most complex and incessantly alert of all the muscles in the body. Hence, the necessity for its more than ordinary care. All the voluntary muscles rest during sleep and at will; the heart never, except for the inconsiderable interval between beats.

In common with all other organs and tissues, the heart is nourished and replenished by the blood-current. "Heart failure" therefore means that the heart muscle has been either starved or overworked until it no longer responds to normal stimuli, and the organ stops flat in diastole simply but unquestionably *for want of breath.*

In most fatal cases of pneumonia the complication most dreaded and most strenuously combatted is heart failure. In case of a starved animal it would be equally pertinent to diagnose "dog failure." The dog fades, but it is the larder that fails.

The primary and fundamental mission of Oxygen is to feed the heart by keeping it supplied with healthy and normal blood. For the performance of this function Oxygen is imperative, indispensable, and without a possible substitute.

But its office as an indirect as well as direct nutrient to the heart muscle is not the only one. Oxygen is the original, the most potent and universal of all the known antitoxins. It has no equal as a prophylactic.

The fatal cases of pneumonia are seldom illustrative of direct apnœa but of toxemia. They are in nearly every instance cases of auto-intoxication, auto-infection — physiologic suicide. The blood becomes a lethal tide loaded with carbon dioxid and other toxic agents, which soon paralyze the respiratory as well as all the other nerve centers.

Here, again, Oxygen is imperative. It anticipates the intoxication, antagonizes the degenerative tendency, antidotes the poisons that result from the morbid processes and interruption of functions that always accompany this disease. In these cases it is primarily prophylactic and secondarily curative.

The office and utility of Oxygen is thus seen to be threefold: It is Prophylactic, Therapeutic, and Antidotal. It prevents degenerative tendencies; it removes abnormal and subnormal conditions, and it antagonizes and destroys toxins and deleterious accumulations.

In every case of heart lesion one or other of these functions, and in a majority, all three, are incisively indicated.

Its use is neither empirical, problematic, nor palliative, but is always rational, radical, and positive. In short, it is not merely permissive and tentative, it is peremptory and indispensable.

A general misapprehension as to its ultimate source and blundering technique in connection with its artificial exhibition have sometimes made its advocacy smack of quackery.

Its sole source, it may be assumed, is the atmosphere, organic and inorganic substances containing it having derived their quota from this original source. The supply usually relied upon in therapeutics is derived from the decomposition of inorganic compounds rich in loosely combined Oxygen is neither accurate nor satisfactory. For this reason the therapeutic use of artificial Oxygen has never commanded adequate appreciation nor attained a popularity commensurate with its importance. Nevertheless it is universally but unconsciously and unintentionally invoked in all these and analogous cases. Thus, in all cardiac lesions and every form of cardiac weakness fresh air is a universal and perfunctory prescription; graduated mountain climbing, which has given such excellent account of itself in Germany, is a means of compelling an increased utilization of Oxygen; hydrotherapy largely depends upon it by accelerating the breathing function and inducing cutaneous absorption of the needed and lacking element. Massage, movements, and all forms of exercise and recreation, bowling, boating, the bicycle, gymnastics, and golf—all these are means and methods of increased elimination, oxidation, and assimilation. All are direct or indirect sources of this universal and almost omnipotent element—Oxygen.

(PUBLISHER'S NOTE.—If any of our readers, appreciating the spirit of the "Brevity Club," would like to become active members—no initiation fees or annual dues—they are cordially invited to address the Editor of the GAZETTE.)

A REFLECTION.

"IN your advertisement," said the man with the suave manner, as he entered the office of the ice company, "you say there are no microbes on the ice that you furnish to your customers."

"Yes, sir," replied the treasurer, as he placed a blotter in front of his diamond stud so that the caller would not have to blink, "and we stand by our assertion."

"I stand by it, too," said the man with the suave manner, "and I have called to say that, and have no fear of microbes, believing they are harmless, I wish you would direct your delivery man to leave at my residence in the future ice of such dimensions that two or three microbes, if they felt so inclined, could occupy it without crowding each other."—Harper's Bazar.

BOOK REVIEW

Progressive Medicine, Vol. IV., December, 1900. Edited by Hobart Amory Hare. Philadelphia and New York: Lea Brothers & Co., 1900.

The volume before us completes the year of this unique and very interesting series. The work is practically without a rival in the entire field of medical publications, occupying a place that has never before been filled. The publishers and the editor have ample occasion to be proud of their work, the fame of which has not been restricted to national boundaries. It stands high with the profession everywhere, and was awarded the grand prize at the Paris Exposition.

If that be possible the present volume is more comprehensive than any of its predecessors. The topics treated are *Diseases of the Digestive Tract and Allied Organs*, by Max Einhorn; *Genito-Urinary Diseases and Syphilis*, by William T. Bellfield; *Fractures, Dislocations, Amputations, Surgery of the Extremities, and Orthopedics*, by Joseph C. Bloodgood; *Physiology*, by Albert P. Brubaker; *Diseases of the Kidneys*, by John Rose Bradford; *Hygiene*, by Henry B. Baker, and *Practical Therapeutic Referendum*, by E. Q. Thornton.

We have noticed this work as each quarterly volume has appeared, and have expressed our approbation of its scope and execution in no unmeasured terms. The final volume, closing the year and the century, not only maintains, but exceeds, the high standard attained by the earlier issues, and this is saying enough.

There is no dearth, rather a glut, of more elaborate and more ponderous works; but the age is incisively demanding concentration instead of elaboration. This is unquestionably the busiest age since time began, and readers, especially medical readers, become impatient over prolix details that can be readily inferred, and minutiæ that have no practical bearing. It is only the essentials that need to be set down in cold type. The practitioner who cannot supply the padding to complete a properly articulated skeleton or outline must belong to a fossiliferous age. The medical spirit moves slowly, but it moves, and the verbose writers, men who occupy twenty pages in saying what could be better said in four, will have to go. Professional men who have acquired either fame, fortune or political prestige still command space in leading medical journals, and hours of time before the medical societies; but their long-winded lucubrations are never read through and are listened to with yawns and empty benches. The conviction is becoming general that, as a rule, medical speakers who exceed thirty minutes are talking against time, and that a four-page essay is worth four times as much as one of thirty pages. We ardently hope that more medical authors will catch the spirit, learn to condense and compress, and thereby earn the heartfelt, if not tearful, gratitude of their listeners and readers.

Poor pepsin is dying hard. In its death struggle dozens of questions that involve doubt are being discussed. It is a sort of "katy-did" and "katy-didn't" discussion. Does pepsin merely dissolve food, or does it perfectly peptonize it, or does it do either? In making tests, what kind of an egg was used? Was it a duck's egg, or a hen's egg? It is said now "that the white of a duck's egg is very considerably more resistive to the peptonizing characteristics of pepsin than a hen's egg." After this has been decided, it, likely, will be necessary to experiment as to the hyper-solubility and digestiveness of the egg of a white duck, or of a brown duck, or of a wild duck, or of a tame duck; of a black Spanish hen, a Brahma, a a Plymouth Rock, a bantam, and so on, to the end. Then after all this has been decided, what relation has the solution of albumen, etc., in a test tube to do with the digestion of food in the stomach, anyhow? —*Medical Gleaner.*

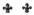

Department of Notes and Queries.

FREEDOM OF DISCUSSION BETWEEN EDITOR AND READER.

THIS Department is designed to furnish a frank, cordial and thorough interchange of ideas between Editor and Reader.

To avoid the conventional pitfall into which so many of these Departments drift, patrons who desire to avail themselves of its privileges are requested to scrupulously refrain from personalities, to make their inquiries and responses brief, to the point, and of general interest. By strict observance of these rules the Department can be made of immense practical value to all our readers.

Query 68. What is the best diet for a stomach which is inclined to over-secretion and acidity?
R. C. G., Ind.

Answer.—Modern experiments prove that fats and fatty foods tend to check the secretion of gastric fluid, and to decidedly lessen the hyperacidity when this quality is marked. An alkaline medium is helpful. Meats should be sparingly used or wholly prohibited in bad cases. Vegetable foods, bread, breakfast cereals, if roasted or thoroughly cooked, milk and most ripe moderately acid fruits usually agree. Potatoes and some other starchy vegetables are apt to cause flatulence. The generous use of olive oil as well as its unobjectionable substitutes, has been found curative of the condition as well as nutritious.

Query 69. In using a milk diet for infants and invalids which is the more desirable and effective process, sterilization or Pasteurization?
G. W. M., Colo.

Answer.—Sterilized milk, much as is said in its favor, is not ideal food. It undergoes certain changes in spite of this process, and it is also much less palatable after this change. For these reasons Pasteurized milk is now given the preference.

Query 70. Is old-fashioned bread and butter, such as our grandmothers handed out to hungry youngsters at all hours of the day, good food for persons whose digestion is not strictly vigorous?
A DOCTOR'S WIFE, Minn.

Answer.—In a general sense, yes. The bread should have been at least twelve hours out of the oven, and it should not be over-fermented. If the butter be fresh and sweet it may be used very freely, and this combination of proteids, carbohydrates and fats is generally well-borne, satisfying and compatible. If the bread be poor, overfermented and much doctored stuff, and the butter poorly made, artificially colored, or frowy, the mess had better be reserved for the neighbor's hungry dog.

In case of weak stomachs and dyspepsia the old German advice as to bread and milk is good. Instead of crumbling the bread into the milk light, white bread twenty-four hours old is to be thickly spread with fresh butter, masticated slowly and thoroughly, and the milk, with extra portions of cream added, is to be sipped slowly along with the bread and butter.

Query 71. What disinfectant is now considered most available and effective in connection with the avoidance and restriction of the infectious diseases?
E. L. H., Miss.

Answer.—The question is pertinent. The medical journals seem to have a habit of decrying from time to time nearly all the substances now used for this purpose. Over and over again it has been announced that the best of them are practically inert and worthless. These statements are for the most part reckless and unreliable. True, some substances have acquired an unwarranted reputation as disinfectants, as, for example, the deodorants, which are seldom disinfectants. But there are reliable disinfectants that are easily used, effective and inexpensive. Sulphurous acid gas, liberated by burning roll sulphur is the old standby, and it is efficient. But it has some serious drawbacks, among which are its bleaching action on colored fabrics. Formaldehyd is a more recent resource and has been both extolled and exploded. It has at last compelled recognition and is probably one of the most reliable substances for the purpose. It has no effect on even delicate colors and does not affect any metal but iron. It is easily exhibited and is effective as regards any material exposed to it for a reasonable time. It does not, however, penetrate as thoroughly as the fumes of burning sulphur. Failures with it have no doubt been the result of a want of care and accuracy in its exhibition.

For general use about sinks and sick rooms nothing has ever supplanted that old reliable preparation, Platt's Chlorides.

For wounds, sores and cavities nothing takes the place of hydrogen dioxid. Corrosive sublimate and carbolic acid (phenol) are germicides, but ought not to be classed with disinfectants. For disinfecting the alimentary canal the sulpho-carbolates head the list. Beta-naphthol and salol are much used for this purpose, but without being any more effective are sometimes followed by untoward accidents.

Editor NOTES AND QUERIES:

Perhaps my question is a little outside your usual line, but it seems to me important and of general interest. If you think otherwise, I have no doubt your waste-basket will hold one more for the current month, and I presume it will not there be lonesome for want of company!

Query 72. Is there any marked virtue in the phosphate of soda treatment for presenility and general debility from advanced age?

Answer.—Once in a great while newspaper therapeutics contain a few kernels of wheat in several bushels of chaff. The reporter is not generally to blame for this accident.

There is nothing either new or miraculous about the use of phosphorus and some of its compounds in the treatment of diseases characterized by failure of nerve tone and a general decline of the vital forces. Every form of wasting disease and of nerve prostration, from phthisis to impotence has been treated with some form of phosphate, phosphite or hypophosphite. It would be easy to name half a hundred preparations of the drug that are familiar to every reader of medical literature and the daily press. Churchill and Winchester set the pace with their sickish and sediment-depositing syrups of the hypophosphites. Their imitators, now numbered by the score, cut a prominent figure in every market, their annual sales mounting high in the millions. The so-called organo-therapy is based chiefly on the use or pretended use of highly phosphorized compounds. It is hardly necessary to mention the names of McArthur, Fellows, Phillips, Wheeler, Hensel or Crosby as a few of the more prominent manufacturers, since these names have long been household words. Within a few years, however, the form of exhibiting this remedy or class of remedies has materially changed. The physiologic chemists have been demonstrating that inorganic salts of phosphorus, as well as of various other elements, are not assimilated to any extent by the digestive organs, but that to be available these salts must be derived from organic nature. The tolerance with which organo-therapy was received was doubtless based on this fact. Among the eligible preparations of the drug the glycero-phosphates have taken high rank.

We do not see the necessity for exhibiting the remedy hypodermically. The phosphates are *foods,* and the stomach is the proper receptacle for food. We do believe there is much in the organic-source theory. Robust organisms are competent to derive their pabulum for growth and repair from chemical and inorganic sources, but robust natures are not in need of such supply. It is the dragged-out and degenerate organisms that need special nourishment.

The recent account of the miraculous cure of a distinguished American by the use of phosphate of soda, hypodermically administered, by a French physician, lost much of its sensational glamor when the "distinguished citizen," on being interviewed declined to corroborate the account and took especial pains to contradict the vital points of the story, which it proved was conceived chiefly in a reporter's brain. Evidently that reporter is not in any immediate need of "highly phosphorized brain food"!

In case of this "distinguished citizen" the treatment administered by a celebrated French physician, when punctiliously repeated by an equally skilful New York practitioner failed to have the expected result. This leaves us to infer that the conditions were different, or, what is more likely, that psychic influence or suggestion had more to do with the result than the phosphate of soda!

In many cases the acid phosphate of lime is quite as efficient as the soda salt. In some cases it is much preferable, because it is more decidedly indicated.

Yes, there is a world of virtue in the phosphates, but let us not forget that it is a *food* and not merely a spur to jaded old men!

THE
DIETETIC AND HYGIENIC GAZETTE
A MONTHLY JOURNAL OF PHYSIOLOGICAL MEDICINE

| VOL. XVII. | NEW YORK, MARCH, 1901. | No. 3. |

A CENTURY'S PROGRESS IN MEDICINE AND SURGERY.

A RÉSUMÉ OF THE REVIEWS.

BY SAMUEL S. WALLIAN, A.M., M.D.

I.

MEDICINE.

THE daily press and the magazines have exhaustively expatiated on the multifarious advances and accomplishments of the Nineteenth Century. Of all these historic records of progress and enterprise none are more interesting or important than those which deal with the advances made in Medicine and Surgery, terms that include all that has been learned of Hygiene, Sanitation and Nutrition, since these are the substratum of scientific fact on which Medicine and Surgery must always be founded. An imposing volume could be, and no doubt will be, made of these wise, interesting and important histories, deductions and inferences. The GAZETTE will spare its readers the reproduction *in extenso* of any of these exhaustive efforts, brilliant as they are, but will endeavor to place before its readers a brief and comprehensive résumé of those that have come to its table.

The progress of the world in material and mechanical directions has been more than wonderful. The utilization of the possibilities of steam and electricity, the harnessing of natural forces has reached a phenomenal stage, and promises to attain to further stages, the scope of which can not yet be predicted. Next to these have been the strides made in the direction of a betterment of the social conditions of human life, in the more general diffusion of education and intellectual culture, and in the elevation of ethical standards. But none of these can compare in importance with the improvements made in the methods of preventing disease and relieving human suffering. In the language of Professor Osler,

"This is the Promethean gift of the Century to man."

Among the definite discoveries that have advanced the art of detecting, diagnosing and treating diseases, some of which were in embryo prior to the advent of the century just closed, are auscultation, percussion, the differentiation of fevers—an accomplishment wholly unknown to the ancients—and the immense value of physiological laboratories for the study of respiration, circulation, digestion, assimilation and excretion. We have learned to localize some of the principal functions of the brain, and to relieve certain injuries and diseases of this organ that were formerly beyond the reach of physician or surgeon.

The advances made in physiology and pathology during the past half century have emancipated medicine from the rut of routine and thralldom of authority in which it had been groveling for ages. An evidence of the expansion of our knowledge is seen in the growth of specialism which was unknown in the preceding century. It is still subject to criticism, imperfections and limitations, but it has yielded some of the greatest triumphs of medicine and surgery. It has developed our knowledge of each of a large class of important diseases to a degree of comparative perfection which otherwise would have still been far off. Instance the improvement in the care and treatment of the insane.

At the opening of the nineteenth century there were but three medical schools in the United States; there were but two general hospitals and three medical journals. Now, medical colleges abound (about 160 in the country) from the Atlantic to the Pacific coast, every city of any size has its amply equipped hospitals, and there are more than three hundred medical journals.

Second to none of these advances, but rather underlying them all, is the immense stride made in the practical study and application of the laws of Hygiene, Sanitation and Preventive Medicine. In a great measure this has been made possible by the overthrow of the theory of spontaneous generation and the development of the science of bacteriology. Crude ideas of animalculæ and living organisms or worms within animal bodies existed prior to the year 1800, but it remained for much more recent investigators to show that these germs are not minute and dangerous animals, prowling about and seeking entrance into human bodies, but that they are all of vegetable origin, are, in fact, microscopic plants, consisting of protoplasm enveloped in a membranous coating very similar to woody fiber, and that while they are very similar in character, scientists have divided them into three principal groups called respectively, *cocci*, *bacilli* and *spirilla*. The first are spherical in form and include the small-

est varieties known, varying in diameter from $^1/_{150000}$ of an inch up. The second are rod-like in form, varying greatly in size according to species and accidental conditions. They measure from $^1/_{25000}$ to $^1/_{4000}$ inch in length, and from $^1/_{125000}$ to $^1/_{10000}$ inch in diameter. Some of them resemble animals, by having organs of locomotion, called *flagella*. The *spirilla* resemble the *bacilli*, except that, as the name suggests, they have a spiral or corkscrew form, or an undulating shape, and are longer than the *bacilli*. Slight variations cause these four species to be subdivided into hundreds of varieties, the special names of which would fill a page or two of the GAZETTE.

In their natural state these organisms are colorless. To make them distinguishable from fat crystals and other formations scientists soon learned to stain them by means of aniline dyes. The method of reproduction of these plants is either by fission or division, or by giving off spores, which latter correspond with seeds in other plants. Under favorable conditions of temperature and environment they multiply at an incredible rate. Assuming that a bacillus that multiplies by fission divides once every hour, a single specimen will increase to over 16,000,000 within twenty-four hours, and at the same rate, if not checked, and if kept in a favorable culture medium, the increase would amount in three days to incalculable billions in number, and to the incredible weight of 7,500 tons!

If there were no natural checks to their rate of increase, and all the conditions were favorable, they would rapidly overwhelm the face of the earth, and swiftly annihilate every other form of life. Nature has effectually forefended the world from such a catastrophe by limiting their food-supply. At a given stage they perish for want of further sustenance, or by surrounding themselves with a preponderance of self-engendered toxins.

Some bacteria are *aerobic*—that is, they can survive in, and possibly require, air; others are *anaerobic*, and die if long exposed to atmospheric influences. All species require moisture, and soon die if deprived of it. Many varieties subsist on animal or vegetable materials, in a sense acting the part of scavengers. Others require living tissues, while a few can flourish on mineral salts, or even the nitrogen of the air. The most favorable temperature for their reproduction is between 60° and 104° F., but some varieties can survive and multiply at or below freezing point and up to 170° F. Ordinary daylight does not interfere with their vigor or growth, but direct sunlight rapidly destroys all forms.

Contrary to popular opinion, these plants have a legitimate mission and are not the universal pests which the early descriptions of them led unthinking people to imagine. They are really an indispensable factor in all the productive processes of nature. They gauge and make possible the farmer's crops; they enable the dairyman to market "prime" butter and cheese, and they destroy or render innocuous impurities in spring, river and lake waters, that without their interference would render our public water supply poisonous and unpotable. Without their presence and activity vegetables, grains, grasses and fruits could not grow or mature, and the science of agriculture would become a dead letter. They are, therefore, not only the farmer's best friend, they are his one indispensable reliance. To annihilate all these microscopic germs would result, as already intimated, in annihilating all life from the face of the globe, and would transform the populous and fruitful earth into a dead planet, uselessly whirling in the solar system. Without doubt these minute plant-lives were the first living forms that were manifested, and that all life, as it now appears, have been evolved directly and solely from them. Germs that are charged with being disease-producing form but an infinitesimal fraction of the several species.

Among the dangerous diseases attributed to microbic origin are *anthrax, leprosy, tuberculosis, typhoid fever, diphtheria, cholera, tetanus, bubonic plague, yellow fever,* *pneumonia,* and *influenza* or *grip.* In this connection it seems fairly incredible that science has failed to prove the microbic origin of the most contagious and infectious diseases known, including *smallpox, scarlet fever, measles* and *hydrophobia.*

Another immensely important fact in connection with germ-infection is, that the human organism is inherently fortified against their inroads. The white blood-cells constitute a standing army or home-guard of defence and repression. Whenever a harmful or virulent germ finds access to the system these corpuscles rush to the rescue, and unless the attack is made in overwhelming numbers, or under conditions of vital depression, they generally succeed in repelling or devouring the foe. They either literally eat up the bacteria or they effectually antagonize the toxins elaborated by them, and thus prevent damage, and overcome diseased action. When they fail in their spontaneous effort, which is the much talked-of *vis medicatrix naturæ,* the vital powers are overborne and the enemy continues to multiply at the expense of the tissues, until the organism succumbs, or until the germs have either exhausted the supply of their peculiar nutrient or die from an overaccumulation of self-generated toxins. The process is a self-limited circle, and an ordinarily robust organism survives all but the extraordinary attacks. When for any reason there is a lack of tone and vigor, when the system of the attacked is exhausted by overwork, exposure or excesses, it is unable to continue the battle to a successful issue, and the result is death.

In these fatal cases it is not necessarily the presence of the germs, in itself, that proves fatal, the chief harm resulting from the toxins evolved or eliminated by the invading organisms. Always fruitful in resources, Nature is not content with fighting the initial battle with the invading microbes, but rallies her forces, by way of causing chemical changes in the accumulating toxins, and by producing counter-toxins or antidotes to the poisons engendered by the germs. A detection and observation of her efforts in this direction led to the discovery of the antitoxin theory of combating certain deadly forms of the infectious diseases. This self-fortification is found to exist chiefly in the blood-serum. Patient and long-continued experimentation with various animals has determined that the blood-serum of the horse—of all our domestic animals freest from constitutional taint of any kind—can be most readily and effectively fortified for the battle royal with germ-life. Hence we have the *serum therapy*. It is not yet universally accepted, since, like all new theories, it must face the opposition that always comes from ignorance of the principles involved, and of prejudice that dies hard. But facts have a way of 'finally overcoming all opposition, and in this case the results bid fair to revolutionize the treatment of a number of very fatal maladies, among which may at present be mentioned *diphtheria, tetanus* and *snake-bite*.

We have not space to recount the modus operandi of the preparation of antitoxic serum, but will summarize it by saying that every step of the process is based on the results of scientific experimentation and observed facts in nature. And as to the opposition with which the theory has been assailed, it matters very little how intelligent and sincere the opponents to any new theory may be, if the facts be against them the facts will remain after the fossils are all dead.

Preventive Medicine comes to the relief of the race in such diseases as *smallpox, typhus and typhoid fevers, cholera, yellow fever, tuberculosis, diphtheria, pneumonia, leprosy, hydrophobia, malarial fever* and *puerperal septicemia*. All these diseases, formerly so destructive and unmanageable, have been brought into line by preventive measures which are constantly being better understood, better disseminated and more intelligently applied.

But of all the advances enumerated, and which seem astonishing when we review them in their entirety, none is more important or more encouraging than the one which the eminent author already cited aptly denominates,

"THE NEW DISPENSATION OF TREATMENT."

As the term indicates there has been a fundamental revolution in the treatment of diseases. From the radical change in our conceptions of the nature and causation of disease this was inevitable. Such have been the progressive changes in the clinical management of diseases, that the physician who still feels compelled to exhibit his polypharmaceutic skill in every case of sickness is not in attune with the spirit of the age. No physician now relies on vomiting, purging, bleeding, blistering, mercury, antimony and opium as his sheet anchors. Few yet cling to the faith that there is a specific drug, if it could only be found, for every symptom and disease, and an implicit faith in the potency of drugs is as rare as it once was common. The battle with polypharmacy is still on, but it is now confined principally to a guerrilla chase of detached bandits, who once prided themselves on their affiliation with the "old guard," but who have lost step and are out of joint with the onsweep of the world about them. The ultra-extremists, who long since lost faith in the old order of things, but who lack intellectual poise and the logic of common sense, are frantically grasping at straws of some form of "faithcure"—a principle that has always done duty with intelligent and successful practitioners—suggestion, "Christian" science healing, massage by a new name, similia, mind-cure, moon-cure, etherialized astrology, or other form of crack-brained ism, revamped and refined forms of the thaumaturgy of the ancients—with which our modern society is afflicted.

All these puerile "sciences" and myth-haunted pseudopathies have an underlying basis of fact behind them or they could not succeed in being recognized; and they must be charitably dealt with until such a time as the microbe of credulity evolves its own lethal toxin, or until a serum of common sense can be so attenuated as to render the great army of susceptibles immune.

II.

SURGERY.

THE contrasts wrought in surgical theories, technic and practice during the century are even more astonishing than those belonging to the domain of medicine.

A hundred years ago, wounded or maimed mortals, lived in a state of overwhelming terror of the surgeon's saw and scalpel. A capital operation was a seventh day wonder, a vital shock from which only a pitiful few of the fittest ever rallied. Now, the cripple and the crushed, or the sufferer from carcinoma, gangrene or necrosis goes to the operating table with all the assurance of one who wraps the drapery of his couch about him and lies down to pleasant dreams. Instead of undergoing untold agonies, that seem as if they would never end, the modern patient fills his lungs and saturates his blood with the sweetish vapor of a volatile liquid, passes into a profound sleep, and wakes in a few hours, entirely unconscious of having been in any way interferred with during his long nap. He even wonders why the surgeon is not at hand and ready to begin the operation. The nurse has hard work to make him believe that his sacred abdomen has been freely ransacked, his appendix, or a batch of gall-stones, or a suppurating kidney removed, without his having realized the touch of a tenaculum or prick of a needle.

Perhaps the most signal advance, amounting in fact to a revolution in surgery, during the past century is evident in the changed methods of teaching the art. At the beginning of the century a medical college consisted of a few dismal recitation halls, from the desks of which serious professors read dry-as-dust didactics to dazed or dreamy students, without so much as a blackboard on which to illustrate the text of their learnedly abstruse lucubrations. Now the student visits a thousand bedsides, and assists at the operating tables of well-equipped college clinics, where every phase of disease, deformity and abnormity is placed immediately before him.

Again, the fees paid by medical students are no longer considered professional perquisites, but are pooled in a fund, from which the professors and demonstrators of the institution are paid a salary, and made independent of patronage and mercenary bias.

To college hospitals have been added laboratories of therapeutics, clinical medicine, chemistry, pathology, bacteriology, microscopy, embryology, physiology, hygiene and surgery. All these branches are now studied by the efficient aid of the most delicate and accurate apparatus, by comparative anatomy and physiology, by vivisection, and by experimentation with human subjects. A hundred years ago there were no libraries of medical books in this country. To-day, in addition to numerous local libraries of great value, the Surgeon-General's Library, at Washington, is the most extensive collection of the kind in existence, and the Index-Catalogue of the same constitutes a monumental contribution to the professional resources of the world.

The discovery of *anesthesia*, in 1846, marked a most important epoch in the history of surgery, perhaps the most important since the dawn of the Christian era. In short it would be hard to point to an occurrence of equal import since the advent of man upon the earth. By way of contrast it is recorded that during the five years prior to that discovery, in the Massachusetts General Hospital, but 137 persons could be induced to submit themselves to the ordeal of the surgeon's table; whereas, during the five years immediately subsequent, 487 persons gladly presented themselves for operation.

True, anesthesia did not rob surgery of all its terrors. For many years after its discovery the after-suffering and disagreeable as well as dangerous sequelæ had still to be reckoned with. Erysipelas, gangrene, tetanus and blood-poisoning made up a formidable list of dangers to be dreaded. Thousands of cases succumbed to one or other of these "accidents," as they were called, that would now be carried through to a safe and early recovery.

Anesthesia, Antisepsis, Antitoxin.—This is the beneficent trio that has enthroned the surgeon, and emancipated his hapless subjects.

Among the advances made and things accomplished during the latter part of the departing century, without attempting to enumerate all, may be mentioned:

1. A marked, definite and considerable decimation of the number of unsolved surgical problems.

2. A vast increase in the number and variety of cases in which surgery is invoked and is successful.

3. Great strides in the range and accuracy of surgical diagnosis.

For example, a quarter of century back, strangulated hernia was comparatively frequent, much dreaded and often fatal. Today it is much more rarely met with, and causes no serious alarm, since it is so safely and readily remedied.

Joint abscesses are less common; clean catheters have done away with the principal cause of cystitis and abscess of the kidney; pyemia and septicemia are no longer considered unavoidable, and tubercular lesions are either of much less frequent occurrence, or are more successfully coped with.

Only a generation back, to open the abdomen, the cranium or the thorax meant almost certain death. Now, every tyro in surgery does the deed with neatness and dispatch, without the least hesitation, and with few casualties. An eminent surgeon estimates that a thousand ovariotomies, under modern precautions, add, on an average, 30,000 years to the lives of women.

Antisepsis completed the revolution in surgical practice. It was the needed lesson in cleanliness, which, in a surgical sense, is not merely next to godliness—it is godliness itself. Only those who lived and observed, in the days of the old surgical régime, can fully appreciate the new, with its sterilized

instruments, sterilized dressings, sterilized operators, and scrupulous observance of asepsis, which implies the making of all these persons, instruments and materials much more than clean to the eye.

Antitoxin, the so-called "serum-therapy," is yet on trial. It has established a few outposts and captured a few pickets, but the results of the general battle are still poised in the balance. We must accept what has been accomplished as an encouraging prophecy of what may be reasonably expected of the coming century.

Was it only a whim of accidental superstition, or was it a vague and rudimentary premonition of the now well-defined theory of antitoxin that inspired our medical forefathers to prescribe the flesh and liver of a mad dog, dried and pulverized, as a cure for hydrophobia?

And was it not "suggestion" pure and simple when one who had been hurt by a weapon was cured by poulticing the *weapon* with "moss from a human skull" and powdered dried blood, mixed with other equally gruesome and ghastly ingredients?

A hundred years ago these things, with a thousand others that might be cited, and on account of which the incorrigibles and iconoclasts are constantly exclaiming that there is really nothing new under the sun, were dreams and chimeras; now, they are scientific deductions.

Organo-therapy has opened up another fruitful field of investigation. Its success is not yet brilliant, notwithstanding some apparently well authenticated results, but it may be that this special study will lead to unsought and unexpected demonstrations in the field of nutrition, namely, a discovery of *how to feed patients and to prevent certain special diseases, by supplying in the diet any lack of the rare and specially needed elements lamely supplied by the new treatment.* These sometimes preposterous claims of the "organic extract" advocates— the strongest of which have been made by commercially interested parties—may indirectly prove the stepping stones to dietetic discoveries of the utmost value to physiologists and sanitarians. Certainly, when special elements of nutrition are lacking in a given case it were better to seek them from direct and normal sources than from second-hand and unnatural ones, that is to say, from dead animals.

And to sum up the whole subject in a sentence:

The future field of medical and surgical progress is comprised in three words, DIETETICS, SANITATION, HYGIENE.

AIDING NATURE.

By A. D. McCONACHIE, M.D.,

Assistant Surgeon to the Presbyterian Eye, Ear and Throat Charity Hospital; Oculist and Aurist to Bay View Hospital, Baltimore, Md.

THE trenchant Hippocratic injunctions that "Nature is the first physician"; "the physician is a servant, not a teacher of nature" and that the physician should "follow nature" are better understood, more generally, consistently and rationally followed than at any period of our art. The master minds of the profession have repeated and emphasized this wisdom throughout the ages of superstition, barbarism, ecclesiasticism and empiricism, in which sorcery, alchemy, mysticism, dogmatism, empiricism, etc., prevailed.

During the Middle Ages the profession was composed of a horde of barbers, bone setters, druggists, midwives, priests, magicians, jugglers, exorcists, butchers, gypsies and other species of quacks and charlatans. The last decade has been a period of advancement in scientific medicine without parallel in the world's history. True scientific methods are being developed by numerous inquiries, keen experimentation and close research. Rational medicine has received its development through scientific research. Scientific medicine will never be fully appreciated until the laity more thoroughly understand scientific methods and spirit of the age. We must now increase their knowledge of and respect for nature

more than formerly, and to have them understand that art is not superior to nature. They must be taught that nature—the sum of all energies—maintains the build up and break down adjustment—metabolism— in health and disease. The old idea that many diseases were due to meteoric influences, the appearances of comets or the visitations of God, must be discarded and assigned to their real causes revealed by increased knowledge in the nature and causation of disease, hence more rational and effective treatment. Increased knowledge as to the cause of disease has led to the adoption of preventive means. Through preventive medicine and the adoption of public health acts by sanitary authorities infectious diseases will soon become unknown in civilized countries and result in increased general health, especially among the poor. To this end individuals and communities must act in accordance with nature's well established laws.

Prevention is the essence of cure. To cure is to prevent. This is the idea, aim and object of medicine in the future. To respect the goddess of health, Hygeia, is our aim. Good health, secured by good digestion and assimilation—the prevention of disease—is fundamental for the physical, mental and moral well being of each and every individual. The physician's object being to prevent disease and thus maintain and secure health, it becomes imperative for him to protest against violations of Nature's laws, as is daily seen in the many heredities, as syphilis, consumption, inebriety, insanity, etc. Prevention is the motto of the future, and this to be secured by a judicious enforcement and rigorous adherence to nature's laws. If we are to follow Nature in order to aid her in combating disease or toxicity, we must comprehend what is meant by *Nature, i.e.,* have a good working knowledge of the means she uses in resisting toxic agents and getting rid of them after they have gained entrance and fully established the phenomena of disease. By the word Nature, as used medically, is meant the natural forces or functions by which a living body overcomes the impressions of foreign agents, and thus prevents the development of disease; or, after disease has been established, is able to neutralize or expel the disturbing factors and restore health. The exact nature of these forces is still obscure.

Biologists have reduced all living bodies into essential elements—cells composed of protoplasm, which is capable of appropriating food material for its growth and multiplication; and utilizing oxygen, by which oxidation and disintegration take place. Thus we see that the protoplasm of all animal life is constantly undergoing changes—metabolism. These changes are the results of life processes. Every cell of the body develops from and inherits the properties of some preceding cell from which it originated. Each cell is thus endowed with the ability to appropriate such matter as is necessary for its nutrition or growth and to refuse all other matter. This inherent power of appropriating or rejecting materials with which it comes in contact is the most important function which cells perform, and enables them to resist the influence of poisonous substances in the higher animal organisms, as man. We find a variety of form, each having a special function, which thus furnish additional means by which poisons may be added from within or appropriated from without, and also meant for their rejection or neutralization. In order that the vital processes of cells should go on harmoniously without disorder of function or structure all that would be necessary would be to keep them in a proper atmosphere and supply them with good food material. All cells, whether muscular, nervous, fibrous or secretive, are nourished or fed from the blood, the quality and quantity of which depends upon the natural activity of the respiratory and digestive organs and the quantity and quality of the material supplied to them. If the digestive organs are supplied with only wholesome food material and the respiratory organs with pure air, the blood product will be normal as to furnish-

ing material for growth and repair of every structure of the body. If the food or air supplied contain unwholesome or toxic materials the blood will be apt to be contaminated with the same, and hence every structure and function of the body disturbed. Fortunately the blood not only supplies nutrition to the tissues, but also is the receptacle of all products of waste, for which special organs are provided, by means of which these waste products are eliminated, as well as other toxic agents which may have gained access from without.

It is thus clear that the natural processes which give to the living human body its resistance are:

First, its intrinsic power of selection and rejection, possessed by each cell of which the blood and tissues are composed.

Second, oxidation, by which tissue change is brought about.

Third, the eliminating processes, by which the metabolic products are carried from the blood and passed out of the system.

The vital resistance of any body will depend entirely upon the harmonious and efficient action of these processes. These processes are best maintained by rest, diet and fresh air, which form the trilogy of rational medicine, and it is on the proper understanding of these that rationalism in the practice of medicine rests. To-day the paramount importance of rest, diet and fresh air, is recognized in each and every diseased condition, without exception.

Physiologic chemistry has pretty conclusively proven that nearly all acute general diseases are caused by toxic agents called leucomains, ptomains, or tox-albumins, resulting either from bacteria introduced from without, or from the retention of exementitious products of metabolic changes from within. It has also proven that these same toxic agents exert their disturbing influence on the blood, interfering with the distribution of oxygen and tissue changes, both nutritive and excretory, and thereby arises more or less disturbance of circulation, respiration, secretion, and the evolution of heat, thus giving rise to fever. All diseases arising from toxic agents have a period of incubation. Now, if the physician could have charge of the patient during this period, viz., securing for him an abundance of fresh air, good water, wholesome food and strict cleanliness, he might so improve the patient's vital or natural resistance as to prevent the development of the disease, or at least render its progress mild and free from danger.

Thus, if we would act in harmony with Nature's own processes, we must study the nature and effects of each toxic agent, as well as the nature and modus operandi of every therapeutic agent we use. A proper understanding of these processes will do away with much of the skepticism regarding the curative effects of drugs. There is no part of the whole field of medical knowledge that needs more thorough research and revision than that which relates to the action of drugs on the living body.

It is apparent that the human system continuously strives to regain its normal tone, when this has been disturbed, and that most diseases are not only self-limited, but, under favorable conditions, self-curative. That a physician should be continuously on the alert to render therapeutic assistance, when such aid is required on rational grounds, is a truism concerning which there can be no dispute. But the indiscriminate and continuous use of enormous quantities of powerful drugs is a procedure which must be relegated to the past. It has been said that, "If all drugs were thrown into the sea, it would be better for mankind and worse for the fishes." This sweeping assertion, although having a semblance of truth, was uttered by a layman and not a physician. We should always bear in mind the tremendous amount of good that can be accomplished in certain conditions without the use of drugs, and the irreparable harm that can be done by the irrational use of drugs. I refer especially to those neurotic conditions amenable to rest, diet, fresh air, etc.

What to do besides the giving of medicine opens a field that would require volumes to exhaust. The first thing to do is to analyze the patient; that is, inquire carefully into the habits of the patient, particularly as to ingestion, excretion, surroundings, habits of exercise, sleep, rest, etc. Very few human beings live correctly. It must be apparent to any one who will stop to consider, that one of the great social problems of our day, which concerns not only the welfare of the home, but of the nation, is how to preserve the highest possible standard of health, physical and mental, among its people. The old philosophical adage, "*mens sana in corpore sano*" has lost much of its force. It should be a motto on the walls of every home in our land. Its neglect, through the spirit of greed and rapacity, has produced a race of dyspeptic money-getters, whose highest ambition is too frequently the almighty dollar, and whose chief concern for health lies in the fact that its possession assists in the procuring of money. This condition of things should be remedied. How? Ignorance and prejudice are the two mighty obstacles to be overcome. The masses are much less informed upon matters pertaining to medicine than in any other branch of knowledge. The remedy lies in a needed reform in the instruction in hygiene and sanitation in our public schools. I believe the physician should be an important factor in our public educational scheme. The coming generations must look to the medical profession as the source of a higher and more rational method of education in the science of healthful living. The physicians' business in the future will be not only to *medicate* but to *educate* the public. They will show the public that it is possible in a great measure to prevent by proper and rational living such diseases as tuberculosis, arterio-sclerosis, rheumatism, gout, syphilis, dyspepsia and a host of lesser ills. There will always be willful sinners against *Nature's laws*, but sinning through ignorance ought not to be permitted in this enlightened age of books. Careless sinning can be lessened by a greater emphasis on these matters in each individual's education.

Why the sale of so many millions of dollars' worth of patent medicines annually? Why so many filthy medical advertisements in the daily press? Why do quacks grow rich upon the credulity of a gullible public? Why is it that suffering humanity is appealed to through the secular and religious press by many and varied agencies for its relief? Why is it that various "faddists"— Christian scientists, divine healers, spiritualists, shriners, faith curists, etc., spring up and flourish? Why is all this except from the utter ignorance as to the simplest laws of their own animal life which prevails among even the most highly educated persons? The majority of people are profoundly ignorant of their own bodies and the proper way to care for them. What is the remedy? The remedy is in one word —Education. The people must be taught through the schools, practically and systematically, the fundamentals necessary in combating disease, viz., a masterly knowledge of hygiene, dietetics, sanitary laws, etc., founded upon the intelligent knowledge of the body in health.

The physician's function is to help Nature and to prevent the occurrence of damaging influences. His labors can be facilitated by a wider and broader culture of the public in the matter of hygiene, dietetics, sanitation and practical domestic medicine.

Our public schools are woefully deficient in such instruction. The employment of physicians as teachers and lecturers in the public schools on subjects of hygiene, physiology and practical domestic medicine, would be the means of saving thousands of human lives, sacrificed by preventable diseases.

The individual will then more reasonably follow Nature's dictates. He will care more for the character of the food that is put into the stomach than for putting medicine into it. Self-denial and self-control will be developed by wholesome exact knowledge. The average man or woman would rather indulge the palate, resulting in an overloaded stomach, and then take a pill, than to apply sense or reason to the subject of eating. The debt of indulgence must be paid, even if postponed by "dinner pills," with interest in the form of rheumatism, gout and other obscure discomforts.

The astute, up-to-date physician knows that a dietetic prescription, rigidly followed, is of far greater value as a rule than a medical prescription in many of Nature's ills. Simple foods in moderate quantity, at proper times, will do much to restore and maintain health. Pastries, French cooking, iced desserts, midnight suppers, irregular meals and gluttony, are absolutely inimical to continued health.

The physician of to-day must remember what rationalism in the practice of medicine demands of him. He must remember the ancient master's aphorism, and still further remember that before all remedies he must place the proper conduct of the patient—his habits—his diet—and the fit ordering of all the conditions surrounding him. He must remember that "the laws of Nature are the words of God," and that it is his duty to direct and enjoin that His laws be kept inviolate. He must remember that the "elixir of life" does not lie in pills and potions; but that the length of a man's life depends upon the sort of treatment the man's body receives at his own hands. Good habits, good morals, a happy and contented home and a clear conscience, are better than all the elixirs the doctors have or will ever discover.

Over the door of one of the most famous operating rooms in Europe the following inscription is engraved: "I dress the wound; God heals it." The "vis medicatrix naturæ" is the science of truth as applied to surgery or medicine. The public must be taught the truths of medicine and frankly told its limitations. An intelligent patient knows or should know that when he has pneumonia or typhoid fever, or, with few exceptions, almost any form of disease, that no physician in the world can cure the disease with medicine. All that the physician can do is to surround him with conditions most favorable for the recovery, and the public must know that the physician cannot cure, that the surgeon cannot heal, that not in the pills, powders, the caustics, the laying on of hands, the salves, the dressings, or the knife is the healing, curing power, but in the Almighty Hand guiding Nature. Civilization still has the problems of death and disease to contend with. There are some who apparently believe that we shall solve all the mysteries of life, but they will be very much disappointed. Let us hope that the twentieth century will witness great improvements in the prevention of disease and the postponement of death; this will be accomplished by increasing the public faith in the teachings and the advice of the medical profession in matters relating to hygiene and to the prevention of disease.

805 N. Charles street.

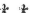

SPRING HOUSE-CLEANING.

By Dr. Harvey B. Bashore,
Author of " Outlines of Rural Hygiene."

ONE of the sanitary customs which we have gotten from our ancestors is the spring house-cleaning, and a vast agent for good it is, the more we understand the science and facts of sanitation.

How we got in the way of a general cleaning in the spring no one seems to know, unless it is the fact that Nature seems to be bent on the same object at this time of the year. James Lane Allen brings this out in his delightful book known as the "Kentucky Cardinal," and I think it will interest all sanitarians to hear his account.

"But most I love to see Nature do her spring house-cleaning, with the rain clouds for her water buckets and the winds for her brooms. What an amount of drenching and sweeping she can do in a day! How she dashes pailful and pailful into every corner, till the whole earth is as clean as a new floor!

Another day she attacks the piles of dead leaves, where lain since last October and scatters them in a trice, so that every cranny may be sunned and aired. Or, grasping her long brooms by the handles, she will go into the woods and beat the icicles off the big trees as a housewife would brush down cobwebs; so that the released limbs straighten out like a man who has gotten out of debt, to almost say to you joyfully, "Now, then, we are right again!" This done, she begins to hang out soft new curtains at the forest windows, and spread over the floor a new carpet of an emeral loveliness such as no mortal looms could ever weave."

Nature does her work well, and what we ought to do is to assist her, in and about our own dwellings.

The cleaning of the house proper should be thorough and effective, and should extend from roof to cellar. Soap and water, sunshine, paint and white-wash are the agents to work with, and the greatest of these is sunshine. The modern house with hard wood finish, waxed floors and a few rugs, is without any doubt more sanitary than the old-fashioned one with soft, thick carpets, yet personally I love the carpeted floors better. When I see a rug on a floor I always think of "Uncle Josh" in the "Old Homestead," and feel like stretching the rug to make it fit the room.

The dry cemented cellar is getting to be pretty general, and is one of the great sanitary improvements of the last twenty-five years, for it can be so readily cleaned, and when cleaned and white-washed it approaches the ideal.

The old-time cellar, if it is dry and well drained, can be kept in fine shape by scraping and plenty of white-wash. I lately saw an old cellar of this sort used for the last 170 years, yet to-day it is sweet and clean. This, too, is an historical cellar, for it was originally the dungeon of Cressap's Fort, which was built during the boundary trobles between Pennsylvania and Maryland.

As much of the wood-work as possible should be repolished or repainted, and roof gutters and spouting should be gone over, for nothing does so much harm to a house as a leaking spout.

The plumbing should be overhauled, re-polished, and exposed lead or iron pipes re-coated with aluminum paint or something else as good. The bath room should be re-papered or repainted, if possible. In the country, where the dry pail system is used, the pails should be exposed to the sun for several days, then scraped and repainted inside and out.

All exposed ground about the house should be dug or raked, unless it is a lawn; soil around a habitation, if not dug over every year and exposed to the sun, becomes, sooner or later, sodden with filth; especially is this so about country houses where the soil is used to absorb the slop waters.

The kitchen sink should be carefully washed out with a hot saturated solution of washing soda; it is astonishing how quickly this will remove the accumulated fat.

Nothing should be allowed to collect from year to year, but every spring all waste should be sorted—if not kept sorted during collection—and disposed in its proper way. Ashes for filling and walks, bottles, tin cans, old rubber, etc., to the junk dealers, old paper and rags to the fire. In fact every-thing which cannot be disposed in any other way satisfactorily and is combustible, should be destroyed by fire; especially is this true of all articles likely to carry contagion, for fire is the greatest disinfectant we have.

THE TONGUE IN HEALTH AND DISEASE.

J. Muller has re-examined this subject. Considering the regularity with which the tongue is inspected, it is not a little remark-able that so little positive knowledge is en-tertained. Müller reminds us that the coat-ing, of variable thickness, on the middle of the dorsum of the tongues of most people in middle life is made up of the filiform pa-pillæ. It is, therefore, a fur rather than a deposit, as is so often imagined. The longer the papillæ, and the thicker the epithelium, the less does the red color of the tongue show, and the whiter or yellower is the sur-face. At times the papillæ reach excessive size, the epithelium is horny, and contains dark pigment, hence the name "black hair-tongue." As the epithelium becomes loos-ened and infiltrated by bacterial growth, the cloudy, yellowish-gray appearance is exag-gerated, and may be further altered by in-gesta, such as berries, chocolate, red wine, etc. Milk causes a white appearance by rea-son of the fat globules. The desquamation of cells and the accumulation of food rem-nants, mucus, leucocytes, and bacteria cause a coat that can be removed by brushing or scraping. In health this sort of coat never becomes excessive because it is removed in the taking of food, but in the morning is apparent on account of the resting of the tongue overnight. The author recommends for obtaining an idea of the activity of epithelial growth in the mouth the examina-tion of sediment obtained by chewing bits of sponge, and squeezing out the fluid (bits of rubber tubing are more convenient). In the morning the sediment may equal one-fifth the column of fluid. There is a marked difference in the growth of the papillæ at different periods of life, with great individ-ual differences at all ages. In old age the atrophy of the papillæ gives the tongue a glistening appearance, as if varnished. The author thinks there is a parallel between the development of the papillæ and of other epi-dermoid tissues, as of the skin. He denies a relation between coated tongue and local diseases of the mouth and throat, except when the former are so severe as to interfere with swallowing. As regards disease, he found a coated tongue by far most fre-quently in cases of acute disease, whether primarily affecting the digestive tract or not. It is less frequent in chronic digestive diseases, and in chronic gastritis does not occur to so great a degree as in healthy people in middle life. The microscopical examination of the coating shows usually a more rich and diverse material than in health, but in general no essential differences exist. The leucocytes appear to be numerous in cancer of the stomach and tuberculosis. The claim of Bernabei, that specific bacteria can be cultivated in certain diseases from the coating on the tongue, the author thinks worth further investigation. The disappearance of a coating of acute origin is a good sign, because it indicates, usually, that food is properly taken. In chronic diseases the disappearances may have another meaning. The best way of keeping down the coating is by chewing hard food, especially bread. For abnormal coating the use of a soft toothbrush is best.—*Münchener med. Wochenschrift*, 1900, No. 33; *Am. Journ. Med. Sciences.*

THE COST OF ALCOHOLISM IN PARIS.

The Paris *Journal de Médicine,* writing on the waste caused by alcoholism, points out that hospital statistics alone show that inveterate drunkenness in itself costs the city at least 2,000,000 francs per annum, through the lost labor of the individual and through the expenses connected with hospital treatment.

RESTORATIVE.—A man dropped his wig on the street, and a boy who was following close behind the loser picked it up and handed it to him. "Thanks, my boy," said the owner of the wig. "You are the first genuine hair restorer I have ever seen."

DIETS FOR EVERY DAY USE.

By J. Warren Achorn, M.D.
Boston.

GENERAL RULES.

ONE should be temperate in the adoption and use of foods named in the diet selected. Change in any one particular is change enough for that day.

It is too much to expect that regulation of the food will promptly revolutionize the habits of a life time.

These diets must be carefully and intelligently followed, if the results claimed for them and expected are to be realized.

No attempt has been made to furnish an elaborate bill of fare.

Health and good digestion are the first considerations sought.

Food known to disagree should be avoided. It may agree later on.

Eating too continuously of one food to the exclusion of others of the same class should be avoided.

Meats should be stewed, roasted or broiled. Fish should be boiled, broiled or baked.

Fried food in any form, especially fried fat, is indigestible.

The best time to drink water or other liquids in amount, is the same in every case —on rising, an hour and a half before meals and half an hour before retiring.

Not more than two glasses should be taken at any meal and but one when soup is indulged in. Drink slowly.

Water should be taken at the close of a meal, milk during the meal: sip after swallowing food. The mouth should be rinsed after drinking milk.

Only liquids should be taken between meals, unless fruit or other food is required for constipation or nourishment.

Constipation must be avoided: it is intimately related to all chronic disorders for which regulation of the foods is indicated.

Properly the heartiest meal should be eight hours away from sleep. If one is at work, however, this rule should not be too strictly adhered to.

DIET IN BILIOUSNESS.

(Copyright.)

TAKE a glass of hot water on rising; add salt, lemon juice, or a teaspoonful of aromatic spirits of ammonia.

BREAKFAST: *Cereals*—Cestus, "cooked gluten," cornmeal mush, oatmeal mush, barley gruel.

Cracked wheat, rolled oats, rolled rye, hulled corn, rice. Eat with cream, Pasteurized milk, butter, salt or prune juice.

Meats (red)—Mutton chops, rump or round steak.

Fish (fine fibered)—Chicken halibut, flounder, smelt, sheepshead, carp; any lake or brook fish—boiled or broiled.

Eggs—Poached, boiled; whites of eggs.

Breads — Gluten, whole wheat, pulled bread, soup sticks, zweizback. Butter in moderation; prune marmalade.

Fruits (f r e s h r i p e)—Apples, peaches, white grapes, pears, strawberries, other berries, cherries, oranges, pineapple juice, canteloupe, other melons.

Drinks—Water, cornmeal water, hot; coffee, clear.

A. M. BETWEEN MEALS: Buttermilk, whey, malted milk, Mellin's food in hot water.

LUNCH: *Meats* (red)—Roast mutton, roast beef, stewed beef, venison, (white) calf's sweet breads; stewed or roasted chicken, turkey, capon, squab; game birds, not too *game*— grouse, pheasant, quail.

Any fish mentioned.

NOTES.

A glass of hot water with a tablespoonful or more of Mellen's Food added makes a good morning drink.

The oil in coffee causes billiousness with some. this is especially true if cream (another oil or fat) and sugar are added.

Coffee is to be preferred to tea, if there is much flatulency, and cocoa to either if there is much acidity, provided the fat of cocoa is well borne.

Strong tea or coffee should be avoided when meat is eaten, especially red meat.

Morbid sensibility of the stomach precludes the use of coffee: the same is true of oils or fats in excess, vegetables, certain cereals and fruits— they may irritate a sensitive stomach and cause excessive secretion.

Dry toast or rusks should be eaten with mushes.

Two slices of bread at a meal should be sufficient.

Dark breads are best, but they have to be watched as they cause indigestion. Bread made from fine, white flour, *may* have to be used. Bread should be toasted and redried.

Farinaceous foods in bilious dyspepsia cause less trouble than meat, especially fat meat; with some people, however, starchy food causes biliousness.

Cracked wheat ferments more readily than dry toast, and so does oatmeal. Hulled corn, corn-meal, and rice are among the best digested cereals.

Red meats. eggs, potatoes, certain fruits, and green vegetables. gluten. oatmeal and concentrated sweets, excite the stomach and may cause excessive secretion. Experience in individual cases should determine, with fair certainty, which of these foods is irritant.

The *best* concentrated sweets are clear honey and pure maple-sugar.

White meats, fine fibered fish, the whites of eggs, rice, cornmeal, hulled corn and wheaten grits are non-stimulating foods.

Gluten, somatose, and nutrose are nitrogenous foods—good substitutes for meat. but they have to be eaten (except gluten) in limited amount, as they disorder digestion.

Acid fruit in quantity delays the digestion of starchy food; soda added to stewed fruit, if acid, saves the need of much sugar.

Foods containing sufficient quantity of fat, such as oatmeal, cornmeal, hulled corn, etc., are to be preferred to *free* fat or meat fat.

Meats in excess, except in individual cases, go badly in this form of indigestion, especially with the rheumatic and gouty.

Lemon juice helps the digestion of fish in atonic conditions of the stomach.

The tongue is an index of the secretions of the *mouth;* it also reflects with fair accuracy the condition of the digestive tract. A *brown,* furred tongue indicates acute dyspepsia or chronic bil-

Any bread mentioned; crusts, Bent's water crackers.

Fruits—Unsweetened apple jelly.

Drinks—Koumiss, matzoon.

Desserts—Popped corn.

P. M. BETWEEN MEALS: Weak lemonade; lime juice in water, slightly sweetened, with a lithia tablet added; raspberry juice.

DINNER: *Soups*—Clear vegetable broths; new corn or split pea soup.

Purees of—Beans, peas, served with *croutons*, pearl barley or okra. Any fish mentioned. The soft part of stewed oysters.

Any meat mentioned. Meat jelly.

Vegetables—Baked potato once a day, or none. Dandelion greens, beet tops, spinach, tender string beans, boiled carrots minced, asparagus, water cresses, plain lettuce, squash, pumpkin, macaroni with tomato, rice with fig sauce.

Any bread mentioned.

Any fruit mentioned. Baked pears, baked ripe bananas.

Any drink mentioned. Pasteurized milk cut with lime water or vichy. Weak tea.

Desserts—Calf's foot jelly, baked custard, blanc mange, sago or tapioca pudding, junket, cottage cheese. Rice with raisins or fig sauce. Rice cooked with peaches, stewed apples with strained cranberr' or cooked with raisins.

9 P. M. Buttermilk, water; an apple.

---

iousness of a septic character; a *yellow*, coated tongue points to an inactive state of the stomach and intestines, a *white* tongue to feverish conditions. A *broad*, pale, flabby tongue, teeth indented, shows a weakened state of the digestive tract and of the whole system. The stomach does poor work in this condition—stimulating food is indicated. A *red* tongue, pointed, with strawberry papillæ showing, denotes an irritated condition of the stomach,—soothing food should be eaten. A *fissured* tongue generally goes with some disease of the mucous membrane of the stomach or with hyper-acidity.

A furred tongue should be scraped daily and a cleansing mouth wash used before meals. Dry food and fresh fruit help to keep the tongue clean. Headache and a bad taste in the mouth show that the products of indigestion are being absorbed into the system.

Gastric fermentation, (not intestinal) is quickest benefited by the exclusive use for a time of meat, toast and lemon juice. If fever and headache are present, only liquids should be taken at first.

Hot water before meals, with a pinch of Carlsbad salts added, helps to sweeten things and stimulates the liver cells.

A diet entirely of fruit for a few days, if it agrees, cleans a bilious tongue and starts up a sluggish liver.

The first stage of acute biliousness is usually evident by a craving appetite, due to stomach irritation; this is followe' by thirst or nausea. *Spring* biliousness is due to winter foods continued into the spring.

The excessive use of fats, sugar, (and starchy food in some cases) is a cause of biliousness; so also is over-eating, or indulging in food hard to digest.

A poor appetite in biliousness is often the result of slow circulation through the stomach, due to "liver torpor." A heavily coated tongue may cause loss of appetite.

Meals in biliousness should be five (or more) hours apart, on account of slow digestion.

A dry diet is indicated if the stomach splashes —one glass of water at the close of the meal may be permitted; a dry, sterile diet should be followed if the bowels are greatly distended and the stools offensive.

Offensive movements indicate putrefaction of material in the large intestine. Flushing the lower bowel twice or three times a week helps this.

In biliousness with marked intestinal symptoms, eggs are contra indicated. They putrefy more easily than meat and are a cause of gases. The fat and iron in the yolk of eggs nauseate many. Nausea is an evidence of irritation of the stomach. The practice of eating eggs regularly every morning should be condemned for those, at least, who are subject to attacks of indigestion.

Butter is a good fat. Cream, cut one-half with hot water, adding five drops of Liq. Amm. Acetatis to each tablespoonful, is usually well borne.

The nervous and thin should take all the fat they can digest—several kinds. One fat free, such as olive oil, will not *fatten*—best taken on an empty stomach between meals.

Vegetables and fruit will have to be eschewed for a time if there is much flatulency. Vegetables

BLEACHING TEETH.

A DIRTY-LOOKING, blue-tinged tooth in the front of the mouth is so disfiguring to the appearance that the subject seeks the aid of the dental surgeon. Such teeth are, too often, recklessly and ruthlessly excised, and an artificial crown attached to the root. The result is brilliant as far as appearance is concerned, and does not call for any great amount of labor on the part of the operator, but, at the same time, it is a question whether the true conservative treatment would not rather be to render the tooth presentable by bleaching and subsequent filling, which is practicable in a large number of cases. The most common cause of staining is the death of the pulp and the infiltration of the dentinal tubules with the products of its decomposition. Another cause, which is much more common than it should be, is the insertion of amalgam stoppings, especially those containing copper, and this stain, unfortunately, appears to be indelible. Two general classes of substances have been introduced for bleaching teeth—oxidizing agents, such as chlorine compounds and peroxide of hydrogen, and reducing agents, as sulphurous acid. The treatment by means of peroxide of hydrogen is extremely simple, and gives good results; but it appears from recent experiments by Dr. Miller, of Berlin, that this preparation acts upon the dentine, remov-

ing the organic matter. Sulphurous acid is also open to a similar objection, in that its prolonged use will dissolve out the lime salts. Generally the chief chemical used for bleaching teeth is chlorine, or some of its compounds. Where chlorine is used, steel instruments are inadmissible, as the salts of iron which would be formed would rapidly discolor the teeth. The instruments must be constructed of gold, platinum, or ivory. In order to prevent the chlorine from passing through the foramen at the end of the root, which would probably cause acute periostitis, the apical third of the pulp canal is solidly filled with gold. The tooth is isolated at the gums, the soft parts being protected by the adjustment of the rubber dam, and the tooth thoroughly dried by means of a warm-air syringe. The pulp-cavity is then washed thoroughly with ether, to remove any fatty material. Various preparations of chlorine have been recommended, but perhaps the simplest is freshly-made chlorine water, as suggested by Dr. Wright, of Richmond, U. S. A., which is forced into the pulp chamber by means of a syringe. Three or four sittings, of an hour each, are usually sufficient to remove the discoloration, when the tooth can be filled in the ordinary way.—*Lancet.*

Dr. Achorn's "diet list" in Bright's disease will be published in the April GAZETTE.

---

resist fermentation better than fruits. Asparagus, tomatoes, strawberries, and grapes should be avoided if the stomach is very sensitive, on account of their seeds and acids. Strawberries, unless perfectly fresh, should not be eaten, even if the *decayed part* can be smothered with cream and sugar.

Sweets cause biliousness by overtaxing the liver, interfering with the production of healthy bile that keeps the bowels aseptic.

Milk sugar is less likely to ferment than cane sugar.

If constipation attends biliousness, and cannot be regulated by the foods allowed, by oil or fruits taken between meals, or by a fourth meal of fruits alone, water by the rectum may be tried. This is better than purgatives or laxatives where the digestion is weak. Purgatives, persisted in,

aggravate indigestion by weakening the digestive tract. Horseback riding stimulates a lazy liver; it is the best sort of exercise for digestive disorders. Medical gymnastics, pool, etc., are good substitutes.

If fermentation or putrefaction are increased by the changes made, the diet is wrong. Putrefaction is more injurious than fermentation.

If the stomach is very weak an *intestinal diet* should be resorted to and the stomach given a rest; it should be concentrated, bland, finely divided, or liquid food, such as milk, if it agrees, Milk Food (Wampole's) meat juice, Mosquera's Beef Meal, Baker's Meat Jellies, calf's feet jelly, somatose, panopepton, finely ground cereals and cream. Rectal feeding may also be resorted to.

This diet meets very well the food indications in intestinal indigestion.

Department of Physiological Chemistry.

WITH SPECIAL REFERENCE TO DIETETICS AND NUTRITION IN GENERAL.

HEADS WITHOUT HAIR.

BALDNESS has become so common with the young, as well as the aged, that an almost equal division seems to have been reached between those who have, and those who have no hair on the top of their heads.

The time was, we are told, when the bald-headed man was looked upon as a curiosity, but, should the ratio in favor of bald heads continue to grow in the future as it has in the past, this stigma, if such it be, is likely to be shifted; the man with the full head of hair will become so scarce, doubtless he will be viewed as the missing link between man and the monkey.

Notwithstanding the frequency of baldness, the man with the full head of hair is still looked upon as the original, if not the genuine article, and the question so often asked, "Why do men become bald?" will not down. All sorts of reasons have been assigned for baldness, and as many remedies suggested for its cure or prevention, but in the face of all reasoning and prolific medication men continue to grow bald, and a head once completely bared from progressive baldness will ever thereafter refuse to grow hair.

Baldness, we venture to assert, is purely a question of nutrition. If the hair were properly nourished, men would not become bald. The hair, as every one knows, is nourished by the blood, as every other part of the body, and if its blood supply were not diminished, or cut off, men would continue to wear hair just the same as they continue to wear fingers and toes. Diminish or cut off the blood supply to the fingers and toes, and they will fall off, too.

If we examine the scalp of one who has a full head of hair, we find a thick integument, plentifully supplied with loose, cellular tissue between it and the skull, thus giving the blood vessels a fair chance to supply nutriment to the hair, but if we examine the scalp of a bald head we find, instead, a thin integument, almost as thin as parchment in some cases, and closely adhering to the skull. The intervening loose, cellular tissue has been absorbed, the blood supply thereby greatly lessened and the hair, for want of nourishment, has departed.

We have said that baldness is purely a question of nutrition. This statement holds true in sudden baldness, resulting from some acute, lingering fever, typhoid for instance, as it does in progressive baldness. The scalp, however, in sudden baldness from severe sickness, has the advantage of having undergone but little or no anatomical change. The conditions for the growth of hair still remain, and, with a fresh supply of healthy blood, a new crop is soon started. But in progressive baldness the scalp undergoes a very great change. The conditions for the growth of hair are very much impaired, if not entirely wanting, and the prospect for a new growth of hair in such cases is very remote indeed.

Many vile practises, we admit, have much to do with hastening baldness, and not one that we know of is more mischievous in this direction than the practice of frequent shampooing the head. This is practised, it is claimed, to remove dandruff. What is dandruff? Ordinary dandruff is nothing more nor less than epithelial scales, which are constantly being shed from the skin, over the entire surface of the body, and, with the ordinary hair brush, they can be removed from the head as soon as they are ready to be displaced. Any undue force made to remove these epithelial scales before their time to drop, such as frequent shampooing the head, leaves the scalp sensitive, tender portions of the hair more or less exposed, and facilitates baldness.

And this is by no means the worst feature connected with frequent shampooing the head. By this practice all the natural oil is removed from the hair, leaving it harsh and dry, and, in order that it may be combed, the barber thrusts his finger in an open-mouthed jar, brings it out loaded with grease, smears it over the palms of his two hands, and proceeds to replace the natural oil of the hair with this vile grease. Is it not surprising that the hair does not instantly become sick or disgusted at such treatment, and drop from the man's head before he leaves the chair?

Much has been said concerning the injurious effects from wearing the hat too much, from tight hat-bands, from keeping the head too hot or too cold, but we doubt that any of these have much to do with the loss of the hair. The frequent applications of medicines to the hair, which is so universally practised, however, is all wrong. Almost every druggist's show-case is covered with hair lotions, hair growers, hair restorers and similar preparations. Unless there is actual disease of the scalp, medicines have no business on the top of a man's head.

From what has been said it will be rightly inferred that we have little or no faith in any treatment to restore hair to a head that has become progressively bald, and that all effort should be directed in the line of prevention. Unless there is some disease of the scalp, every child starts out in the world with a full head of hair, and there is no sane reason why, under proper management, he may not continue to wear hair till the end of his days.

The chief objects to bear in mind are the conditions of the scalp requisite for the growth of hair, and then make the effort to perpetuate, and, if possible, improve these conditions. A thick integument, loosely adhering to the skull, plentifully supplied with intervening cellular tissue, so that the blood may have free access to the roots of the hair, are the requisite conditions, and these can be maintained, or restored, if only partially lost by massage. We mean by massage a gentle but firm manipulation of the scalp over the entire head, at least once a day, preferably, just before retiring. This manipulation, or massaging the scalp, is accomplished by placing the fingers of the two hands at different places, on opposite sides of the head, and pushing the scalp, with a lifting motion, to and fro over the skull. This should be continued, by changing the fingers from place to place, until the entire scalp has been massaged. By this procedure the scalp will be kept loose, encourage the deposit of fatty tissue between it and the skull, and thereby facilitate the flow of blood to nourish the hair.

There is but little or no danger from carrying this treatment too far. We have in mind one young man, with a scant head of hair, who persevered in this treatment until his scalp become so loose that he could move it about over his head to the extent of much resembling the shifting of a wig. and, with it, the hair grew as thick and luxurious as that upon a dog's back.

The question is frequently asked why women do not become bald like men. Women, as a rule, are better supplied with adipose, fatty tissue, under their scalps, as well as under the skin over their entire bodies, than men, and this is doubtless one reason why they do not so readily lose their hair. But the chief reason is, we fancy that women, unconsciously, practice everyday the treatment here given whenever they comb their hair. Holding their long and heavy tresses in every conceivable direction above their heads, when running the comb through them, has the tendency, much the same as massage, of lifting the scalp loose, encouraging the deposit of fat between it and the skull and thus facilitating the nourishment of the hair.

Much more could be said on this subject, but sufficient has been said, we think, to encourage thought and practice in the right direction.

THE MEDICAL PRESS ON DIET.

A MAJORITY of the medical journals of the day are giving more than usual attention to the subject of dietetics, but that the most of them feel a little uncertain on their feet when they essay to talk on the subject is quite evident from the tenor of a recent editorial in our bright contemporary, the *Medical Council* of Philadelphia. After making the statement that the subject of diet "may truly be said to be a prize seed for the sprouting of crankism, and that few subjects are so hackneyed and done to death, *ad nauseam,* entire periodicals being devoted to the consideration of matters pertaining thereto," the editor proceeds to ask: "But how many physicians out of ten will agree on the question of diet, and why is there not more harmony on this subject?"

We would modestly inquire whether the question itself does not imply a general lack of thoroughness in studying the subject, and we would continue our catechism by asking how many physicians out of ten will agree on the subject of medicine, and why there is not greater harmony on this subject? If compelled to testify, the editor of the *Council* will agree with us that nutrition is quite as important as medication, and that if more than three hundred journals in the United States are "entirely" devoted to a discussion of the subject of medicine, there surely should be room for a few devoted "entirely" to that of dietetics. And when this editor feels constrained to apply such uncomplimentary epithets to the study of diet—"prize seed for sprouting crankism," "done to death, *ad nauseam*, etc.," we cannot help wondering how he himself found time or courage to wander outside the domain of medicine.

"The fact is," continues this editor, "that all our errors are based on a misconception, which is, that all stomachs, at certain ages and under given conditions, are alike. This is fallacy. Nowhere in the body do we notice greater divergence of peculiarity than in this very organ. Its digestive capacity for different things varies greatly, at times enormously, between individuals, often much so in the same person."

"Some stomachs are peculiarly affected by articles of food that are usually devoid of any noticeable effect. What one will retain with ease another rejects with unmistakable vigor. And we are now speaking of stomachs that otherwise give their owners no trouble—of normal stomachs. But the divergence becomes greater when this organ becomes diseased. Its vagaries are sometimes past comprehension. Why it is so is due to the simple enough reason that it is an extremely complex organ of heterogeneous parts and functions. We do not understand so many of it vagaries because it is impossible to do so. Years ago two of us made a series of experiments and observations upon this very subject, extending over a period of three years, and our harmonious conclusion was that, in most instances, man's stomach knew better what was good for it than a doctor could know. And the lesson from this is that we should confer with the patient about his diet before deciding what he had better take, leave alone or cautiously try."

This sounds well, but if we are not at sea in our anatomical reminiscences, it is into this same "extremely complex organ of heterogeneous parts" that we introduce medicines; and if it behaves so badly at times under the natural stimulus of food, what may we not expect of it under the influence of a foreign substance that is neither flesh, fish nor fowl, a medicine, which may be strictly necessary, but not intended for the sustenance and repair of either bone, nerve or flesh? We venture to say, and the editor of *Council* will, no doubt, admit that no two stomachs comport themselves exactly alike when they are presented with a given dose of medicine. Nor does the same stomach act the same at different periods, and under different conditions. Is this a valid reason for not studying medicine?

The popular idea of a busy doctor is that he has little or no time to eat, sleep, or say his prayers; and we cannot help thinking what a trying ordeal it must have been for the doctor, and his friend, to spend three weary years eating by rule, and for experimental purposes. What a relief it must have been when this period of dietetic penance finally ended!

"Milk is not," he continues, "one of the most easily digested of foods, though it usually causes no trouble. In some, however, it painfully and persistently disagrees. In others it causes constipation. When told by a patient that milk is not well borne, the statement should be taken carefully into consideration. Prepared foods are upon the market in almost numberless abundance, and nearly all of them the result of patient study and expensive research, for which it is claimed that they supply all kinds of nutriment, without digestive requirement, and ready for immediate absorption into the blood current, and yet they quite often disagree. Thus we have one patient, a consumptive, who promptly gets diarrhea if she takes a malt preparation (sweet) or any of the peptonized foods. We have a three-and-a-half year old child who would be poisoned every time she ate an egg. Another, a man, has only to take the smallest amount of buckwheat or eat oysters, and he gets as red as if poisoned by belladonna, and purges and vomits until worn out, being compelled to keep his bed twenty-four hours.

"These are instances. The reader can recall others from his own experience. They mean something, they convey a moral, and this should be heeded. It is, again, that stomachs differ, that hard and fast rules governing feeding are impracticable, because the parts to which they are to be applied are too complex and too varied to be fully understandable and amenable to fixed rules. The best practice in feeding or special dieting is to be governed: (1) By what is nourishing and should be good for the patient; (2) by what the patient's own experience tells him of his stomach peculiarities. When upon uncertain ground, always move tentatively. Give small amounts, well prepared, at sufficiently long intervals to be on the safe side.

"At no time is careful dieting as important as it is during the hot season. The necessary thing to remember is that food should be seasonable to insure good gastric function, and always as nearly applicable as possible in diseased states. Acute diseases of short duration, like tonsillitis, require little or no feeding. Rheumatics can eat fruit with impunity, nay, with benefit, though acid, because they enter the blood and remain there till eliminated as alkaline carbonates, in which form they leave the body. Ice-cream is good food for most fever cases, being refreshing and nourishing.

"Coffee is not only a stimulant, but it is also a food, and yet it is a rank poison to some. It is a routine practice to stop tea and coffee in sickness, without any regard to the necessities of the case. It is safe to follow the rule that customary stimulants should never be withdrawn except to depress the patient. Of what use is it to withdraw customary and needed coffee, thereby depressing the heart's action, which is then stimulated by whiskey or some other remedy, whereas it might not be required at all if the coffee had not been withdrawn? But these are merely straws that point the way —only suggestions to encourage consideration along lines bound to prove profitable alike to doctor and patient."

We have thus given the editor of the *Council* plenty of rope, and leave our readers to decide for themselves whether he has committed, logical, or, rather, dietetic suicide. He begins by saying, "give the stomach just what it craves; the doctor who would dictate its foods is an ass," or words to that effect. He ends with some quite sane advice as to the exercise of good judgment and great discretion in selecting a dietary for sick or well.

As to his reckless first advice, it, too, is based on a "fallacy." Even a normal and healthy stomach can only be trusted to dictate its own regimen when it can be made certain that its tastes have not been seriously perverted by early parental example and long-continued, wrong-feeding habits. It has been our observation that a large majority of so-called "normal stomachs" have been thus perverted, and should no more be turned loose at the loaded dinner table than we should turn our invalids loose in a well-stocked drug store, and tell them to help themselves. It is true some of our patients are doing this, but it is not with the direct sanction of their medical advisers. On the other hand, a goodly number of the most intelligent practitioners are rapidly getting out of the rut of promiscuous drug-prescribing. They are feeding better, and trusting more to nature. We are sure our friend, the editor of the *Medical Council*, is not one of the exceptions, but that he is in the front ranks of the body-guard of the van of progress. However, if we measure him by the editorial quoted, we are forced to the conclusion that either he has not read the GAZETTE with sufficient care and faith or that our work has not been as thorough and convincing as it ought to be.

But we do not despair, and a realization of our past short-comings shall spur us to increased diligence in the future. This editor will probably agree with us that of the three hundred and odd medical journals in this country the DIETETIC AND HYGIENIC GAZETTE is the only one that is strictly devoted to a scientific study of the laws of dietetics, hygiene and sanitation, *minus the fads and "crankisms."* It is hardly necessary to assure him that we are making encouraging headway in our effort to enlighten the profession in regard to the all-important subject of feeding the people, sick or well.

In the nearly seventeen years we have been in this field we have labored hard to make it unnecessary for the editor of the *Medical Council*, and his friends, to experiment on themselves in order to reach such an unsatisfactory conclusion as he reports, and the latter part of the editorial before us would indicate that he is under conviction. The field we are working in is as wide as the world. At first our class was very small. Doctors did not appreciate the subject. Most of them were, at that time, inclined to be pharmacomaniacs. They had

a childlike and almost limitless faith in drugs, and had a dozen "elegant" prescriptions with which to attack each symptom. Now, they are giving more attention to feeding, disinfecting and exercising their patients, relying on a few well-selected, scientifically prepared and thoroughly tested drugs, and leaving assisted Nature to do the rest. Especially are they dwelling on the potency, for good and evil, of diet. But they are not permitting their patients, with demoralized stomachs and morbid tastes, that have been confirmed by years of bad habits and worse examples, to dictate their own food and drink. They are beginning to study the underlying principles of dietetics with an interest they have never before experienced, and they are learning that the well man, or sick man, who is not regularly and constantly supplied with a fairly balanced and intelligently selected dietary is already, or is bound to, become a chronic invalid and a lifelong sufferer.

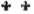

NOTES ON FOODS.

As a general rule, says Harvey Snyder, in *Sanitary Home*, too little attention is given to the subject of foods. We frequently eat those which are either unwholesome or not suited to the demands of the body. If more attention were given to the study of foods and less attention to the study of fads, we would all be better off health-wise and financially, except, perhaps, some doctors and undertakers.

A perfect food should supply all of the demands of the body. (1) Heat for warming the body and producing mechanical energy, and, (2) material for renewing worn-out tissues.

Some foods contain more heat-producing, and less tissue-renewing, materials than others. The potato, for example, is an excellent heat-producing food, but is deficient in the nutrients most necessary for vital purposes. The egg, on the other hand, is rich in the albumin or proteid nutrient—the tissue-renewing material. Neither food alone will supply all of the demands of the body, but jointly they are capable of doing so.

A great many of our foods are overestimated in value, while some are underestimated. Let us consider a few examples.

Cream and Skim-milk.—Cream is generally considered the most important part of milk, while skim-milk is considered of little account. What is cream? Its principal material is butter fat, a valuable heat-producing food, but deficient in nutrients essential for vital purposes and for the general repair of the body, Skim-milk contains these compounds. Of the two, skim-milk, strange as it may seem, will sustain life much longer than cream.

If a healthy child were fed entirely on cream, it would be starved for the want of proper bone, muscle, and tissue-forming food. I do not desire to underrate cream, but I do desire to give a different impression in regard to the value of skim-milk. More skim-milk should be used in the preparation of food. In bread-making it results in producing a more nutritious bread.

As to the use of milk it can be said that it is not economy to purchase meat, even at 15 cents a pound, in preference to milk at 5 or 6 cents a quart.

While milk comes nearest to being a perfect food, the mistake should not be made of confining a growing child too closely to a milk diet and not giving any solid food. A child's digestive apparatus is weakened if some solid food is not given at the proper stage of its development.

Prof. Davenport, of the Illinois Experiment Station, conducted some interesting experiments in feeding calves. While they are not human babies, these bovine babies nevertheless illustrated the point in question. All solid food was withheld, and nothing but milk was given. At first the calves grew, but, after a time, even with an abnormally large amount of milk, they failed to grow, became weak, were unable to stand, and finally died—even when fed a generous amount of pure, whole milk. They died simply because they were unable to get some solid food to develop the various organs. Some of the calves were fed a little solid food, after they were partially paralyzed, and they soon recovered.

Sugar is another article of food which deserves our attention. Many regard sugar simply as a food adjunct and not as a true food. This is a mistake; sugar is just as much of a food as flour. Every adult should use, on an average, two ounces per day of sugar—it is a part of his food, the amount for young children should, of course, be proportionally less. A child should not be deprived entirely of sugar, neither should he be allowed to eat excessive amounts. An ounce to an ounce and a half per day is not an excessive amount for a child of twelve, and three ounces per day for a hard working man is only a liberal allowance.

The small boy who comes in and asks for a slice of bread and butter, with lots of sugar, is simply expressing a want of Nature. I do not mean to say that the "lots" of sugar should be given. When children receive their normal amount of sugar regularly with their meals, there is not that natural craving for candy, which generally is an indication of mal-nutrition.

Rock candy is the least objectionable kind of candy, because of its purity. Pure sugar will not form crystals when any amount of glucose and other impurities are present.

Wheat and Graham Flour.—We hear a great deal about the comparative values of graham, entire wheat, and other kinds of flour, and we read in some of our popular magazines that white flour is all starch, and is not nutritious, and that entire wheat flour is preferable, etc. What about it? The fact that some one says so and so does not prove anything. Where is the proof? I do not wish to underrate the value of genuine entire wheat and graham flours, but what I wish to say is that most that has been written upon the subject is guess work, and that a good deal of it is nonsense. Entire wheat is valuable for persons of sedentary habits,

but it cannot be said to contain any more total digestible nutrients than good white
flour, made from our hard northwestern
wheat.

Many of the flours sold as whole wheat
flour and bread are not genuine. A mixture of dark-colored flour, with some products of the bran or shorts, is frequently
made to resemble entire wheat flour. Such
a combination, however, has less actual food
value than genuine high-grade white flour.

When bread is only 5 cents a loaf, it
might seem as if it were cheaper to buy the
bread than to make it at home. Let us consider this matter. · When a pound loaf of
bread is made, at least a quarter of a pound
of water and milk are added—so that a
pound loaf of bread is made from less than
three-quarters of a pound of flour, which
would ordinarily cost about a cent and a
half. Making the liberal allowance of a
cent for the milk and yeast, it will be seen
that the bread can be made at home (not
counting fuel or labor) for at least a half
as much as is charged at the baker's. It is
not economical for a family in moderate circumstances to buy baker's bread. You can
buy at least two barrels more of flour for
what it would cost at the bakery to get the
bread from one barrel of flour. Not only
is bakers' bread expensive, but that from
some bakers is liable to contain undesirable
materials, as alum and ammonium salts.

Breakfast Foods.—The question of breakfast foods is also an important one. In
place of the old time rolled oats and oatmeal
our grocers carry a large number of mixed
cereal products. The breakfast foods prepared from oats or wheat are of more value
as foods than those from other grains. A
great many of the breakfast foods are composed largely of corn, and while corn is a
good food it is not equal in food value to
oats or wheat, and there is no reason for
paying five times what the corn is worth.

In order to get the full value from oatmeal and rolled oats they should at least be
cooked four hours.

COCOA; ITS PROPER PREPARA-
TION.

THE consumption of cocoa is steadily increasing in the United Kingdom, and there
are indications, says Dr. Goodfellow, in
The Epicure, that it is gradually replacing
coffee as a breakfast beverage. And yet
how few people know how to prepare a cup
of good cocoa! In five cases out of six, a
considerable portion of the powder is left at
the bottom of the cup, and so wasted; while,
if properly prepared, the cup should be comparatively clean.

Cocoa differs materially in its composition and properties from tea or coffee. In
the latter we have always the tannic acid,
while in the former it is practically absent. With tea or coffee the beverage consists of the liquid portion of the mixture,
the insoluble matter, in the shape of leaves,
being left behind; but with cocoa we take
both the soluble and insoluble constituents.

Cocoa does not form a solution with water, but really a very fine physical mixture,
and the art of preparing cocoa lies in the
operations which produce so thorough a
mixture that it resembles an actual solution,
both in appearance and effect on the palate.

The following hints may be useful in this
direction:

(1) Start with a pure cocoa of undoubted quality and excellence of manufacture, which bears the name of a respectable
firm. This point is important, for there are
many cocoas on the market which have been
doctored, either by the addition of alkali,
starch, malt, kola, hops, etc.

The treatment of cocoa with alkali is to
render it more miscible with water, and,
therefore, a cocoa which seems to dissolve
very freely should be regarded with suspicion. If the cocoa thickens very much in
the cup, even though only a small quantity
is used, it probably points to an addition of
starch, which lowers the nutritive value of
the beverage. The addition of other constituents is unnecessary, and has no good
effect, but, on the contrary, may be positively harmful.

(2) With a little warm water or milk, thoroughly reduce the powder to a fine, thin batter, carefully crushing down all lumps.

(3) Pour on actual boiling water, as quickly as possible, stirring rapidly. It is necessary that the water should be really boiling; if just below the boiling point, a perfect mixture is not obtained. If milk be employed it should also be at the boiling point.

(4) If milk be added, it should be *hot*. If cold, the difference in temperature throws a sediment.

Cocoa prepared in this way forms, with water or milk, a perfect mixture, and drinks smoothly on the palate, leaving no sediment in the cup. It is a good plan to stir the contents of the cup now and again between the intervals of drinking.

If cocoa is to be prepared in large quantities for catering, the best plan is to bring the water to the boil, and then gradually add the powder to the boiling water, constantly stirring.

Many people who taste cocoa for the first time form a dislike to it, and in the majority of cases this is caused by improper preparation.

Pure cocoa is so fine a beverage that it is a matter for regret that in so many cases it is spoilt in the making, and I hope that the few hints that I have given may lead to an improvement in this respect.

THE DIGESTIVE GLANDS.

OF late years Prof. Pawlow, the head of a large laboratory in St. Petersburg, has devoted his whole energies, says the *New York Lancet*, to the study of the digestive glands, and in eight lectures, recently published, has summed up the work which he and his pupils have done, and which, though already set out in many communications to Russian journals and societies, has not, owing to its being in that language, become widely known. It is the most important treatise on the subject which has appeared for many years.

In order to obtain the effect of eating, without that of food in the stomach, the esophagus is severed and its two ends united, separately, to the wound in the neck. Then "mock-feeding" (Schien-fütterung) can be carried on, the food escaping through the lower end of the upper part, which excites gastric secretion. Dogs so treated have been kept alive and in good health for years by artificial feeding. To investigate the nervous arrangements of the process of digestion, elaborate sections of the vagi and sympathetic, at different levels, were performed, and the dogs again kept alive for a considerable time—weeks or even months. Although some of the experiments are carried out at the time of operation, in which case section of the cord below the medulla obviated the effect of shock, yet, for the most part, the animals are kept until all effect of operation has passed off, and no experiments on their secretion carried out until the general health is re-established. With such dogs, pure gastric juice is obtained, and the isolated, small stomach is found to reproduce exactly the condition obtaining at the time in the walls of the true stomach. This has been sufficiently established, by means of fistula into the true stomach, as well as into the artificial.

The results are very remarkable. Gastric juice is secreted in considerable quantity with "mock-feeding," and equally when the dog is shown food, but does not eat it. This "appetite secretion" is large in quantity, and as powerful in quality as that produced by true feeding. But this secretion does not last more than two hours, if no food is received in the stomach, although it can be reproduced by the same stimuli as before. On the other hand, if food be introduced into the stomach unknown to the dog, as when he is asleep, and without awakening appetite, the secretion is, from the first, small in quantity, but lasts for a much longer time. Natural secretion is the sum of both effects.

Different kinds of food vary much in

their power to excite secretion. In a dog whose esophagus is intact, meat, milk, and bread are, at different times, given in quantities representing the same equivalent of albuminoids. The meat produces a free flow, the milk a scanty flow, the bread a scanty flow of very powerful juice. The acidity of normal gastric juice does not vary with the pepsin, but remains the same unless neutralized by mucus. Food introduced unawares into the stomach also produces a variable secretion. Bits of meat excite secretion to a certain extent, but egg albumen, bread, and milk, not at all. All meat extracts produce the effect of meat. Mechanical irritation produces no secretion whatever. Experiments have proved that in meat there are some bodies already existing which provoke secretion, and that similar bodies may be produced in the other foods by the act of digestion itself, so that, once started, as by the "appetite secretion," the process is kept up.

Both stomach and pancreas are under the control of nerves. To both, the vagus certainly, and probably the sympathetic, too, acts as a secretory nerve. Inhibitory fibers likewise exist, which run in the vagus. "Appetite secretion" is excited through the vagus, and stops directly if, during the secretion, the vagus be severed. Contact secretion, from the food in the stomach, is likewise a reflex act, and is not due to any direct influence upon the peptic glands.

Pancreatic secretion, studied by a pancreatic fistula, shows similar variations in quantity and quality. It is little if at all affected by appetite. Its chief excitant is the acidity of the chyle, which acts reflexly through the duodenal mucous membrane. Starch excites pancreatic secretion no more than water, but fat has a marked effect. Yet the little pancreatic juice that is produced by feeding with bread has a much greater amylolytic power than that produced by meat feeding. Fat produces both a considerable amount of juice, and a juice that has strong fat-splitting powder.

ADVANTAGES OF STERILIZED MILK.

In discussing this subject at a recent meeting at the Academy of Medicine, Dr. A. D. Blackader said: The gastric digestion of infants is imperfect, in that microbes, which find their way into the digestive tract, are not as readily destroyed, and thus rendered harmless, as in the adult. This barrier to the entrance of bacteria into the system not being present, sterilization of the food material supplied becomes absolutely necessary. Cow's milk is never sterile, even under the most favorable circumstances. If it is obtained from the cow with as great attention to cleanliness as possible, and then immediately put on ice and kept at a low temperature until used, very few bacteria will be found in it. If these precautions are not taken, it may easily swarm with germs of various kinds. Some method of removing the bacteria is absolutely necessary. Pasteurization kills 99.8 per cent. of the microbes in full milk. It has been said that cream is more resistant to Pasteurization. Microbes that escape destruction are all of them spore-bearers. The older the milk, the more difficult it is to Pasteurize it.

Preservation of Milk.—Pasteurized milk will remain unchanged for a considerable length of time, especially if it is kept at a temperature just above 0° C. If it is not kept at this low temperature, however, fermentations are set up, and these disturb infantile digestion. This liability to fermentation also occurs even in sterilized milk that has been heated up to 100° F. While Pasteurization is quite as effective as sterilization, it has no more advantages than the other process.

Bacterial Destruction.—All the now known pathogenic bacteria succumb to Pasteurization. The bacillus of yellow fever, of typhoid fever and of diphtheria have been shown, by a number of experiments, to be destroyed. Tubercle bacillus was thought to be more resistant, but Smith showed that the bacilli of bovine tuberculosis are destroyed at 140° F. if proper precautions are taken. The pellicle which forms over milk protects them, so that this must be removed, or the milk stirred, during the heating process.

Changes Due to Heat.—When milk is heated certain changes, which interfere with its digestibility, take place. It is possible, also, that unheated milk may contain ferments which are an aid to digestion. In fresh milk the presence of a trypsin has been noted, which is destroyed by heating. In recent years it has been found that immunity to disease in animals is not conferred upon their young by direct heredity. If the young animals are suckled by a mother, who is immune to disease, they acquire that immunity. The substances in the milk which confer this immunity, however, are destroyed by a heat of 60° C. These disadvantages of heating milk are now well recognized. It is necessary to choose between the two evils of a milk containing germs, and one the digestibility of which has been impaired. It would seem, however, that the evils consequent upon Pasteurization are much less than those due to sterilization at a high temperature, and that practically none of the pathogenic bacilli are left alive. The changes induced in the milk by Pasteurization are not very great.

FOOD PRESERVATIVES.

THE following paper was published in the *Brooklyn Med. Journ.*, more than ten years since, and, judging from the numerous papers recently appearing in the various medical and health journals on the poisonous adulterations of food and drink, it is as appropriate to-day as when first published:

The use of preservatives for articles intended for food and drink is an important one, both for the manufacturer and the consumer. From a sanitary point of view, it is doubtful whether any of the preservatives ordinarily added to articles intended for human consumption ought to be encouraged. Laws exist in continental European coun-

tries prohibiting the use of certain of these preservative agents. Salicylic acid is prohibited by most of them, and the manufacturers are there beginning the use of benzoic acid, which is preservative in small amount, and is not easy to detect. After a discussion, at a convention of chemists at Speyer, Bavaria, on the 10th of September, 1888, the conclusion was reached that boric acid, as a preservative for foods, is to be regarded with caution. Sanitary authorities have generally spoken in stronger terms of the use of boric acid, and yet it enters into the composition of a large number of the preservatives in the market. Hirschsohn (*Chem. Ztg. Repertor.*, 1889, p. 46) gives a description of several different boroglycerides which he recommends for preserving foods. Boro-glycerin is prepared by heating glycerin with boric acid, in the proportion of 124 of the former to 190 of the latter. He also recommends sodium, calcium, and magnesium glycero-borates. These compounds are mostly tasteless, and quite soluble in water and alcohol.

Magnesium borate is recommended as a remedy in throat affections.

A. R. Rosen recommends the following method for preserving meats: Boric acid or its salts are dissolved in water and the solution is then frozen. The article to be preserved is then covered with this ice, with the result that the meats are preserved after the ice melts.

Dr. E. Polenske (*Kaiserlich Gesundheitsamt*, 1889, p. 198) has made an examination of ten commercial preservatives intended for meats. Three of the ten contained sulphurous acid or sulphites; two contained borax, and five boric acid; one each contained alum, arsenious oxide, salicylic acid, and free phosphoric acid; two contained glycerin, and two boro-glycerin; three contained niter, and six common salt. The one containing arsenious acid (1⅔ grains per quart) was sold under the name of "Stuttgart Preserving Fluid for Meats." (Translated.)

This was the only one actively poisonous, but several of the others were decidedly objectionable. Indeed, we should object to the addition of anything to our meats which is not a natural ingredient of food or cannot be converted into a compound natural to the human body.

FOOD BEFORE SLEEP.

MANY persons, though not actually sick, keep below par in strength and general tone, says Dr. Cathell, and I am of the opinion that fasting during the long interval between supper and breakfast, and especially the complete emptiness of the stomach during sleep, adds greatly to the amount of emaciation, sleeplessness, and general weakness we so often meet.

Physiology teaches that in the body there is a perpetual disintegration of tissue, sleeping or waking; it is, therefore, logical to believe that the supply of nourishment should be somewhat continuous, especially in those who are below par, if we would counteract their emaciation and lowered degree of vitality; and as bodily exercise is suspended during sleep, with wear and tear correspondingly diminished, while digestion, assimilation, and nutritive activity continue as usual, the food furnished during this period adds more than is destroyed, and increased weight and improved general vigor is the result.

All beings except man are governed by natural instinct, and every being with a stomach, except man, eats before sleep, and even the human infant, guided by the same instinct, sucks frequently day and night, and if its stomach is empty for any prolonged period it cries long and loud.

Digestion requires no interval of rest, and if the amount of food during the twenty-four hours is, in quantity and quality, not beyond the physiological limit, it makes no hurtful difference to the stomach how few or how short are the intervals between eating, but it does make a vast difference in the weak and emaciated one's welfare to have a modicum of food in the stomach during the time of sleep, that, instead of being consumed by bodily action, it may during the interval improve the lowered system; and I am fully satisfied that were the weakly, the emaciated, and the sleepless to nightly take a light lunch or meal of simple, nutritious food before going to bed, for a prolonged period, nine in ten of them would be thereby lifted into a better standard of health.

In my specialty (nose and throat) I encounter cases that, in addition to local and constitutional treatment, need an increase of nutritious food, and I find that by directing a bowl of bread and milk, or a mug of beer and a few biscuits, or a saucer of oatmeal and cream, before going to bed, for a few months, a surprising increase in weight, strength and general tone results; on the contrary, persons who are too stout or plethoric should follow an opposite course.

THE NUTRITIVE VALUE OF CERTAIN FOODS.

SPEAKING roughly, says London *Health*, a quart of oysters contains, on the average, about the same quantity of actual nutritive substance as a quart of milk, or a pound of very lean beef, or a pound and a half of fresh codfish, or two-thirds of a pound of bread. But while the weight of actual nutriment in the different quantities of food materials named is very nearly the same, the quality is widely different. That of the very lean meat or codfish consists mostly of what are called, in chemical language, protein compounds, or "flesh formers"— the substances which make blood, muscle, tendon, bone, brain, and other nitrogenous tissues. That of the bread contains but little of these, and consists chiefly of starch, with a little fat and other compounds, which serve the body as fuel, and supply it with heat and muscular power. The nutritive substance of oysters contains considerable amounts of both the flesh-forming and the more especially heat and force-giving ingredients. Oysters come nearer to milk than almost any other common food material as regards both the amounts and the relative proportions of nutrients and their food values, of equal weights of milk and oysters—*i. e.*, their values for supplying the body with material to build up its parts, repair its wastes, and furnish it with heat and energy would be pretty nearly the same.

MODIFICATION OF MILK.

DR. TOWNSEND sums up as follows:

1. The modification of cow's milk, with a knowledge of the percentages, is preferable to the guesswork feeding of infants.

2. Percentage feeding can be carried out by a milk laboratory, or by home modifications.

3. Milk laboratories are unavailable to many, by reason of their absence, or on account of the expense.

4. Laboratory modifications do not, in the experience of the writer, agree with infants as often as home modifications.

5. Laboratory modifications are necessarily subjected to more handling and transportations than home modifications.

6. Milk that is fresh, clean, and from cow's free from tuberculosis, is preferable uncooked, or, in other words, pasteurization and sterilization, although sometimes essential, are to be avoided if possible.

7. The method of home modification and of calculating percentages should, and can be, made extremely simple, and such modifications are sufficiently accurate and uniform.

8. The addition of cereals to the milk, in the form of barley or oatmeal water, is generally advisable after the seventh month, and is desirable before that age in some cases, as an aid to the digestibility of the milk.—*Boston Medical and Surgical Journal.*

REGENERATION OF THE ORGANS.

WITH many of the lower animals the regeneration of certain organs, either in part or entirely, says the *National Druggist*, is a common and well known phenomenon. The crawfish or crab, for instance, from which a claw has been torn away, will usually soon grow another in its place. This phenomenon is also seen, but to a certain extent only, with animals of higher organism, but the regenerative power is here always very limited.

No one has ever observed a paw, or even a single claw or toe, to grow on any higher animal which had lost a member of the sort; but while the bony skeleton and the muscles are but little adapted to regeneration, some of the internal organs are so in quite a high degree. Thus, for instance, several glands, after partial excision, are known to be regenerated, and some of them very rapidly. Rabbits, dogs and cats, from which as high as three-fourths of the liver have been removed, have, within the course of five weeks, reproduced the organ in its entirety. The same is true as to the thyroid, the suprarenal capsules, the pancreas, the ovaries, and the salivary glands, but always under the condition that a portion of the organ has been left intact, apparently no matter how small. The kidneys, in the dog at least, are another regenerative organ, which has been known to restore itself even after three-fourths of it have been removed. Very recently M. Vetzon has demonstrated that the monkey's brain is capable of at least partial regeneration. All these facts are of the highest interest, and may become of the highest value to the surgeon of the future.

TEA AND COFFEE AS A CAUSE OF INSOMNIA.

SIR JAMES SAWYER, Birmingham, Eng., lecturing recently on insomnia, said: "The effects of the consumption of tea and coffee in causing sleeplessness are well known.

This effect is so obvious that patients usually remedy it for themselves. As you well know, tea in the form of an infusion or of a decoction is generally used in civilized countries as the daily beverage of the people. Tea leaves contain an alkaloid which has been called theine, and coffee seeds contain caffeine, and theine and caffeine have been shown to be identical, and both these leaves and these seeds contain only principles. With regard to tea, what may be called its physical action appears to depend upon the joint action of its theine and of the volatile substance which tea leaves contain. What is called green tea is produced by drying the fresh leaves on a heated iron plate, until they become shrivelled; while black tea is manufactured by placing the leaves in heaps and allowing them so to lie while they undergo a kind of fermentation, after which they are dried. Green tea and black tea are powerful cerebral stimulants, exciting the mental faculties and the cerebral circulation, and tending to prevent sleep. Coffee, too, is a cerebral stimulant and antisoporific. It is sometimes used in need for these properties, to counteract the effects of opium and its derivatives, and of other narcotic poisons. Some people are extremely susceptible to the sleep-preventing effects of tea and coffee, others by use do not feel such effects, even when considerable quantities of the beverages are consumed. In all cases of bad sleeping you should make sure that tea or coffee is not taken to excess near bedtime.—*Medical Record.*

KOUMYSS AS A THERAPEUTIC AGENT.

C. Fleuroff has, during the past six years, noted the folllowing action of koumyss, or fermented mare's milk: (1) In anemia, neurasthenia, and hysteria, amelioration of general condition and all symptoms; (2) in some cases of hepatic and renal colic, increase of the pain; (3) in diseases of heart and blood-vessels, negative results; (4) generalized tuberculosis, negative results; (5) in incipient and early phthisis, improvement of appetite, of digestive functions and of the general condition, increase of weight, diminution of cough, amount of sputum, fever, etc.; (6) treatment by koumyss should be long continued; (7) diseases in which it is contraindicated are: Atheroma of blood-vessels, heart diseases, abdominal plethora, rheumatism and gout, cerebral hyperemia, the later stages of pulmonary phthisis, hemoptysis, hepatic and renal colic.—*Med. Record.*

BUTTER WITHOUT SALT OR OTHER CHEMICALS.

Mrs. C. F. Z. writes to the *National Druggist* that, during her recent visit to Europe, Germany and France, butter was put on the table perfectly fresh and guiltless of salt or other chemicals, and wishes to know how this can be effected. We are not advised, says the *Druggist*, as to the methods employed in Germany, but believe that the people who sell fresh butter in the market places bring in only sufficient butter to supply regular customers, with a slight excess for sale to transient customers. The oversupply is kept in cold cellars, or salted for cooking purposes. In Holland, the north of France, and probably in other parts, the following process is said to be employed: The butter, after churning, is washed and worked until nearly every particle of water has been removed. It is then formed into prisms or blocks, which are at once covered with a layer of simple syrup, applied hot, by means of flat pencils, made especially for the purpose. A strong syrup is made with white sugar, and, while still hot, it is applied to the surface as stated. The heat melts a very thin layer of the butter, in cooling, which forms with the syrup a sort of hermetical envelope, which protects it from the rancidifying effects of the air for some time, especially when kept in cool, dark cellars. Butter thus preserved is said to preserve a flavor and fragrance quite unknown to the salted product, especially when the latter is kept on ice, which quickly destroys the aroma.

A COLOR NUT FOR PSYCHICS TO CRACK.*

WHEN intently listening to certain, but by no means all, eminent speakers, and to a few operatic singers of great renown, I have, for some years past, distinctly detected, or rather have involuntarily become conscious of, an emanation of color from the head of the speaker or singer with each distinct tone of the voice. The more impassioned the words and tones, the more intense the color, and the larger the visible aureole or color area. The color has thus far been limited, with a few exceptions, to a transparent and ethereal but decided blue. It emanates suddenly with each explosion of sound, passes upward like a thin cloud of smoke, and fades like a swiftly dissolving view. I noticed it for the first time while listening to Prof. Felix Adler, later on when listening to Colonel Ingersoll, faintly over the head of William Winter; again quite distinctly in case of General Sherman and General Horace Porter, faintly in case of some other public speakers, including Anna Dickinson, Helen Potter, the elocutionist, and some eminent divines, but not at all in case of President Cleveland and some other equally prominent public men.

In cases of singers, the most noted instances I can recall are the De Reszke brothers, Jean and Edward; Mme. Emma Eames, Lilli Lehmann, Mme. Albani, Vogel, and Gudehus.

In case of Mme. Lehmann the blue color verged towards a liquid green, and with Albani it was a pale sheen of silver vapor. In case of Vogel, the tenor, the aureole was an evanescent and very pale straw color.

* Extract from a letter in "Science."

In Mme Mielke the blue became a velvety purple or violet. Mme. Nordica emitted an aureole of pale, translucent gold; Emma Juch gives me the impression of a delicate and liquid pink, while Patti seemed to emit no distinguishing color, but rather a kaleidoscopic blending of many colors.

DENTAL CARIES AS A FACTOR OF DISEASE.

HUNDREDS and thousands of people are going about with rotten teeth, carrying with them so many small cesspools in their mouths, filled with fetid abominations of stinking food *débris,* with its teeming population of micro-organisms, and the resulting toxines as concomitants, and daily swallowing these putrefactions, and absorbing the pus. Many cases of septic disease are due to dental caries, and to that alone. Its effects may be manifested in multifarious ways. The author reports a case of persistent spasm of the right hand, of two years' duration, the diagnosis having been tetany or hysteria. Finally, two septic molar teeth were observed and removed, with the result that the spasm disappeared, not to return. Many of the so-called "scrofulous" scars of the neck have had their starting-point in carious teeth. The usual complaint by patients that fresh air will give them face-ache, is in most cases due to uncared-for carious teeth. Many laryngeal and pharyngeal troubles have their origin in the same cause. A man with a decayed molar hardly ever has a clean tongue. Insufficient mastication of food is another effect of dental caries. Teeth should be cleaned twice a day and always the last thing at night. A toothbrush should be considered as a conglomeration of toothpicks, and used accordingly. Children should never be allowed sweets or biscuits on going to bed. And the teeth should be inspected by a dentist from time to time as a matter of routine.—*Dr. J. R. Leesown, in N. Y. Medical Journal.*

RUSKIN'S VIEWS ON COOKERY.

JOHN RUSKIN, who, in the domain of letters, will doubtless ever be referred to as one of the foremost of those of the Victorian age, has endeared himself to the women of the English-speaking people from the evident interest he has taken in all that pertains to their domestic sphere. No man ever was truer, says *Food and Cookery*, to what was commendable in woman than was he, whether it was in laudation of the patronage of a Catherine de Medici, or in the superior roasting of mutton by Mary Stone, the servant in his father's house. That Mr. Ruskin knew something of cookery may be inferred from the charming manner in which he defends the term. "Cookery," he says, "means much tasting and no wasting; it means English thoroughness, French art, and Arabian hospitality; it means the knowledge of all the fruits and herbs, and balms and spices; it means carefulness, inventiveness, and watchfulness; the economy of our great-grandmothers, and the science of modern chemistry; in fine, that the wife is always to be a lady, or loaf-giver, and see that everybody has something nice to eat."

CARE OF THE TEETH.

AT a meeting in Berlin, last spring, of the German Association of American Dentists, the best means of preserving the teeth were discussed, and Dr. Richter, of Breslau, said: "We know that the whole method of correctly caring for the teeth can be expressed in two words—brush, soap. In these two things we have all that is needful for the preservation of the teeth. All the preparations not containing soap are not to be recommended, and, if they contain soap, all other ingredients are useless except for the purpose of making their taste agreeable. Among the soaps, the white castile soap of the English market is especially to be rec-ommended. A shower of tooth preparations has been thrown on the market, but very few of which are to be recommended. Testing the composition of them, we find that about 90 per cent. are not only unsuitable for their purpose, but that the greater part are actually harmful. All the preparations containing salicylic acid are, as the investigations of Fernier have shown, destructive to the teeth. He who will unceasingly preach to his patients to brush their teeth carefully shortly before bedtime, as a cleansing material to use castile soap, as a mouth wash a solution of oil of peppermint in water, and to cleanse the spaces between the teeth by careful use of a silken thread, will help them in preserving their teeth, and will win the gratitude of all who follow his advice. Tooth brushes should have bristles of unequal length, the latter to dislodge particles of food collected between the teeth. The same view is taken by Paschkis, who in his "Kosmetik," advises not to employ even the finest tooth-powder oftener than about once in two weeks.

SUNSHINE AND SLEEP.

SLEEPLESS people—and there are many in America—should court the sun. The very worst soporific is laudanum, and the very best is sunshine. Therefore, it is very plain that poor sleepers should pass as many hours as possible in the sunshine, and as few as possible in the shade. Many women are martyrs, and yet they do not know it. They wear veils, carry parasols, and do all they possibly can to keep off the potent influence which is intended to give them strength, beauty, and cheerfulness. The women of America are pale and delicate. They may be blooming and strong, and the sunlight will be a potent influence in this transformation.— *Pub. Health Journal.*

POTATOES IN DIABETES MELLITUS.

A. Mossé answers the mooted question as to whether potatoes may have a place in the dietary of the diabetic, in the affirmative, and cites two cases in which the wisdom of such addition to the fare was evidenced by a prompt decrease in the amount of sugar execreted in the urine. The potatoes should be given to the amount from two to three pounds daily, as a substitute for the whole or a part of the bread allowed. The cases which seem to respond best to such management are those of medium intensity and of the arthritic type.—*Klinisch-therapeutische Wochenschrift*, October 7, 1900.

THE FIRST "BILL OF FARE."

It is not generally known that the originator of the "bill of fare," says *Food and Cookery*, was Duke Henry of Brunswick, who was first observed, in the intervals of a banquet, to scan carefully a long strip of paper by the side of his place. When the curious guests ventured to inquire into the nature of his studies he explained that it was a sort of programme of the dishes he had commanded from the cook, to the intent that if some delicacy which especially appealed to him were marked for a late stage in the repast, he might carefully reserve his appetite for it. This, according to history, occurred in the year 1845. The menu card, from that moment, became an institution, and has since then attained a world-wide popularity.

COLD AIR ON DRAUGHT IN THE NEXT CENTURY.

During the coming century, says the *Ladies' Home Journ.*, hot or cold air will be turned on from spigots to regulate the temperature of a house, as we now turn on hot or cold water from spigots to regulate the temperature of the bath. Central plants will supply this cold air and heat to the city houses, in the same way as now our gas or electricity is furnished. Rising early to build the furnace fire will be a task of the olden times. Homes will have no chimneys, because no smoke will be created within their walls.

When the sun is pouring down its rays upon the ocean at noonday, none of them penetrate to a depth of over 200 feet. Could a diver descend below that depth, he would find himself shrouded in darkness as profound as though he were immersed in a sea of ink.

It is said that a physician in Richmond, Va., writes the age of the patient on his prescriptions. We cannot help wondering how large a female clientage he has.

Husband—I see they're advertising bargains in patent medicines at Kutt & Price's drug store.

Wife—Isn't that too aggravating? There isn't a thing the matter with any of us.—*Philadelphia Record.*

Department of Hygiene.

WITH SPECIAL REFERENCE TO STATE AND PREVENTIVE MEDICINE

THE SPITTING NUISANCE IN PUBLIC CONVEYANCES.

Now that the authorities have actually made an example of a spitter, in this city, the public is aroused to a more vivid sense of the importance of abating this universal nuisance. How best to practically accomplish this result is not a simple matter. It is not enough than an enforceable ordinance is in existence, and that the penalties are commensurate. The warning notices of the Health Board are conspicuously displayed, but evidently the spitting public does not yet take them as being seriously intended for any but confirmed consumptives, or "the other fellow." Some of the notoriously unobserving may never have noticed them at all. A wilful and brutal few, which, in a city of the size of New York, means a really large number, boldly sneer at these notices, looking upon them as dead-letter sentimentalisms, and continue their careless and evil habit. They flout the ordinance as a sanitary whim, that can be disregarded with perfect impunity. It will require a more rigorous and general resort to legal prerogatives and punitive examples to convince this class that the authorities are really in earnest.

Every one who has occasion to ride daily, in either the elevated or surface cars, is aware that if every infraction of the ordinance led to an arrest there would have to be wholesale additions to the police force on duty, and a multiplication of criminal courts all over the city. We presume it is about the same in all the other large cities. The remedy at hand may be legally competent, but it is not easy of application. Guards and conductors cannot possibly take the time to follow up complaints and provide evidence, nor can they even warn offending passengers on crowded trains. Even if they were so disposed, the work would be interdicted by their superiors, as seriously interfering with their regular and imperative duties.

For observant passengers to assume the offensive by making themselves complainants and constables, is not only disagreeable and distasteful, it is also often out of the question for them to break all their own engagements in order to follow the cases to court and supply the necessary evidence. In many cases, and these the very worst, it would involve personal abuse that would sometimes amount to personal danger, and, at the very least, would subject them to a degree of unenviable notoriety.

A friend of the writer, who uses the west side elevated roads from two to four times a day in conducting his business, has recently resolved himself into a missionary society for the suppression of spitting in the cars. His present stint is to warn at least one observed transgressor of the ordinance daily, calling his attention to the menace to public health, as well as to the penalty to which every offender subjects himself. He reports that his average experiences are not equal to a night at the opera or a supper at Sherry's, and, on the advice of his family physician, he has decided that his nervous system is not good for a greater strain than one passenger per day. That they may not be wholly unprepared, he has notified the members of his family that he may be brought home on a shutter at any hour of the day or night, and warns them to keep bandages, arnica, and a trained nurse ready to meet the emergency.

He should have vigorous co-operation;

and, to make this work more feasible and less trying to the nerves, he suggests that either the health authorities or some philanthropic individual, who is interested, shall provide a liberal supply of cards containing the essential features of the ordinance, the sanitary reasons for its enactment, and the penalties attached to its non-observance. It would be much easier, and less obtrusive, to hand one of these cards to an offender than to personally address him in the hearing of other passengers, and it would be much less likely to offend a bully to the fighting pitch. Will some one move in the matter?

COMPULSORY DISINFECTION IN TYPHOID FEVER.

THE discovery of the cause of an infectious disease, says the editor of the Boston *Med. and Surg. Journal*, should have as its principal result the prevention or limitation of that disease. This is the greatest benefit which such knowledge can bestow. In general our boards of health have been quick to take advantage of these advances in medical science. In typhoid fever, however, although our increased knowledge of the cause of the disease has led to much, it has led to less in the way of prophylaxis than should be the case.

Bacteriology has shown that the infectious material may be destroyed much more easily in some diseases than in others. For example, in diseases of which diphtheria is a type, the infectious material is so disseminated from the patient that it is impossible to prevent persons and objects in close proximity from becoming infected. In such a disease isolation of the patient must be carried out, but if this is done thoroughly there is little danger of the infection being carried to persons at a distance.

Typhoid fever is an illustration of a disease of a very different type. Here practically all the infectious material is in the urine and feces, which are received in a receptacle by the attendant. In that receptacle all the bacilli may be destroyed and almost all danger of infecting others easily removed, by the addition of some suitable disinfectant. If this is not done, articles of food or the water supply may be infected, and the disease thus carried to persons at a distance. Nearly every case of typhoid fever that occurs has been infected from the excreta of a typhoid patient. To prevent typhoid, therefore, we have only to disinfect the excreta of every case.

These simple facts are understood by all practitioners. We mention them here only to emphasize their simplicity as well as their importance. It is hard to see how the control of any disease could be more completely in the hands of man. We should, therefore, expect that our boards of health would endeavor to insist that disinfection should be carried out in every case. In reality, however, we find that practically not much is done by health officials in this direction. Circulars have been issued, notably one by the Boston Board of Health, giving valuable instructions and inculcating good advice. A few physicians and most of the hospitals insist on disinfection, but this is not enough to have any appreciable effect in stamping out the disease. To this end, not merely must the gospel of disinfection be preached, but some means must be sought and, if possible, be found for enforcing its precepts.

As a result of our indifference to these precautions, typhoid, though most distinctly a preventable disease and though less prevalent than formerly, is constantly present in the community. It attacks chiefly those who are in the prime of life, and most needed for the support of the family. It takes away from the community and from public life many of those who can least be spared. Even in modern warfare it destroys more than the enemy's bullets.

The constant presence of typhoid in our midst is probably the cause of our comparative indifference to the disease. Cholera is spread in a similar way, and is probably not a more serious disease; yet the very name is sufficient to make the public shudder, and boards of health do their utmost to prevent it spreading from the cases that have occurred. What are the precautions which are taken in cholera? The same which should be taken in typhoid, a disease of similar origin and spread in a similar way, namely, a thorough disinfection of the excreta from the patient and of everything which may be contaminated by them. As a result of these measures, cholera is stamped out of every civilized community, and only occasionally gets a foothold through the neglect of proper precautions.

At the time of an epidemic of typhoid our health officials frequently display very great thoroughness and energy in tracing out the source of infection. The reports of these investigations, and of the following up of each clew, afford as interesting reading as a detective story. They fill us with admiration for the skill of the investigators, whose efforts, unfortunately, are seldom of more than a restricted benefit. On account of the long incubation period of typhoid the cutting off of the discovered source is merely locking one door of the barn after the horse is stolen. Direct this same energy toward securing disinfection in all cases, and the disease will soon become extremely rare.

The remedy for this condition is to be found in legislation. The question of disinfection should no more be left to local boards of health in typhoid than it is in diphtheria and scarlet fever. There should be no local option in such matters. It is not sufficient that disinfection should be done in the city or town where we live. It is much more important that it should be done in the country places from which come our water and milk. Our Massachusetts law might be amended so as to require disinfection of the excreta in every case of typhoid within the borders of the Commonwealth. The public statutes now require disinfection after diphtheria, smallpox, scarlet fever, or any other infectious or contagious disease dangerous to the public health. In compliance with this law, our local boards of health carry out expensive formaldehyde disinfection of the infected rooms, although probably in those diseases the infection takes place in various ways. How much more important that disinfection should be done in typhoid, where every chance of infecting others may be removed by the destruction of all the bacilli!

The public statutes might require the local boards of health to send their agents or inspectors to every case of typhoid that is reported, to convince themselves that the dejecta are being properly disinfected. When necessary, disinfectants might be furnished free. If it is found that the directions of the board are not being complied with, they might have authority to remove the patient to a hospital, where disinfection will be done.

The initiative for any steps toward securing disinfection in typhoid fever must come from the medical profession. The medical societies ought to take up this question. It should be agitated and brought before the Legislature. Let us hope that very little of the twentieth century will have passed before measures will have been taken to stamp out the disease. May it no longer remain a reproach to our profession and to the intelligence of the age.

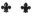

HYGIENE OF THE HANDKERCHIEF.

WE are making our pockets into nests of microbes by using handkerchiefs as we do—so we are warned by M. Vallin, in the *Revue d'Hygiene,* translated for *The Literary Digest.* What we ought to do, says M. Vallin, is to carry detachable india-rubber pockets and disinfect them at intervals, never using the same pocket both for clean and soiled handkerchiefs. The *Revue Scientifique,* in a notice of this article, says:

"The spittoon is without doubt very useful; . . . but it has been demonstrated that expectoration hurls out to a distance of a yard or more virulent vesicles that remain floating in air like little soap-bubbles. On the other hand, the handkerchief is a repugnant object, and the Japanese make fun of Europeans who carefully preserve in their pockets the execretions of their noses, mouths, throats, and bronchial tubes. . . M. Jorissenne remarks that the same handkerchief does service in wiping dust from the face or in removing sweat or tears from it; and in rubbing off a spot of dirt from one's clothes after moistening it with saliva; we shake it in token of joy, adieu, or admiration. . . .

"But, says M. Jorissenne, we do not limit ourselves to these eccentricities. You put your dirty handkerchief in one of your pockets, not always the same one, perhaps, with other articles. And ladies, who usually have only one pocket in a dress, thrust it in among the collection of small articles that seems to be a necessity to them. This is done by the most careful people, by those who are most easily disgusted, by the most intelligent men as well as by the foolish. Later, when it is thought necessary, the soiled handkerchief is replaced by another, a clean one, which you slide into the pocket that all your soiled handkerchiefs have previously occupied. You still regard it as a clean handkerchief when you take it out of your pocket, and you offer it to the first friend who is in need of it. Have you thought what a bacteriologist would say to this? This handkerchief that is supposed to be clean will soil your hands when you use it. Your pockets are receptacles where, in a warm, dark, and moist environment, there accumulate the germs collected by your handkerchiefs. Ah! it is not wonderful that the origin of diseases is so difficult to discover in the majority of ordinary cases.

"Our fathers' handkerchiefs were huge, many-colored cloths, that dried for weeks in their vast pockets before being washed. In the time of Louis XIV. everybody did not use them, and they were regarded as luxuries; sometimes there was only one to an en-

tire family. The Japanese are ahead of us; they have little paper handkerchiefs, made at home, and used only once; but after use they are thrown anywhere—on the floor, out of the window, in the garden, wherever it happens. These contaminated handkerchiefs are agents of propagation for a host of diseases, and so we may turn the laugh on the Japanese.

"Two forms of remedy present themselves; a small bag, easily opened and closed, or a similar pocket, impermeable and susceptible of being disinfected without rapid deterioration. India-rubber would be the most convenient material. The pocket could be fastened by a button or other device, whence it could be removed for disinfection. Clean handkerchiefs of small size, could be kept in a pocket not less clean, separate, and used only for this purpose. They could be contained or not in a protective case, and should be sufficient in number for a day's needs.

"M. Vallin observes that there is a great amount of truth in all this, with a certain degree of exaggeration. It will be a difficult task to alter our customs in this regard. Although the fashion has somewhat changed, let us not forget that, thirty years ago, ladies at a ball were accustomed to hold in their hands a lace handkerchief, worth several hundred francs. Was not this a singular idea—to exhibit such an object as a measure of the good taste and the wealth of the one who carried it, and who, besides, took good care not to use it? An ingenious critic of the period suggested that it be replaced by paper—that is to say, a bank note."—*Translations made for The Literary Digest.*

INGRAHAM enthusiastically recommends the use of heat in cases of pneumonia. He says there is but one agent that will produce the desired effect, and that is heat, the king of all remedies as regards results, immediate and permanent.

DIABETES MELLITUS—ITS ETIOLOGY AND TREATMENT.

By Adrian D. Williams, M.D.,
Brooklyn, N. Y.

During the past two years our progress in the successful medicinal treatment of diabetes mellitus has been far in advance of the information gained during the past decade regarding the pathological conditions which cause the disorder.

The presence of glucose in the urine is not always pathological. Glycosuria is induced by the ingestion and assimilation of large amounts of peptones and the excessive consumption of carbohydrates. Some believe that these dietetic errors, oft repeated, will cause true diabetes. The administration of such toxic agents as chloroform, morphine, amyl-nitrite, and phlorizin, frequently causes glycosuria, probably because they so act upon the hepatic cells as to lessen their glycogen retaining power. It has long been known that irritation of the floor of the fourth ventricle will cause the presence of sugar in the urine—due to increased flow of blood through the liver in consequence of the vasomotor paralysis. This would argue that the disease is a disturbance of the glycogenic function of the liver. Another class of cases (though more rare) is accompanied by lesions in the pancreas, causing certain circulatory changes in the organ. In these we find atrophy, cirrhosis, cancer, and the like. I recall a case which was severe and rapid in termination —the autopsy revealing a remarkable fibroid change in the pancreas—being practically a mass of fibrous tissue. What then is the relation of the pancreas to diabetes mellitus? The pancreas evidently serves some purpose aside from its digestive function. The pancreatic blood, hurried into the portal circulation, evidently contains some agent vital to the economy, and, like the ductless glands, possibly supplies an internal secretion. Extirpate the pancreas, and severe diabetes is apt to occur. Retain a small portion of the gland, and normal metabolism proceeds undisturbed. With so complete an analogy in the relation of thyroid to myxœdema, we are justified in this conclusion. Unhappily, however, the good results shown in myxœdema by thyroid treatment are not paralleled in diabetes by the administration of the pancreas, either in the form of the gland itself, its extract, or of transplanted grafts. Nor is it determined as to what percentage of cases of diabetes may arise from pancreatic lesions. The true cause of diabetes has eluded the research of the pathologist and clinician. We recognize that it is a disturbance of metabolism—more especially of glycogenesis. We know that the disease is associated with lesions of the cerebrospinal axis or of the pancreas; that it is more common in some localities than in others, shows a marked predilection for certain classes, and that heredity plays an important part. It has been claimed (though not shown) that it is co-existent in husband and wife. This, however, seems to be purely accidental. Bacteriologists have shown that the majority of diseases have as their fundamental cause some micro-organism. Sheridan and others argue the existence of a specific germ in diabetes mellitus. The writer inclines to that belief and an examination of the etiology of the disease favors this view. Many of the symptoms seem to be due to toxines in the blood, which have been elaborated by some undiscovered micro-organism. This theory is compatible with our present knowledge, though its exactness has not been established. The symptoms of the disease are familiar. The presence of sugar in the urine, abnormal thirst and hunger, loss of flesh, debility. We find secondary and complicating lesions in the lungs, kidneys, brain, and other organs, such as would be noticed in diseases having germ origin. Pulmonary tuberculosis frequently associated with diabetes is rapid and deadly in its course. The possibility of mixed infection thus suggests itself. We know that such cases always fare the worst. In that dread complication, diabetic coma, with all its protean manifestations, we know that it is a toxæmia due to some poisonous material circulating in the blood. Its exact nature is the subject of speculation. We are thus very much in the dark so far as our definite and exact knowledge of diabetes is concerned.

In the treatment of diabetes, we have, however, made decided progress. We have learned the value of hygiene, diet, and proper medication. Hydrotherapeutic measures aid in the elimination of toxic materials, keeping the skin and kidneys in good order. Proper surroundings and exercise give occupation to the patient's mind, exercising a good psychical influence. Massage is of value to tissues and stimulates the circulation. In the matter of diet, each case requires special decision. Some require a strict diet of fat meat; with others it is not permissible at all. Some patients should be permitted a diet of carbohydrates; with some we should exclude all starches and sugars, yet in other cases a small amount seems advisable. Hydrocarbons and proteids sometimes induce gastric intolerance; hence, the necessity of carefully watching each individual patient. As to the medicinal treatment, the writer begs to report several cases. Opium has been urged as of value in diabetes mellitus, and, while it would be folly to deny the value of codeine in many cases, still, under its administration, the continued use of the narcotic should be the last thing to which the practitioner resorts. We must admit that the greater number of morphine habitués are started in this enslaving habit by the incautious exhibition of opium. Having administred the narcotic, when the time comes to withdraw it, we are confronted with serious and even dangerous symptoms; thus, while we use opium, the fact should be borne in mind that the physician should carefully consider its extreme advisability before subjecting the patient to the treatment. In vigorous patients, especially those who are gouty or rheumatic, the use of alkalies has been followed by excellent results. The urine should, however, be carefully and continuously watched. Arsenic is mentioned by almost all authorities as being of value in diabetes, but the forms in

which arsenic has hitherto been obtainable have not been such as could be borne by the stomach where administered in large quantity and for a long continued period. Several months ago my attention was drawn to the use of arsenauro in diabetes. I was impressed by the statement made by Stucky that the combination of the bromides of gold and arsenic, as in arsenauro, gives rise to a chemical compound, wherein the original ingredients are robbed of some of their objectionable properties, while the therapeutic value of each is, to some extent, accentuated. We know that this holds true in the case of many drugs. We may, for instance, combine two griping cathartics, calomel and jalap, the result being an agent which does not gripe, but produces a comfortable and effective movement. The writer has demonstrated to his satisfaction that the arsenic in arsenauro possesses far less irritant properties than arsenic in any other form, and can be administered in fuller and more effective doses. The cases cited will show that we have a valuable agent in arsenauro. The writer, however, does not assert that it will cure all cases of diabetes. There are many which baffle our skill, no matter what the treatment. I believe that arsenauro is possessed of marked antiseptic properties. We know that it is a powerful tonic and conclude that it exercises a specific action in diabetes mellitus. The first case cited is fairly representative; not a severe one, yet not mild.

Case I.—John W., aged 35, machinist, consulted the writer. He had an itching eruption on the chest; yellowish, xanthomatous appearance; patient married: two children. He had ravenous appetite, drank large quantities of water, had to rise at night to urinate, passing large quantities of urine. Patient said sexual power declined considerably and that his mental activity was much lessened. He weighed 156 pounds, had not noticed any loss of flesh: was a moderate drinker; family history negative. Examination showed sp. grav. 1031, reaction acid, and the glucose present, as determined by both Fehling's reaction and the phenyl-hydrazin test, approximately $3\frac{1}{2}$ per cent. He was passing between fifteen and sixteen pints urine daily. Was given general directions regarding hygiene, placed on a nitrogenous diet with limited carbohydrates. Administered arsenauro, 10 drops, in one-half goblet of water four times daily, instructions to gradually increase, warning being given as to possible toxic symptoms. One week later there was no perceptible change. He increased dose of arsenauro, then taking 18 drops three times a day; amount of sugar in urine seemed, however, to be slightly diminished, was standing the restricted diet very well; was instructed to continue treatment. One week later his condition was substantially the same. Two weeks later a marked change was noticeable. Examination of the urine showed but a trifle over 1 per cent. of glucose present. Polyuria had diminished; appetite much less; patient stated that he felt far better, physically and mentally. Was at that time taking 32 drops of arsenauro t. i. d.; no toxic symptoms, no irritation. The dose was increased, steady improvement was manifest, and at the end of six weeks the urine was free of sugar, polyuria had ceased, and the patient weighed 164 pounds. Three months have elapsed and at the present time patient is using arsenauro, 60 drops t. i. d. He claims to be perfectly well; examination and appearances certainly confirm his statement. In this case the patient was not put upon a rigid diet, being allowed small proportion of starchy food. We must note the fact that as the dosage of arsenauro was increased, the signs of improvement were manifest. In this case the point of saturation was never reached, nor were there any unfavorable physiological symptoms, even though the patient is now using over three drams daily.

Case II.—Mrs. N., aged 56, married; has had six children, four of whom are living. Family history of diabetes, her father having died of the disease. She was stout, heavily built, had lost considerable flesh,

and when consulting me, September 26th, weighed 138 pounds. Had been indisposed for a year, her loss in flesh accompanied by loss of strength; unable to do her housework. Complained of severe pruritus vulvæ, which she attributed to an ovariotomy performed in 1897; said she had never been a well woman since that time, and had developed very favorable opinions of gynecologists in consequence. Patient has highly neurotic temperament, the writer taking up her treatment very reluctantly. Directions regarding treatment same as in Case I., particular stress being laid upon hygienic measures and the employment of hydrotherapy. The pruritus received local attention. This patient was a source of endless annoyance; complained of diet and the trouble which the hydrotherapeutic measures entailed. She, however, took her arsenauro regularly, increasing the dose as directed. First examination she was passing three gallons of urine daily; glucose, 4 per cent. This condition continued for a month without any improvement. About November 1st, however, quantity of urine was diminished, percentage of sugar remaining substantially the same. On November 6th she exhibited a commencing gangrenous process in two fingers of the left hand. One of my colleagues suggested the employment of mercauro instead of arsenauro. Amputation of the two fingers was resorted to, the patient placed on mercauro, the arsenauro being temporarily withdrawn. The result was quite astonishing. In ten days' time the quantity of urine had fallen to eight pints and the glucose to 1 per cent. Coincident with this was the general improvement physically. At the present time the quantity of urine is normal and practically free from sugar, patient weighs 154 pounds, is able to do much of her housework; instead of being a confirmed invalid she is apparently on the road to complete recovery.

Case III.—Nellie L., age 16. This case is particularly interesting because of the youth of the patient. First seen October 3d, presenting the usual symptoms of diabetes. Had an insatiable appetite and her mother stated that the amount of water she drank was "simply enormous." An attempt to restrict this resulted in her resorting to various devices to obtain water surreptitiously. Symptoms had been present since last spring; patient much run down, skin dry and harsh, suffered from constipation and severe headache. Examination showed sp. grav. of urine, 1036; glucose, 5 per cent.; she passed daily 30 pints of urine. Placed patient on a rigid diet, and carbohydrates were strictly interdicted. As in other cases, patient was given careful instructions regarding hygiene, exercise, frequent bathing, cold spinal douches, and Turkish baths. Arsenauro was prescribed, beginning with 10 drops in one-half goblet of water three times daily, instructions given to gradually increase the dose. Contrary to expectation, patient took kindly to restricted diet; hygienic measures recommended were carried out faithfully. The patient was seen twice each week, an examination of the urine made each time. For two weeks no great change occurred, although the girl said she felt much better. Hunger, thirst, and polyuria reduced. On October 21st, however, the percentage of sugar had fallen to a trifle less than 3 per cent., quantity of urine remarkably lessened, patient taking her treatment faithfully, dose of arsenauro having reached 28 drops three times a day. From this time there was a steady decrease in the quantity of urine and of sugar. There was a marked improvement in the general condition of the patient. November 4th, glucose is absent for the first time. Weight of patient increased from 92 pounds (when first seen) to 100 pounds; skin softer, is healthier looking, bowels acting well, headache had ceased; still passing abnormal quantity of urine, yet much less than two weeks previously. Patient taking 40 drops arsenauro t. i. d., no physiological symptoms had developed, and as patient was steadily improving, she was instructed to continue at that dosage. November 10th

small quantity of sugar was detected, although the patient's condition was steadily improving. Next examination no sugar was found and I allowed the patient a limited amount of carbohydrates—a change she welcomed. Since that time no sugar has been found. The weight of the patient, now on a more liberal diet, is 108 pounds; is feeling in good physical condition, parents stating that the change in her disposition is most marked. Her appetite continues a trifle greater than that of most girls her age, but the excessive thirst and polyuria have ceased.

Case IV.—G. R., clergyman, age 56, family history negative. For sixty days had passed abnormal quantity of urine, his rest at night being frequently disturbed; always a large eater, did not think his appetite greater now than formerly. His hair (turning gray) is falling out rapidly; notices marked change in his mental powers; finds difficulty in memorizing his notes and concentrating his attention. Large, well-built man, inclined to corpulence. Sp. grav. of urine, 1036; slight amount of albumen; sugar, 4 per cent. Pulse somewhat of a high tension, the second aortic sound being accentuated. No apparent valvular lesions. His weight, 198 pounds; no loss of flesh or strength; daily excretion of urine, twenty-two pints. He was a man of regular habits, instructions regarding personal hygiene being superfluous. Was placed on restricted diet, but allowed some carbohydrate food. Medicinally, arsenauro was again relied on exclusively, beginning with 15 drops t. i. d. The case ran an uneventful course. In thirty days the urine was free of sugar, polyuria materially decreased, being no longer a source of annoyance. Mental condition much benefited, memory decidedly improved. First he complained of pruritis; this had disappeared. Skin now in good condition. Trace of albumen had disappeared, not having been noted for some time. The arterial tension still high. At one time patient was taking 85 drops of arsenauro three times a day; now using 60 drops t. i. d.; no physiological intolerance has developed.

Case V.—R. J. H., age 38, German, lens grinder by trade. Family history shows three cases of diabetes besides himself. Patient is fully aware of his condition, having been previously treated for the disease. Presents the classical symptoms and, in addition, a well-marked acne pustulosa. Is unable to do his work satisfactorily. His appearance evidenced extreme debility, being just able to go around, no more. Sexual power gone, patellar reflex absent. Patient weighs 126 pounds, having lost twenty-five pounds in the last five months. Examination of urine shows sp. grav., 1041; 5 per cent. sugar; passes daily large quantity of urine. Gave same directions regarding hygiene as in Case IV. Placed on rigidly restricted diet; acne given appropriate treatment. This patient previously treated with codeine and moderately restricted diet. Polyuria and glycosuria were but slightly affected. The writer is strongly inclined to attribute the extreme debility to the large doses of codeine which had been taken. Aside from the depressing effect, the codeine had acted very badly upon his stomach. The patient was placed upon arsenauro, beginning with 15 drops t. i. d., with instructions to increase the dose from day to day. Without giving tiresome details, it is sufficient to say that patient, after eight weeks' treatment, shows great improvement. Quantity of urine considerably diminished, though still contains about ½ per cent. of sugar. The hunger and thirst, which, at the beginning, were extreme, are now materially lessened; weight, 137 pounds (a gain of eleven pounds); patient feels stronger and better than in months: is now taking 60 drops arsenauro t. i. d., having been reduced from 84 drops, at which point physiological symptoms were manifested. Patient has shown slow but steady improvement. There is every reason to conclude that the case will go on to complete recovery.

These five cases show a few interesting facts. In every one the course of the disease has been favorably influenced and the symptoms checked. The results cannot be attributed entirely to dieting, for in three of the five carbohydrates were allowed in limited quantities. The case of the young girl might have been expected to fare badly, yet the termination was most satisfactory. One cannot fail to note also that with the increasing doses of arsenauro, the symptoms were modified. The patient who had previously been treated with narcotics was the only case in which sugar was found after six weeks' adminstration of arsenauro, yet the percentage of glucose in that case has greatly diminished. He now excretes less than 1 per cent. of sugar, as compared with 5 per cent. when the treatment was begun. The writer has three other cases under treatment, which are progressing favorably, though no definite conclusions can yet be reported. From the five cases quoted, however, it is evident that we have in arsenauro a most valuable agent in the treatment of diabetes mellitus. The writer does not, as yet, feel in a position to state positively as to the exact manner in which the arsenauro acts, but has some views as to its therapeusis, which he hopes to present later. An essential point seems to be the administration of the drug in sufficiently large doses. The maximum effect is thus obtained as well as maintained.

OYSTERS AND DISEASE.

THE *Boston Medical and Surgical Journal* says that with the advance of our knowledge of the subtle and unexpected ways in which disease may be transmitted, suspicion has, from time to time, and not unjustifiably fallen upon the oyster. It has been easy for a somewhat vivid imagination to picture the contamination to which oyster beds may be exposed, and to conceive of the possible multiplication of pathogenic bacteria or other agents inimical to health within their shells. Admitting these facts, it is a short step to imagine the effect upon man of eating such oysters and to add another terror to the constantly increasing number with which we are surrounded. Fortunately, in this, as in many other matters, an appeal to experiment does much to clear the way for a calmer and more rational interpretation of the facts. This service has lately been rendered by an exhaustive and painstaking study on the general subject of oysters and diseases, undertaken by Prof. W. A. Herdman, of Liverpool, and Prof. Robert Boyce, also of Liverpool, and both of University College. Their work is published in full, with plates, in the second volume of the Thompson Yates Laboratories Report, and well repays a careful perusal. The conclusions of these investigators are of moment, and should be generally known both by the raisers and consumers of shellfish. In general their experiments, in common with those of others, go to show that oysters and other shellfish, used as food, must, from their nature and the circumstances of their cultivation and sale, be regarded as liable to contamination from pathogenic and other organisms, or their products.

Recognizing this fact, the following statement made by the writers is sufficiently self-evident:

Shellfish must not be taken as food from grounds where there is any possibility of sewage contamination; after removal from the sea, while in transit, in store, or in market, they should be carefully protected from any possibility of insanitary environment; they should not be kept longer than is absolutely necessary in shops, cellars, etc., in towns where, even if not running the risk of fresh contamination, they are under conditions favorable to the reduction of their vitality, and the growth of their bacterial contents—the fresher they are from the sea, the more healthy they are likely to be; finally, only absolutely fresh shellfish should be eaten uncooked, and those that are cooked must be sufficiently cooked, raised

to boiling point, and kept there at least ten minutes."

Among the details of their experiments several matters of great interest were brought out. The vexed question of "greening" in oysters was one. The investigation showed that there are several perfectly distinct varieties of greenness, some being entirely healthy, and others indicating an excess of copper; in certain American oysters, for example, it was distinctly proved that their green color was due to copper, and also that the copper is situated in the blood cells, or leucocytes, which are much increased in number. This condition they call a green leucocytosis. On the other hand, experiments in feeding oysters with weak solutions of copper and iron salts gave no clear evidence of any absorption of the metals accompanied by greening.

The investigations on the presence of typhoid bacilli in oysters is also of much importance. They did not find the bacillus in any oysters obtained from the sea or from markets, but were able, experimentally, to inoculate the oysters with typhoid, and recover the organism from their bodies, up to the tenth day. It appears, however, that the bacilli do not increase in the body or tissues, and probably die in the intestine. Sea water was found inimical to the growth of the bacilli, and the washing of infected oysters in a stream of clear sea water led to a great diminution, or, in some cases, a total disappearance of the bacilli, in from one to seven days. The colon group of bacilli is frequently found in shellfish, but probably not in those living in pure sea water. It is unsafe, however, to infer from this that the presence of colon bacilli invariably indicates sewage contamination. Further investigation on this point is desirable.

The writers inform us, with reference to the negative results regarding typhoid, that their samples of oysters were, in no case, so far as they were aware, derived from a bed known or suspected of contamination with typhoid.

As a result of their investigations they

feel amply justified in sounding a warning note regarding the raising and selling of oysters. They urge the greatest possible care in the prevention of contamination, and for the regular inspection of the grounds by qualified persons.

Foreign oysters should be as carefully inspected as those raised at home, and a systematic quarantine established.

The report is, in a general way, reassuring, and yet, throughout, it recognizes a real danger, provided the utmost precaution be not taken to guard the oyster beds as we would any other source of food supply. It is well that we should be fully aware of all the facts, and insist upon the legal enforcement of close inspection. When this is done, we may, no doubt, still enjoy our oysters, with the practical assurance of their harmlessness.

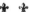

AMONG THE MICROBES.

THE microbes are much like the woman's numerous progeny, of whom she said she "could neither live with them, nor without them." The bacteriologists have been insisting that the microbes are the cause of all our diseases, and now they say that we cannot live without them, either. Dr. Kijanizin has proven this by putting animals into chambers supplied only with sterilized air, and then fed them on sterilized food. They were thus robbed of all chances to contract any disease from the microbes, but they all died in one and a half to five days. Why they did not live to a hoary old age was for a time a great puzzle, but an elaborate series of analyses finally showed that the animals became poisoned with their own products of respiration and digestion. The doctor has come to the conclusion that certain micro-organisms of the air are absolutely necessary to life and to normal respiration. They are introduced into the blood during the process of respiration, and are then developed into oxidizing ferments, which prevent the acumulation of leucomaines in the blood and the self-poisoning of the animal. Without these the poisons accumulate, digestion of food is hindered, and the animal dies. Then a German investigator has tried similar experiments upon certain plants, growing them in sterilized soil and sterilized air. The plants grew, but not nearly so vigorous as under normal conditions, and the seeds remained undeveloped. He concludes that the microbes are necessary to vegetable life also.

So the ubiquitous microbe is not altogether an obnoxious neighbor after all, and perhaps it is well for us that he cannot be frozen out, even by liquid air. Even when kept in liquid air, at a temperature of 310° F. below zero, for a week, the germs will come out in good condition and ready for business. We cannot freeze him out, and it is not easy to make it too warm for him without burning ourselves, too.

On the other hand, none of the pathogenic bacteria can survive contact with the earth very long. A belief has prevailed that the microbes of infectious diseases retain their virulence and vitality, for long periods, within dead and buried bodies. This has lately been disproven, and it is found that the infective power is lost, usually within a month, in a body buried either in a coffin or wrapped in a cloth. Other experiments have shown that the soil bacteria make war, on sight, on the pathogenic germs, and, whereas typhoid germs, for instance, will live for a long time in sterilized soil, they disappear within twenty-four hours in ordinary germ-filled earth.

There is a rebellion developing against the idea that the germs are the great cause of disease. Prof. Kueppe leads the opposition in the theory that diseases are inherent in man, and the disease germs act merely as liberating impulses. Disease is innate, and only requires the advent of a morbific stimulus to set it free. Therefore, disinfectants and antiseptics are not to be used to cure diseases, but only to prevent them. They may prevent a disease breaking out, but they cannot, in any degree, cure it, because the germs are not the generators, but only the liberators of, disease. This is the opposite view of what commonly prevails, and leads to the view that man's tendencies and not the evil-mindedness of the germs are to blame for sickness. The ideally perfect animal would be immune to disease, and might nurse all the germs freely without harm.

Some force is lent to this view by the fact that in a number of instances the same germ appears to be at one time pathogenic and at other times not. At least certain pathogenic bacteria have been shown to be identical with certain other non-pathogenic and widely-distributed bacteria. The germs seem to enjoy a change of work, and they change their duties at times. This causes the bacteriologist lots of trouble, and keeps him guessing as to just what a particular germ is going to do, or who his near relations are.

It is not easy to distinguish the germs solely by their appearance, they being so extremely minute, and so their characteristic properties are taken into account also. But a muddle seems to be developing here, in that these properties may depend upon conditions and environment, and, therefore, they cannot be depended upon. Like many men, the character of the microbe depends upon the influences around him.—*Prof. W. L. Scoville, in The Spatula.*

FORCED PROPHYLAXIS.

HENRY C. NIERMAN, an employee of the Adams Express Company, was fined $25 by Justice Jerome, in Special Sessions, yesterday, for insistent expectorating in a Ninth Avenue elevated train, in violation of the ordinance of the Health Board prohibiting such practices. This is the first conviction under this ordinance, which, although the fact is not well known, makes spitting in street cars and ferryboats a misdemeanor. The notices of the Health Board, posted in surface and elevated cars, heretofore have merely prohibited spitting in the aisles, without mentioning the penalty which may be inflicted. These placards have been superseded by new ones, stating specifically that spitting in cars is a misdemeanor, and will be punished to the full extent of the law.

Henry W. Hardon, a lawyer, of 313 West Seventy-first street, who was formerly an instructor at Columbia University, was the complainant against Nierman. Upon the stand yesterday Mr. Hardon stated that he had taken a seat beside Nierman in an elevated train, last Saturday, and that Nierman had spat repeatedly on the car floor. Mr. Hardon called Nierman's attention to the sign prohibiting spitting, and was told to mind his own business, and that the ordinance was a dead letter anyway.

The guard's request that the expectorating cease was also insolently disregarded. Nierman's arrest followed. Nierman pleaded guilty in court yesterday, and his counsel asked that leniency be shown his client. Justice Jerome, imposing sentence, said:

"The public should be grateful to you, Mr. Hardon, for your action in this matter. Expectorating in cars and on the streets is the cause of many tubercular diseases, and many subsequent deaths. I wish to emphasize this offense, and it is well for the public to know that this health ordinance will be rigorously enforced. This spitting practice in cars and in public buildings is entirely too prevalent, and must be stopped. The ordinance is a wise and salutary one."

Nierman's explanation was that he had catarrh, and was compelled to expectorate freely. He paid the fine.

WATER PURIFYING.

OF the various branches of public works connected with the pollution of water supply, says *The Sanitarian*, there is none in which such substantial progress has recently been made as in water purification.

Ten years ago information upon this subject was very meager, and comparatively few plants were in operation. During this period English sand-filter plants had been increased from about 1.5 to 19 acres, with respective normal capacities of about 4,000,-000 and 57,000,000 gallons daily; and the American, or mechanical filter plants, have been increased from about 12,000 to 90,000 square feet, with respective nominal capacities of about 36,000,000 and 270,000,000 gallons daily. Projected plants for some of the largest cities in this country showed that in the next few years there would be very rapid development in the application of both of the leading methods of purification.

Of the various processes for the purification of water supplies, there were two general methods which had shown distinctly their practicability—namely, the English method of slow sand filtration, and the American method, employing rapid mechanical filters. For those waters which never possessed more than a slight or moderate amount of turbidity, or dissolved vegetable color, the English method was somewhat more efficient, and, as a rule, was slightly cheaper for such waters. For those waters which, for a long period of time contained excessive quantities of either finely divided clay, or of dissolved vegetable matter, there was now no practical method of purification without the use of coagulates and subsiding basins. While coagulants could be successfully used in connection with the English method of sand filtration, the American method, in which coagulants were imperative, yielded somewhat more efficient and economical results as a rule.

Dr. F. H. Newell, Government Hydrographer, contributed a paper, showing some results of the investigation of stream pollution which has been made by the United States Geological Survey. He said that the Government, realizing the importance of public water supplies, and their conservation and protection against pollution, has established a special division, or branch of the geological survey, under the title of "Board of Hydrography." Its duties are to ascertain the amount of water flowing in the various important streams in different parts of the country, to survey reservoir sites, examine geological conditions which govern currents of water under ground, and to prepare maps and charts showing the depth at which water can probably be had in different localities. He referred to the work of this kind, which, he said, is being done with rare delicacy and thoroughness under the direction of Dr. Charles O. Probst, of Ohio, secretary of the Association.

In the discussion of Dr. Newell's paper on government investigation of stream pollution, Dr. Josiah Hartzell, of Canton, President of the State Board of Health of Ohio, said that in his State investigations of streams will be continued until every watercourse and water-shed is thoroughly understood. He said that the investigation, as it has thus far progressed, has revealed an astonishing degree of pollution of the public water supplies of the State. When Dr. Lee, of Pennsylvania, was asked by President Bryce for an expression on this subject, he raised quite a laugh by saying, laconically: "Just at present, so far as my State is concerned, I would rather not say anything about stream pollution."

BRITISH CONGRESS ON TUBERCULOSIS.

A BRITISH Congress on Tuberculosis, for the prevention of consumption, will be held in London, on July 22, 1901, and will continue in session five days.

Every British colony and dependency, says the London *Health*, is invited to participate by sending delegates; while the governments of countries in Europe, Asia, and America are invited to send representative men of science and others, who will be the distinguished guests of the congress.

The information already gained, both at home and abroad, shows that consumption and other forms of tuberculosis, although preventable and controllable by intelligent precautions, still remain the direct cause of a high rate of death and sickness. In the United Kingdom alone, some 60,000 deaths are recorded annually from tuberculosis, and it is stated on good authority that at least thrice this number are constantly suffering from one form or another of the disease.

The knowledge of these facts, and the recognition that the disease is peculiarly amenable to open-air treatment, has aroused profound international interest in the question; and in many countries public authorities have been led to put in force preventive measures directed against the propagation of consumption between human beings, between animals, and between human beings and animals.

The object of the forthcoming congress is to exchange the information and experience gained throughout the world as to methods available for stamping out this disease. Papers will be read, and clinical and pathological demonstrations will be given; while the museum, which is to be a special feature of the congress, will contain pathological and bacteriological collections, charts, models, and other exhibits.

Authorities in this and other countries will be invited to supply documents bearing upon the historical, geographical, and statistical aspects of the subject; while as a result of the papers and discussions, practical resolutions will be formulated, which will serve to indicate the public and private measures best adapted for the suppression of tuberculosis.

ALCOHOLISM: A CRIME OR A DISEASE?

In a paper read before the Medical Association of Central New York, Dr. F. E. Fronczac said:

"This is the age of prophylaxis. The highest and most eminent branch of the medical science is the teaching of hygiene, or preservation of health and prevention of disease. The preventive measures for the fracture of a limb, I suppose the surgeon would name: 'Do not fracture it.' The preventive measures for alcoholism, I answer, 'Do not expose yourself to alcoholic influences.' And this we must leave to the solons of the legislatures of our different States, and the nation, who are supposed to pass such laws as will bring about this condition. But when one does expose himself to the morbid condition following alcoholic indulgence, whether this condition is chronic or temporary, I believe the members of our profession owe it a duty to themselves, and to mankind, to step in and use their power to bring the patient to his former condition, as much as this is possible.

"Alcoholism is classed among the nervous and mental diseases, and the pathology, as studied by various author's, shows most marked changes in the nervous system; various nerve cells are changed and disintegrated, capillaries are dilated in the entire central nervous apparatus; in one word, there is an abnormal condition in that system after each and every alcoholic debauchery. These are the physical conditions we are to rectify, and not simply the moral one, which the penal code provides for the treatment of this so-called crime.

"Drunkenness is not a crime, it is a disease, and should be treated as such. This is an opinion of men of eminence in law and medicine, and, therefore, let us begin to treat it as such, in this the closing year of the nineteenth century of our era. Insanity was considered a crime but a short time ago, but now the civilized world considers it a morbid condition of the mind, and provides proper hospitals for its cure. Let us, therefore, give the alcoholics, like the insane, proper surroundings, and proper treatment and cure. We do not liberate the insane before he is considered cured, by proper authorities; let us, therefore, on the same basis, put alcoholics where they properly belong. Give the alcoholics, meaning the chronic drunkards, the men who compose the majority of the prisoners on the blotters at the police stations, and who occupy the greater majority of the cells in the penal institutions, proper hospitals, proper surroundings, and proper treatment and care, and a large percentage of chronic alcoholism will disappear. Alcoholism, like smallpox through vaccination, or typhoid fever through hygienic prophylactic measures, will slowly cease to be an endemic disease in certain localities, and many a medico-legal case will thereby be eliminated from the dockets of our criminal courts."

IMMUNITY.

It is not unusual in the experience of bacteriologists, at one time or another, when raising the virulency of a strain of bacteria by passing the virus through a series of rabbits, to find, every now and then, certain of them which are unaffected by the inoculation. This individual immunity is often noticeable in man, for in any serious outbreak of diphtheria, plague, smallpox, or typhoid fever there will be found those who not only may be in attendance on infected cases, but may also be in far from good health themselves, and who yet do not contract the disease. The cut-and-dried explanation of the above, generally given, is that the reason they do not suffer from the epidemic is that they are naturally immune, leaving, however, the question of why it is so unanswered. It has been lately shown that the Arabs, as a race, are immune from enteric fever, and the theory has been advanced that the immunization is attained by reason of the fact that the Arab in childhood is habitually accustomed to drinking foul, unwholesome water. It has been further pointed out by those who support these views that army medical statistics show that diseases of the digestive canal are twice as frequent among European troops as among the native soldiers in Algeria and Tunis. In traumatic infections the serous membranes of the Arab are very resistant, and particularly the peritoneum and the pleura, which prob-

ably accounts for the very exceptionally favorable results in abdominal surgery among the Arabs.

In striking contrast, however, with the above, it is found that Arabs, as a race, are singularly subject to pulmonary affections, and exhibit a very marked susceptibility to pneumococcal infection. Exceptions in regard to infections are very interesting studies, but it would seem difficult to establish the fact that there is such a condition as absolute racial immunity. In the case of anthrax, though it is very fatal for ordinary sheep, Angora sheep are not affected by it, and in the same manner ordinary rats are susceptible to anthrax, whilst white rats are immune, but these statements do not apply if the animals are placed under abnormal conditions.—*Medical Press.*

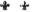

A RACE OF IMMUNES.

The Arabs are practically immune to typhoid fever, and to all diseases of the serous membranes, so we are informed in a paper read by Messrs. Tostivint and Reutlinger, before the Paris Society of Biology. There are always compensations in Nature, and hence we need not be surprised to learn that the race is also prone to pneumonia and diseases of the lungs. We quote an abstract of the paper, given in the *New York Medical Journal*:

"It seems that army medical statistics show that diseases of the digestive canal are twice as frequent among European troops in Algeria and Tunis as among the native soldiers. This is true of diseases of all parts of the intestinal canal. Affections of the liver also are much less common among the Arabs than among Europeans. On the other hand, all pulmonary affections are more prevalent among the natives. These peculiarities, the authors think, are due, the one to immunization in childhood by drinking unwholesome water, and the other to the fact that the Arab's lungs, accustomed to the pure air of vast solitudes, are little fitted to struggle against the germs encountered in the air breathed by multitudes.

"As to the resistance of the Arab's serous membranes to infection, the authors say it is observed in case of all those membranes, but particularly of the peritoneum and the pleura. . . . In consequence of this resisting power, abdominal surgery among the Arabs is attended with the most favorable results. Rheumatism is exceptional, and metastasis [shifting] of infectious diseases to the synovial membranes of the joints and to the other serous membranes is very rare. The only serous affections that are met with as frequently among the Arabs as among Europeans are those occasioned by Koch's bacillus, or the pneumococcus; the Arabs' very decided susceptibility to these two micro-organisms contrasts sharply with the general resisting power of their serous membranes. This resisting power . . . . seems to be a peculiarity of the primitive races. The peritoneum of the lower animals, it appears to be added in support of this theory, grows less and less resistant to infection the higher the creature is in the scale of living beings.

"Race peculiarities in regard to morbid susceptibilities are always interesting subjects of study, and much may be learned **from their investigation.** It is to be hoped, however, that the theory of intestinal immunization by the habitual drinking of foul water in childhood will lead to no attempt to introduce the practice into preventive medicine, for, to our mind, it could result only in the survival of the toughest, like the 'hardening' process."—*Literary Digest.*

CIDER VINEGAR, administered a few minutes after swallowing carbolic acid, is the antidote. Dilute one-quarter or one-half,

BORIC ACID, mixed with linseed meal poultices, is highly recommended in the treatment of erysipelas.

THE NATURE TREATMENT OF TUBERCULOSIS.

R. O. BEARD says that the study of the warfare waged between the human tissue cells and the bacillus tuberculosis teaches us the lesson that the task of the public sanitarian and the physician is largely one of prevention, and that cure—a secondary and short-lived possibility in the course of the disease—is best accomplished by extending the principles and methods of prevention to the assistance of the tissue cells. Only now are we learning that but two prime factors are essential to make localities favorable to the tuberculous patient—purity and dryness of atmosphere, in whatever latitude, at whatever altitude, on plain or mountain, in forest or on ranch. Consumptives should be isolated. Tuberculosis should be quarantined in our towns as effectively as yellow jack. As to the creation of the Minnesota park, the nature treatment of tuberculosis in this available region will repay the nation in men more than it can gain in timber by its destruction or in navigation by its saving. As nearly complete physiological rest as possible should be attained by the consumptive. Forced feeding is also an important element in treatment. The gradual increase of food is well endured, even in advanced cases. The combination of all these measures should brighten the hope of control of this most destructive of the diseases of civilization.—*Med. Record.*

ASAFETIDA, in doses of sixteen grains, administered four times a day, is said to completely break up the worst case of grip at any stake of its development.

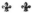

IN cases of vomiting, from almost any cause, one-quarter grain doses of codeine usually answer exceedingly well.

Department of Physical Education.

WITH SPECIAL REGARD TO THE SYMMETRICAL DEVELOPMENT OF THE BODY.

SYMMETRICAL DEVELOPMENT.

E. STUVER, in the *Journal of the American Medical Association*, for December 22d, considers the question whether or not our present school system develops the highest powers of the pupils.

He says that the physical, intellectual and moral powers of the pupils should be developed at the same time.

Parents and teachers should thoroughly appreciate the fact that in its development the child is an epitome of the development of the race, and possesses many of the impulses and passions incident to the savage, barbarous and semi-civilized phases through which the race has passed, and that, in order to attain the best results, the instruction must be carefully adapted to the ever-changing, ever-varying needs, and to the comprehension of the child.

As "teaching is the art of promoting human growth," the successful teacher must understand his own powers and limitations; he must understand the growing pupil, and be able to put himself in the latter's place, and he must have a thorough knowledge and grasp of the subject taught. Teachers should have a more thorough and comprehensive knowledge of the laws of mental development, a better understanding of educational methods and the best means of imparting instruction. To insure such knowledge and teaching power, the rank and file of teachers should have a more thorough education, a more professional training and preparation for their work, and, last, but by no means least, they should be better paid, and thus encouraged to make teaching their life work.

We need more enthusiasm and less routine; more original investigation and search after truth for the truth's sake, and less cramming for examinations; less talking and lecturing on the part of the teacher, and more time devoted to training pupils in systematic and logical analysis, and in clearness and accuracy of expression.

Then, too, not so many studies should be pursued at the same time, but the work should be more thoroughly done, and a stronger grasp of the fundamental principles, on which all true education depends, should be secured. To get time for such training, the number drill and arithmetic, together with other formal and abstruse work, should be greatly curtailed, or entirely omitted from the primary grades, and the children should be given greater opportunities to study natural objects, in their natural surroundings. The study of flowers, trees, rocks, birds, animals, insects, etc., in their actual conditions and environments, is of infinitely greater value to the pupils than the fragmentary conception of such things that can be given to them in the school room, in the midst of artificial surroundings. In addition to imparting more exact information, the outdoor excursions furnish healthful exercise, inspire enthusiasm, rest and strengthen the brain and mind, and elevate the pupils morally, while the indoor study of such objects soon becomes a drudgery, and is of comparatively little benefit.

More time and attention should be given to manual training. This training of the muscles develops the motor centers in the brain, discharges the accumulating nerve force in the motor centers, develops and strengthens the association fibers between the various brain centers, and permits the higher brain centers to develop normally, and store up power.

This gives the student a richer sensory content, a more harmonious physical and mental organization, and a better balanced moral nature.

Greater care should be exercised in promoting the health and proper physical development of the pupils.

THE ELEMENT OF PLEASURE IN PHYSICAL EDUCATION.

To make physical education popular among all classes and all ages it is necessary, says the editor of *Mind and Body*, that it combine work with pleasure. Physical training, as taught in most of the schools and gymnasia, in this and in other countries, is nothing but an additional burden for the pupil. The time allotted for it is consumed in administering a series of well-arranged lessons, which require close attention on the part of the pupils. The consequence is that the gymnasium hours are, at times, regarded with even less favor than is any other hour for certain other studies.

This is not because the child does not like gymnastic or athletic work, but because of the almost total absence of the element of pleasure from the program, and because the strict adherence to so-called educational rules is not to the taste of the pupil, as *e.g.*, a child may be fond of music, but dislike taking lessons.

Music and physical training cannot, however, be judged on the same standard. The latter possesses the happy characteristic of being practised without much preparatory education, while the former involves a great deal of practice. In gymnastic work it is not necessary to master a certain degree of technique in order to perform at all. Even a class of beginners is well capable of going

through a large amount of physical exercise, and of deriving a great amount of benefit from it. The fault seems to be with the teachers of physical education, who teach their pupils in gymnastics as they would teach a pupil in the mastering of a musical instrument; impressing them with a lot of little insignificant details, of very little practical value, and making them disgusted with the subject proper.

What we want is wholesome exercise that builds up and perfects the body, but no monotonous drills.

If we are unable to interest the pupil, our cause is lost. We have but one way to create interest, and that is by combining actual pleasure with the hardship of the work.

Prof. K. Moeller, of Altona, Germany, in an address to an educational society recently, expressed this sentiment as follows:

"We live in an age of hyper-culture. There is no lack of instructions as to how we should live properly, but we are far from living according to Nature's ways. In our efforts we must not overlook that most important element, pleasure. For the pleasure derived from them, we take up such exercises as bicycling, swimming, etc.

"Only, when combined with pleasure, physical exercises are performed with vigor. In a great many places physical training is made one of the ingredients of the school curriculum, and is thereby robbed of the glamor with which the natural instinct for physical exercises are performed with vigor. Whenever possible it should be undertaken in the open air, and the arrangement of lessons should be such as to favor the development of the general vitality (the lungs and the heart) in preference to the building up a powerful muscular system.

"Running, games and contests must have a prominent place in physical training, since these seem to meet these requirements more than a monotonous, strictly scientific gymnastic lesson."

DEEP BREATHING.

DEEP breathing, says Dr. J. H. Pryor, cannot be overestimated, because in modern civilization few of us, after childhood, breathe deeply. Yet this full lung function means, first, all the proper oxygenation of the blood, and its therapeusis is, in brief, the same as oxygen in the system. At any time of life, and for either sex, better lung action would be undoubtedly of great value; and in disorders of the blood, in which purification and added tone are required, it will, on trial, be found a great adjuvant of other rational therapeutic means. Among such conditions are to be mentioned chlorosis, anemia, and the depreciated states after severe illnesses. When the lungs intrinisically show deficient action, as in the muscularly feeble, or when, after disease, especially the various forms of pleurisy, pneumonia and bronchitis, their sequelæ and complications, they are found imperfect in function, it is exceedingly probable that most or entirely all of the difficulty can be eradicated or compensated for by training in forced voluntary respiration several times each day. In children very likely the deformities of the chest, incident upon rickets and similar disease, could be, in part, neutralized by proper breathing gymnastics. In the sub-acute forms of bronchitis and pneumonia we have the air vesicles glued together with exudate. By opening these, absorption and even discharge of the exudate, by expectoration, will be initiated and stimulated. In some of the old, semi-consolidations of pneumonia a like process obtains, added to the advantage of general stimulation by this process. It is closely analogous to the similar results of massage of joints. This might be called lung massage. Cough is not a contraindication; in fact, has the advantages of expelling exudate. For the inhalation, various soothing remedies can be added to the air. The patient should repeat this exercise several times daily.

MASSAGE IN SPRAINS.

No TWO masseurs are alike by Nature, nor in skill, tact and education, and the one who knows his anatomy and physiology well, says *Health,* when called to a recent acute sprain, will not begin at once to masseur tne injured joint, but at a distance above it, on the healthy tissues, by gentle stroking or effleurage towards the heart, gradually proceeding nearer and nearer to the painful place. This has a soothing effect, and pushes the flow along in the veins and lymphatics, making more space in them for the returning currents coming from beyond, and carrying away the fluids that have leaked out of the vessels. The same should be done on the part of the limb beyond the joint, for the circulation is hindered both in going out and coming in by reason of the swelling.

Next, the masseur who knows his business will begin again, at a safe distance above the injured joint, and use deep rubbing, kneading, or massage properly so-called, one hand contracting as the other relaxes, alternately making circular grasps, with the greatest pressure upward, and this should be done on the parts above and below the seat of sprain. By this procedure the effects of the previous stroking, or effleurage, are much enhanced, an analgesic or agreeably benumbing effect is produced upon the nerves which extend to the painful place, and the retarded circulation is pushes along more vigorously, making room in the vessels for the swelling, the effusion, the embargo caused by the landslide of blood and lymph that is inundating the surrounding territory with exudates farther up the stream, to float off, and preparing the way for the next step in treatment. At the end of fifteen or twenty minutes of this manner of working, gentle, firm pressure can be made immediately over the swollen and, but recently, very tender parts, which in a few seconds can have circular motion, with the greatest push upward added to it; and this, if sufficient tact is used, will, in all probability, not hurt, but be positively agreeable.

MASSAGE A SCIENTIFIC THERAPEUTIC MEASURE.

MANUAL training for disease has, to a certain extent, says Dr. C. S. McDonald, in the *Indianapolis Polyclinic,* existed since the creation. Man had, by instinct, acquired the art of manipulation long before Nature yielded her secrets in medicine. This is still the practice among natives in Sweden. Even at the present time certain manipulations are used among the peasants for cramps and swellings.

The Swedes seem never to have lost the art. The priests of Egypt used some manipulation, in the form of kneading and friction, for rheumatic pains, neuralgias and swellings.

The Greeks were the first to recognize gymnastics as an institution. In the fifteenth and sixteenth centuries well known physicians recommended gymnastics.

Fuller and Tissot wished to combine the movements with the study of medicine. In the early part of the nineteenth century a therapeutic system of gymnastics acquired a reputation heretofore unknown, in movements based upon a certain action between operator and patient.

The Swede, P. H. Ling, 1776-1839, and his predecessors, erected the first scientific system, in which they adapted the new medical science, making the movement treatment a perfectly scientific remedy.

The word "massage" is a deviation from the Greek "massein," or, in the French, "masser," which means to knead.

Massage is a scientific treatment, by certain passive systematic manipulations, upon the nude skin of the human body.

Dr. Mezger, of Amsterdam (now practicing in Wiesbaden, Germany), and his two pupils, the Swedish physicians Berghman and Helleday, were among the first to apply the massage treatment scientifically. Their methods are now used throughout Europe. According to Mezger, massage is a scientific treatment, based upon the anatomy and the physiology of the human body. His manipulations are certain—that is,

given or fixed—so that an uninstructed person cannot pick up the treatment.

It is an art that cannot be self-acquired. All manipulations are passive, and are also systematic. Massage treatment is divided into four principal manipulations—effleurage, friction, petussage, and tapotement. It depends upon the nature of the case which you have to treat as to the manipulation.

EXERTION.*

IN his work on dietetics Dr. B. W. Ideler wrote, in 1858, "The exertion of an organ is the fundamental law of its development." Another sentence reads: "Physical training embodies nearly all laws of health depending upon the will."

Does it not seem as though our weak and nervous race had forgotten the importance of exertion? There are, indeed, circles in society where all and every possible exertion is avoided for fear of detrimental results. The incredible plan is even said to have been made, to practice gymnastics without exertion. By exertion we understand, first of all, muscular movement. Life is movement, and wherever it manifests itself in mechanical expression it results from muscular movement. All the functions of our body, as respiration, circulation, digestion, and certain excretions, require muscular activity. These vital processes are intensified and stimulated through general and voluntary muscular movements. Nature has implanted in every animal an innate impulse to move, and made it hereditary. This of itself is sufficient proof of what importance muscular exercise, *i.e.,* exertion, is for our well-being. The products of inactivity are relaxed, slender muscles, weak nerves and a pale, cold skin; symptoms which, sooner or later, work great common reasoning will lead to the conviction that all organs are strengthened by well regulated muscular movements, and are harm upon our will and character. Even

* Translated by Carl L. Schrader, for Mind and Body.

thereby rendered more capable to assist one another. This undisturbed working in harmony of all parts, as it were, is the very foundation of health. This will become clearer to us when we examine the results of muscular exertion in another than merely casual way.

That muscular exercise does strengthen the nervous system is made evident through experiences in our daily life. These experiences go to show that thousands of people who, through mental strain, have become fatigued, find relief in taking light exercises, such as walks, gymnastic exercise, riding a wheel, etc. Healthy children, after the close of their school hours, relieve themselves, preferably, by running games. Muscular activity enhances the benefits of recreation, since it increases the circulation and provides the fatigued brain more rapidly with oxygenized blood. One can hardly conceive of a better standard to measure poor health than nervous energy. Strong nerves are the foundation of the condition known as "laughing health." Those persons are classified as healthy whose body is neither characterized by laxity nor by a lean hardness. This condition of the body is the result of enhanced metabolism, and this is present to a higher degree in an active than in a passive muscle. Uninterrupted metabolism is the resultant of systematic physical exercise. The renewal of worn-out, organized matter, and the organic restoring of youth, is the essence of health. The muscular system is by far the most extensive in the entire body, and for this reason its activity is the most effective means of bringing about an increase of vital energy. Schreber writes: "Physiological experiments have sufficiently proven that man, when continually active, renews his entire body in about four to five weeks, whereas an inactive person, under like conditions, will require from ten to twelve weeks for this renewal."

Metabolism is life, interruption of it is disease, and total arrest of it is equivalent to death. Continuous metabolism imparts to the body, in all its parts, the power of full activity, of elasticity, and of re-creation. Since it is but the result of exercise, it is self-evident that exertion is the real nucleus of dietetics. The fruit of muscular exercise is not only strength, endurance, and speed, but also higher quality and increased quantity. The untrained person wastes more muscular energy than is necessary; he works at a disadvantage, and his movements necessarily appear awkward. By means of exercise the movements become easy. Judicious selection of exercises, the interchange of exercises of strength with those of endurance and of speed, and the alternation of arm movements with those of the legs and trunk, contribute to a symmetrical development of the entire musculature. If the exertion of simple muscles or of groups of muscles be greater, either by the occupation of the individual or by one-sided physical exercise, than is that of others, the development of these particular groups will have been achieved at the expense of the latter, and the symmetry of the body and its movements will have been disturbed. This is prominently the reason why systematic physical training is not only an absolute necessity for the welfare of those people to whom, through their occupation, all physical exertion is denied, but also of those who, through their daily occupation, are destined to develop only one-sidedly. But how many persons are not cocksure that they can enjoy lasting health without this continuous muscular activity! Do they not see innumerable people, who reach old age without it, if they only avoid the well-known dissipations?

That this so-called well-being is synonymous with perfect health is very much to be doubted. One is not healthy simply because he is not exactly ill. The great demands of modern life, with its innumerable obligations, can only be satisfied with the greatest expenditure of intellectual and will power. To be sure, the organism, owing to the lack of exertion, does not possess the strength of health; it settles into a fever-like condition, which ultimately gravitates toward the nervous system. This abnormal condition of constant nervous strain also impairs digestion, heart action and nutrition.

Thus we see multitudes about us with overtaxed nerves on the one, and a relaxed musculature on the other, hand. This abnormality is known as nervous constitution; it exercises its detrimental influence upon the character, whose manifestations alternate betwixt overstimulation and relaxation. Hence this frequency of weakness of character, this frequent change in mentation and volition, this superficial but rapidly sinking assiduity, this hunting and chasing after idols of an eccentric imagination. Weak nerves are one of the principal causes of human ills, and with increasing effeminacy and relaxation this evil must necessarily grow greater.

Too often man learns only through loss. Or he would realize that through ignorance and indolence he places his life in direct opposition to one of the fundamental laws of Nature. To prevent a one-sided, sickly condition, Nature endowed man, from childhood on, with an untiring desire for activity, necessary for his development. We must keep awake and alive this natural craving for activity, the manifestation of which has never yet been erased from any healthy boy or girl, lest it grow weaker as the years go on; we must see to it that through uninterrupted exertion it gains in strength and endurance, so that the sum total of life may reach the maximum energy. Our race will have to overcome this abhorrence of exertion if it wants to be healthy.

If you practise gymnastics, beware of overdoing it; especially in the beginning, but do not allow interruptions to occur on account of trivial causes. The systematic exercises must be part of our plan of life, like eating, drinking. and sleeping. All exercises. even the simplest, should be executed with military precision, with the greatest of accuracy and exertion. Exertion to the point of fatigue is an implicit requisite of success, but it later on must be compensated by rest.

Many believe to have satisfied Nature's demand if they daily exercise in a gymnasium for a half hour, in a haphazard sort of way, or if they roam about in the open air for a half or whole hour. The determining factor, however, is what exercises, in what manner, in what order of succession, in what length of time, and in what quantity they were performed. Even the free exercises, so frequently scorned, should be so dealt with that one is warmed up by them. We can only expect a systematic development, muscular strength, an improved digestion, and healthier sleep, etc., if we give due credit to the importance of exertion; for Nature permits every organic function only to reach the fullest and lasting development through exertion. Nature has taken ample and wise precautions that the limits of exertion are not too easily overstepped. The feeling of fatigue is a safeguard. If no fatigue results, the purpose of exertion has not been accomplished. Yea, in order to assist our organs to acquire their best possible function, and highest state of energy, one may occasionally go beyond the limit set by Nature.

SOME REASONS FOR DAILY EXERCISE.

ANY man who does not take time for exercise will probably have to make time to be ill.

Body and mind are both gifts, and for the proper use of them our Maker will hold us responsible.

Exercise gradually increases the physical powers, and gives more strength to resist sickness.

Exercise will do for your body what intellectual training will do for your mind—educate and strengthen it.

Plato called a man lame because he exercised the mind while the body was allowed to suffer.

A sound body lies at the foundation of all that goes to make life a success. Exercise will help to give it.

Exercise will help a young man to lead a chaste life.

Varied, light, and brisk exercise, next to sleep, will rest the tired brain better than anything else.

Metal will rust if not used, and the body will become diseased if not exercised.

A man "too busy" to take care of his health is like a workman too busy to sharpen his tools.

THE TREATMENT OF BRONCHIAL DISEASES BY POSTURE.

DR. O. JACOBSOHN speaks favorably from his experience, of Quincke's suggestion of treating bronchitis and bronchiectatic processes by posture. In acute processes in which the mucous membrane is hypersensitive, the measure is useless, and even harmful. In chronic cases, however, in which the bronchial mucous membrane has lost its reflex excitability and the smooth muscles of the bronchioles their tone, good results may be achieved. Abscesses of the lung, empyemas which have broken through, and similar processes, are not benefited by the postural treatment. In cases of fetid bronchitis, the relief obtained is marked. The purpose of the treatment is to drain the secretions from portions of the mucous membrane which are not irritable into areas which still retain their irritability, and by the force of gravity to cause an evacuation by coughing. The posture is the dorsal one, with the foot of the bed gradually raised by means of bricks. It is practised morning and evening, for an hour each. In fifteen minutes some result should be achieved; if no sputum is obtained by this time, the procedure is usually useless. In ordinary cases, the entire day's secretion may thus be evacuated.—*New York Med. Journ.*

THE BENEFICIAL EFFECTS OF AMUSEMENTS.

REALIZING that there are more sides than one to every important question, and that if all sides are given a hearing the correct solution is more likely to be reached, *The Spectator* discusses the effects of amusements, in the following manner:

"The increase of the desire, not so much for games as for seeing games, reading about games, talking over games, is admitted on all hands, and is condemned by a good many moralists as a sign that the nation is deteriorating, and giving up both work and thought for frivolous forms of recreation. The moralists are right in part, but, as often happens when social questions are discussed, they perhaps read in a social change more evil than there is in it. It is quite true that the nation is a little more frivolous than it was; that it is under the influence of a mood which it has betrayed several times before, a mood in which it is impatient of hard thinking— wants everything short, even its stories, likes no plays that are not exciting; gossips without gusto, principally about the great, whose movements fill columns, even in grave papers; and, in fact, is keenly desirous of any distraction which does not burden its mental powers. All this is regretable, if only because there is in it such a dissipation of energy, of which there is never too much for the increasingly heavy demands that fall upon every class and every country in the world. We should not admit, however, having some notion of what society was like in the eighteenth century, that the public is more vicious than it has ever been; it certainly drinks a great deal less than it did; and, though its desire for amusement has increased, the kind of instrument is almost infinitely less barbaric.

There are causes at work in favor of amusements, and especially of non-sedentary amusement, which in themselves are by no means to be regretted. One is undoubtedly increased prosperity among the masses of the people. We all talk about "depression," and none but the bad question the existence of terrible suffering from poverty among us, but the majority are so much better off that they are inclined, with the sanguine temperament which is part of our national character, to be a little wasteful of money. More is spent upon diet, much more upon clothes—God only knows how the children of working households are turned out so trig—and more, therefore, upon amusements. Just look in an evening at the crowds of bicyclists who pass, watch their dresses and faces, and explain, if you can, on any theory except that of the workingman's prosperity, how they get their machines. They do not, of course, pay the quoted prices—the rich, in fact, in bicycling as in surgery, being taxed a good deal for the benefit of the poor—but if they want one they always contrive to get it. Whoever is ruined, the steady workers are not, and, after all, in this country, though there are loafers at every street corner, and though the mass of what must be described as the precipitate of humanity is enormous, still the steady workers are in an overwhelming majority. We should not think a curate very wild who bought a bicycle, and the well-to-do artisan is much better off than he is. The universality of the power of reading, too, must be allowed for, and then there is the greatest cause of all, the spread of education. The fanatics of education will exclaim at that, but we have not a doubt that education is responsible for much of the new interest in amusement. The steady, if imperfect teaching of one generation—for all men and women of thirty can now read and write, and would be horrified at the idea of their children growing up letterless—has had many varied effects, not all of them good effects, but one of them has undoubtedly been to increase the national cheerfulness.

We, who are not fanatics of education, and do not believe that it breeds all the virtues, can say with the strongest conviction that it has lifted a sort of dull cloud from the national mind. The common folk are becoming distinctly better tempered. They are much more "cheeky," the boys especially, and much more given to acid criticism, but the dull moroseness that we can remember as a kind of note among a large section of those who worked, has, to a perfectly amazing extent, passed away. It exists, of course, and always will exist, but the old sullenness has been immensely softened and decreased. Naturally, with that change has come an impatience of monotony, a wish for interests that are disconnected with the daily work, and as the mass of men are not intellectual, and never will be, that means a new and keen interest in all excitements, and especially in the excitements that have in them the elements of contest.

We can see the progress of this impatience quite as much among the cultivated as among the handicraftsmen, though the former have, from circumstances, a method of taking their distractions in lumps—holidays, they call them—which the latter are unable to follow, and we can certainly testify that the cultivated are no worse. The old professional men, merchants and manufacturers, who used to boast that for thirty years they had never been absent from their offices on a single working day, were by no means universally saints in conduct. We regret, and, perhaps unconsciously rather despise, the modern craving for distractions, but we doubt, when we think it over, whether it means serious mischief.

HYGIENE OF THE CYCLIST.

Just Lucas-Championnière states that cycling, like all exercise, should be taken up moderately. The heart should be carefully watched, not because this exercise is more harmful in this respect than others, but because it can be indulged in much longer without giving a sense of fatigue. Vicious attitudes, such as a crooked posture, although not being so important as is generally supposed, nevertheless, ought to be avoided. In a long journey the position in which the body is moderately inclined is best for the organs of respiration and circulation. The position in the saddle is hard to decide upon for every case. Practice shows that the perineum accommodates itself to the saddle better than would have been supposed. Moderation in eating is a necessity in muscular work, as is also abstention from alcohol. The bicycle should vary in details for the man, the woman, the child, the racer, and the invalid. In the case of a man, the perineum, with its component parts, should be carefully watched. As to the woman, this exercise is easier for her than for the man, since she is more supple. It causes far less fatigue than walking. Its effects on the pelvic organs are good. The exercise should be suspended during menstruation, and it is not to be recommended during pregnancy. The child does not feel so much fatigue as the adult, but it should use the bicycle with the greatest moderation. As a rule the courier understands his limitations well. He should, like all athletes, possess perfect organs. As to the invalid, many ailments are improved or even cured by the use of the bicycle, *e. g.*, gastro-intestinal troubles, deformities of the vertebral column, etc. Indeed, the author believes that this branch of the subject is so extensive as to deserve a special chapter.—*Gazette Médicale de Strasbourg, Med. Record.*

UNHEALTHY SCHOOLROOMS.

According to *Treatment* for November, says the *Charlotte Med. Journal*, Schmidt-Maunard of Leipzig has been occupied for several years in making observations on the health of children in schools. It is, of course, very difficult to obtain exact information as to the manner in which attendance at school affects the growth and weight of children, but he is able to affirm that during the first year at school the growth, both as regards height and weight, is less than during any preceding year. He is of opinion that the well-being of the children, and incidentally their growth, is injured by the

ill-health caused by imperfect sanitary conditions, especially inadequate supplies of fresh air and light. In the higher schools in Leipzig, Dr. Schmidt-Mounard found that headaches, sleeplessness, and nervous ailments were frequent, especially among girls. Schools in which the pupils are obliged to practice gymnastic exercises every afternoon had a much smaller proportion of children suffering from insomnia than those in which study went on all day. Further, he claims that children who do not go to school until they are seven years old become stronger, and are in all other respects better developed than those who go to school a year sooner.

Dr. Schmidt-Mounard would doubtless agree with the dictum of Sir James Crichton-Browne, "First make your son a good animal."

HOW TO AVOID COLDS.

DRINK A LOT OF COLD WATER, AND USE A HORSE BRUSH ON THE SKIN.

A woman who for years suffered from violent colds, which several times threatened to end fatally, claims to have attained immunity, says the *Washington Star*, by the use of pure cold water as a medicine and an ordinary horse brush, for currying, as a morning and evening exercise. Owing to a severe nervous breakdown, she was obliged to consult a New York physician, famous for his original and simple methods of treatment. After laying down the law on the subject of diet and fresh air, he said: "You will also go to some big department store, and purchase, for 35 cents, a horse brush, with which you will give your whole body a thorough rubbing each morning, before you bathe. As soon as you arise you will fill a quart pitcher with drinking water, and sip it slowly, while dressing. At night, do the same thing over again, omitting, of course, the bath."

The cold water was easily managed, and soon became indispensable, but at first the horse brush seemed to tear the sensitive skin. Having absolute confidence in her physician, however, the patient persisted, at first barely touching the bristles to her body. Within a few weeks she was not only able to do the currying most vigorously, but really anticipated it with pleasure. The signs of the first winter cold drove her in haste to the doctor. The great man of medicine refused to supply her with drugs. He questioned her as one would a child, as to leaving her windows open at night, as to drinking water regularly and taking her exercises, upon all of which she passed a fair examination. He said: "Then you have been indulging in holiday overeating. Whenever you eat a heavy, rich dinner, and let it be as seldom as possible, omit the next meal, and substitute a quart of water. You can't take cold unless you get into condition for it."

This she did, and the cold failed to mature, and although she has frequently left undone those things which she ought to have done, and *vice versa*, and paid a penalty proportionate to her carelessness, she has never since suffered from a really violent cold.

Of course, any system of living which builds up a well-nourished body is inimical to colds, as well as other forms of disease. Cold water taken in this manner simply washes the stomach, carrying off the injurious acids which generate there and which, allowed to circulate through the blood, impoverish it, thereby weakening the vitality of the person. After washing the blood clean, as it were, the next thing is to induce circulation. This is done by means of the vigorous currying, which, besides bringing the blood to the surface to resist external chill, also opens the pores, allowing impurities to escape. Then the daily bath finishes the work.

The woman who has banished colds by means of water drinking and currying claims to require much less clothing than formerly. In terror of her health, she built breastworks of flannel, which proved utterly useless when the assault came.

Since she has gone in for the home-made product in heat, she finds that she is now much warmer with less clothing.

Those who intend to put this simple cold cure in practice, and it is a remedy for many another evil, should remember that water taken with meals does not count at all, or if it does it is rather to be added to the side of the enemy. It must be taken before breakfast and again just before retiring, and a whole quart must be sipped within, say three-quarters of an hour. If cold water chills one, the temperature may be raised a little until this difficulty is overcome. Some good, cheap distilled water is best where there is any question of the purity of the water supply.

There is one other essential point to be remembered by those who would escape colds, as well as drugs. By the free circulation of the blood much impurity is thrown off through the pores. It is, therefore, important, when the presence of the cold indicates some impurity in the blood, that in addition to the daily bath the clothes worn next the skin should be changed frequently to prevent reabsorption to the skin. Of course, clothing worn during the day should never be worn at night.

URIC ACID.

THERE is hardly any factor more insidious in its evil doing, more metastatic in its manifestations, more hydra-headed in its stubborn resistance to treatment, more lethal in its results and yet more ignored by the medical profession than uric acid. Every stage of life, every condition of existence is susceptible to lithemia. We can scarcely conceive a disorder which, having baffled all attempts of research and treatment, is not due to this pathological cause. Early excreta of tissue decay constitute an array of powerful toxics, and if not eliminated from the system produce serious disorders, often with fatal results. Nitrogenous waste creates a condition incompatible with health. Remaining in the blood, it exerts an influence upon the nervous system which we call auto-infection, causing neuralgia, impaired vision, gout, rheumatism, eczema, constipation, dyspepsia, bronchorrhea, diabetes mellitus and insipidus, chronic lithiasis, etc. When the uric acid is properly neutralized and eliminated through the urinary and alimentary tract all these ailments produced by faulty metabolism disappear. Therefore, Kutnow's Improved Effervescent Powder has gained such a favorite position with the most prominent practitioners throughout the world. For it is composed of the health spending mineral salts obtained direct from the waters of the most celebrated European mineral springs, with the additional advantage of being perfectly palatable, gentle and efficacious. It will be found an unexcelled alkaline and saline, a cholagogue and diuretic, and most reliable in all hepatic, nephritic and stomachic disturbances, especially indicated in the lithemic and uric acid diathesis.

THERAPEUTICS AND HYGIENE OF OBESITY.

At the recent International Congress at Paris, Deschamps read a paper with the above title (*Le Bulletin Médical*, August 8, 1900). We should not content ourselves with a mere momentary reduction of weight, but should aim at securing physiological equilibrium between the ingesta and egesta. Diet, calorification, and muscular exercise are the most important elements to consider in the hygiene of obesity. The dietetic regimen should guarantee the patient sufficient food for all his needs, which includes the maintenance of all the gastro-intestinal functions. The regimen of choice is one in which vegetables predominate. and from which farinaceous and feculent articles need not be excluded. Water, pure or slightly alkaline. is the only drink to em-

ploy, and enough should be taken to quench the thirst. In certain cases it may be necessary to recommend an excess of water. Physiological calorification plays the chief rôle in reducing the weight of the corpulent. This is effected by prolonged bathing, the temperature of the water ranging from 33° to 36° C., and the duration. one to two hours. The static-electric bath is an adjuvant of incontestable utility, as it also favors organic combustion. Muscular exercise cannot be imposed on the obese beyond a certain. point. It is useful when regulated, but dangerous when it goes beyond the endurance of the individual. The temporary loss of weight obtained by its agency is more than offset by disorders of function which are set up.—*American Medical Review of Reviews.*

THE INCUBATOR CHICKEN.

Backward, turn backward, oh, time, in your
    flight,
Make me an egg again, smooth, clean and
    white;
I'm homesick and lonely, and life's but a
    dream,
I'm a chick that was born in a hatching
    machine;
Compelled in this world sad and lonely to
    roam—
No mother to shelter, no place to call home,
No mother to teach me to scratch or to
    cluck;
I, alas! scarcely know if I'm chicken or
    duck.
My brothers and sisters have all gone
    astray;
If a pullet I prove, I will loaf around all day,
And never a bit of an egg will I lay.
So backward. turn backward. yet once more
    I beg;
Reverse the new process—and make me an
    egg.
        —*Boston Gazette*

CONDENSED WISDOM.

No man is a really accomplished physician or surgeon who has not made dietetic principles and practice an important part of his professional education.—*Sir Henry Thompson.*

THERE are but two bodies in the field of medicine, physicians and the *paths.* Try to make the public understand this. If you must have some name, let it be that of a common-sense doctor, who, brought face to face with the problems of life and death, is willing to save life in any way, who acknowledges no boundaries, no sects, no schools, but who searches heaven and earth to find means to relieve suffering and cure disease.—*Prof. H. C. Wood.*

THE happiest man is one who has enough in his own inner wealth, and requires little or nothing from outside for his maintenance; for imports are expensive things, reveal dependence, entail danger, occasion trouble, and, when all is said and done, are a poor substitute for home produce.—*Scopenhauer.*

WHEN Socrates saw various articles of luxury spread out for sale, he exclaimed: "How much there is in the world that I do not want!"

WERE the world full of happy homes, all other things could look out for themselves.—*Rev. M. J. Savage.*

SUICIDE may be regarded as an experiment—a question which man puts to Nature, trying to force her to an answer. . . . It is a clumsy experiment to make, for it involves the destruction of the very consciousness which puts the question and awaits the answer.—*Scopenhauer.*

THERE is no man who is not, at some-time, indebted to his vices."

"THE soul says, eat; the body would feast."

"WARS, fires, plagues, break up immovable routine, clear the ground of rotten races and dens of distemper, and open up a fair field to new men."

"THE sun were insipid, if the universe were not opaque."—*Emerson.*

"EVERY parting gives a foretaste of death, every coming together again a foretaste of the resurrection."

HE invited the celebrated virtuoso to dinner, and then, as though struck by an afterthought, he added:
"You can bring your violin with you, if you like."
"Thanks, for myself," answered the artist, "but, as for my fiddle, it never dines."

A PRACTICAL little Hebrew boy was asked by his teacher: "Jesse, if one orange costs eight cents, how much will two oranges cost?"
He looked up brightly, and replied: "Don't you think, teacher, we ought to get two for fifteen cents?"

A TRAMP applied to an Oakland woman for something to eat, and was asked how a chop would suit him. He thought a moment, and looked up, suspiciously, "Mutton, or woodshed, lady?"—*American Kitchen Magazine.*

MR. NICEFELLOW—What do you think is the proper age for girls to marry?
Miss Lena—Oh, about nineteen.
"Indeed! And how old are you?"
"Oh, about nineteen."—*Town Topics.*

DR. GOULD AND THE "PHILADELPHIA MEDICAL JOURNAL."

MUCH comment, of a rather mixed nature, followed the sudden rupture of the apparently satisfactory and successful relations existing between the founder and distinguished editor-in-chief of this virile weekly, at the opening of the century and the year. We have hitherto refrained from commenting on this quite unexpected, and, to outsiders, unaccountable change of front, hoping to receive some more plausible and valid assignment of reasons than has yet, so far as we know, been proffered. A few rival medical journals indulged in covert sneers and uncomplimentary compliments, of the "I told-you-so" sort, which were neither dignified nor enlightening.

Dr. Gould is nothing if not aggressive, and, therefore, it would be strange if he had not made some enemies and piqued some critics during his career as a medical editor. For our own part, we have no quarrel with the aggressives. Medical journalism needs more of them. They are the men who lay the axe at the foot of the forests of shams and charlatanism that still abound in the profession.

We opine that Dr. Gould has displayed too much professional, and not enough commercial, zeal to suit the mercenary spirit of this commercial age. But why should there have been any disappointment from this source? It is exactly what was announced as the original purpose of the new venture. It is exactly what Dr. Gould proposed and explicitly announced, exactly what he promised, and exactly what he accomplished. Had the effort been designed and undertaken as a commercial venture it would not have needed nor asked Dr. Gould to become its oracle. There could have been no misunderstanding. His light has never been hidden under a bushel, nor have his principles or opinions been suppressed or dissembled. Every man in any way associated with the enterprise knew its object, and knew that Dr. Gould had never surrendered to the delusive spirit of compromise. They were thoroughly well aware that no corporation or private interest had ever dared, or ever would dare, directly or indirectly, to approach him with a bribe.

Well, the *Philadelphia Medical Journal,* as an exponent of what might be called the higher criticism in medical journalism, has had its day. It may live in name, but its spirit has passed over to a proposed new medium, which we understand is well under way, and from which it is confidently hoped all doubtful elements have been eliminated. When it makes its maiden bow to the profession, we may have occasion to mention it again.

✤ ✤

DR. O. W. HOLMES, the doctor, poet, and philosopher, once closed his little chat "Over the Teacups," in *Atlantic Monthly,* as follows:

"If all the trees in all the woods were men,
And each and every blade of grass a pen;
If every leaf on every shrub and tree
Turned to a sheet of foolscap; every sea
Were changed to ink, and all earth's living tribes
Had nothing else to do but act as scribes,
And for ten thousand ages, day and night,
The human race should write, and write, and write,
Till all the pens and paper were used up
And the huge inkstand was an empty cup,
Still would the scribblers clustered around the brink,
Call for more pens, more paper, and more ink."

✤ ✤

EXERCISE the mind with contemplation and the body with action, and so preserve the health of both.—*Confucius.*

✤ ✤

SECOND BRIEF OF THE BREVITY CLUB.

NOTE: Announcement was made in the February GAZETTE of the origin of the "Brevity Club," its laconic history, and the publication of a paper read at its first meeting. The object of the Brevity Club is to attract a membership of "brevity" thinkers and writers, men and women who have useful ideas to express but do not care to go into lengthy details. On most subjects punctillious details are no longer in demand; let the reader do the padding.

If the publishers of either literary or scientific journals, standing on the threshold of this new century, have had one lesson more insistently and vividly burned into their consciousness than any other, it is the lesson of brevity, directness, aptness and condensation. Everywhere, and in all fields of literature, editors and authors are being sharply admonished to condense, compress and eliminate. Even the churches no longer tolerate the old-time, long-drawn-out, sleep-inducing sermons.

It is not obligatory upon the members of the Brevity Club that they shall attend its meetings. Let them send in their papers; they will be read and discussed before the club, and then published in the GAZETTE.

The first paper of the club was devoted to "Air." This one touches upon

WATER.

Normal man is 90 per cent. water. Civilized habits have desiccated him until he is about 25 per cent. water and 75 per cent. nerves. Hence the predominance of a neurotic tendency in all modern diseases. Think of the list: Nervous dyspepsia, neurasthenia, neuralgia of a hundred varieties, epilepsy, hyperesthesia of this or that tissue or surface, insomnia, syncope, shock, hemicrania, hysteria, enteralgia, gastralgia, proctalgia, coxalgia, neuritis, neuratrophia, neuralemmitis, neuremia, psychalgia, and the well-nigh endless catalogue of the real and pretended psychiatrists.

Nothing in the organic world can be formed or compounded without the aid and presence of water. Not even the crystalline rocks that rib the earth can take form without the presence of their water of crystallization. Every structure and substance, muscle, nerve, brain and bone, food and drink, wholesome drug and deadly poison, starch and strychnin, protoplasm and prussic acid, chops, corn and chloroform, sugar salt and sulphuric acid, all are based on this bland element, water, and none of them could exist without it. Moreover, with its slight addition or substraction, and a turn of the chemist's wrist, blandness is turned into virulence, food into poison, and *vice versa.*

Its preponderance in Nature and in man's physical organism proves it a principal and indispensable source of supply and repair. Necessary as it is, most of us avoid its internal use almost entirely, except when it is contaminated with some extraneous taint of caffeine or chicory, mead, malt or meat juice, alcohol or other aboriginal admixture. *A hint from Nature might forefend a hundred hurts from Art!*

(PUBLISHER'S NOTE.—If any of our readers, appreciating the spirit of the "Brevity Club," would like to become active members—no initiation fees or annual dues—they are cordially invited to address the Editor of the GAZETTE.)

GOING to bed hungry is a relic of the misconception of the laws of hygiene following physiological investigations in the early part of the last century. Man is the only animal who was ever foolish enough to voluntarily go to sleep while hungry. Judging from the advice now given by thinking physicians, the practice will soon become a mere tradition.

Department of Notes and Queries.

FREEDOM OF DISCUSSION BETWEEN EDITOR AND READER.

Query 73. How do medicines act? In other words, do medicines act upon the system, or does the system act upon the medicines?
J. S., Harrisburg.

Answer.—Your "how" question is one upon which oceans of ink have been expended. Some medicines act mechanically, to a certain limited extent—that is, by their mere presence, ponderability, specific gravity, bulk, contact, incompressibility and other physical or material qualities. In case of Mark Twain's jumping frog it was the simple law of gravitation that got in its "depressing" work. In that particular case the bird-shot or lead would have to be called a "depressant."

Some medicines act chemically, but in the presence of the vital forces the laws of chemical affinity are very much modified. Living tissues are largely composed of hydrocarbons, yet they stubbornly refuse to oxidize in the presence of the usual oxidizing agents, at least until after the contact has been made unusually intimate and persistent. Otherwise, organized beings would soon succumb to the chemical agents by which they are more or less constantly surrounded.

A respectable volume might be expended on the second part of your query, and still leave unsolved issues for further discussion. The nihilists in medicine insist that medicines *never* act on the system, but are *always* acted upon by the life forces. In a sweeping sense this is true; but to our short-sighted perceptions there are very decided and unmistakable exceptions. For example, a few drops of hydrocyanic acid placed on the base of the tongue cause almost instant death; yet even the most incorrigible of the therapeutic iconoclasts will hardly assert that the system *killed itself*, on account of a few drops of HCN. So of strychnia, aconitia, and other powerful poisons. Just how these potent alkaloids do their deadly work remains a chemical as well as physiological conundrum. We say, in the absence of any more satisfactory explanation, that this or that one paralyzes the spinal cord; but this is one of the thousands of explanations that do not explain.

Turning to the ordinary drugs used as medicines, there is no gainsaying the fact that the system or organism into which they are introduced either utilizes them as food or expels them as poisons. Take the case of an ordinary cathartic.

When introduced into the stomach the sentient vital forces at once discover that it is inimical to the welfare of the tissues. It is therefore quickly enveloped in a coating of protective mucus, and by a copious secretion of fluids on the part of the intestinal glands is sent hurtling along to its exit from the system. In providing a protective medium for the intruding matter Nature appropriates such material as is at readiest command, and thus frees herself of foul and injurious accumulations and excretions that have, perhaps, already been too long retained. The benefits are in proportion to the amount of offending material removed. Your pharmacomaniac is sure his aloes and podophyllin and calomel *act.* The therapeutic nihilist is equally certain that the *vital forces* do all the acting— Nature kicking out an intruder. Technically, even food does not *act;* the system dissolves, disintegrates, absorbs and assimilates it. The food itself is entirely passive. It is the system that selects and utilizes what it needs, and rejects and eliminates refuse material that it can not use.

Our language is full of expressions quite as misleading as the one to which our correspondent evidently objects. We all say, and even the almanacks tell us, that "the sun rises"; and yet every schoolboy can demonstrate that, so far as this planetary system is concerned, the sun has no motion. It is the stupid earth that is doing all the hustling. There is no such thing as a "rising tide." The tides are playthings for the magnet moon and the synergist sun. The river flows, smoke rises, stars shine and trees grow. All these are inaccurate expressions, but they are too firmly established to be thrown aside for others that might be exact truth without being expressive or intelligible to ordinary mortals. We shall have to tolerate the expressions as they run, on account of their antiquity; but there is no reason why we should not more fully realize that living Nature is, for the most part, superior to dead matter; that in a general way the living forces do all the acting, and that ordinary medicines are as passive as the water that runs down hill.

Query 74. How is the infection of smallpox disseminated? It seems to me we are much in the dark concerning the spread of this loathsome disease. No scientist has announced its germ, if it have one, and its mode of propagation seems to be a matter of speculation.　G. R. A., Iowa.

Answer.—According to the latest researches a number of the infectious diseases are usually spread by the same. means, namely, by the movement of infectious dust. In the list thus disseminated are included consumption. diphtheria, pneumonia, scarlet fever, influenza, whooping-cough, measles and smallpox. If some way could be devised by which all buildings inhabited by human beings could be constantly freed from the dust nuisance, if our inventors would turn their attention to devising dust-consumers as well as smoke-consumers, which latter have been made a success, it would be a boon to humanity. Few persons, even though they be medical men, realize the danger that constantly menaces us in the dust of the street and of our apartments. The principal avenue of entrance for communicable diseases is the nose. Through this useful but much abused organ there passes from 1,000 to 1,200 cubic inches of air every hour, or about 28,000 cubic inches every twenty-four hours. Even in the most carefully kept of our living rooms this air is constantly filled with floating but most of the time invisible dust. It cannot be otherwise than that an almost incredible quantity of dust is thus constantly taken into the system. This dust at all times contains germs, most of them harmless, but some of them capable of setting up diseased action unless vigorously and effectively combated and repulsed by the defensive powers of the system. When such germs find an exposed surface, a little patch of mucous membrane that is abraded or inflamed and thereby weakened in its capability to defend itself, the opportunity is promptly seized and disease results. That all persons who are exposed to them are not attacked by the most virulent of the infectious diseases proves that not all are at all times susceptible to the infection. It has happened in several instances that persons suffering from smallpox in the most communicable stage have passed in public conveyances from one end of the city to the other without perceptibly spreading the disease. Robust health is at all times the chief condition of immunity. The mouth is another avenue of entrance. Mouth-breathers are considered rather more liable to infection than those who breathe normally and constantly through the nasal passages. Germs reach the air and mingle with floating dust, from the breath and from the sputum of an infected person. Flies and other insects frequently carry infection from sputa, from wounds visited, from sores and excreta. They may convey it directly to another person through a sore or abrasion, or by depositing it on articles of food, which if not rendered innocuous by cooking may convey the disease to a susceptible partaker. Thus some infectious diseases are taken with the ingesta. The eyes are another but rarer means of ingress for pathogenic bacteria. Normally they are provided with an antiseptic lubricating fluid which destroys hurtful bacteria, but in case of congestion or slight inflammation this fluid may fail to act with sufficient promptness, and living germs then find their way into the nose, through the lachrymal ducts, and thus reach the general system. Smallpox is no doubt conveyed by all these methods at times, but chiefly, it is thought, by inhaling the volatile *materies morbi*, whatever that may be.

Query 75. Is formaldehyde a reliable and safe disinfectant, and what is the simplest way of using it?   E. M. H., Wis.

Answer.—The value of this agent has been frequently called in question, but it has been finally settled that its failures have not been owing to the gas itself, but to the faulty methods of procuring or liberating it. At first it was assumed that the decomposition of wood alcohol by heat was an effective source; but it was discovered that much of the spirit was merely vaporized, and hence failed to supply the disinfecting gas.

Really, no expensive apparatus is necessary. Sprinkling a 40 per cent. solution of formaldehyde on cotton sheets hung in a room, from an ordinary sprinkling pot, is all that is actually required. One must do the sprinkling rapidly, and get out of the room in a hurry, to avoid the stifling vapors that are rapidly evolved. Eight ozs. of this solution suffices to disinfect 1,000 cubic feet of room-space.

Query 76. Will the GAZETTE give its readers a comprehensive definition of the word *Hygiene?* It has come to be used very promiscuously and, it seems to me, at times, indiscriminately.
      J. L. F., Conn.

Answer.—The "Century Dictionary" gives this: "That department of medical knowledge which concerns the preservation of health; a system of principles or rules designed for the promotion of health; sanitary science."

Dr. Henry B. Baker, long at the head of the Health Department of Michigan, says:

"Progress in hygiene consists in advancement of knowledge (1) of the causation of disease, (2) of the modes by which communicable diseases are spread, (3) of the modes of entrance into the body of those diseases which are communicable, and (4) of the best measures for the avoidance, for the restriction, and for the prevention of diseases."

In a word, we will add, that *Hygiene means the How of Health.*

THE
DIETETIC AND HYGIENIC GAZETTE

A MONTHLY JOURNAL OF PHYSIOLOGICAL MEDICINE

| VOL. XVII. | NEW YORK, APRIL, 1901. | No. 4. |

HOW SHALL WE DISPOSE OF OUR SEWAGE?

BY R. M. BUCKE, M.D.,
London Insane Asylum, Ontario, Canada.

THIS is one of the most vital and important questions at present before the hygienic world. By way of making a small contribution to the discussion of it I will state here the experience of this institution and show to what conclusion it has led us.

The London Asylum was opened for patients in November, 1870. At that time the sewer opened into a small creek a few hundred yards to the east. This creek runs nearly or quite dry every summer, and its condition after having received our sewage for a few years may easily be imagined. In answer to the clamors of the farmers, whose lives we were constantly threatening, and sometimes taking, a filtration plant was put in. The sewage was now supposed to be made innoxious by passing through a few feet of a mixture of gravel and charcoal. The worst of it was it was found impossible to keep our filter in order; the attempt to do so involved much labor and some expense for material, neither did it wholly remove the nuisance when it was kept at its best. Something more and better had to be done, but what? At last it was decided to adopt what is called the "Intermittent Downward Filtration" system.

A piece of sandy land some four acres in extent a few hundred yards west of the main asylum building was chosen for the experiment. The field was graded to a perfect level. It was then very elaborately under drained, which doubtless in some cases is necessary, but was in our case a waste of tile and labor, as the water from the sewage has never, any of it, entered the tile in question but has passed away by diffusion into and through the sand. After being leveled the field was graded to a series of beds and depressions so that when done these were alternately running east and west across it, first a bed ten feet wide, then a depression with sloping sides eight feet wide at top and two feet wide across its level bottom and eighteen inches deep. Then another exactly similar bed and depression, until the whole field was thus graded. At the east end of the field a plank runway somewhat similar to a mining sluice and provided with little simple iron gates conducts the sewage to and into the depressions in the field.

All the sewage of the asylum, including waste water from the laundry and kitchen, is collected by sewers into a central tank placed underground, arched over, covered with earth and then grass and ventilated into the tall boiler house chimney. Once a day this sewage, of which there may be sixty, seventy or eighty thousand gallons, is thrown by a centrifugal pump into a shallow concrete well at the northeast angle of the sewage field, from which it runs into the depressions as already described. By means of the gates it is directed day by day to the depression or depressions where wanted.

Within two to six hours after pumping the sewage has disappeared into the soil; it never has time to ferment, and there has never been any smell of sewage in any part of the institution since this method of disposal was adopted. At first what has now been told was supposed to be the whole story. There was no question of making any use of the sewage, and indeed the asylum was instructed by the government to plant nothing on the beds between the depressions. But after a few years the temptation became too great to be longer withstood and I began planting the beds. My report for that year shows that in 1893 we grew on these beds 110 dozen watermelons, 216 dozen muskmelons, over 10,000 dozen cucumbers, besides squash, pumpkins, celery, peppers, tomatoes, peas, radishes, chillies, and that the total value of the crop on the four acres was over $750.

Latterly we have extended the beds and depressions to about seven acres instead of four, not for purpose of sewage disposal, but so we could irrigate the beds, and attached to the sewage field a few acres of other land adjoining that had been lying waste. The result has been that last year on this sewage field we raised asparagus, beets, beans, cabbage, cauliflower, carrots, celery, lettuce, melons, onions, peas, rhubarb, strawberries, sea kale and tomatoes, to the value of $1,840.15.

The field converted into the sewage field was high, sandy and barren; it is now perhaps the most fertile field in Ontario; not only so, but the fruit and vegetables grown upon it are much superior in quality to those grown elsewhere, on our land at least.

Further, the barren sandy field, which had no beauty that one should desire it, is now as beautiful as it is fruitful. It has no unpleasant odor at any time, not even when the sewage is being pumped, there is nothing to offend the eye, for the sewage is converted by the centrifugal pump which handles it into a homogeneous fluid having very much the appearance and smell of dishwater.

It is needless to say that the patients and caretaker who work on the sewage field are as healthy as any other people about the institution, or that the fruit and vegetables grown on this field are as wholesome as those grown elsewhere; in fact whatever prejudices existed in this regard at first it is now universally acknowledged that the produce of this field is in every way superior to that grown elsewhere on our farm or garden.

It seems to me that we have here in a nutshell the solution of the sewage difficulty. Wherever men upon the land are massed together permanently upon a given area—whether in city, town, village, or institution, this method can be practised and not only by it can absolute and cleanly disposal be accomplished, but at the same time a large return of the best products of the earth may be had in exchange for a product which if not used is certain to become dangerous.

If we run our sewage into streams or bays we pollute the water, waste the sewage, and cause disease. To treat it with filters or chemicals is never perhaps absolutely safe from the point of view of health, is more or less expensive and the sewage itself is wasted. But if we return the sewage to the earth, to which it belongs, we obtain clean wholesome and absolute disposal at a nominal cost and at the same time secure the value of the sewage—a very considerable item.

WE move in a cycle. In the words of the humorist:

"A certain man caught a fish with a worm
　　That did eat of a king;
Then did he eat of the fish
　　That did eat of the worm."—

To which we might add:—

Thus in eating the fish
　　He ate also the worm,
And in eating the worm
　　He ate also the king.

SOME PLAIN TALK ABOUT THE STOMACH.

BY C. F. ULRICH, A.M., M.D.,
Wheeling, W. Va.

THE stomach occupies a very important position in the animal economy. However, it is not our intention to speak of the stomach of the lower animals, but only of the human stomach. This organ has been gradually developed from a simple, almost straight tube in some of the lower animals which feed upon a single article and require no complicated system of digestion. As the animal rises in the scale of living creatures and consumes a greater variety of food, the alimentary canal is elongated and lies in numerous folds, studded from one end to the other with glands, secreting and giving out fluids such as are necessary to work up the nutrient material, preparing it for the process of assimilation, *i. e.*, of converting such parts of it as are suitable into the different tissues of the body, leaving the superfluous material to be carried off by the emunctories.

Originally the alimentary canal did not differ very greatly in diameter throughout its length, as the animal fed almost continually, and the nutrient material, in its various stages of digestion, was regularly passing from the oral to the anal extremity, giving off such portions as were to be assimilated. But, as the animal rose higher in the scale of being, and began to engage in other employments besides eating and sleeping, there arose a necessity of eating a considerable quantity at one time, which had to be stored up as in a reservoir. This receptacle was developed by the expansion of the canal, near the upper end, just below the thoracic cavity, where there was room for expansion. This formed the organ known as the stomach, which is found in the greatest perfection in man and the highest order of mammals.

Many of the laity are still laboring under the erroneous belief that the stomach is the sole organ of digestion, not being at all aware that the intestinal tract has anything to do with that important function; supposing that its only business is to carry off the waste material. This degree of ignorance is gradually being dissipated since the public schools are teaching physiology and the people are beginning to investigate Nature, learning more and more about the human body with its complicated machinery.

The stomach has a twofold function. It serves as a reservoir or storehouse to receive, and temporarily store up the food that is taken at stated intervals between the periods devoted by man to his avocations, amusements and rest. As has already been stated, it is an expansion of the alimentary canal, lying transversely across the upper part of the abdomen, immediately below the diaphragm which divides it from the thorax. Its shape is determined by the space into which it can stretch itself, while its size depends upon the amount of food habitually taken at one time. Thus a heavy eater will be found on dissection to have a large stomach, while that of a light eater is found to be proportionally small. The infant has a very small stomach and spends most of its time, when not asleep, taking nourishment from the mother's breast or the nursing bottle. It has a most remarkable facility for disgorging its food when it has taken too much, which proves the diminutive size of the stomach. From this storehouse the alimentary canal draws the material for the work of digestion and assimilation, while the man (the word man must be understood to apply to both sexes) is engaged in his various avocations, or resting from labor.

The second function of this organ is to perform the work of digestion in one of its stages. This work begins in the mouth, consisting of mastication with the teeth, reducing it as near as possible to pulp, during which process it is mixed with the product of the salivary glands, whose function it is to prepare the food for its reception in the stomach. The inner surface of this organ is studded with numerous little follicles which pour out the gastric fluid that mingles with the food to prepare it for the action of the fluids found in the duodenum and other parts of the intestines.

Since I am not writing a work on elementary physiology I shall not enter into any details of the process of digestion. The main object of writing this paper is to give some hints to the readers of the GAZETTE as to the proper care of the stomach, which organ is perhaps more abused than any other part of the human body.

The size of the stomach depends, as I have said, on the quantity of food that is habitually taken at each meal, since it will naturally stretch to make room for excessive quantities of ingesta. Now this stretching process necessarily diminishes the efficiency of the organ. You may ask: How? The number of follicles is not increased, but frequently diminished, since many of them are obliterated by the stretching. Now we have an enlarged stomach, industriously kept filled, yielding a diminished amount of gastric fluid. What is the result? The work of gastric digestion is only half accomplished, and the imperfectly digested food is rushed into the other compartments of the human tissue factory in an unprepared state. This incompleteness goes on increasing until the entire process of digestion and assimilation is botched; the emunctories or human sewers are clogged with undigested material, so that diseases which should be unknown to the system attack the various organs and good health becomes impossible. From this source arise habitual constipation, gastritis, enteritis, typhlitis, appendicitis, and many other diseases that torment the human race.

The first lesson, therefore, to be learned in regard to the care of the stomach is not to eat too much; regulate the quantity by the needs of the system. Do not let your appetite run away with your discretion, causing you to overload your stomach so as to stretch it out of shape and ruin its efficiency. The consequences of such incautious procedure do not stop at the stomach itself, but involve all the abdominal organs, and indirectly the entire body. Dyspepsia with its train of physical and mental suffering (for what an unhappy, disagreeable, pessimistic being the chronic dyspeptic is we have all doubtless observed); persistent constipation, with its annoyances and terrors; Bright's disease of the kidneys, with its awful sufferings, its complete upsetting of all the functions of the body, harrowing of the mind and the premature death following in its wake; all these and many other dire effects result from the habitual overloading of the stomach.

Another lesson to be learned is to know what to eat. There are many articles of food that, although palatable and stimulating to the appetite, do not in any way contribute to the growth or maintenance of the human body.

I have no space to enumerate the suitable and unsuitable articles of diet, but will refer my readers to the columns of the GAZETTE, where they will find ample intsructions along that line. A good rule to observe in the matter of diet, which I always inculcate in my patients during and after convalescence, is to observe closely, when eating anything, whether or not it agrees with them; whether they feel comfortable after eating it, with all the functions continuing in good working order, or whether there ensue disturbances of any kind. In the latter case I tell them not to touch it again. This rule, of course, applies to articles of doubtful utility, and not to such as are known to be injurious.

It is also very important to pay attention to what we drink; for liquids must be absorbed in abundance if we do not wish to dry up and be mummified. Water is by far the best liquid to take into the stomach, and should be used constantly and abundantly. It is true much has been said and written about the diseases caused by the use of polluted drinking water; but, notwithstanding this trouble, it is perferable to any other beverage. If it is not pure it can be rendered innocuous by filtering and boiling. The filtering should always precede the boiling, because this removes much of the coarser impurity, thus improving the taste and, by that means, tempting us to drink it in greater abundance. No other beverage can successfully supplant the use of water, although some of them may be taken in small quantities without injury. Coffee and tea are almost universally used, but should be taken with moderation and caution; great care being exercised to have them always freshly made, never allowing them to stand any length of time on the grounds or leaves, as this develops a principle that is irritating to the stomach and injurious to the system. Alcoholic beverages are now generally condemned by many of the profession. Yet there are circumstances under which they would be advisable in very limited quantities; but they should never be used as an habitual beverage. Water is the only drink that is safe for habitual use. Excessive consumption of coffee or tea is generally injurious, although I have known persons who drank two cups of coffee three times a day during their entire life and lived high up in the eighties. But I would not advise any one to follow their example.

Excess in the use of alcohol is to be avoided at all times, since it causes gastritis, with the final result of destroying the efficiency of the stomach. Some of the secondary results are cirrhosis of the liver, followed by jaundice, dropsy and premature death; Bright's disease of the kidneys and many other diseases; all of which can be avoided by taking proper care of the stomach and not filling it up with noxious and deleterious substances.

It is not my province, in this paper, to speak of the terrible effects of the excessive use of alcohol on the brain, the intellect and the moral character of man; this being only a dissertation on the care of the stomach. Neither can you allow me sufficient space in your valued journal to enter into particulars in explaining how these evil results are brought about. So we will have to content ourselves with a mere allusion to them.

I will close this article with a brief recapitulation. The function of the stomach is two-fold: for storing up food to serve as nutriment for the body, allowing it to pass out gradually, as it is needed; and for performing the preliminary work of digestion. For the care of this important organ certain rules are to be observed: Avoid excessive eating, taking only such an amount of food at one time as can be conveniently worked up by the digestive apparatus. Be careful to ingest no deleterious substances into the stomach, which might derange the functions of the digestive tract and result in disease. if not in direct poisoning. Drink plenty of water; filtered and boiled, or distilled to be preferred. This can be taken hot or cold. to suit the circumstances, or the condition of the system at the time. Avoid excessive use of stimulants; coffee, tea, alcoholics. etc. You may observe I use the term *excessive*, because there are many circumstances and conditions where a moderate use of these articles would be useful. Moreover, the coddling of the human body by absolutely abstaining from everything, that is thought or said to be injurious, sometimes does nearly as much harm as the excessive use of them. Moderation in all things is advisable. Excess, even in temperance lectures, crusades and " smashing of joints " is to be deprecated; for excess begets excess, without accomplishing any good. To all who may complain that I have been too general in my remarks and have not entered sufficiently into particulars, I would say: Read THE DIETETIC AND HYGIENIC GAZETTE, where you will find all these topics treated with fullness, acccuracy and precision. I advise my lay friends of the more intellectual class to read that journal, as it will enlighten them on all questions and save them much trouble and suffering.

ARE THE TEACHINGS OF SCIENCE REGARDING FOOD ECONOMY PRACTICAL?

By A. P. BRYANT.

Storrs Agricultural Experiment Station.

AMONG the different lines of scientific investigation that have been followed during the last century those dealing with the food and nutrition of man are of vast practical importance. Probably none would deny this, and yet in an article on the nutritive value of different foods, published in a popular magazine some time since, this statement appears, " From the practical, not the scientific standpoint." Is there, then, so marked a difference between theory and practice; between the deductions from scientific investigations and their practical applications to the conditions of every-day life?

It was not so very many years ago that the teachings of science regarding agriculture were by many likewise considered impractical, and yet to-day among our successful farmers there is scarcely one in a thousand but profits by the practical applications of such teachings. Agricultural papers are constantly showing how the products of the farm may be increased or improved by the application of the teachings of scientific investigations. There is, however, a prevalent impression that in its relation to human nutrition science is frequently not practical. One reason for this is perhaps the ruthless way in which many of the results of scientific research disprove some of the most cherished ideas, such, for instance, as the belief that fish is particularly valuable as a brain food, or that beef tea furnishes concentrated nourishment. Some of the beliefs that still find adherents are on a par with the notion that potatoes must be planted on a particular phase of the moon in order to ensure a successful crop.

Another reason for the feeling that the teachings of science are not always practical may be found in the hasty assumptions and unwarranted conclusions reached by some who call themselves scientists, or misrepresentations of the facts by those who fail to get a just comprehension of their bearing. To this latter class belongs perhaps the following statement, presumably disclosing some of the teachings of science: " Apples especially are said to be an excellant diet for those who work with their brain. They supply positive brain food." And yet there is probably not to-day a physiologist or chemist who has any clear conception of what "brain food" really is.

If one were asked in a few words to contrast the teachings of science and of practice it would be difficult so to separate these that one would not encroach more or less upon the other. In a general way some of the teachings of scientific research may be contrasted with those of every-day observation as follows:

. From scientific investigation we learn:

1. The different kinds of nutrients in food and their rôle in the nutrition of the body.

2. The composition and digestibility of different food materials.

3. The food requirements of the body.

From practical observation we learn:

1. The peculiar therapeutical properties of different food materials and their application to different bodily conditions.

2. The proper preparation of food to render it most palatable and digestible.

3. The proper regulation of diet in health and disease.

Avoiding any detailed or technical discussion of the subject it may not be out of place to still further contrast the character of the information which is derived from the two sources, science and practice. Science tells us that foods are composed of four classes of nutritive materials: protein and mineral matter for the building and repair of muscle, bone, brain, and sinew; fats and carbohydrates for fuel. Science tells us that the leaner cuts of meat, and cheese, milk, beans and peas, and foods made from oats and wheat furnish large amounts of protein for keeping the running gear of the human machine in good order, while fat meats, butter, lard, sugar, and all cereal products yield large amounts of fuel for running the machine; the vegetables and fruits as a rule, contain so large a proportion of water as to be a dilute food although furnishing fuel ingredients and considerable quantities of mineral matters.

Taken in connection with the teachings of science practical observation indicates what are the food requirements of the body, as regards the different classes of nutrients, and what particular kinds of food materials best serve for the diet of persons under conditions other than normal. Scientific investigation shows what are the starchy foods; practical observations aided by such teachings provide diets for diebetics. Practical observation also shows that vegetables and fruits have a value in the diet far beyond that derived from their content of protein and fuel ingredients.

The practical applications of the teachings of science and practice. Even when times are the most prosperous there is a large class of people with whom the problem of subsistence is ever present in its most gloomy and uncompromising aspect. These people live from hand to mouth and too frequently cannot tell at the close of one meal from whence the food for the next meal is to come. The crying need of the day is such teaching, scientific or practical, as will show these people, in such simple and taking way how they can get the most healthy and nutritious food for the least cost. Many attempts have been and are being made by charitable organizations and otherwise to bring about this end, and with the most encouraging success. But the great mass of the poor are as yet not reached to any extent.

One way by which these people may be benefited is by teaching them some of the simpler and more easily comprehended facts concerning food and nutrition. All of these facts must be eminently practical; that much is certain. Some will be based upon practical experience, others will be derived from the teachings of modern science. These latter, should, however, be tested in every instance by experience.

Starting with the knowledge derived from the study of the composition and digestibility of different food materials, and taking into account their cost per pound, an effort has been made to put scientific food economy upon a practical basis by comparing the relative value of different food materials as a source of nutriment, both as regards protein and fuel ingredients. It is such classifications that are probably referred to in the quotation at the beginning of this article. Of course the best classification of food materials must be based upon the knowledge of the amounts of nutrients which they contain that are actually available for use in the body and the physiological or therapeutical action of different foods. Such classification is difficult to make owing to the widely different physiological effects attributed to various food materials by different writers.

Many studies of the actual amounts of nutrients found in the diets of people under different conditions of age, sex, and occupation have been made. These are called dietary studies. A few years ago a considerable number of such studies were carried on among the poor in New York City. In these investigations it was found that many famlies had little or no conception of the actual nutritive value of the different foods purchased, but acted entirely upon the dictates of the appetite or upon the passing whim. The investigations showed that some of these people were paying much more per pound for the same kind of food materials than were others, and that some might have, by wiser selection of food obtained much more nutriment for the same expenditure of money. There was one poor, underfed sewing woman in particular who obtained not more than three-fourths the actual nourishment in her food which she might have obtained had she bought as cheaply as some other families and made different selections.

Scientific research fails to find any greater amount of nutritive material in the more costly cuts of meat than in the cheaper cuts, and wheat flour or bread has been shown to constitute one of the most nutritious as well as economical sources of nourishment that can be found. The dried legumes, such as beans and peas, are a most economical and nourishing food. In fact they furnish one of the cheapest sources of protein or muscle food that can be found and are at the same time one of the most inexpensive forms of fuel.

I recently overheard a generous hearted woman, who out of her own scanty means gives and does much for the relief of the destitute, say to a friend, " Poor woman! She did not have enough to eat, so I gave her twenty-five cents and told her to get some porterhouse steak." When asked why she did not tell her to get "top round," instead, since it was quite tender, just as nutritious and much cheaper, she replied: "What, do you mean to say that porterhouse steak is not more nutritious than round steak?" She was much surprised to learn that the difference in price went to pay, not for a more nutritious food, but for a more tender, and, as ordinarily considered, a more toothsome one.

On the other hand practical observation shows that in sickness the value of a food may be entirely out of proportion to its actual content of nutriment. A savory, appetizing dish frequently has a value far beyond that which its nutritive ingredients would imply.

Many who look at the matter from the practical side, while recognizing the wholesomeness and nutritiousness of the cheaper kinds of meat do not agree as to the practicability of using the dried legumes to any great extent as meat substitutes. When meat is unusually high in price it becomes desirable for the poor man to reduce his butcher's bill if this can be done without impoverishing the diet.

A little experiment was undertaken in a private family in order to see whether meats could be almost entirely substituted by dried fish, and dried beans and peas, and still have a reasonably appetizing and palatable menu. The result was very satisfac-
tory. For a week and a half meat was purchased but once, and then nothing but a cheap boiling piece. In its place for dinner was served salt codfish prepared simply in various commonly adopted ways, and baked beans. For the other meals codfish cakes, codfish on toast, and the old fashioned bean porridge afforded variations. Although no other changes were made in the diet the cost of the food was reduced about one-third. The diet was agreeable, and appeared to be just as well fitted to the needs of the different members of the family as that which contained more and expensive cuts of meat. In short the experiment proved eminently practicable. It is not to be inferred for an instant that any such extreme diet would be selected for constant use. It would, without doubt, soon prove monotonous and distasteful with an accompanying decrease in its actual nutritive value. It is certain, however, that a considerable saving can be effected in the living expenses, if such is required, by the proper selection of the cheaper cuts of meat, and the use of a certain amount of meat substitutes such as salt fish and dried legumes.

It cannot be gainsaid that the results of scientific research are of great practical value in the realm of human nutrition as elsewhere. The inferences drawn from these results are not necessarily correct, neither are the inferences drawn from practical observation. The results of scientific investigation interpreted with the aid of practical observation and experience form the basis upon which true economics of nutrition must be founded.

WHEN TO KEEP QUIET.

When you feel that ideas are crowding your brain
  And struggling for ardent expression;
When impulses come which you scarce can restrain
  To arise with some charge or confession;
When your inmost emotion persuades you to speak
  Opinions which fairly run riot;
When the thoughts come so fast that your soul yearns to shriek—
  It's a mighty good time to keep quiet.
             —*Indianapolis Journal.*

WHAT THE CENTURY HAS TAUGHT US ABOUT LIVING.

BY SAMUEL S. WALLIAN, A. M., M.D.

I.

A WORD PRELIMINARY.

WE have weathered the Old and welcomed the New Century.

Life is better worth living to-day than at any time since our ancestors hunted with clubs, wore furs and fig-leaves and lived on nuts, roots and fruits.

It is a good time to review the vital and social situation, and take an inventory.

The progress made in the Old has been extolled by poets, paragraphers and reviewing essayists until there are no more adjectives at hand. The impetus gained will undoubtedly make the movement of the New so much more rapid and satisfactory that all that has gone before will seem slow and commonplace. Because of this momentum any forecast of the future, based on the experience of the past, will be incompetent. Above all, we have learned that LIFE IS NOT AS WELL WORTH LIVING AS IT CAN BE MADE.

The Typesetter has unhorsed the Knight; the caravan has crystallized into the commonwealth; the Citadel has been remodeled into the Common school.

The Prophets have taken in their signs and capitulated to the Printing Press; the telegraph, telephone and aerograph have signaled the death-knell of distance; and the phonograph has rendered the voices of the dead immortal.

With the victories, discoveries and failures of the past century before us we should be unfaithful stewards if we should fail to make much more revolutionary and startling advances in the coming years.

As a sure foundation for all progress we must *build better habitations; breath better air; eat better food; sleep in better beds; wear more sensible clothing,* and then it will be easy to *live better lives.*

The physician of the future will be compelled to become a conservator of health instead of a patcher and repairer of perverts; a pilot to Hygiea, instead of a recruiting sergeant for the hospitals and purveyor to the undertaker; and his study of prophylaxis will be in the field of sanatory science rather than in the delusively fascinating realm of bacterio-pathology.

To this end the coming medical college must endow a chair of Domestic Economics and make it the substructure of its entire curriculum.

THE HOME.

The Anglo-Saxon of the word is *ham,* the German *heim,* from which we have the English forms, *Allingham, Birmingham, Cheltenham,* etc., also the diminutive *hamlet;* and the German, *Altenheim, Hochheim, Mannheim,* etc.

The original or aboriginal man was a nomad. His place to lay his head was doubtless just where night overtook him.

The difference between barbarism and civilization is merely a question of homes. Compare " a club, a spear, a mat and the twentieth part of a shed to sleep under," with the ordinary appointments of a modern residence!

The home is the magnetic field, drawing everything within its magic circle. Without this central lodestone there can be no accumulation of either wisdom or wealth. From it spring all the finer needs, tastes, ambitions and capabilities.

The nomads sought safety from the attacks of wild beasts and the inclemency of the weather in natural caves, or built themselves rude huts wherever they decided to tarry for a week or a month. They realized few wants, ambitions or possessions, formed few attachments, felt no sentiment of patriotism, and had no conception of home. They needed only the rudiments of speech, since they neither read, wrote, printed, painted nor used the chisel.

Homes are the external evidences of Civilization, and Culture. Society, Education, Literature, Art, Music, Religion, Science and Recorded History all have their origin and foundation in the Home.

Consequently the highest human ambition is to possess a Home, first, in the substantial present, and finally, in the mysterious to be. Not to possess a home in the now is to be semi-nomadic; not to hope and pray for one in the hereafter is to be a heretic. The saddest, sweetest song yet sung or heard was wrung from the heart of a man without a home! The modern renter is a semi-nomad. Every Mayday, for him, the caravan or its counterpart is revived. Dislocated so often the Lares and Penates are never quite enthroned, and soon lose most of their sacredness.

A home, however humble, is a whole locker of anchors to windward. In a home the man has something to work for, improve, embellish; something to love and become attached to; an object in life, a realm for realizations, a nursery in which to develop manhood and womanhood, an asylum in which to hide from the cankering cares of the world, a rallying center and an heirloom to hand down to his children and his children's children.

Every human being is by instinct a home-builder, not a walking, migrating exponent of the compound interest tables. To own a corner of the earth and to eat your own bread, under a roof that neither leaks nor is covered by mortgages, is to feel yourself a full-fledged citizen.

The home is the basis of the commonwealth, the corner stone of society, the nursery of morality and the .1ope of humanity. Every step in the progress of the race has been measured and punctuated by the betterment of the homes of the people. Education, refinement, culture, the pursuit of science, literature and art—all these are made possible by and keep even pace with the establishment and improvement of homes.

What a master stroke of statesmanship and public policy it would be for the government to organize a National Home-Building and Loan Association, which, at nominal interest, would induce every family in the land to build and beautify its own homestead! Such a scheme, practically founded and honestly managed, would do more to establish habits of thrift in the citizen, advance public morals and *purify the political pool* than any or all possible legislation looking toward governmental or municipal ownership of private franchises and industries.

The most pitiable and pathetic orphan in the world is the man without a country. Next to him is the man without a home. For him every gulf of crime yawns, every pitfall of poverty is open. He is at sea without an anchor, and in a rudderless craft that is beyond his control. He it is who is drenched and driven by every tempest and tornado that sweeps across the ocean of life. It is easy to say, *Heaven pity him!* It would be far better if some mundane power would *picket* him!

It is the nomads, the Wandering Jews, the unhoused tramps in every community that constitute its dangerous element. It is from these that originate the lawless mobs that surge to the front in every labor strike and race riot, and that replenish the criminal ranks and people the penitentiaries. It is only the man without a home to whom "every door is barred with gold and opens but to golden keys," and who is sooner or later driven to crime, either against society, his neighbor or himself—only that he has no neighbors.

To multiply homes would be to decimate the ranks of the unthrifty and improvident. It would give the courts a long vacation. It would make two-thirds of the magistrates, lawyers, constables and policemen a superfluity. It would relieve the congestion of all our great cities, double the products of the farms and factories, and in time reduce pauperism and crime to a minimum.

CHOOSING A CLIMATE AND HOME-SITE.

From the standpoint of the sanitarian the first question to be considered by the home-builder relates to climate and general surroundings. The former may be the result of accident or circumstances which it is not feasible to escape or undo. All climates yet investigated have their peculiarities, and some of these, to certain individuals, become serious drawbacks. "Ideal" climates exist on paper and in the advertisements, but not on the face of the prosaic earth. There are, however, decided differences and marked preferences. The recent expansion of our national domain has made available to our citizens every variety of soil, scenery and climate that the world can afford, from the Arctic bleakness of Alaska to the tropic isles of the far Pacific. If you are not permanently anchored, but are inclined to seek a new climatic environment, do not be over-persuaded by *ex parte* and interested evidence. Study the conditions for yourself. If you have need to provide for an invalid or semi-invalid, the sanato-economic promise of a proposed climate becomes of paramount importance.

A few guiding rules, deduced from extensive observation and established data, will be of service.

1. To be salubrious a climate should be dry rather than moist. Even excessive dryness is preferable to excessive moisture. It is better to dry up and blow away than to drown.

2. Except in a small minority of cases, excessive warmth or extreme equability are neither of them specially desirable. This contravenes popular belief, but some decided alternations of heat and cold, without sudden or severe transitions to either, are favorable to the maintenance of the fighting tone and vital equipoise of the human organism.

3. For those in normal health the question of altitude may be practically ignored. A moderate altitude above sea-level, with rather high average barometric pressure, is generally preferable. Some invalids need to climb the heights in order to secure the best results.

4. Warmth and permeability of the soil are prime essentials.

5. High winds and severe storms, if frequent, are a dismal drawback.

6. There should be an abundance of unimpeded sunshine. It is the most potent antiseptic and disinfectant in the universe.

But in studying locations do not pin your faith to the "reports," to the readings of somebody's lying dry-bulb thermometer, nor yet to the uninterpreted tables of the Weather Bureau. There are plenty of localities where the "mean" annual temperature and the "mean" annuals of every kind are *mean* in a double sense and with a big M.

Unfavorable locations are to be found, and are to be shunned in all climates. Ignoring this precaution, life becomes an incessant battle with fate, in the guise of a horde of invisible foes. Thus, to remain in a vicinity that is incurably permeated with paludal influences imposes a vital handicap that no display of patience, industry or pharmaceutic prodigality can overcome.

Edison, Tesla and Marconi have harnessed the lightning; locomobiles promise the faithful horse a long vacation; liquid air may eventually finish solving the problem of heat, light, refrigeration and power, and the wonder-workers may sooner or later learn how to modify the harsher features of changeable and uncongenial climates. By and by we shall learn how to warm the air of our apartments without vitiating it.

Look to the natural drainage. Keep away from *cul de sacs* from which the rainfall is not promptly absorbed or carried away. See that the streams are free flowing, and that there is no stagnant or semi-stagnant water in the vicinity.

In facing the house be guided by the topography and climatic characteristics. If sunshine is at a premium, as it is in most of the Eastern States, the living rooms should have preference. Except in a decidedly hot climate, do not banish that laboratory which must supply the motive force and determine the physiological integrity of the entire household—the Kitchen, to a damp or cold and unrelieved north side.

The next installment of this series of papers will take up the subject of the construction and arrangement of the home.

⚜ ⚜

ARTIFICIAL PERFUMES.

THOSE who regale themselves with " real fruit juices" at the soda fountain and those who buy the essences of divers blossoms for their handkerchiefs may flatter themselves that their favorite flavors and perfumes are derived from the vegetable products whose name they bear; but this is naturally far from the case. Modern chemists are so skilful that if they can not manufacture the actual odorous principle that they want, they can at least make something that passes for it. In a recent note, the *Revue Scientifique* (Paris, January 12) speaks as follows of this industry:

" During these last years France seems to have made great progress in the industry of manufacturing perfumes by chemical synthesis, and at the Paris Exposition this branch of chemistry appears to be the only one in which the French exhibit was equal to that of Germany. * * *

"In the perfumery industry there are three principal methods; the extraction of odors from the products where they occur in Nature; the artificial preparation by synthesis of odorous compounds that occur also in Nature; and, finally, the fabrication of compounds that have odors similar to those possessed by natural substances.

" The odoriferous principle of oil of bitter almonds is one of the first that was isolated and afterward made synthetically. In 1832 Liebig and Woehler separated benzyl aldehyd from this oil, and now it is prepared no longer from almonds, but by the hydrolysis and oxidation of benzyl chloride. Unfortunately there remain some traces of this latter substance, whose odor is penetrating and disagreeable, so benzyl

aldehyd serves only to perfume common soaps.

" Vanillin was prepared artificially in 1874 by Tiemann and Harmann by the oxidation of coniferin; but now it is generally extracted from eugenol, which when treated with soda gives isoeugenol, which by oxidation becomes vanillin. This synthetic vanilla has altogether replaced the vanilla-bean in perfumery and the manufacture of confectionery, and it now costs only about one one-hundredth of what it did in 1876. Piperonal, under the name of heliotropin, has replaced the .essence of heliotrope, whose odor it has. It is extracted from safrol, an ether of the oil of sassafras or of camphor; in twenty years its price has fallen 99 to 100 per cent. * * *

" As the artificial perfume industry is evidently only in its infancy, we should expect interesting discoveries from the chemists who are at work in this line of investigation. They will be very bounteously rewarded, and, considering the prices paid for work in pure science, we can but congratulate them."—*The Literary Digest.*

⚜ ⚜

DO WE THINK WITH ONE HALF OF OUR BRAIN?

Is it not possible that in a healthy, normal condition we do all our thinking with one-half of the brain? In a recent number of *The American Journal of Insanity* it is contended that we do. Says the writer:

" The brain is, anatomically, a double organ, yet mental processes are single. *A priori*, we should expect in a double brain a double mind. A sufficient number of cases have been recorded to make it certain that a man can retain his personal characteristics and mental activity in whom one-half the cerebrum has been destroyed. Physiological arguments in favor of this view are found in the following facts: While coarse movements can be performed nearly as well by one-half of the body as by the other, whenever it becomes necessary to carry out movements involving speed, dexterity, and accurate judgment, Nature organizes one-half of the brain much more fully than the other. Righthandedness is not an accident."

We are told that the phenomenon of "double consciousness" means nothing more than a large increase in the activity of the half of the brain which usually has no part in conscious life. The theory makes explicable many of the most puzzling abnormal mental states. Among other conclusions, the author presents this:

"Anything which tends to make the ordinary quiescent half [of the brain] assume control tends to impairment of mental processes and the damage of the individual. If this be true, the attitude of those who advocate a cultivation of ambidexterity is thoroughly illogical. Instead of trying to make a right-handed person less right-handed we ought rather to try to make him more right-handed. Conversely, the attempt to make a left-handed boy right-handed is a physiological crime. Every effort ought to be made to make the left-handed boy more left-handed."—*The Literary Digest.*

THE POSITION OF THE HEAD IN SLEEP.

Custom has imposed the use of the bolster and the pillow, but it does not of necessity follow that they are advantageous or conducive to sound sleep. Physiologically, we are entitled to entertain a doubt, seeing that physiologists are still unable to sleep authoritatively whether the brain in sleep is congested or anemic. The general experience is that the lower the head the deeper is the sleep, and *vice versa.* Apart from morbid conditions which render it impossible to some persons to sleep with the head low, conditions which vary *ad infinitum* from mere preference for a thick bolster to positive orthopnea, habit, and, possibly, physiological conformation, render the head-low position in bed intolerable to some. It is urged against the use of these supports

that they inflict a constrained position of the neck, which interferes with the passage of blood to and from the brain, and contracts the thorax. On the other hand, unless one lies on the back, it is obvious that the neck must be uncomfortably curved in the absence of a pillow, far more so than would result from even a very thick bolster. On the whole, it would seem that in order to obtain sleep as deep and reposeful as possible, we ought to aim at having the head as low as is consistent with actual comfort. To submit to actual discomfort, in view of a problematical and much-disputed advantage, is not an experiment that will commend itself to the majority of mankind.—*Med. Press and Circular.*

NOTHING EASY.

I received a letter from a lad asking me to find him an easy berth. To this I replied: "You cannot be an editor; do not try the law; do not think of the ministry; let alone all ships, shops and merchandise; abhor politics; don't practice medicine; be not a farmer nor a soldier nor a sailor; don't study; don't think. None of these are easy, Oh, my son! You have come into a hard world. I know of only one easy place in it, and that is in the grave."—*Henry Ward Beecher.*

"If to do were as easy as to know what were good to do, chapels had been churches and poor men's cottages princes' palaces. It is a good divine that follows his own instructions; I can easier teach twenty what were good to be done, than to be one of the twenty to follow mine own teaching. The brain may devise laws for the blood, but a hot temper leaps o'er a cold decree; such a hare is madness, the youth, to skip o'er the meshes of good counsel, the cripple."—*Merchant of Venice.*

You will find the mere resolve not to be useless, and the honest desire to help other people, will, in the quickest and most delicate way, improve yourself.—*Ruskin.*

DIET IN BRIGHT'S DISEASE.

(Copyright.)

On rising take a glass of hot or cold water, or milk with a pinch of salt and soda added, or of milk and vichy hot.

Breakfast: *Cereals*—Bisbak, farina, shredded wheat, cracked wheat, hominy, rye mush, oatmeal with cream and a dash of sugar, with milk alone or with salt or butter.

Meats (red)—Mutton chop, lamb chop, steak, bacon and tripe, pepper and salt.

Fish—Cod, haddock, chicken halibut, smelt, flounder, butter fish, scup, bass, cunners, perch, pickerel, trout or other lake or brook fish.

Eggs—The yolks of eggs, soft boiled or scrambled, twice a week.

Breads—Gluten bread, whole wheat, rye, French bread; Cestus brown bread, butter.

Fruits—Orange, lemon or pineapple juice; stewed or roasted apples; raw ripe apples; grape fruit or white grapes sparingly; raw ripe peaches, apricots, pears, the same prepared; cherries, berries, cantaloupe, other melons; stewed prunes, stewed figs, when indicated.

Drinks—Milk flavored with tea, coffee or caramel; Phillip's digestible cocoa; Vigor chocolate; hot water, milk and vichy hot. Irish moss tea.

A.M. Between Meals: Water, hot or cold, hot or cold milk diluted; buttermilk, clam broth, weak lemonade. Fresh fruit, cooked or raw, when indicated.

Meats (red)—Veal, lamb, beef. fat ham; (white) chicken, breast of turkey, capon, squab, quail, woodcock, partridge, grouse and prairie chicken.

Lunch: Any fish mentioned. Sardines in oil.

Any vegetable mentioned.

NOTES.

Drink milk or water freely four times a day, unless advised to the contrary—alternate.

Milk can be made palatable, usually, if cut with Saratoga, Vichy, Val's, French Vichy, or carbonic acid water; flavor to suit individual taste.

An exclusive milk diet calls for from four to six pints a day, at least.

If milk causes a feeling of heaviness in the stomach, sip it from a spoon, that the saliva may be mixed with it. Patients may be taught to like it eaten in this way—a teaspoonful every fifteen minutes, at first. Try junket for a change.

A milk diet should be established gradually in chronic Bright's disease, replacing an article of food by a glass of milk—it should also be discontinued slowly.

Milk should be the chief source of proteid in acute and chronic renal disease; the nearer the disease is to being acute the more milk required. On the other hand it should not be the only source of proteid, lest it prove insufficient to maintain body strength. Reducing nitrogenous food should not be carried to the point of sub-nutrition or uremia will result from cardiac failure.

If dropsy has occurred the amount of liquid ingested should not exceed two and a half pints daily, especially if dysnea or heart failure threaten. Arterial degeneration may follow too great tension from liquid in excess.

If milk cannot be taken as milk, it should be incorporated into every prepared diet.

If milk cannot be taken, in any form, gruels. cream, olive oil, butter, fruit, and vegetables will have to be depended upon.

Gruels made of arrowroot, barley flour, strained oatmeal and rice are substitutes for milk. Plasmon may be tried, or Wampole's milk food.

Irish moss tea is a very soothing drink on account of the mucilage it contains.

Buttermilk or skimmed milk go well if the patient harbors a lazy liver.

Milk increases the elimination of urea and decreases the albuminous waste.

Milk decreases intestinal putrefaction and by lessening auto-intoxication, indirectly relieves the kidneys.

Carbo-hydrates and fats are indicated in this form of disease in the acute stages, if well borne. The waste of these foods is eliminated by the skin and lungs chiefly; nitrogenous waste, on the other hand, passes out by way of the kidneys.

Starchy foods and fats will need to be eaten in moderation if the liver is sluggish, the patient constipated or obese.

The best fats are butter, cream, olive oil, vigor chocolate. ham fat, and Terraline.

Salt should be excluded as much as possible from the foods allowed, unless the urine is over acid; it is eliminated entirely by the kidneys.

Fleshy people may use skimmed milk, buttermilk, milk diluted or water; if fleshy and rheumatic water is to be preferred.

Lean people may use milk or cream; if lean and rheumatic, cream diluted meets the indications.

In cases of obesity, constipation, or flatulency, potatoes must be excluded from the list.

Avoid sweet fruits.

Almonds, walnuts, and filberts make, with crackers or fruit, a suitable lunch. Masticate thoroughly.

Chestnuts diminish albumen on account of the tannin in them.

Bisbak is especially recommended on account of its easy digestion and elimination.

Any bread mentioned. Cestus, phosphated crackers, pilot bread, French bread, Bent's water crackers; bisbak and milk, rice and milk.

Any fruit mentioned.

Any drink mentioned. Irish moss tea.

Any dessert mentioned. Nuts.

P. M. BETWEEN MEALS: Same as A. M. Lime juice and water slightly sweetened, adding a lithia tablet if rheumatic.

DINNER: *Soups* (purees)—Of potato, corn, young peas, squash, celery and onions, adding milk when possible or agreeable. (soups) Milk, thickened with arrow-root, tapioca, vermicelli, sago, rice, flavored with lemon, grated orange peel, fruit jelly or current jelly, unsweetened.

Any fish mentioned. Oysters, stewed or raw; Little Neck clams; plain lobster.

Any meat mentioned.

Vegetables—New string beans, new peas, cooked celery, artichokes, beet tops; French string beans and French peas. Haricot beans, minced carrots, cauliflower, turnips, parsnips, squash, pumpkin and cucumbers. Baked potato once a day.

Salads—Lettuce with oil, lettuce and grapé fruit, lettuce and white grapes, cream cheese and lettuce.

Any bread mentioned. Cream toast, milk toast.

Any fruit mentioned. Ripe bananas.

Any drink mentioned. Irish moss tea, soda lemonade.

Desserts—Rice, apple tapioca, Indian and farina puddings; blanc-mange, orange charlotte, gelatin; ice cream eaten slowly.

9 P. M. Hot milk and Vichy, hot water.

Cheese and eggs increase albuminuria.

Chicken and veal are poor in albumen.

Vegetables, cheese, milk, and eggs contain no uric acid.

A diet of vegetables, eggs and milk will lessen uric acid.

Avoid eating meat, also liver, sweet breads, or other viscera, except as specified—they contain uric acid. Meat extracts contain uric acid.

Tea, coffee, and cocoa contain uric acid; these beverages are permissible in selected cases.

If the stomach or heart are irritable white meat is to be preferred to red and fish to either. Fish is an albuminous food.

Elderly persons or any anemic patient may require red meat once a day in order to maintain nutrition.

Alcohol in any form is to be avoided, unless required to sustain the heart. Avoid ginger ale.

A purely vegetable diet decreases albumen but is apt to increase dropsy; it decreases arterial tension, but if long continued anemia will result.

Chronic heart or lung disease may cause albuminuria, so also overstrain, overwork, worry, and errors of diet.

People suffering from Bright's disease usually have sensitive stomachs—foods not too stimulating meet the indications in the majority of cases.

Maintaining good digestion and nutrition are prime essentials in chronic nephritis, even if the albumin is increased; over-working the digestive apparatus, however, is to be avoided, as the waste from indigestion or over-digestion irritates the kidneys, having been imperfectly handled by the liver.

In false Bright's disease (oxaluria) apples, pears, rhubarb, sorrel, tomatoes, and asparagus in excess should not be eaten.

In chronic nephritis with profuse albuminuria and marked dropsy, vegetable food with milk should predominate—milk and vegetables are not to be taken at the same time.

Where there is little dropsy, little albumen, and great weakness or marked heart changes, a mixed diet, not too stimulating, with as little liquid as possible consistent with the rules laid down, should be used; if uremia threatens, however, milk is the best food, provided cardiac compensation holds good.

Urea is the *white ash* of complete proteid combustion, uric acid is the *clinker* in the grate. Uric acid is due to the ingestion of foods containing it—the proteid derived from animal sources, and to incomplete combustion of other foods.

Albumin is the chief source of proteid; it is a vital constituent of the blood. Its presence in the urine usually indicates congestion, irritation from failure of elimination, or loss of function by the kidneys. It increases the acidity of the urine. Patients may lose forty grains of albumin a day without serious harm if strength and nutrition are maintained.

The elimination of urea is diminished in all forms of Bright's disease, in gout, intestinal indigestion, and where the absorptive power of the intestines is diminished.

If the urine remains abnormally acid, gastric juice is not being secreted in sufficient quantity. It should be kept *alkaline*.

If there is an excess of hydrochloric acid in the stomach, the chlorides in the urine will be greatly diminished.

Excess of chlorides in the urine means excess of salt in the foods eaten.

A teaspoonful and a half (ninety grains) of soda-bicarbonate, taken the first thing in the morning, will neutralize the acid in the system, if normal, the urine remaining alkaline for two or three hours.

Citrate of potash and benzoate of soda lessen

THE HYGIENE OF HIGH ALTITUDES.

It is well known that the chemical composition of the atmosphere differs but little, if at all, wherever the sample be taken; whether it be on the high Alps or at the surface of the sea, the relation of oxygen to nitrogen and other constituents is the same. The favorable effects, therefore, of a change of air are not to be explained by any difference in the proportion of its gaseous constituents. One important difference, however, is the bacteriological one. The air of high altitudes contains no microbes, and is, in fact, sterile, while near the ground and some 100 feet above it microbes are abundant. In the air of towns and crowded places not only does the microbic impurity increase, but other impurities, such as the products of combustion of coal, accrue also. Several investigators have found traces of hydrogen and certain hydrocarbons in the air, and especially in the air of pine, oak and birch forests. It is to these bodies, doubtless consisting of traces of essential oils, to which the curative effects of certain health resorts are ascribed. Thus the locality of a fir forest is said to give relief in diseases of the respiratory tract. But all the same, these traces of essential oils and aromatic products must be counted, strictly speaking, as impurities, since they are not apparently necessary constituents of the air. As recent analyses have shown, these bodies tend to disappear in the air as a higher altitude is reached, until they disappear altogether. It would seem, therefore, that microbes, hydrocarbons and entities other than oxygen and nitrogen, and perhaps we should add argon, are only incidental to the neighborhood of human industry, animal life, damp and vegetation.—*The Lancet.*

PROGNOSIS IN THE HEART DISEASES OF CHILDREN.

It has impressed me, as it must have impressed every physician who has had the opportunity to see sick children, that when they suffer from diseases of the heart the prognosis should generally be more hopeful than when adults suffer with heart disease. This is partly because they are more elastic than adults, whose tissues are stiffer and may almost be said to be brittle, and most of all, perhaps, because children who have not attained their full growth have the opportunity for repair during growth. Injury, or any distortion of the heart that is caused by disease may be efaced as the organ increases in size, for the usual tendency of Nature is toward the production of an ordinary type.—*Dr. A. V. Meigs,* in *Journal American Medical Association.*

Dr. Achorn's "diet list" in Heart Disease will be published in the May GAZETTE.

---

the acidity of the urine and the irritability of urates and uric acid by preventing their crystallization.

A good daily drink in Bright's disease is an infusion made from Juniper berries (one pint) to which two tablespoonfuls of bi-tartrate of potash have been added.

Indican in the urine is an evidence of constipation, or of obstruction in the small intestine, albuminous putrefaction of undigested food.

Cream of tartar water is indicated if there is constipation—a teaspoonful to a pint of boiling water, flavored with lemon juice, and sweetened, if allowed, with Maltose or milk sugar.

The constipation resulting from a milk diet may be relieved by stewed prune juice or the inside of baked apples, strained oatmeal or Phillips' milk of magnesia.

If the bowels are loose use lime water or barley water in the milk.

Wear wool next the skin. Wear an abdominal band. Bathe in tepid water. Avoid dampness. Keep the feet dry. Walking is the best form of exercise.

This bill meets fairly well the dietetic indications in gout.

Irish Moss Tea—Wash, add water and cook slowly until the goodness is all extracted; then add water until thin enough to drink; flavor with lemon.

Department of Physiological Chemistry.

WITH SPECIAL REFERENCE TO DIETETICS AND NUTRITION IN GENERAL.

IS CHEESE WHOLESOME?

WHEN we think of the thousands of tons of this product of the dairy that are annually consumed, and of the shiploads of it that are imported, the question of its digestibility and wholesomeness looms up as an important one. It has been adopted as a part of the army ration, every grocer and provision dealer makes it an important item on his list of standard food products, and nearly every family has it occasionally if not constantly on the table.

That it is nutritious, that is, that it is chemically rich in the proteids, hydrocarbons and "calories" no one can dispute. All the analyses and food tables agree as to that. That nine-tenths of all that is consumed is positively unfit to be introduced into the human stomach and may be charged with its share in the production of a nation of dyspeptics could no doubt be proven by proper investigation.

What is the matter with the cheese?

Simply this, that it has come to be an almost universal belief that coagulated casein and butter fat, which are its constituents, must be "cured." This "curing" process is chiefly accomplished by time. It is not considered fit to eat until it is old enough and rank enough—from gradual processes of decomposition—to be buried. The average palate has been gradually educated to relish cheese after it has undergone butyric acid fermentation and is, in fact, putrid. This is plain English, and it flies in the face of the reigning authorities on gustatory standards. Certain brands of the stuff, as Roquefort, Limberger and several other varieties, sell at enormous prices simply because they represent ideal degrees of rankness—putridity.

This butyric acid fermentation has its proper bacillus, and in case of the special varieties present in Limberger and other delectable brands, the characteristic odor is vile enough and strong enough to bar all attempts at counterfeiting or substitution. The flavor comports with the smell, and either one would cause a respectable canine to drop his astonished tail and sneak out of the rankest soap factory or tan yard on the face of the earth.

Every normal stomach rebels at it, and every normal palate repudiates it at sight, taste or smell. Years ago, when all the small dairymen made a little cheese for their own use, if not for the market, they began to eat it before it was a fortnight old; ate it as freely as they did bread, and never thought of it being difficult of digestion. Nor was it.

To put such compressed casein before a lover of Limberger would be to offer him an unpardonable insult. And yet, from a health standpoint, it is the only cheese that can be approved.

Of the semi-putrid, rank-smelling and acrid-tasting stuff now sold for cheese many persons cannot partake with impunity; and those who do eat it are compelled to be very sparing in their indulgence, making it a relish or condiment rather than a food. This is because it belongs with other antiques. It belongs with "embalmed beef," mouldy bread and gangrenous "game," for which palled palates either possess or profess a gusto.

Among the gourmands all this protest is the rankest heresy. Nevertheless, it is the truth, and no amount of gustatory pettifogging can change it.

If the creameries would try the experiment of making little "cheeses," weighing from two to five pounds each, and send them to market as soon as they will hold shape—say not to exceed two to four weeks from the press, it would not take long to create a market for their product that would grow to untold proportions, because people would learn to eat cheese at every meal, and as freely as they now devour cake or crackers.

In time the taste for butyric acid, putrid casein and the concentrated stinks of the Augean stables would be superseded, and the market for this major item of dairy products multiplied a hundred fold.

VEGETARIANISM AND INSANITY.

IRA IBSEN STERNER, an unfortunate young student at Harvard, is confined as a lunatic. He had been working extremely hard, and leading the life of a vegetarian.

He was poor. The amount of money at his disposal might have kept him properly nourished had he not hit upon the unfortunate and, in his case fatal, idea of vegetarianism.

There is no doubt that vegetarianism would be an ideal dietetic condition. There is something repulsive in eating huge pieces of meat, murdering our fellow-animals to obtain them. But, constituted as at present, meat-eating is an absolute necessity, especially when hard mental effort is required.

Our teeth are arranged for meat-eating, as well as for the eating of vegetables. Our stomachs are arranged for meat-eating. Our nerves crave meat, and this craving increases enormously with increase of mental activity.

The huge Egyptian propelling a dhow on the Nile may live on a few handfuls of grain. But the Egyptian priest, who measured the Nile's waters, predicted the floods and provided for the welfare of the people, did not confine himself to vegetables.

The time will come, perhaps, when we shall with safety respect life, and refuse to devour meat. That time has not yet come.

Meanwhile, on behalf of the meat-eater, it may be said that the animal which is not butchered always dies tragically, since in the animal kingdom there is no such thing as a " natural " death. All animals fall a prey to some other when age or illness exhausts their strength.

In addition, it may be said that there is no proof that vegetables which we eat so gayly are any less sensitive about death than are the lower animals. We sympathize with the boiled lobster because we share his particular kind of animate life.

There may be just as good cause to sympathize with the cabbage boiled alive as with the lobster boiled alive.

Anyhow, when you boil a cabbage you destroy thousands of minute animal lives.

If a live ant happens to be boiled in the cabbage leaves, you destroy in that ant a brain far superior to the brain of any sheep or ox.

(All this is simply puerile.—Ed. GAZETTE.)

It is to be hoped that chemical combinations will ultimately relieve us from the necessity of devouring other living creations, animal or vegetable.

For the present, while you have a big body inherited from ancestors fed on meat, and which itself demands meat, give it the meat that it must have.

Don't follow the example of the unfortunate Harvard student. Don't follow the example of Tolstoi. He made himself ill for lack of meat, and then gave up vegetarianism.

Live sensibly. Don't eat too much meat, but eat enough. Anyhow, as we have said before, remember that, while you may torture your own body with vegetarianism, you have no right to impose it on your children or others dependent upon you.—*New York Journal.*

WE have frequently commented on newspaper therapeutics. It is a subject on which much that is amusing is written. Perhaps most of this kind of literature is harmless, but occasionally it is decidedly baneful, in that it influences the habits of uninformed and unthinking people, a species that at present numbers an overwhelming majority of the human race. The above flippant and only superficially plausible editorial from the *Journal* may be classed with the baneful variety. It contents itself with citing the silly examples of a couple of cranks of the most pronounced type. It is idiotic to hold up the examples of fanatics who attempt to live on three crackers and a pint of cold water, or on a crust of sour bread, a cruet of bran mash and a pudding of crushed corn cobs, as a warning to sane people who do not need to be told that all the food of the race must come from the vegetable kingdom. To eat it in the form of flesh is to take it at second hand and subject to a greater or less degree of contamination, during its transmigration through one of the lower animal organisms.

As we understand the case, the Harvard student must have been weak in the upper story at the outset, and starved himself into full-fledged insanity, the variety of his food having little to do with the matter. As to Tolstoi, every intelligent reader knows that he is an incorrigible cynic, a social iconoclast and a religious fanatic of the most pronounced and uncompromising type. His philosophy would turn every happy home into a domestic hell and eventually depopulate the world. Judged by his writings there is not a more despicable or dangerous lunatic at large.

The GAZETTE has never joined the army of cranks who howl themselves hoarse under the banner of impracticable vegetarianism, but it most emphatically decries such "smart" but inconsiderate efforts as the foregoing to urge the "necessity" of consuming larger quantities of flesh-meat upon a race and an age that is already suffering from chronic uremic poisoning and the rheumatic diathesis through over-indulgence in the flesh-pots of Egypt. Nothing is more certain than the fact that the American people eat too much "meat," as all

flesh is improperly called. Instead of flesh-eating being "an absolute necessity" for brain workers there is no gainsaying the claim that the highest type of intellectual vigor is perfectly compatible with a diet intelligently selected from the vegetable kingdom.

A PLEA FOR RAW MILK.

THE objection to the raw-milk feeding of infants is based, according to Dr. Louis Fischer, upon the contamination of milk with various pathogenic bacteria. Such risk, however, is reduced to a minimum when all the principles of modern hygienic measures are rigidly enforced. It is a well-known fact that the prolonged use of sterilized or boiled milk will produce scurvy, and when scurvy exists, both sterilized and boiled milk must be discontinued, to give place to fresh, raw milk. Does it not seem more plausible, in the face of such clinical experience, to commence feeding at once with raw milk rather than risk the development of scurvy, and be compelled to discontinue all other forms of feeding, excepting raw foods? There is a certain deadness, or, to put it differently, absence of freshness in milk that is boiled or sterilized. It seems to be the lack of this same element of freshness which, in the absence of meat and green vegetables, will produce scurvy in the adult. Speaking of the development of scurvy in children fed on sterilized or boiled milk, Rundlett says that changes take place, not in the albumen, fat, or sugar, but in the albuminate of iron, phosphorus, and possibly in the fluorine, vital changes take place. The albuminoids are certainly in milk, derived as it is from tissues that contain them, and are present in a vitalized form as proteids.

On boiling, the change that takes place is due simple to the coagulation of the globulin or proteid molecule, which splits away from the inorganic molecule, and thus renders it as to the iron and fluorine unabsorbable, and as to the phosphatic molecule un-

assimilable. This is the change that is so
vital, and it is this only which takes place
when milk is boiled. It is evident that children require phosphatic and ferric proteids
in a living form, which are contained only in
raw milk.

Cheadle says that phosphate of lime is
necessary to every tissue. No cell growth
can go on without earthy phosphates; even
the lowest form of life, such as fungi and
bacteria, cannot grow if deprived of them.
These salts of lime and magnesia are especially called for in the development of the
bony structures.

WHEY-CREAM MODIFICATIONS IN INFANT FEEDING.

F. W. WHITE and M. Ladd (*Philadelphia Medical Journal*, February 2, 1901),
from their work in this line, have arrived
at the following conclusions:

1. By the use of whey, as a diluent of
creams of various strengths, they are able
to modify cow's milk so that its proportions
of caseinogen and whey proteids will closely
correspond to the proportions present in human milk. They, therefore, render it much
more digestible and suitable for infant feeding.

2. The best temperature for destroying
the rennet enzyme in whey is 65.5° C. Whey
or whey mixtures should not be heated
above 69.3° C., in order to avoid the coagulation of the whey proteids. The amount of
whey proteids in the whey obtained by these
observers was 1 per cent., while in the analysis of the whole milk approximately
three-fourths of the total proteid was caseinogen and one-fourth was whey proteids.

3. On the basis of these analyses they
were able to obtain whey cream mixtures,
with a maximum of 0.90 per cent. and a
minimum of 0.25 per cent. of whey proteids, in combination with percentages of
ceseinogen varying from 0.25 to 1; of fats,
from 1 to 4 per cent.; of milk-sugar, from
4 to 7 per cent.

4. The emulsion of fat in whey, barley-
water, gravity cream, and centrifugal cream
mixtures was the same, both in its macro-
scopic and microscopic appearances. The
combination of heat and transportation, such
as sometimes occurs in hot weather, partially
destroys the emulsion in all forms of modified milk, but this disturbance can be prevented by the simple precaution of keeping
the milk cool during delivery.

5. Whey cream mixtures yield a much
finer, less bulky, and more digestible coagulum than plain modified mixture with the
same total proteids; the coagulum is equaled
in fineness only by that of barley-water mixtures. The coagulum yielded by gravity
cream mixtures and centrifugal cream mixtures is the same in character.

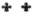

A NEW KIND OF BREAD.

A SOCIETY has just been formed in Paris
to promote the establishment in all the
large French towns of combination milling and baking-houses, worked by machinery known as the "Schweitzer system." This has for its object the making
of 100 kilograms (220 pounds) of nutritious and digestible white bread from 100
kilograms of grain at the lowest cost of production. The United States consul at Rou-
baix, as quoted in *Popular Science*, says
that the model establishment, which is at
La Villette, Paris, opened its doors to the
public on June 15, 1899. Says this paper:

" At a meeting of the society in December last, a report was made concerning the
success of the effort to supply good bread
at a low price to the Parisian public In
the bakery at La Villette, and the branch
houses, sales are rising daily. Official analyses by the National Agronomical Institute and by the Municipal Laboratory of
Paris, demonstrate that the Schweitzer
bread contains more nutritive nitrogenous
properties than ordinary baker's bread, and
more than double the phosphates in the latter.

" The bread known as *pain de ménage* is sold to the working classes at about 1¼ pence [2½ cents] per pound, considerably less than the usual price. The Villette establishment is a building of iron and stone, about 515 feet long, situated on a canal, and constructed at a cost of about 40,000 pounds sterling [$200,000]. The wheat arrives in a boat, which is moored in a canal, elevators hoist it into bins, whence it is carried by an immense elevator to the top of the mill, and turned into the different cleaning and separating machines. After all foreign substances have been removed and the grains of wheat have undergone a thorough brushing and washing, they are clean and shining; but the grooves of the wheat sometimes retain a little dust.

" This is completely eliminated by a Schweitzer appliance, which, seizing each grain lengthwise, splits it exactly in the groove. The wheat thus cleansed passes into the mill, composed of flat circular steel grinders, grooved in such a manner that they accomplish the decortication of the kernel and its granulation into meal at the same time. These grinders are movable, but do not touch, so that instead of crushing the wheat and producing a flour in which the starch only is retained, the outer and harder portion of the wheat, containing gluten and other nutritive properties, is retained in the flour. The bran alone is expelled. Attached to the mill are the works for kneading the meal, water, and yeast into bread.

" All this is done mechanically, the works being separated into three stories. Special yeast is prepared in the upper story in rooms heated in winter and cooled in summer. The yeast, flour, and the salted water are carried down by machinery into kneaders, in the form of half-cylindrical tubs, rotating on two pivots placed in the axis of the kneading-troughs, so that the tubs may be placed at a lower or higher angle, in order to accelerate or retard the kneading. The wheat, salted water, and yeast automatically enter one end of the tub, and dough, in an endless skein of pale yellow,

issues from the opposite end. This dough finally falls on tables on the ground floor, where it is weighed and made into bread of every shape and dimension. In connection with this model establishment is a laboratory for the chemical examination of the samples of wheat submitted for purchase. These are, upon arrival, ground and passed through a sieve by a small hand-bolting mill, which determines immediately the nutritive volume of the grain in gluten and nitrogeneous matter."—*Literary Digest.*

THE BABY'S DIET.

THE problem of artificial feeding, says the *Georgia Journal of Medicine and Surgery*, is one of growing importance, especially to the family physician and obstetrician; the latter of these is especially derelict in his duty if he fails to inform himself upon the great advances which have lately been made in this direction. The cause of much of the indigestion, inanition and marasmus seen during infancy is laid during the first few weeks of life, but the importance of starting the diet right from the very outset is not yet sufficiently appreciated. An attack of indigestion must be regarded as a serious misfortune for a child; the younger the child, the greater the misfortune. A single careless feeding may produce an acute indigestion which will be the starting point of a long series of digestive disturbances. A few weeks of improper feeding may so derange the digestive processes that the infant does not regain its normal digestive power during its first year.

The error is quite too common of looking upon the body as a machine, any derangement of which will be set right by simply removing the cause. The human body is not a lifeless machine, but a combination of living tissues, each of which has its own functions to perform. Stopping the original cause of disturbance does not, therefore, usually stop the symptoms. A child that has been improperly fed can rarely be set right at once by the administration of proper food. If the indigestion is due to bacterial action, or to a vegetable ferment, it will probably continue for a certain time under the most favorable feeding, because the germ or the ferment remains to act upon everything that is introduced into the stomach. An intestinal catarrh, once begun, is *very* slow and difficult of cure, and will prolong the indigestion.

When the digestive secretions are impaired, or undergo any decided change, they do not at once recover themselves or adapt themselves to changed conditions, even if those conditions are perfection itself. The nervous system, notably that portion which presides over the digestive functions, readily acquires habits and peculiarities of action which continue after the causes which generated them have been removed. The debility and anemia which quickly follow in the train of improper diet are felt by the digestive organs in common with the rest of the body, and impair their action long after the cause is removed.

The younger the child, the less is its resisting power, and the more potent do these various factors become. There is no more difficult task than the remedying of an impaired digestion in a young infant. In no place is the old adage that an ounce of prevention is better than a pound of cure more true than in medicine; in no place in medicine is it more true than in the management of early infancy.

Error is constantly being made in allowing new-born babies to have too much food, to have it at irregular intervals, and without proper preparation. One of the most common errors is the use of too strong milk mixtures. During the first two weeks, the baby should be fed every two hours by day and should not have more than two feedings between 10 P. M. and 7 A. M. With the beginning of regular feeding on the third day, the amount of each feeding should not be more than one ounce, which may be increased to two ounces by the fourteenth day. In exceptional cases two and one-half ounces may be given.

Even in the case of breast-fed babies, the doctor has an important duty to perform in giving rigid instructions regarding regularity of nursing, the duration of each feeding, and the management of the breasts. The importance of engendering right habits in the breast-fed infant is almost as great as in the case of the artificially fed. The well-being of the infant, as well as the well-being and comfort of the mother, depend greatly upon the habits formed during the first few weeks. Whether the baby be breast-fed or bottle-fed, the physician is derelict in his duty if he neglects to start the diet right.

FEEDING OF INFANTS IN HEALTH AND DISEASE.

IN a paper read before the West London Medico-Chirurgical Society, on this subject, says *The Hospital*, Dr. H. Campbell Pope said: The subject was one which, from its inherent simplicity should be easy to approach and handle, but it was also one which, by the evolution of our civilization, had attained an added complexity, requiring no little patience and much technical knowledge to unravel and elucidate. The problem as presented by Nature was simply that of maternal feeding, which required no more care than due respect to the mother's health and the sanitary condition of her person. One of the chief difficulties confronting the practitioner was the willful shirking of nursing by mothers in a good station, and the compulsory abstinence from nursing enforced upon many who had to earn their daily bread. Supposing artificial food were a necessity, three courses were open—the rule of thumb, the guidance of the patent food manufacturer, or a physiological and scientific system. Owing to the efforts of Holt and Rotch, ably seconded by Cautley, Pritchard and others in this country, adequate scientific knowledge on the subject was now available. Rotch set forth two principles: One, that the infant's physiological requirements as to quantity and quality of milk must be met; and, secondly, that by proper treatment cow's milk could be so modified as to approximate very nearly to human milk or to any required standard, when by reason of some idiosyncrasy or pathological condition a departure from the normal was indicated. The four important elements of milk were fat, proteid, sugar, and salts. Pritchar says a milk mixture can be prepared by simple means containing these elements in any proportion, and a table had been constructed which contained the percentages, which were applicable for infants of all ages and tallied with those of human milk at the corresponding stage of lactation. In America special dairies, known as Walker-Gordon milk laboratories, were largely used, and they had one of them in London. At this laboratory all the modifying of the milk was done, and it was supplied daily to the children, of appropriate strength to their age, but by means of Pritchard's table and the Soxhlet sterilizer, the same thing could be done at home. If an infant did badly on its food, three points should be noted—the weight, the character of the motions, and the absence or presence of vomiting. In weight, for the first six months, an infant should show a weekly increase of 5 to 8 ounces. A critical examination of the motions would show which element of the food was disagreeing, and the quantity of such element must be modified in the milk supplied to the infant. The usual cause of vomiting was excess in the quantity of food given at each feeding, and the quantity appropriate to the different ages of infancy was worked out in Pritchard's table. The commonest cause of rickets was overfeeding, and generally in one element of the food, namely, the carbohydrate. Rickety children recovered most rapidly on fresh foods not subjected to boiling. Virol, being a non-cooked food and also anti-scorbutic, from its containing eggshells dissolved in lemon juice, was a valuable addition to the food in such cases. When milk disagreed entirely, a food of meat-juice or egg-albumin in water would be found to meet the difficulty.

Overfeeding.—The mother-fed baby ran least risk of overfeeding. In choosing a wet-nurse, overfeeding might be produced by selecting a strong, florid woman to nurse an infant of a pale and delicate mother. Discretion was needed in approximating the foster-mother to the physiological requirements of the nursling. Where the mother's milk was too abundant, it should be drawn off and supplied in measured quantities. The danger of predigested food lay in its easy absorption, and consequent absence of symptoms of overfeeding. When a baby began to perspire much, especially at the back of the neck, it was time to limit its food and see that it obtained more fresh air. In patent foods, the carbohydrate element was generally in excess. Diarrhea and vomiting were caused by excess of fat and proteid. Only careful watching of the weight and muscular and bony development would indicate when the physiological limit of fat deposition had been reached, showing that the carbohydrate element was in excess.

Weaning had sometimes to be accomplished rapidly. In such cases a modified milk diet, adapted to the exact age of the child, should be employed; preferably, weaning was a gradual process. One bottle at night might be given, and at the end of three days, two; and three at the end of six days. Rotch strives to get the infant as rapidly as possible to cow's milk by commencing on modified milk appropriate to the age of the child. Pritchard, on the other hand, says the child should not begin with food appropriate to its age, but on food of a lower standard, whether weaning was intended or not. The nightly bottle should be begun at six months, and weaning should be commenced at the ninth month, even when the child was doing well. Weight should be recorded every week, either by means of Cautley's baby chart or Pritchard's physiological nursery chart.

Nursery Milk.—The possible contaminations between udder and mouth were very numerous. Possibly the cow had a sore teat or teats contaminated with fecal matters. The milkman might have dirty or unhealthy hands and the barn gallons were without dust-protectors—an improvement urgently demanded—and might not be efficiently scalded. Empirical quantities of preservatives were added when the milk reached London; some tablespoonfuls of dirt and dust would be found in each barn gallon; the milk was then served into nursery cans, not always properly sterilized. The danger of non-sterilization was most real. Dr. Pope had seen both scarlet fever and diphtheria patients drinking out of such cans. The tube of a tube-bottle was almost certainly foul within, and a nurse or mother, possibly with carious teeth, drew the bottle first. Lastly, a pacifier was picked up from the floor and wiped, as likely as not, with a dirty pocket-handkerchief and put into the baby's mouth.

Feeding of Infants in Sickness.—Most important was the examination of the motions to see which element of the food was disagreeing, and then modifying the milk in accordance. A sick infant, like a sick adult, should be put on a lower scale of diet. Frequently the opposite was done, and the infant, which only began with a slight cold, developed bronchitis from the irritation produced in the bronchial membrane by the excess of metabolic products. Bronchitis was the commonest cause of death in West London, and he had little doubt that improper feeding, both in young and old, had far more to do with the matter than exposure to cold or any other cause. The infant, when it cried and wished to suck between its meals, was thirsty and wanted water, not food.

Method and Simplicity.—It had been perceived, in 1883, in France, that more method was required in feeding, and the tube-bottle was universally execrated. Notwithstanding that fact, the tube-bottle had yearly massacred more innocents than Herod. An artificially-fed infant must be fed, and not allowed to feed itself. Its food must be apportioned to its physiological needs, not only in quantity and quality, but in the number of feedings per diem and the proper intervals between such feedings. The system of the Walker-Gordon Company, by having the milk bottled at the farms in sterilized bottles, avoided pollution in transit over long distances, and was the model of the plan which should be adopted in feeding infants. The modification, however, could be done at home, and by using one method for all children simplicity was obtained. Last of all, they must not overlook that maternal nutriment was the best, but in its absence the system advocated was founded on true scientific principles. The first three months of life were of tremendous import to every human being; if the machinery were started wrongly, all vital processes might be vitiated until the end.

MUSHROOMS AS FOOD.

NONE of the edible fungi is worth much in a nutritive sense, according to Dr. Andrew Wilson, an English dietary authority, however useful they may be as luxuries for varying ordinary diet. A British society for the better understanding of fungi has been formed, and Dr. Wilson has given the society his opinion on the subject.

Mushrooms, he says, contain 93 per cent. of water to begin with. Of tissue-building material they contain only 2 per cent., of fat and of starch practically none; but they contain two kinds of sugar-making elements, together about 1½ per cent. For the rest there is about 1 per cent. of cellulose, which is found in all plants, a little less than 1 per cent. of minerals and a little less than 2 per cent. of other material valueless to the human system.

Truffles contain a little more nitrogenous matter and starchy and sugary elements, but they are of little more account than mushrooms as food. Moreover, neither is easy of digestion.

✢ ✢

WHY DON'T I GET WELL?

THE above question is asked more frequently, says Dr. S. F. Meacham in *Suggestion*, than almost any other one by those suffering from chronic ailments of all kinds. It is almost the first thing asked of the physician. Next to, " Can you cure me," it is beyond doubt the most common refrain of all.

It is not as commonly known as it should be that the answer to the first question is found in the very nature of the second one, Can you cure me? The very question shows an entire misconception of the nature of cure and of its source.

What does it really mean to cure? Almost every one know what that means 'till asked, then but few can really tell what it is. But that there is a very widely mistaken view on the subject I am thoroughly convinced.

I shall use the word to mean to restore to health, to re-establish equilibrium, to re-establish ease. The usual definition " to destroy disease," " to remove disease " contains a key to the whole misconception, both as to remedies used and also to a satisfactory answer to the question at the head of this article.

It is plainly impossible to remove any*thing* unless there is some*thing* to remove. It is just as impossible to destroy a disease if it is not a *thing* to destroy.. The attempt to cure is usually embodied in the above ideas, and also the attempts to get well.

Disease is only a wrong or imperfect life work. What we need is correction, improvement, not destruction. Destruction would be impossible if attempted. The organism is all there really is that is destructible, and I am sorely afraid that in the too vigorous attempts to destroy some*thing*, this is what is often destroyed. If life is really eternal, then the *life* cannot be destroyed. The *form* in which it works can be destroyed, and often is, but probably *not* the *life*. While this latter is only a guess, it is *no more a guess than its*

opposite, and I prefer this one.

But we do not escape by claiming that life is a derived something, for motion can no more be destroyed than can matter. All those who claim that life is derived, claim at the same time that it is derived from matter and motion, and that both these are eternal. But, if they are eternal they cannot be destroyed. So here we are again where we can easily see that *change* is what we want, not destruction or removal. So I am going to claim that disease is a life process just as much as health is; that it simply is much narrower in its adjustment both in time and space, and hence not desirable.

I am also going to assert my belief that life itself is indestructible, that the form alone *can be destroyed.* Again, that the acting forces in each organism is all the source we know of the organism itself. That is to say, life alone can repair the organism in which it resides.

This life in man becomes conscious and possessed of a certain degree of spontaneity by means of which it can, to a degree, adjust its actions so as to be in harmony with environment. That all correct methods of adjusting an organism to the needs of its existence must take the resident life force into account and act in harmony with it, endeavor to aid and remove obstacles from its path.

So in the light of the above, let us answer the question, " Why don't I get well?"

First, because you don't know how.

Second, because you have never tried to know how. You have simply tried to find some one, or some*thing* that would cure you, but you have not tried to find out *how to get well*, which is quite a different thing. You have not tried to find out *how to live a* correct life, and most of you have rebelled against all methods of instruction as *preaching*, or as interfering with your personal liberty. Remember that there is no liberty save in health; disease is limitation. It is bondage. It is hindrance, so that instruction is what is always needed. *No ignorance, no disease.* Write that sentence on a conspicuous place in your consciousness and never forget it, and if you are sick, it is because you are ignorant. What is the remedy? Knowledge plus rational living.

Many things and many courses of action may relieve, but knowledge alone can lead to a cure. I say *lead* to a cure because even after we know, we must do.

Remember that in matters of disease, in matters of law, in matters of cause and effect, there can be no vicarious atonement. Have you set in action the cause, then you must suffer the effect. We may at times, if we learn of our mistake in time, set a counter cause in action and thus escape suffering the full penalty, but the above statement is a general rule with *few* exceptions —none if not interfered with.

If we are sick, we have simply been living at cross purposes with Nature. The fact that we have been moral and unselfish is not to the point. These things are good as far as they go and simply exempt us from suffering on these planes, but how should we ever learn of physical order, and the necessity of obedience here also, unless we suffered when we ran counter to those laws? If God is immanent he is in what we call physical as much as in what we call spiritual. The one word *substance* unites both the other terms into one, and physical nature and its laws are seen to be brothers of spiritual nature and its laws, and the whole world is unified and substantial.

Let us cease at once trying to degrade, or ignore our relations to the material world, including our bodies, for they are one segment of the world, and not an unimportant one at that.

Each one has a course of action that, if adopted, would lead through life with comparative comfort, and *it is the business of life to find that line of action and unwaveringly adopt it.* So, the one diseased is far out of the correct attitude of mind when he asks his physician, " Can you cure me? " If properly informed, he would ask, " Can you point out the way? " " Can you help me to get on my feet again? " And the physician is also far behind the van who

undertakes to *cure* his patient's ills. The one who imagines he can cure does not feel sufficiently the need of instructing, and the real fact is that nine-tenths of our patients need nothing but encouragement and advice.

It is well for each sufferer to keep in mind that no external help can take the place of individual adjustment to the active nature around him and in him. It is incontestibly true that such external aid is often needed. It is certainly true that our relations are reciprocal and that times come when we are all heavy leaners, and for the time, poor lifters, but even so we can never strengthen either mental muscle or physical muscle by sitting passively on the shoulders of some friend or physician. We are each expected, nay demanded, to grow by effort, by action, not by trust alone. It is practically impossible to overestimate faith, yet faith without works is dead. We desire what we desire because we are what we are, and our correct place to begin is within, by changing our thought life, and through this our active life, and finally our life of desire will change also, and our real character modify so as to lead to correct adjustment, which means at the same time health. It can be readily seen that getting well means work and will; means the correcting and improving of our thought life, our life of love, our active life, and all these require effort, heroic effort. Idle dreaming, or faithful hanging-on to externals, can do nothing save possibly to temporarily modify conditions.

You truly then, do not get well because you do not know how, and you have just as truly not tried in the correct manner to learn how.

Go to your physician and demand instruction as to how to become able to stand alone; demand that you be told the real source of your trouble and the best way to overcome it. If he refuses and endeavors to convince you that all you need is to take his potions and trust him, change doctors, for he is not the one you need. Life alone is the healer. The life incarnated in each tissue can alone repair that tissue. The above cannot be too frequently repeated. It cannot be too firmly believed or relied on. Take it with you to your physician as a measure of where he stands, and if he is found wanting you are better off alone than with him, so quit him and find a teacher who can at the same time give the external aid needed, for remember that a child must, at times, be held by the hand, must be aided, but it must be taught, or at least be permitted to learn to walk. This requires individual effort on the part of the child, and, all, courses of action that hinder this, defeat its own end. So if you wish to get well, straighten your back-bone, adjust the jaws and go to work to do whatever is possible, and widen as far as may be the reach of that word, possible.

You are all familiar with what was at one time accomplished by the vigorous use of a jaw-bone. Well, the time has not passed for the use of that weapon. A firm jaw and an erect and stable spine are two of the most powerful therapeutic agencies known to-day. I feel perfectly safe in stating that nine-tenths of all human ills would yield to a vigorous application of these two agencies.

Renunciation is a word we need much to study in this connection. We cannot *get* well; neither can we long remain well if we will persist in carrying the burdens of years past on the shoulders of to-day. Neither is it possible to sail *peacefully* the sea of life while the sails are constantly being filled with the winds of personal passions, personal desires, personal demands. I do not wish to imply, or teach, that *individuality* must be sacrificed. I am contending for just the reverse of this, but it is nevertheless true that we must cease to concrete every desire, we must cease to affix our whole attention to one little wavelet of life's ocean, and learn to view it as a whole and take our course and trim our sails from this larger view-point.

While we are individuals, with a work that none can do for us, and which nothing but ignorance, laziness, or cowardice

can possibly lead us to wish them to do for us, we are at the same time members of a great co-operative whole, whose relations are reciprocal in many ways.

While it is probably true that each has a *destiny to fulfil*, it is at the same time true that each has a *fate to conquer*. Law rules, but it need not enslave. To illustrate, one cannot plant corn and reap wheat, but no law under heaven can prevent the sowing of wheat where corn has been, nor can any law hinder the plowing up of weeds and planting flowers in their places.

So we may be better fitted by capacity, character and will to do some things than others. We may even be unfitted by Nature to even desire to do many things. This is what I mean by each having a destiny to fulfill. But, after choosing, and choosing correctly, the line of destiny, that does not necessarily mean that there shall be no fate to conquer on that path.

Adverse circumstances are really opportunities to a determined spirit. Let us then renounce once for all the idea of personal ease and *present* comfort as our ideal, and choose progress and soul advancement in knowledge and power of adjustment instead, and our changed view-point will soon revolutionize our lives.

Stiffen the spine, set the jaw and go to work at your task, which in the case of this article is overcoming physical weakness. I do not mean to do the above in a spirit of fight or even contention, but of a determination to hold correct ideals and to work individually for self advancement. In choosing your road to health, remember that the cause must be found and attacked. Here again we have great misconception to deal with. Our custom has been to look outside for the causes of disease. The real cause of disease is always our individual ignorance of law and how to utilize law as our friend and helper. The occasion of disease may be outside, but the cause is inside.

The full stomach of the gormand is the occasion of the pain, but abnormal and uncontrolled appetite was the real cause, and the cause that no emetic nor cathartic can remove. Teaching, or acquiring self-control, can alone suffice for permanent health to him, and so on throughout the long list that I have no time to view now.

It is here that the suggestionist is pre-eminent. He is nothing if not a teacher. By suggestionist, I mean all who make teaching the basis of treating.

Change your attitude to-day. Stop trying to get cured and commence learning how to get well. Learn to renounce and dare to conquer. *Fulfill* destiny if you must, but *conquer* fate. Fall in love with difficulties, for they are opportunities. Wrestle with the devil and, when conquered, you will find that he was really an angel.

PROBLEMS IN FERMENTATION BY YEAST.

ACCORDING to the *Revue Scientifique*, says the *Phila. Med. Journ.*, the subject of the fermentation of sugar by the action of the yeast-plant has recently been investigated, with some interesting results. The subject has interest for physicians, because, as will be seen, it tends to throw light on some allied problems in bacteriology. The fermentation of sugar, as is usually taught, is caused by a low vegetable organism, known as the yeast-plant. This plant takes in the sugar and gives off carbonic acid and alcohol. In 1897, Büchner, a German investigator, announced that fermentation was not dependent on the actual presence of the growing yeast-plant, but that the process was maintained just as well by a liquid extract, which he had made from the yeast-plant itself. This extract is called a zymose. More recently some English experimenters have gone over this ground, in order to determine whether the fermentation caused by this zymose is identical with that caused by the yeast-plant itself; and especially whether the usual products—alcohol and carbonic acid—are obtained in the same proportions, and whether the amount of sugar trans-

formed is in exact proportion with the quantities of these substances produced. They have found that the proportion between the alcohol and carbonic acid varies greatly, and that the exact proportion between the amount of sugar that disappears and the quantities of carbonic acid and alcohol that are produced is not maintained. In other words, a large quantity of sugar disappears and is not accounted for. This would seem to show that the yeast-extract, artificially produced, is not so potent as the yeast-plant itself, and that its potency is only maintained for a while. This whole process, as can be readily perceived, is analogous to what occurs in the case of many pathogenic bacteria. These minute organisms probably act by producing toxins, which are analogous to the yeast-extract, and these toxins become gradually reduced in strength. By taking advantage of these facts pathologists are able to obtain a preventive serum.

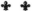

THE CHEMISTRY OF TEARS.

TEARS have their functional duty to accomplish, like every other fluid of the body, and the lachrymal gland is not placed behind the eye simple to fill space or to give expression to emotion. The chemical properties of tears consist of phosphate of lime and soda, making them very salty, but never bitter. Their action on the eye is very beneficial, and here consists their prescribed duty of the body, washing thoroughly that sensitive organ, which allows no foreign fluid to do the same work. Nothing cleanses the eye like a good, salty shower bath, and medical art has followed Nature's law in this respect, advocating the invigorating solution for any distressed condition of the optics. Tears do not weaken the sight, but improve it. They act as a tonic to the muscular vision, keeping the eye soft and limpid, and it will be noticed that women in whose eyes sympathetic tears gather quickly have brighter, tenderer orbs than others. When the pupils are hard and cold the world attributes it to one's disposition, which is a mere figure of speech, implying the lack of balmy tears, that are to the cornea what salve is to the skin or nourishment to the blood.

The reason some weep more easily than others, and all more readily than the sterner sex, has not its difference in the strength of the tear gland, but in the possession of a more delicate nerve system. The nerve fibers about the glands vibrate more easily, causing a downpour from the watery sac. Men are not nearly so sensitive to emotion; their sympathetic nature—the term is used in a medical sense—is less developed, and the eye gland is, therefore, protected from shocks. Consequently, a man should thank the formation of his nerve nature when he contemptuously scorns tears as a woman's practice. Between man and monkey there is this essential difference of tears. An ape cannot weep, not so much because its emotional powers are undeveloped, as the fact that the lachrymal gland was omitted in his optical make-up.

HOW FROZEN MEATS DETERIORATE.

MEATS frozen and kept in cold storage for long periods do not undergo organic changes in the ordinary sense—that is, they do not putrefy, soften, or smell bad, but they certainly do deteriorate in some intangible way. After a certain time frozen meat loses some life-principle essential to its nourishing quality. Such meat lacks flavor; it is not well digested or assimilated. Its savorless condition cannot be remedied or successfully disguised by the use of sauces and condiments. Those who eat cold-storage food for any length of time develop diarrhœal disorders, lose in weight, and would eventually starve to death unless a change of diet was made. The same reasoning applies to tinned fruits and vegetables. They should not be used after a certain period has elapsed. Especially should people be warned against using stale eggs and old milk and cream. Milk and cream are kept for days, rancid butter is washed and treated chemically, but all food, and especially cold-storage food, is damaged by long keeping, and will not nourish the body properly. There is the greatest abundance of food, but it does not satisfy.—*Sanitary Record*.

WON'T EAT THEIR OWN DISHES.

THE fact that cooks rarely have much appetite for the food of their own preparation is illustrated nightly at a well-known up-town chop house. There may be found the chef and several of the assistant chefs of one of the first hotels in New York. These men can have anything they want from the kitchens in which they are employed free of cost. The greatest luxuries of the market are at their disposal, and furthermore, they know that everything is beyond reproach. The kitchens are supplied with all the latest improvements, and are so clean and appetizing that visitors are taken through them. As for the cooking, the fact that many of the best-known gourmets of the city have forsaken their old resorts for this one is ample recommendation. Yet the men who are responsible for all this go nightly to a simple chop house, where they have to pay the same as other customers for their suppers. The chef gave this explanation:

"When a man is constantly surrounded by food suffs he gets tired of the sight of them. It is so with any other business. It is all right while you are at it, but when your work is done you want to get away from it. We come here to forget our work, and to eat things we have not seen nor handled."—*New York Sun*.

FEEDING THE INFANTS OF THE POOR WITH UNSTERILIZED COW'S MILK.

DR. PALMER, in the *New York Medical Journal*, September 8, 1900, claims that pasteurization or sterilization impairs the food value of milk, making it difficult to digest, at times producing alimentary disturbances and causing disorders by reason of malnutrition. No amount of boiling will purify a foul milk; not even a temperature of 356° F. will destroy the bacterial products in the milk; if the milk contains any pathogenic bacteria, it will be impregnated with their toxines before steriliation ordinarily begins. If there are present comparatively few bacteria—for all milks contain some bacteria—and the milk is used a reasonable time after milking, the result will be more favorable than if the milk is used after sterilization. Sterilized milk is more easily contaminated than raw milk, and the ordinary housekeeper cooks the milk either too much or too little, in the former case diminishing its dietetic value, and in the latter making it an ideal medium in which the bacteria present may multiply.

Accordingly, if it is possible to obtain a fresh and pure milk, to pasteurize or sterilize it is very objectionable; if the milk is not too foul, given in the raw condition it is less deleterious than after pasteurization or sterilization; if it is altogether foul it should be entirely discarded, for sterilization is then useless. Modification of the milk is of little importance compared with its purity.

PHYSIOLOGICAL REMEDIES.

THE most important measures which can be employed in dealing with the sick may be said to be baths, exercise, and diet. The chronic invalid can be made well only by being reconstructed. The sick man must be transformed into a healthy man by a process of gradual change. Little by little the old tissues must be torn down and new tissues built in their place. By means of exercise the movement of the blood is accelerated and the old diseased tissues are broken down and carried out of the body. Exercise always diminishes weight. Warm baths increase the elimination of waste substances, and cold baths stimulate the destruction of tissues, increase the activity of the heart and of all the tissues, encourage the formation of the digestive fluids, and increase the appetite for food. A dietary consisting of pure food substances, of a character to be easily digested and assimilated, is the proper material with which to construct a new and healthy body. Thus, baths, exercise, and a natural dietary, constitute a therapeutic trio, each member of which is a complement to the others.

Health-getting, for the chronic invalid, is simply a matter of training, of health culture under favorable conditions, which include the discarding of all disease-producing habits, such as the use of tobacco, tea, coffee, and all irritating, indigestible, and disease-producing foods.

THE NERVES NEVER GROW OLD.

COMMENTING on the common causes of nervous disorders, Prof. W. H. Thompson says: "The message of modern science about the nervous system has a greater store of reserve vitality than all the other bodily systems put together. It is the only texture that is found not to have lost weight after death by starvation, as well as after death by any cause. It is the last to grow old; and as to the mind, it need not grow old at all, provided it be steadily applied with that mighty spiritual element in us which we call interest. Even the muscular system can be wonderfully sustained by interest; for should a man attempt the same muscular work on a treadmill which he lightly endures along a mountain brook after a trout, he would faint dead away. But the mind will, by interest, grow steadily, even while bone and sinew are wasting through age.— *Practical Review.*

CONSANGUINEOUS MARRIAGES.

CONSANGUINEOUS marriages are thought by a recent writer upon the subject to be undesirable, not because they originate disease, but because they intensify existing disorders or diathesis. It being almost impossible to find a family without taints, we rely upon the process of natural selection to counteract the bad effects of this taint. Close selection should therefore be discouraged. If the diseased and degenerate insist on getting married, it is their duty to posterity to mitigate their innate unfitness by the selection of suitable consorts. The practical inference from this seems to be that the feeble must marry the robust, and the neurotic the level-headed, but at the same time the robust should not marry the feeble-minded or the level-headed the neurotic. Nature is essentially haphazard in her workings.—*Medical Age.*

STARCH DIGESTION IN INFANTS.

IT has long been the custom to say that no amylaceous substances should enter into a young infant's food, because it has from Nature at an early age no ferment capable of digesting starch. The saliva of a newly-born child—and it is wrong to say that there is no saliva at this age—will dextrinize starch, as any one who wishes may prove for himself.—*A. Jacobi.*

THE Scotch are the greatest dyspeptics on earth, largely owing to their use of half-cooked oatmeal and soft bread. Next to the Scotch are the Americans, and no single thing has contributed more to American dyspepsia than half-cooked oatmeal mush for breakfast. In rural France, where dyspepsia is practically unknown, hard bread and vegetables, with a moderate amount of meat, comprise the chief items of the bill of fare.—*The Sanitary Home.*

COLORS AND THE MIND.

"THAT colors affect the mind with different force," writes C. de Kay, in the *New York Times,* "has been known for ages, but it is curious that artists who deal with colors professionally, have done little or nothing to formulate the impressions that different hues produce. The ancients believed that certain kinds of music roused certain emotions, and it was part of their theories of medicine that music ministered to a mind diseased. But we have no evidence that they tried to influence people consciously by surrounding them with different colors. Perhaps they did, since we have only the merest fragments of the various systems of cure for melancholy and other mental troubles practised by physicians, who may have failed to put theories in writing, or, having intrusted their professional secrets to paper, never had the luck to reach the reading world of modern times.

"When we enter certain houses we are immediately affected by their air, without being able to assign a cause; rarely do we think of the general color of the room or try to discover the reason for the pleasant or disagreeable impression in the tone of the physical surroundings. Yet we are fully aware of the influence of stained glass of certain kinds in church, and can hardly avoid noticing an exhilaration that comes with a sudden sight of a hillside clad with the ruddy hues of our autumn leaves. Doubtless there are people peculiarly sensitive to color impressions, as there are others in whom the sense of smell or hearing raises them in that respect far above their fellows. Sometimes an injury makes one sense abnormally acute.

"A patient in one of our insane asylums, who was there temporarily because of an injury to his head in the football field, told his attending physician that it was all he could do to prevent screaming aloud when he saw red. Long ago Chevreuil drew attention to the exciting effect of red and orange, and the calming effect of gray, green, and greenish-yellow. Since then we have had the "blue-glass" craze, and some attempts were made at an insane asylum of Paris during the seventies to investigate the effect of red rooms and blue rooms on patients. Lately some German investigators have been experimenting on workmen confined most of the day at their work in rooms hung with red and other colors. One conclusion reached is an apparent increase in the rapidity of work carried on in red rooms. A club in New York, which has olive green and dull gold for the chief colors of most of its apartments and galleries affects some people very agreeably; they say it is restful. Others, on the contrary, complain that the gold on the walls is not enough to counteract the melancholy of the green. The conclusion is fair that we have to do with different temperaments, the lymphatic instinctively desiring the excitant colors, while the sanguine find the restful colors soothing.

"It is pretty certain that black is a melancholy color; instinct, as we may call a reasoning that does not reach consciousness, has naturally selected black as a sign for mourning the dead. Death and night are naturally associated, since the sun dies every evening and the tomb is dark. The Chinese use red as a symbol of joy, perhaps with an unconscious groping toward symbolism, owing to the red sunrise; perhaps because ripening fruits and the cheeks of young people are ruddy. At any rate, this is the color they use for marriages. Yellow is the favorite color for the robes of Indian priests, as if they felt, rather than argued, that yellow belongs to autumn and old age—to the sunset and the ripened fruit. White is common everywhere for extreme youth and innocence; it is the color of the dawn, and of many flowers that bloom or open only at night, and would be observed, therefore, in the earliest morning hours.

"There is thus a symbolism in colors which seems to have been followed by mankind long before people set their wits to work reasoning why one color rather than another should have been employed on this or that occasion for this person or for that. It is still worth while for hospitals and asylums to hang and paint rooms in different colors, and assign patients to them according to the character of their disease or mental troubles. Plainly the youth who felt like screaming when he saw red was a patient fit for a room hung with pale green or gray, or greenish-yellow; then the color might soothe him. But a melancholy, lymphatic patient might find in red surroundings a constant stimulus, a quiet but persistent prompting which would help him to greater activity of the brain, and form a minor element in his cure which it would not be well to disdain.

"The painter also should study the impressions that color masses make on different people. He would soon find that certain colors are slightly attractive and certain slightly repulsive to the same person. He can look about him among his comrades and see how a given painter has a natural predilection for a certain color, or certain groups of colors. It might lead him to investigate his own taste and perhaps prove of use to him in his profession. And to the decorator-artist who has to arrange schemes of color for interiors it will be of a certainty useful to realize that he can produce effects on people in this or that direction, according as he makes this or that color, or combination of colors, predominate in his scheme. Perhaps the dark-paneled dining-room is a mistake, on the principle that cheerfulness at meals is a good thing. It is not by wine alone that a dinner party can be set in a good humor; that is a coarse method compared with the action of colors on the unconscious subjects of a properly managed interior. Perhaps in time the value of color will appeal to the architect also, and some attention be paid to its application to buildings. Meantime it is for scientists and painters to work at the problem.

Department of Hygiene.

WITH SPECIAL REFERENCE TO STATE AND PREVENTIVE MEDICINE.

WHY IS THE MEDICAL PROFESSION TRADUCED?

THE medical is probably the worst and most unreasonably traduced profession in existence. In view of the jests, jokes and jibes so constantly hurled at clergymen and lawyers this is a very strong assertion; but it is warranted, as a glimpse at the subject will demonstrate.

We are constantly charged with being only pseudo-scientific, and we are compelled to admit that all our deductions are virtually based on empiricism. Other charges are, want of faith in our own weapons, insincerity, hypocrisy and cant, in that we do not resist the temptation to fall into routine ruts of makeshift, by palliating thn pains and assuaging the feelings of our patients, assuming but really neither hoping nor caring to cure them; that when we are honest we frankly admit that the more we study the nature of disease and the unreliability of medicines the more positively are we convinced that our real knowledge does not extend beyond prophylaxis and conservative surgery. We are pointed at by scientists in other fields of physics as being the only learned body claiming scientific attainments and yet being without science. Everywhere we find the scripture text, Physician, heal thyself, staring us in the face. In corroboration of all this it is boldly charged that many of our brightest lights have practically turned "states' evidence" against us, so that we are self-convicted.

We are plied with disrespectful epithets. Physicians are " Pillbags," "Deaths' heads," or " Quacks " and " Undertakers Allies." Surgeons are " Sawbones," " Butchers," and " Bloodsuckers." Our very forbearance in not noisily resenting these current and chronic aspersions is cited as proving that they are founded in fact. Our critics tauntingly ask us to admit that we are only a little more dignified than the other vendors of nostrums and " wonder cures," inasmuch as we do not quite so unblushingly use the columns of the daily and weekly secular and *religious* press! They do not hesitate to charge that we do use the reporters in divers covert ways, and indirectly say to the world, " Behold my unparalleled success with phthisis, cardiac troubles or catarrh!" Or, "What can compare with my wonderful instrument for rapid lithotomy, my natural curve, double traction forceps, my never-failing method in tracheotomy," my " quick lunch " process in talipes vulgus and lithotomy, or my unparalleled success in appendicitis!"

"I was the first surgeon to transplant the tricuspid valve from the heart of a sheep to a human being! Of course the patient died from shock; but the operation was a beautiful success."

And have not many of us invented new diseases, new anatomical parts, new operations? Witness Basedow's, Bright's, Addison's, Graves', Potts' and dozens of others; the Circle of Willis, Fissure of Rolando, Island of Riel, Poupart's, the Pons Varolii, and even the Pons Asinorum! Add to these the long array of proprietary operations. requiring ten pages in Foster's Dictionary to describe and name them.

That we do better than the outspoken and unblushing quacks and charlatans, who do not pretend to do well, and who assume no virtuous scruples concerning questions of ethics, is not saying much for us, while we continue to lend our names and voluminous titles to aid in puffing every sort of remedy, food and instrument in the market.

Possibly we deserve some of this universal abuse and detraction.

THE NEW YORK LEGISLATURE AND THE PSEUDOPATHS.

THE GAZETTE is not on the warpath against the " paths," except as they demand special privileges on account of their special methods or supernatural origin. There has never been a time in the world's history when fakirs in medicine and religion have not flourished, simply because they have always found plenty of gullibles and susceptibles to patronize and applaud them. To abolish quackery it is only necessary to educate the masses out of their ignorance and superstition. The process is a slow one, but it is the only effective one.

But when the " Bony-paths " and " Science-Healers " demand privileges and immunities denied to those who do not harp on a single physiological string, invoke the supernatural, or adopt the rôle of miracle-workers, it is time to call " time ! "

This the *Medical Record* of this city does, as follows:

" These people," says *The Record,* " who practice under these peculiar names possess no knowledge which educated physicians do not possess. Whatever is known of disease, its causes, manifestations, and treatment, is taught in every medical college. The peculiar effects of the mind in producing physical derangements ; the effects of massage and manipulations, the therapeutic value of notes—all these are known and taught in medical colleges, and practiced by educated physicians."

The *New York Times* adds:

" The quacks trust to a single remedy for the cure of every disease, and, working under some other name than that of doctor of medicine. they have hitherto found it easy to evade the laws governing medical prac-

tice. As described by its advocates, the bill now pending in the State Legislature simply imposes on all who hold themselves out as competent to cure diseases the necessity of proving that they have the knowledge entitling them to a license. Some think it does more than that, but, however that may be. *The Medical Record* is entirely right when it asks what conceivable reason there can be why one class of practitioners should pass an examination more rigid than another class, or why any class should be allowed to enter upon the practice of so important a calling—one dealing with human life, human health, human honor—without any examination, simply because they practice some peculiar method under some mystifying or unusual name.

TOPICS OF THE TIMES.

IN the address read by Surgeon General Wyman at the recent Pan-American Medical Congress, something approaching discouragement was expressed at the small degree of success yet attained in the suppression of diseases known to be suppressible. Referring, among other diseases, to smallpox, Dr. Wyman said : " In vaccination we have an absolute preventive, and in the glycerinized lymph we have a safe inoculating material absolutely devoid of the danger of exciting undue inflammation. Thus a mere scratch or a needle puncture insures, without discomfort, protection from one of the most loathsome and disfiguring diseases known. Even after smallpox has become epidemic, the methods by which it may be rapidly and surely suppressed have been so frequently demonstrated as to become now almost a matter of mere routine." Yet, as New Yorkers know only too well, there are modern cities where smallpox can linger for months, claiming new victims day after day, just as if its banishment were the very reverse of " a matter of mere routine." Why? " The answer," declared the Surgeon General. " is plain. It is that sanitary administration has not kept pace with scientific knowledge. It is also evident that the scientific knowledge is not so widely diffused as it should be, even among those of whom we have a right to expect it. It is evident that we are not making ' use of those means which the God of Nature has placed in our power.' " This puts the responsibility directly on the Board of Health in cases when, as in New York at present, a disease both preventable·and conquerable, not only makes its appearance, but gains a firm foothold and spreads steadily though slowly through a considerable part of the city. Our "sanitary administration" might be, and, indeed, has been, worse than it is; not a little is accomplished by it, and the general disposition among competent critics is to praise rather than to blame the health officials; but the existing situation is proof that, for one reason or another, it may be lack of highest competency or the existence of laws out of harmony with scientific knowledge, New York is not protected as it should be, and as it might be.

RELATIONS OF INFLUENZA AND APPENDICITIS.

A FRENCH DISCLAIMER.

SOME of the prospectors for pathological novelties have been discovering that there is a relation between grip and appendicitis. Jumping at a conclusion the press has been crediting the suggestion or " discovery " to a French professor, who promptly and chivalrously disclaims in favor of our own Dr. Keen, of Philadelphia.

We reproduce the *Herald's* version of the professor's remarks, from which it will be seen that he takes us Americans to task for our pro-cannibalistic proclivities. Perhaps it is quite as rational to associate excessive flesh-eating with the causative factors in appendicitis as to charge it to influenza. It seems to us that both are coincident rather than causative.

Dr. Lucas Championnière sends a letter to the *Herald* regarding his communication to the Academy of Medicine regarding the relations of influenza to appendicitis.

"I regret," says the doctor, "that the citations from my communication published by the *Herald,* which were necessarily incomplete, have raised contestations by eminent American doctors and surgeons. I never attributed to myself the discovery of the relations of influenza to appendicitis. I confined myself to saying that I regarded the thing as proved, and gave my reasons for saying so.

"I added that I thought that excess of animal food predisposed to intestinal troubles, and, in consequence, to appendicitis. I said that this condition might explain, in a certain measure, the extreme frequency of appendicitis in England and America, where animal food is much more largely used than in France.

"I cited, to show the frequency of appendicitis, the opinion of Dr. W. W. Keen, of Philadelphia, who in a brochure which he had already done me the honor to send me, said we must assume that nearly one-third of all adults have had one or more attacks.

"Though appendicitis is becoming more and more frequent in France, and though I almost consider it like a new malady, we do not admit that it is as common as that. We therefore find it quite natural that the most interesting reports on this malady have come to us from America. We regard them as particularly valuable and instructive, and I cited several of them in my communication to the Academy.

"You will understand the regret I feel to see my communication reproduced as if I had taken no account of these labors."

IS WETNESS OF SOIL A CAUSE OF PHTHISIS?

For a long time back it has been held that a damp soil is provocative of phthisis. Dr. Bowditch, so far back as the year 1862, says the London *Hospital,* laid it down that a residence on or near a damp soil was one of the primal causes of consumption in Massachusetts—probably in New England, and possibly in other portions of the globe. The late Sir George (then Dr.) Buchanan, as the result of very careful investigation of the subject in regard to England, came to much the same conclusion. He was more especially concerned with inquiring into the health results of the various sanitary improvements which had been carried out in certain English towns. These had largely consisted of drainage works, and the result of the inquiry was to show that in many towns in which drying of the subsoil had been effected the mortality from consumption had very considerably declined. Nevertheless, as pointed out by Buchanan himself, there were exceptions. Some of the towns in which undoubted lowering of the ground water had taken place had failed to reduce their phthisis mortality, while others, in which hardly any change had been effected in the condition of the subsoil, had improved markedly in regard to their consumption statistics. After this Buchanan investigated the variations in the prevalence of phthisis in different districts in the counties of Surrey, Sussex, and Kent (the area in question covering 3,182 square miles and embracing a population of 1,118,372), with direct reference to geological considerations, especially to perviousness of soil and contour of land. Putting the results of the two inquiries together, he came to the conclusion that "wetness of soil is a cause of phthisis to the population living upon it," and for many years past this view has been generally accepted. Still, a good many observers have doubted whether the above dictum expressed the whole truth, and they have laid especial stress upon the exceptional cases, holding that, in the absence of any obvious disturbing cause, such exceptions ought to invalidate the generally accepted conclusions.

Recently Dr. Arthur Newsholme has discussed this question afresh. He asks: "Is there an essential relationship between wetness of soil and phthisis mortality among the population living on such soil, or is the common excess of phthisis on wet soils rather due to the fact that a lower class of the community, worse housed and worse fed, are likely to be found dwelling on a wet soil?" and he answers that "it appears probable that much of the benefit ascribed to drying the soil has been due really to other factors of improvement which commenced to operate about the same time as the former." It has to be remembered that the essential cause of phthisis, viz., the bacillus tuberculosis, has been discovered since the days when Buchanan formulated his proposition on the subject, and we have to ask how our present knowledge as to the prime cause of tuberculosis fits in with the wet-soil theory. Like overcrowding and insufficient nourishment, the wet soil, he says, must be placed among predisposing causes; and it must be placed, furthermore, in a much lower position than the above-mentioned causes. Wet soil implies greater loss of heat by evaporation, more easy provocation of catarrhs, especially when, as would commonly happen, it is associated with cold and wet houses. But a house even on a wet soil can be effectually protected, and then the phthisical patient or the person predisposed to phthisis need not suffer.

The conclusion is arrived at that much of the improvement in the phthisis mortality, which had seemed to Buchanan and others to be due to drying of the soil, was really to be attributed to the coincident improvements in the social condition of the people in regard to housing and food, which had taken place in the same period. Dr. Newsholme's view is that "personal infection is the main cause of the spread of phthisis, and that this occurs chiefly where people are most closely agglomerated and live an indoor life; that deficient nutrition is an important favoring cause of phthisis, and that wetness of soil operates in a minor degree by favoring catarrhal conditions of the respiratory mucous membrane."

NATURE'S ALKALINE TREATMENT OF GOUT AND RHEUMATISM BY THE USE OF NATURAL ALKALINE THERMAL WATERS.

IN a paper read before the International Medical Congress at Paris and printed in *The Lancet,* Dr. Carl H. Brandt said: My only excuse for attempting any addition to the already overdone subject of rheumatism and gout is that in an experience of a number of years in the treatment of these conditions solely, certain clinical facts have been impressed upon me to so great an extent that I feel that the lessons learned by clinical work may be of some value to those of the profession who are called upon to deal with the subacute and chronic forms of so-called gout and rheumatism.

To go into the theories that have been advanced in the past is not my purpose, but merely to try to show why and how results are obtained by the use of natural alkaline thermal waters, internally and externally, in a large number of cases where all other means had failed. That such is the case can, I am sure, be testified to by almost all the leading medical men of the day, and my only surprise is that they fail to understand how such results are obtained. No treatment gives rise to so much disbelief as the use of water as a therapeutic agent, and the idea that after the use of all the drugs, the so-called specifics, the alkalies and the salines, relief should be given by the use of water is by many considered absurd, and the man who advocates such treatment is dubbed a fanatic.

The profession, as a rule, may be said to be satisfied that the most approved treatment for these conditions is the so-called alkali treatment, and yet they express surprise that good results should be obtained by the use of alkaline waters. Have they ever stopped to consider that, after all, the so-called water cures or treatment for gout or rheumatism are nothing more or less than the alkaline treatment, differing only in the fact that the alkali is, on the one hand, supplied by the druggist, and on the other by Nature? Such is the case. All the water cures for these conditions consist in the use of alkaline waters, not only internally, but also in the form of baths.

The use of the alkaline waters is but one factor in the proposition. Another is that when properly used we have the application of the alkaline treatment under the best circumstances and with the best possible surroundings. Quite possibly the patient's physician at home will have laid the fullest stress upon the proper diet, exercise, mental rest, etc., that the patient is to have, in addition to the medication advised, but (and herein lies the kernel of the nut) the patient does not follow these instructions. He will take his pill or teaspoonful of medicine with absolute precision and regularity, but he has no time for exercise and dieting. After finishing his business and following his pleasure he may give these a half-hearted attention for a day or two, but there it, as a rule, ends. These are not conditions to be helped solely by medication.

On the other hand, when taking a so-called cure, he not only has his medicine, *i. e.,* alkaline water internally and externally, but having no business to attend to, no pleasures to follow, his one occupation is to conscientiously carry out in every detail his régimé as laid down for him by his adviser, who has him constantly under observation. Given then, the alkaline treatment, *i. e.,* in this case supplied by the use of alkaline waters, good air, a carefully regulated diet, proper exercise, absolute cleanliness, free action of the skin brought about by the use of the alkaline baths, and free action of the kidneys and bowels due to the internal administration of the alkaline waters— added to the knowledge which the patient has that he is doing that for his condition which is best—can any patient fail to improve?

The first clinical fact which has been impressed upon me is the absence of any clearly defined line of demarkation between the symptoms of cases which have presented themselves, in which a diagnosis of either rheumatism or gout has been made. I have been unable to demonstrate to my own satisfaction any different pathological condition in these so-called diseases, the clinical picture in either case being practically the same. The diagnosis, it would seem, is most often settled by the exciting cause. On the one hand, if the initial attack followed exposure to cold, dampness, etc., we are most frequently told that it is a case of rheumatism. If, on the other hand, the primary attack was apparently induced by excesses at the table or by indigestion, we are said to have a case of gout.

The absence of difference in the symptomatology and pathology of the many cases which have come under my observation of so-called rheumatism and gout has led me to discard the terms rheumatism and gout and bring these conditions under the one general head of uric acid toxemia, my own belief being that in the absence of any clearly defined pathological condition neither rheumatism nor gout are true diseases, but are groups of symptoms arising from improper metabolism, or, in other words, the effects produced by the retention in the system of the products of metabolism or waste. I am strengthened in this belief by the observance of two clinical facts: First, that in all cases which have come under my personal observation, in which a diagnosis of gout or rheumatism has been made, the retention of uric acid has always been readily demonstrated. Secondly, that immediately the free excretion of uric acid was brought about the symptoms have disappeared, irrespectively as to whether the diagnosis has been rheumatism or gout.

My universal experience has been that on presentation the so-called caes of rheumatism or gout is found to be excreting less than the normal amount of uric acid, and after being put under treatment this amount gradually increases, and with its increase a diminution of the symptoms. The amount of uric acid excreted under treatment is frequently found to be twice or three times greater than before treatment was begun,

and then gradually diminishes until the normal mark is reached, at which it remains so long as the patient continues so to conduct his life and habits as will insure his maintaining a proper relation between waste and repair. The ground being taken that uric-acid retention is the indication at least, if not the prime factor in the causation of such condition or conditions, which I name uric acid toxemia, it follows that the knowledge of the exact amount of uric acid daily excreted is most essential. The ordinary routine of instructing a patient to bring his medical man a bottle of urine, with no instruction as to amount or how and when the same is to be collected being given, is useless.

Neither a qualitative analysis nor a microscopic determination will suffice—the first owing to the fact that that particular portion of the daily amount of urine may contain a greater or lesser percentage of the entire output of uric acid; the second owing to the fact that the drop or drops examined may contain all or none of the crystallized uric acid present, and thus lead to error in judging the amount excreted.

Obviously, a quantitative analysis is necessary. My procedure is as follows: A thoroughly clean glass vessel, large enough to contain the output of urine for twenty-four hours, is given the patient, with instructions to collect all urine passed for the following twenty-four hours. He is also instructed to first empty the bladder whenever having a bowel movement, so that no urine may be lost. From this a quantitative analysis is made, no change of diet having been ordered up to this time.

From the evidence gathered from this first analysis treatment is the following day begun, and the patient is instructed as regards diet, exercise and the use of the waters. On the day following, a second analysis is made, the treatment as regards diet, baths, etc., being changed in accordance with the results of uric-acid excretion as shown by said analysis. Analyses are continued every two or three days throughout the treatment, which is ended when the excretion of uric acid has reached the normal, the patient then being allowed to return to his home, after having been instructed as to his manner of living so as to maintain a proper excretion of uric acid. A record of the amount of uric acid excreted is kept in each case from day to day, and on this record, as I have said, is based any change in diet, baths, etc. It is not claimed that the use of the alkaline treatment as supplied by Nature is a specific, but that its employment, owing to the conditions by which it is surrounded, gives a larger percentage of good results.

In my experience, I may say that next to the internal administration of the alkalies and their external application in the form of baths, diet plays the most important part, and by which Haig has shown, and my own experience has proved, uric-acid excretion can be controlled. A dietary is to be carefully followed, not by any set rule to be applied to all cases alike, but by suiting the new diet to each patient in accordance with the indication as shown by the urinary analysis, remembering the importance of personal individuality.

The utility of the alkaline bath has been a vexed question, many practical men holding that there is no absorption of the mineral contents of the water, and many experiments have been made to prove this. My own experience leads me to believe that the taking of the alkaline baths alone will induce an increased uric-acid excretion, my theory being that we here again have applied that old physical law of exosmosis and endosmosis, an acid condition of all the tissues, an alkaline medium, *i. e.*, the bath, and an animal membrane, *i. e.*, the skin, intervening.

The alkaline treatment, as supplied by alkaline thermal waters, I use in the following manner: A patient is given a daily alkaline bath, varying in temperature from 90 degrees to 105 degrees F., for a period of from five to twenty-five minutes. He is given none but alkaline water to drink, a portion being taken on an empty stomach. He takes from two to four hours' active exercise daily, and his diet is specifically ordered for him. No form of alcohol is permitted, all the different factors of the treatment being regulated by the excretions of uric acid as shown by the analyses. The results in an experience of a number of years have been most satisfactory.

I would call attention to the following essential points in the use of alkaline water for the treatment of uric acid toxemia: 1. Frequent quantitative urinary analyses. 2. Changing the diet, the amount of exercise and the amount of water taken until there is a free excretion of uric acid. 3. The taking of sufficient exercise for the thorough oxidization of the foods taken. 4. The putting aside of all mental work. 5. A specific diet ordered, not depending upon the patient's knowledge as to what contains or does not contain the proximate principles which are to be avoided. 6. To teach the patient what Nature's laws are as pertaining to his health and well-being and how to follow them.

In conclusion, let me deny the statement that has so often been made, that there is a great difficulty in making patients follow stringent rules. Such has not been my experience when I have had ability sufficient to impress them with the importance of these restrictions. This treatment, as I have tried to show, is in no way specific. It is not claimed that there is any magic in the waters used, but that it is merely an application and use of the recognized utility of the alkalies, augmented by the surroundings and conditions possible when the patient is so placed as to be constantly under the observation of his physician.

The treatment is a rational one, and a true exponent of the practice of physiology, a step I trust towards brushing away some of the mysteries which, unfortunately, have surrounded many medical measures. I hope in the near future that it may be said of our profession, "They practice physiology and not medicine."

STAMMERING.

THERE is no subject of more interest to the stammerer than his own impediment. Indeed, if he be seriously afflicted the study of it, says a writer in *The Phono-Meter,* is a means of cure. A full and perfect understanding of the cause and symptoms and their removal is a sure foundation for a cure. Speech is articulate sound. Whenever the easy flow of articulate sound is broken or emitted in spasmodic jerks, stammering ensues, or more correctly, this is stammering. To easily understand the cause of this interruption it is necessary to possess a clear knowledge of the position and formation and uses of the organs essential in the production of speech. The vibrations causing the sound we call voice are produced in the larynx, or voice-box. This is a hollow box-shaped organ, composed mainly of cartilage, and situated at the upper end of the trachea, or windpipe. The lower end of the larynx opens freely into the trachea, but the upper end is closed with the exception of the glottis, a chink-like opening an inch long. The front part of the glottis is at the base and back of the tongue, with the opening shelving toward the rear, and is neither horizontally nor perpendicularly in the throat. The sides of the opening are bounded by two fibrous membranes, the vocal chords, by the vibration of which sound is produced. These chords are more like pads than elastic tissue, and project into the larynx, leaving only the glottis between them. All breath going to and fro must pass through the larynx and glottis. In quiet breathing the chords remain undisturbed, but when placed in the right position and breath expelled they are set to vibrating, and the vibrations being transferred to the out-flow of air, voice is produced. The pitch and tone of the voice depend upon the length of the vocal chords and their tensions. The loudness of sound depends upon the force with which the breath is expelled. By separate or combined action of the nose, palate, tongue, teeth and lips the voice is changed into articulate speech. This flow of sound must be continuous during articulation or else there is nothing to make speech. As long as breath is expelled easily and the formation of sound permitted to go on uninterrupted, articulation can be performed without difficulty. The stammerer, in his efforts to articulate, stops the flow of breath either entirely or partly, or he lets a portion of it escape, causing snatches of words or syllables, which in his efforts are repeated many times. The cause of his trouble lies in the lack of will power to control articulation, which must be simultaneous. Here is where the stammerer's troubles begin. The production of voice is as easy and natural to the child as breathing. The child, at an early age, hearing conversation around him, tries to imitate what he hears, and his efforts are soon followed by syllables and words. He continues trying, and thus gradually acquires the vocabulary of his associates. As the child gains confidence in his ability to form words he begins to talk more rapidly, joining words into longer sentences. When the child is of somewhat nervous, high-strung temperament, or has naturally a weak control over the speech organs, it is easy to see how a slight thing may induce hesitation. Association of stammerers with such children cause an unconscious imitation of the impediment. Stammering is sometimes one of the attendant results of disease in children; of such diseases as cause a great weakening of the vitality and nervous forces. As the child grows older and realizes that his speech is different from his play-fellows and his attention is frequently called to the impediment and by them in a curious or jesting manner, he begins to fear to talk at all. The trouble gradually grows worse, and each attempt to speak but increases his nervous fear. To such life becomes unbearable, society is shunned, ambitions perish, energy is lost and all hopes of happiness fade away. This is not the life of all stammerers. Many struggle on, hoping for a cure. A few realize their impediment, which is slight, have will power and entirely overcome it. The mental agitation produced by the continual stammering can but impair the health and the nervous system of the stammerer, in proportion as he is troubled. Loss of sleep, dissipation of any kind, mental worry, all of which requires an extra effort of the will to counterbalance their effort, tend to lessen the stammerer's control over his organs of speech. The stammerer nearly always lacks self-confidence. This is partly on account of his impediment and constant fear of being unable to talk. He should get hold of an idea that he must talk. Very few people, except singers and elocutionists, have placed any foundation on the cultivation of the voice and speech; but the people are beginning to see the lack of teaching correct habits in respiration and articulation in our public schools. It should be enforced the same as other studies; then stammering would be robbed of its horrors and become very much less aggravating.

ON THE DEMONSTRATION OF NITROUS ACID IN WATER BY MEANS OF ERDMANN'S AMIDONAPHTHOL-K-ACID METHOD.*

By Dr. H. Mennicke.

The number of reagents for the detection of the extremely important nitrous acid or nitrites in drinking water is not small; but they almost all have the disadvantage of keeping badly and depending upon a readily misunderstood color reaction. As the result of my experiences and researches I believe that the Amidonaphthol-K-acid, recommended by Erdmann, is the very best of them all, and enables us to decide upon the chemical and bacteriological properties of a water. Comparative experiments with this and zinc iodide and iodide of potash-

* Abstract from the Zeitschrift für angewandte Chemie, No. 10, March 6, 1900.

starch solution of drinking, waste and distilled waters, lead me to the following conclusions:

1. The reaction always appears when nitrous acid is present.

2. The color reaction cannot be misunderstood, and does not occur under other conditions, such as the presence of chloride of iron, nitric acid, and other oxiding agents, alone. When any one of these, as the iron salt, is present in larger quantities, the reaction still occurs, only its color is a deeper claret.

3. The grade of sensitiveness of the reagent for a sharp eye is 1 : 300,000,000 (calculated for nitrite of sodium).

4. When there are only traces of nitrous acid present the test is best made by daylight.

5. The reaction is more delicate than that of the other tests, and appeared where these latter were no longer seen. Thus the limit of the iodide of potash-starch test was at 1 : 1,000,000, calculated also with sodium nitrite.

6. I found it very convenient to be able to combine the qualitative test with a quantitative determination, by comparing the color tint, after the lapse of one hour, with that given by known dilutions of normal nitrite solutions.

7. The maximum depth of the claret color was attained in half an hour.

The unreliability of the zinc iodide and iodide of potash-starch reactions need not be recapitulated. No disturbing influences were found to affect the demonstration of the presence of nitrous acid by the Erdmann test, not even the presence of oxidizing combinations.

The author then gives two tables embodying his results with the test with pure water, very dilute sodium nitrite solutions, and ordinary drinking and drainage waters. They show that positive results were obtained in the presence of nitrites in cases where, for example, the iodide of potassium-starch test failed entirely. The reaction undoubtedly enables us to make a rigid examination of any questionable water.

THE USE OF BROMIDES IN HYSTERIA, DELIRIUM, ETC.

By J. S. Murphy, M.D.,
Sullivan, Ind.

Considerable has been written on this subject, which has all the respectability of ancient lineage, and like most other obscure things, has received no stint of authoritative attention.

The etiology of hysteria has never been satisfactorily explained. For a long time it was thought to be in some way related to uterine disturbances. But while it is not denied that sexual disorders may have a bearing on the primal cause of the phenomena, still it is also claimed that the ailment attacks both sexes. We have progressed not further than this.

The treatment at best has been attended in most cases with disappointing results. We are confronted with a "loss of due balance between certain of the high functions of the brain, spinal cord and sympathetic system." The treatment obviously should be, then, to restore this balance. Rest is a very essential feature. By rest is meant *restraint* of overaction of certain of the spinal nerve centers. My experience has taught me that nothing gives better results than the combined bromides; and these should be of the very purest obtainable. For this reason I have availed my professional self of Peacock's, not only for their purity—freedom from bromates and carbonates, so common to the commercial bromides—but on account of their ideal synergic effects and the fact that they are neutral in reaction, which permits of combining certain alkaloids in the solution without fear or danger of precipitation.

In various forms of neurosis I have found Peacock's Bromides invaluable as an all-round agency of alleviation and cure. They have never disappointed me. In obstinate cases of epilepsy, where the treatment is necessarily protracted. I find them particularly useful in that their administration is not followed by the too common symptoms of bromism. And I would specially urge their utility in instances of delirium following alcoholic excesses.

Anything that conserves the vital forces, that does not depress any organ, as for example, the cardiac center, anything that gives the rest of normal sleep when repair is greater than waste, anything that tends to restore the nervous equilibrium, soothing the exciting centers, whatever and wherever they may be, must benefit the entire organism when each separate organ, then, of course, will receive its needful quota of help. And since local treatment is out of the question, I cannot conceive of better procedure, or one more infallible to the successful management of hysterical cases.

FIRST MUNICIPAL CREMATORIUM IN GREAT BRITAIN,

The first crematorium erected by any municipality in England was opened in Hull, Yorkshire, in the first week in January. The cremating apparatus is a furnace of the regenerative type, designed by the late Mr. Simon, of Manchester. The degree of heat can be regulated in the most exact manner. There is no smoke, and little visible flame before the body is introduced, and if the coffin is made in accordance with the regulations, there is no smoke and no noise during cremation. The process occupies about an hour, at the end of which there remain only the inorganic bases of the bones, in the form of silvery-gray, pumice-like fragments. These are removed by passing an asbestos brush through the chamber, which causes the remains to fall through an opening into the urn which is to receive them. Undoubtedly graveyards in or near great cities, says the *Med. Record*, are more or less a menace to the health of the inhabitants. Cremating is, in every particular, a more sanitary mode of disposing of the dead than earth-to-earth burial. It is probable, when the public become conscious of this fact, and when prejudices arising from religious scruples and sentiment have died, that cremation, in towns at least, will take the place of the older method.

THE PUBLIC SPITTING NUISANCE.

It is a source of gratification, says the *New York Med. Journ.*, that at last some steps have been taken, by the arrest and finding of one offender, to show that the ordinances of the health board of the city of New York are meant to be complied with, and are not merely the vaporings of a few harmless enthusiasts. Let the duty of taking steps to prevent the nuisance be responsibly imposed upon officials, and the filthy practice will soon be checked. It is scarcely fair to expect the private individual, however disgusted he may feel at the habits of his hoggish fellow-passengers, to risk the unpleasant notoriety of creating "a scene"; though the same individual would doubtless experience no difficulty in carrying out his express orders were he in an official position. It might be a good plan to have a number of small cards printed, with the legend, "You are required, under penalty of a fine, to abstain from expectorating in public vehicles or in public buildings," or some other suitable formula. One of these cards might be unobtrusively handed by the official in charge as a reminder, whenever he observed the commission of the offense, thus sparing the feelings of the possibly thoughtless offender, and at the same time placing him in the position of a deliberate recalcitrant, deserving of no consideration should he repeat it.

OZONIFEROUS ESSENCES AS ANTISEPTICS.

Listerine possesses essential properties analogous in their effects to the ozoniferous ethers so highly recommended by Dr. Benjamin Ward Richardson and others as deodorizers and disinfectants for the sick-room, and should be used in the same way—sprinkled over handkerchiefs, garments, and the bed-linen of fever cases. Mantegazza, "On the Action of Essences and Flowers in the Production of Atmospheric Ozone, and on Their Hygienic Utility" (*Rendiconti del Beale Instituto Lombardo*, vol. iii., fasc. vi.), as quoted by Fox on Ozone, reports that the disciples of Empedocles were not in error when they planted aromatic and balsamic herbs as preventatives of pestilence. He contends that a large quantity of ozone is discharged by odoriferous flowers, and that flowers destitute of perfume do not produce it. Cherry-laurel, clove, lavender, mint, lemon, fennel, etc., are plants which develop ozone largely on exposure to the sun's rays. Among flowers, the narcissus, heliotrope, hyacinth, and mignonette are conspicuous; and of perfumes similarly exposed, eau-de-cologne, oil of bergamot, extract of millefleurs, essence of lavender, and some aromatic tinctures. He also points out that the oxidation of the essential oils, such as nutmeg, aniseed, thyme, peppermint, etc., are convenient sources of ozone, and concludes that the ozoniferous properties of flowers reside in their essences, the most ozoniferous yielding the largest amount of ozone. It is of such aromatic essences that Listerine is composed, and hence its efficacy under the circumstances indicated.—*The Sanitarian.*

A DANGEROUS CLASS OF PEOPLE.

Dr. E. D. Frear writes in the *Philadelphia Medical Journal* concerning the dangers to communities visited by the "pestiferous pack peddlers." "This class of mendicants," he says, "is usually composed of an undesirable class of aliens, whose ideas of hygiene, or even of common cleanliness, are very limited. Whenever they can gain admission to a house, their packs, which are generally made up of fabrics which are good conveyors of diseased germs, are opened and spread over sofas, beds, and other convenient articles, and are promiscously handled by the members of the household. The air of the room may be impregnated with the desquamations of variola or scarlatina, the exudations of diphtheria, or the expectoration of tuberculosis. The goods are carefully repacked and carried to the next home, or several homes, where the germs are distributed. Without going into details, I have seen two developments of scarlatina and one of diphtheria, in each case a clear history of the contagium being carried in this manner. I recognize the fact that our cities and more populous communities are spared this nuisance, but it is in the country, wnere the population is sparse, and where, in many cases the disease is in so light a form that a physician is not called, that this danger exists."

THE COCAINE HABIT.

COCAINISM, says G. W. Norris (*Philadelphia Medical Journal,* Feb. 9, 1901), is the most insidious of all drug habits. The use of the drug being unaccompanied by disagreeable after-effects—headache, nausea, vomiting, etc., which are met with after the ingestion of opium or alcohol—the vice is readily and rapidly established.

Cocainism is occasionally acquired by the local use of the drug in diseases of the nose and throat, teeth, etc., but more often as a substitute for opium or alcohol.

Cocaine is eventually tolerated by the system in huge doses. (One case is recorded where 60 grains daily was consumed.)

A relatively large number of habitués are found in the medical and dental professions (it is said 30 per cent.).

The continued indulgence in cocaine invariably, and usually soon, leads to marasmus, with mental, moral, and nervous degeneration.

The smallest fatal dose on record is one-third grain hypodermically.

While many cases of acute intoxication are being continually reported, there are relatively few fatal cases. The majority of such are the result of large doses injected into the urethra and bladder—*e. g.,* in two cases, five or six fluid drachms respectively of a 5-per cent. solution into the urethra.

The amount of cocaine sold yearly is rapidly increasing, and its self-prescribed use among the laity and lower classes is becoming proportionately more frequent.

"EUCALYPTUS ROSTRATA" IN SEA SICKNESS.

IT may be of interest to some of your readers, especially that portion who, like myself, have been employed as ship surgeons, to have my experience of the above.

From time to time, at sea, I have been driven nearly to my wits' end endeavoring to relieve that most distressing vomiting which takes place in some cases of seasickness, especially in the case of delicate or strumous females. I have tried amyl nit., camphor, cocaine, bismuth, chloroform, morphine, caffeine, bromides, and most of the other treatments usually employed, but, I must confess, with very little success. At length I was induced to try the effects of the "red gum." I got the idea from an old "gold digger," who was a passenger under my care, saying that it always cured him. I have made several experiments with it, and am very pleased with the result, as it almost invariably gave relief where the more orthodox modes of treatment failed. I think the most convenient mode of administration is in the form of lozenges (trochisci eucalypti gummi, gr. i, in each). The patient can thus easily carry about a few in the pocket, and take one when he feels the sickness coming on. By using them in this manner, I have found three or four during the day sufficient: and, I may remark, I have never heard any of my patients complaining of the treatment producing constipation.— *Dr. W. M. Russell, Brit. Med. Jour.*

THE NATURE AND TREATMENT OF GASTRALGIA.

GASTRALGIA is a symptom of organic disease of the stomach in some instances, as in gastric ulcer or cancer. Again, it appears as one of the symptoms of locomotor-ataxia. But very often the disease presents itself independent of these affections, and is a functional neurosis, which bears no relation to any organic disease of the stomach. It is this expression of the disease which shall receive consideration here.

Most of the patients who are afflicted with gastralgia are those who have neurasthenia; hysterical women, women about the menopause, and men of the nervous temperament. Gout, or malarial poisoning, hyperacidity of the stomach, lead poisoning, excessive employment of tobacco, over-indulgence in tea, and other influences, tend to establish the disease.

The symptoms of gastralgia are generally well marked. Patients complain of a boring, tearing, burning pain in the region of the stomach, which is at times so severe as to be almost insufferable. This pain often radiates around the waist. Frequently the patient tells us that the pain seems to fill the side, and when the side is pressed upon we elicit pain. Vomiting is rare, and these patients experience a degree of relief from eating. When an exacerbation of pain is on the abdomen retracts and the patient assumes a fixed position. The attacks may last from a few minutes to two to five hours, and may recur with irregular intervals. As Lockwood has put these attacks recur with such regularity that malarial infection may be expected. In nearly all cases of gastralgia we shall find that the patients are of decided neurotic temperament.

The diagnosis is to be made by the exclusion of organic disease, and a general consideration of the case, which will show the patient to be neurasthenic or hysterical in most instances; but occasionally we shall experience great difficulty along this line. The treatment is a matter of course of the greatest importance. When an attack is on we can serve the purpose of bringing about relief greatly, having hat clothes applied over the epigastrium. Often mustard plasters bring relief. Of course, proper relief must come from correct internal medicine. Daniel's Conc. Tinct. Parsiflora Incarnata, in doses of two teaspoonfuls every two hours, exerts a most happily influence in these cases. It is a reliable and prompt anodyne, and if it be taken regularly the patient does not have attacks. In fact, it is very rare to have an attack of gastralgia come on while this remedy is being taken. By the action of this remedy the patient, whose nervous system is dun down—who is, in other words, a sufferer with neurasthenia, is given exemption from pain, and the nervous system has time to recuperate, and recoveries will follow, which would not have been failures by any other system of treatment. Daniel's Conc. Tinct. Passiflora Incarnata will bring us better and more speedy results than any other remedy in the treatment of gastralgia, and that it will be welcomed as one of the great therapeutic needs in this affection, to say nothing of its value in other diseases.

MOSTURO JONES, M.D.

Nova Scotia.

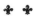

CATARRHS.

As a general remedy in the treatment of all kinds of irritated mucous membranes, nothing gives me more satisfaction than hydrastis. As a local treatment in most cases of catarrh, I want nothing better than equal parts of non-alcoholic fluid hydrastis, glycerine and listerine, acompanied by such general treatment as may be indicated.— *Chi. Med. Standard.*

DEATH-RATE IN THE STATE OF NEW YORK.

THE number of reported deaths from all causes in this State for the year 1900 was 128,468. Add to this 1,600 deaths occurring during the year but not reported in time to be included in the official list, gives an actual total of 130,068, which is 7,247 in excess of the returns for 1899, and 9,600 more than the average of the past five years. Of these deaths 1,948 were from typhoid, which is 350 more than the average, and does not argue well for the vigilance of the local health officers. There were 1,333 deaths from measles, which is at least a thousand more than it ought to be. On the other hand there was a decrease below the average of 500 deaths from diphtheria, while grip is charged with 1,500 fatalities.

SOME WAYS OF IMPROVING THE COMPLEXION.

YOU want to keep your skin nice all summer? Well, then, here are some rules for you:

Don't bathe in hard water; soften it with a few drops of ammonia or a little borax.

Don't bathe your face while it is very warm, and never use *very* cold water for it.

Don't wash your face when you are traveling, unless it is with a little alcohol and water, or a little vaseline.

Don't attempt to remove dust with cold water; give your face a hot bath, using plenty of good soap; then give it a thorough rinsing with water that has had the chill taken off of it.

Don't rub your face with a coarse towel; just remember it is not of cast-iron, and treat it as you would the finest porcelain— gently and delicately.

Don't use a sponge or linen rag for your face: choose, instead, a flannel one.

Don't believe you can get rid of wrinkles by filling the crevices with powder. Instead, give your face a Russian bath every night; that is, to bathe it with water so hot that you wonder how you can stand it. and then, a minute after, with cold water, that will make it glow with warmth; dry it with a soft towel, and go to bed, and you ought to sleep like a baby, while your skin is growing firmer and coming out of the wrinkles, and you are resting.—*The Nightingale.*

DR. W. C. COOPER gets at the heart of things as follows:

"There are a number of axioms underlying therapeutics which are as inflexibly true as those fundamental to mathematics. Thus,

" 1. No morbid effect can be dissipated except by a removal of its cause.

"2. What will make, or tend to make, a well man sick will make a sick man sicker.

" 3. Medicine is medicine, food is food.

" 4. Each drug has a specific affinity (kindly or not) for a particular nerve center. (A fairy tale.)

" 5. A drug, to be remedial, must not, at least in the long run, oppose natural reparative effort.

" 6. A drug's capacity for doing good, when indicated, is invariably less than its capacity for doing harm when not indicated.

" 7. A drug is double-edged, so that however much it may cut in the right direction, it will cut some in the wrong direction.

" 8. There is no such thing as a drug tonic—drugs are heterogeneous to the animal organism.

"9. Hygiene is the big brother of drugs, physiology being included in this branch."

"Some Medical Philosophy" is Dr. Cooper's late prize paper in the literary contest of *Merck's Archives.*

POSITIONS THAT AFFECT SLEEP.

ACCORDING to Dr. Granville, the position affects sleep. A constrained position generally prevents repose, while a comfortable one woos sleep. He says: "Lying flat on the back, with the limbs relaxed, would seem to secure the greatest amount of rest for the muscular system. This is the position assumed in the most exhausting diseases, and it is generally hailed as a token of revival when a patient voluntarily turns on the side; but there are several disadvantages in the supine posture which impair or embarrass sleep. Thus, in weakly states of the heart and blood-vessels and certain morbid conditions of the brain, the blood seems to gravitate to the back of the head and to produce troublesome dreams. In persons who habitually, in their gait or work, stoop, there is probably some distress consequent in straightening the spine. Those who have contracted chests, especially persons who have had pleurisy, and retain adhesions of the lungs, do not sleep well on the back. Nearly all who are inclined to snore do so in that position, because the soft palate and uvula hang on the tongue, and that organ falls back so as to partly close the top of the windpipe. It is better, therefore, to lie on the side, and in the absence of special disease rendering it desirable to lie on the weak side so as to leave the healthy lung free to expand, it is well to use the right side, because when the body is thus placed the food gravitates more easily out of the stomach into the intestines, and the weight of the stomach does not compress the upper portion of the intestines. A glance at any of the visceral anatomy will show this must be. Many persons are deaf in one ear, and prefer to lie on a particular side; but, if possible, the right side should be chosen. Again, sleeping with the arms thrown over the head is to be deprecated; but this position is often assumed during sleep, because circulation is then free in the extremities, and the head and neck, and muscles of the chest are drawn up and fixed by the shoulders, and thus the expansion of the thorax is easy. The chief objection to these positions is that they create a tendency to cramp and cold in the arms, and sometimes seem to cause headaches during sleep, and dreams. These small matters often make or mar comfort in sleeping.

PRACTICAL HOME METHODS OF BATHING IN TYPHOID FEVER.

DR. S. BARUCH recently discussed this phase of this subject. He said that the first impression of cold upon the skin was the so-called shock; it was really a physiological irritant. The impression lasted a longer or shorter time, depending upon the method of procedure and its duration. The friction stimulated the contracted arterioles to dilate again, and performed the important normal function of propelling the blood, thus keeping up a proper peripheral circulation. The latter was usually so crippled in typhoid fever that the heart was compelled to beat faster and more forcibly. By the proper use of cold water the pulse diminished in frequency and gained in force. The skin assumed a rosy hue because its arterioles had been dilated in a tonic fashion. The countenance lost its apathy, the respirations were deepened, and the kidneys were aroused to renewed activity. Friction should always accompany the cold-water treatment—a fact which even at this late day needed reiteration and emphasis. As an illustration of how the cold-water treatment should not be applied in typhoid fever the speaker mentioned the abdominal ice coil, still so popular with many physicians. This was a direct violation of the fundamental principle of all hydrotherapy, that cold applications must be accompanied by frictions. In home practice the ablution was the simplest procedure. The patient was stripped, a blanket was placed underneath him, and first the back and then the anterior surface of the body treated to the ablution. It should be given with considerable friction, the temperature

of the water being reduced from time to time until the temperature reached 60° F. The abdominal compress was another useful method of applying cold water. This consisted of three folds of toweling wrung out of water at a temperature of 70° F. and applied snugly, being covered with thin flannel. It should be renewed hourly. When the temperature persisted in remaining at 103° F. or above, the towel bath was appropriate. A towel was dipped into water at 85° F. and laid dripping and smooth over the entire back. Water at 70° F. was dipped up with a cup and poured on the upper left part of the back, and then this part was rubbed with the hand. This was done three times, and then the other parts of the back were successively treated in the same way. The water on the sheet was mopped up with a sponge, and then the anterior parts were similarly treated, care being taken not to use pressure over the iliac region. The temperature might be reduced five degrees each time until the temperature of the water for the towel reached 60° F. and that in the cup reached 50° F. The "sheet bath" was still more potent, and was very useful when objection was made to the full bath, or the latter was impracticable. An old linen sheet or tablecloth should be dipped in water at 90° F., and wrung out very lightly. The patient having been wrapped in this, water at a temperature of about ten degrees lower should be poured successively upon different parts of the body, and each part rubbed with the hands until it no longer warmed up. The typhoid fever patient should be given internally from four to six ounces of water at 40° F. every two hours, and this should be alternated with the same quantity of milk.
—*Medical Record*, Dec. 8, 1900.

MUSIC AS A CURE FOR THE INSANE.

RECENTLY music has been introduced "as a method" in the detention hospitals of Chicago. The result is being watched with great interest by nerve specialists.

THE GRAPE CURE.

Gazeta Medica Lombardi contains an account of the grape cure. This method of treatment is recommended by Dujardin-Beaumetz and others for cases of dyspepsia, especially when accompanied by constipation, and in the gouty. It is also valuable in chronic diarrhea, of dysenteric origin, and Tissot tells a story of a regiment of soldiers decimated by dysentery, which vanished in a marvelous manner on encamping among vineyards full of ripe grapes. Chronic cystitis is benefited by the alkaline carbonates developed by the vegetable acids of the fruit, but in such cases care must be taken that the grapes are not sour. Cardiac affections are relieved by the laxative and diuretic action, while almost all patients are benefited by the fresh air, exercise, and early rising which the rules of the "cure" involve. Grapes grown on volcanic soil are said to have a more markedly stimulant and diuretic action than others. As to the amount, Dujardin-Beaumetz recommends patients to take as much as they possibly can without exciting disgust, while others advise a gradual increase to a daily maximum of four kilos. The duration of the cure is from one to three months.—*Medical Magazine.*

WOMEN'S CLUB VS. MOSQUITOES.

As the mosquito has no greater enemy than the fair sex, the fact that the women of certain towns are forming clubs to fight it is news of direful import for *Anopheles quadrimaculatus*. At Richmond Hill, near New York, they got a scientist to explain the value of kerosene oil as an exterminator of the young of the mosquitoes. They explored the country around their town with boys provided with oil cans, and wherever there was a puddle, ditch, pond, or marsh, they poured oil generously on the surface. The result has been, we are told, that the residents of Richmond Hill enjoyed sitting out on their porches last summer, having almost complete immunity from mosquitoes.

Department of Physical Education.

WITH SPECIAL REGARD TO THE SYMMETRICAL DEVELOPMENT OF THE BODY.

A WORD WITH OUR READERS.

The Gazette has never adopted the practice indulged by so many of its contemporaries of publishing the many good words said of it by its friends, preferring to let the work it is doing and the matter presented each month do the talking for it. Often these kindly commendations are so extremely " handsome " and enthusiastic that we are sorely tempted to insert them. Some of them are from editors who appreciate our efforts from the standpoint of those who know what it means to conduct a successful medical journal.

The papers of our Boston contributor, Dr. Achorn, are commanding, as they certainly should, a wide-spread attention. In one instance a foreign journal has begged the privilege of reproducing the series.

Other papers are meeting with a similar reception. It is our purpose to follow these papers with others of equal or even greater practical interest. Without infringing our custom, we desire, in one sweeping sentence, to thank all our good friends who have taken pains to tell us that they are both pleased and profited by the monthly *menu* we place before them, and to assure them that their kindly words are not lost, but that every such genuine expression of approbation strengthens our ambition to deserve all the good things said of us. All the time we are aware that if we do not *earn* the applause of our growing family of readers no amount of egotistical boasting will help the matter. For ourselves we are not satisfied unless we succeed in making each issue of the Gazette worth all we charge for the full year's subscription. If we manage to give every subscriber *twelve dollars' worth for one dollar*, and if each subscriber will undertake to send us one or two new subscriptions during the year, there is no reason why we should not end the first year of the New Century with 100,000 readers, keep a clear conscience and enjoy refreshing sleep!

In several primary schools in Paris, Colonel Bérué, Inspector General of Physical Education, says London *Health*, has been carrying on experiments to determine the value of physical training in the development of children with marked physical defects. The children were all weak, anemic, poorly developed, with consumptive tendencies or otherwise afflicted. Those motions of the limbs and body which require little or no effort constituted the greater part of the exercises ; trunk movements, marching and respiratory gymnastics were included. The boys were instructed in the savate, the French style of boxing, in which the feet as well as the hands are used. The physical deformities of the children were lessened, the resistance to disease apparently increased, and inherited and acquired defects largely remedied. Eleven pupils became exceptionally well developed, their growth exceeding the average of children of their age. One boy grew four centimetres, and three other sickly pupils became rapidly healthy. In every case a manifest impulse toward development and good health was given. For the benefit of children suffering from more severe maladies or deformities, a special course of medical gymnastics was held under the constant supervision of a physician at a primary school in the Rue Bolivar. Children were measured and treated, that the flexibility of shoulders and spinal column might be increased, the habitual deforming postures corrected, and the condition of the various organs, especially of the bones, muscles, and nervous system, improved. As a result, the Municipal Council of Paris has decided to establish a regular course of gymnastics at one of the leading primary schools.

MASSAGE OF THE STOMACH.

ACCORDING to Gustaf Nortröm, on account of the deep situation of the stomach and the slight resistance of the deep plane on which it rests, only a limited portion of the viscus can be reached in dorsal decubitus. For dilated stomach the author kneads at first from left to right with patient on back, the knees bent and head raised. After a few minutes he has patient lie on right side, and petrissage is performed with both hands alternately, from pylorus toward cardia. Gentleness is necessary during the séance. The sittings should last about fifteen minutes for stomach alone, and as much more time for the intestine, if there is constipation. They should begin two or three hours after a meal. The benefit most often shows first by a returning appetite, then by the disappearance of the rumblings, eructations, gastric pains, headache, vertigo, etc. At the beginning of treatment the diet must be light and limited in quantity. · Besides dilatation of the stomach, massage is of benefit in chronic gastritis, dyspepsia, essential gastralgia, gastralgia due to neurasthenia or anæmia, pyloric cramp, etc., but it may do harm in ulcers or tumors of the pylorus.—*Medical News.*

PROF. JOSEPH MCFARLAND, M.D., a recognized teacher and authority on bacteriology, has engaged himself with Messrs. Parke, Davis & Co., of Detroit, Mich, for purely scientific research in connection with their biological laboratories.

THE HOPE OF THE NATION— PHYSICAL EDUCATION.

I KNOW I am advancing a very startling, very unorthodox, proposition when I state, says John R. Stevens in *Physical Culture,* that the hope of future distinction for our nation lies in physical development. A whole army of disputants and objectors will arise to clamor against this sweeping statement. The religious element will say to me, " Where is Providence and the prayers of the just? Will they not avail anything?" The university man will wildly and wordily expostulate: " But the mind—education, what about that? If we ever achieve a leading place among nations, depend upon it, it will be learning that elevates us." Scientists will arrogantly claim the honor for themselves, and hazily prophesy of some discovery of dazzling importance. Then will come the jester, with his flings about the race of prize-fighters, football cranks or golf players. But in spite of all that I am hard-headed enough to maintain the proposition: The hope of the nation lies in physical development—better, more general, more scientific development than we have at present.

To the hopeful Christian I would answer, " God helps those who help themselves. Physical perfection is a thing we have fallen away from through our own faults; it is a condition we must get back to by our own efforts." To the man of letters I would say, " The most perfectly balanced mind, the one capable of really great feats, demands a sound bodily habitat— physical vigor is a necessity before intellectual prowess." The scientist I would silence by asking him if he knows any formula for producing muscle and preserving health except Nature's grand law of exercise. As for the jesting, scoffing crew, let them sneer; even a prize-fighter of the worst type is better than a narrow-chested, spindle-legged, pessimistic degenerate.

The nations that are lowest in the world's congress as producers, as inventors, as warriors, those that have the fewest statesmen, smallest resources, are those in which the physical development of the individual is lowest. We have but to glance over a few of the recent pages of history for proof. France, Spain and Italy are clearly the weakest in the European concert, and their population, taken collectively, presents the fewest specimens of superb physical development. Volumes have been printed about the degeneration of the so-called Latin races, among which those mentioned must be included. What is this degeneracy? It is of morals, of intellect, and of virility, all following in the train of lessening physical powers. In all these countries men and women have become weaker, less powerful to resist, less able to labor, during the last two centuries.

There is a pretty firmly established law of heredity which here has operated backward. A weak generation has been followed by a weaker, with no concerted attempt to remedy the evil until the national existence is threatend.

Against these we have powerful contrasting types in that great trio of European powers—England, Germany and Russia. The strength, stability and activity of these nations are at their greatest, yet they are no younger than the first mentioned. When we seek for a reason, we find it in the national habit of exercise and outdoor life.

England's strength for centuries has reposed in the hearty, hale, bluff "John Bull" type. The men of the shires—the squires who live most of the time out of doors; the general custom of activity which makes every Englishman a sportsman, and of nearly every Englishwoman a pedestrian and horsewoman. The blood has not been tainted by any infusions, and the race retains virility after a national existence of a goodly number of centuries.

Germany shows a race that has advanced instead of retrograded. The system of gymnasiums and the compulsory military service have made a robust, resisting male population. It is the leading country to-day in the matter of physical development—in fact, the only one in which the government has undertaken to develop the physical powers of its citizens.

Russia, with its broad territory and its half-savage customs, is the one nearest the primitive, or savage, state which produced the strongest men—physically. Her people, hardened by a rigorous climate, by active outdoor lives, are among the strongest, hardest, on the earth to-day; and they may be depended upon to play a prominent part in the history-making of the future.

And America—where does she rank? How do her people stand? Patriotism shouts at once, "In the van!" But do we? We have a population in which there is a perplexing blend of racial strains. The infusion does not seem to have produced any very notable types. It has given us a most nervous, restless population, but physically it is not, as a whole, comparable to some of the races I have mentioned. We have passed the stage when the conditions of living were such as to produce superb physical development. The habits of the generation that is growing up are not such as are calculated to produce splendid physical types. Our boys are encouraged to strive for early entrance of professional or business life rather than directed to pursue a course that will result in perfect physical manhood. Our girls are encouraged in habits positively injurious to health. There is no concerted effort to train and develop muscular power along with the intellectual. Already the signs of warning are appearing. In our cities hordes of narrow-chested, sallow-faced, cigarette-smoking young men crowd the streets and places of business. Nine-tenths of our female population are afflicted with some functional disorder, and a host of doctors and druggists and vendors of nostrums grow wealthy every year by preying on the weak. Sanitariums and asylums are becoming crowded. He who runs may read the signs, and the wayfaring man, though a fool, ought to be able to see where it is all leading to.

There is a chance for the Land of Freedom to always be the leader of nations;

but prayers won't keep it there—the intellectual drill given in schools and colleges will not insure it this proud distinction. Just one thing will, and that is general physical development. The signs of weakness should be heeded, parents and teachers should spread the eternal truth: Activity is life, and stagnation means decay and death.

DO NOT SLOUCH.

ERECTNESS of bearing has a moral and a mental as well as a physical effect, says *The Outlook*. When the mind is alert, the head goes up and the shoulders are squared. So also when the spirits are high and the heart is full of pure aspirations. Physical well-being absolutely demands that we should not stoop. If we lean forward we contract the chest, and the lungs have not wholesome full play. When we start out to do anything that is brave and noble we do not slouch; we look danger, when we are brave, straight in the face and go at it with head high and shoulders back. That is the way soldiers march; that is the way the bridegroom leaves the church when the solemn words have been said and he goes out into the world to meet the sweet responsibilities of life. Erectness of bearing is the sign of courage, the evidence of hope; slouchiness indicates decadence and is evidence of incapacity. One dandy in this busy world is worth half a dozen slovens. The dandies are more prompt, they are braver, they are more courageous, they are more self-respecting, they are in every manly quality finer and more worthy of the respect of both men and women. The slovenly man who slouches through life is a severe trial to men who must be thrown with him; how women can put up with him is one of those inexplicable things past finding out.

WORDS are like spectacles; they darken whatever they do not help us to see.

A PLEA FOR THE EDUCATION OF THE BODY.

BY C. E. EHINGER, M.D.

IT was Plato who said: "To educate the mind and neglect the body is to produce a cripple."

Theoretically, no fact is more generally admitted than the necessity of a substantial physical basis for all educational effort. The veriest tyro knows that if the organic processes are performed in a lame or halting manner, or the bodily structures fall below a certain standard, life becomes a burden and a misery, and educational effort seriously restricted or absolutely interdicted.

Every parent, guardian or educator may glibly quote the Latin maxim which inculcates a sound mind in a sound body. The majority of our boarding schools, seminaries and colleges, in their announcements, are careful to state that the physical welfare of their students is carefully looked after. School authorities point with pride to the gymnasium or the athletic field as guarantees that the physical interest of their students is not neglected. And yet, with all these indications of an intelligent care and forethought for the physical welfare of our youth, I make plain to say that the whole subject of physical training and hygiene is still in a most chaotic and immature condition, and betokens a short-sightedness, ignorance or disregard which ill befits our vaunted claims for educational progress.

I do not wish to be understood as minimizing the good that has been accomplished, and yet candor compels the admission that little more has been done than to clear the ground for intelligent action. The popular clamor for gymnasia, athletic fields, outdoor sports, and the introduction of systems of physical training in our schools and colleges is, indeed, a healthful indication; but it must not by any means be taken as the measure of what has really been accomplished. for much that passes current as physical training and hygiene is not worthy of the name. It is only fair to say that the lay and educational mind is not yet fully alive to the great need of the introduction of such branches as physiology, hygiene and physical training into the school and college curriculum. The attempts made, and the somewhat meager results thus far attained, have been in response to the popular or superficial newspaper agitation along these lines, and not to a well grounded and thoroughly understood need. It is because of an always dimly felt, but now rapidly growing recognition that the home, the school and the college have erred in this particular.

No permanent good can, however, be accomplished until a more vigorous and healthful sentiment has been aroused in favor of an early, persistent and intelligent reverence for and care of the human body. It must be no longer ignored, abused or relegated to a secondary place. The training of the body must become the chief concern of education.

What a travesty on education that the student may come from the school or college training not only no better physically than when he entered, but often vastly worse, and not seldom, alas, such a wreck that no amount of medical advice and treatment, travel or rest can fully atone for the physical sins committed. Such a course is not simply permitted, it is encouraged; nay, more, it is often actually demanded.

I make bold to say that this question is not a trivial or an unworthy one; indeed, in its highest sense, it is not a material question at all; it is a religious question, and the cause of morals and religion cannot progress at a steady and adequate pace until the world pays due respect and reverence to that most beautiful and wonderous of structures, the human body. A great obstacle which stands in the way of this movement is the prevailing unwillingness to realize and acknowledge our personal responsibility in conditions of physical weakness, deficiency and disease. We fail to see that much weakness and most diseases are self-imposed, and that it is not so much what others can do for

us—in a medical way or otherwise—as what we can and must do for ourselves, that counts for our bodily condition and welfare. The most needful thing is the right personal attitude, the willingness to put forth individual effort in our own behalf. Physical righteousness, like virtue, must be self-evolved; it cannot be imputed or imparted.

The general superstition and ignorance is still such as to render us prone ever and again to attribute physical weakness, infirmity and disease to some mysterious dispensation of Divine Providence, and not, as it properly should be, to palpable violations of well-known or easily-ascertained laws. It seems so difficult for us to learn that weakness and disease are not arbitrary inflictions or accidental phenomena due to chance contact with the specific contagium, that lies in wait for its innocent and unsuspecting victim. The faith that some mysterious germicide will vet be discovered, which will put to death these lurking enemies, and so forever banish weakness and disease, still persists and influences, to a marvelous extent, both the lay and the medical mind. Such views are but vestiges of the ancient belief in magic, relics of the dark ages, when it was the function of the priest to minister to both the physical and spiritual needs of the people, and this by means of magic, charm, incantation and ceremonials. It took ages to arrive at the belief that there could be such a thing as a natural cause for our physical infirmities, and even to-day we are reluctant to ascribe them to modes of life, vicious habits and unnatural practices, and expect that they may be removed by swallowing drugs rather than by ceasing our evil ways. We are just beginning to see that the physical, to a great degree, conditions and determines the mental, the moral and the spiritual, that all attempts to separate these, or to consider the one less worthy than the other, have brought, and will ever continue to bring, discord and disaster. To those who would look upon this as a species of materialism and an inversion of the true order, I reply that it is clearly the ordained course of Nature, and every violation of it, even in the name of religion, has been fraught with the saddest results. " First, that which is natural, then that which is spiritual." The physical is prior to the mental in the order of development, and must, therefore, be given the first and foremost consideration. In modern educational phraseology this is expressed by saying that the education of the senses must precede the education of the mind and the spirit. Let this not be understood as any denial of the mighty influence of the mind and spirit upon the body; such belief has my fullest sympathy and recognition. I am merely contending now that Nature's order of teaching be followed, and that we cease to abuse or ignore that which, though called " natural " or " material," is still a part of and indispensable to the expression of the spiritual.

But you ask, " What is the evidence that there is this imperative need of physical training and care of the body?" For, strange as it may appear to some of us, this question is still asked. For answer, let me cite to you, first, not to the physiologist and physician, but one who gave his chief efforts for the spiritual needs of mankind. Henry Drummond, in his " Ascent of Man," with a clearness which is characteristic, foresaw and explained this need. He says: "Civilization—and the civilized state, be it remembered, is the ultimate goal of every race and nation—is always attended by a deterioration of some of the senses. Every man pays a definite price or forfeit for his taming. . . In an age of vehicles and locomotives the lower limbs find their occupation almost gone. For mere muscle, that on which his whole life once depended, man has now almost no use. Agility, nimbleness, strength, once a stern necessity, are either a luxury or a pastime. Their outlet is either the cricket field or the tennis court. To keep them up at all, artificial means— dumb-bells, parallel bars, clubs—have actually to be devised. Vigor of limb is not to be found in common life; we look for it in the gymnasium; agility is relegated to the hippodrome. Once all men were athletes: now you have to pay to see them. More or

less, with all the animal powers it is the same. . . So everywhere the man, as animal, is in danger of losing ground. So great, indeed, is the advantage of increasing mechanical supplements to the physical, rather than exercising the frame itself, that this will become nothing short of a temptation, and not the least anxious task of future civilization will be to prevent degenerafion beyond a legitimate point, and keep up the body to its highest working level. For the first thing to be learned from these facts is not that the body is nothing and must now decay, but that it is most of all, and more than ever worthy to be preserved. The moment our care of it slackens, the body asserts itself. It comes out from under arrest, which is the one thing to be avoided. Its true place by the ordained appointment of Nature is where it can be ignored. If, through disease, neglect or injury, it returns to consciousness, the effect of evolution is undone. Sickness is degeneration, pain the signal to resume the evolution. On the one hand, we must ' reckon the body dead '; on the other, we must think of it in order, not to think of it."

It will hardly be charged that this man, whose whole life and teaching gave evidence of a transcendent spirituality, was guilty of undue worship of the body.

Let us remember that it is not the inanimate body which we speak of, but the living, breathing body, pulsating with all those mysterious powers and possibilities that inhere in that marvelous thing we call vital force. In this age of machinery, when every hour brings forth some new marvel of mechanical wonder, no product of the time is even worthy of comparison with this perpetual wonder, the self-directing, self-repairing, reproducing, thinking machine.

Permit me, again, to quote Drummond. He says: " Science is charged, be it once more recalled, with numbering man among the beasts, and leveling his body with the dust. But he who reads for himself the history of creation as it is written by the hand of Evolution, will be overwhelmed by the glory and honor heaped upon this creature.

To be a man, and to have no conceivable successor; to be the fruit and crown of the long-past eternity, and the highest possible fruit and crown; to be the last victor among the decimated phalanxes of earlier existences, and to be nevermore defeated; to be the best that Nature in her strength and opulence can produce; to be the first of that new order of beings who, by their dominion over the lower world and their equipment for a higher, reveal that they are made in the image of God—to be this is to be elevated to a rank in Nature more exalted than any philosophy or any poetry or any theology have ever given to man. Man was always told that his place was high; the reason for it he never knew till now; he never knew that his title deeds were the very laws of Nature; that he alone was the Alpha and Omega of creation, the beginning and the end of matter, the final goal of life."

Is it possible that we can be guilty longer of abusing and disregarding the needs of such a structure? Let us have done with those false and wicked conceptions, the products of an age of darkness; let us glorify and ennoble this marvel of all marvels; make it one of the leading aims of our life to bring it to a perfection of development which shall render it a worthy receptacle of an immortal spirit.

Shame upon that person who says he has not the time to take exercise or care for the body. As well say that he has not time for prayer or religious worship.

Who can estimate the moral value of good health; and good health, be it known, is not the result of chance, but must be earned by struggle, either voluntary or through the stern necessities of our existence.

Man, by nature, is a country dweller, and when living under primitive conditions, in rural or sparsely settled communities, enjoys immunity from a large number of physical deficiencies and disorders which afflict the city dweller. He cannot congregate in cities and subject himself to all the unsanitary and unhygienic conditions of such a life, without inevitably suffering the consequences.

I am not contending for a return to primitive conditions, and am by no means unmindful of the great progress that has been made, especially in sanitation and preventive medicine; but I do maintain that this has been more than counterbalanced by harmful, artificial habits and unnatural modes of living. In this field, as in all others, sudden and radical changes of life are always disastrous. New and more specialized occupations, changed methods of caring for and educating our children, the stress of social and business life, and the sudden acquisition of wealth, have wrought grave physical disaster. In the young and the old the emotional side of life has been unduly cultivated and excited. The whole trend of modern life—in this country, at least—has been toward premature and continued over-development of the nervous system, while but little time or opportunity has been afforded for adjustment to these new and trying conditions.

The feverish unrest apparent in every avenue of life betokens an intensity and diversity of effort which sadly militates against the proper functioning of the great organic processes.

It is one of the laws of life that growth and repair only take place during periods of rest; that while activity is indispensable, the alternating periods of repose are quite as imperative. With life always at fever heat and faculties keyed up to their highest pitch, true repose becomes finally impossible. It is not only our business, professional and domestic affairs that are carried on at this high-pressure rate, but it characterizes every pursuit of life, and, sad to relate, is as much in evidence in our sports, so-called recreations, educational methods and religious observances as elsewhere.

It would seem as though, with the advent of steam and electricity, that we became possessed with the idea that speed was the great requisite of life; that the spirit of the times demanded not only that people, but ideas and measures, must also have "rapid transit." Everything, from a congressional bill to a missionary scheme, must be "railroaded through." There is no longer time for repose, contemplation, poise, leisure; the very terms are becoming outgrown and obsolete. In vain are the feeble protests that are uttered now and again; they are inaudible above the tumult and rush. Before the words have died from our lips, we are again caught in the swiftly-moving stream and hastened onward with the speed of the "limited." No, I am not pleading for a return to the stage coach. I merely desire to remind you that while speed is often necessary and rapid transit a great boon, even in this rushing age, the law still holds that activity must be followed by repose. Action creates friction, friction causes waste, waste demands repair, and repair can only take place during rest. I would further call to mind the fact that waste is directly proportional to speed; that it is, indeed, in a very literal sense "the pace that kills."

Physical weakness and disease are so common that I fear we have come somewhat to look upon such conditions as our natural heritage, necessary conditions attendant upon life processes. The truth is the very reverse; health is our normal heritage, weakness and disease are incidental, wholly unnecessary and entirely preventable. No doubt, so stated, this sounds optimistic to the point of absurdity. But if this is not true, I maintain that we have no right to speak of an "all-wise Creator." To my mind, it is impossible to conceive of an all-wise and all-loving Creator establishing a condition of physical inharmony. No, weakness and disease are not a penalty nor an infliction visited upon us because of our spiritual transgressions; not the result of "Divine Wrath." They come because the conditions necessary for their production have been complied with; they come because of, and in response to, law; not as punishments, but as kindly suggestions, promptings, admonitions, warnings. How blind we are not to see that it is impossible for us to feel pleasure without at the same time being capable of experiencing pain. No, health is impossible without its negative counterpart—

disease. It is not necessary that we suffer disease, but it is absolutely essential that we be capable of becoming subject to it.

All the aches and pains, and the manifold diseases, which come to thoughtless humanity, are but the warning notes, the necessary protests of Nature, which we unthinkingly disregard and foolishly attempt to still by resort to paralyzing drugs.

I desire especially to enforce the thought that, in reality, disease is our friend, and this not simply in the old, narrow, theological sense of a permitted affliction for spiritual discipline, though doubtless this may sometimes result. We are justified in studying disease, not because it is a positive, natural process, but because it is a morbid state or deviation from the normal, and we should be able to recognize it in order that we may avoid it. be familiar with its features, that it may not come upon us unawares.

I regret to say that it has been too much the tendency of the medical profession, no less than the laity, to look upon the unusual, the abnormal, rather than the normal. In other words, too much time has been spent in studying the phenomena of disease, and not enough in becoming familiar with the more attractive and positive conditions of health.

Dr. H. Lahman, a German medical writer, in commenting on the sad condition of the health of his people, recently said: "But we cannot expect to see any great improvement in this respect until the subjects of health and hygiene, the very foundation of life and wisdom, are taught to the rising generation in our schools. Only thus can we render possible a real prevention of disease and a perfect development of the body and its functions." He thinks that as bodily misery and disease grow less, physicians, though finding less employment as such, will become teachers of hygiene and protectors of health. He says: "To-day the ordinary work of a doctor is 'mending work.' His patients merely use him to help them to sin again against Nature."

Now let me cite the views of Eustace H. Miles, M.A., an English university teacher, who, though not a physician, is a student of this subject, and a noted athlete, being champion of England in two of their most popular sports. He speaks as follows: "Another crying evil is the almost universal ignorance of all classes on the subject of health. That there is a desire for health on the part of most people can hardly be denied, but education at present does practically nothing in the sphere of health. In my own case, I may say that I never received a word of instruction on health throughout my whole education, which means about six or seven years of private school life, about five years of public school life, and about four years of university life. This is an evil of the day scarcely inferior to any, and it will do much to account for the physical degeneracy of which many so constantly complain."

In pleading for the education of the body, I am merely asking that it be included in the educational scheme. In the past we have appeared to proceed upon the assumption that man was but a brain, a bodiless something for the acquisition of facts, a sort of memorizing machine, which was so unfortunate as to sometime require the services of a gross and corrupt medium—the body.

But some one says there is, after all, something higher than the body and its needs; may we not be making it a fetich? True enough, and far be it from me to deny the possibility, but so far as this remark applies to the rational needs of the body, I think we have no reason to fear that such a condition will be brought about by its intelligent study and care.

No, the person who, through intelligent study, painstaking and persistent effort, attains to a knowledge of the bodily structures and functions, and strengthens it through physical conquest, acquires a true reverence for its beauties and uses that make it impossible for him to be a sensualist or a materialist. Self-mastery begins with overcoming and controlling the lower appetites and propensities, thus paving the way for, and leading to, the same mastery in higher spheres.

In this way we may say, with David Starr Jordan: "The perfect man will be master of the world because the perfect master of himself." He has learned the lesson which that greatest of coöperating communities—the human body—can teach: That we serve ourselves best when we serve others, and we serve others to the greatest degree by keeping our own body up to its highest working level.

Although my paper already exceeds the prescribed limits, I would be recreant to my duty did I fail to point out that this ideal training of the body, the new gospel of health, must include the fundamental principles which lie at the root of the problems of sex-life, ignorance of which produces untold misery and unhappiness.

Only the great mind of a Tennyson could have conceived these thoughts and clothed them in such fitting expressions: "We reverence God's holiest sanctuary when we reverence ourselves. Self-reverence, self-knowledge, self-control—these three alone lad to sovereign power."

Perhaps no more fitting thought could be chosen to close my plea for the body than Montaigu's: "It is not a mind, it is not a body, that we have to educate, but a man, of whom we are not to make two beings."

REST A NECESSITY.

THE necessity for an occasional rest from labor, and more particularly for some outdoor recreation, is shown by some interesting experiments recently conducted at Munich, which demonstrate that the system loses oxygen to the amount of one ounce as the result of a hard day's work. It has been found that the laborer does not recover during the night the oxygen he has thus overdrawn, but that an occasional day of rest intervening at the right time will serve completely to restore him. It is equally the case in other kinds of labor, whether mental or physical. A complete day's rest gives renewed vitality and renewed energy to recommence work.

THE CHINAMAN'S DREAD.

ONE of the things that a Chinaman fears most is that he will die away from home and his body will not find its way to a resting place beside those of his ancestors. The ship on which the New York *Sun's* correspondent went to China carried a number of Chinamen as steerage passengers. One day one of these passengers died.

"We'll have a burial at sea," said a first-class passenger to the first mate.

"Not on your life," said the mate. "Do you think we'd throw away $25? Not much."

"What do you mean?" asked the first-class passenger.

"Mean," said the mate, "mean what I say. That passenger is worth $25 more dead than when he was alive. The doctor gets $12 and the ship $13."

"How?" demanded the passenger.

"Why," said the mate, "no Chinaman wants to be buried away from his ancestors, and one of the things that the Chinese Six Companies in San Francisco does is to insure Chinamen against that. When a Chinaman lands in America or in Canada he pays a certain amount to the Six Companies, and that insures that his body shall reach home if he dies. The Six Companies has a contract with the steamship company, and it pays $25 for every dead Chinaman we deliver in China. So we never bury them at sea. The doctor embalms the body and the company allows him $12 as his share. Yes, sir, a dead Chinaman is worth $25 more to us than a live one."

"Where in China do you deliver the bodies?" asked the passenger.

"Wherever the corpse's ticket calls for delivery," said the mate. "If he bought a ticket through to Canton we take him there, or if he bought a ticket inland we deliver him at his destination."

PERFECT language is like a perfect pane of glass, not seen.

MADE A SCOTCH-IRISHMAN OF HIM.

FOR fiction displaying the most vivid qualities of invention an ordinary American newspaper is hard to beat. The following incident of the war, says the London *Hospital*, has escaped the notice of all our war correspondents, but it is told in the *New York Herald* as the experience of a doctor who had been in South Africa. We give it as the surgeon is said to have told it to some acquaintances at a club: "There's one incident, which occurred at Pretoria, which I had almost forgotten, but which, I think, might interest you. It was really the most remarkable operation I ever saw. In a skirmish an Irishman, whose regiment I forget, was riddled with dumdums. His name was Patrick O'Hara, and he was one of the best men in the corps. He died like a hero and was carried to the rear. I happened to see the body as it was carried past me, and remarked on the fine physique of the man. Not long afterwards I was in the thick of the fight, in which were engaged also a body of Highlanders. One of the men I knew, and called out a few cheery words to him as I passed by. 'Eh, dochtor,' he replied, 'but we'll pound the deils afore munelicht,' and he rushed on with a bravery which every one knows the Scotch possess. I thought no more of him until I came back, when, to my sorrow, I found my old friend Angus MacTavish—for that was his name —on a stretcher, with his upper lip clean blown off by one of the guns of the enemy. He was a horrible sight, and I was more than concerned what to do for him. Suddenly a thought struck me, which I immediately carried into effect. I found the body of Patrick O'Hara, which was still warm, and, giving MacTavish an anesthetic, I sliced the top lip off Patrick and stitched it under the nose of MacTavish. The operation was perfect, though you may think me conceited in saying so. A month or so afterwards I was in Pretoria, not having seen MacTavish since the operation. One day I came across him and was delighted to see him looking so well. Evidently he was quite convalescent. I stopped him and said, 'Well, Angus, how goes it, my man?" To my astonishment he replied, in the richest brogue, 'Begorra, Dochtor, I'm as roight as I can be, and faylin' illigant.' You see, the fact of the lip being transplanted had transferred the accent also."

WHY THEY STEAL THERMOMETERS.

" IF you want to keep a thermometer in Guatemala, you have to set a guard over it," said a New Orleans man who has just returned from a visit to Central America. " It's a fact, I assure you. Shortly before I started for home, I made a trip from Port Barrios to Guatemala City. The weather was broiling hot, and when we got to Guatemala, which is about the biggest town on the road, I thought I'd see what the temperature really was. So I strolled out of the hotel to locate a thermometer, and after a long search I found one hanging on the porch of a residence. To my astonishment it was surrounded by a cage of wire netting heavy enough to hold a young bear. It was a cheap thermometer, not worth over 40 or 50 cents, and such a precaution seemed all the more remarkable because petty household pilfering is practically unknown in that country. People think nothing of going off and leaving their houses wide open, and why a thermometer, which was apparently the last thing on earth anybody would want to steal, should be so carefully guarded was more than I could understand. On my way back to the hotel I saw two others, both protected in exactly the same manner, and my curiosity was highly excited. When I questioned the landlord he smiled and assured me that the screens were absolutely necessary, to prevent the natives from breaking the instruments to get out the mercury. 'They suffer from

torpid livers,' he said, 'and they regard mercury as a specific. How the belief became current the Lord only knows,' he went on; ' but it is universal all through the interior, and if an outside thermometer is left unprotected over night it is morally certain to be broken and drained.' I couldn't credit the story at first and thought that he was ' kidding ' me for a tenderfoot; but later on I learned that it was absolutely true. An English surgeon at Zacapa told me that he had seen scores of natives suffering from chronic rheumatism brought on by swallowing raw mercury, and I dare say the dose is occasionally fatal; but they still cling to the superstition. When a European settles in the country he is pretty certain to hang a thermometer somewhere outside of his house, and, after losing two or three, he generally concludes that it would be cheaper to buy a piece of netting. I doubt whether you could find an unprotected instrument between Port Barrios and the capital."—*New Orleans Times-Democrat.*

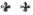

COULDN'T BELIEVE IT.

GOVERNOR W——, of Virginia, was a splendid lawyer, and could talk a jury out of their seven senses. He was especially noted for his success in criminal cases, almost always clearing his client. He was once counsel for a man accused of horsestealing. He made a long, eloquent, and touching speech. The jury retired, but returned in a few moments, and, with tears in their eyes, proclaimed the man not guilty. An old acquaintance stepped up to the prisoner and said:

" Jim, the danger is past; and now, honor bright, didn't you steal that horse?"

" Well, Tom, I've all along thought I took that horse; but since I've heard the Governor's argument, I don't believe I did!"

BOOK REVIEWS.

THE AMERICAN YEAR-BOOK OF MEDICINE AND SURGERY FOR 1901. A Yearly Digest of Scientific Progress and Authoritative Opinion in all branches of Medicine and Surgery, drawn from journals, monographs, and text-books of the leading American and foreign authors and investigators. Arranged with critical editorial comments by eminent American specialists, under the general editorial charge of George M. Gould, M.D. In two volumes—Volume I., including "General Medicine," octavo, 681 pages, illustrated; Volume II., "General Surgery," octavo, 610 pages, illustrated. Philadelphia and London: W. B. Saunders & Co., 1901. Per volume: Cloth, $3.00 net; half morocco, $3.75 net.

THE issue of the Year-Book for 1900 in two volumes met with such general approval from the profession that the publishers decided to follow the same plan with the Year-Book for 1901. This arrangement has a two-fold advantage. To the physician who uses the entire book it offers an increased amount of matter in the most convenient form for easy consultation, and without any increase in price; while specialists and others who want either the medical or the surgical section alone, secure the complete consideration of their branch, without the necessity of purchasing considerable for which they have no special use.

When Dr. Gould edits a book or a medical journal, those who are familiar with his professional *timbre* have a sufficient guaranty that the work will be well selected, thoroughly digested, and concisely stated. The volume before us only confirms the inference. Not à page in the volume is either humdrum or hackneyed. Each author has been made to say what he has to say, without wasting time in circumlocution and non-essentials. The volume is more comprehensive than any of its kind that has reached our table. With its aid the busy practitioner can make a hasty and, at the same time, quite satisfactory review of what the past year has contributed to his professional armamentarium. It is a whole century ahead of its early predecessors, issued a decade ago, and is alike creditable to editor, contributors and publishers.

EXCURSION TO THE ROCKY MOUNTAINS AND CALIFORNIA.

THE Editor of the DIETETIC AND HYGIENIC GAZETTE has planned an excursion to Southern California, to include a side trip in the Rocky Mountains, starting about the 20th of April or 1st of May and returning at the option of the party. Having resided seven years in Colorado and five in Southern California he is thoroughly familiar with the best features of each, and will act as escort and medical attendant for a select number of ladies and others who desire to make the trip for health or pleasure. Spring is really the most delightful season to visit either Colorado or Southern California, and this outing can be made extremely profitable and entertaining to those who need a change.

For particulars address
EDITOR D. & H. GAZETTE,
No. 503 Fifth avenue,
New York.
References exchanged.

THE blood of an adult male human of average size and weight measures 4,400 cubic centimeters, equal to nearly nine and one-third pints. If the corpuscles were spread out side by side they would cover 57,000 square feet of surface, equal to nearly an acre and a third.

It is rather startling to think that a man can be spread all over a good sized villa plot without at all disturbing his solid parts.

If his blood disks thus arranged would cover so much surface, to what world-wide dimensions would he extend if every cell in his body was duly flattened and the whole spread out to their fullest extent? Would he cover and eclipse the entire American continent and lap over Behring's Straits into Russia?

TRANSACTIONS OF THE BREVITY CLUB.

Third Paper.

CAUSATIVE, OR EXECUTIVE?

THE atmosphere about us is at all times permeated with germs, many of them being so-called "pathogenic." Healthy organisms inhale, ingest and imbibe them every day and every hour, in numbers sufficient to overstock the entire realm of animated nature, and yet only a comparative few become attainted. Every robust nature and normal organism repels or destroys them. Seventy-six millions of people, in the United States, are daily exposed to the germs of tuberculosis. By means of infectious floating dust and otherwise these invisible and insidious organisms find ready access to the lungs, stomachs and mucous membranes of every individual member of the census total. About fifteen or twenty out of each thousand develop some form of the disease. The rest are exempt, immune.

Let us pursue the thought.

Unquestionably the ultimate and original source of all organized matter, from mollusk to man, poor little helpless, vegetating germs, as innocent of any evil design as the bland and passive elements that combine to form water or wind, merely obeying the law of propagation and preservation, who shall champion their cause? That they have an absolutely indispensable mission to perform all our later researches prove beyond question. Is it not a more sweeping, radical and comprehensive mission than any of us have yet divined or admitted?

Their existence is as legitimate as that of their would-be destroyers. They are a primal and necessary part of all the great processes of the creative force of the universe. Without them the soil would be unfruitful, plants could neither grow nor fructify, and all animal life would forever cease. They constitute the creative unit. All these established facts tempt us to ask,— are not these so-called "pathogenic" germs the means adopted by inexorable Nature to eliminate the unfittest?

Faulty nutrition weakens the defences; coddling habits, shut-in living and reckless excesses undermine the physical vigor; and then, the stoical and mercilessly merciful creative force again takes the field, and says: "*This organism has forfeited its opportunity. Let it be put aside, to make room for a fresh effort.*"

Nature cares absolutely nothing for individuals, everything for genera and species. She manifests no whit of sympathy for the sorrowing survivors, but strides on, to the ultimate accomplishment of her grand purpose, indifferent to obstacles and oblivious to pain. However frantically we interpose our boasted germicides, our pre-digested foods, cod liver oil, creasote and corrosive sublimate, to stay the demoralization and slay the germs, we only briefly defer the final catastrophe, since the slaughter of a few millions, more or less, of microscopic organisms, that have a habit of multiplying at the rate of countless billions in a day, is but an insignificant drop in the bucket. It is an attempt to dip the Atlantic with a teaspoon. The ranks of the germs are unbroken, and they sweep on undaunted and practically undiminished.

The "cure" lies in keeping the individuals immune, fortifying in advance of the attack, overcoming susceptibility, preserving the integrity of the organism and maintaining the vitality at normal tone. To accomplish this Nature has but one chemic symbol—H. N. S., which being extended reads, HYGIENE, NUTRITION, SANITATION.

Fourth Paper.

THE BLOOD OF THE MARTYRS.

THE history of religious martyrdom is familiar reading, but the martyrs have not all been pious monks and overzealous devotees, or sinless saints, ready and willing to die for the sake of their faith. Every department of science has its victims. Innovators in Art, Music or Medicine have all been punished. Every author of a new school in painting has been declared a lunatic and starved to death. Wagner was driven from country to country, traduced, ostracized and vilified. Harvey lost his business through his enthusiasm concerning the circulation of the blood. Lady Mary Wortley Montague suffered in her reputation for introducing smallpox innoculation; and for the greater boon of vaccination the theologians of his day denounced Jenner as the real Antichrist referred to in Holy Writ.

The same spirit, somewhat differently manifested, has followed the ages and exists at the present day.

We have not yet learned to accept a candidate for what he *is* and what he *knows*, but hold him at a stand-off until it is determined where he found out what he knows, and to what particular paleozoic period the fossils who yawned over his examination papers belonged. A wave of logical protest has begun to roll shoreward on the ocean of conventional conversatism with which society is surrounded, and the time will no doubt come when what a man shows himself to *be* will be made the crucial test, and will outweigh that which any man, any set of men, any college faculty or theological board may *say* he is. When that time arrives, *character* will be recognized as the real thing, *reputation* a fashion or mere appearance that may be put on or off at will, the paper money that ought but too often does not stand for the genuine coin.

When that day arrives it is evident that the possession of a bit of parchment, duly signed and countersigned, will not necessarily furnish an unquestioned passport to cultivated society, whether social, political, literary or professional. Nor will the want of such formal credentials be made a permanent bar to any who possess the genuine diploma of actual attainment, culture and character.

And in this connection we must bear in mind that *the blood of the martyrs has ever been the seed of the church.*

A CLERGYMAN WHO IS ELIGIBLE TO MEMBERSHIP IN THE BREVITY CLUB.

DR. LYMAN ABBOTT, as an advocate of the blue pencil in the construction of sermons, rather startled the students of the Boston University Theological School when he said:

"The trouble with most sermons is not that they are too long, but that they are too lengthy. We are living in a time when everything tends to condensation. It is an age of steam and electricity, and we must think like steam and act like electricity. It is much better for a young preacher to say 'Can I ever get what I have got to talk about into one hour?' than to wonder how he can get out so long a sermon with so small a text.

"We should leave out introductions and start right in at the beginning. How many newspaper editorials you begin at the second paragraph, as the introduction is a preliminary with nothing in it.

"The minister should have an idea for every word, and illustrations should not be given to such an extent that they will distract the mind from the object in view. One must find time to read and study and thoughts acquired should be put in writing.

"The young preacher should at all times be himself. He should buttonhole his congregation, as it were, and talk with a specific object in view. The minister is not in the pulpit to tell his hearers what he learned in a school of theology, any more than a doctor is called to the bedside of his patient to tell what he was taught of anatomy at the medical school.

"The minister's purpose is to win a vote for the great cause, and to be a father to those needing enlightenment and soul salvation. He must doctor in the spiritual sense, and to do this he must first have among other requirements that great essential—a firm belief in good order."

Department of Notes and Queries.

FREEDOM OF DISCUSSION BETWEEN EDITOR AND READER.

TO CORRESPONDENTS.

We receive many inquiries without the signatures of their authors. It is a time-honored editorial edict that such communications shall be consigned to the waste-basket. Occasionally, when a question is unmistakable as to its perfect good faith and it is evident that the name is withheld from a sense of diffidence, we ignore the rule and publish the query. We much prefer to adhere to the rule, and reiterate the request that every communication shall contain the real name of the sender. Those who do not find their inquiries answered in this Department will understand the reason.

Query 77. What is your editor's opinion of the various brands of antiseptic soap advertised in the market? Are any of them reliable as disinfectants or as antiseptics?
M. B. M., Delaware.

Answer.—A good quality of soap is itself detergent, disinfectant, and moderately antiseptic. Soap, hot water, sunshine, and towels were the only antiseptics used by Lawson Tait, and we all know how wonderful were his surgical results. Various scientists have experimented with the several varieties of so-called antiseptic soaps, and have arrived at the conclusion that the attempt to combine corrosive sublimate, salicylic acid, and the other antiseptics of general repute with soap has not proved a success. They have even demonstrated that the addition of these powerful antiseptics to soap destroys the antiseptic properties of the latter, and that the antiseptics themselves are thereby rendered practically inert.

It follows that good soap without any of these admixtures is a more effective and reliable disinfectant and antiseptic than any of the much-vaunted group.

There is, however, a great difference in soaps. Such as are made from impure and unclean animal fats are unfit for surgical or toilet use. When made from pure vegetable oils, especially fresh olive oil, by a process that ensures perfect saponification, so that there is no excess of alkali remaining in the product, the result is a bland, non-irritating detergent that is at the same time disinfectant and antiseptic. Imported white castile soap is presumed to be all this, but sometimes falls short of the mark by containing an excess of unsaponified alkali.

Query 78. I have for a long time noted, particularly in the columns of the medical journals that regularly reach my table as "sample copies," an intemperate reiteration of the statement that there is no such disease as hydrophobia or rabies. In one case a gentleman offers a premium of $100 for an established case of this dreaded disease. Can the editor of the GAZETTE throw any light on the subject?

Answer.—We have heard of the $100 man. He belongs in the city of Washington, which, as we all know, is a favorite rendezvous for an annual assortment of political adventurers, ranging all the way from wise men to visionaries and lunatics.

It is a great pity that even professional men can still be found who honestly, let us assume, believe that all the now well-authenticated cases of rabies, either in humans or animals, have been cases of mistaken diagnosis. They believe that scientific men deceive themselves when they decide that certain mysterious, agonizing, and otherwise unaccountable symptoms are attributed to the bite of a "mad dog." They insist that these manifestations are but an obscure and very aggravated form of hysteria or other neurotic explosion.

If these incredulous enthusiasts would stop to think they would probably recall the fact that but a few years ago hysteria itself was considered an imaginary disease. Those who so considered it have learned more about it, have closely investigated some genuine manifestations of the disease, whether in men or women, and have changed their opinions. The only thing they lack in case of hydrophobia is the unmistakable evidence. Cases are rare, and they have not yet investigated any but those of either feigned or extremely doubtful character. When the gentleman who had $100 to burn was offered facilities for studying a genuine case of rabies, by the Secretary of the Committee on Animal Diseases, etc., he promptly subsided, and has not since been heard from.

We have no doubt but that some of the many anti-rabies "professors" have made capital out of the popular dread of this fatal malady, and have done some profitable "faking" with "madstones" and other bogus "cures." But this does not alter the fact that rabies is a very real, a very terrible and a very fatal disease. As yet there is no record of a genuine case having recovered, although competent and thoroughly honest observers believe that prompt treatment by attenuated virus has succeeded in preventing the occurrence of the disease, in humans who have been bitten by rabid animals.

Query 79. Can you mention the infallible symptoms of cancer of the stomach in language that a layman can readily understand?

B. C., Minnesota.

Answer.—As a rule the symptoms of any disease are not uniform and "infallible." In the early stages of cancer of the stomach the diagnosis is always obscure. The prominent points to be noted are as follows:

Cancer of the stomach usually occurs between the ages of forty and sixty, and more frequently in men than in women. The first symptoms do not differ much from those of chronic indigestion, viz., poor appetite, pain at the lower portion of the organ, slow digestion, vomiting, at first of the food, but later on of a substance that resembles coffee grounds. Sometimes blood is vomited, but it is always very dark, almost black, and would not be taken for blood by any but a physician. The pain becomes constant, is dull and gnawing rather than sharp, and very soon a well-defined tumor can be felt at the outlet or pylorus. If all these signs are present and do not yield to rational treatment but continue to grow more severe, and if the patient "runs down" and acquires a complexion that resembles tallow, that is, of a creamy paleness instead of a clear white, it may be inferred that the disease is cancer.

If cancer is suspected there should be no time lost in consulting the best surgical talent in the vicinity, since the only possible "cure" is *early removal,* and happily this is now quite feasible and safe.

Query 80. Dear Editor: I enjoy the GAZETTE and gain valuable information from each number received.

Will you please answer the following:

Is there any harm in the use of powdered borax? I keep it on my wash-stand and use it freely for softening the water to bathe in. Will it in time roughen the skin? Please tell me what scientific or hygienic objections there are to such use of it, if any, and oblige,   ——? Ga.

Answer.—Any reasonable use of borax in the way and for the purpose mentioned is not only harmless, but beneficial. It is much less liable to irritate or dry the skin than soda or ammonia. It very rarely roughens the most sensitive skin, and in these rare cases an inunction with fresh olive, cotton-seed or cocoanut oil, or liquid vaseline to be applied with plenty of rubbing, after a hot bath, will prevent all trouble of the kind. In fact, a weekly inunction is a luxury and of great benefit to lean or debilitated persons. The skin will readily absorb two to four ounces of oil at a rubbing.

Query 81. (Note. This correspondent's question comes under the head of personal advice. The answer requires expert surgical knowledge. It will be referred to a competent surgeon, and will be answered if at all by personal letter.)

Query 82. Will you oblige me by giving me the name of any work that gives an analysis of the different foods and shows the proportion of *inorganic salts in each?*

I should be much obliged to you for this information, or a suggestion as to where to apply for it.   E. J. B., Brooklyn.

Answer.—We take it that you mean *earthy constituents* when you say "inorganic salts," since these salts as found in vegetables, grains, fruits and the like are properly *organic.*

You will probably find what you want in some of the following standard works, any of which you can consult in the large libraries:

Yeo, on FOOD, published by Lea Brothers;

Burnet, FOODS AND DIETARIES, P. Blakiston's Sons;

Blyth, ANALYSIS OF FOODS, William Wood & Co.

The Agricultural Department at Washington is also publishing some very instructive tables, reports and analyses of foods.

For these, address the Secretary of Agriculture, Washington, D. C., and also apply to the Storrs Agricultural Experiment Station, at Storrs, Conn. They are sent free.

THE

DIETETIC AND HYGIENIC GAZETTE

A·MONTHLY·JOURNAL OF·PHYSIOLOGICAL·MEDICINE

Vol. XVII.   NEW YORK, MAY, 1901.   No. 5.

DIACETIC ACID, DIET, AND DIABETES.

BY CHARLES PLATT, M.D., PH.D., F.C.S. (LOND.),

Philadelphia.

WE test diabetic urine nowadays for acetone, diacetic acid, etc., realizing that these substances have a bearing on the prognosis of our case. In fact, this unfavorable prognosis, recently commented upon in the journals, has long been recognized by physiological chemists, and much has been done, in an experimental way, to clear up the true significance of these substances in the urine. Incidentally much has been learned as to the cause of sugar in the urine, and it is of moment to examine these recent experiments with a view of bringing our treatment of diabetes more in line with physiological knowledge.

Practically many have already discovered that it is not advisable to cut off all carbohydrates from the diet, and, indeed, in many cases it has been observed that so to do not only fails to reduce the amount of sugar in the urine, but also results disastrously for the patient. The old idea, that the sugar in the urine constituted the disease, has now been superseded by the knowledge that the sugar is but a symptom, and that it is, moreover, a symptom belonging in common to any of a dozen or more different conditions, to disease of the liver, pancreas, lungs, brain, or general nervous system, etc., etc. We now know that, though some sugar may be derived from the carbohydrates of the food, the usual source is to be found in proteid matter, normally in the circulatory proteids, abnormally in the tissue proteids. We know that the sugar may appear in the urine as the result of overproduction, or as the result of deficient transformation.

With the knowledge that we have in diabetes to deal with proteid katabolism—witness the emaciation—we know that our first aim should be to maintain metabolism at as near a normal as possible. This, we know, can not be done by giving a grossly improperly-balanced diet, made up of proteids. To preserve the body in health we require a certain sufficient amount of nitrogen, and, with this, enough carbon to act as fuel. Nitrogenous food alone can not maintain body-substance, energy, and temperature, or can do so but for a short period. On a continuation of the unnatural diet the attempted excretion of the excess of nitrogen puts the kidney under a strain, the assimilative powers lessen, and the body wastes, for, having no fuel added, and fuel being necessary, that required is drawn from the body tissues, from the proteids.

The sugar then comes from the proteid, the complex proteid molecule yielding a carbohydrate radical in what seems to be a physiological decomposition. As we continue the starving of the patient, however, the manner of proteid decomposition changes, and, finally, we get abnormal poisonous products, among them B-aminobutyric acid, CH_3 CH NH_2 CH_2 $COOH$, a substance capable of producing all the phenomena of diabetic coma and probably the cause of this serious condition. This lately discovered compound is eliminated in the urine as B-hydroxybutyric acid, CH_3 $CHOH$ CH_2 $COOH$, a forerunner of diacetic acid or aceto-acetic acid, CH_3 CO CH_2 $COOH$, and of acetone $(CH_3)_2$ CO. Historically, the last-named substance has long been suspected of being associated with the coma, though it was early proven to be in itself harmless. Diacetic acid, too, has been held up as the coma-producing agent. Neither acetone nor diacetic acid are themselves poisonous, but in their progenitors, the two derived butyric acids, we have poisons capable of profound action on the nerve centers.

Is not the significance of the acetone, diacetic acid, etc., clear from the above? Is it not natural that these substances should be regarded as inclining toward an unfavorable prognosis, coming direct, as they do, from an abnormal proteid katabolism? Could we expect a good prognosis, when, instead of endeavoring to save the tissues, we force their consumption by removing available fuel from the diet? And if this be so in those cases of diabetes where sugar excretion can be influenced by the diet, how criminal is our attempt to cure the disease by removal of food in those conditions not influenced by diet. Experimentally, as is well known, we can simulate a renal glycosuria by administration of phloridzin, or of other toxic substances; now, have we not cases of a like nature in practice, depending, not upon phloridzin, but upon some glucoside or leucomain of body origin? In these cases, so far as the sugar eliminated is concerned, it matters not whether the patient receive a normal diet or one containing no carbohydrates, but as regards the prognosis, it does make a difference, for most certainly we can expect the worst results only if we limit the patient to nitrogenous food.

As before mentioned, I am aware that, clinically, many have long ago discovered the advisability of a more liberal diet in diabetes; the above is an endeavor to justify such a course from physiological and scientific grounds. I do not advocate, be it understood, a continuance of the excessive carbohydrate diet of which most Americans are guilty, but rather a regulation of the dietary with the aim of conserving and of furthering a normal body metabolism. I condemn the misuse of the diet in an attempt to remove the symptom, sugar.

ITEMS FROM A RECENT ADDRESS BY PROF. WILEY.

The coloring matter of green peas is chlorophyl. A little age changes this to zorophyl, which is yellow. If *yellow* "green peas" were offered for sale, the purchaser would imagine they were spoiled. So, the canners add a pinch of either copper or tin salt to each can. The result is the intensely "natural" green found in all "good" brands of green peas!

It is a popular impression that it is oxygen that destroys things, causes wood to rot, etc. This is a mistake. It is a ferment that rots wood. Of course, the air may supply this ferment.

Lavoisier discovered the principle of Pasteurization nearly a century ago.

All the baking powders are bad and for that matter there is little difference in them. The cheapest ones are apparently just as wholesome as the dearest. (They are cheapened with starch or flour.—Ed. *Gazette*.)

Doctors ought to be promoters of health and longevity, even as a matter of business. They can reap quite as much income from the man who lives eighty years in fairly good health, as from one who dies at forty from a lower degree of health.

The so-called "embalmed beef" of the

army was most of it all right. The trouble was the soldiers did not know how to use it. It needed to be used up promptly as soon as opened, especially in the hot climate of Cuba. It acquired germs and decayed very rapidly as soon as exposed to the air.

Oxygen destroys nothing that has been sterilized.

ECONOMICS OF HEALTH.

By Alexander Wilder, M.D.

The preservation of health is one of the highest duties which the individual owes to himself and to community. The person who is disabled is a drawback upon the energies of those around him, and to that extent a source of weakness to the general body. While consuming the proceeds of the labor of others and rendering little or nothing in return, he requires care, assistance and protection.

It is plain that one who is of no benefit to those around him has little moral claim to their good offices. The great law of the universe is reciprocity. A community that is burdened with an undue number of unproductive members can not long sustain itself. In the event of war, it is at the mercy of the enemy; and even in peace it is crippled, unable to carry on productive industries ample to nourish those belonging to it, or to make due advancement in social, material. moral and institutional pursuits.

In many savage tribes, and in countries with customs that differ from ours, the problem has often been summarily solved. Every form of society has its outlaws, for whom many seem to regard it as a merit not to care. The prison and the scaffold are monuments of the failure of society and its institutions to properly do their duty. But crime has been only a solitary evidence of outlawry. Those who fall short of meeting the requirements in regard to the general defence, whether as the result of mis-

fortune or wrong-doing, have also been thrust outside the pale. Under the pretext that self-preservation is the first law of Nature, the feebler members of community have been first to suffer when there was impending danger. If the means of subsistence were hard to procure, the new-born children were put to death, females, the sickly and deformed being first sacrificed. In some communities the infirm and the old have been doomed to a similar fate. The veneration which was paid the father of a family sometimes spared him from the general slaughter; but childless men, old and sickly servants, and other dependents, were seldom permitted to live to a reasonable old age. Classic literature abounds with evidence that the practice was so common as not to elicit condemnation or censure.

Wrong-doing, however, is infallibly certain to produce its own Nemesis. Crime implies and includes within itself its own punishment. The destroying of children has always been followed by its natural consequences. The adult population became too few to defend their country, as well as unpatriotic from being enervated by luxury. Sparta, where child-murder was prescribed by statute, and the slaves were systematically massacred, to keep down their number, went eventually to decay. Palybias declares, a scarcity of men caused the cities of Greece to be deserted and left the fields uncultured. Tyre, Sidon and Carthage were destroyed because they had not citizens of their own to defend them. Rome, in her turn, became the prey of her barbarian legions. Italy and Northern Africa were depopulated of their own yeomanry, so that their invaders, the Northerners and Moslems, found little difficulty in overrunning the lands that had once produced a Julius Cæsar and a Hannibal. The statesmanship which deprecates the increase of human beings, and regards animals and material wealth as more desirable, if not arrested in its course, will always terminate in destruction. Human life is the great end and purpose of the Creation. and whatever cheapens it. or in any manner detracts from its utility and enjoyableness, militates against the order of the universe. Political economy, rightly understood, is not merely the science of wealth and national prosperity, but includes the welfare of the entire population. Failing in this last and most essential particular, it is defective throughout.

Civilization differs from savagery as widely as the North Pole from the South. It is the art of living in society as neighbors and brothers; the savage is the wild one, his hand against everybody, and everybody's hand against him. Political economy cannot rise to the dignity of a science, except by its superior regard for human life and human welfare. The very least, whether a babe, a cripple, or houseless wanderer, is recognized as entitled to care and protection. It contemplates no waste or destruction of life, but the ending of a policy which shall cripple oportunity for any one, but shall open to every one a career of activity and usefulness. Hence it may be stated as an axiom that the care taken in a community of its various members is the index of its advancement.

It is by no means the perfection of statecraft, however, to provide armies, maintain order, facilitate enterprise, and encourage popular education. More important than costly schools and productive industries, than arms and armaments, is the existence of wholesome sanitary conditions. It is impossible to create or assure prosperity, where there is not salubrity of the atmosphere and physical vigor among the people. Health is the important factor in individual and national greatness.

In the history of nations this has been forcibly illustrated. In early times the seat of empire was by turns upon the Euphrates and the Nile. Egypt, we are assured by Herodotus, was the most salubrious country of the world, and Babylonia appears to have been the traditional paradise of Eden. War and conquest, however, put an end to the former happy conditions, and all the countries of the Orient have long been deserts, the rendezvous of wild beasts, or the hot-beds of pestilence. Syria, Armenia, Asia-Minor, and the neighboring countries, whose people have become servile and impotent from misgovernment and the plague, take their sorrry revenge by evolving pestilence and transmitting it to the other regions of the globe.

Once the Campagna was full of cities and alive with human activity. The Tarquins made Rome habitable by constructing the famous Cloaca, which drained a lake and converted a large area of marsh into a wholesome district. But after their overthrow the Romans became a conquering people and destroyed all the public utilities about their city. This intolerable rapacity has been followed by an exemplary vengeance. Like the unborn spirit that had gone out, the malaria, the chilly damp of marshy regions, returned to its former abiding-place, and the last condition became worse than the first.

For a thousand years the population of Europe was stationary. Wars passing, and pestilence recurring as regularly as the seasons, prevented human increase, and arrested the progress of civilization. The people became little better than savages. Hardship, privation and disease kept every country sparsely inhabited and wretched. The surface of the continent was covered with forests, and the lowlands were undrained and reeking with the deadly dampness. The cities of London and Paris were mere collections of wooden houses, unfloored and abounding with filth and vermin. A pile of rubbish and garbage stood at every door. Personal cleanliness, even among the dignitaries of the State and church, was utterly unknown. The first Stuart King of Great Britain, and Thomas â Becket, of Canterbury, were notorious for being unwashed and lousy. The inordinate use of perfumes was resorted to in order to conceal the body odor.

The conflict of races and religions which existed for centuries, was frightful, from its massacres and atrocious cruelties, but the encounters with disease and pestilence were infinitely more terrible. There seemed to be an apocalypse of the rule of Death and the insatiable Grave, with power given them over a fourth part of the earth to kill with sword, with hunger, with fatal disease, and with wild beasts. For ten years, from 1345 till 1355, the Black Death ran riot over Europe and destroyed a fourth of the population. In 1348 it entered France and exterminated a third of her people. The ensuing three centuries constitute a history of successive pestilences. An array so formidable blanched the very hearts of men. They became mad in their despair, and snapped the ties of social life. Many forsook their families for the convent, and others plunged into excesses too horrible to be described, and from the sequences of which the world has not yet wholly recovered.

It was termed the plague, or the Great Death, that so often depopulated Europe. But the exact or specific diseases which were so denominated have not been accurately determined. Sometimes it was a malignant form of variola, "the black smallpox," which is represented as having come from Arabia and Africa with the Moors. Again, it was a typhoid seizure, typhus with buboes, which was one of the "diseases of Egypt," which foreign invaders had transplanted into that once healthiest of countries. These are maladies, however, that, like fungi, have repeatedly sprung up spontaneously in foul places, as, for example, where armies were long kept together, or the population was too densely congregated. No importation of contagion is required in such conditions for any of these visitations. The Thirty Years' War originated smallpox and distributed it over Germany. After the Black Death came syphilis. It may have been some other malady raging like an epidemic, hidden from sight and perpetrated under the name of plague. It appeared four centuries ago, among the Spanish troops in Italy, and rapidly spread to every country of Europe. Kings, nobles, the clergy, all, from highest to lowest degrees, and common people alike contracted the pest, and its victims died in countless numbers. There is every reason to believe that the taint of blood from that one cause alone is not yet eradicated, but that many disorders now common are among its consequences.

The rapid acquisition of wealth which has characterized our modern period, has been the wonder and admiration of students of political economy. The working capital of the world has tripled in a generation.

Another index of prosperity has been the rapid increase of population. In the earlier periods, every country of Europe was impoverished and bereft of male population. When William the Conqueror held the sceptre of England, the country had about two million inhabitants; five centuries later the number had doubled; since that period the increase has reached ten times that number. The average length of human life four hundred years ago was less than eighteen years; it now exceeds thirty-six. In the better governed countries of the European continent there has been a like increase, the result of a general improvement of conditions.

The great factor contributing toward this fast progress is manifest to every intelligent person. Political changes have only aided it; science was but a minister. This marvelous increase of wealth, this prodigious achievement, this general amelioration of human conditions, all these, in advance of all these causes, are due to the general exemption of the civilized world from pestilence, to the better health that prevails, and to the longer average term of human life.

No country in which the permanent conditions are insalubrious can attain and maintain prosperity; to acquire wealth, an individual must be steady, industrious, thrifty, and, above all, healthy. If he is enervated by his surroundings, or an invalid, he can not acquire; and when quite prostrated by sickness, what he has earned and saved must be expended. In a sickly family, no matter how great the industry, thrift is impossible, poverty inevitable. Sickness is impoverishing wherever it exists. What is true of individuals and families is infinitely more so of communities. No sickly community can be prosperous.

War did not keep Europe poor for so many centuries. Modern campaigns are vastly more expensive than were the protracted contests in former times. The countries of the Old World might have prospered without the use of the precious metals and the advantages offered by machinery. It was disease that spread the pall of poverty over Europe. Every family was wasted and enfeebled by sickness, besides having to meet several times in each century the unsparing conscription of pestilence. The diminished capacity for production, the waste by sickness and the recurring plagues, which were worse than a prohibitory tariff in interrupting commercial intercourse, all combined to check effort and keep all the people destitute.

We, of the United States, have had our lessons. Cholera, and other deadly epidemics have been periodical in their visitations. They will overleap any quarantine when insalubrious conditions invite their inception. We remember the disorder which many contracted who visited Philadelphia during the Centennial season. New England has attained the bad repute of being the hot-bed of pulmonary consumption. The influence of this fact upon her commercial prosperity is manifest. The city of New Orleans has been an incubus on the prosperity of the Southwestern States for the recurring epidemics of yellow fever and other infectious and deadly diseases.

When an epidemic rages, business is paralyzed. The pecuniary losses by pestilence far exceed those by fire. Savannah had an epidemic of yellow fever, lasting but a few months, yet was brought to the verge of bankruptcy. A visitation upon New Haven, many years ago, entailed a depressing result, from which the city has never fully rallied. Philadelphia was so disabled in resources by the yellow fever of 1795, as never to regain her commercial and metropolitan supremacy. She lost more than thirty millions of dollars in the last century from an epidemic of smallpox, which proper sanitary and hygienic precautions might have prevented.

There is unprecedented competition at the present time among the nations. The best evidences of statesmanship are put forth to extend and maintain commerce and productive industry. Every country having special advantage is in a way to prosper, but is liable by any temporary misfortune to be left behind in the race. There is, therefore, an intense anxiety in regard to every possible drawback. The individuals or public journals, that report the appearance of an epidemic in the city of New York, have often incurred severe censure for the commercial injury they have caused. The presence of cholera has sometimes been actually conceded, for business reasons. Some of the arbitrary requirements by way of precaution taken in large mercantile and manufacturing houses, senseless and useless though they are, afford indisputable evidence of existing business apprehension.

The bubonic plague, which has devastated large districts of India, is watched with trepidation, but it finds a foothold on Western shores; yet the fact that a city or a country may be efficiently protected was illustrated by the late General B. F. Butler, when in command at New Orleans. If his administration had been extended over all the lower valley of the Mississippi, for a term of years, yellow fever, cholera and other filth diseases might have been effectually excluded. No prevention is possible to any pestilential visitation, except by throttling the cause. A Waring may arise and do this intelligently and efficiently. The nucleus of epidemic diseases should be destroyed wherever found. Human abodes and everything about them should be cleansed of whatever is unwholesome and impure. No disease will be contracted, whatever the current epidemic, except in the presence of an abnormal state of body, a vital depression, which induces a receptive condition.

In short, true political economy places health foremost as an essential to the prosperity of a people. Popular education, social advancement, and national greatness are attainable only upon this condition. Whatever achievement or excellence may exist or be possible beyond, if not primarily and solely due to it, is nevertheless largely dependent. Physical efficiency results in more or less of moral power, the capacity to originate, and the energy to accomplish. It is these qualities that enable individuals and the commonwealth alike to realize their ideals.

WHAT THE CENTURY HAS TAUGHT US ABOUT LIVING.

By Samuel S. Wallian, A.M., M.D.,

(Copyright 1901.)

II.

OF THE HIVE ITSELF.

It is not intended to make this series of papers a treatise on architecture, but it is a palpable fact that altogether too many modern houses in every community, and especially in cities, are being constructed with a very bold, a very careless or a very ignorant disregard of the fundamental edicts of the sanitary engineer. The aim is either conventional, commercial, or both—the greatest number of cubic feet of space and the largest degree of external display, for the least possible expense.

Tastes and means vary so much that it would be idle to discuss detailed plans from any general standard; besides, your country house built over a vegetable cellar, with lot room going to waste all about it, is one thing, and your city dwelling, with its site limited to a definite number of feet and inches "front" and "deep" is quite another.

For the country house cellars are now quite generally condemned as unsanitary, as direct breeders of colds, fevers, rheumatism, diphtheria, and even consumption. As usually constructed and mismanaged the criticism is merited; but it does not follow that cellars are necessarily evils. If the earth emanations or "ground air" be effectually excluded by a layer of asphalt, and this covered with a coating of good cement; and if the walls are also made impervious, or, better still, built with an airspace, like the outer walls of brick buildings; and if the latter are frequently treated to a fresh coat of sharp, caustic lime whitewash, and a rational system of ventilation be provided for, there is no reason why the cellar should, *per se,* breed disease. But it must be kept scrupulously clean, and free from any form of decaying vegetation. The danger lies in neglect of some of these precautions.

In the country, it is better to store all perishable products in a cellar built on purpose, at a little distance from the main building. It need be but half underground, and can be made frost-proof in any climate.

LIGHT, VENTILATION, CONVENIENCE.

This is the sacred trinity on which the builder of the future must base all his work, or it will not pass inspection at the court of Hygiea. The site selected, building material used, height of ceilings, arrangement of rooms, warming facilities and all other appointments must be made secondary and subservient to this Court of Appeals.

As to building material, brick is probably, all things considered, the best building material now in common use. Composed of unobjectionable elements and subjected to the ordeal of fire, it is thus thoroughly sterilized and made aseptic. It is quite permeable to air and does not furnish a culture ground for any hurtful form of germ life.

But for a greater or less degree of porosity and permeability inherent in all varieties of building material, doubtless the human race would have long since become extinct, from actual suffocation. Brick, wood, stone, plaster, paper, cloth, felt—all these are, in varying degrees, permeable to air. This fact is well illustrated by the old trick of blowing out a candle through a thick piece of tanned buckskin.

Sanitarily considered, wood is second best as a building material. It is porous, economic, everywhere available and is necessarily relied on for inside work, whatever other material is employed for the body of the building. Its keeping qualities are much enhanced by the modern use of "fillers" and varnish, at the expense, however, of a considerable degree of its porosity. Its greater inflammability is an objection, but less serious than is generally supposed, when we reflect that complete destruction generally follows every fire of a serious nature, regardless of the structural materials of the building. Decaying wood is always a menace to health.

Stone is perhaps third on the list. There are no sanitary objections to properly constructed stone dwellings. This means that they must have double walls, enclosing an air-space as a non-conductor of heat, cold and moisture. The sense of substantialness afforded by stone structures is, to many persons, a source of satisfaction.

The color of dwellings is usually decided by the taste, or want of taste, of the builders, or by some prevailing fashion. It has recently been shown that colors have much more significance than merely that of being either negative or agreeable. This fact has long been instinctively recognized, without yet being intelligently defined. Black is depressing. It is the symbol of darkness, night, death; and colors that approach it are proportionately depressing. The careful study of the effect of color-masses on the minds of different people brings out facts that have a more or less important bearing on health. These effects are being tested, more particularly in hospitals, and will be referred to in connection with the discussion of the decoration of rooms and the selection of furnishings and clothing.

Some colors are naturally exciting, and others are distinctly soothing. This applies more to interiors than to mere exteriors; but there is much to be studied in deciding prevailing colors for the outsides of dwellings, barns, outhouses and fences. The architect and builder is apt to fall into the way of following the prevailing fashion, as to his color specifications. Sometimes these are strictly in good taste and unobjectionable, and sometimes they are incongruous even to hideousness. A rational guide is found in the colors donned by the vegetable kingdom. The soft greens and grays of spring verdure, the creamy white, pale gold, and countless shades of brown of autumn tints are all harmonious and pleasing. No eye tires of them when they are properly blended. None of them are glaring, none of them depress or excite the mind. The ethereal blue of the sky is equally delightful, but it is never more than bunglingly imitated by the painter. The deep blues and greens approach too near to black and are suggestive of melancholy and "biliousness." The intensity of a "blood-red" sunset is too evanescent and too unusual to be copied as a permanent coloring for every day in the year, but the mellow rose of a summer dawn is always inspiring. White is too glaring as a house color, unless the structure is so situated as to be perpetually masked and modified by masses and shadings of green or gray or brown. Hence it is better to discard white for mass-color on exteriors. Colors affect different individuals so differently that it is not best to select exterior colors according to the fancy of any one member of the family, but to compromise on a tint or shade that will not offend any. The modest creams, grays, drabs and various stone tints best answer this requirement, and afford considerable latitude for the exercise of taste. Human life is sombre enough without the addition of sombre surroundings, when these can be avoided. Even the cemeteries would be made less depressing and less appalling to the living if the tendency to enshroud them in funereal colors could be overcome.

As succinctly stated by a recent writer, "Clear, delicate blues are found to exercise a sedative or calming effect, even upon those suffering with very violent manias. Yellows are exceedingly efficacious in combating melancholia or extreme depression. Scarlets and vivid reds will raise the drooping spirits of many depressed and mentally disordered individuals. Bright, tender, spring-like greens will cause life to take on a new aspect and become worth living to insanity victims with suicidal tendencies. Violets are soothing, browns and grays dulling in their effect, while black is distinctly and generally bad. Some insanity experts even go so far as to forbid the attendants upon their patients to wear black at any time."

To secure a sufficiency of light in all parts of the dwelling and at the same time not seriously interfere with the architectural edicts and internal arrangements always taxes the ingenuity of the most expert designers. Generally there is more or less subservience to custom, fashion and convenience, as well as a practical study of the item of expense. No argument based on any one of these items should be allowed to interfere with the hygienic requirements. Let there be light, abundance of light, everywhere in the house, at whatever cost of custom, architectural conventionality or cash.

In providing for light much can be done to make ventilation ample and efficient. This is the stumbling block of the architects. They talk about it and contrive various make-believe schemes for "scientific" ventilation, but they do not ventilate. A perfect system of ventilating living apartments ought to be within the reach of the modern builder; but such a system is nowhere in vogue. The requirements are that all the air in a room shall be changed at intervals regulated by its cubic contents and the number of persons occupying it. A further condition is that the new air supplied must be pure and of proper temperature. Proper ventilation also includes the constant removal of the floating dust of the room. In winter, when fires or warming facilities are required this can be accomplished more or less perfectly by means of open grates; but the tendency in cities, and to a great extent in recently built country houses, is to do away with local heating apparatus and to rely on either steam or hot-air furnaces located in the cellar. In case of steam there is no provision for changing or renewing the air, but merely for warming it up to a requisite degree. In case of hot air, the volume sent up from Tartarus below must necessarily displace some of that in the room; but the warmed air that takes its place is often contaminated with combustion gases and dust, and at best is little better than so-called "dead air."

A system of house-warming for cities and villages where illuminating gas is used, has been announced, by which the air of the room can be constantly changed, and at the same time the floating dust is drawn into the burners and cremated. It is a plausible and practicable method, and if not already economic and satisfactory in its working details will no doubt eventually be made so, and may be, in time, generally introduced. Sanitary appliances in other directions are constantly multiplying, but it would seem that less inventive energy has been expended in connection with hygienic heating and ventilation than in any other department of sanitary science. Not that there is any lack of devices, but that none of them are adequate. Most of them are more ornamental than useful. When people rush their furnaces and deoxygenating heaters; seal up their windows with rubber weather-strips, and muffle them with upholstery, and then build storm doors over the outside entrances, so that there shall never be a ghost of a "draft" admitted, they are not ventilating, they are conducting culture-rooms for *bacilli tuberculosis.* Pale-faced anemics, starved bodies and souls in the midst of plenty, the only wonder is that these souls and bodies manage to remain so long in partnership!

Our ancestors lacked much of our sanitary knowledge. They had not even dreamed of "sanitary plumbing," wore linsey-woolsey, and had very crude notions as to what constituted "good form." They, however, were not toothless at twenty-five, and bald at thirty. Most of them could read their Bibles without glasses at seventy-five, and they lived to be centenarians, without ever having puzzled themselves over a printed *menu*, in French, Choctaw or Hindoostanee.

But they lived in houses that were as open as a hospital tent, spent their days out of doors and their evenings before great fireplaces as big as a barn door and furnishing prompt exit for "dead air," dust and animal exhalations as fast as these accumulated. They had not heard of the *comma bacillus*, but they held in reserve a substantial stock of hard common sense. They didn't know enough to blood poison their poor horses and then bleed them to death for the sake of turning their blood-serum into ducats, at fifty dollars a quart, warranted to out-toxin some other toxin; and they didn't die of suffocation or surfeit. Their own blood serum was charged with its own antitoxin, derived from its intimate contact with the oxygen of the air. It was not surcharged with carbonic acid and ammoniacal gases, produced by those retrograde vital processes of which we now talk glibly as "morbid metabolism." In other words, with all their scientific short-comings, their houses were *homes*, while many of ours are charnel houses—simply for want of FRESH AIR.

HOUSE PLANNING.

In planning a house, there is every latitude for the display of individual taste; but it should not be forgotten that its general convenience will add much to its healthfulness.

First of all, especially in cities, the kitchen is almost universally slighted. A dark and damp basement, or a cramped corner that is of little use for anything else is generally considered good enough for the kitchen. There could be no more fatal mistake. The Kitchen should be spelled with a big K. It is the vital laboratory, the engine room that furnishes the motive force of the household and largely molds the character and destiny of coming generations. It should be large, light and airy, with facilities for absorbing a glint of sunshine every day that the sun

is on tap. It should be so redolent of comfort and cheer that it will be attractive to the entire family, the scene of informal and enjoyable reunions—taffy pullings, popcorn parties, rollicking games, domestic visitings and family picnics galore. This was the kitchen of our ancestors of a hundred years ago. It not only held all the family, numbering perhaps a dozen children, but on occasions it accommodated the members of a neighboring family, at apple-paring bees, and other neighborhood reunions. It had no resemblance to the modern cookery-closet with its reeking odors of onions, turnip-tops and burnt fat. In the Model Kitchen, which science will surely provide us in due time, none of these unsavory and unhygienic conditions and concomitants will be tolerated. With the advent of the perfected steel ranges already being supplied, including their greatly improved appurtenances; with better culinary appliances and kitchen facilities of every kind to comfort, burnt steaks and sputtering fat will become things of the past, all disagreeable odors will be conducted directly into the flue—a modern substitute for the old-fashioned fireplace, and perfect ventilation will make the Kitchen as sweet and wholesome as the dining-room or parlor.

To those who are about to build, who hope to build, or who think of rebuilding, the best possible advice is to plan the Kitchen first, and plan it on an extravagantly liberal scale. Every dollar's worth of extravagance indulged in this direction at the outset will be ten dollars' worth of economy in the future. Breaking away from stingy and shortsighted precedents, let the room be of generous proportions; let at least one side face the sun at some portion of the day, and on this side build a roomy, projecting window, with ample window-seat and shelving for plants.

When the kitchen of the future country home shall have come and the housewife of the future aligns herself to preside over it, there will be no more cringing to a false pride that now handicaps the race, and no bowing to the edicts of an irrational and pseudo-æsthetic social standard. To continue the hackneyed figure, the Coming Woman, whose name has been so much bandied about—not the dear, restless, ambitious, unsatisfied and unhappy being who is now passing through a painful and trying, but absolutely necessary stage in her process of evolution—really emerges from the trammels of fashion, custom and a semi-barbaric past, the society, of which she will be an integral factor instead of a stipendary and plaything, will hold it in higher esteem to be thoroughly and scientifically accomplished in the vitally important Art Culinary, the Art of Living, than to excel at the piano, to compete in the professional arena, or to be apt at dispensing the superficial graces of the reception room and salon. Just now she is exercising the saddle horse —not always on a senseless side-saddle!— making century runs awheel, graduating at Vassar and Wellesley, and golf, elbowing men in business offices and editorial sanctums, filling chairs in scientific and literary schools—developing both brawn and brain, both of which she sorely needs in order to successfully grapple with the problems of her impending and inevitable mission. When she really finds her niche, she will be neither a drudge nor a wall-flower. Then the drawing-room will no longer absorb the virtues, the vices and the vital force of the entire estate. Then, the Kitchen will become the Throne Room of the domestic empire, and the reigning queen will rule her realm with quite as much dignity, intelligence and pride as she now displays in presiding over a meeting of the suffragists, or a literary reunion of Sorosis. The Millenial Kitchen will compete for the title of "Best Room," and will cease to be a domestic dungeon, banished to sunless and depressing basements, where weary and overworked housewives and domestics are treated to an earthly foretaste of purgatory.

Nature evolved and embellished the country; man has heaped here and there a blotch, and calls it a town. He builds up walls that shut out the sweet sunshine and air of heaven, piles unsightly masses, and calls his work architecture. Nature spreads out landscapes with lavish hand and crowds them with restful outlines and glintings of delight, of which only the morbid eye tires. Man hangs his walls with dauby and unsatisfying imitations, and calls it art.

Life in the country may be made a perpetual idyl; life in the city is a compromise, a sickly substitute. The restless urbanite must have props and prods. He burns midnight oil and midday nicotine. He eats "quick lunches," and then chokes on a "digester," as he rushes to his office or the poolroom. He never *lives*, but he *exists*, at the same pace that he eats, smokes and rushes to business.

It would be useless to make any suggestions to him as to where to locate his kitchen, dining-room or parlor, since he has but a transient acquaintance with either of the trio. He is a moral and social derelict, and no man can predict as to his comings up or his goings down.

In warm climates, and for summer use in almost every part of the country, where plenty of ground-room is to be had without asking, it is feasible to adopt a radical innovation in the general domestic arrangements. To this end erect, at a distance of thirty to fifty feet from the main building, a kind of Executive Annex, connected with the house by a covered, latticed and vine-embowered promenade. Dedicate this structure, which may be in the form of a Moorish cottage, a Chinese pagoda, or any other style to suit the taste of its owner— to the purposes of kitchen, dining-room and pantry. Let the division between the two principal rooms consist of a wide hallway or court, open at both ends and furnished with rustic seats, hammocks and camp-stools, so that the entire family and friends can spend an hour or two in the cool of the evening, lounging at will and enjoying themselves, oblivious to the restraints of all conventionalities.

Such a structure admits of the most perfect lighting, ventilation and drainage, and with due precautions can be made to effectually banish the odor and housefly nuisances, from the balance of the premises.

In cities a wise compromise or substitute can be resorted to by transporting the culinary and dining departments to the top of the house. This plan has been introduced, but is not yet common or popular. It has every hygienic and æsthetic argument in its favor. On this floor ample room is usually at command, lighting and ventilating facilities are ample, and disagreeable odors are dissipated in space; they do not descend.

Next in importance is the living room. This should be the grand rallying center— a sort of compromise and composite of kitchen, dining-room, library and parlor, with the cooking, dining and prim-propriety functions omitted. This room should be large, light, airy, and full of everything that conduces to comfort and good cheer,— books, music, pictures, flowers, couches, easy chairs, and a reasonable sprinkling of happy children! Here, again, is opportunity and plenty of logical excuse for extravagance. The room cannot be too large, nor too light, nor too full of unostentatious but thoroughly substantial furnishings that at all times invite to rest, reaction, and amusement, and that are never too good to be used.

Of the drawing-room or "parlor" little need be said. It has its conventional uses, and makes a good lumber or storage room for bric-à-brac that is seldom looked at, except when it is dusted! If there is a room in the house in which the doctor is not interested it is the parlor. Social ambition and inbred conventional pride will in most cases determine its location, size, shape, and appointments; but if possible one should avoid making it an artistic dungeon, "o'erwhelmed with a dim, religious light," into which conventional but not "best" friends are inveigled and regaled for half an hour, with suboxidized emanations of foreign tapestries, and the semi-suffocative punctiliousness of the prescribed proprieties. Fortunately, if "good form" is their

highest conception of godliness, they do not stay long, and they do not come very often; therefore, both the entertained and the entertainers will survive an ordeal that is inimical to health and depressing to spirits in exact proportion to its length and frequency. Perhaps evolution will eventually eliminate the room, or transform it into a picture gallery, music chamber or recitation room. It is no longer accepted as an exponent of its owners' taste, culture or financial pretensions. The word itself is from the French *parler*, to speak, and hence signifies the talking room—in blunter English, the *gossip room*. None too sentimental in its origin, it is being rapidly vulgarized by innovation and association. We already have "misfit," "tonsorial" and "oyster" parlors, "billiard," "smoking," and "gambling" parlors, "parlor" maids, mantels, and matches, "ice-cream" and "lunch" parlors—the list is already extensive and is constantly lengthening. No one need be surprised to hear of "beer parlors," "bootblacking" or even "chewing-gum" parlors.

Now that the name is lapsing into disgrace it would be more appropriate to call this perfunctory apartment and traditional appendage the "show room." Under this name we could consistently embower it in all the tawdry, germ-harboring hangings, conventional pictures, hung in Dutch-gilt frames, bizarre bric-à-brac—everything called for by prevailing fashion and permitted by our means, or our mortgages! A few ambitious people are straining to transplant or imitate the Paris *salon*, but this presupposes a degree of wealth, art and culture quite beyond the reach of ordinary mortals. It calls for mansions and millions, for architects and artists, and for social and literary queens, who are not yet overwhelmingly in evidence, but all of which and whom are being aped and cultivated on this side the Atlantic. We are rapidly accumulating the millions, and we are building the *Maisons d'Or*. Later on in its swiftly changing history, what this American democracy, with foreign and "plutocratic" tendencies, will evolve along social and æsthetic lines no living seer can foretell.

SURGEON-GENERAL GEORGE M. STERN-
BERG has fully accepted the mosquito theory
of the transmission of yellow fever, and in
his official capacity has issued an order to
the army treating the conclusions of the
physicians who made the recent experiments in Havana as demonstrated facts, to
be used as the basis for all governmental
action against the disease. The General's
course will evoke a howl of protest from all
the people who, from timidity or self-inter-
est, are opposed to any change in the present
methods of disinfection and quarantine, but
he will have the support of many and high
scientific authorities—of all, indeed, who
have any appreciable right to speak on the
subject—and his prompt acceptance and
practical application of the new discoveries
deserve the warmest commendation, especially from those of us who, two years or so
ago, were applying to General Sternberg
adjectives not remarkable for kindliness. In
an address which the Surgeon-General delivered this week before the American Social
Science Association, in annual session in
Washington, he presented the mosquito
theory in all its details, and thoroughly
justified the immense importance which he
and others familiar with the results attained
ascribe to it. He credited Dr. George Finley, an American long resident in Havana,
with having been the first to suspect the
relation between yellow fever and mosquitoes. Now, Dr. Finley was undoubtedly
the first to give the matter serious attention,
and the investigation which he made fifteen
years ago certainly forms the beginning of
real work in this line, but the insects were
suspected long before that. A friend informs us that not much, if any, later than
1847, he heard Dr. J. K. Mitchell, father
of Dr. S. Weir Mitchell, tell of an experience on the African coast that set the doctor to wondering whether litoral fevers and
mosquito bites did not somehow go together. The ship he was on lay long in a
river mouth, but no fevers developed among
the crew until off-shore winds began to
blow, bringing clouds of mosquitoes with
them. The phenomena did not seriously
impress Dr. Mitchell, but he remembered it
and more than once made it a subject of
conversation.—*New York Times.*

DIETS FOR EVERY DAY USE.

BY J. WARREN ACHORN, M.D.,
Boston.

THE question of foods and their application to the individual for the relief of acute
diseases or chronic disorders, with our present accurate knowledge of their composition,
compatibility, time and place of digestion,
action and effect, has passed the stage of
experimentation and is on a successful scientific basis.

Physicians should be able to write their
prescriptions to the baker-chemist, to-day,
with as much knowledge and confidence as
they write prescriptions for medicine to the
druggist. Double prescribing should certainly secure more speedy and permanent relief for a patient than either method practiced alone, and it *does,* but of the two, regulation of the system through regulation of
the food should come first, unless the severity of the symptoms for a time calls for the
heroic use of medicines.

Putting drugs into a stomach or system
that is at a standstill affords little satisfaction to an intelligent physician, even if done
for the purpose of starting that system up,
unless dietetics are also applied for the same
purpose, and the *after* purpose of securing
permanent results. The doctor knows that
the majority of cases he is called upon to
treat, aside from infectious diseases and
acute disorders of whatever nature, are due
to the improper use of our "every-day
foods" and bad habits.

If his knowledge of the use of food is as
clever as his knowledge of drugs, and he has
the best interest of his patient at heart, he
will write a diet list instead of a prescription
and the result will sustain the practice. By
the time his patient is well he will have been
taught a good habit and gotten rid of a bad

one, to his everlasting credit and relief. Or, if drugs are adhered to, because that is the way most of us have been trained and upon what we have been taught to depend, regulating the food with skill and care will certainly help their action.

It takes just as much of a machine, in working order, and imposes just as much strain upon it, probably, to assimilate drugs, as foods prescribed to accomplish the same purpose. Hypodermic medication may be made the exception.

Leaving patients to continue doing the thing that makes them ill, only to have them relapse regularly, while the doctor repeats his medicines for their temporary relief, is not the best that physicians can do.

There are schools where men are taught to run locomotive engines; there certainly ought to be schools or gymnasia, where a man can go and learn how to run himself.

What older physicians have acquired from experience, young physicians might be taught; that food and drink are an integral part of the treatment of disease. This subject should be as thoroughly a part of medical education as our present knowledge of the subject warrants.

NOTES.

Liquids should be distributed evenly through the day.

Limitation of liquids lessens the work of the heart.

A small amount of fluid beyond the needs of the system may overtax the heart; a small amount less than needed, by lowering the pressure and allowing the blood to thicken in the capillaries, increases resistance and lessens elimination.

The quantity of urine, the edema present, if any, the force of the heart's action and the arterial tension are guides to the action of liquids and the amount required.

The stimulating properties of hot water in heart disease, with many, is equal to that of alcohol.

Hot water four hours after meals starts a flagging digestion and washes out the stomach.

One or two eggs should be sufficient for breakfast; if not eaten at this time one may be taken with the evening meal.

A dinner should consist of not more than three courses; at most two vegetables are allowed.

Supper should be the lightest meal of the day.

A typical diet in heart disease should be mainly nitrogenous—"cooked gluten," gluten bread, almond meal, almond milk, milk, peas, string beans, other lentils, eggs and meat.

In heart disease of not severe type, onions, asparagus, lettuce, water cresses and tomatoes may be eaten.

DIET IN HEART DISEASE.

(Copyright.)

ON rising, take a small cup of hot water, adding a little aromatic spirits of ammonia, if desired; sip slowly.

BREAKFAST: *Cereals*—Cestus "Cooked Gluten," other gluten, shredded wheat, biscuit powder, milk arrowroot; strained oatmeal or oat porridge with cream—a saucer full.

Meats—Scraped meat ball, top of the round steak, mutton chops, tripe; pepper and salt.

Fish—Weak fish, sole, haddock, chicken halibut; trout, perch, pickerel; boiled or broiled. Other fine fibered fish, not fat.

Eggs—Soft boiled, poached or scrambled—one.

Whipped eggs.

Breads—Gluten bread, pulled bread, soup sticks, pilot bread, zwieback; whole wheat or stale bread, toasted and redried—one slice. Butter, prune marmalade.

Fruits (raw ripe fruit)—Apples, pears, peaches, white grapes, well

Nuts with toast and fruit make a substantial dinner, or some of the nut foods may be tried. Masticate thoroughly and not impatiently.

Fats, starches and sugar are the enemies of heart disease; fats are badly absorbed in severe cases, while sugar and starches ferment.

A preliminary exclusive milk diet for two weeks or longer is beneficial in some cases of cardiac dyspepsia—it rests the stomach, lowers arterial tension and by its diuretic action regulates the circulation.

A weak heart, whether due to valvular disease, fatty degeneration, dilatation or some exhausting disease, hinders digestion by checking absorption from the stomach. A dry diet is indicated.

If patients are very thirsty on a dry diet, hot water may be sipped between meals.

Milk and lime water, soda bi-carbonate, sour lemonade and dilute phosphoric acid relieve the thirst incident to a dry diet.

In valvular disease, if compensation is good, the extremities nourished and warm, no strict dietetic treatment is indicated, no matter how loud the murmurs.

Valvular disease, cardiac enlargement, fatty degeneration do not require different forms of diet, except in so far as is necessary to meet special symptoms or satisfy complicating diseases.

In valvular disease with gastric and intestinal catarrh a light diet is indicated—white meats, fine-fibred fish, whites of eggs, arrow-root, rice, corn meal, wheaten grits and milk.

cooked fruits, the inside of stewed
prunes, stewed or minced figs.

Drinks—Almond milk, infusion of
cocoa nibs, milk and lime water, milk
and hot water, cream and seltzer, cereal
coffee. Or, a small cup of hot water at
the close of each meal.

A. M. BETWEEN MEALS: Almond milk, buttermilk, weak lemonade; grape fruit if
constipated.

DINNER: *Soups*—Light, clear consommé.
Purees of tomatoes, asparagus, fresh
peas, sweet corn, celery, onions, and
squash.

Any *fish* mentioned. Pounded fish.

Any *meat* mentioned. (red) Roast
lamb, roast mutton, rare roast beef;
(white) broiled chicken, pounded
chicken, chicken wings, sweet breads,
game birds.

Vegetables—Spinach, tomatoes, stewed celery, baked potatoe, macaroni.

Any *bread* mentioned. Toast with
butter.

Any *fruit* mentioned. Hazel nuts,
almonds, chestnuts.

Any *drink* mentioned. Milky cocoa
without sugar.

Desserts—Milk pudding, cottage
cheese, renét custard, blanc mange, junket, sponge cake.

P. M. BETWEEN MEALS: A small glass of
hot water; a cup of weak tea with
cream and sugar. Irish moss tea, meat
juice, warm or cold. Lemon juice for
thirst. No solids.

SUPPER: Oysters, raw or stewed, the soft
part.

Eggs—If they have not been eaten in
the morning.

Vegetables—Baked potato—best in
the morning in place of cereals.

Breads—Toast, one slice. Bread and
milk alone.

Fruit—Any mentioned. Unsweetened apple sauce. A baked pear.

Drinks—China tea, almond milk,
Irish moss tea.

Desserts—Whites of eggs custard,
gluten custard.

9 P. M.—A small glass of hot water.

Valvular disease with veinal obstruction, causing congestion of the liver, is apt to produce
nausea, loss of appetite or vomiting even—whey,
milk, lime water and soda are useful here.

If compensation is very bad and digestion
greatly interfered with, liquids must be depended
on, taken in small amount and often repeated.

Acute attacks of indigestion in valvular disease
call for laxatives, whipped milk, whipped eggs
and broth, every three hours for the first few
days, with a gradual return to solids.

Valvular disease in itself does not preclude the
use of alcohol.

Coffee and cocoa are better than tea in valvular
disease, generally.

Palpitation may be due to dilated stomach, irritation of the sympathetic nerves from displace-
ment of some of the viscera, to disease of the
heart itself or blood vessels, to alcohol, morphine,
tobacco, sexual excess, uterine disease, tea, coffee
or red meat.

Palpitation due to dietetic errors is easily remedied—by a light diet, small meals, non-flatulent
food, the avoidance of tea, coffee and tobacco or
any other habit recognized as detrimental. Palpitation and dyspnea occurring suddenly, only
small amounts of food at a time are to be permitted.

Laxative food and fruits are indicated in palpitation.

Hypertrophy is usually associated with some
other lesion—in severe cases, rest in bed and non-
stimulating diet is best.

Well cooked fruits are admissible in hypertrophy and valvular disease.

Sudden dilatation calls for bed and a milk diet;
dilatation calls for the use of alcohol. In dilatation of long standing, small meals and a dry diet
may prove beneficial.

Fatty heart in the obese calls for the avoidance
of fats, sweet wines, milk and sugar—liquids
should not exceed a pint and a half in twenty-four
hours.

Arterial degeneration calls for a vegetable diet;
the condition of the kidneys must be known.
Tufnell's diet may be tried. Port wine or claret
may be used by old people.

Arterio-sclerosis calls for a milk diet—no meat
or alcohol. Oysters are to be avoided. A milk
diet relieves at once the headache and insomnia.

In angina pectoris the evening meal must be
small; the indications are to decrease the arterial
tension—a vegetable milk diet does this.

In an acute attack of angina, from over-eating,
the stomach pump is indicated.

Ulcerative endocarditis calls for broths, eggs,
pounded meat.

Myocarditis, if recognized, calls for alcohol.

In pericarditis of rheumatic origin stimulants
should be avoided; if associated with Bright's
disease, the condition of the kidneys determines
the diet.

Rapid heart is a neuro-muscular disorder and
not related to gastric disease; mere frequency of
the pulse is not trachycardia.

Slow heart or irregular, is seen in nervous
dyspepsia, splashing stomach, dragging stomach,
retention and ulcer. Strong excitation of the
gastric mucous membrane slows the heart's
action; if gastric catarrh or any of the diseases

INHERITANCE OF ACQUIRED TENDENCIES.

VERY much study has been given to the subject of the inheritance of the peculiarities of the ancestors. It has been accepted now as a working axiom, says the Canadian *Practitioner and Review*, that there are many characteristics of the ancestors that may skip a generation, or more, and then reappear. These characteristics are fixed in the germ-plasm of the species, and, though they may not always appear, they are always potentially present. It is in this way that unexpected peculiarities, or powers, may be found in a person, no trace of such being noted in the near ancestry. These are spoken of as latent powers, or features, and account for instances of atavism, or reversion. The crossing of races tends strongly to bring out these latent ancestral characteristics.

But when one passes to the consideration of acquired characteristics, the ground is not so secure. Many have argued with great energy that acquired characteristics can be transmitted. This has again been as strongly denied. If acquired characteristics cannot be transmitted, then nothing that was not in the first germ-plasm can be passed on from one generation to another. Something less may be, but nothing more can be. By this view the first germ-plasm must have been endowed with every potentiality that any member of the race has yet manifested, or may ever in the future manifest. But there are great difficulties in the way of this theory. Take, for example, the variations due to environment, as in the color of different races. Here the peculiarity appears to have become perfectly fixed, and the germ-plasm of the race has been so modified by the somatoplasm that the color has become a certain feature in the heredity of the race. If acquired characteristics cannot be transmitted, then every possibility of color, genius, disposition and activities must have been provided for in the first germ-plasm. But it is known and admitted that as a given race advances in civilization, the children are born with greater capacities and mature with larger brains and more comprehensive powers than their remote ancestors.

When one turns to the study of disease, some of the strongest arguments are found for the view that acquired characteristics are inherited. If Weismann is correct, that the somatoplasm does not affect the germ-plasm, and that every potentiality is found in the germ-plasm, how can the inheritance of acquired disease and disease tendencies be explained? It is well recognized in pathology that a certain mode of life produces gout. Several generations of this mode of life fixes the gouty diathesis very firmly in the family history. It becomes then a question of great difficulty to eliminate this gouty tendency, and even though a member of such a family lives in a most appropriate manner, he may not escape. He then has an acquired condition, and one that in the first place acted upon the somatoplasm, has modified the germ-plasm so as to make the diathesis hereditary, even though efforts are made to neutralize this tendency. This line of argument could be pushed much further. All in all, it would appear the acquired characteristics may become hereditary, and this is the view of many eminent scientists.

✠ ✠

Dr. Achorn's "diet list" in Bronchitis will be published in June GAZETTE.

mentioned is present, a non-stimulating diet or one to meet the indications is in order.

In slow heart with no recognized disorder of the stomach a stimulating diet goes best—red meats, eggs, potatoes, some fruits, green vegetables, gluten, oatmeal and concentrated sweets.

In senile heart five hours must elapse between meals and no solid food be taken in the interim.

If oatmeal and cream are eaten nothing else goes with it. If the heart is feeble or dilated,

half an ounce of brandy or Holland gin may be taken at lunch time in three ounces of water.

Constipation is to be avoided by the use of the pulp of cooked fruit, or vegetable purees, taken at meals, or between meals.

Almond milk.—Remove the skin of twenty almonds by scalding, powder in a mortar, add to a pint of boiling water, allow to stand over night. Filter through a cloth. Use one part of emulsion to two of milk.

Department of Physiological Chemistry.

WITH SPECIAL REFERENCE TO DIETETICS AND NUTRITION IN GENERAL.

NEXT!

WHAT has become of the Ralston Club? We do not hear much of late concerning this once popular organization. It flourished for some years most remarkably, numbered its members by millions, and possibly still flourishes, since it is semi-secret. Its name has been hitched to various articles of merchandise, from footgear to food products, and from coffee substitutes to water stills. Its founder and his immediate disciples must have retired on a competence, for his scheme caused money to flow like water, and his converts did not waver in their enthusiasm. Along with its folderol it inculcated many hygienic rules that were sensible and sadly neglected. This was the secret of its success, and there is no disputing the fact that the orgaonization did a sight of good to the world. It invented some special terms for its dietetic and other semi-mysteries. "Glame" was the potent principle in any food product that made it valuable and nutritious. According to the philosophy of these physico-pious saints, the average dietary was not selected with due regard to the "glame" it contained. Some things contained "glame" when perfectly fresh but soon lost it with age. For example, fresh honey contained "glame;" old honey was glameless, and so on. They taught people to bathe, which is a good thing, and to breathe, which is even more necessary. A hundred forced inspirations at a dose, and two or three times a day, at specified hours and in the open air, wasn't the prescription of a fool, and has no doubt put new life into thousands of stingy breathers. . . . There was a lot of nonsense mixed in with their sensible teachings, but no more than the populace on its present plane demands.

Every member became a veritable walking delegate and preached his aggressive gospel on all possible occasions. As a result, no similar movement or organization of which we have any record has made such rapid progress in proselyting the public. Nor was it content with merely making converts. It arranged a system of degrees and promotions in pseudo-scientific occultism through which members were induced to progress until they should attain to some promised thirty-third degree of perfection, after which they were to be able to navigate the air or remove mountains. Of course this is not a literal statement, but it was something equally sublime and impossible. Everything they taught was decorous, virtuous and smacked of genuine piety; and hence it is more than likely that from the ranks of this club came all the aftercrop of mind-curists, Eddyites and Christ-science cranks, who now hold the boards.

These, too, will change, for the modern mind craves novelty and always wants it cloaked under some far-fetched or taking name. It is not likely that any of the new names will achieve any marked permanence or immortality. Scores of later names have been suggested, but in this matter the old adage will prove true. Many names will be called but few will be chosen, because only a few have the genuine staying power.

Schlatter, who created such a flutter of excitement a few years ago, and was reported to have gone into the wilderness of New Mexico and suffered translation, leaving only his bones and those of his old white horse behind, has returned; but he now has no more prestige than any one of the several hundred soothsayers and "spirt" mediums that advertise their necromancy in the yellow journals.

Next !

MEAT RATION IN THE TROPICS.[1]

UNDER the above title, Dr. Egan, Surgeon U. S. Army, publishes in a recent number of the *Boston Medical and Surgical Journal* a rather remarkable paper, which we herewith reproduce. We give space to this paper, not because we agree with its arguments or coincide with its conclusions. We are quite ready to agree with Dr. Egan, that the dietary of the Porto Ricans should be reformed in very essential particulars, but we do not believe that its principal lack is *chuleta de cerdo*, or *"Char-r-rones."*

In short, we hold the doctor's views to be the result of superficial observation or prejudice, or of both, and that his deductions are distorted and unreliable. We trust that the wide publicity given to the paper will provoke profitable discussion and result in bringing out the bottom facts. The pernicious anemia to which Dr. Egan calls particular attention may be the result of a poorly selected vegetable regimen, or it may be caused by any one of a dozen other unhygienic conditions, not one of which is hinted at by the author. Dr. Egan writes:

Following the late Spanish War, American soldiers were scattered from the Arctic Circle to the Equator. Speculation as to their requirements under these new surroundings soon became rife. The necessary clothing alterations were sufficiently apparent, but the requisite food is still a matter of discussion. In the first days of the occupation of Porto Rico an officer of the line wrote home that his principal food consisted of crackers and milk, and that he was in excellent health because he avoided all heating diet.

Physiologists had for a long time observed that there was a rise of body temperature of nearly one degree in the tropics;

[1] Read before the Lyceum, Fort Douglas, Utah, January 2, 1901.

that the pulse-rate was lowered; that respiration and blood pressure were diminished; and that there was a marked languor and tendency to depression. Proteids and fats increased heat production, and should, it was stated, be abandoned or used very sparingly. They also proceeded to analyze the diet consumed by the Negro in the Antilles, the Hindoo in India, and the Malay in the Eastern Archipelago, and to point out a great diminution of the proteids and fats in his dietary. But they also discovered that the carbohydrates were diminished to an equal degree; or, in other words, that their diets were those of chronic starvation, a condition that exists to some extent in most tropical countries where the rate of increase of population is so great that the country is unable to raise sufficient produce to feed them, and where, as in India, famines are now beginning to be regarded as inevitable. Overlooking these facts they declared that there was need of more sugar and tropical vegetables, and less meat and fat to reduce our dietary to their standard; that is, to the standard of those who are unable to procure nourishing food. But coming nearer home, these same physiologists would not for a moment declare that because the Crofter lives on oatcake, and the cotter on potatoes, that the diet suitable to Scotland was oatmeal, and to Ireland, potatoes. Yet, guided by their theories, some, like the line officer, lived principally on crackers and milk, and others believed, like Major Louis Livingston Seaman, surgeon to the First Volunteer Engineers, who is reported as declaring before the board of officers on the tropical ration that what should have been a delightful outing for his regiment was turned into a tragedy because of the heating foods his troops had to eat. When they landed in Porto Rico not a man was on sick report. In less than three months nearly one-third of the regiment was on the sick list, and the rest were scarcely able to carry their personal belongings when they reached New York. Dr. Seaman said that all had suffered from bowel irritation, and that when they needed delicate food they had to use that which had inflamed the intestinal tract and had produced symptoms like a catarrhal condition, making the patient peculiarly subject to attacks of typhoid and other fevers. He also said the food used was diet food, and not the regular rations. However, few of the persons who have had extended experience of the tropics agree to the so-called heating effects of the proteids; nor does the diet of the natives who can afford other than starvation fare tend to support this theory. The late governor, General Henry, of Porto Rico, wrote, in December, 1899: "The better class live and dress like ourselves. The food of this class is, for the early meal, coffee and bread for breakfast; at noon, coffee, vegetables, eggs, meat and dulces, or sweets. The night meal is about the same. They are great meat eaters, it being cooked in various ways."

Duty has taken me at one time or another, since the first day of the American invasion, into almost every town from Ysabella, on the northwest coast, to Humacao, on the east coast, and then up the military road to this capital. In the districts of Guayama and Southern Humacao it was part of my business to investigate the cause of deaths among the natives. Everywhere I found the main cause assigned to be anemia and phthisis. Everywhere I went I was struck by this ever-prevalent anemia. The pale, yellowish, waxy skin, the bloodless lips, and the swollen, puffy features, formed a picture never seen by me outside of tropical Porto Rico. Yet I soon found that these people had been living on rice, beans, maize, dried codfish and fruits. Meat very rarely entered into their diet. On the other hand, I soon discovered that the people who lived in the towns and could afford it, ate two hearty meals daily. These people, I believe. use more meat than we use in American cities, and there is no doubt in my mind that I have used more meat and felt more need of it since I have been here than ever in the same time in the United States. Yet I am one of the few who did not have to go home for ill health, while the natives that eat in

the hotels with me, and as freely as I do, are perfectly healthy individuals, and show not the least trace of anemia. Only a few days since, a native informed me, with much gusto, that one of the best things that Porto Rico afforded was *chuleta de cerdo* (pork chops), surely one of the most unsuitable articles of diet for a tropical climate, as our physiological friends will tell us, and yet the absence of which, in my opinion, made the native anemic to a noticeable degree. These observations are so common in this climate, and have been so forcibly impressed on me, that I feel more and more the wisdom of going very, very slowly in urging alterations in the ration.

Major Stephenson, Surgeon U. S. Army, made the following statement: "My personal experience of a year in Tampa, Porto Rico and Santiago was that I craved and ate as much meat of all kinds relatively to all food eaten in cooler climates. I believe that meat consumption among the natives of hot climates is limited to their purses, not to their tastes. In Cuba and Porto Rico I found the noon and evening meals in private houses and restaurants prodigal of meats of all kinds."

The absurdity of arguing from theory and not from experience was forcibly impressed on me as I read on a balcony in San Juan the essay that gained the hundred dollar prize given by Major Louis Livingston Seaman for the ideal tropical ration. As I reached the part that discussed the "distaste for fats in considerable quantities, so early acquired in the tropics," I was aroused by the cry of the "Char-r-rone" vendor. For more than a month I had noticed that same cry every afternoon. I had tried faithfully during that time to detect what he was calling out. but had as signally failed. until one evening I was fortunate enough to have an Englishman. educated in Spain. along with me when he made his rounds. Then I learned that "Char-r-rone" was the Porto Rican abbreviation for "chicharrones," and that this was Spanish for pork fried crisp with the skin on it. For twenty centavos I obtained a piece about a foot square. I found that, while the outside was crisp, the interior of my piece, an inch in thickness, was simply cold fat pork, with a very little lean through it. The man sold it as a bonne bouche through the streets every afternoon. A couple of mouthfuls was all I desired to test, but the rapidity and relish with which my four little Porto Rican girl friends devoured it gave me a striking example of the "distaste for fats in any quantity, so early acquired in the tropics," and of the value to be attached to theories derived from analysis of "jibaro" dietary, as to what constitutes a suitable food for the tropics. On the other hand, it is now being claimed by some writers that the depression and languor of the tropics call for increased food and vinous stimulants, and this idea seems to be warranted by the large amount of meat, and of claret, or water with a dash of rum, used twice daily by the better classes of the population.

The board before which Major Seaman made his plea has recently, according to the public press, reported to the Secretary of War that, "The recommendation that the fresh meat ration be reduced in quantity was so opposed to all the teachings of experience, both in our country and in Cuba and Porto Rico, that the board was unable to accept the recommendation as conclusive without further investigation. Two members of the board have served in Cuba and the third in Porto Rico, and their personal experience has been that as much meat has been desired and eaten as in the United States, and with no deleterious effect on the health of the men. The natives of these countries are also large meat eaters when they are able to secure it, and the meat eaters are noticeably stronger and healthier looking than the poorer classes, who from necessity are mainly vegetarians. The board also interviewed a number of officers and other persons who had been in the Philippines, and, taking all sources of information together, the board is of the opinion that it would be a mistake to make any fixed reduction in the meat ration." The criticism of General Henry in the above quoted

article that, "The objection to the meat (of Porto Rico) for an American is, that, having no place to keep beef after being killed, it has to be put in the pot in a hot, quivering condition; and I believe this made many an American soldier ill," is in part well applied. Porto Rican beef cannot be cooked American fashion and be other than tough and unpalatable, as it is killed about 3 o'clock in the morning, and eaten by 11 or 12 o'clock the same day. I had so fully recognized this fact that for more than a year before leaving the island I refused all "bifstek" or "rostbif," as presented by the seductive native. Only Swift or Armour refrigerated beef can in Porto Rico be prepared American fashion. Native beef, however, prepared by native cooking, is tender and palatable, devoid of this objection, and is habitually consumed with only the best results. In fact, when they ask us to replace the meat ration by vegetables we should not forget the Spanish motto that says: *Bellotas y tostones hacer malos trabajadores.* (Acorns and toast make bad workmen.)

✢ ✢

SOME CURRENT ABSURDITIES IN DIET.

In an address on the subject of chronic Bright's disease, recently delivered before the Halifax Medical Society, Dr. Alfred Barrs pointed out, says *The Hospital,* how absurd were some of the restrictions as to diet, which are sometimes imposed upon patients suffering from this disorder. In laying down a diet for such a case one must remember, he said, that chronic Bright's disease is a very chronic disorder, and when properly managed is not incompatible with much usefulness, and not a little enjoyment of life, and we ought to take care that such usefulness and enjoyment are not unnecessarily curtailed by anything we may do. We do not keep all patients suffering from this disease in bed to the end of their days, neither ought we to keep them continuously on restricted diets.

To limit the input of proteid material so as to bring the work of the kidney within its capacity, is to act on scientific lines; but we know so little of the more remote stages of nitrogenous metabolism that, beyond this very general statement we cannot safely go. Yet there is no disease in which the tyranny of diet has been so recklessly practised. To live for weeks and weeks on a purely milk diet is not necessary, is indeed distinctly harmful, and there is no clear evidence that it meets the scientific indication. It has been shown that the output of nitrogen is greater on a purely milk diet than on an ordinary mixed diet, so that as far as the urea output is concerned, there is no theoretical advantage in such a diet, and clinical experience in chronic Bright's disease shows the same thing. Dr. Barr's rule is simplicity itself. He says that if the bowels are acting freely the patient may live on such ordinary mixed diet, including meat, as he has an appetite for and can digest. Patients who are confined to bed and suffering from uremic vomiting or diarrhea, and are getting towards the end of the disease, cannot, of course, have any appetite, and the difficulty is to contrive food of any kind for them. The distinctions, again, which we draw between different kinds of meat in dieting cases of renal disease and gout are ridiculous. A patient may eat chicken and fish, and not mutton, mutton and not beef, and so on. There is no reason for this. Pork, which is white, and, in the case of Alexis St. Martin was shown to be the most digestible of meats, is usually entirely forbidden. Van Noorden mentions the case of a patient with chronic parenchymatous nephritis, who took half a pound of poultry daily for five days, during which he excreted the same amount of nitrogen, and a trifle more albumin than he did in the next five days, in which, instead of poultry, he took an equivalent amount of nitrogen in beef. Water and other fluid sustenance should be taken freely, but alcohol is perhaps as well avoided if cardiac failure does not require it.

✤ ✤

CAMEMBERT is no doubt the best and most salable of the soft and fancy cheeses which have become so popular during the past few years, and instructions as to the method of making them will, no doubt, be appreciated. About five gallons of good new milk are required, says *London Health*, to make one dozen cheeses, and the curd is made in two batches, half of the milk being set in the morning and the other half in the evening. The temperature of the milk used ranges between 80° and 84° F., depending on whether the day is hot or cold, and rennet is used in sufficient quantity to cause a fairly firm coagulation in three hours. The rennet is always measured with a cubic centimeter pipette, which is much better than the ordinary method of measuring, as small and exact quantities have to be used.

Let us suppose that it is required to make one dozen cheeses. Twenty-five pounds of morning's milk would be required, and if the natural heat is in the milk, so much the better. The temperature is raised or lowered to, say 82° F., the milk being set in wooden tubs, which conserve the heat. We add to this milk two cubic centimeters of Hansen's rennet, mixed with a little water, and stir occasionally the first half-hour. In about three hours the curd will be ready to ladle out into the moulds, which are perforated tin cylinders five inches high and as many broad.

These moulds are placed on straw mats, which assist drainage, and give to the cheese a nice surface. In ladling out, care must be taken not to break or smash the curd, or loss of fat will result. In the evening the same quantity of milk is taken, and treated in exactly the same way, except that perhaps a little more rennet would be required, the evening's milk being richer. By the time the evening curd is ready, that made in the morning will have sunk considerably, which enables us to fill in the other curd, having previously broken up the top of the first curd, so that the two will join properly. By the evening of the second day the cheeses will have settled, and be sufficiently firm to turn on to fresh mats, when they are slightly salted on the upper surface and left for twelve hours, being then turned and salted on the other surface and sides, and the moulds removed.

The cheeses remain in the making room for four days, when they are placed on shelves covered with straw; in a room where they can get currents of air, which ensures partial drying. While here they become covered with a fine white fungus or mould, peculiar to Camembert, and which is absolutely necessary in order to obtain the proper flavor, as the mycelium of this fungus strikes down into the cheese and causes changes in the substance equivalent to ripening. If a half-ripe Camembert is cut in two, the peculiar effect of the fungus can be seen, as we have, as far as the roots of the mould have penetrated—a yellowish, creamy substance, while the center will be neither more nor less than unripe curd. After the cheeses have been in the drying room about a week a fine blue mould will make its appearance, which is an indication that they are ready to be removed to the cellar or cave to perfect ripening. This cellar should be cool (about 50° F.), and dark, with very little ventilation and a fairly moist air, and provided with shelves covered with straw, on which the cheeses are placed. Turning is done each day, and in the course of three or four weeks they will be ripe, which condition is known by their assuming a reddish tint, and the body of the cheese on pressing being soft and yielding. A ripe Camembert weighs about eleven ounces. They are sent to market in packages of six, wrapped in straw, which keeps the cheeses in shape.

TABLE TALK.

THERE is a happy medium between garrulity and reticence at table: but, like the Scriptural narrow path, "few there be that find it!" And yet, the household dinner should serve up an attractive intellectual *menu*. Why not? Are we to bank the fires of intellectual energy as soon as we begin to eat? If the stomach becomes absorbent is that any reason why the brain should grow dormant? I have noted over and over again that clever people are anything but clever while dining. I have sat out public dinners where the conversation fairly driveled, only to hear those same drivelers speak with force and pertinency when the cloth was removed. It is much the same in the household on the average scale. Papa in his library chair, with lighted cigar, grows amiable and entertaining; but, at mealtime, he will not shake off the repressive coil of taciturnity. Being the chief actor on the boards, in his own estimation, at least, he gives the cue to wife and children. Is it strange that they are more concerned about the dish of gravy than they are about an interchange of ideas. I suppose it is our American habit, fostered by high pressure, compound-engine speed in getting through with a given task. We are unlike the German, the Frenchman, the Italian, and even the Spaniard. Consequently, we find color, life, buoyancy, effervescence on tables other than our own. The physical result is that indigestion in America touches high-water mark. If every member of an American household were forced at table to tell a story, propound a conundrum, recite a current event, or even to box the compass—why, the time gained would make the gastric juices to leap for joy!

Now Nature's order is that of corruscation of brains co-incident with mastication of food. Where do you find some of the most brilliant sayings in literature? In monologues? ·Not at all. Rather in the reported table talk of great minds. There is something in good cheer that promotes good fellowship. And good fellowship ought to loosen tongues more quickly and certainly more safely than champagne. We utterly fail to appreciate this fact in our ordinary domestic intercourse. It is a curious thing that Americans, so keenly alive to humor as a class, should sit down at the home table with the gravity of pall-bearers! The voice of the prattling, even "bumptious" child, is not infrequently a welcome diversion. It breaks an exasperating silence only relieved by the clashing of knife and fork. It may be that simpler fare would remedy the evil. The American meal is not infrequently a hecatomb of dainties. And between the task of eliminating what one does not wish from that which one desires, the mind is quite preoccupied. But, whatever the reason, the absence of table talk hits hard the virtue of conviviality and the blessing of perfect digestion. At heart, in spite of our adaptability, we are a pretty serious people. Most middle-class households would be momentarily upset by the advent of a genuine *bonvivant* of the Brillant-Savarin type. In France he creates no surprise. We take our food seriously, and, if Max O'Rell is to be credited, take our pleasures penitentially. The joyous, bright, unhindered flow of talk at dinner is the exception, not the rule. In rural commuities taciturnity is appalling. I know because in my early career as a preacher I have exhausted every topic from oats to oasis in the vain effort to elicit reciprocity! In cities the case is not so bad, but it is still obvious, this paucity of table comment, badinage, discussion, and repartee. If all the clever things said by clever people after dinner were said at dinner, the dreadful awkwardness between courses, now so conspicuous, would disappear. Somebody remarked not long ago that what we most needed in culinary affairs was a revival of table talk and not the refinement of a *menu!* That somebody was right. The more one talks at dinner the less one eats, and that is not an unmitigated calamity since more graves are dug with the teeth than are opened by what we commonly term dissipation.—*Frederick Stanley Root.*

✤ ✤

THE TOBACCO HEART.

AMONG the various causes by which the action of the heart may be disturbed, says *The Hospital,* tobacco occupies an important place. It is of especial interest in that the effect of tobacco can be studied unhampered by many of the complicating circumstances which tend to make the investigation of some other cardiac poisons, such, for example, as alcohol, so difficult. Alcohol undoubtedly poisons the heart, but at the same time it produces a widespread effect on all the tissues, often an actual degeneration, so that in studying the operation of alcohol on the heart, we are in most cases studying its action in a diseased organism. But in tobacco we have a poison which shows its effect upon hearts still sound, and in constitutions otherwise apparently uninjured, and we are thus able to inquire how far a merely temporary toxic agent may be efficient in producing symptoms of cardiac disease. In the Lettsomian Lectures, recently delivered, Dr. Mitchell Bruce says that the uncomplicated effects of tobacco on young healthy hearts, as they present themselves clinically, are palpitation in every instance, a sense of irregular action, poststernal oppression and pain in half the cases, and in one out of every eight sufferers either angina or uncomfortable sensations in the left arm. Faintness or actual faints occur in one-third, and giddiness and a feeling of impending death in a smaller proportion. In 50 per cent. of the cases the heart appears to be of the ordinary size, in a few it is very slightly enlarged; the precordial impulse is often very weak, but occasionally increased in force and frequency, and almost as often irregular as not; the pulse tension is nearly always low. Out of twenty such cases complaining of the heart, not one presented a cardiac murmur beyond a weak systolic bruit varying with posture or cubitus. So much for the cardiac symptoms produced by tobacco in the presumably healthy heart. Now let us turn to the man over forty. In such cases, while palpitation is still the common complaint, pain, including angina, is put forward more prominently, and so are faintness, actual faints, a feeling of impending death, and a sense of cardiac irregularity, each intermission being accompanied with a sudden stab through the precordia. In these subjects the heart is more frequently found to be large and feeble, the same weak systolic murmur as has been mentioned above is to be heard occasionally, the radial pulse is often irregular, and the vessel wall is thick. Thus we have a combination of symptoms and signs sufficient to alarm the casual observer. But if we study them in the light of what we know about the tobacco heart in young subjects on the one hand, and of what we know about the normal condition of the heart arteries at sixty years of age on the other hand, we may be able to reassure ourselves. Every cardio-vascular change which is found in great smokers must not be put down to tobacco, but *vice versa*, precordial pain, angina, faintness, and irregular pulse, in a man sixty years of age with a full-sized heart, are not to be hastily regarded as evidences of grave disease without further inquiry as to his habits. The cardiac enlargement and large pulse may be nothing more than the result of a life of bodily and mental activity; the precordial distress and the other symptoms may be the result only of tobacco. Dr. Mitchell Bruce relates several cases in which well-marked angina was clearly the result of tobacco and ceased to trouble when the tobacco was given up. The moral of this is important, and extends far beyond the question of the tobacco heart, for if tobacco can by itself do so much damage, and if in cases of cardiac disease, or when, without the actual presence of disease the heart is merely getting older, the addition of tobacco poisoning can produce so marked a simulacrum of severe cardiac disease (all of which may vanish on removing this superadded cause), we must in all cases of heart disease look out for the superadded and possibly remediable cause by which the present condition has been produced, and not be content with ascertaining the more or less permanent disorder with which the heart has been more or less successfully struggling perhaps for a long time. We are all apt, says Dr. Mitchell Bruce, to overlook in diagnosis, and still more in

treatment, the fact that, whether in an ordinary senile heart, or in a heart that is the seat of chronic valvular disease, or in arterial degeneration, something more than the pathological changes have to be regarded—usually some entirely adventitious disturbance which alone calls for treatment, such as indigestion, flatulence, worry, a bronchial catarrh, or it may be free indulgence in tobacco, tea, or coffee.

STRAWBERRIES AND GOUT.

A WRITER in *Nature* speaks of the cruel medical tyranny which banishes the strawberry from the diet of the gouty, and quotes what Linnæus had to say about the curative properties of this delightful fruit. The great naturalist was persuaded to take strawberries during a severe attack of sciatica, with the result that sweet sleep ensued, and when he awoke, the pain had sensibly subsided. On the next day he ate as many strawberries as possible, and on the following morning the pain was gone, and he was able to leave his bed. Gouty pains returned at the same date in the next year, but they were dispersed as soon as Linnæus was able to get strawberries. Although strawberries are forbidden to the gouty by some authorities, by others they are permitted, the fruit being regarded as a useful food for such persons on account of its richness in the salts of potash, soda and lime, and its cooling, diuretic and laxative qualities. The analysis of the strawberry shows it to be particularly rich in sodium salts, and in spite of the high percentage of water this fruit excels all other common fruit in the amount of mineral salts. The chemistry of the strawberry, therefore, would teach that this fruit is likely to be beneficial in gouty states.

CLEAN FOOD.

THE importance of making clean all fruit, meat and vegetables that come to us from market is receiving, says the New York

Sun, special attention just now. The dangers from such articles when unclean are very great. Their possibilities for uncleanliness are tremendous. Think of the many hands they pass through, the dust and the filth with which they are brought in contact, the opportunities they offer to the enterprising migratory microbe. All this is especially true with regard to fruit and vegetables. Many a household for years past has had its fruit and vegetables carefully washed before cooking or serving; now-a-days few of them stop short of disinfecting. Fruit bought, as many an average household buys it, upon the street corners, is gradually becoming famous as a carrier of disease. The parents and the physicians of the children who were stricken and died with diphtheria not long ago were at a loss to know how the disease originated. Careful examination failed to reveal anything at fault with the plumbing and drainage; the children had not been associated with diphtheretic patients; in no way could their illness be accounted for. A few days after the last death the father again repaired to his office, and, as he often did, stopped to chat with the Italian fruit vender on the corner. "I haven't seen ye fo' a long time," said the fruit vender. The father admitted that it was so and told why. "It is the sore throat, ye mean?" cried the Italian, and in his turn told how his little family, some time before, had been attacked in the same way and died too. The mystery was explained. At the very time that the Italian's children must have been at the height of their "sore throat" the father had bought and carried home to his own children some oranges.

CAUSES OF HEADACHE.

THE common headache of every-day life is the one we desire to call attention to. We think we are safe in saying that all simple acute headaches are caused by indigestion, which is produced by the use of inferior food or an inability to use good food. Also almost all chronic headaches are caused by dyspepsia, constipation, and disorders of the liver, and these troubles are very closely related. Constipation is always associated with dyspepsia. The liver, the greatest depurating organ of the body, is obstructed and diseased in cases of dyspepsia. So it ought to be understood by all who wish to be informed on the subject that the stomach, bowels, and liver belong to the digestive system, and that one cannot be diseased without more or less involving the others. These are the blood-making organs. About one-sixth of the blood of the body circulates in the head, and when this blood is loaded with impurities and improperly elaborated, then the brain and its structures are irritated and painful. This is called headache. The depurating organs—the bowels, liver, skin, kidneys, and lungs—have failed to carry out the waste of the system from some cause. There has been too little exercise, sitting or working in ill-ventilated rooms, too little or poor quality of food, or partaking of too much wholesome food—overeating. Over-excitement in business or sad and depressing news are among the common causes of disturbances in the system that result in headache.—*Health.*

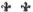

SUN BATHS IN THE TREATMENT OF TUBERCULOUS JOINTS.

MILLIOZ (*Thèse de Lyon,* 1899), unlike Finsen, of Copenhagen, who used the ultra-violet rays of the spectrum in the treatment of lupus, has employed all the rays of sunlight to act on tuberculous joints. He disapproves of the systematic fixation of the limb in which the tuberculous lesion is situated. The patient is placed on a suitable couch in the sunniest part of the garden or other open place, with the affected joint fully exposed to the rays of sunshine. To protect the head of the patient, some sort of sunshade may be improvised. If the upper limb is the seat of the disease, the patient may preferably be allowed to walk about in the garden. The duration of the sun bath should be several hours a day. During the intervals the joint is covered with wool, and rather firmly bandaged. Sometimes after the first or second bath the joint becomes more painful, but this soon passes away in most cases. If it should continue, it may be necessary to intermit the treatment for several days. Rapid pigmentation of the skin by the sun's rays has been noticed to coincide with comparatively quick recovery. The joints are said to become smaller, the skin healthier looking, the discharges, if such be present, less purulent, and the fistulæ close. Such results, however, may require months of treatment.—*British Med. Journal.*

Dr. E. F. Brush, of Mount Vernon, N. Y., in 1892, read before the American Medical Association, at Detroit, Mich., a paper entitled, "The Relation of Food to Scorbutus in Children." In part, Dr. Brush concluded as follows: "Every living creature requires for his proper nourishment some raw, living food. Every young living creature needs living food. The mammalia all take it direct from the living fountain, and young feathered tribes are supplied by their parents with living creatures for food. Even the young fishes consume living animalcula, and man seems to be the only son of God's creatures who thinks he knows better. The artificially-fed infant gets its food from the knowing chemist, or must, according to prevailing fashion, have all life sterilized out of it, if it gets any as Nature supplies it without the intervention of the chemist. I am positive that there is more in organism and the vitality that holds it together than is dreamed of in our advanced chemical knowledge."

THE RECENT CHRISTIAN SCIENCE MIRACLE.

As those of our readers who have access to any of the leading New York papers,

are already aware, "Second Reader" Lathrop of the recently completed "Christian Science" Church in upper New York, announced on Easter Sunday that the corner-stone of that sacred edifice, erected to science and dedicated to the holy St. Eddy, was originally inscribed with a name which did not accord with the wishes or æsthetic taste of "Mother Eddy"; but that, without the touch of visible hands, during its transit from the Vermont quarry, where it was wrought and engraved, that inscription was changed by the simple power of concentrated prayer and mental effort on the part of the faithful. The *New York Times* reviewed. the incident in language that everybody, even an Eddyite, could understand. This drew out Mr. Lathrop with an explanation, to which the *Times* responds as follows:

"We are in receipt of a holographic—that's such a good word!—of a holographic letter from Mr. John Carroll Lathrop, the 'Second Reader' of the new Eddyite Temple on Central Park West, and in it—the letter—Mr. Lathrop presents what he says are the exact facts in regard to the cornerstone miracle described by him to gaping multitudes the day the temple was opened. This version of the episode differs in several rather important details—we will not say from what Mr. Lathrop said, for that would be unkind—but from what every one of the large number of reporters who attended the opening exercises thought they heard him say. It turns what happened to the stone from an out-and-out miracle into not much, if anything, more than a queer and fortunate accident of the sort, duplicated once or twice at least in the experience of us all. As told in the letter, there is nothing quite incredible in the story, and nothing very ridiculous except the importance which the writer attaches to the occurrence and his belief that it illustrates the working of a mystical power. It would, therefore, be to the interest of 'Christian Science' to have the letter published, but we hesitate to print it, and for a very curious reason. Mr.

Lathrop writes a pretty and ladylike hand, but his—well, to be frank, his spelling—is just the least bit peculiar. For instance, he twice writes the word 'Baptist' as 'Babtist.' As a rule we are willing to correct little things like that in communications otherwise acceptable, but we can hardly venture to edit the 'copy' of so important a personage as a 'Second Reader,' of a personage that is, who has won acceptance as a leader of men and women and the adept expounder of a new and precious philosophy. There is, however, a way out of the difficulty. Let Mr. Lathrop and his associates give the manuscript a little 'absent treatment.' No doubt they can exert their all-compelling influence on the misspelled words and bring them under what he calls 'the rule of infinite Harmony.' As they stand at present they jangle terribly with that rule as crystallized in the dictionaries, and surely it ought to be as easy to edit a bit of paper as it was to edit a big block of granite. Then think what an effect it would produce in this office if the letter, while safely in our possession, should suddenly become 'copy' of the sort to which our compositors are accustomed! Why, it might even change the tone of the 'Christian Science' paragraphs in this column. Mr. Lathrop should set his thinker to work at once."

A HOSPITAL FOR THE UNBORN!

ACCORDING as one does or does not believe in heredity as the main factor by which the progress or the decadence of the race is determined, so is one inclined to regard critically or kindly the efforts of physicians to cure the sick. For humanity's sake, in the cause of charity, and, it may be added, with a laudable desire to earn a living, we do our best to cure diseases and cocker up sick folk. Yet if we look beyond the individual and consider the race, we can hardly doubt that all this tinkering of invalids is a direct interference with well recognized "laws of Nature," and that just so far as we succeed in setting on their feet those who, without our aid, would have been eliminated as "unfit," we lower the racial stamina and spoil the breed. But the question must sometimes arise whether this duty of saving life, which we have undertaken as our daily task, may not be carried to an almost undue extreme, and probably many will think that this question very properly arises in regard to the proposal to found hospitals for the unborn! No one who recognizes how largely the dangers of childbirth are due to conditions which might be discovered, and might indeed sometimes be guarded against, were the expecting mother to be under medical care for some time before her hour of trial, need hesitate in admitting that in hundreds of cases it would be the kindest of charities to take these women into well-organized hospitals or homes, where, during the later months of their time, they might at the least have rest, and where steps might be taken to minimize the risk of what every woman regards as the most dangerous event of her life. But when we are urged to found such hospitals, on the plea that they would tend to the conservation of fetal life, that is of fetal life which Nature would destroy, the matter assumes a somewhat different aspect. There are certain diseases and deformities and monstrosities which Nature eliminates by the simple method of preventing their propagation. For the sake of the race it is well that this should be so, and the question is, Ought we to interfere? In regard to sentient mankind we put on one side all considerations of race and posterity, and in the name of humanity do our best to relieve suffering. But in regard to the unborn, ought we to help these immature, deformed and sickly ones to pass the portal at which Nature would destroy them, and let them come into the world carrying with them, as we believe, all their tendencies to produce immature and deformed and sickly offspring in their turn? When as an illustration of the sort of case in which such a hospital might be used we are told of a woman who was truly a "monstripara," a producer of monsters, a woman who had already brought three monstrous fetuses into the world and had had several abortions, we may well ask whether it is wise, even were it possible, to interfere with Nature's ways of preventing the multiplication of "sports" and monsters. Let the poor woman stand aside and let the task of peopling the world be left to those who are more fitted for it.

We take the foregoing from the (London) *Hospital* for April 13. This movement and agitation are not confined to the Western States, whose legislatures are wrestling with the subject of unfit marriages. Physiologists, sanitarians, and students of sociology no longer question the propriety, nay, the necessity, of its serious consideration. The Spartans were no doubt extremists, but they were on the right track.

Some years ago we published a paper on the benign mission of the bacillus tuberculosis in eliminating the unfit. It called down a storm of criticism, but it was not half as crazy or inconsistent as some of its critics.

A CATERER CORNERED.

WE reproduce the following as a bit of literary dessert, from the columns of the *New York Times:*

"Got anything here beginning with a 'K' that's good to eat?" inquired a new customer in a Sixth avenue grocery store and meat market the other day.

"How would pickled kidneys answer?" replied the clerk, after a moment's thought, "or, maybe, a mess of kale—"

"Say no more," interrupted the strange patron enthusiastically, as he fervidly wiped the band of his hat with his handkerchief. "Give me a dozen cans of pickled kidneys and a basketful of kale. The kitten's life is saved. I told my wife when I left home this morning that if I failed to send home a kangaroo, dead or alive, before 2 o'clock, I should expect to find the kitten served for dinner in the latest Chinese style. But your happy thought has saved her."

In reply to the pitying glances of the grocer's assistant, the peculiar customer went on to explain himself.

"You see, we all got tired eating the same things day after day," he said, "and I got into one of those fool arguments with my wife about the domestic and culinary arrangements, and it led up to the alleged difficulty experienced by housewives in thinking up what to have for dinner. My wife took the ground that the mere matter of deciding from day to day what to put on the table was a downright wear and tear on a woman's system. The statement made me tired, and I said so, at the same time calling attention to the fact that in this city there are vast hordes of people whose principal daily cause for anxiety is whether they will have anything at all to eat. I took such high moral grounds and went on at such a rate that my wife threatened to cry about it, and said she just wished I would do the marketing for about a month, and I'd soon change my tune.

"Well, the upshot of it all was that I agreed to do the marketing myself for a few weeks. I became reckless and went further. I agreed, just to show how easy the thing was, that we would begin and eat up (or rather down) the alphabet, taking one letter a day, with bread, potatoes, tea and coffee thrown in as staples. Furthermore, I agreed that if I didn't succeed I'd buy a new piano for the front parlor.

"And say, continued the customer, confidentially, as he settled himself on a barrel of cabbages and took a pinch of sauerkraut out of an open cask, "between you and I, I'm rather glad I left that staple clause in the agreement.

THE NEW DIETARY SYSTEM.

"Well, I inaugurated the dietary system with a bill of fare which, although bountiful, was to a certain extent vegetarian. We had apples in many forms, apricots, pickled asparagus, artichokes, almonds and the staples. The next day's menu was considerably more substantial, consisting of beef, beans, black bass, bacon, biscuits, bluefish, butter milk, beets, bon bons, butter and batter cakes. My wife and family protested that the dinner lacked homogeneity, so to speak, and bordered on the erratic, but this was just what I was striving for. Originality, I declared, was my watchword.

"The next day was even better. We fairly rioted on chicken, cucumbers, codfish balls, celery, curry, clams, cheese, cauliflower, crabs, cabbage, cake, carrots, crullers, canned currants, crackers, caviar, corn, canned cherries, consomme, catsup, calf's head, and candy. It looked like a cinch for me. My wife hinted at dyspepsia and indigestion, but I retorted that she was envious.

"We calmed down a little the next day, partaking of roast duck, doughnuts, and dumplings. We made a regular Easter of the next day with eggs in every conceivable form. I added variety with a dish of eggplant and a liberal allowance of fried eels, so that after all it was really a variegated menu.

"On the following day I wanted to make a regular fish day of it, but my wife arose to a point of order. She pointed to the fact that we had already exhausted a portion of the fish family in the way of codfish balls, bluefish, eels, crabs, and the like, and that under the rules I couldn't go ahead and spring the whole piscatorial connection on her during one day and then be coming along with scattered tribes afterward. So I got along with baked flounder, frogs' legs fritters, finnan haddie, and Frankfurters. It was a weird and lonely sort of day. I was beginning to feel the need of vegetables, and I had tried on this day to sneak in with a few mushrooms under the head of 'fungi,' but my wife sprung the rules on me again. She said mushrooms were mushrooms. She was afraid that under the letter 'M' I might want to send around the entire contents of a butcher's shop under the head of 'meats.'

"Next day brought the scurvy nearer to our door. But as for meats, we were very well supplied. There was roast goose, broiled grouse and baked guinea hen with gooseberry sauce and grape fruit.

"The succeeding day began to tell on me, owing to the vegetable famine. Our meals were provocative of extreme thirst, consisting of ham, hominy hoecakes, herrings and many different kinds of hash.

"I realized, however, that my troubles were just beginning when I tackled the 'I' menu. I thought over the 'I' problem for two days beforehand, and offered a prize of $3 in four groceries and meat markets in the neighborhood for an edible dish under this head, but all in vain. One man told me that in South America the natives roated the succulent flesh of the iguana and devoured it with a relish, but I could not procure an iguana in time for dinner. A learned friend of mine told me that 'inconnu' was but another name for the fish of the salmon family. Oh, with what a light heart I told my wife that we would have a nice salmon for dinner, but that aggravating woman wouldn't hear of it. A salmon was simply a salmon, she said, and certainly came under the letter 'S' or not at all, so on that day we breakfasted, dined, and supped on ice cream and the ever faithful staples.

A DAY OF DESSERTS.

"And yesterday was also a day of desserts. We had jellies of every conceivable flavor, color, and consistency, and as an offset to this we had jam. It was the best I could do, and I was about to lose heart. It was a gay day indeed.

"But to-day your happy kidney and kale suggestion saves us from starvation, and to-morrow—ah! to-morrow we will make a feast of it indeed. We will luxuriate on liver, lamb, lobster, lettuce, lentils and leeks, and anything else you can think up in the eating line that begins with 'L', just you send it around.

"And, oh, please help me to look ahead to the 'X' and 'Z' menus. I'll try and get hold of a zebra by that time, but as for 'X,' I'm afraid I'm up against it there.

"A queer thing about my new food departure is the number of things it has led us to put into our mouths that we have never thought of before. But say, don't you ever advise anybody to tackle this problem. I'm going to take a vacation after I get through the alphabet."—*N. Y. Times.*

GERMANY, up to date in everything scientific, has started a movement that might well be copied in every other country. Two superintendents of schools in cookery in Berlin have organized special courses of study and instruction for medical practitioners, in which the scientific properties of food and the character of food that may properly be offered to invalids, are studied.—*The Chef.*

THE TREATMENT OF CONSUMPTION IN ENGLAND.

THE London *Spectator* says: "The cure of consumption has undergone a complete transformation as to the theory of its origin and distribution. The first great revolution was the discovery that it could be treated with far better promise of success in the high Alps than in the warmer regions to which doctors of an older generation had been in the habit of sending their patients. It was as a result of this discovery that Davos Platz rose into fame. The success of the new plan was remarkable. Patients who seemed not to have twelve months to live, found that by passing every winter in Switzerland they might hope to go on for years. Now, however, further investigations and experiments have led to a fresh discovery. What is so valuable in the Swiss treatment is not the air of the Alps, but the air. People who in England would have been shut up in their rooms all the winter, have been encouraged to be a great

deal out of doors, and have gained fresh life and strength by the process. Air is the secret of the cure, and experiments carried out in districts so unlike as Edinburgh, Norfolk, and Ireland, have convinced the medical profession that treatment, which at Davos or St. Moritz is of necessity costly, may be had at home at a comparatively small outlay. Sanitoriums are about to be built at London and at York, and by and by, doubtless, they will be as common as hospitals. Further experience will doubtless suggest fresh developments of the open air system, and will make it possible for patients to profit by it in their own homes. The association has abundance of work before it, but it begins its labors with the most encouraging prospects.

CAR SANITATION.

AT a recent meeting of the *American Public Health Association* Dr. S. H. Woodbridge of Boston read the report of a committee which ought to have received more attention than was shown it. The following are the leading ideas urged by the committee: (1) When a passenger was known to be contagiously ill, he should be isolated in a compartment appropriately equipped and ventilated in such a manner as to separate it from the rest of the car. Through trains should be provided with rooms for the sick, as well as state-rooms, interchangeable in use. (2) The interior of passenger cars should be plain, finished with hard, smooth, and polished surfaces. (3) All furnishings should be as non-absorbent as possible. (4) Coaches should be furnished with effective means for continuously supplying not less than one thousand cubic feet of warm air an hour for each single seat, and for distributing and removing the air without troublesome draught. (5) The temperature should be regulated. (6.) The cleaning of cars should be frequent and thorough. (7) Floors and sanitary and laboratory fixtures should be frequently treated with a disinfecting wash. (8) All fabrics in cars should receive sterilizing treatment. All bed and lavatory linen should be thoroughly sterilized in the process of laundering. (9) Sewage tanks and earth closets should be provided under the cars. The practice of disposing of excreta by scattering it over roadbeds was dangerous. (10) Water and ice should be obtained from the purest available sources. The use of tongs in handling ice should be insisted upon. (11) The water tank should be frequently cleansed and periodically sterilized with boiling water or otherwise. (12) The public should be educated to use individual cups. Paper paraffined cups might be provided by a cent-in-the-slot device. (13) The use of canned goods in buffet-car service makes careful inspection of such goods imperative. Fruits and all eatables before and after purchase should be stored with care to avoid unnecessary exposure to street and car dust. (14) The filthy habit of spitting on car floors should be dealt with in a manner to cause its prompt discontinuance. It should be punished as one of the most flagrant of the thoughtless offences against the public right to health. (15) Station premises should receive attention directed to general cleanliness of floors, furnishings, air, sanitaries, lavatories, platforms, and approaches, and should be plentifully supplied with approved disinfecting material. The recommendations of the committee were concurred in by the association.

HOUR OF DEATH.

DR. PILGRIM, Superintendent of the State Hospital for the Insane at Poughkeepsie, has made a careful study of the statistics of that institution for the last decade and finds that 20 per cent. of the deaths occur between 3 and 6 P. M., and the next highest rate was between 3 and 6 A. M., though the fewest deaths in any one hour were between 4 and 5 A. M. And it is not an un-

common thing to notice a clearing up of the clouded brain a few hours before the final change; especially is this true of those dying of phthisis, or after surgical operations, or from acute intercurrent diseases. Dr. Pilgrim also remarks that the number of cases diagnosed upon admission as acute melancholia are about two and one-half times as great as that of acute mania. This not only proves that it is the rule for insanity to begin with depression, but it also shows that cases are sent to the hospital much earlier than formerly, before the later stage of mania has had time to develop.

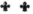

COFFEE DRINKING IN BRAZIL.

"MISS WARD writes from Brazil," says *Omega*, "that the whole country is perpetually in a state of semi-intoxication on coffee —men, women, and children alike, and to babies in arms it is fed from a spoon. It is brought to your bedside the instant you awake in the morning, and just before you are expected to drop off in sleep at night, at meals, and between meals. The effect is plainly apparent in trembling hands, twitching eyelids, mummy-hued skin, and a chronic state of excitability, worse than that produced by whiskey."

REST A MEDICINE.

DR. DIET and Dr. Quiet are two of the best physicians. It would surprise many sick folks if they knew just how much rest has to do with their restoration to health. All the doctors in creation cannot cure a sick person unless he will *rest*. In many instances if the rest were taken in season there would be no sickness. A woman has a splitting headache, and is obliged to go to bed. She rests half a day, and the headache is cured without doctors or medicine

EXCURSION TO CALIFORNIA.

THE Excursion announced in the April number of the GAZETTE has been postponed to meet the convenience of a majority of those who desire to go. The exact date of starting will be arranged by personal correspondence with applicants.

The most delightful month at Coronado Beach is June, and this is true of many other of the coast resorts.

There is no extra expense connected with the trip. This point seems to have been misunderstood.

Address, Editor DIETETIC AND HYGIENIC GAZETTE, 503 Fifth Avenue, New York.

MENTAL EXERCISE CONDUCIVE TO LONGEVITY.

THOSE people who have been accustomed to the continued disciplinary use of their brains daily, and who have placed their nerve power under a highly developed constitutional training, are enabled by these very means to escape the so-called early decay and to avoid those alarming accidents to health from which so many apparently health men succumb. People who use their brains and observe ordinary hygienic care of their bodies resist disease in the first place ; and when the are actually ill they prolong their lives or recuperate sooner than do those who have lived less intellectual lives. Thus there is given a new force to the assertion that you may kill a man with anxiety very quickly, but it is difficult to kill him with work. Whether the brain can actually give power to the muscles is not certain, though the enormous strength sometimes developed in a last rally looks very much like it. That it can materially affect vitality is quite certain, and has been acknowledged by the experienced in all ages. —*London Speaker.*

REACTION AFTER THE BATHING.

REACTION must follow cold bathing always (Dr. Baruch) or the purpose of the bath is rendered abortive. We might think that emphasis need not be placed on this point in our day. Consultation of some of the text-books, however, shows what mistaken notions may be conveyed by ill-given directions. Lauder Brunton, the distinguished English therapeutist, in his textbook of therapeutics, edition of 1898, says that when the patient's temperature reaches a certain point he should be placed in the bath and left there until his temperature comes down. When he is first put in the temperature of the water should be about 65 degrees F. and this may be reduced by additions of colder water or ice to 40 degrees F. It is no wonder that he concludes his directions with the advice to remove the patient from the bath before his temperature becomes quite normal, because it may sink still lower after the patient is put to bed, and symptoms of collapse may ensue. The main purpose of the bathing is neglected if these directions are followed and no friction is employed during the bath No wonder under such circumstances that the bath should prove an unpopular remedy.

Department of Hygiene.

WITH SPECIAL REFERENCE TO STATE AND PREVENTIVE MEDICINE.

THE THERAPEUTIC VALUE OF CLIMATE, WITH A WORD CONCERNING SOME AMERICAN CLIMATES.

PSEUDO "Science-Healing," under various semi-sacred or sacrilegious names, is one of the current playthings with which fakirs and faddists are amusing themselves, leading their dupes and lining their pockets; but we hear little or nothing concerning the science of climate in its relations to the healing art. There are a few ancient and threadbare saws to the effect that, "Change of climate is equivalent to rebirth," or, "No man can farm against climate," but beyond the annual hegira of a few thousand consumptives, dyspeptics and physical derelicts, not much progress is being made in the study of climatic possibilities. At the same time "Change of Climate" was early adopted as a reformatory resource, the first recorded instance being that notable prescription in the Garden. It was designed as a bit of moral discipline, resulted in the exodus of the pair, and was responsible for the inauguration of the fashion of furs, fig-leaves and feminine blushes! The little army of occupation, through stress of circumstances over which it had forfeited control, became the army of evacuation, and filed out into the wilderness of the Annexed District to the time of the Rogue's March.

Doubtless Adam shivered—possibly he swore—and Eve, realizing that the rôle of Godiva had been permanently expunged by the management, became hopelessly hysterical and sent for a costumer! Thus Adam became the first man-milliner sixty centuries before Worth was born.

Since that primeval episode of compulsory emigration the decendants of Eve have never for a moment ceased to do battle with the elements—the weather! Rich or poor, wise or witless, sane or silly, man, monkey or microbe—nothing mortal can escape it; and when we can no longer endure the climate about us or escape to a better one—lights out, curtain, and the crematory!

Warmth hatches and harbors; extreme cold depresses and destroys. Animal life is conceived at fever heat; when the temperature of its environment rises above or falls below the vital limit, its career ends.

"Climate is to a country what temperament is to a man—Fate." Climate determines temperament, hence climate is fate; and back of all other causes stands climate as the final umpire in determining human longevity. It decides the character, composition and varieties of food human beings shall eat, the air they shall breathe, and the range of diseases to which they must be subject. All endemics and most epidemics are originated, disseminated and territorially limited by edicts from Nature's Weather Bureau; and the distribution, virulence, persistence and subsidence of all the infectious and contagious diseases are definitely determined by meteorologic influences and climatic boundaries. It has dictated the rate and direction of the progress of civilization, and continues to dominate the doings of universal humanity, from the root hunt of the Digger Indian of the western deserts, to the forlorn expeditions of the scientific lunatics who continue to commit ice-cold suicide in the vain and useless search for the mythic North Pole. Throughout all time, everywhere and forever, it has held and holds the individual members of society in abject thrall, as its unwilling vassals.

Bringing down the record, another evening and another morning were the Eighth Day, that is, the modern day; in which heaven knows what hasn't been done and made in the matter of costumes! Men still lean toward millinery; bare-skin is still in vogue—at the opera—while blushes have become a drug in the market, are sold by the jar and quoted in the lists with other toilet preparations.

It is the hospitable weather of the temperate zones, especially of the North Temperate zone, that has evolved all the energy, enterprise and culture of the civilized world.

True, the glassblower and ironmolder, in time, inure themselves to the white-hot flames of their respective furnaces; and the human animal is tough, managing to adapt itself, more or less imperfectly, to violent extremes; but these strange adaptations ultimately cost quite all they are worth, in vital expenditure, and are also subject to definite limitations.

Molière was right as well as sarcastic: "If you are dissatisfied with your physician, I will procure one from across the way who will condemn him."

Medical men proverbially combat each other's theories, and agree to disagree as to practice; but they have at last almost unanimously subscribed to the admission that the only treatment in any sense approaching a specific for that universal scourge, consumption, is the treatment by climate. Hence the verdict of the last International Medical Congress, emphatically reiterated by the recent congress of tuberculosis experts, that *there is no known medicinal specific for tuberculosis of the lungs.*

And this in the face of the thousand and one "great discoveries," whose impossible virtues are heralded in all the cheap prints and emblazoned on every blank wall that can be stolen or hired for the purpose of "cheating the sick of a few last gasps as he sits to pestle a poisoned poison behind his crimson lights."

And what an army is involved! Twelve hundred thousand in our own country, and in the world not less than ten millions of doomed prisoner victims, hopeless of reprieve, clutching at straws, or stoically awaiting their inevitable fate!

And yet this somber sky is not without its bow of promise and hope. The same experts assure us that probably not quite all but a very large proportion of these smitten sufferers are now or were at one time in the history of their baffling malady amenable to treatment, that is, *curable by climate!*

The human animal manages to survive under the widest divergence of climatic conditions, and sometimes succeeds in adapting itself to the most violent extremes of temperature; but these adaptations are not economic, sometimes costing life itself.

All endemics and most epidemics are originated, disseminated, controlled and finally limited by climatic and thermometric laws.

The emphatic reiteration of this consensus of medical opinion that there is positively no known medicinal specific for this fatal disease, ought to be a sufficient admonition to the great and growing army of sufferers from tuberculosis. Those who delude themselves by listening to the panacea venders and catching at "great discovery" straws are wasting valuable time, if not inviting their own doom and throwing away their last opportunity.

Among the irregular and apparently contradictory effects of a residence in hot climates are an increase of the appetite, increased activity of the skin and kidneys, a tendency to precocity, enlargement of the liver, loss of body-weight and tendency to leanness, notwithstanding the increased consumption of food. The man from either of the temperate zones who removes to, or for the first time sojourns in the tropics, must expect to do battle with the demon of "biliousness," and to always live next door to dangerous diseases of the digestive tract.

As to Arctic climates, no man goes to Alaska or volunteers to discover the North

Pole strictly for his health! The unfortunate dweller in polar regions is Nature's slave and beggar. He has neither time nor incentive for thought beyond the painful necessity of procuring to-day's dinner and providing against to-night's frost.

The North Temperate zone has been the cradle of all the aggressive and progressive branches of the human race, and it is the climates of this zone that we need to study. Within the boundaries of this zone are found all those varieties and modifications of climatic environment that are directly contributory to human evolution and advancement.

Americans do not need to go abroad for climatic variety. The United States fairly overflows with climates. There are so many varieties and they shade off into each other so gradually that one can traverse half a dozen during a three-days' journey by rail. We Americans have an unenviable reputation for annually spending millions at foreign shrines without in a single instance finding anything better adapted to our needs, climatically speaking, than we could find within our own borders, with twice the satisfaction and at a quarter the expense. Ignoring foreign Meccas, we deem it quite within our province to devote a little attention to some of the more desirable of our home climates, the advantages of which to a large class of invalids are not sufficiently well-known.

Beginning with Colorado, it required an even century of the Republic before she lined up for Statehood. Topographically she is the *Apex Americanæ*, the crown and dome of the continent. From this dome the waters flow to all points of the compass, north, northeast, southeast, southwest and west. The counterpart of this configuration is not duplicated on this continent. Nowhere else are there mountains in such massive groupings.

The writer spent several rather eventful years in Colorado, at the critical stage of her transition from territorial savagery to progressive statehood. To his feeling that he may have modestly contributed toward her internal development and outside repute, must be ascribed any apparent over-enthusiasm in statement that may follow. At the same time he assures the reader that no item will be wilfully exaggerated.

In material resources Colorado corresponds with her physical outlines. For example, any mineral that can be named she can supply, and her general mineral wealth is inexhaustible.

She probably has not yet tapped the Mother Vein. (This prediction is ventured as a revelation of the Oracle!)

Anything that will grow in the ground outside the tropics and even some tropic trees and plants, with little coddling, she can grow.

When the ghouls of the scientific schools would add a particularly rare specimen to their paleontologic treasures they have but to repair to her eocene graveyards and delve deep into her fossiliferous storehouses to find it. Here was the pristine playground of the sportive megalosauri and other giants of the genus lizard, with bodies as long as an ocean steamer, and tails that had to be reefed or wholly removed when the animal wobbled into the Ark.

Gold, silver, tellurium, cinnabar, zinc, lead, iron and coal; mountain masses of obsidian, seams and scintillations of rock crystal, rubies, agate, jasper, garnet and chalcedony—"What will you have," quoth God, "dig here and find it!"

Lakes that sparkle and shimmer in the sunlight, hemmed in by mountain barriers ten thousand feet above the sea; forests that climb the mountain sides a thousand feet higher than they can live in regions where the weather and winds are less propitious; a climate that compasses all varieties, from that of sunny and congenial valleys, to that of summits where the snows and ice of one season blend with and perpetuate those of the next, and where the Frost King relaxes his grip but for a few hours a day in midsummer.. You choose to your liking; pitch your tent on the borders of the Great Plains, or in one of the lower valleys, at an altitude of 4,000 feet; locate in one of the elevated parks, each as large as an ordinary State, at 8,000 feet, or climb to mountain retreats as much higher as prudence permits. Wherever you locate, Nature incessantly lends her aid and labors in your behalf. She invites you to a closer intimacy and woos you, if you be an invalid, toward the one thing which can accomplish your physical salvation—*an active out-door life.* She bathes you in antiseptic sunshine, fans you with mountain breezes, makes you hungry, and brings you profound and refreshing sleep. She will ward off your annual paroxysm of hay fever, cure your asthma, allay your cough, and stay the insiduous inroads of the gnawing but invisible destroyers within you; and if you be not already moribund she will rejuvenate you and send you back to a life worth living and to a future worth fighting for.*

The soil is warm, dry, porous; the air is tonic, aseptic, ozonic, full of e lectric energy. There are gushing springs without number, hot springs, cold springs and springs of every conceivable composition, from *aqua pura* to *aqua sulphurosa,* and from simple pure water to compounds so mysterious and complex as to baffle the analytic chemist and astonish the imprudent imbiber. Springs so cold that one wonders if they emerge from a fountain of liquid air, and springs so hot that they will do an egg in three minutes, or cook a speckled trout while you bait the next hook!

To the man with the rod and gun she offers game of every size, nature, and variety, from the speckled beauties of the mountain stream and the chattering pine squirrel to salmon trout that try the stoutest line, and to antelope, black-tail deer, mountain sheep, elk, mountain lion and grizzly.

The influences of her climate on the human race are already in evidence. Her people are full of the spirit of push and progress. Politically, while other States

*I said something like this, in 1871, and the present editor of the Denver Times declares he will never forgive me for inducing the deluge of invalids that followed. As thousands of them still live to testify in my behalf I shall live out my days in spite of his (selfish and inhuman!) indictment.—Ed.

have hesitated to experiment with new ideas, she has tested Populism (and condemned it), and is now quietly watching the results of woman suffrage. Commerically, she has made strides that distance and dumfound the would-be "hustlers" of other communities. She is gridironed with railways; her mines of gold and silver are yielding more than any other region, not excepting the Klondike; and her capital, the proud, aggressive and audacious Queen City of the Plains—there is nothing in Chicago, New York, London or Paris that can not be quickly duplicated in Denver, from French millinery to opera houses; and from chambers of commerce to Chinese hells, and hells that are not Chinese.

Not content with her present water system which supplies 5,500,000,000 gallons of the best water used by any city in the world, Denver is now constructing a dam which will be the highest structure of the kind in existence, rising 250 feet from bed-rock to summit, and is to be *faced with waterproofed steel plates.* It will form a lake miles in extent, mirroring mountains 13,000 feet high, and impounding 35,000,000,000 gallons of water, wholly derived from melting snows. It is an engineering feat that would appall the boldest engineer who had never witnessed western daring.

"Above me, skyward, towers the rocky steep;
Beyond me the illimitable sweep
Of distance, there the city's far-off gleam;
Beyond, the plains, soft fading as a dream,
Farther and fainter, till the utmost edge
Of hazy purple—seen from this high ledge,
Wrapped in the distance—seems some shoreless sea
Upon the border of Eternity."
—Mrs. Cora M. A. Davis.

Of what use to quote stupid statistics? In a community without prototype or precedent there can be no standards of comparison. As to temperature, rainfall, humidity and the other meteorologic items, all these depend on where you betake yourself; whether on the plain or on a mountain side;

and whether exposed or sheltered; in the sunny valley, or high up among the eternal snows of the Continental Divide. You choose your own site and conditions, for they are all here, and very near each other—all except "equability!" Nothing here is equable, nothing is "consistent" with anything elsewhere; nothing is quite compatible with anything but itself. Nothing is passive, imitative or stagnant; but everything is individual, unique, and stands to challenge criticism as its own exemplar.

Reverting to the word "stagnant," can any man who has never been west of the Mississippi credit the statement that there is not a gallon of stagnant water in the whole State of Colorado? Yet it is literally true.

The summers are delightful in a sense so different from the conventional one that only those who have experienced them can realize it. The winters, barring an occasional and unlooked-for spasm of severity, are mild and enjoyable, the air being always dry, crisp and bracing, and sunny days predominating. It is idle to compare the climate with that of Switzerland or any other land. It is a climate *sui-generis*. You may find any climate you desire, unless it be tropic or sub-tropic, and if you stray into the Arkansas Valley, along the southern border of the State, in midsummer you can experience a taste of the latter, omitting the item of humidity.

You put a poser if you ask for what ailments the climate of Colorado is especially favorable. The advertising cure-all man of the hour, too busy counting his "ten-for-five-cents" orders to be interviewed, insists that his shotgun prescription "will help you no matter what ails you." If it were bottled Colorado climate he dealt in, there would be hope that he would escape the lake whose fires, according to tradition, are never to be quenched—at least, not till she experiences a change of climate by falling below freezing point!

This may sound extravagant, but it is not; and to corroborate this estimate the railroads are perfectly willing to return your money—or your body!—"for one first class fare"—if you don't get well, with return tickets at excursion rates if you do. What more can you ask of a "heartless corporation?"

"Age cannot wither her nor custom stale her infinite variety."

WANT OF TOUCH BETWEEN THE PROFESSION AND THE PEOPLE.

ELSEWHERE we publish the comments of the *New York Times,* on a somewhat remarkable address of Dr. Andrew H. Smith at a recent meeting of the Academy of Medicine. Dr. Smith has struck a key-note that will find an echo in every medical community throughout the land. It has crystallized into a proverb that the medical profession is the most conservative and slowest to move with the tide of progress of any of the so-called learned professions.

The laity know a good deal more than was formerly known about medicine, and much that they do not know they think they know, which is immeasurably worse than simple ignorance. This is getting to be true of all branches of science, as well as of religion. Educated people now glibly talk the "higher criticism" and read medical journals, while the lay press everywhere dabbles in medicine. Proprietary medicine venders publish, in attractive form, and lavishly distribute, well-written statements of advanced theories and recent scientific demonstrations in pathology, therapeutics and dietetics, and are, to-day, doing more to illustrate and popularize current advances than is the profession itself. It is a humiliating fact that many physicians get their first intimation of important discoveries and announcements through this irregular and irresponsible source.

To illustrate the contrast between the methods adopted, the proprietary men do not rely upon lay statements, nor content themselves with publishing the scientific versions that may be culled from the cyclopedias; they pay liberally for expert investigations and employ the best available professional talent in putting the acquired knowledge into the most attractive and convincing literary form. It is true that behind all their work there is a business axe to be ground, but the weapon is no longer of the cheap and disreputable kind that formerly was so common in the advertising world.

The strictly professional way of disseminating knowledge is not very democratic or effective. The members of a medical society get together at infrequent intervals, straggling into the place of meeting an hour or more behind the appointed time, and with an air as serious as if a funeral was the order of business, and with a frigid semi-observance of parliamentary rules, proceed to discuss, not invariably, but very frequently, far-fetched and abstruse questions in which not more than one member in twenty is directly interested, the very evident object in a majority of cases being to advance the fame and financial prospects of an individual practitioner, operator or consultant. But all these conferences are virtually executive sessions behind closed doors. If on rare occasions some member feels the thrill of a progressive impulse and prepares a practical paper on some living issue of vital importance to the entire community, unless it has reference to desired legislation, he runs against the "time all occupied" excuse of the president or censors, which is the mildest form of putting a rejection. If such a member tries to wait his turn he finally grows disgusted and burns the paper, or publishes it in one of the medical journals, lucky if "leading" weeklies or monthlies do not politely return his MSS. with a similar apology.

If an intelligent layman should accidentally straggle into one of the sessions of the decorous professionals, and should make an inventory of the surroundings, while he sleepily listened to the learned dissertations,

his first remark would probably be, *sotto voce,* "how the devil can these fellows survive for two hours in this stuffy atmosphere?" Here these assumed exemplars of hygiene sit, session after session, in a room without any discoverable facility for ventilation. There is not an outside window or door opening into it; no visible outlet for bad, or inlet for fresh air, and yet the essayist of the evening avers that the only cure for consumption and other wasting diseases is fresh air!

And when the speaker or essayist of the evening, and those who have been previously elected and foreordained to combat or corroborate, under the head of "discussion," all conventionally togged in claw-hammer coats and expansive shirt-fronts, like society dudes aping the Four Hundred, have duly subsided, a movable partition glides slowly upward and discloses an ample dining-room with extensive tables spread with a bounteous "collation." Thither these scions of science and exponents of the laws of life repair and indulge in indigestible salads, sandwiches and sardines as a further insult to stomachs that haven't yet recovered from the overload of a heavy seven-o'clock dinner.

Little wonder that so many city physicians are bald at thirty, or that they have, as a class, acquired a reputation for dying a dozen years before their time. They shed their hair on account of impaired nutritive processes, and die of atheromatous arteries. They preach little and practise less hygiene, and their attitude toward the laity is practically that of the elder Vanderbilt toward the people—"the laity be d——d."

It is this attitude that drives the people to the quacks and nostrum vendors. It is this that is making such fearful inroads in the income of average physicians, and that is causing so many well-equipped practitioners to turn their attention to other and more remunerative avocations.

If doctors will descend from their dignified stilts, come down from their pseudo-ethical perch and begin to make themselves useful as well as ornamental, they may be able to check a popular and very wide-spread movement that bids fair to leave them, in time, without an occupation.

STATE SANATORIA FOR CONSUMPTIVES.

FROM a very suggestive address under this title, delivered by Dr. H. L. Taylor, of St. Paul, before the Minnesota Legislature, and published in the April number of the *St. Paul Med. Journal,* we extract the following:

Tuberculosis is the leading cause of death in all civilized lands. No country, no climate is entirely free from it. It is the greatest and most dangerous pest still to be conquered by civilization. Yearly it numbers its victims the world over in the millions. In the United States it carries off 150,000 annually. In the State of Minnesota it claims a tribute of 1,500 men and women every year, as shown by the records of the State Board of Health for the past decade. This is almost twice as many deaths as are due to any other disease, which is sufficient to show the importance of the subject.

It is a contagious and hence a preventable disease. It is communicated from man to man, from man to animals, from animals to animals, and from animals to man. The manner in which this communication takes place is thoroughly understood. It is the exceedingly minute bacilli, found by the thousand in the expectoration of consumptives, that carry the disease from one to another. These little intruders obtain an entrance to the system in the dust-laden air that we breath, in the contaminated milk, butter, cheese, or meat that we eat, or they may have been deposited on any article of food or drink by the hand of some sufferer from this disease, or in the ever-present dust that has settled upon it. The dust found in the house in which a careless or ignorant consumptive has lived and died, often contains virulent germs months after his death, and infects some member of the family that has moved into the dwelling.

The infant child of consumptive parents raises the bacilli-laden dust as it creeps across the floor, and, breathing it in, acquires the poison that is usually supposed to have been inherited. When it has grown older it deposits myriads of bacilli in the school-room dust; there the restless feet of the school children stir it up and it is inhaled by teachers and pupils alike. We can follow it from the school to the work-bench, the office, the store, or any of the numerous places where men and women work, and there the deadly germ finds new victims; or such a child may live on a farm and help to care for the cattle.

*   *   *   *   *   *

It is not only a preventable disease, but it is also a curable disease. Post-mortem examinations of people who have died with some other complaint show that a large number who have been consumptive, at some time in their lives, have entirely recovered, although the fact that they have been tubercular is easily proven. It is this fact that has been known for years, that has encouraged us to seek for some method of treatment that will help the man who is unable to resist the inroads of the disease. It has been found that life in a sanatorium, with its rest, discipline, fresh air, and generous diet, is the most successful method. It succeeds in a remarkably large percentage of cases, when we consider the usually hopeless lot of a poor man who has acquired consumption. From two-thirds to three-fourths of those admitted are returned to their homes and to their work after an average residence in a sanatorium of from three to nine months. Now, gentlemen, this pest has been shown to you as the leading cause of death, as a communicable or contagious disease, but fortunately also as a curable disease. Another fact of interest is that it is in middle life, the period of the greatest activity and wealth production, that it is most prevalent. Two-thirds of all the deaths from consumption occur between the ages of twenty and fifty years. While it is distributed through all the ranks of society, it is the poor who suffer the most. The poor man can not quit his work when this insidious enemy first fastens itself upon him, and take that rest which is so essential to his recovery. He is obliged to keep on at his work until compelled by weakness and fever to give it up. In this way the golden time is lost when his recovery was possible. The course of the disease is so long that all the savings of the family are required for the urgent needs of the invalid, and after his death poverty and destitution are the only estate he can leave them.

It is the duty of the State to protect the well from a dangerous disease, and by doing this the sick will, at the same time, be restored to health and to the work that both enriches the State and supports their families. Just as surely as the invalid and old age insurance companies of Germany have found that they made money by supporting sanatoria in which their consumptive members could be treated, and some of them saved, just so surely will the State be the gainer in the end if it gives its wealth-producing citizens the advantages of sanatorium treatment in the early stages of this disease, the time when scientific care offers the most chances of recovery.

MORTALITY.

In a recent health report, the mortality from diphtheria and scarlet fever is noticeable. In 719 diphtheria cases, 149 deaths occurred, and in 719 cases of scarlet fever, only 46 deaths. Antitoxin is credited with lessening, to some extent, the mortality of the former disease, while in the latter the marked decrease indicates that recovery is largely dependent on the antiseptic treatment in vogue, viz.: the increasing use of the chloride solution known commercially as "Platt's Chlorides," both locally and for general disinfecting purposes.—*N. Y. Medical Examiner*, March, 1901.

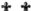

CHLORETONE IN PRACTICE.

By Louis F. Bischof, M.D.

My experience with chloretone has served to convince me that in this product of acetone and chloroform we have a most satisfactory general hypnotic, free from the distinct dangers which have become familiar in the use of narcotics of the opium group, or the coal-tar derivatives, and quite lacking in unpleasant after-effects. In the present group of cases I submit some results of my use of the drug upon persons who are normally in a sound and healthy state, but who, for temporary reasons, rather than constitutional ones, stand in need of a sleep-inducing agent. It will be readily understood that such cases may arise from excessive muscular exhaustion, from over-excitement of the brain centers, or from any one of several other causes. It is these cases which call for the most careful treatment. We need here an agent which will induce a natural sleep, rather than one which will compel a forced and unnatural sleep. In these cases we must seek to avoid any agent for the production of sleep which entails gastric troubles, or the depression of reaction, and thus compel the patient to pay in the morning, by physical distress, for the repose which he has had over night.

An object particularly to be desired in these, as, in fact, in all cases where sleep is sought, is to avoid every tendency toward the causation of a drug addiction, a sort of habit which is most to be feared in those who are normally in a sound state. In this connection we must recognize the widespread inclination on the part of patients to repeat, when away from the physician's care, the prescription which has already given relief, and for this reason we should seek an agent which, while effective, shall be harmless when used under conditions where medical supervision is lacking. My experience with chloretone shows that this valuable agent fulfills all these necessary requirements; that it gently induces a sleep most closely approaching the normal, that it does not produce uncomfortable symptoms, or the depression of reaction, that it is safe up to the most exaggerated doses given by the most unskilled hand. From my case books I select the following few interesting cases in which I have used chloretone where sudden emergency has arisen in the normally healthy person.

Case 1.—Mr. N., age 28 years, perfectly sound in mind and body, could not sleep. Gave one dose of chloretone, 10 grains, and induced sleep charmingly.

Case 2.—Mrs. W., age 70 years, sleepless. Gave three grains of chloretone with excellent results. The patient was otherwise in good health.

Case 3.—Miss E., age 24 years, healthy, sleepless. Gave five grains of chloretone. which acted splendidly, and almost immediately produced wholesome and refreshing sleep.

Case 4.—Mr. H., age 30, healthy, wakeful, and had been in the habit of taking brandy to secure sleep. Cut off the brandy and gave him nightly five grains of chloretone, which acted nicely and soon established the habit of normal sleep without further need of recourse to stimulants; a highly satisfactory case.

Case 5.—This case is of a different type from the foregoing, but I include it because of its interest. Miss W., age 20 years, chronic myelitis complicated with convulsions, two a month for several years, and, therefore, to be considered of a chronic nature. Gave one grain chloretone twice a day for three months. During this period she had only one convulsion, and that of a mild tone; all other symptoms have improved. The chloretone is continued, and there is every reason to expect a satisfactory cure.

❧ ❧

MUST THE FAMILY DOCTOR GO?

Obliquity of view and extravagance of expression (*Philadelphia Medical Journal*) are among the venial sins of some of the modern newspapers. To deal in paradox is their specialty, and they exercise this privilege nowhere more rashly than on the subject of medical practice. For instance, one of our metropolitan dailies (by which expression we mean, of course, a New York newspaper), recently wrote a sort of obituary notice on the family doctor. On the authority of a fashionable specialist, this newspaper announced that the days of the general practitioner are numbered, and that in the near future the specialist and the trained nurse will monopolize the field. Even as it is, the functions of the family doctor, it thinks, can be performed just as well, if not a little better, by a well-trained nurse. Moreover, the specialist to occupy the field will be the surgical specialist—the man who stands ever ready with knife in hand, because, according to our New York newspaper, the day is rapidly approaching when all, or nearly all, diseases will be cut out bodily. In this promised golden age, all that will be necessary will be for a well-trained nurse to recognize the disease and call in the surgical specialist, who will proceed to cut it out and hand over the patient again to the nurse, who will keep him aseptic and return him to business in due time.

All this sounds like persiflage, and was probably written by a man with his tongue in his cheek, but we take note of it because it represents superficially a kind of criticism that is growing too common. The family doctor is not doomed to extinction. Far from the day of his decline having come, the day of his greatest usefulness is only just beginning. It is evident, however, that he must, in one sense, be a specialist himself, *i. e.*, he must have special alertness of mind to recognize disease, and to know what remedy is needed. But the field of preventive and domestic medicine is largely his own, and will continue to be his. He will always occupy a position of great advantage, for he stands at the threshold. He will continue to dispense his patronage to the specialists, and they will know him when they see him. But he must be thoroughly trained for this work.

FRESH AIR AND TUBERCULOSIS.

FROM the Report on State Hygiene, by Dr. Granville P. Conn, President of the N. H. State Board of Health, published in the *New England Medical Monthly*, for April, we extract the following:

The public is becoming very much interested in reports from foreign and domestic sources regarding the possibility of obtaining substantial relief from the effects of a disease that for a long period has increased the mortality rate in this and other States more than any other one malady.

There is nothing that more nearly concerns the individual, the corporation, the municipality, the State and the nation, than health, and consequently it is but natural that the people should be ready to inquire into any means looking to the alleviation of so fatal a disease as tuberculosis.

It is very true that the profession and the people have a far more intelligent appreciation of pulmonary disease than formerly. We realize to-day that of two persons inheriting the same tendency to this disease, the one living most nearly in the open air will probably live the longer, and enjoy the better health. Our grandfathers in medicine did not realize this. It was the custom, even less than two generations since, to protect such persons from the fresh air, fearing they would take cold. Such patients were coddled in feather beds and imperfectly nourished, but were given plenty of medicine.

To-day, we consider the cardinal means of the treatment of pulmonary tuberculosis to be: (1) The maximum of pure, fresh, dry air and sunshine; (2) abundance of nourishing food; (3) rest physically, and

freedom from nervous care and worry. It does not matter so much where the patient is being treated, only that these prime requisites to good health, or its restoration, shall ever be present in unlimited quantities.

In a few States money has been appropriated to aid in carrying out these ideas, and philanthropic people have contributed largely from their means to assist those who would otherwise be unable to take advantage of the modern treatment of this disease. Other States have directed committees or commissions to report to the next legislature the expediency of the State becoming a party to this work. The Massachusetts Board of Charity is expected to report to the next legislature on this subject, and all New England may be said to be waiting with great interest to learn the recommendation of so experienced a commission. Discussions and investigations in this line of thought cannot be other than useful, as it will prove educational to the public. The rich and the poor alike will learn that in the treatment of tuberculosis, as in other forms of disease, the old is giving way to a new order of reasoning, and ultimately but few will be left in ignorance of the value of pure air, sunlight, good food, and a dry, unpolluted soil, to assist the inherent power of Nature in the elimination of all disease.

POISONED BY SHOE-BLACKING.

THEY put poison in our foods, the hair dyes are full of it, medicines are frequently adulterated, and finally shoeblacking is brought up as a culprit. The following is translated from the *Journal des Practiciens* by the *Philadelphia Medical Journal:*

Six children in one family, all of whom had worn shoes fresh from the shoemaker, upon which the aniline polish had not yet dried, were attacked suddenly with symptoms of *poisoning*. Their ages ranged from two to fourteen years, the youngest being the earliest affected. First, pallor of the face, a bluish discoloration of the skin, and a violet color of the lips and nails were noted, then dilatation of the pupils, headache, vertigo, absolute muscular weakness, transitory paralysis, followed by unconsciousness, slowing of the pulse, and arhythmia, with cold extremities. Slight convulsive movements occurred in two cases, besides. In from one to three days all signs disappeared, including the faint trace of albumin found in the urine. Another case occurred later, in a child of six. A thorough investigation revealed the fact that in each case the shoes worn had but just come from the shop, and the polish was not yet dry. Chemical examination of the polish used showed *aniline*. Experiments were made upon guinea pigs, in which the polish produced precisely the same symptoms as in man.

PERSONAL HYGIENE IN DISEASES OF THE NOSE AND THROAT.

FROM a paper on the above subject in *Health* for March 9th, we extract some pertinent suggestions. Says the writer:

"The balneo-therapeutic side of this question of hygiene, is, perhaps, the most important of all. We have only to recollect two facts to show this: One is, that mucous membrane of the upper respiratory tracts, especially of the nose, is most affected of all by derangements of function in other excreting organs; and the other is that of the total amount of water and other excretory products, the skin furnishes 80 per cent., amounting to about two pounds daily. A graphic illustration of the importance of this function is furnished by an incident which took place during the ceremonies of the installation of one of the mediæval Popes. In the fancy of the times, an angelic cherub was supposed to bring to the new-crowned Pontiff the greeting of the heavenly host. A boy of ten years was chosen to represent the cherub, and, that

he might be in heavenly fashion, was covered from head to foot with gold leaf, laid with a coating of varnish. The boy fulfilled his part in the show, and within a few hours went to join the heavenly host, whose messenger he was supposed to be. While we do not see cases of this extreme nature, de do see many cases where inattention to proper bathing was the chief cause of catarrhal troubles.

"In the middle and poorer classes it is customary to stop giving children their daily bath at about four years of age, and this is also the time at which many begin to develop catarrhal diseases. There seems to be an intimate connection between these facts.

"The regulation of diet properly comes under this discussion. There are certain states or local conditions which may be directly traceable to a general diathesis, as, for instance, a rheumatic or gouty pharyngitis. The relation between obstruction of the portal circulation, the movement of the bowels, and the condition of the tubinated bodies, is very close, and very frequently cases resembling a chronic hypertrophic rhinitis with nasal obstruction, headache and ocular symptoms, will speedily be relieved by a brisk cathartic, followed by laxatives."

THE LAITY TO THE RESCUE.

A GOOD many people and a good many American papers have championed the cause of the medical fakirs. The people do it ignorantly, or else as instigated by the saffron-colored sheets. The latter are actuated wholly by meritricious motives. The fakirs advertise, and the papers share the blood money.

It is reassuring to meet with laymen who do not abet the faith-shriekers, and with newspapers that handle the subject without perjuring their consciences or surrendering to the swindlers. There are many such laymen, and there are some journals that are not "going straight to perdition, in the vulgarest way," as Carlyle bluntly charged Anthony Trollope with doing. Among the latter is the Leadville (Colorado) *Herald-Democrat.*

In referring to a bill to regulate the practice of medicine, before the Colorado Legislature, this fearless editor, among other good things, said:

"The bill that has been the subject of attack aims to keep the individual who knows nothing of the science of medicine and surgery from attempting to practice the profession and to secure money under false pretenses. This is declared to be interference with the liberty of the citizen and an effort to create a trust. Both claims are in a manner correct. Protection would be given to those who need to be protected, the little child, who is offered as a sacrifice at the altar of ignorance or deceit, and the adult who entered the world without a sufficiency of brains to protect himself. It would place the regular practitioners in a reputable, honest position and the others where they belong.

"The land is filled with the leeches who profess to be able to work miracles, who not only rob the gullible, but do much harm to the profession. A month seldom passes in which there is not a new Cagliostro abroad in search of victims, and as human nature is at present constituted, it requires statutory protection.

"Medicine and surgery are not exact sciences; an exact science is largely a myth. The science that progresses and is advancing with the age cannot be called 'exact,' because it has to dispense with pre-conceived notions as they are found to be incorrect; and we know of no science that has progressed with the same earnestness and certainty, with the same devotion to the cause of humanity, that has done more for humanity and the allied sciences, as the science which treats of the constitution and care of the human body. Subtract the discoveries that have been made by members of the medical profession and there is left a great vacuum in the much vaunted progress of the nineteenth century. Philosophy and invention must ever be dependent on the advances made in biology and physiology. And yet we do not wish to be understood as upholding solely the material as against the spiritual; the power of mind over matter, which is not very well understood yet, must be given greater and greater recognition, but its scientific application and exploitation must not be left to the illiterate fakir, but to the learned professions, to the practitioner in surgery and medicine, to the student and the experimenter, to the person who has been educated in the school of science and logic.

"No great discovery of any value whatever to the human race was ever made by the class of persons who oppose the recognition of medicine and surgery and who are benefited by existing conditions. The world would be poor, indeed, had it to depend on the outcasts of the medical world for its succor from the evils of the dark ages."

Speaking of the entire ilk, from the sacred "Scientist," metaphysical "Healer," Indian Mahatma, Chinese snake-dung doctor to the hoodoo negro, who emits sparks of medical magnetism, this writer adds, that: "all are united against the profession of medicine as recognized by the reputable colleges and universities of the civilized world; and there are people who ought to be better employed, because they know better, who throw reason and logic to the winds and grasp at necromancy or any of the fallacies that have done service since mankind began to worship the snake and the totum. These people take the position that while the world has advanced by leaps and bounds in all other directions, the profession of medicine and surgery has remained at a standstill or degenerated, despite the fact that the best intellect of the world is engaged in the profession and in the study of medicine and surgery and in the communication of its learning to others." He ends by saying, in a general way, that all these "mental" and "suggestive" processes "will undoubtedly help those who imagine that they are ill, but humanity is far from that stage of beatitude and purity where the mind can be made to kill a diphtheria germ or heal a broken leg. When a child falls ill, and a child has not the misfortune to imagine illness, and it is placed in the care of fakirs and schemers and illusionists, the individual and the State should be held responsible for what befalls. This cannot be done under the present laws."

And here is another view of the same topic, with some variation of the treatment suggested, which we find in the *New York Sun:*

"It is a curious characteristic of human nature, or of a great deal of human nature, that people who would grudge paying a cent to a regular medical practitioner will cheerfully pay a great deal of money to an irregular medical practitioner. Go where you will and you will find the quack prosperous. His rooms are full of patients, and his patients are full of faith. Men and women will buy wondrous remedies from traveling mountebanks who do not disdain to sing a comic song on the wagon from which they peddle their nostrums. Natural bonesetters, and long-haired 'Indian doctors,' and botanic doctors ignorant of botany, and faith healers of many kinds, abound; and the trade of most of them is good. The world likes to be healthy, but it loves to be humbugged. If a thousandth part of the blind, unhesitating faith that cleaves so readily to incompetent, and often illiterate, practitioners of fantastic means of healing were bestowed upon religion, there would be no complaints that the churches are not filled. But often those who are full enough of doubts of the supernatural so far as it relates to their souls are quick to believe in an almost or altogether supernatural gift of quack salves to cure the body. Legislation can do but little if anything to interfere with the gains of the medical pretenders or of the professors of visionary and semi-religious medical 'science.' You cannot legislate away a state of mind; and the state of mind of thousands, perhaps millions of persons, is one of crass credulity in humbug. Their delusions and illusions can be removed only by experience and a wider knowledge. They take their own lives and the lives of their families in their hands when they neglect the methods and the agents of modern medicine and surgery and resort to the moonshine of Christian 'science,' or to any other crank system, or to any individual quack. But you cannot prevent people from killing themselves if they have the will; and you will only stimulate faith in quackery by giving it a chance to yell 'Persecution!' A private arrangement between patient and 'healer' will nullify any provision of law forbidding the 'healer' to heal for a consideration. A gift can take the place of a fee; and 'gratuitous' treatment can be acknowledged with a gratuity. The best way to deal with a delusion is to let it alone. Common sense must win in the end."

THE ROLE OF PETROLEUM IN THERAPEUTICS AND WHY IT IS PRESCRIBED.

(Synopsis of Research Experiments made by G. Burbidge White, M.D., Diplomate State Medicine, University Dublin, F.R. C.S.I., etc.)

PETROLEUM has of late become a most popular remedy; it is a comparatively new drug and not much information is forthcoming respecting its therapeutic action. That which has been available has been somewhat confused and misleading. I may be able to throw some light on the subject by the brief remarks which follow.

The name, Oil of Petroleum, may convey the idea to the average medical reader that it is a fluid fat having all the characteristics of fat, and behaving like one when swallowed and subjected to digestive action, and the most likely fat for it to be confounded with is the well-known cod-liver oil. This error may be accentuated with the fact that both substances are to be found in the form of emulsion, about the same strength, and it is frequently stated that petroleum is a substitute for cod-liver oil. If we examine the chemical and physical characters of these two substances we ought not to again confound them. Cod-liver oil is a true fat, consisting chiefly of olein, containing an active principle, termed morrhuol, and traces of I. Br. with phosphates, etc. It behaves like a fat when digested, being emulsified, partly saponified, absorbed to be assimilated and when it enters into the body metabolism, the great objection to its use being that while undergoing digestion the fatty acids are set free and cause the usual eructations, also its smell produces nausea. It is not a good vehicle, as it soon becomes rancid. Furthermore, it offers concentrated nourishment for bacteria, and therefore serves as a culture medium for the growth and multiplication of micro-organisms, thus producing gastric and intestinal fermentation and auto-intoxication from absorption of toxines from the intestinal tract. Petroleum, the absolutely pure residue after complete purification of the crude substance, is a fluid hydro-carbon, not a fat or oil, the formula C. Hn. representing a type of the series. It is devoid of chemical substances or salts in solution, cannot be digested nor assimilated, nor can it enter the body metabolism. It is unchangeable, organisms will not grow in it, and it does not become rancid. Therein lies its superiority as a vehicle over perhaps any other substance used for this purpose. That it is capable of producing great clinical benefit cannot be denied. I now proceed to point out how it acts:

Besides acting as an ideal vehicle, petroleum rivals belladonna in its numerous applications and therapeutic actions. It has been largely recorded of it that it increases weight, relieves dyspepsia, flatulence and constipation without aperients, diminishes cough, catarrh of the mucous membranes of the respiratory, intestinal and genito-urinary tracts.

In some experiments I made with Angier's Petroleum Emulsion upon digestion and absorption, I satisfied myself of the following effects: I found that certain proportions of the Emulsion rendered peptones and fats (chyle) more miscible and diffusible, and that a quicker and more complete absorption of the weight-giving nutrients took place in a given time under its influence. This effect was enhanced by solution of thick impure mucus covering the wall of the bowel, while increased peristaltic action favored digestion, and also presented constantly new flesh portions of the finished products of digestion and absorption, while as additional action it was proved that the Emulsion is a perfect intestinal antiseptic, inasmuch as it completely inhibited the growth and action of putrefactive bacteria such as inhabit the alimentary canal. Peptic and tryptic digestion was hastened and rendered more complete.

The well-known clinical fact that Angier's Petroleum Emulsion favors natural bowel movements, even in cases of chronic constipation, was proven in my experiments to be due to the fact that petroleum acts as a well-distributed lubricant to the intestinal mucous membranes and induces natural mild peristalsis, which persists for several hours after death of the animal.

To put the matter shortly, petroleum, properly purified and prepared, is a substance that renders the digestion of all classes of food-stuffs, albuminoids, carbohydrates and fats, more thorough than occurs without petroleum, and favors the complete absorption of the finished products of digestion into the system. It thus acts as a true nutrient, providing the tissues with exactly the character of material required to repair waste and, by thus maintaining normal nutrition, it antagonizes the progress of morbid processes, such as tuberculosis, scrofula, inanition, marasmus, etc. Furthermore, Angier's Petroleum Emulsion was found by actual experiments to exert a more promptly beneficial influence upon the inflammatory conditions of the respiratory tract than any combinations of expectorants and cough sedatives. It exerts this influence without inducing gastric disturbances of any kind; indeed, it was noted that these disturbances, when present as a complication of the disease, were invariably overcome, and the processes of digestion reinforced to a most pronounced extent. In pulmonary tuberculosis, and in both acute and chronic bronchitis, not only was the cough rendered less severe and less frequent, but expectoration of retained secretions was easy and free from effort on the part of the patient. The symptoms of catarrh of the respiratory organs promptly disappeared, and proved that Angier's Petroleum Emulsion has a *selective action upon the larynx, bronchi and pulmonary alveoli.* In all cases the disappearance of the local symptoms was accompanied by improvement in nutrition, manifested by increase of appetite, ability to digest and assimilate food, and a rapid and progressive increase in body weight.

SMALLPOX IN THE UNITED STATES.

ACCORDING to the *Public Health Reports* there has been more smallpox in the United States during the past fall and winter than during the corresponding period one year ago. The total number of cases reported up to March 29th was 11,964, as against 7,279 for approximately the same date last year. What we wish to call attention to especially is the astonishingly low death rate. As we pointed out last year in these columns, smallpox has been prevailing in widely separated parts of the United States, but almost everywhere it has presented itself in an exceedingly mild type. Thus there were but 157 deaths among the 11,964 cases—little more than 1 per cent. Some of the results are still more striking when the figures are analyzed. Thus, in Wisconsin 560 cases were reported with only four deaths. In Virginia there were 257 cases without a death; in Tennessee 308 cases with 4 deaths; and in Oklahoma Territory 690 cases without a recorded death. In Minnesota there were not less than 1,985 cases reported, and yet out of all these cases there were rceorded but three deaths. In Colorado there were 1,190 cases without a death. In Louisiana the disease appears

this year, as last, to have prevailed in a more malignant type than elsewhere, for out of 157 cases there were 37 deaths. This is about 23 per cent. This mortality rate for the whole United States would have given about 2,760 deaths instead of the 157 deaths reported. This serves to show, as graphically as figures can, how mild a type of smallpox has been prevailing in the country at large. In the large Eastern States, New York and Pennsylvania, there has been but little smallpox this winter; in the former 416 cases; in the latter only 102. Pennsylvania had but three deaths against New York's 67.—*Med. Times.*

ANTI-MALARIAL PHILOSOPHY.

THE new learning in regard to the origin and dissemination of malaria will disparage many of the ancient preventives. Professor Celli, of Rome, in a recent summary of the matter, alludes to the influence of trees, such as the pine and eucalyptus, and dismisses their anti-malarial powers by saying that trees afford shelter for the insects of the air and are a danger. Now that the rôle of the mosquito is thoroughly understood in the propagation of malaria, on the other hand, some herbaceous plants, mostly of the composite kind, and from which are prepared the so-called insecticide powders, are effective in killing larvæ in water and mosquitoes in the air, and it is suggested that these should be cultivated on a large scale; and it might be possible that a malarial swamp could, by this means, be made to free itself from the malaria by which it is infected. As a means of preventing infection being conveyed by malaria, the protection of the house by netting answers very well. For protecting the bodies of those who have to remain in the open air during the evening and night, it is found that soaps, pomades, and perfumes are of no use. Mechanical contrivances, such as veils and gloves, must be used. Celli seems to think that he has discovered some cases of immunity, though he professes that he does not yet know the means by which this immunity is secured. He has found that the daily administration of half a gramme of eucanin makes a man capable of bearing with impunity the injection of a large quantity of very virulent malarial blood. There is no doubt that the vast interest awakened in malaria by the new doctrines of its origin will lead to very definite results in its prevention, and it may be reasonably expected that Italy will very shortly be entirely free from this scourge.—*Medical Age.*

"AMERICAN MEDICINE."

WE have received the initial number of Dr. Gould's new weekly. We are both pleased and disappointed. Pleased at its virile attitude and appearance; disappointed that its founder did not include in his enterprise an authoritative and suggestive example for all other medical journals as to the size of type. Dr. Gould is an expert oculist. He well knows how many, even young physicians, now wear glasses. He knows that they read when they are tired and when the ocular functions should be subjected to the least possible strain. The type used for editorials and original papers is beautifully clear, but is moderate in size. That for general situations, book reviews and the like is smaller and set solid. It is all wrong and nobody knows this better than the accomplished editor of *American Medicine.*

The title is ambitious and expressive. There is not in this country a medical editor more competent to stand as a faithful exponent of American medical science; although it is in our opinion a mistake to attempt to localize knowledge on any subject. Knowledge belongs to the world, not to any nationality.

The number is a plethora of good things and an apoplexy of advertisements.

The first fifty-two pages are advertisements. Then there are six pages of Prospectus and names of patrons, followed by forty-eight of regular reading matter, six more of subscribers' names, ending with fifty-eight more of advertisements.

Six pages are devoted to editorial matter, three in small, close type to the review of twelve different books, four to American News and Notes, three to Foreign News and Correspondence, twenty-one to Original Papers, two to Practical Therapeutics, eight to Latest Literature and one to the Public Service.

There are three pages at the end devoted to what we call Covert Eulogium. It seems to be necessary in this commercial age, but we hardly expected to find it in *American Medicine.*

The editorials are crisp and to the point. None of them are verbose. The excerpts are well chosen, and if any of our readers are restricted in the number of medical magazines to which they can afford to subscribe, we advise them not to leave *American Medicine* off the preferred list.

What we have said that may sound a shade derogatory is only intended as our modest protest against the too prevalent custom of small type, *but we mean every word of it!*

DIOXOGEN.

IT is with much satisfaction that we call attention to the new announcement in our advertising pages, by the Oakland Chemical Company. This company's product of that sterling pharmaceutical preparation, of which the chemical formula is H_2O_2, but which has been called by a dozen names—oxygenated water, peroxide of hydrogen, dioxide of hydrogen, "hydrozone," "pyrozone," sauerwasser, and what not, and the repute of which has suffered much at the hands of shyster manufacturers, is henceforth to be known by a distinctive title. Those who use this agent, and who are familiar with this company's product, will now have some assurance that their orders for it will not be filled, as has too often been done, by irritating and inferior substitutes.

Department of Physical Education.

WITH SPECIAL REGARD TO THE SYMMETRICAL DEVELOPMENT OF THE BODY.

TREATMENT OF OBESITY BY MASSAGE.

HIPPOCRATES says: "A physician must be experienced in many things, but assuredly also in rubbing; for things that have the same name have not always the same effect: for rubbing can bind a joint that is loose, and loosen a joint which is tight. "Hard rubbing binds. Soft rubbing loosens. Much rubbing makes them grow." He also adds, that "rubbing can make flesh and cause parts to waste." Celsus, too, suggests the use of friction for the removal of deposits in the tissues, and especially for the relief of pain. Among the Chinese written allusions will be found, dating back to a period 3,000 years before the Christian era, and their oral traditions are of still greater antiquity. The Chinese manuscript of Kong Fan, the date of which is 3,000 B. C., seems to have contained detailed accounts of these operations. Closely allied in their nature and mode of action are the sarchuna of the Persians, the Greeks, and the friction of the Romans. Much useful information respecting its early history will be found in the works of Hippocrates, Celsus, Galen, Oribase, Caelius, Aurelianius, and other writers, both ancient and modern.

Dr. Maurice Steinberg says: "During a part of last century there is reason to believe that the true massage was practised in France, but it was carried on secretly, and the professors of the art were but little inclined to impart their knowledge to casual inquirers. It is to Dr. Mezger, of Amsterdam, that we are indebted for much of our knowledge of the modern phase of massage. His thesis was published in 1868, and is entitled, "Die Behandlung von Distorsio Pedis mit Fricties." In the preface he states that he commenced studying the subject in 1853, and that he has modified it and practised it constantly since 1861. I may mention incidentally that Mezger has published no large work on the subject, and that his reputation rests chiefly on the undoubted success which he has attained in treating his private patients. He is not now connected with any hospital, and some time ago declined a professorship in the University. In Holland very little is known about massage. As an example of the ignorance which prevails on the subject, it may be noted that in a well-known dictionary of medicine, it is stated that massage, shampooing, kneading, and medical rubbing are synonyms, and it is defined as a process of treatment by rubbing, which consists in deep manipulations.

"The so-called massage, practised by medical rubbers and nurses, is not massage at all, as the term is understood on the Continent, and little or nothing in common with it. In the words of the *Lancet*, 'It is as absurd to suppose that rubbing and shampooing is massage, as it is to say that a daub of paint is a work of art.' There was at one time a deep-rooted objection to massage, as a method of treatment, but this has gradually disappeared, and it is now admitted that it is really a useful and scientific mode of cure, not unworthy of the notice of even the most orthodox physician or surgeon. More than ten years ago it received in Germany the adhesion and support of such distinguished authorities as Billroth, Esmarch, and Langenbeck. It is not free from the taint of quackery, but as a recent writer says: 'Quackery does not consist in the thing that is done, so much as the spirit in which it is done. The most time-honored and orthodox remedies may be employed in such a manner, and by men boasting of the highest qualifications, as to be fairly chargeable with this taint. That we should be debarred from the use of such potent therapeutic agents as massage, or systematic muscular exercise, or electricity or hydrotherapeutics, and for the like, because in unworthy hands they have been abused, seem to be almost worse than absurdity.'

"Massage, as already stated, is a scientific manipulation in treating different diseases. The individual muscles or groups of muscles are picked out or isolated, and stimulated to contraction mechanically. The movements must be made in the direction of the muscle fibers, and the tips of the fingers must be carried along the interstitia, so as to promote the flow of lymph and increase tissue metamorphosis. In addition, an attempt should be made to stimulate mechanically the various motor points, in order that the muscles may be made to contract by a stimulus conveyed along the nerves. The manipulations are carried out systematically in definite order, and with a definite object. In ordinary medical rubbing, these conditions which are essential to massage, are considered to be of no importance, and the operator simply rubs or pummels the patient without any regard to the anatomical arrangement of the parts, and usually without any very definite object.

"There is as much difference between massage and shampooing as there is between playing a difficult piece of music and striking the keys of the pianoforte at random."

THE PURPOSE OF GYMNASTIC TRAINING IN A RATIONAL EDUCATIONAL SYSTEM.

NEVER before, not even in the days of ancient Greece, writes Frank H. Curtis in *Mind and Body*, has the physical side of education received so much careful scientific study from educators as at the present day. The recent researches in the fields of psychology, pedagogy, and child-study, have demonstrated the fact that first of all a student should be a healthy animal, and that a high degree of intellectual advancement is seldom attained, and cannot be sustained, except it rest on a healthy physical basis. Recognizing this fact, nearly all of our great universities and colleges either have erected or are now erecting and equipping gymnasia for the use of their students, and are requiring a course in physical training as a part of the regular college work.

This growth of physical training has not been one of mere sentiment, nor the cultivation of a fad. Even in some institutions in which it was introduced merely in acquiescence to a popular demand, it has been demonstrated that the time lost from classes by the students on account of sickness has been materially reduced; in some instances, as at Amherst, over 40 per cent. Moreover, a decrease in rowdyism and destruction of property, on the part of a certain class of students, has been frequently noticed and commented upon. The superabundant energy with which the college students give vent to the healthy animal instinct of play has been, in a great measure, diverted from personal encounters, hazing, "Class scraps," and other forms of disorder into definite gymnastic and athletic training, which, while allowing the buoyant animal spirits full expression, yet turns them to the furtherance of the individual's education.

But while physical training thus, indirectly, raises the moral standard of the student by furnishing a safe outlet for his physical energy, by giving him something to do, of far greater importance is the direct educational effect it has on the brain itself.

Modern psychology has demonstrated that we cannot consciously move a muscle without the nervous impulse actuating it first arising in a center located in one of the motor areas of the brain. Physiology asserts that "function makes structure." That is to say, that the constant use of a certain part of the body causes it to grow and develop. Thus by constantly using the muscles they grow and become developed. But to use those muscles means also a constant use of their nerves and of the brain centers controlling them. There, therefore, follows a development of the nerve fibers themselves, and of the brain centers as well as of the muscles involved.

Grace of movement results from the coordination of many separate groups of muscles. The use of a certain part of the body naturally involves the use of other parts more or less closely associated with it because of the peculiar constitution of man's nervous system, which he inherits from ancestors that lived under very different conditions from those now confronting us. The movement of some of these associated parts may not be wanted in the result now desired, and consequently some have to be controlled and others inhibited. It may also be necessary at the same time to move several different parts not directly or closely connected naturally; so we find that a variety of impulses must come at one time, may-be from several different centers, and all must be harmonized to produce the desired result. When this harmony is attained we say that the movements were co-ordinated. Lack of co-ordination produces awkwardness.

It is only by repeated practice that co-ordinations can be brought quickly and with the least expenditure of energy, and thus control and grace of movement established. It is one of the aims of physical training to give practice in making co-ordinations; for with proper co-ordinations correctly learned right action tends to become habitual, and one of our foremost authorities has said, "The ends of exercise may be characterized in a general way, as, first, the promotion of health, and, second, the formation of correct habits of action."

In applying these principles in a practical way in the gymnasium the student begins with the most simple and fundamental movements. He is shown exactly what movements to make and how to make them, and is then practised in these until they are thoroughly learned. Each succeeding lesson is progressive, and is so arranged that the student continually advances, using the work already mastered as a foundation for the next lessons. In this manner new and increasingly difficult co-ordinations are constantly made and mastered until the student can execute with ease the seemingly impossible combinations of the trained gymnast.

To execute even a simple exercise, however, demands a certain amount of will power. This may be little enough at first, but as the exercises become more complicated a greater and greater demand is made upon the will for their execution, and thus its power is gradually but definitely developed. Without further explanation it will easily be seen that along with will power goes the development of such qualities as attention, self-reliance, courage, self-control and other qualities of mind that go to make up character.

Character may be defined, in a general way, as the sum total of our habits: habits of thought; habits of speech; habits of action. Physical training drills the body and mind in correct habits of action until they become so natural as to be well nigh instinctive. These habits of action have a powerful influence and play an important part in the formation of character. And, after all, the aim of all true education, life itself, in fact, is the formation of character.

It may seem strange to some readers that little or nothing has been said about the development of muscle. This has been done because it is of less importance than the educational side of the subject. Muscular development does not indicate the strength or power of the individual. That depends not so much on the cross-section of the muscle as on nerves and nerve centers supplying it with energy, and back of these yet it depends upon the will power. Muscular development is merely one of the results, you might almost say a by-product, of the physical training. It comes, to a certain degree, as a matter of course from that training, and hence is not made its aim or end. Increase in the size of a muscle amounts to little unless there comes also an increase in control and usefulness.

However great the educational value of physical training, the first and most fundamental aim must always be the promotion and maintenance of health. The exercises given are arranged with a view to increase the circulation, deepen the respiration, and stimulate the processes of secretion and of elimination. The teacher who strives to develop muscle merely teach tricks on apparatus, or special feats in athletics, without knowing and keeping in mind the effect of such work on the health of the participants is guilty of negligence quite inexcusable in these days of scientific gymnastic training. It is on this very point that college athletics have been so severely criticised in the last few years. And justly so, in many cases. The average athletic "trainer" does not understand the physiological significance of his work, and therefore cares nothing about its scientific aspect. He claims to be intensely "practical." That is, he will make his men win their races even if they do become unevenly developed, or if they are weakened for life as a result. To the scientific teacher, however, the health of the individual, present and to come, is fundamental, and all the student's exercises are arranged to meet his needs in this respect. In other words, the modern physical trainer cares less for teaching tricks or winning races than for securing for his pupil healthy vital organs and a body subservient to the will.

GENERAL MASSAGE.*

By Haldor Sneve, M.D.,
St. Paul.

This is the form of massage which is most commonly administered by masseurs and nurses, when prescribed by a physician; in fact, this is what a physician usually means when he orders massage; I shall

* Lecture delivered at the University of Minnesota, Feb. 5, 1901.

therefore enter into some detail as to the preparation for and administration of this form of massage.

Preparation of the Operator.—The dress should be loose and free, and no corset should be worn; remove rings; prepare the hands and nails as if for an operation, using a stiff brush and green soap; now anoint the hands with a little cocoanut oil perfumed with a little oil of rose or rose geranium, if desired.

Preparation of the Patient.—The patient should, the day before or on the same day, have had a warm bath, in order to avoid having the bacteria of the skin rubbed into the glands and follicles; the patient should be in a room with the temperature at about 70° F., and should be placed on a narrow bed accessible from both sides; the patient should be placed between woolen blankets, and only the part of the body being operated upon should be exposed. We first begin each manipulation of a limb with medical gymnastics.

In this connection we mean simply the so-called Swedish movement or passive motions. In the case of the upper extremities we begin by rotation of the shoulder, flexion and extension of the elbow joint, pronation and supination of the forearm, rotation, flexion, and extension of the wrist and fingers, each manipulation being performed from six to nine times. In the case of the lower extremities we perform practically the same manipulation as with the upper extremity. The reason for using these movements, first, is, that because through these movements we cause a greater activity in the circulation of the blood streams, both to and from the limb, and also increase the current in the larger lymph vessels; this is accomplished by the alternate compression and relaxation exerted on the vessels running in the flexures of the larger joints, and by the mechanical effect upon the muscles. It is not of much consequence whether we begin this treatment with the upper or lower extremity; it is customary to begin with the lower extremity.

Place yourself on the right side of the patient and grasp the right leg just above the ankle with the right hand, place the left hand over the patella and rotate, or better, circumduct, the limb at the hip six times in each direction, being careful not to bring the knee beyond the middle line. Next we administer the massage proper of the thigh by grasping the upper part of the thigh as high up as possible, with both hands, and rolling and kneading the muscles; when we arrive at the knee joint we stroke firmly upwards from the knee to the hip, paying particular attention to the course of the larger vessels on the inner anterior aspect of the thigh.

We now grasp the patient's ankle, as in the other movement, with the right hand, and place the left hand upon the knee, and flex and extend the knee joint, including also the hip joint, by bending the knee as far up on the abdomen as possible, and then bringing the limb down straight, repeating about six times. Then with the thumbs and the inner border of the hands we massé around about the knee joint; next we manipulate the leg from the knee to the ankle, as we did the thigh; then we grasp the leg just above the ankle with the inner side of both hands, one behind the other, and pressing firmly, wring the soft tissues upwards and around the limb, working circularly in opposite directions with the two hands, upward to the inguinal region, once or twice, following this with upward strokings, at first firm, then lightly with the palms of the hands. We now sit down facing the foot of the bed and grasp the leg just above the ankle on its anterior aspect with the left hand, and bring the leg across our left knee, grasp the end of the toes, then circumduct the foot about six times in opposite directions; then we flex and extend the foot upon the leg about six times. With the inner border of the hands and thumbs we perform friction and kneading of the foot, after rising and facing the patient; finally, we stroke the whole limb from the toes up with the flat of the hands; after both limbs have been treated in this way, keeping the body covered, we go to the upper extremity. We stand with our left side toward the patient's head and grasp the right arm just below the elbow on its outer aspect with the right hand, and place our left hand upon the shoulder; we now circumduct the shoulder joint with as large excursions as possible, six times in each direction. Beginning as far up on the shoulder as possible, we perform the same manipulations as on the thigh. Grasping the arm just above and underneath the elbow, we take hold of the wrist with our fingers on the anterior, and our thumbs on the dorsal side of the wrist with the right hand, and proceed to flex and extend the elbow joint about six times; then taking hold of the patient's hand with the right hand as in shaking hands, we pronate and supinate the forearm about six or eight times. We massé the forearm in precisely the order and manner as we did the leg. Grasping the hands and wrist, as we did the foot, perform circumduction, flexion and extension, afterwards "masséing" the hands and fingers as we did the foot, finishing up just as we did in the case of the lower extremity. The left arm is to be treated in the same way, after bringing the patient to the left side of the bed, to which we have transferred ourselves; the patient is now put in the prone position; if desired, a pillow can be placed under the abdomen, and we now massé the back.

For this manipulation we use, first, the tips of the fingers of one or both hands, describing little circles, and stroke thereafter downwards from the neck along the sides of the vertebræ to a level with the top of the hip bones; beginning at the top of the thorax, we stroke downward and outward, following the curve of the ribs with the tips of our fingers, applying them as far as possible in the inter-spaces of the ribs; the tissues can be pinched up with the fingers and thumbs, and stretched and rolled lightly, and the other stroking varied by stroking downwards and outwards with the palms of the hands. The buttocks are manipulated with the tips of the fingers in the same manner, but the stroking of the lower part of the back should be made upwards and outwards. Those who have learned the manipulation should now perform hacking all over the back; those not familiar with this manipulation should perform instead a light clapping with the palms of the hands; the manipulations are finished with light palmar strokings of the whole surface; the patient is then returned to the supine position, and practically the same manipulations are practised on the chest as were practised on the back; finally, we finish the treatment by manipulation of the abdomen.

Standing or sitting on the right side of the patient, we knead the abdomen with the hands placed flat upon it, and finally stroke the abdomen, following the direction of normal peristalsis in the large intestine; to do this, we apply the fingers, first of the right, then of the left hand, over the cecum and stroke upwards to the ribs; then we place the left hand just at the border of the ribs at the right side and stroke firmly straight across the abdomen with the flat hand or the heel of the hand, to the lowest point of the ribs to the left side, here we change hands and stroke downwards along the left side of the abdomen with the palm of the right hand, moving it across to the lower part of the abdomen to the cecum, in one motion; this concludes the treatment. Should the patient appear nervous or excitable at the conclusion of the manipulations, a very light stroking of the whole body may be performed with the palms of the hands barely touching the skin, peripherally, in just the opposite direction to the former stroking described; this has a sedative, soothing effect. At the conclusion of the treatment, which occupies thirty minutes to one hour, beginning with the first period of time and working up to the last mentioned, the patient should be warmly covered up, the blinds carefully drawn, and the patient instructed to sleep from one-half to one hour, unless treatment has been given in the evening, which is the best time for it,

under which circumstances the patient will probably sleep all night.

Indications.—General massage is used in many conditions and diseases. Its physiological effects are, in a general way, to increase metabolism in all the tissues. Observations by Dr. Eccles, of London, show that the bodily temperature is increased temporarily, from 1 to 4° F., which lasts for a short time, and then the temperature falls below what it was when the treatment was begun. In other words, a reaction occurs. On the respiration it produces an increase in both depth and frequency. The bodily weight is increased, as shown by Dr. Gopodze and others, except in the case of very stout individuals, otherwise healthy, in whom a decrease in weight occurs. General massage increases the number of red blood corpuscles circulating in the blood, as shown by Dr. John Mitchell, although no increase in hemoglobin occurs. An increase in the amount and a change in the character of the urine always occurs. In neurasthenics, leucomains in the form of phospho-tungstates, are increased, as hown by the tests of Von Poehl. Uric acid is also increased, as is also the amount of water. Active exercise produces both fatigue and, at times, aching, but the general massage above described relieves fatigue and does not cause pain. The increased amount of oxidation, or, better, metabolism, results also in the setting free of toxic substances, which, being thrown into the circulation, produce a greater or less degree of poisoning of the large nerve centers. Thus we can account for the desire to sleep after a treatment.

It follows from the above short synopsis that this treatment is useful to improve malnutrition, resulting from any cause. To relieve insomnia, to prevent atrophy, to hasten convalescence, favor elimination, and act as a restorative. Like tonics and reconstructives, it is useful in manifold conditions. It is useful in diseases of the blood, such as anemia and chlorosis. In nervous diseases, especially where nutrition is below par, we find it of great value, especially in the form of the Weir Mitchell rest-cure, or in the modified rest-cure.

Some Points.—The treatment is usually given but once a day, but may be employed with advantage morning and at bed time.

Always cover up each limb well after it has been manipulated.

Do not use, as is recommended by some authors, an alcohol or other bath after massage, because you will be defeating the purpose of the whole treatment; when the treatment has been given in the morning, and the patient wishes to be relieved of the cocoanut oil or other fat, this should be removed an hour or two afterwards by means of a little bay-rum, eau-de-cologne, or alcohol on a rough towel.

Avoid unnecessary talking. Do not use enough force to hurt your patient.

DR. GERMAIN SEE ON EXERCISE.

THIS eminent French physician recently summarized in "La Gymnastique Française," the following excellent rules relating to exercise, the translation of which we quote from the *American Physical Education Review:*

"Football is a dangerous exercise without value. Lawn tennis is an innocent game. Foot races are of moderate value. Races with burdens merit thorough disapproval. Bicycling is a very remarkable exercise, but racing should not be encouraged, since serious consequences to the heart and to those forces actively called into play are to be feared. Instead of popularizing these contests, therefore, we should restrain and prevent them.

"Active and passive gymnastics ought to be encouraged in so far as they facilitate respiration and help the muscular system.

"Fencing deserves the heartiest approval, as it develops the strength.

He apportions exercise appropriate for the various ages, sexes, individual constitutions, etc., as follows:

"(a) For children up to twelve years of age, I prescribe very easy sports without effort, as lawn tennis. I permit quick walking, but not racing. I prohibit bicycling. If one goes beyond these prescriptions, the heart is dilated and weakened.

"(b) For adolescents from twelve to sixteen or eighteen years, bicycling and rowing are excellent. Fencing should be moderate and horseback riding insignificant in amount.

"(c) For adults eighteen to thirty-five or forty years of age, with a tendency to obesity, or with large, inflated, gaseous stomaches, bicycling is desirable, since it decreases the bodily weight without diminishthe strength. For a large stomach it is useful, though not always efficacious.

"(d) For fleshy adults with thickening of the heart: The moment the heart is attacked and becomes fatty, bicycling is bad. Walking up an incline is preferable; and if at the same time one decreases the amount of food and drink taken, and abstains from alcohol in all its forms, this form of exercise may prove very efficacious.

"(e) For affections of the heart: No one should be permitted a bicycle unless a careful examination of the heart has been made. I have seen, as I have shown at length in my book, "Sur le Traitement Physiologue du Cœur," the most grave accidents result in the case of those who have the least lesion of the heart. For them, bicycling should be absolutely prohibited.

"(f) For persons with diseased lungs: Asthmatic patients may bicycle to advantage if the heart is sound, but consumptives cannot. In any case the patient should not be allowed to bend over.

"(g) For persons with nervous disorders: Bicycling and hydrotherapy are very useful.

"(h) For persons with feminine weaknesses: In the case of women in general, and of young girls with chlorosis or anemia, bicycling is exceedingly injurious. Fleshy women may bicycle if they have no disease of the heart, blood or feminine organs."

SPINAL CURVATURE FROM WRONG SITTING POSITIONS.

CAREFUL investigations made in various European cities have developed the startling fact that in most schools a large proportion of the students, even at an early age, have developed curvature of the spine as the result of the wrong attitudes assumed in sitting while at their studies.

In Dresden, for example, Professor Kunig found lateral curvature in twenty-four per cent. of the pupils in the common school. This is truly a terrible spectacle—one-fourth of all the boys and girls in the public schools deformed before they have reached maturity. Many more girls are affected than boys, in the proportion of about five to one. This would make forty per cent. of all the girls deformed. Apparently the only curvatures considered in these investigations were lateral curvatures. Posterior curvature of the upper part of the spine, giving rise to so-called "round shoulders" and the consequent flat chest, is a condition much more comon even than lateral deviation of the spine. The habitual posture, whether sitting or standing, constitutes a mold by which the body is shaped, especially during development.

Curvature of the spine is a matter of importance not only from a histological standpoint, but because of the direct relation between external deformities of this sort and internal displacements of the viscera, such as prolapsed stomach, movable kidney, and prolapsed liver and bowels. It is strange that among civilized people so little attention is given to the development of a good physique and erect carriage of the body. Among many half-civilized tribes, as the Arabs, for example, great attention is given to this matter. Children are taught from earliest infancy to walk, sit, and stand erect, and as a result spinal curvature is practically unknown among the children of the desert.—*Modern Medicine.*

THE BUSINESS OUTLOOK IN MEDICAL PRACTICE.

THE ratio of physicians to total population in the United States is rather more than 1 in 600. The 120,000 physicians are dying at the rate of about 25 to 1,000. To make good the deficit of physicians by death, about 3,000 should be graduated annually. The population is also increasing at the rate of about 1,300,000 annually, and this increase could accommodate some 2,100 additional graduates in medicine annually. In 1899, according to statistics of the Bureau of Education, all of the medical schools of the country graduated not quite 5,000. Thus, statistically considered, there is a very slight favorable tendency toward the reduction of a tremendously overcrowded profession.

On the other hand, it should be remembered that as a country increases in density of population, it can support fewer physicians. For instance, European countries with a ratio of approximately 1 to 2,000 of physicians to population, support their medical professions even more poorly than does the United States. Moreover, sanitary science and medical and surgical skill, as well as more wholesome modes of living, are markedly reducing the work of the profession. The well-known fact that a fifth or sixth of graduates do not practise is little comfort, as this has always been the case, and it simply denotes the unfavorable conditions against which the medical man has to contend. Thus, it is the urgent duty of every physician, by fair argument and reasonable means, to create a sentiment against the entrance of young men upon medical studies, unless they are especially fitted for their pursuit.—*Philadelphia Medical Journal.*

✤ ✤

CHANGE OF ADDRESS.

THE Eastern office of the Abbott Alkaloidal Co. in New York City has been removed to 100 William street. The new quarters are located more conveniently, are much more commodious, and afford better facility for the handling of the rapidly increasing business of this office. Eastern patrons of the Abbott Alkaloidal Co. will kindly note this change of address.

ELLA WHEELER WILCOX'S GOWNS.

"I HAVE always rebelled against the slavery of fashion," said Mrs. Wilcox. "I remember a gown one season which I knew made me look like a guy, only it was fashionable. When I scolded about it, my friends comforted me by telling me it was a most stylish costume. One day at a Turkish bath, when the attendant knotted a sheet about me, I thought, 'Now, here is comfort, common sense, and the most graceful lines imaginable.' Next day when I went to my dressmaker I carried a fine linen sheet in my bag. I took it out and draped it about myself. The woman stood looking at me in amazement. Her amazement turned to consternation when I told her I wanted a gown made exactly after this style. She declared she could not do it. She would be wasting material, ruining her reputation and making me look perfectly ridiculous.

"'Very well,' I said, calmly, 'I can find somebody who will make it.' She relented, and my first loose street gown was the result. The public of our little shore resort was shocked as much as the dressmaker, but gradually they ceased to look their wonder. With one gown after another improvements have been made, till now I have all my clothes, house, street and evening gowns, cut after the same comfortable, graceful style. I also consider myself the pioneer in another emancipation. I was the first woman—in this part of the country, at least—to bid defiance to style and don a short skirt, such as you find to-day in nearly every feminine wardrobe. I had grown perfectly tired of the combination of country life and trailing gowns, so ten years ago I had a skirt made that just reached my shoe tops. What freedom! What exhilaration! The woman of to-day realizes the comfort of it as I did."—*Good Housekeeping for May.*

EXTRAORDINARY FECUNDITY.

ONE of the Italian journals has recently recorded an extraordinary case of fecundity of which it guarantees the authenticity. Flavia Granata, who it appears is well known at Rome, has recently given birth to her sixty-second child. This woman is now fifty-nine years old. She was married at twenty-eight years of age, and has successively given birth to a daughter, then six sons, then five sons, then four daughters, and then a long series of twins annually, and ended recently by having four sons. It is much to be regretted that this interesting woman did not marry earlier, as she thus lost ten precious years of her life, and so missed the distinction she might have enjoyed of being the mother of a hundred children.—*Medical Age.*

THE GRAND PRIZE FOR ARTIFICIAL LIMBS.

THE medical profession should note the fact that the firm of A. A. Marks, 701 Broadway, New York, was awarded, at the Paris Exposition, the grand prize for the excellence of their artificial limbs. When it is borne in mind that the basis on which the award was made was, that it took twenty points of merit to entitle the exhibitor to this much-to-be-envied prize, it can be readily understood how great is the award, and what a magnificent showing A. A. Marks must have made to be entitled to such distinction. We congratulate the firm upon the very high position to which they have attained in this industry. It speaks volumes for the character of their work.—*Canadian Journal of Medicine and Surgery.*

ELECTRICAL INSTRUMENTS FOR PHYSICIANS AND SURGEONS. Chicago: R. V. Wagner & Co., 308 Dearborn Street.

Catalogues are generally classed with Patent Office Reports and proprietary almanacs. One does not take to their perusal in lieu of the Sunday paper or the latest novel. In fact, most catalogues that come to the editorial table are tossed into the waste basket without a sympathetic glance, and with disrespectful haste. A few manufacturers, and the number is rapidly multiplying, have caught the spirit of the hustling age, and are putting out handbooks that, while they contain price lists, and are, in that sense, commercial, are real works of art and brimful of interest and information. Of this kind, the one before us is a notable example. There are plenty of electrical companies in the field, some of them advertising extensively, with bargain counter inducements and ponderous catalogues that have scarcely been revised in the past twenty years. They practically ignore the marvelous advances that have characterized the last decade. Scores of medical men who once availed themselves of this potent agency in their practice have grown tired of the antiquated, inaccurate, and unreliable forms of apparatus in vogue, and although conscious of its immense power and importance, abandoned its use for all but emergency practice, and relegated their batteries to the lumber room. We had realized this in a vague way, but it required a practical demonstration to bring the situation and contrast home to us in such a way as to arouse our interested attention.

On a recent visit to Chicago we visited the works of this company, and, while the catalogue tells a good story, it scarcely tells the half that might be told. To say that we were surprised is putting it mildly. As we passed from one department to another, our surprise deepened into astonishment at the radical advances made in the technics of electro-therapeutics.

In turning the pages of this fascinating little work, it is refreshing to note the absence of the stereotyped cuts of cells, batteries and electrodes that have been staring us in the face from the advertising pages of the medical journals for the past quarter of a century. Every illustration is suggestive of the touches of a master hand in the designing and adaptation of improved and up-to-date forms of apparatus. There are no bargain-counter goods turned out. It is the trashy instruments, of which there are millions in the market, that have well-nigh brought the use of electricity into disrepute with professional men. We call special attention to wall plate No. 10, on page 22; to shunt coil, with switchboard, No. 44, on page 27; to the direct-current transformer, No. 34, on page 39, and to the 16-plate static machine on page 78. This latter is the ideal static machine of the new century. Nothing more elaborate or efficient could be desired.

Attractive as is this catalogue, a visit to the establishment is far more satisfactory, and those physicians who can make it in their way to inspect the works will be inclined to discard all their old makeshifts in the electrical line, and to leave their orders for a new equipment with which they can confidently resume work in a department of the healing art that is just now undergoing its Renaissance.

FOR years I was annoyed by the quickness with which plaster of paris "set" before my work was finished. One day I was using it in a room where a painter was at work, and he asked, "Why did you not mix that plaster with glue water?" Since then I have had no trouble, and find it an easy matter to mend anything, from the setting of a stationary washbowl to a hole in the plaster. I take one-half teacup of glue, soak till soft in lukewarm water, and then add enough cold water to moisten one-half pound of plaster of paris.—*Good Housekeeping for May.*

WISDOM OF MARCUS AURELIUS ANTONIUS.

"Elegies and quoted odes, and jewels five words
  long,
That on the stretched forefinger of all time
  sparkle forever."

REMEMBER to put yourself in mind every morning, that before night it will be your luck to meet with some busybody, with some ungrateful, abusive fellow, with some knavish, envious or unsociable churl or other. Now all this perverseness in them proceeds from their ignorance of good and evil. . . I am satisfied the person disobliging is of kin to me. . . I am likewise convinced that no man can do me a real injury, because no man can force me to misbehave myself, nor can I find it in my heart to hate or be angry with one of my own nature and family.

As for your body, value it no more than if you were just expiring. For what is it? Nothing but a little blood and bones; a piece of network wrought out of nerves, veins and arteries twisted together. . . . Now consider thus: you are an old man; do not suffer this noble part of you under servitude any longer. Let it not be moved by the springs of selfish passions; let it not quarrel with fate, be uneasy at the present, or afraid of the future.

Do not let accidents disturb, or outward objects engross your thoughts, but keep your mind quiet and disengaged, that you may be at leisure to learn something good, and cease rambling from one thing to another. There is likewise another sort of roving to be avoided; for some people are busy and yet do nothing; they fatigue and wear themselves out, and yet aim at no goal, nor propose any general end of action or design.

When the longest and the shortest-lived persons come to die, their loss is equal; they can but lose the present as being the only thing they have; for that which he has not, no man can be truly said to lose.

Nature never does any mischief.

Hippocrates, who cured so many diseases, himself fell ill and died. The Chaldeans, who foretold other people's death, at last met with their own fate. Alexander, Pompey and Julius Cæsar, who had destroyed so many towns, and cut off so many thousands of horse and foot in the fields, were forced at last to march off themselves. Heraclitus, who argued so much about the universal conflagration, died through water by a dropsy. Democritus was eaten up by vermin; another sort of vermin destroyed Socrates. What are these instances for? Look you: you have embarked, you have made your voyage and your port; debark then without more ado. If you happen to land upon another world there will be gods enough to take care of you; but if it be your fortune to drop into nothing, why, then you will no more be solicited with pleasure and pain.

Put yourself frankly into the hands of fate, and let her spin you out what fortune she pleases.

Every man's life lies all within the present, which is but a point of time; for the past is spent and the future is uncertain.

To have the senses stamped with the impression of an object is common to brutes and cattle; to be hurried and convulsed with passion is the quality of beasts of prey and men of pleasure—such as Phalaris and Nero —of atheists and traitors, too, and of those who do not care what they do when no man sees them.

I will march on in the path of Nature till my legs sink under me, and then I shall be at rest, and expire into the air which has given me my daily breath; fall upon that earth which has maintained my parents, helped my nurse to her milk, and supplied me with meat and drink for so many years; and though its favors have been often abused, still suffers me to tread upon it.

THE saddest ignorance in this world is not to know the pleasure that comes from self-sacrifice.—*Ram's Horn.*

BOOK REVIEWS.

HYPNOTISM. A Complete System of Method, Application and Use, Prepared for the Self-instruction of the Medical Profession. By L. W. De Laurence, Instructor at the School of Hypnotism and Suggestive Therapeutics, Pittsburg. Chicago: The Heneberry Company, 1901. Price, $1.50.

We have copied the title-page of this work in full, for the reason that a careful reading of its 256 pages has failed to reveal any evidence, except its complimentary dedication to a doctor, that its "preparation" included any but the most superficial recognition of the needs of the profession. There is plenty of dogmatic assertion that hypnotism is the underlying science of all sciences, and the true secret of all successful medical practice. Now, this may be true, but Mr. De Laurence has not advanced any such evidence as medical men are in the habit of weighing, to prove that it is even a pseudo science.

The book is written from the standpoint of a layman, yet avowedly for the profession. Here and there a medical term creeps into the text, probably at the instigation of the medical friend to whom the work is inscribed, but they seem, for the most part, lonesome and out of place. Constant references to methods for impressing an audience compel the reader to the conclusion that the author aimed his effort principally at those who desire to join the ranks of the peripatetic "professors" who care nothing for science but everything for the tricks of the trade, with which to draw and awe a gaping crowd.

The author is voluble to the extent of his vocabulary, but is compelled to repeat his leading ideas and assertions, none of which he stops to prove—in order to pad out his pages and round out his paragraphs. Had the forty chapters of the book been winnowed of redundancy and repetitions, fifty pages would have more than held the whole. In short, the volume is palpably commercial rather than professional. If any of our readers propose to go "on the road" as exponents of hypnotism, mesmerism and mind healing, this book will give them "suggestive" aid. But if they seek a scientific exposition of these subjects, they will be disappointed.

PROGRESSIVE MEDICINE, VOL. I., 1901. A Quarterly Digest of Advances, Discoveries and Improvements in the Medical and Surgical Sciences. Edited by Hobart Amory Hare, M.D., Professor of Therapeutics and Materia Medica in the Jefferson Medical College of Philadelphia. Octavo, handsomely bound in cloth, 430 pages, 11 illustrations. Per annum, in four cloth-bound volumes, $10.00. Lea Brothers & Co., Philadelphia and New York.

The first volume of the 1901 series of this unique and valuable quarterly has reached our table. The marked excellence of its predecessors in 1900 imposed upon its editor, contributors, and publishers, the necessity for maintaining the high standard heretofore set up. Accordingly this volume is brimful of practical matter that is up to date and concisely put.

In the first section, Dr. Da Costa handles the subject of the surgery of the head, neck, and chest, in his usual masterful manner. The articles on plastic operations about the face, surgery of the lungs, and the latest methods of dealing with pericardial effusions are given special prominence.

Dr. Packard's article on "The Acute Infectious Diseases" dwells on the important subject of typhoid, and makes good use of the rapidly accumulating material relating to this still by far too prevalent disease.

We note the not at all unusual but quite unwarranted use of the word "malaria." This putting the name of a cause for the name of the disease produced has become so common that it seems useless to protest. In other words, we shall have to accept "bad air" as a disease and not as a cause—Foster and all the philologists to the contrary notwithstanding!

The disorders of childhood, and the practice of surgery upon children, are ably presented by Dr. Crandall.

Pathology receives attention at the hands of Dr. Hektoen, to the extent of eighty pages, some of the special topics treated being of great importance, particularly that relating to immunity.

In the section devoted to Laryngology and Rhinology Dr. Logan Turner devotes six pages to a discussion of the tubercular diseases affecting the nose and throat, a somewhat neglected topic.

Otology receives very practical treatment at the hands of Dr. Randolph, and the volume concludes with a very full index.

IN RE THE BREVITY CLUB.

An occasional contributor recently asked the publisher whether the Brevity Club had come to stay, or was intended as an ephemeral joke, a gentle reminder to authors and general contributors.

To the publisher's emphatic assurance the godfather of the club has been requested to add his solemn affirmation.

This gives the godfather an opportunity to air his most aggressive thought without further apology to publisher or readers. Let the apostles of verbosity brace up for the onset!

The godfather loves the GAZETTE. He would have it assume its rightful position in the very van of the spirit of this busy, hurrying age, and be read and supported by every physician in all the English-speaking communities. It has steadily grown and improved ever since its modest birth, seventeen years ago. It must go on growing and improving, and, at the risk of being called a growler, the godfather of this club ventures some of the suggestions that have been haunting him for many months.

Imprimis, as to the GAZETTE itself: Its name—let it stand. It is good; it is significant. To shorten might weaken it.

2. The "Gazette Publishing Company," let it be banished. It is too long; every reader and subscriber would rather feel that he is dealing with a human being, and not with a cold-blooded corporation. Expunge it!

3. Compress the pages: make them less in number, rather than more. Compression of matter would mean expansion of real thought and multiplication of readers. Let sixty-four be condensed into forty-eight, and everybody will say "amen."

4. Kick out the small type. Good eyes are the exception. Let not a "Hygienic" advocate follow any custom that tends to make them worse. Let the small type go and stay. The ruin of eyes will go on, through the detestably small and indistinct type of the daily newspapers.

5. Do away with the "Departments." Health knows no classification. Let every paper be a curiosity or a surprise. In other words, sandwich the subjects and bunch the editorial matter. Other journals now have hard work to distinguish what your editors have to say from selected matter.

6. Adopt aggressive tactics. Say something that is wilfully wicked, or notoriously not so, for the sake of calling out somebody's bottom logic, and waking up the sleepers.

7. Offer a handsome prize to the author of the most health wisdom in the fewest words, keep the competition open throughout the year, and award the prize as a New Year's present, Jan. 1, 1902.

[The Godfather, as he calls himself, of the Brevity Club, has had his "growl," and he seems more inclined to *snarl* at the publisher than any one else. Let him do all the fault-finding and make all the suggestions he likes, and we will profit by them, if we can.—PUBLISHER.]

Department of Notes and Queries.

FREEDOM OF DISCUSSION BETWEEN EDITOR AND READER.

THIS Department is designed to furnish a frank, cordial and thorough interchange of ideas between Editor and Reader.

To avoid the conventional pitfall into which so many of these Departments drift, patrons who desire to avail themselves of its privileges are requested to scrupulously refrain from personalities, to make their inquiries and responses brief, to the point, and of general interest. By strict observance of these rules the Department can be made of immense practical value to all our readers.

Query 83. What about mosquitoes and malaria? Is the connection between the two another medical bugaboo, or do the varmints really have a hand in spreading intermittent fever? And if so, what can be done to eradicate them?
W. M. T., N. J.

Answer.—When this theory was first announced we were quite inclined to ridicule it as a vagary of the scientific brain. Further and quite exhaustive investigations have seemed to prove that certain species of mosquitoes are capable of conveying the germ of intermittent fever from one person to another, or rather of acting as an intermedium for the development of the germ embryo. Many species have however been acquitted of harm in this direction. In fact, but one species is as yet charged with being *particeps criminis*—the *anopheles.*

Various methods are advised for destroying these pests. The most efficient one seems to be the use of petroleum on ponds and marshes wherever they propagate. It is also asserted that a small quantity of permanganate of potassium, crystals or solution, thrown into any standing pool that harbors this insect will effectually destroy the larvæ. If people living in malarial localities will combine in the matter no doubt this source of infection can be reduced to a minimum. In the long run prevention will be a source of economy. It will save drug bills, funeral expenses, shivers and profanity.

This mosquito theory is not strictly novel. The subject was broached by writers as early as the beginning of the Christian era. Among early American writers who studied the question may be mentioned Nott, of New Orleans (1848), King, of Washington (1883), Mitchell, of Philadelphia, and others.

A recent writer observes:

"The fact that the malarial parasite is paludal in its habits, and that the mosquito is a blood-sucker and also paludal in habit, is extremely suggestive of this connection. The idea, however, did not take definite form until Patrick Manson, in his Goulstonian lectures, delivered in 1896, set forth a definite hypothesis, based on certain well-established facts, namely, that the malarial parasite possessed a flagellating phase, that this phase is developed from the mature parasite, that it is evolved only when the parasite is outside the human body, that the flagellæ, when formed, break away from the parent parasite, and that, when free, the flagellæ were capable of living as independent organisms. He was thus led to believe that the flagella was the extracorporeal phase in the life history of the parasite. As it was impossible for the latent form in which this organism originated to escape from the human body by itself, it was necessary to invoke the assistance of some outside agency. The most probable agent was the mosquito, and Manson supposed that the flagellated body was sucked, in its latent form, into the stomach of the mosquito and developed therein. The flagellæ then broke away from the central sphere, and in virtue of their locomotive power traversed the blood in the mosquito's stomach, penetrated the stomach wall, entered some cell and started the "outside-of-the-body" life of the malarial parasite. Manson still believed, however, that malaria could be air or water borne, for he supposed that on the death of the mosquito the parasite was liberated, and either inhaled from the air or carried into the system in drinking water.

"Sulphur has been recommended to prevent the bites of certain insects, and it is probable that it will prove more or less effective against the bite of the mosquito, thus forming a prophylactic against malarial fever.

"Laveran says that in Italy the belief is common that fever may be prevented by eating garlic, and Prof. Celli, of Rome, says that the Sardinian peasants protect themselves by rubbing garlic on their skins. The essential oil contained in the garlic contains a large percentage of sulphur in combination as allyl sulphide. D'Abbadie mentions some investigations by Prof. Silvestri of Catania, in Sicily, showing that the workmen in sulphur mines situated at low levels in malarious districts are almost exempt from malaria. The percentage of miners suffering from fever averaged 8 to 9 per cent.; while among the inhabitants of the vicinity following other occupations, over 90 per cent. suffered from malaria.

"Fougué says that the village of Zephyria, in Greece, has become depopulated, owing to the fever, which is very severe in that locality. The depopulation is said to have begun when the sulphur deposits ceased to be worked. A similar instance is reported in the district of Catania, in Sicily, where a village had to be abandoned owing to the prevalence of malaria. The only people who are able to reside there are a small colony of men who work the sulphur mines. These facts furnish valuable corroborative evidence of the use of sulphur as a prophylactic against malaria."

Query 84. I have met with a stumper in the word *bacteriolysins*. Will your editor of *Notes and Queries* enlighten me concerning the meaning of this term?   G. L. T., Ky.

Answer.—Of making many words there is no end. Our correspondent is quite excusable for his lack of knowledge. The word has been coined by the germ hunters since Gould, Foster and the "Century" had passed their final revisions. The rapid advance being made in the study of germs and their products has necessitated the invention of new terms to name and describe the newly discovered micro-organisms, their media, laws of development, excreta, toxins and anti-toxins. This particular word is applied to certain complex substances containing a peptic ferment combined with a bacterial derivative. These substances seem to have the power of dissolving certain bacteria and also possess digestive activity, on account of the peptic ferment referred to. They are accredited with a specific action which is supposed to explain the destruction of micro-organisms in the animal body, and by this means conferring a degree of bacterial immunity. In time scientists will doubtless be able to clear up the yet unexplained reason why some persons are immune to certain infections while other equally robust individuals are quite susceptible and perhaps readily succumb to them. We are slowly making progress in this direction, but there is much for us to learn before we can speak with much confidence or authority.

Query 85. Do you consider hypnotism and hypnotic suggestion of very much value to the practising physician?   F. R. H., Idaho.

Answer.—Yes, it has always been of inestimable value to practitioners of medicine, and the most successful physicians are the ones who consciously or unconsciously use it most adroitly. Thousands of otherwise competent physicians fail because they lack hypnotic faculty.

This does not endorse all the rhodomontade that is now being paraded under the name of hypnotism. It is a case of *nascitur non fit.* Hypnotists as well as poets are chiefly born, not made

by mail! At the same time the faculty can be cultivated, and there is little in it to be afraid of, popular opinion to the contrary notwithstanding.

Query 86. What breakfast foods are now considered most wholesome and most reliable as to quality?

Do you consider mushes of any kind strictly proper in a well-regulated dietary?

Answer.—We answered a similar question, in this Department some months since, (see Sept., 1900, issue of the GAZETTE), but will venture a little further discussion of the subject on the presumption that our querist is a new subscriber.

The list of breakfast foods now clamoring in the various advertising mediums for recognition as "the best" in the market is quite bewildering. In popularity, crushed oats heads the list. Of this product there are dozens of competing brands put up in packages, while immense quantities are sold in bulk. Among the package brands the range is from the original "A. B. C.," through the alphabet to—well, perhaps not quite all the letters have yet been appropriated!

Originally this "A. B. C." brand was all that could be desired. Latterly it seems to have fallen from grace. The "H. O." brand has had a great run, and there are several other brands that have become more or less popular, sometimes more by advertising enterprise than from real merit. We try them all from time to time, each new claimant as it appears, but we invariably fall back upon the brand called "Quaker Oats," as more uniformly maintaining its qualities and its cleanness from smut and other seeds.

Of wheat preparations there seems to be no end of new names. The uncooked crushed wheat is not as popular as it would be if it did not require so much cooking to make it satisfactory to delicate or weakened digestive organs.

This objection is also applicable to many brands of prepared oats. All these grains should be thoroughly steamed or roasted. This process accomplishes two purposes; it sterilizes, thus promoting the keeping qualities, and it insures a sufficient transformation of the starchy element. When this pre-cooking is well done it is impossible for the careless or ignorant cook to send the morning dish to the table in an entirely unpalatable and indigestible condition.

"Germea" for a time was the leading wheat preparation. Its success was so immediate and unprecedented that scores of rivals and imitators have crowded the field, and competition has had the usual effect of lowering the standard of quality. Every few weeks a new candidate is announced. Among them all "Parched Farinose" and "Granose Flakes" are far in advance of any others that have come to our knowledge. We are surprised that the parching idea has not been more generally adopted. It is better than steaming, because it gives the product a nutty flavor not otherwise attainable, and palatability is a paramount quality in all these breakfast cereals. If manufacturers would give us parched corn, oats, wheat, rye and barley, properly cleaned and *granulated* instead of being ground fine, there would be fewer dyspeptics and fewer complaints as to the indigestibility of these foods.

As to the second part of your question, it is partially answered in the foregoing. The objection to mushes in general comes chiefly from the fact that they are insufficiently cooked and are almost universally, since they need no mastication to render them easy of deglutition, swallowed without due insalivation. To obviate this objection, which is a serious one. they should be made of firm consistence, not gruels, and as a further precaution, bits of zwiebach, dry toast or "grape nuts" should be eaten with them.

Query 86.   W. P. of Decatur, O.

Answer.—Your inquiry is rather too comprehensive as well as too technical for reply in this Department. See also remarks in April number of the GAZETTE concerning unsigned communications.

Query 87.   I am deeply interested in Dr. Achorn's diet tables, and especially in his "Notes." (I can't quite understand why they should be banished from the body of the work and set up in smaller type.) The GAZETTE is to be commended for providing its readers with this striking and instructive series, at once so comprehensive and so scientific. I do not feel competent to formally criticise any of Dr. Achorn's essential statements, but it seems to me that if he errs at all it is on the side of leniency and liberality. For example, the dietary prescribed in Bright's, in the April number, includes and permits almost every item that any one but the most exacting epicure and gourmand could desire.

In this respect does he not to some extent clash with the general tenor of the teachings with which you have all along been educating your readers?
                                        D. C. F., Washington.

Answer.—To this and all similar queries that are coming to us we desire to reply comprehensively that it is only justice to our esteemed contributor that all criticisms of his positions should be passed over to him, so that at the close of his series of papers he can in his own way consider them in detail. Our readers are cordially invited to the freest and frankest expression of their views, whether approving, inquiring or dissenting. We shall be glad to publish all such brief inquiries and criticisms as shall reach us, if couched in courteous terms and actuated by the spirit so evident in the foregoing. In all cases when a paper is read and discussed before a medical body the author, both by custom and courtesy, has the last word.

This querist is referred to a short paper in this number of the GAZETTE, taken from *The Hospital*, of London, "Some Current Absurdities in Diet."

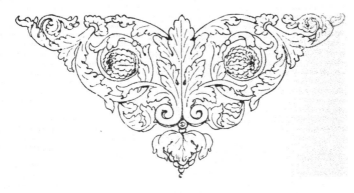

THE

DIETETIC AND HYGIENIC GAZETTE

A MONTHLY JOURNAL OF PHYSIOLOGICAL MEDICINE

Vol. XVII.   NEW YORK, JUNE, 1901.   No. 5.

WHAT THE CENTURY HAS TAUGHT US ABOUT LIVING.

By Samuel S. Wallian, A.M., M.D.

(Copyright 1901.)

III.

THE SLEEPING ROOMS.

NEXT in importance are the sleeping rooms, a statement or admission that will be promptly and emphatically disputed by the sagacious sanitarian, since one-half our lives are spent in bed. Intelligent people are beginning to realize this fact, but too many otherwise sensible people, especially in large cities, where the masses live, that is, they exist, spend their lives in "flats" and "apartment" houses, and put up with little six-by-nine closets, that are called bedrooms. These "cubby holes" are ventilated by a transom that merely opens into another room, or by a dismal window in a dark air-shaft. Even in the country there are too many sleeping rooms that are almost hermetically sealed, as far as regards the ingress and egress of fresh air. To this cause can be directly traced a large percentage of the admitted increase of the "Great White Plague," tuberculosis, and some other chronic diseases. So many people have an ingrained and instinctive horror of "drafts!" Coddling makes them susceptible, they "take cold," and at once try to recall some real or imaginary exposure to a "draft."

The bugaboo of the present generation is "taking cold." To this vague and misunder-stood accident it has become a chronic and almost universal habit to attribute more than half the ills, aches and pains that flesh is heir to. Our ancestors did not shudder at sight of their own shadows, nor did they swathe themselves in Jaeger woolens or Alaska sealskins. They slept for the most part in large open rooms that were not sealed with double-sash windows, rubber weather strips, and air-tight doors. Their chimneys and fireplaces were as wide as a city "flat," and as roomy as the throat of a blast-furnace. These were their ventilators, and they did the work effectually. With a blazing fire and a good "draft" all the impurities and floating germs of the whole house were drawn into the chimney and cremated. They had no acquaintance with Wilton, Axminster or velvet carpets, but, barring a few removable rag rugs, lived on bare floors, that were regularly scrubbed with home-made soft soap and sharp white sand. Without knowing it they were antedating Lister and Tait, by practising both asepsis and antisepsis, with the result that epidemics of influenza, scarlatina, diphtheria, pneumonia and other fatal disorders were not half as prevalent or virulent as they are under our more "civilized" theories and practice. Of course many of their habits were different from ours, but there is no kind of doubt that the foundation of their greater immunity and surpassing virility were chiefly due to the fact that they lived, moved, had their being and said their prayers, day and night, in a better atmosphere. Furthermore, they inured themselves to the ordinary vicissitudes of the climate about them, went out freely in all weathers, did not overburden themselves with an excess of fine and fluffy flannels, breathed with their cutaneous mouths as well as with their lungs; and, although they bathed occasionally, they did not keep their skins water-soaked and hypersensitive by too frequent hot bathing and superabundant clothing. It is said they ate more simply, and this is true in a sense; but often their dietary was crude in the extreme, and would have sorely tried a modern stomach. They not only endured but relished it with a zest to which we are strangers. Furthermore, they exercised more freely and breathed more deeply, thus securing a degree of oxidation not otherwise obtainable, and as a consequence *digested* what they ate.

Until recently the doctor has been content with making the acquaintance of the sickroom, with occasional invitations to the parlor to consult with a brother physician, or to be confidentially catechised as to the invalid's actual instead of nominal progress and prospects. That time has gone by. His province has been broadened until now he must begin his inspection and inquisition in the kitchen and cookroom. He can no longer close his eyes to the fact that the success of his treatment can be seriously impeded and even radically overcome by bad living habits, by unhygienic housing, feeding, nursing, and general environment. It is a new dispensation that he is called upon to interpret. His Praxis has been merged into Prophylaxis. He must first of all forefend; mending only when it is too late to prevent. To do this he needs a more comprehensive education than under the old régime. He must look after the grounds, and when

every unsanitary feature of these has been corrected he must enter the Kitchen. The *chef* will have to don a fresh frock—not merely a clean apron to hide the dirt of a soiled working suit—must scrub his hands, arms, and finger-nails with a stiff scrubbing brush and antiseptic soap. He must "clare up" the cookroom, purge all the dark corners, dump out all the accumulated trash, disinfect the walls, sinks, and cupboards, and take a fresh course in culinary cleanliness, which now means much more than shining china and glassware and unwrinkled linen.

The doctor is no longer a mere pharmacist and dispenser of drugs. Henceforth the most advanced and intelligent practice will be based on Sanitation, Hygiene and Dietetics.

When he has made the Kitchen all that it should be and directed and properly regulated the daily *menu*, he must proceed to the living room, the library, and not pause until he has reconstructed the sleeping apartments.

In a sweeping and emphatic manner, but not a whit too emphatic, it may be laid down as a rule that no room that is not amply and efficiently ventilated every hour of the day and night, regardless of the season and of the weather, is fit for a well-bred dog, let alone a human being, to sleep in. Yet how many people imagine they are ventilating a room when they open a transom or set the door ajar into another apartment, itself equally as pent up and foul as the one they are in. The most dangerous "cold" one can take is the one of which he is wholly unconscious at the time. It does not come from a "draft," but chiefly from breathing impure air. It is then that we ingest too much and eliminate too little, and this regardless of our most rigorous attempts at abstemiousness. *Fresh air and forced feeding are "curing" more cases of confirmed consumption than all other treatments combined.* But forced feeding without fresh air to correspond is a fatal failure. The food must be brought into direct contact with its full requirement of oxygen or there can be no appropriation or assimilation, and it will harm instead of help.

It is much easier to be forehanded by preventing tuberculosis and other devastating forms of chronic disease, than to overcome them after once established. It is a case in which an ounce of prevention, that is certainly available, is worth a ton of cure, that at best is uncertain.

WHAT TO PUT IN THE HIVE.

The furnishings of the home are very properly beginning to absorb more attention than ever before in the history of the race. Following the agitation of the last few years of the old century, in connection with "sanitary plumbing," the impression is gaining headway that there is a certain degree of danger in unsanitary furniture, fittings, hangings and decorations. Every new fact adduced in connection with the identification and biologic history of microorganisms emphasizes the conviction that there can be no thorough immunity from germ infection until we cease to make our dwellings the convenient and congenial harbors of all forms of germ life. Granted that the human organism is naturally fortified, to a definite degree, against all ordinary morbific influences, the exigencies of human life are such that no one can predict when some member of the family, through carelessness or some unavoidable cause, will fall below the normal standard of health, and lose the power of resisting and repelling the initial approach of disease through infection.

Exposed to the light of modern sanitary science, many of the old-time fittings of our dwellings, of hotels, public conveyances, and, in a lesser degree, of public halls, school-buildings and churches, are either passively or positively bad.

Beginning our inspection at the foundation, the floor-coverings have almost universally been ready and constant accumulators of that most insidious and prolific source of disease, infectious dust. An old carpet becomes a veritable reservoir and magazine of invisible, insinuating and incessantly moving filth. It is a saturated storehouse of impalpable, impermeating and yet invisible particles, largely composed of germs, spores and ethereal animal exhalations, that float at a touch and are inhaled at every breath. These insidious particles attach themselves to all the moist mucous surfaces with which they come in contact as they pass along the respiratory tract, and the great wonder is that human beings escape contamination as long as they do. Every footfall, every movement through the room, opening of doors—even the lifting of a chair, or movement of a curtain, starts invisible eddies and fills the room with countless millions of microscopic atoms, from which there is little hope of escape. What is wanted is dust annihilators. There are plenty of devices for the coarser "renovation" of rooms and fabrics, and plenty of corporations ready to guarantee the clearing of the premises of rats, mice, roaches and all other kinds of vermin; but the man who will devise an effective and universally applicable system of removing domestic dust will deserve to head the list of the canonized of all the ages. Such an invention would cut the current deathrate in two, within the first year of its general adoption.

Sweeping and, iconoclastic as the statement may sound, carpets are, in the eyes of the sanitarian, an unmitigated and inexcusable nuisance. Scrupulous care can mitigate the evil, but can not radically cure it. Carpet-sweepers take up the coarser accumulations, but they set the finer and most dangerous particles to whirling at will throughout the air, not to be deposited again for hours. If carpets were to be first sprinkled with wet sawdust, and this quickly removed, by the patented sweepers, and committed to the fire, it would prove a wonderful stroke of hygienic and preventive economy. But this suggestion will be deemed infeasible by an overwhelming majority of those who stand most in need of its benefits.

Movable rugs for room-centers, with the

borders of the room bare, waxed, oiled, or finished with some one of the floor dressings, varnishes, or "hard oils," involves a great improvement over carpets, simply because they present less surface of absorbent material, and because they can be carried out of doors at frequent intervals and thoroughly cleaned. There is a choice as to the best kind of rugs to buy. The best rug—barring fashion, fad, and fancy—is the one that will harbor the least dust, and that will yield that little most readily to beating, sweeping and other cleansing processes. Those with a firm and close-woven underbody and short, stiff pile, but not reversible, are the best, the grades called Wilton and Axminster being representative examples.

Mattings are much preferable to carpets, but this assertion must be qualified. Mattings permit the dust to sift through them to the floor, where it is temporarily concealed and prevented from circulating; but these coverings are apt to be left in position too long, thereby gathering such quantities of this fine filth that it begins to be given back to the air, as busy feet pass over it. Some housewives wash it periodically with strong solutions of common salt, which more or less mitigates its evils.

Wall coverings are an item of equal or greater importance, and one to which too little attention is paid. The almost universal use of paper in "decorating" the walls of modern dwellings can not be unequivocally endorsed by the sanitary expert. The designing and manufacture of hangings has been carried to a high degree of perfection, as far as artistic effects are concerned; but while the manipulators of paper pulp, and the color-artists may be chemists in their way, it is evident that they waste no time in studying physiologic chemistry, and some of the "effects" attained are incidental rather than intended. This subject has been frequently agitated, and its evils often exaggerated, in the public press and in medical literature. Some of the processes and pigments used are, no doubt, indictable before the High Court of Health. Perhaps no cases of directly fatal poisoning have

ever been traced to this source, but even slow or partial poisoning is not a result that intelligent people knowingly care to invite. Some colors are more detrimental than others, but the harm does not all lie in the ornamentation or printed design. The chemicals used in preparing the blanks or stock are often as pernicious as the print-colors—the occupation itself shortening the lives of the operatives, it is said, by an average of ten years. Aside from the poisonous chemicals and pigments used in their manufacture, all papers are more or less absorbent, the glazed varieties less so than others; therefore, for these several reasons, wall paper, sanitarily permissible only under the utmost possible precautions, can never be made to figure as an ideal lining for living or sleeping rooms. Cloth hangings—not draperies—are free from some of the objections pertaining to paper, and are beginning to come in vogue, especially for halls and dining-rooms. The draperies now becoming fashionable in the palatial drawing-rooms of some of our millionaires are very effective, from an artistic point of view; but they can, by no stretch of leniency, be recommended by the strict sanitarian. They, too, harbor too much. Fresco painting, tinting and ordinary painting can be successfully resorted to in all the rooms in common use. In this way walls and ceilings can be made quite acceptable to the most exacting sanitary critic, and at the same time not offensive to good taste and the artistic sense. Glass mosaics for wall coverings are announced and may prove a sanitary boon. For halls, dining-rooms and kitchens, ceiling with wood, which is to be treated to "filler" and varnish, or with paint, makes a good finish, and is becoming more and more popular. Panelled and patterned walls and ceilings, after the fashion of the Mosaic or parquet floorings, would be a sensible innovation. Steel ceilings are also a safe refuge, and admit of artistic effects. To those who are compelled to make the best of whatever surroundings they already enjoy, or endure, these suggestions will doubtless prove valueless.

With many it will not be a question of how to build but how to readjust, ameliorate and modify. In some instances, perhaps, little can be done to improve existing conditions. A small kitchen can be enlarged, an extra window—possibly a wide, projecting one for plants—can be inserted. The walls and ceilings can be renewed, recovered, ceiled or painted. A poor range can be discarded and a good one installed. Shelving and cupboards can be made more convenient, and the water-supply and drainage more efficient.

Whether building or repairing, do not forget the matter of the bathroom and the numerous closets. Let the bathroom also be roomy, the tub a modern one, and its arrangement suitable and convenient. If the floor is a common one, full of shrinkage cracks, let it be re-covered with tile, parquet flooring or linoleum; have the walls wainscotted four feet high, and then finish this and the flooring, if of wood, with two good coats of a hard varnish—one of the best now in the market for this purpose being called "marble finish."

Of course, every sleeping-room should have its closet, and a closet off either the hall or dining-room will be a great convenience.

A mere hint as to general furnishings must suffice. For the practical living rooms, as already intimated in what has been said as to floor coverings, avoid absorbent fluffiness. Leather coverings for chairs and couches is preferable to any kind of tapestry. "Pantasote" is one of the newer substitutes for leather. Brass, or enamelled iron or steel bedsteads, casings and framings that harbor as little dust as possible; curtains selected on the same principle, and shades that are not too dark or somber—all these suggest themselves. Inside blinds are not so desirable as outside, the latter permitting proper ventilation in all weathers.

As a suggestion and aid to those who have yet to provide, or who are prepared and inclined to improve their culinary equipment, it has been deemed best to omit all mention of particular items or preferable patterns and manufactures *en passant*, and instead of the merely casual mention that would be appropriate in this place, to devote a few final pages to a more detailed description of all the leading appliances and utensils that go to make the kitchen more complete, to render its results as nearly perfect as may be, and, at the same time, to make its cares and labors as light as possible. In this direction great advances have been made within a few years. By means of new and improved utensils as fast as introduced, the lot of the modern housewife has been made much more endurable, and the health of the household has been relieved of many sources of minor menace. It will be the aim to make this final *Index Rerum* a helpful guide to those who are not yet familiar with the more recent advances in the manufacture of kitchen furniture and improved utensils which will do so much to ameliorate the trials of the housewife.

Besides the scores of labor-saving and helpful utensils and appliances, there are many food preparations in the market which are proving their practical value, both as labor-savers and health-promoters. It looks now as though the next generation would be able to live with very little effort in the way of cooking, and on a much more wholesome and sensible dietary than is now in vogue.

Descriptions of these newer food products, with an estimate of their nutritive and economic value, as far as these have been reliably established, will be included in the list referred to.

There are now, and rapidly coming to be more, things 'twixt heaven and earth, Mrs. Horatio, than were ever dreamt of in our grandmother's philosophy. The day is not far distant when the endless paraphernalia, now considered so necessary to kitchen and dining-room, will be reduced to a fourth part of the present array, and the labor and care of the household proportionately reduced.

THE KITCHEN ARMAMENT.

The first article of importance is the range or cook-stove. A poor range is the dearest article of furniture any house can contain. If I were a prospective bride I would have the quality of this indispensable item—which is either the Housekeeper's Best Friend or Housekeeper's Horror—guaranteed in the m a r r i a g e contract! No family is so poor as to be able to afford an inconvenient fuel-wasting, food-destroying makeshift or monstrosity called a stove or range. The better class of manufacturers are no longer turning out this grade of goods, but there are plenty of such in use. There are still plenty of women, both in city and country, who have never known the comfort and luxury of doing their work over one of the perfected and easily managed ranges which have been designed and supplied by various competing firms within the past decade. It is safe to say that by the aid of these improved appliances the work of the cook-room can be done with one-half the fuel, one-fourth the labor and a hundredth part of the worry and exasperation that it once required.

The difference in the cost of an ordinarily bad, a regular woman-killing and wasteful range, and one that combines modern facilities and working qualities, is not much in dollars, but it is immense in the matter of comfort, convenience and good health. In whatever families such a relic of barbarism remains, let there be a domestic insurrection. Seize the ax, borrow a sledge-hammer, unhorse the thing and break it into a thousand pieces, lest some other deluded family shall try to "get along with it for a few more years"! The only broils it is capable of doing to perfection are family broils. It savors of domestic discord, it drives husbands to drink, and wives to the divorce court and the missionary society. It breeds disappointment, dyspepsia and despair. It has transformed many a sweet-tempered maid into a frowzy termagant. It has soured the dispositions and the stomachs of as good husbands as ever knelt at the altar and took the oath of marital allegiance. Charity begins at home—when it begins at all. Begin it at the hearthstone by procuring the best range the market af-

fords, and see what a multitude of domestic sins it will—not *cover*, but avert. There is more to beget genuine charity, which the "Higher Criticism" tells us means love, than in whole volumes of doctrinal sermons, or the Nicene Creed. If the money for a new one is not at hand, borrow it, commit highway robbery, or buy on time, and pay in instalments. You will more than save the instalments in the cost of fuel, food and fury! It will be the most profitable investment you ever made. In buying, don't be penny-wise and pound-foolish, as to a few dollars' difference in the first cost. Get the best, and with it get the best furniture, copper wash-boiler, agate ware and nickeled steel and other *best* varieties of modern cooking utensils. These are light to handle and will not taint your food.

There is no escaping the fact that a faultless, up-to-date range and full complement of first-class appurtenances and accessories, is a positive moral force in the household. Indulging a little harmless hyperbole, it will prove a means of grace and present help in time of need. It promotes domestic sunshine, daily harmony and all the sweet amenities of life. It cultivates peace of mind, amiability and serenity of temper that diffuses itself throughout the entire household. No one can appreciate its manifold blessings who has not succeeded to it after years of misery and domestic nightmare with its counterpart.

Kitchen Furniture in Detail.—Without good tools the best of carpenters fail to turn out good work. Still more the housewife needs a complete and convenient armamentarium. Aunt Chloe, in "Uncle Tom's Cabin," was, no doubt, a picture from real life. With meager kitchen facilities she could, on state occasions, produce culinary wonders—measured on the table!—but the appetites of the guests would not have been improved by a glimpse of her soot and suet-smirched cook-room, redolent of all the odors that ever emanated from Cologne, Hunter's Point, or Chicago (before she reformed her Stygian Pool)!

We have said enough about the range,

which answers for the engine of the establishment. The next item in order, when gas is not used for fuel, is the tender, the fuel provider. Do not waste ten per cent. of your time, temper and muscular strength carrying fuel from a distance, even though that distance be but a dozen steps. A fuel hopper, occupying but trifling space, and yet holding a day's supply, can be deftly arranged within easy reach of the range or stove. If coal be the fuel used, an upright storage box or bin, with a trap door at the bottom, of a size to admit the fire shovel, is the most convenient. It need not be larger than twelve or fourteen inches square on the floor, by three feet high, to hold a full day's supply.

There are a score or more of small accessories to the kitchen which it would not be necessary to mention in detail, except that they contribute so very much to the completeness of the room. A small table or stand, without drawers, that can be moved about on easy rolling casters, will be found of great utility. All cupboards should be ventilated by the insertion of end openings between each of the shelves, to be covered by brass or galvanized wire gauze. For summer use, and in warm climates, it is an excellent way to imitate the California practice of building "food safes" into the north kitchen wall, making them project a foot or more into the air outside. These projections are to be closed at the back, while the ends are covered with the same wire gauze, so that the winds of heaven can freely blow through them at all times. The Californians substitute these wire-enclosed safes for the usual ice-boxes and refrigerators used in other parts of the country, and find that vegetables, fruit and cooked foods of all kinds keep both longer and better than in closed refrigerators. They might be utilized even in winter by providing removable doors with but minute air-openings, sufficient for cold-weather ventilation. In all cupboards designed for the storage of food, plate glass shelves are ideal, when they can be afforded. Over the sink should hang its rubber-edged shovel, a wire pot-scourer, and a generous container for soap and sapolio.

Next in importance is the kitchen sink. Generous size, accessibility, and perfect drainage—these are the essentials. Adjoining it should be a table or broad shelf, in constant demand as a temporary receptacle for dishes and utensils. This table is not to be considered a passable makeshift for the regular working table, now becoming common in the market, with drawers, drawshelves, and hinged meal-hoppers, its lower part divided into convenient compartments for holding the several grades of floor and meal used in cooking.

The ordinary ice-box or refrigerator, as usually arranged, is a menace to health. It is next to impossible to keep it sweet and clean, and the least neglect in this direction soon makes it a source of contamination and infection. The more recent models of this kitchen appendage are a great improvement on those heretofore in use. They are better constructed, better ventilated, and some of them are lined with glass, porcelain, or thoroughly glazed earthenware, and are without open seams and hidden recesses for harboring dirt—in the kitchen, dirt and germs being usually synonymous. If this useful apparatus could be thoroughly scalded and sunned for a couple of hours, every few days, even the wooden varieties could be kept wholesome; but they are so heavy and cumbersome that this is out of the question. When from necessity these closed refrigerators and food safes are used, in addition to scrupulous cleanliness, the best substitute for sunlight is to burn a bit of sulphur, half the size of an egg, first moistening it with a little alcohol and placing it in the bottom apartment of the food safe, in an iron skillet or other metal container, closing all the doors and lids while it is burning. This fumigation should be repeated at frequent intervals—at least once a month.

PROGRESS IN THE SANATORIUM TREATMENT OF TUBERCULOSIS.

PROGRESS in the sanatorium treatment of tuberculosis is shown in the third annual report of the Free Hospital for Poor Consumptives of Pennsylvania, from which we epitomize the following:

In Germany, there have been established during the last few years nearly 100 sanatoriums for the treatment of consumptives, with a combined capacity of 5,000. This has been established partly through the government, partly through private charity, and largely through the life insurance companies. In Germany, the life insurance companies find it profitable to send their insured who have tuberculosis to sanatoria for treatment, because of what they can save in the payment of insurance money with those who get well, and the deferment of such payment with those whose lives are prolonged. They also profit by the prevention of the spread of the disease.

In England, prior to the present movement on behalf of consumptives, there were already hospital accommodations for consumptives to the extent of about 2,000 beds. Since this movement began many new sanatoriums have been opened, and the old ones have been improved. England has probably 3,000 beds for consumptives at the present time.

In France, about 2,800 beds for tuberculous subjects existed when the present movement began, and since then sanatoria either have been built, or are being built at Lyons, Paris, Orleans, Bordeaux, Nancy, Lille, Havre, Canet, and Cimiez. The French Government is about completing a sanatorium at Agincourt, at an outlay of over a million francs.

In Russia, under the leadership of the Tsars, five sanatoriums have already been established and a number are underway.

In Italy, sanatoriums are being established at Arizanno, Padua, Umbria, Naples, Messina, Tarent, Cadore and Milan. A law has also been passed requiring existing hospitals to set aside wards for the treatment of consumptives.

In Norway, since 1897, three sanatoriums have been established, and two are under way—all under the government. A number of private sanatoriums have also been opened.

In Denmark, a hospital for consumptives, with 94 beds, was opened in 1900 for the use of the entire country, and another with 110 beds for the use of the city of Copenhagen only.

In Sweden, a large sanatorium for consumptives is at present being built as a Jubilee memorial.

In Switzerland, there are already seven sanatoriums for poor consumptives, and a number of others have been projected.

In Austria, a sanatorium has been established at Alland, and similar institutions are projected in Bohemia, at Maehren, and at Steiermarck.

In Hungary, a sanatorium for consumptives is at present being erected as a memorial to the late Queen Elizabeth.

In Poland, three sanatoriums for consumptives have recently been erected.

In Spain, under the leadership of the royal family, a large national sanatorium for consumptives has been opened at Porta Cœli.

In Portugal, Queen Amelia has recently given 20,000,000 reis for the establishment of a tuberculosis hospital.

In Holland, the popular young Queen of Holland within a year has given a large sum of money for the establishment of a sanatorium for consumptives.

In Canada, there are as yet but two sanatoriums for consumptives with a combined capacity of seventy-five beds. The Government of the Province of Ontario has, however, recently passed a bill encouraging the establishment of sanatoriums by providing legal machinery for raising revenue for the same. Under this act any municipality can, with the consent of the general government, establish a sanatorium, and raise revenue for its maintenance.

United States.—The National Government has established sanatoriums in New Mexico for the treatment of tubercular marine hospital patients, and for consumptives of its army.

The State of New York has at present ten sanatoriums for consumptives under private management, and one projected sanatorium to be supported by the State. These have an aggregate capacity of about six hundred beds. The State of New York appropriated $50,000 during the last session of the legislature for a hospital site, and is asked to appropriate $100,000 during the present session of the legislature for buildings and maintenance. The City of New York appropriates $75,000 annually for maintenance of consumptive patients in the Spuyten Duyvil Hospital on the Hudson.

Massachusetts has five hospitals for consumptives, one of which has been established by the State. The combined capacity of the five hospitals is about three hundred and fifty beds. The State of Massachusetts appropriated $150,000 for the establishment of its hospital.

Illinois has one hospital for consumptives in operation, and two projected—all in Cook County. The three will have a combined capacity of about five hundred beds.

Colorado has three private sanatoriums for pay patients.

Maryland has one hospital for poor consumptives with a capacity of one hundred beds.

Ohio has one hospital for poor consumptives, with a capacity of one-hundred beds for consumptives.

Alabama has two sanatoria for consumptives, one for pay patients, and one for consumptive prisoners of the State.

New Mexico has three small pay sanatoriums for consumptives and one large one projected.

Connecticut has one small pay hospital for consumptives.

Pennsylvania has three tuberculosis hospitals with a combined capacity of about one hundred and twenty beds, and nearly one-half of these beds are in wards of general hospitals, supported by the Free Hospital for Poor Consumptives.

Other States.—Sanatoriums for consumptives have been projected in New Jersey, Ohio, Minnesota, Michigan and Rhode Island, and probably in many other States. Rhode Island has under consideration a bill appropriating $200,000 for a tuberculosis hospital.

The contagiousness and the prevention of pulmonary tuberculoss are as certain as that the hospital treatment of the poor afflicted with this disease is at once the scientific and the humane way of preventing the spread of the disease. The late Professor J. M. DaCosta, shortly before his death wrote:

"The lot of the consumptive poor is indeed a terrible one. Constantly losing strength and power; feverish and in distress; shut out from hospitals because their accommodations do not permit them to receive any large number of cases likely to be of very long duration, because, too, it is now recognized that it is not fair to others to admit into the wards what will be a source of infection; shunned and neglected, and ever growing weaker, while yet obliged to labor incessantly for the daily bread of himself and family—the poor consumtive is the most pitiable figure in our midst. Help him where you can; labor for him."

✦ ✦

GETTING AT THE CAUSES.

WE do not belong to the pessimists who, with Scopenhauer, insist that human life, stripped of sentiment and illusion, becomes either hell or a hospital. Nor do we appreciate the efforts of the opposite extreme, the optimists, who hold that life is a great privilege for which we should daily go on our knees and return thanks. We are here either without an invitation or without having had the privilege of declining an invitation. We may go further and admit that invalidism is the rule, health the exception. This is practically confessed in the inevitable salutation on meeting. "How do you do? How are you? How is your health, and how is your family?" This form of greeting is more particularly Anglican and

American. The French say, *Comment vous portez vous?*—How do you carry yourself? Or, *Cava tout bien, ce matin?*—Goes everything well, this morning? Your caballero greets an acquaintance with a similar inquiry. The Italian varies the salute, but is more anxious to know whether heaven has been propitious than whether the doctor needs to be summoned. It may be that the foreigners quoted are quite as frequently "knocked out," in a physical sense, as Americans or English, and that here this condition of perpetual invalidism has merely come to be more universally admitted and more habitually remembered. On meeting a friend, after even a brief absence, it is considered quite discourteous and an evidence of inexcusable indifference not to make minute and detailed inquiry as to the physical condition of each member of either or both families, with reiterated expressions of sympathy—and some prescriptions—for this or that one who is reported as unusually ailing.

No doubt habit has much to do with this sort of conventional circumlocution, but fixed habits are generally an expression of either immediate or remote causative conditions.

In an ideal state of human society each individual's heritage should be a balanced mind in a vigorous and well-developed body. In an endeavor to determine the various causes that conspire to make a nation of semi-invalids it is not necessary to become pessimistic by denouncing every home as Sheol in embryo, or else a hospital; but an earnest inquiry into the principal causes operating to undermine the health of communities and commonwealths is essential to any intelligent effort to overcome them.

Beyond question environment is a potent factor, but there is an unwarranted tendency to attribute too much to climate, surroundings and heredity, since underlying all other causes is that of faulty and ill-regulated dietetics. We are a nation of bad cooks, and we are bad feeders, even when the cooks do their whole duty. Losing sight

of first principles and natural ways we have drifted into a thousand unhealthful and unthinking habits of living. With a superabundant supply of the very best materials in the world at command we have come to transforming the simplest viands into complex, unhygienic, irritating and innutritious dishes that do not cater to normal palates, but to acquired and morbid appetites and tastes. Instance the bread supplied to even the best tables. In the face of the fact that we raise the best wheat, corn and other grains of any nation on earth, and that we have devised the most perfect milling machinery, we really eat poorer bread than do the peasants of Norway or the Bedouins of Arabia. With neat cattle and sheep grazing to satiety over our myriad hills and throughout our countless valleys, with poultry farms and yards alive with every strain of cultivated fowls, forests abounding with the finest game, and waters teeming with representatives of the finny tribe nowhere equalled, we manage to utilize these abundant and unsurpassed materials in such a clumsy manner as to invite hydra-headed dyspepsia and all its train of disaster, discomfort and disease. The motto seems to be: The best flour, and the poorest bread; the best bullocks, but the poorest beefsteaks. So poor and insipid is our average baker's loaf that very many people have begun to look upon bread as a traditional appendage of the dietary, an item that is neither essential, attractive nor appetizing.

Whereas good bread contains nearly all the essentials of perfect nutrition, its degenerate modern substitute is little more than a puffy, over-fermented, over-salted and underbaked conglomeration of starch-cells, not much more nutritious than cotton batting, or solidified sea-foam. Instead of being the staff of life, the modern loaf, the loaf of the professional baker, consists of the devitalized remains of the annual booty from robbed grainfields. It is neither palatable nor satisfying, and as to nutritious properties it is a dietetic delusion. Those who rely upon it as a principal article of diet gradually starve, finally lapsing into some form of wasting disease—marasmus, inanition. Their mouths become the rich prey of the dentists, who thrive by myriads everywhere; their teeth finally succumb to caries, chiefly for lack of vigorous use, and at last they fall out. They shed their ill-nourished hair, and their bones grow brittle and prone to fractures and dislocations. If they procreate, their children are but half-endowed, mentally, morally or physically. If they manage to survive the vicissitudes of childhood, with its dentition and diphtheria, measles and meningitis, its croup, cholera infantum and chickenpox, they develop into scrofulous, precocious and over-susceptible youths, turning into withered women and decrepit men before they have fairly reached the age of adolescence, and dying young of tuberculosis or semi-marasmus. Some of them beget a few still more degenerate specimens of the race, and thus help to people the asylums and homes for paretics and imbeciles.

This picture is more especially true of the denizens of large cities. In the country, thank heaven, there yet remains a little more kitchen sense—another name for common sense. Thousands of families still make their own bread; but the baleful and enterprising baker is rapidly encroaching on the rural districts, so that in all the villages of any size other thousands are losing the knack of bread-making and already rely upon the conscienceless and chemically idiotic baker for their daily supply of this principal table resource.

Nor is the evil restricted to cities and villages. Every year finds more and more country housewives falling into the dietetic rut. The bread bowl is being surrendered to the kitchen maid. Often the latter is a decided improvement on the city baker, but she expends brawn rather than intelligence in her manipulations, while her prejudices overwhelm her discretion, and the results are anything but uniform or satisfactory. Or, if she be semi-intelligent she, too, succumbs to the inevitable, falls into the rut of passive acquiescence

and becomes an unthinking routinist in the matter of selection. She uses whatever material is supplied by the nearest tradesman, without question, makes up the flour he brings her into a stereotyped form of baked dough which she calls bread, regardless of its constituents, nutritive qualities or digestibility. She sees no object in discussing the value or qualities of proximate principles. To her mind starch belongs in the laundry, and gluten is a hypothetical quantity which has no legitimate place in the domestic equation.

And then, every household in the land keeps on hand a supply of machine-made starch-alum-ammonia-baking-powder, froth solidified, called "crackers" by courtesy, pale, unsubstantial and innutritious, so that children and those who happen to be on the invalid list need not be without the "light diet" so frequently prescribed but so rarely realized. The result is that thousands of the little dears, especially the strumous and scrawny ones, learn to make half their living from these delusive makeshifts, and a sorry half-living it certainly is.

Thus the city baker, with his rank brewer's yeast and his alum-saline-starch bread, cakes, crackers and cookies, insinuates his innutritious and demoralizing wares into all our homes, and we feed them to our babes and invalids and then wonder why they are the victims of rhachitis, pernicious anemia and tuberculosis.

The vegetarians are no doubt theoretically right, but so long as they are content to swallow such unsubstantial trash and call it bread they are practically wrong, and their enemies exult over their stumbling and failures. There are wholesome bread-stuffs in the market, but they are used by only an insignificant minority, and are either unknown or indignantly rejected by the masses. Tastes have been so long schooled to the use of shams in the food line that nothing else is relished or tolerated. If the one item of bread could be made universally good instead of indifferently bad, nutritious instead of insipidly negative, wholesome and satisfying instead of constipating and cloying, it would do more toward emancipating the race from prevailing degenerative influences and tendencies than any or all other dietetic reforms combined. This is strong language, but it is not too strong.

We have no spite against the bakers as a class; they are catering to an established appetite and fashion which they did not originate. A majority do not know any better than they do. What is wanted is a College for Cookery; and no *chef* should be allowed to practise his art without a diploma from an established institution of domestic science. Licensing physicians to practise the art of patching and healing is unimportant in comparison. When the doctor's clients are properly fed they will have less need of his services. Already his field of operations is undergoing a process of metamorphosis. His prime effort will soon be Prophylaxis; prevention will largely supersede the necessity for cure, and he will become a conservator rather than a repairer. Already his Pharmacopœia has been relegated to an upper shelf, while he is filling its place with the advanced and rapidly multiplying works on Physiology, and he is subscribing for "Systems of Physiologic Therapeutics."

INFANT FEEDING.

THE normal breast milk is the best and safest nourishment for an infant. According to Southworth, 97 per cent. of infant mortality from gastro-intestinal disease occurs among infants not nourished exclusively from the breast. The official statistics of the German Government show that, of artificially fed infants, 51 per cent. die during the first year, while only 8 per cent. of those exclusively nursed perish during the same period. In view of such facts, and also of the increasing proportion of artificially fed infants, due largely to the ignorance of mothers, Southworth considers it incumbent upon the family physician and the obstetrician to enlighten this ignorance. It becomes his duty to instruct the mother as to the proper diet, exercise, etc., necessary to promote the secretion of nutritious milk for her child; also the necessity for its regular nursing at proper intervals. He emphasizes the fact that there is very often a great lack of fluids taken into the system by the mother, and that it is essential to drink water freely during lactation; or, better still, milk, the gruels, and cocoa, which have definite food and milk-making possibilities. An extended experience has convinced Southworth that it is important to conserve the maternal milk, even if it is not sufficient for the child, stimulating its increase by proper diet and supplementing by artificial feeding; as such a course is more conducive to the child's healthy growth than to be completely bottle-fed. Modifications of cow's milk are usually vastly superior to infant foods.

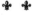

DIFFERENCE BETWEEN NATURAL AND ARTIFICIAL FEEDING OF INFANTS.

T. ESCHERICH, (*Wiener Klin. Wochenschrift*, Dec. 20). Is it possible, Escherich queries, that mother's milk contains some unknown substance which stimulates metabolism? This assumption would explain the inconsistencies observed and the results of natural feeding, which in some cases indicate an almost specific reaction of the infantile organism to the mother's milk. The presence of such a ferment in mother's milk would include the child in the mother's metabolism somewhat in the same way as during placental circulation. It renders futile all our present efforts to approximate mother's milk in artificial feeding, but opens a path for future research which may yet lead to important results.

DIETS FOR EVERY DAY USE.

J. WARREN ACHORN, M.D.
Boston.

TAKING cold is nothing but a *vulgarity*.

It is from this cause primarily that most bronchial affections arise.

Habitual colds are due to an ill-kept skin on the outside and depraved mucous membranes on the inside, coupled with carelessness.

For one whose digestion is right and whose skin is bright, who takes common sense precautions when exposed to unfavorable conditions, colds have little use.

Grooming, hardening, common sense, proper food and pride of person are the foundations upon which a cold cure must rest.

The man who occupies the bath room every morning for three quarters of an hour to the detriment of everybody else, who can be heard sporting and splashing in the shallow water, is usually the healthiest one among the *boarders*.

A cold sponge one to three minutes long, with a brisk rub immediately before and after it, is all that is necessary to keep the cutaneous circulation alive and the skin reactive to sudden changes of temperature. Never bathe when cold; rub warm first.

If the cold sponge or shower cannot be taken in the morning for some *mighty* reason, although the whole procedure should occupy less than eight minutes' times, it may be had at night before retiring.

For those unaccustomed to cold water, tolerance can be gained in three weeks' time, by the use of water at any comfortable temperature, making it one degree colder each day, until it can be employed without dread, as cold as it will run.

For cold feet, wading ankle deep before retiring, in water in the bath tub, for one or two minutes, or until the feet begin to pain, should be practised.

Rub hard afterwards.

If reaction does not set in, wrap the feet in blankets and let them alone; they will soon thaw out.

Do not use water bottles or other debilitating heat.

A month or two of this sort of hardening will effect a cure.

Cold hands may be treated in the same way—cold clammy hands.

Salt may be added to the water for its stimulating effect, or alcohol; witch hazel is also useful.

Tuberculosis is no contra-indication to the use of cold water. The more delicate the person, the greater the care required, but the more brilliant the results.

Cold water intelligently used, does not steal vitality, but fosters it. It stimulates the nerves that control the calibre of the blood vessels and regulates the cutaneous circulation. It is a respiratory stimulant.

Hot water should be employed once or twice a week when a full bath is taken and soap used. The duration of the bath should not exceed ten minutes, except for the obese, and end with a cold sponge.

If catching cold results from dust or disease in the nasal passages, they may be washed out regularly with some tepid alkaline solution and with as much satisfaction as one brushes the teeth. This procedure is properly a part of the morning toilet for those at least who suffer from catarrh in the atmosphere of great cities.

Operative interference on the nose and throat may be required for deflections, deformities, or diseased tissues acting as an exciting cause.

The inside and outside skins of the body are so much in sympathy, so dependent upon each other, that disorder of the one is sure to react upon the other; and this is as true of the bronchial mucous membrane, as it is of the alimentary canal and the cuticle.

Over-eating when tired, over-eating in connection with over-exertion, over-eating anyway, indulging in things known to disagree, that cause headache in this case or palpitation in that, biliousness, or insomnia, that precipitate an attack of asthma, hives or piles, or aggravate an existing cough or skin disease, are among the *habit* causes of colds; for taking cold is nothing but an attack from without, that succeeds, made upon the outside skin when not properly supported from within or from lack of tone, its own, or carelessness on the part of the man that wears it.

A healthy digestion and a healthy skin acting and reacting in harmony, coupled with purpose enough on the part of the owner, to discover the cause that ushers in the unwelcome visitor or with common sense enough to "keep moving when rained on," reduces the liability of having this guest to entertain regularly to a shadow knocking at the door. One should never stand on a street corner in winter if chilly or cold, but keep moving and *breathing*. Work the lungs as bellows till the perspiration (fire) starts.

The person who keeps moving when wet and moving and breathing *deep* when chilly, will seldom have a chance to complain about taking cold from getting soaked through, while standing on a street corner at night waiting for a car.

It is by care in eating and drinking, by controlling bad habits and cultivating a healthy skin, we are enabled to banish colds and regulate the circulation through the lungs and bronchial tubes.

NOTES.

When milk is freely used, the mouth, tongue and teeth must be cleaned before each feeding or the appetite will become impaired.

Red meat should be eaten sparingly if the bronchitis is associated with rheumatism, gout, rheumatic nerves, heart disease, Bright's disease, or other complicating disorder or disease contra-indicating its use.

Fish are useful in bronchitis on account of the oil they contain.

If associated with gastric disorders, only fine fibred fish or those known to agree should be eaten.

Breads, cereals and vegetables in this affection should be eaten sparingly.

Irish moss tea acts favorably in bronchitis on account of the mucilage, sulphur and iodine it contains.

Koumiss should not be drunk in bronchitis associated with or due to heart disease, plethora or old age (arterial change), because its use increases the solids in the body and would simply aggravate the condition present.

Soups, broths and purees serve their best use in acute bronchitis, or where fever is present. They also act favorably in chronic bronchitis when aggravated by a common cold.

The first day or two of a common cold is best

HOT milk cut one half with Em's water. Taken every two hours to the exclusion of everything else, for several days, this form of treatment in both acute and chronic bronchitis is often very effectual. German seltzer, French or Saratoga Vichy may be substituted for Em's water when the latter is not available.

BREAKFAST: *Cereals*—Oatmeal or wheaten grits with lemon, tamarind or prune juice. Hominy, farina, or rice with cream. Rye mush, corn meal mush, flour of maize.

Meats (red)—Mutton chops free from connective tissue, loin chops with fat, lean beef sandwiches, scraped meat ball, breakfast bacon with dry toast. Pepper and salt.

Fish (oily)—Shad, blue fish, salmon, mackerel, eels, if they agree; (fine fibered) cod, haddock, halibut, cunners, etc.; any lake or brook fish. Lemon juice.

Eggs—Raw, whipped with hot milk, the yolks lightly boiled or poached.

Breads—Whole wheat, malted bread or biscuit, zwieback or rusk. Stale

treated by liquids, *hot;* especially if there is loss of appetite. One may "stuff a cold," on the other hand, if the appetite is good and digestion prime.

The heaviest meal should be in the earlier part of the day, when digestion is vigorous.

Dinner should not be had later than 2 o'clock in the day if there is any tendency to cough at night.

Too much starchy food must not be allowed at supper, and red meats must be avoided at this time in all cases, where there is a tendency to asthmatic attacks or stuffiness.

If the cough is very bad, only liquids should be taken for supper and at least three hours before retiring.

Coffee goes better than tea in disease of the bronchial tubes. Clear coffee will often abort an asthmatic attack.

Light nourishing food is the rule in acute bronchitis, and an abundance of fatty food of the disorder is chronic, and without complications.

Bronchitis if associated with emphysema calls for non-flatulent foods easy of digestion.

In bronchitis due to Bright's disease, gout, diabetes, heart disease, the diet in the main follows the exciting cause.

An acute attack of bronchitis is often best relieved by going to bed and living on hot milk and Em's water.

bread toasted. Butter, clear honey, Meltose.

Fruits—Grapes, olives, peaches, pears, apples, oranges, plums and blackberries.

Drinks—Irish moss tea, almond milk, Vigor chocolate, Philip's digestible cocoa, water, milk, and Vichy hot. Coffee clear.

A. M. BETWEEN MEALS: Lemonade, orangeade, koumiss; egg water, flavored with lemon; hot milk and Em's water with a tablespoonful of sugar of milk added to each glass.

DINNER: *Soups*—Clam broth, barley broth, clear chicken soup with rice (adding a little pounded chicken if the tongue is clear), mutton, veal, lamb or oyster broth. Cream of rice, asparagus or peas. Vegetable purees of—(clear) onions, lettuce, spinach, peas, beans, celery and lentils.

Any *fish* mentioned. Oysters raw, sardines if they agree.

Meat (red)—Roast mutton, rare roast beef, free from connective tissue; (white) stewed or roasted chicken, squab, woodcock, quail, turtle dove or partridge.

Vegetables—Raw tomatoes, lettuce with oil, new string beans, new peas, asparagus tips, macaroni or vermicelli with fruit pulp or jelly.

Any *bread* mentioned.

Any *fruit* mentioned. Use inside of either stewed prunes, apricots or plums.

Any *drink* mentioned.

Desserts—Custard Pudding; sago, rice, tapioca, arrow-root with fruit pulp or unsweetened jelly. Custard blanc mange, wine, orange or coffee jelly, junket and cream. Devonshire, Spanish or Bavarian cream.

P. M. BETWEEN MEALS: Hot lemonade, tamarind tea, barley water sweetened with licorice, linseed or hempseed tea.

SUPPER: A little clear soup.

Fish—Oysters raw. White fish.

Eggs—Soft boiled, if not eaten in the morning.

Meat—Pounded; white game.

Vegetables—One baked potato with butter.

Breads—Bread and milk alone. Milk toast, cream toast, stale rolls with plenty of butter.

Fruits—The inside of baked apples and cream, stewed fruit pulp.

Drinks—Weak tea, whey cut with Em's water.

Creams—Whipped orange, tapioca, cream of rice. Cup custards, boiled custards with float, apple float. Orange or lemon sherbert, junket.

9 P. M.: Hot water.

In cases due to pleurisy with effusion, if the diet consists of soups, water, milk and tea and is less in amount than two pints a day, the outgo should be greater than the intake and absorption should follow. Easily digested solids, however, best meet the indications.

Very little liquid goes with a meal, and where liquids alone are taken the amount should be moderate each time, sipped slowly.

Half an hour before meals a small cup of hot water, adding soda or a pinch of Carlsbad salts, helps settle things. A little cayenne pepper in a glass of hot water an hour before meals relieves tightness and has a stimulating effect.

Hot milk and German seltzer with a dash of brandy in it an hour after meals acts as a tonic: equal parts of glycerine and whiskey, the white of an egg sucked through the shell, often serve to allay or loosen a cough.

Hempseed tea is soothing, having a beneficial effect on the bronchial mucosa and vocal cords.

Alcohol in large doses increases vascular engorgement and protracts this disease.

Whey, the pulp of cooked foods and finely divided vegetables, should be represented in the bill

of fare where bronchitis is complicated by obesity.

Grapes go well in abdominal obesity or plethora; when used extensively starches and fats should not be. They act well on gastric catarrh, and are somewhat laxative in effect.

Hot water a half hour before retiring helps some.

The stomach is a morbid point in the vicious circle, from which colds, bronchitis and asthma may start.

Egg water is made by shaking the whites of eggs in water (an egg to an ounce of water) until dissolved. Filter, flavor and serve cold. Most agreeable in acute bronchitis where fever is present.

Hemp seed tea is prepared by adding a spoonful of crushed hemp and crusted oatmeal to a pint of milk. Cook thoroughly. Strain, flavor and serve hot.

Large comfortable shoes with thick soles are a help in chronic bronchitis.

This diet carefully controlled, attention to individual idiosyncrasies being also recognized, meets the indications in asthma due to dietetic errors or dyspepsia.

THE PROBLEM OF EVIL.

THE question of an explanation, scientific or otherwise, of the problem of evil in the world, may seem at first thought somewhat remote from the interests of the readers of a journal devoted to the practical science of medicine. Yet it is certain that, historically, the popularly accepted explanation of evil has had immense influence upon the development of that science. There were long centuries during which doctors of physic were looked upon askance, and a knowledge of drugs was believed to be evidence of relations with the evil one; and the more effective these drugs in relieving pain the more conclusive was thought to be the evidence of witchery, for, so it was reasoned, evil, of which pain and sickness are a part, comes from the devil, and therefore that which relieves it must come from the devil also.

In modern times we have discarded the idea that evil is the result of sin, and have attempted now and then to give to it a rational or scientific basis, one consequence of which has been certainly a much more rapid development of the science of medicine than could otherwise have been possible. But it does not follow by any means that any generally accepted explanation of the problem of evil has been established. Indeed, there is, perhaps, less unanimity of opinion on that point now than there was when the theological explanation satisfied every one save, perhaps, a few individuals who were less simple or more disagreeable than ordinary folk. Some tell us that evil is a mystery not to be explained; others that it is possible only in a world governed or misgoverned by blind force; still others console us with the thought that the individual is sacrificed to the race, and that evil for the individual is necessary for race perfection; while we have recently been assured by a brilliant and versatile writer that evil is, after all, merely a relative term—that good, in other words, is only a lesser evil, and evil only a lesser good.

Recently there has appeared a new solution of the problem of evil which is not without interest. M. Bourdeau, writing in the *Revue Philosophique* on the "Cause et Origine du Mal," suggests a solution which is somewhat as follows: Every organ is an aggregate of simpler organisms co-ordinated into a whole, and is itself a part of a still larger aggregate. There is, therefore, in each organism two principles working in opposition—the principle of harmony and the principle of strife. The principle of harmony is due to the co-ordinating influence of each organism over the smaller organisms which compose it; the principle of strife is due to the egoistic opposition of each organism against the larger organism of which it is a part. Each organism has a keen sense of its own needs and tendencies, but a less keen sense of the needs and tendencies of the organisms of which it is composed, or of the organism of which it is in turn a part. This inevitable discord is the cause of evil—it *is* evil. It is a conflict which is universal, and the constant expression of which may be seen in man, in Nature, in society. Last and most intolerable evil of all is death, which is nevertheless the necessary foundation and condition of life.

This surely is interesting, but what, after all, does it tell us of the cause and origin of evil? It shows us, rather, that evil is the result of the conflict, perhaps the necessary conflict, of forces. That we knew before. But what causes this conflict, and why is it a necessary one?

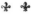

Dr. Achorn's "Diet List in Eczema" will be published in the July GAZETTE.

Department of Physiological Chemistry.

WITH SPECIAL REFERENCE TO DIETETICS AND NUTRITION IN GENERAL.

YOUTH AND YEARS.

HOLMES—there never has been but one Holmes who could say such things in the way he said them—once remarked: "My friend, over there, is eighty years young!"

That remark hints at a whole volume of practical philosophy.

Sweet natures never grow old. Years may blanch the hair and gradually lessen the elasticity of the gait, but they should have no dominion over the heart.

Keep step! Never "retire from active life." Never say, "at my age." Keep in the swim! Do to-day whatever you have been in the habit of doing, only do it with a little more circumspection and judgment than heretofore.

Time enough to die when there's nothing more to live for. One of the sweetest natures and most womanly woman I ever knew made it an invariable rule to choose the very best of everything at her command for each day's use, never saving the best for to-morrow; and so she always lived on the very best she could afford. When she went to the bin for apples she always picked out the largest, plumpest and soundest, instead of selecting the "specked" ones, and leaving the best to be "specked" to-morrow. Every day she had the best fruit the bin afforded, and thus if any rotted before it could be used, it was the nurliest and not the fairest. She also believed in thoroughly living in the immediate present. "To-day is our opportunity," she would say. "The past is gone. Only its lessons can avail us, and they are with us now. The future is not ours, and may never be. To talk of the past is to linger in the shadows. It is to waste the day in foolish regrets for the night. Let the dead past bury its dead! I am going to live as long as I can see anybody else live; and when the change comes I will meet it boldly, face to face, and not looking over my shoulder. I will greet death as the right and proper thing to be attended to at that particular moment!"

She died ripe in years, universally beloved and without a hesitant fear of any kind.

So many people, advanced in years, begin to say, "When I was young." It is a great mistake. Be young now, every day. Keep up your interest in all the things that interest young people. Cherish your young acquaintances, join in their studies, their readings, their games. Throw stilted dignity to the dogs. Unbend on every possible occasion. Heads up, shoulders erect; no stooping nor stupidity. Mind clear, muscles active, no laziness, no limping! Don't be an ogre; play with the children, take an interest in the babies, and kiss the sweet young girls. Keep the wrinkles out of your face, the cobwebs out of your brain and the ice-water out of your heart. Patronize the opera, go to the theater, laugh at the comedians and the minstrels. Keep in touch with all your nieces and nephews; and while you remember all their birthdays forget your own. It's of not the slightest possible consequence whether you are forty or seventy-five. Make no birthday parties or birthday presents. Once old enough to vote you are always the same—old enough to vote! That's enough for anybody to know. Even the census man has no right to pry into your private affairs. Let there be no "golden weddings," not even a tin or wooden wedding. Taboo the reminders, and go on living in the immediate present, the actual *to-day*, which is all the time you are sure of.

Never give a thought to the advent of the "sere and yellow leaf," but if a grandfather be a "Foxy Grandpa" out and out, and show the youngsters that some things can be done as well as others if not a little better.

These rather random thoughts have been suggested by the quaint and interesting paper of Mrs. Thorpe, which will be found in another column. We are not going to tell our readers how old a girl Mrs. Thorpe is, for the reason that girls are always sensitive on this subject, but we are sure that if she lives to be a hundred she will still be a girl.

WHITE BREAD *VERSUS* BROWN BREAD.

What passes for "science" in popular publications is not always "up to date." A ten-cent magazine with a very large circulation contains, in its February issue, an article which deals with diet and kindred topics. The author, who is a physician, says: "Our white bread contains little else but the starchy or carbonaceous matter, which supplies only heat and energy." He makes no reference to gluten, but tells us that "we pay a dear price for having *white* bread on our tables. The wheat grain contains phosphates . . . nitrogenous matter . . . and carbonaceous . . . matter. All these should be contained in our bread; but instead, the flour is passed through a bolting cloth," and almost everything but starch is removed by that process.

Let us look at the other side of this question. An ounce of experiment is worth more than a ton of hypothesis. Within four or five years the bread question has been thoroughly investigated by Dr. Lauder Brunton, of London, England, whose report was published in either the *Lancet* or the *British Medical Journal.*

While it is true that whole-meal bread contains more nitrogen than white bread, it is necessary to remember that the nitrogen found in cereals exists in two forms: the coagulable and the non-coagulable albuminoids. The latter are almost useless for purposes of food, because they consist of alkaloids and nitrogen salts. The fine portion of the flour contains some coagulable nitrogen; the other parts of the flour contain nitrogen, which has very little value as food. There is, in addition, another point of importance. However finely whole-wheat flour may be ground by the use of steel rollers, it contains gritty particles, which irritate the alimentary canal and lead to the evacuation of partially digested food. As a result, whole-wheat bread has a laxative property which may have some value in cases of chronic constipation so often due to the insufficient consumption of water. But the claim that the so-called Graham bread (or brown bread or whole-wheat bread) is a better food than the white bread is nothing short of a fallacy, because the latter contains all the available nitrogen that is found in the wheaten grain.

PARTHENOGENESIS (VIRGINAL REPRODUCTION).

A couple of months ago I received a letter from a gentleman, a physician, who asked me to inform him of some form of life which reproduces its species both parthenogenetically and also by sexual fertilization. The facts are as follows: Reproduction without fertilization is not known among mammals. In the insect world, however, it is very common. Aphides (plant lice) reproduce both ways. During the summer there is a constant production of females, which are viviparous (born alive), without any fertilization upon the part of the mother. The progeny have, as a rule, no wings. But the reproduction of these insects is so rapid that the plants upon which they live would be destroyed if another form of the species did not arise. Occasionally, therefore, a female is produced which has wings, and she, taking herself to another plant, starts a new colony. The progeny of these "colonial" aphides, in turn, resemble their grandparent, in the fact that wings are usually absent, though the preservation of the species is provided for by the occasional appearance of a winged individual. (The phenomenon referred to —the likeness of the insect to its grandmother, and not to its mother—is known as metagenesis, or the alternation of generations.)

As yet no male has appeared upon the scene. But colder weather and the scarcity of food result in the birth of males, which fertilize the females, and eggs are then laid. These eggs do not usually hatch until spring.

The relation between sex and feeding can be easily demonstrated with tadpoles. If they are fed upon meat, and plenty of it, the percentage of female frogs will be about eighty. Upon the other hand, if the tadpoles are given little albuminous food, the percentage of female frogs will be less than forty. Semi-starvation must be avoided, for it is likely to prevent the metamorphosis, and to keep the tadpoles indefinitely in the sexless stage.

The life-history of aphides sounds like a romance, but it is well authenticated, and not particularly difficult to prove.

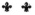

SUGAR AND THE DOCTOR.

UNDER this heading Dr. Edwin W. Pyle protests, in the *Medical Summary*, against a very widespread evil and one which is, we believe, far more serious than is generally admitted. Says Dr. Pyle:

"We object to sugar in medicine for the reason that, in our efforts to help the sick or fallen, we would not add to their burdens by throwing a weight upon them. Dr. Albert R. Leeds has very properly observed that cane sugar is not fitted for assimilation without hydration; that it will not pass into the circulation until every large molecule is broken up into two smaller dextrose molecules by the absorption of one molecule of water, which chemical change extracts just so much energy for the work performed. In health the human system has a surplus of energy and is equal to the many tasks imposed, but when the doctor is called, impaired function and general debility demand the withholding of all products that unnecessarily tax the strength of the patient.

"It may be mentioned here, however, that grape sugar, fruit sugar, and pure honey are dextrose in character—that is, predigested—and therefore not so objectionable. But let us inquire into the clinical facts respecting the use of cane sugar:

"First. We observe that in apparent health many cannot digest it without distress; that it has had a large share in the increase of stomach disorders; that children become irritable from reflex ailments when food is too much sweetened; that in sickness sugar is the first article rejected; that the profession is unanimous in discarding it from the sick dietary; and that it is particularly contraindicated in all disorders of assimilation and in the exhaustion of continued fevers.

"Second. What are the drug-store facts?

"That syrups are made by boiling down twelve pounds of sugar in eight pounds of water until a teaspoonful of syrup represents a teaspoonful of sugar; that an elixir contains only 10 per cent. sugar, but 20 per cent. alcohol; that the high per cent. of sugar in the first and the low per cent. in the second, reinforced by the alcohol, are expressly to make these preparations stable while in the druggist's possession, disguising taste and preserving medicine being secondary considerations.

"Therapeutics were made for the sick, not for the convenience or monetary interests of the commercial world. There is a gruesomeness in the suggestion of concentrating sugar, or adding one-fifth alcohol, to preserve *outside* the body, to let Nature wrestle with the problem and pay the penalty when put *inside*. There is no hygiene in therapeutics that stops short of consideration as to what takes place in the human economy. When we look over the formulæ of dispensatories, the prescriptions appearing in journals and as presented to pharmacies, we do not wonder at the tide of therapeutic nihilism that has turned so many into other methods of treatment.

"There is a vast amount of accumulated trash in the old-time drug shop, authorized still by our Pharmacopœia, that should be swept out of existence. No medicine should be administered that abstracts energy or whose beneficial action cannot be readily demonstrated. Syrups are no longer in accord with practical therapeutics, but an enormous quantity is still consumed, and particularly by proprietary recommendations. Through the public press medical knowledge is becoming part of a general education. When the people come to a right knowledge of the uses and abuses of cane sugar, and thoroughly comprehend what *has been* and *is* given them under the guise of 'syrups' and 'elixirs,' they will settle the question themselves, without waiting for unanimity among doctors.

"The trend of modern medicine is to study a few remedies scientifically and to apply them rationally. Experience has well demonstrated that the sick need only a few simple measures. The physician who makes disagreeable work of prescribing has something yet to learn of vital interest to his patient and not a little to himself. Rarely is it necessary to use a menstruum other than cold water."

MEDICAL USES OF FRUITS.

A LONDON physician has a very interesting paper on the uses of fruits in the relief of diseased conditions of the body. "To us," says *Health*, "this article is worthy of careful perusal, coming, as it does, from one who has made the medical uses of fruits a study for nearly a generation. The physi-

cian says that he does not want it understood that edible fruits exert direct medicinal effects. They simply encourage the natural processes by which the several remedial processes which they aid are brought about.

"Under the category of laxatives, oranges, figs, tamarinds, prunes, mulberries dates, nectarines, and plums may be included. Pomegranates, cranberries, blackberries, sumac berries, dewberries, raspberries, barberries, quinces, pears, wild cherries, and medlars are astringent; grapes, peaches, strawberries, whortleberries. prickly pears, black currants, and melon seeds are diuretics; gooseberries, red and white currants, pumpkins, and melons are refrigerants; the lemons, limes, and apples are refrigerants and stomach sedatives.

"Taken in the early morning, an orange acts very decidedly as a laxative, sometimes amounting to a purgative, and may generally be relied on.

"Pomegranates are very astringent, and relieve relaxed throat and uvula. The bark of the root in the form of a decoction is a good anthelmintic, especially obnoxious to tapeworm.

"Figs, split open, form excellent poultices for boils and small abscesses. Strawberries and lemons, locally applied, are of some service in the removal of tartar from the teeth. Apples are correctives, useful in nausea, and even seasickness and the vomiting of pregnancy. They immediately relieve the nausea due to smoking. Bitter almonds contain hydrocyanic, and are useful in simple cough; but they frequently produce a sort of urticaria or nettle-rash. The persimmon, or diospyros, is palatable when ripe, but the green fruit is highly astringent, containing much tannin, and is used in diarrhea and incipient dysentery. The oil of the cocoanut has been recommended as a substitute for cod-liver, and is much used in Germany for phthisis. Dutch medlars are astringent, and not very palatable. Grapes and raisins are very nutritive and demulcent, and very grateful in the sick-chamber. A so-called grape has been much lauded for the treatment of congestions of the liver and stomach, enlarged spleen, scrofula, tuberculosis, etc. Nothing is allowed but water, bread and several pounds of grapes per diem. Quince seeds are demulcent and astringent; boiled in water, they make an excellent soothing and sedative lotion in inflammatory diseases of the eyes and eyelids."

A BEAUTY BREAD.

OLD-FASHIONED "CORN DODGERS."

"ALL MAH young ladies' been eatin' dis bread, ever since dey was li'l bits o' chillern," explained the quaintly turbaned "Mammy," who reigned supreme in my Virginia hostess' big, raftered kitchen.

"Dat's why," she continued proudly, pouring another cupful of corn meal into the yellow bowl, "dat's why dey's all got sech soun' white teef, and skin laik peaches and cream. I tell yo', honey, dere ani't nothin' better'n good old cawn meal dodgers," and she chuckled complacently as she deftly flirted a pinch of salt across the corn meal mound.

It didn't look promising, the mixture before me of corn meal, salt and water. But thirty minutes later, when it came from the oven in crisp, smoking-hot little dodgers, a fascinating brown without and as mellow as mush within, I was ready to vote these the most delectable morsels Chloe's culinary skill had yet produced.

Such a breakfast that was—slices of golden brown bacon as sweet as beech nuts, and with them Mammy's famous corn dodgers. No soggy, yeast raised dough there. Each bite of the tasty dainties one felt would carry with it the nourishment and good digestion so necessary for bright eyes and clear skins.

My hostess told me that in her family, as in nearly all Southern households, corn dodgers were the favorite bread. Her daughters had been faithful to them ever since their little teeth were strong enough to nibble about the edges, and, with Mammy Chloe, she believed they owed much of the beauty of their healthy, fine-grained skins to this corn meal fare.

Asked for the recipe, Chloe, who was flattered by my interest in her specialty, offered to teach me every quirk of dodger-making, and, simple as the proceeding proved, I found its entire success lay in rigid adherence to that very simplicity.

I have tried to teach a five-dollar-a-week cook to make these dodgers only to find that she invariably spoiled them as soon as my back was turned by slily introducing a lump of butter, a dash of yeast powder, a few pinches of sugar or the beaten yolk of an egg. Now the real corn dodger, the dodger, with which Dixie cooks woo your palate, consists of nothing but corn meal, salt and water. In Southern kitchens they have a decided preference for white meal, but farther north I have found the choice is given a brand as yellow as a bar of gold. White or yellow, provided the meal is wholesomely sweet, the toothsome little cakes will be a success.

For a family of four take a heaping cupful of corn meal. Place in an earthen bowl and sprinkle with half a teaspoonful of salt. Then scald with a cupful of boiling water. Poured over the meal this brings it to the consistency, when well mixed, of what Mammy so aptly termed "chicken feed." Stand the mixture aside until quite cold. Then add enough hot water to reduce it to a soft, mushy state, "runny" enough, in fact, to be dropped off the spoon in small portions on buttered tins. The tops of these cakes generally have a macaroon-like roughness which is very appetizing. With a brisk fire in thirty minutes or less they will brown prettily. Served hot and well buttered within, they will convert even the skeptical to an admission of their tastiness.

The old-fashioned corn dodger while cheap enough to appeal to the most economical housewife, is delicious enough to satify an epicure.—Dorothy Maddox, in *Table Talk*.

THE FOOD OF FISHES.

Many are Vegetarians and Many Others Enjoy a Dish of Greens.

A WRITER has recently distinguished animals as those which derive their food from the soil and those which live on other animals. The fact is, however, that all animal life is supported directly or indirectly from the soil. The food of all animals is vegetation or other animals which live on vegetation. Thus all animal life rests on a vegetable basis.

Many persons have the idea that the food of nearly all the fishes is animal life found in the sea. This is probably true of many varieties, but not a few fishes are vegetarians and there are a good many fish that vary their meat diet with more or less vegetable food. A little while ago an English naturalist who was dissecting a bream found in its stomach in addition to a crab, a considerable quantity of two kinds of seaweed, though the bream is reputed to live on animal life. Some of the text-books say that the gray mullet, a popular fish in British waters, feeds only on the animal matter it obtains by straining sand or mud in its mouth. This is not a scientific conclusion. No biologist of a European university could convince a practical Cornwall fisherman that the gray mullet does not eat seaweed. He knows that this is so for he often finds the fish's stomach full of seaweed.

There is a great deal of vegetable matter floating around in the sea. Everybody knows of the eddy in the Atlantic Ocean, where the currents whirl for hundreds of miles around a great center, the Sargasso Sea, into which seaweeds drift and remain in the quiet waters within the swirl until they become water-logged and sink of their extra weight. It has been found that the enormous quantities of seaweeds, algæ and other vegetation that cover the surface of the Sargasso Sea with vivid green are mostly torn by the waves from the shores of Yucatan and other Gulf of Mexico coasts and drift for many hundreds of miles before they find lodgment in the Sargasso. Vast quantities of vegetation also drift out to sea that never reach the currents whirling around this grass-covered part of the ocean. Thus vegetation from the land has wide distribution over the sea and it has been proved that it is relished by many varieties of fish.

The scientific work of Dr. Nansen in Arctic waters proves that a large population of fish is introduced into the cold seas from the west, and that the food supplies to support this vast marine population come mainly from the east. He says that the Siberian current flowing to the northwest is of great importance in conveying a constant supply of nourishment to the pelagic animals of the north polar basin. This nourishment consists of microscopic algæ, some of the smallest specimens of vegetable life. They are chiefly diatoms which are found to abound from the east. He says that the Siberian Sea, though gradually diminishing in quantity westward, apparently owing to their being largely fed upon by various pelagic animals. Indeed, without such a constant conveyance of nourishing matter there could be no such rich fish and other animal life in the polar seas. We have read accounts by Arctic explorers of the dark bands and discolorations exhibited by ice in northern waters. They are mainly due to those minute and lowly plants on which the northern fish feed to a considerable extent.

Of course, the sea is full of a great variety of food. Fish not only prey upon one another, eat seaweed, algæ, and other forms of vegetation, but they are also able to vary their diet with worms, jellyfish, seaweed, and many kinds of shellfish. The fish must have a delicate stomach, and a most exacting palate that cannot find in the myriad forms of animal and vegetable life pervading the sea materials for a tempting meal.

"A TRUST is a large body of capitalists, wholly surrounded by water."

THOMAS B. REED.

"RUBBISH TEA."

A serious charge, according to *London Hospital,* is being brought against the ingredients from which we brew the cup that cheers yet not inebriates, for we are told that the fine art of tea blending, by the proper exercise of which flavor and strength are judiciously combined, is being prostituted for the purpose of giving a false appearance of wholesomeness to rotten leaves. According to the methods of the modern planter, who makes large use of machinery, a good deal of tea is spoilt in the making, and it is easy to understand that the commercially successful blender is the one who succeeds in making his well-flavored leaves bring him full value for as much of his "rubbish" also as may be. The seriousness of the matter is that the consumer, buying his pound or his half-pound at a time, is practically helpless in the matter. All he knows is that the tea does not agree with him. The stuff looks clean and well rolled, and in the packet or the handful it smells nice enough; but it is a mixture in which the rottenness of the rotten is covered up by the flavor and the aroma of the good. Mr. Brownen, F.C.S., in a letter to the *Times,* says that quite recently there has been a meeting of planters in Ceylon, at which it was stated that teas known to be unfit for human consumption had been exported, and he adds from his own knowledge that recent samples of tea obtained in this country contain leaves which, although dried, are perfectly rotten and full of the microbes of decomposition. He maintains that, although the consumer cannot easily detect these defects in the blended article as he buys it, nothing could be simpler than for the Government to stop the importation of such stuff.

For one tyrant there are a thousand ready slaves.

W. Hazlitt.

VEGETABLES AS MEDICINE.

Asparagus is very cooling and easily digested.

Cabbage, cauliflower, Brussels sprouts, and broccoli are cooling, nutritive, laxative and purifying to the blood, as a tonic; but should not be eaten too freely by delicate persons.

Celery is delicious cooked, and good for rheumatic and gouty people.

Lettuces are very wholesome. They are slightly narcotic, and lull and calm the mind.

Spinach is particularly good for rheumatism and gout, and also in kidney diseases.

Onions are good for chest ailments and colds, but do not agree with all.

Watercresses are an excellent tonic, stomachic and cooling.

Beetroot is very cooling and highly nutritious, owing to the amount of sugar it contains.

Parsley is cooling and purifying.

Turnip tops are invaluable when young and tender.

Green neute shoots, if gathered in spring and cooked as spinach, form a most delicate and wholesome, blood-purifying vegetable.

Potatoes, parsnips, carrots, turnips and artichokes are highly nutritious, but not so digestible as some vegetables. Potatoes are the most nourishing, and are fattening for nervous people.

Tomatoes are health-giving and purifying, either eaten raw or cooked.

Chili, cayenne, horse-radish and mustard should be used sparingly. They give a zest to the appetite, and are valuable stomachics. Radishes are the same, but are indigestible, and should not be eaten by delicate people.

Cucumbers are cooling, but are indigestible to many.—*Pub. Health Journal.*

Apply sulphuric ether to insect stings.

THE DIETETIC VALUE OF SUGAR.

THE *British Medical Journal*, April 27, 1901, has the following: H. Willoughby Gardner gives the following as the chief points about sugar as a food: It is easily digested and absorbed. It is readily stored up as glycogen, forming a reserve of force-producing material. It is in this form readily available when required. It becomes completely oxidized without any waste and leaving no residue. Under certain circumstances it can be converted into fat and so produce heat and force. It can be called a proteid-sparing food. It is pleasant to take, acts as a relish, and stimulates the activity of the digestive processes. So it should be an admirable food for producing heat and energy. It is necessary for growing boys and girls, and their nutrition often suffers owing to a popular prejudice against it. It is valuable in cases of anemia and for the aged. Sometimes sweets harm the teeth, but on account of impurities. Cane sugar is apt to cause an undue secretion of mucus. Those who are gouty and fat must avoid sugar as they would poison. Thin gouty patients may use it. [See "SUGAR AND THE DOCTOR."—ED. GAZETTE.]

ALCOHOL AND INFECTION.

THE *Journal of Inebriety* has the following: "It has been shown by Abbott and others that alcoholic animals are more susceptible to infections with various organisms than normal animals. And Laitinen, after having studied the influence of alcohol upon infections with anthrax bacilli, tubercle bacilli and diphtheria toxin, in dogs, rabbits, guinea-pigs, fowls, and pigeons, reaches the same general result, and this with certainty and directness. Under all circumstances alcohol causes a marked increase in susceptibility, no matter whether given before or after infection, no matter whether the doses were few and massive, or numerous and small, and no matter whether the infection was acute—anthrax, or chronic—tuberculosis, or more the nature of an intoxicat.on—diphtheria. The alcoholic animals either die while the control remains alive, or in case both die, death is earlier in the alcoholic. Without going into details in connection with the experiments—and there is room for further work here—it may be said at this time that the facts brought about by the researches of Abbott, Laitinen, and others, do not furnish the slightest support for the use of alcohol in the treatment of infectious diseases in man.

INFLUENCE OF LIGHT ON THE SKIN.

"THE influence of sunlight on the appearance of the skin can hardly be overrated," says *The Family Doctor*. "Recent experiments with the electric light, which, of all artificial illumination most nearly resembles sunlight, have shown how important a part light plays in promoting growth. It has long been known that plants deprived entirely of light soon droop. Some time ago the beneficial action of light was forcibly illustrated. At the close of a public lecture it was found that some buds which had remained on the table had actually blown under the influence of the electric light, while others which had been kept in the dark had made no progress whatever.

"Animals, too, are well known to have similar susceptibilities, and it is certain that much of the pallor observable in the faces of those whose lives are passed in our gloomy courts and alleys and underground work shops, is due to insufficiency of light. No wonder that children reared in badly lighted nurseries. and æsthetic people who delight in small windows. with colored glass which still further dim the entering light. should pay the inevitable penalty in pale face and impaired health. Certain skins are very susceptible to the direct action of the sun's rays. Freckles, or small spots of discoloration, are due entirely to an exceptional formation of pigment in the favoring light of the sun, and sometimes fade as rapidly as they come. The heat rays of the sun act in just the same manner as a fire or mustard plaster, causing general pigmentation or sunburn. Absence of light is said to stimulate the cells in which pigment exists, causing them to contract and so hide the pigment; hence the surface becomes lighter in color, returning to a darker tint again on the reaction of light."

THE deleterious effects arising from the habit of coffee-drinking are discussed by Leszynsky in the *Med. Record.* One-third of the coffee crop of the entire world is consumed in the United States. He points out the fact that children are especially susceptible to the effects of coffee, tea, etc., and believes that these drugs are frequently the unsuspected cause of insomnia, night terrors, and some intellectual precocity. He distinguishes between acute and chronic coffee-poisoning. "When taken in sufficient quantity by those unaccustomed to its use it produces excitability even to the point of delirium. In the chronic form it gives rise to a depressive form of neurasthenia. It closely resembles chronic alcoholism, for which it is frequently mistaken and with which it is sometimes associated. Guelliot has studied carefully this form. He states that digestion is first deranged. At times there is epigastric pain radiating to the dorsal region. It was similar to the other neuralgic pains from which these patients suffer. The pulse is slow, soft, and compressible. The tremor which is present, at times, disappears after a dose of coffee, just as in chronic alcoholism. Sexual impotence in the male and profuse leucorrhea in the female are prominent symptoms. It has been observed that confirmed coffee drinkers have a slow pulse (from 40 to 60). In treating the condition, which is frequently not diagnosed, the stim-

ulant should not be absolutely withdrawn, but a morning cup of coffee allowed. The author recommends nerve sedatives and tonics, and at times the rest cure is necessary. Most cases recover in from three to six months."

FATTY FOODS.

"THE fat man," according to the *Med. Sentinel,* "is generally the contented man, and the lean man is generally the restless man, and while in this, as in most other things, a happy medium is the most desirable, mental sufferers need the merits of fat-producing agents exploited before them more generally than the merits of the anti-fat agents, and to produce fat in the mentally afflicted, I know nothing better than the good American hog and his products. The merits of good bacon and good salt pork, properly prepared for food, need to be preached by the missionary physician.

The use of pure olive oil as a food, with the meals, should be indulged by both the mentally depressed, and the abnormally excitable. It helps nutrition, and gives a gentle aid to elimination. If it can not be taken with food preparation, a teaspoonful or two can be taken regularly at the close of each meal.

INCREASING LONGEVITY.

"FREE institutions," says *The Inter-Ocean,* "have made greater progress in the last hundred years than ever before. There is more tolerance in the world than ever before. The religious and political convictions of individuals are respected as never before. The rights of persons and things are held to be more sacred than ever before. Freedom's ultimate triumph shows clearer and clearer. Suspicion of brute force and confidence in enlightened thought grow stronger and stronger. There are more opportunities for the man with the large brain, for the man with the developed moral convictions and the dwarfed prejudices than ever before.

"Mr. J. Holt Schooling, an English actuary, makes a statement in a business way which gives strength to one phase of optimistic thought, but which in many respects has a bearing upon all others. When Victoria became queen the average male life was under forty years. To-day it falls little short of forty-six years. The life of the average woman was forty-two years. To-day it exceeds forty-eight years.

"Similar statements have been made by American actuaries. They are based upon scientific observation. They mean that physical drudgery and mental anxiety are not wearing out the human machinery as formerly. They mean that the masses of the people are better fed than they were sixty-five years ago, and that they are more contented. They mean that we are progressing—that humanity is making gains; that not only have comforts and pleasures increased, but the capacity for enjoying them has increased. They mean in addition to all this, that the common level of mankind is becoming higher and higher with every decade, and that the only class that in making no headway is the croakers."

REPOSE AND HEALTH.

WE cannot, says one of our exchanges, write or talk too much of repose, in this busy, hustling world, where people are keyed to such high nerve tension. More mental quiet is an unconscious demand of the race to-day.

On every side we meet with this mental unrest, this struggle with burdens of some variety or other, until from the expenditure of nerve force a large number are among the never well, always tired, class; after which follows the morbid and finally the insane.

The marvelous power of the nervous system to wreck or build is startling. Where the mind force that rules the body is scat-

tered and disorderly, the consequent lack of repose is almost sure to result in disease. This mental unrest is most subtle, and therefore a sure health destroyer; it may quietly work for years, yet it will accomplish, with no apparent effect, in time some form of bodily disorder.

The majority are not trained to mental quiet; even the children are not receiving such discipline.

Every healthy child is brimful of active life, but it is not restless, only under artificial conditions. If repose is power, then we cannot too early train the child to observe times of daily silence, short intervals when both body and mind rest.

Our public schools should cultivate more repose on the part of both teacher and pupil, for in the school lies much of the moulding of the race. The schools would send home fewer tired nerves if relaxation and energizing were more frequently alternated during the day.

INTELLIGENT DIRECTION OF ENERGY.

"INTELLIGENT direction," says *Public Policy*, "requires knowledge and judgment. Its purpose is to secure the largest results with the least expenditure. All earning comes by working, but all work does not result in earning. Energy expended with greatest diligence may be destructive instead of productive, through lack of knowledge and judgment. The more deficient men are in knowledge and judgment, the greater is their need of combining with others in an organization by means of which they can secure the directing supervision of those who are most capable to perform such service. If the energy they are capable of exerting is directed by a knowledge and judgment superior to their own, the earning value of their energy will be increased by the value of superior ability employed for direction. The larger the number is of the persons combined, whose energy is directed by a knowledge and judgment superior to their own, the larger will be the portion of the extra earning value of their labor, on account of superior direction, that they can retain for themselves. Thus if a superintendent directs the work of twenty men working 300 days in the year, and his salary is $1,200 per year, it is equivalent to 20 cents per day taken out of the extra earnings on account of superior direction. If, however, a superintendent directs the work of 200,000 men working 300 days in the year, and his salary is $1,000,000 per year, it is equivalent to less than 67-100 cents per day taken out of the extra earnings on account of superior direction. If all of the extra earnings on account of superior direction divided between the workmen and the superintendent, it is very clear that those workmen who are combined in the largest organizations, under the direction of the highest paid superintendents, will receive the highest wages. This fact is equally true when the element of capital is admitted into the equation. Capital requires a larger per cent. for its use and profit when invested in small amounts in small undertakings. The larger the investments become the smaller is the per cent. capital will require for its use and profit, and the larger will be the share of extra earnings absorbed by workmen and superintendent. The bonds of the largest corporations can be issued at par, with an interest rate of from 3 to 4 per cent. and their stocks will sell at a high premium if they can be depended upon for dividends of from 6 to 8 per cent. On the other hand, the securities of small corporations can be handled only with difficulty, if at all, at rates twice as great as these.

Superior knowledge and judgment, applied to industrial undertakings, is the factor of greatest economic value. Instead of antagonism there should be the cosiest fellowship between the power to labor and the power to direct. The compensation of the latter is only obtained by increasing the earning power of the former.

REV. DR. WILLIAM S. RAINSFORD, in a speech at the last gathering of the New York Credit Men's Association, said: "The tendency of modern life, in which we are active to a point of exhaustion at times, is to bind too many blinkers on a man. We may deplore it. We cannot evade it. The tendency of modern life is to force us all towards specialism. We recognize in our own life, with the long hours of work and toil of the day, the weariness that follows our concentration of attention under the gulfs of condensation under which we all toil, leaves us very little time for anything but the duties of our business. Men who are taken up with the affairs of life need to make time for a kind word, a kindly act. The key-note of to-day is association. Those trades, those men, those interests that combine will lift those away that have not sense enough to combine, and they will fall. The only way to build up this great country —there is no profession to which a good man puts his hand yet that has no profound basis to it, not that we shall simply have a great nation of seventy-five millions of people, but a greater nation under liberal institutions—is to make the darkness less dark, and make truth, honor, and manhood more evident to the wide world."

A COLD QUESTION.

DOES artificial ice under like conditions melt more quickly than natural ice? It has been positively asserted that it does.

The *American Grocer* says:

We understand that an interesting test of the melting properties of natural and artificial ice was recently made by Professor Denton, of Stevens College. He used for experiment three fifty-pound cubes—lake, river, and artificial ice, respectively. All were submitted to like conditions of exposure, temperature, etc. The artificial and river lots melted simultaneously; the lake more quickly dissolved by two pounds. Practically the time of liquefaction was the same.

For water to solidify, a certain quantity of heat must be withdrawn, and we could never see why it should not require just as much heat withdrawal, under like conditions, in the artificial freezing as in the natural. Granting the heat-withdrawal is the same in each, the heat-impregnation must be the same for each, resulting, under similar conditions, in simultaneous melting.

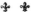

COCAINE DEBAUCHERY.

BILLS to forbid the sale of morphine and cocaine without a prescription of a physician, says the *American Druggist*, are now up for passage in the legislatures of the States of Alabama, Georgia and Tennessee. The chief of police of New Orleans has issued an order to all police commanders of the city, calling attention to an ordinance relative to the sale of cocaine. The order reads in part:

"You are directed to notify the force under your command to use extreme diligence in enforcnig the city ordinance against the use of cocaine and to make arrests. You will make a written report to this office of each offender arrested, and from whom the drug was purchased, whether from a druggist or pedlar."

The complaints against the abuse of cocaine have been very loud for some time, thousands of persons, mainly negroes, using the drug and injuring themselves physically and mentally by it. Some drug stores confine themselves almost wholly (?) to the sale of cocaine, but the bulk of it is sold by pedlars in either pellets or in powder to mix with wine.

Cocaine is used extensively by the negroes of Atlanta, the *Constitution* of that city reports, as a substitute for alcoholic stimulants. A preparation of the drug in the form of a powder, which can be inhaled through the nose. thus rendering unnecessary a hypodermic syringe, has done much to facilitate the use of "coke," as the negroes term it. The drug is now used as openly as snuff. Negroes can be seen at any time on the streets or in the police court snuffing the white powder. A few drugstores are growing rich selling cocaine in 10 cent. boxes. The law requires that druggists register the purchasers and place a number on the box, and so the druggists do not violate the law.

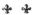

PERSONAL HYGIENE AND THE SALINES.

THE use of aperient waters dates from time immemorial. The ancients flocked to their mineral springs and held the waters in sacred veneration.

The annual rush to the numerous Carlsbads of the Old and New Worlds is a rush of multitude. These cleansing waters are one of Nature's most effective methods of physical renovation. With sensible and educated people they take the place of the thousand and one nostrums that are annually responsible for so many ruined constitutions and premature deaths. They clear up the system, without leaving behind a wake of unliquidated damages. They make it feasible to rewrite the old Portuguese saw:

"Joy, temperance and repose,
Slam the door on the doctor's nose,"
until it now reads:

Joy, temperance and Sprudel salts,
All help to hide the doctor's faults.

Thousands are learning to purge themselves of bile, brickdust, bilgewater bogies and the blues, without the expense of a long journey to far away fountains. The active ingredients of the most famous springs have been made available so that, at nominal expense, every household can set up its own mimic Carlsbad and Aix-les-Bains. One of the best of these preparations is Kutnow's Effervescing Saline. which can be found at every pharmacy.

TESLA'S NEW SUNLIGHT.

NICOLA TESLA has given to the New York *Sun* a statement concerning his new experiments in the production of light, from which we quote as follows:

"The lamps are glass tubes. I most generally use a rectangular spiral, containing about twenty to twenty-five feet of tubing making some twelve to fourteen convolutions, with a total illuminating surface of from 300 to 400 square inches. The ends of the spiral tube are covered by a metallic coating, and provided with hooks for hanging the lamp on the terminals of the source of oscillations. The tube contains gases rarefied to a certain degree, determined in the course of long experimentation as being conducive to the best results.

"The process of light production is, according to my views, as follows: The street current is passed through a machine which is an electrical oscillator of peculiar construction and transforms the supply current, be it direct or alternating, into electrical oscillations of a very high frequency. These oscillations, coming to the metallically-coated ends of the glass tube, produce in the interior corresponding electrical oscillations, which set the molecules and atoms of the enclosed rarefied gases into violent commotion, causing them to vibrate at enormous rates and emit those radiations which we know as light. The gases are not rendered incandescent, or hot, like an incandescent filament.

"High economy results from three causes: First, from the high rate of the electrical oscillations; second, from the fact that the entire light-giving body, being a highly attenuated gas, is exposed and can throw out its radiations unimpeded; and, third, because of the smallness of the particles composing the light-giving body, in consequence of which they can be quickly thrown into a high rate of vibration, so that comparatively little energy is lost in the lower or heat vibrations. The lamps need not be renewed like the ordinary ones. as there is nothing in them to consume. The illuminating power of each of these lamps is, measured by the photometric method, about fifty candle power, but I can make them of any power desired, up to that of several arc lights. Given a certain quantity of electrical energy from the mains, I can produce more light than can be produced by the ordinary methods. In introducing this system of lighting, my transformer, or oscillator, will be usually located at some convenient place in the basement, and from there the transformed currents will be led as usual through the building.

"It is a remarkable feature of the light that during the day it can scarcely be seen, whereas at night the whole room is brilliantly illuminated. When the eye becomes used to the light of these tubes, an ordinary incandescent lamp or gas burner produces pain in the eye when it is turned on, showing in a striking manner to what a degree these concentrated sources of light which we now use are detrimental to the eye.

"I have found that in almost all its actions the light produces the same effects as sunlight, and this makes me hopeful that its introduction into dwellings will have the effect of improving, in a measure now impossible to estimate, the hygienic condition. The light produces a soothing action on the nerves, and also improves vision, exactly as the sunlight, and it ozonizes slightly the atmosphere. These effects can be regulated at will."

Tesla further declares that he can and does operate this apparatus without any wire. so that the lamps can be carried about freely. like candles, the energy being conveyed through space. But a number of improvements must be made yet before it can be generally introduced.

ORDINARY NOSE BLEED.

THE following very sensible remarks concerning a very common accident we take from a paper by Dr. E. W. Pyle, of Jersey City. Dr. Pyle says:

The practice of plugging the nares to relieve the ordinary forms of hemorrhages should be condemned. It subjects to aural dangers; it makes a superficial clot that is not reliable; it imposes a foreign substance that sets up excessive secretion, occludes the nostril and shuts out the hemostatic influence of the inspired air.

The bleeding point is almost invariably just within the vestibule, on the cartilaginous septum near its junction with the floor. A knowledge of this fact should simplify the subject and clearly point out the method of procedure.

Intelligent work of this character cannot be done in the dark. In the absence of a head mirror, the strong sunlight or the direct rays of a lamp should be utilized to locate the hemorrhage. The nose should be cleared of all clots and a speculum used to dilate the vestibule. Then, seated directly in front of the patient, with the lesion well in view, and armed with one or more nasal applicators or wooden toothpicks, upon which cotton is firmly wound, direct pressure should be made with the cotton-tipped point upon the bleeding spot, to form a deep clot in the vessel. When the hemorrhage has ceased the surface should be lightly touched with the solid stick of nitrate of silver, which secures the clot or binds the lumen of the open vessel and prevents the return so characteristic of the other method, which forms a superficial clot only.

This is the simple rationale of action. With a little skill it can be so cleverly accomplished, in most instances, as to obliterate to the eye the seat of lesion. The plain, dry absorbent cotton answers better than when moistened with any styptic. Occasionally it becomes necessary to change quickly for a dry point and to continue the pressure, it may be, until the arms are tired.

To succeed is always possible, and the advantages over the usual method are appreciated best by the patients themselves. To stop hemorrhage and, at the same time, maintain function, is a triumph.

CREMATION.

WE emphatically endorse the following from the *N. E. Med. Monthly:*

"The rite of cremation, whose revival is one of the encouraging features of our latter day cvilization, has made on the whole, satisfactory progress during the past year, though there still remains some latent opposition and an ill-defined prejudice which, no doubt, time will overcome.

"In America and Europe there are said to be at the present time sixty-five crematories, of which twenty-six are located in the United States, while several more are in process of construction. In Boston during the past year there were 327 cremations, which, when compared with the annual death rate, speaks well for the increasing popularity of incineration, and it is not surprising that among those who make a study of social conditions the opinion as to its advisability is most unanimous.

"The conditions of existence at the present time favor the reform in question, and with the increase in population and the status of affairs in congested districts, there are sanitary reasons which will help to turn the scale.

"We hope to see in the near future an extension of the movement in question and the establishment in every large city of a proper plant for crematory purposes, and we feel sure that such a project, if properly carried out, would meet with generous support."

LEEUWENHOEK AND HIS MICROSCOPE.

UNDER this head *Popular Science Monthly* has this to say:

"Leeuwenhoek seems to have been fascinated by the marvels of the microscopic world, but the extent and quality of his work lifted him above the level of the dilettante. He was not, like Malpighi and Swammerdam, a skilled dissector, but turned his microscope in all directions, in the mineral, as well as the vegetable and animal kingdoms. Just when he began to use the microscope is not known; his first publication in reference to microscopic objects did not appear till 1673, when he was forty-one years old. He gave good descriptions and drawings of his instruments, and those still in existence have been described by Carpenter and others, and, therefore, we have a very good idea of his working equipment. During his lifetime he sent as a present to the Royal Society of London twenty-six microscopes, each provided with an object to examine. Unfortunately, these were removed from the rooms of the society and lost during the eighteenth century. His lenses were of fine quality and were ground by himself. They were nearly all simple lenses of small size, but considerable curvature, and needed to be brought close to the object examined. He had different microscopes for different purposes, giving a range of magnifying powers from 40 to 270 diameters and possibly higher. The number of his lenses is surprising; he possessed not less than 247 complete microscopes, two of which were provided with double lenses and one with triplet. In addition to the above he had 172 lenses set between plates of metal, which gives a total of 419 lenses used by him in his observations. Three were of quartz or rock crystal, the rest were of glass. More than one-half the lenses were mounted in silver, three were in gold."

HARMONY IN NATURE.

NATURALISTS say that when examined minutely with a microscope, it will be found that no creature or object in Nature is positively ugly; that there is a certain harmony or symmetry of parts that renders the whole agreeable rather than the reverse. So the most disagreeable tasks in life, when viewed in their proper proportions, reveal a poetic, an attractive, side hitherto undreamed of. Turn on the sunlight of good cheer, the determination to see the bright as well as the dark side, and you will find something pleasant, even in the most dreaded task.

EVERY DISEASE HAS ITS ODOR.

DR. McCASSY, declares—*Doctor's Magazine*—that every doctor should be able to diagnose measles, diphtheria, typhoid fever, consumption, and even epilepsy, by the smell, as every one has an especial odor when disease is present. Thus in the case of favus, the patient exhales the odor of mice; in rheumatism, there is an odor of acid that is very easily recognized. In cases of pyemia, the breath is nauseating in its smell; in scurvy, too, there is a putrid odor. In peritonitis, the odor is like musk; in case of scrofula, like sour beer. In ordinary fever there is an ammoniacal odor. In intermittent fever, the odor is like that of fresh baked bread. Among hysterical women there are many delightful odors, violet and pnieapple being most manifest.

THE HEALTH OF NEW YORK STATE.

ACCORDING to the report of the State Board of Health, there were, during March, 11,913 deaths in the State from all causes, and a death-rate of 19.2; a decrease from a daily rate of 394 in February, to one of 384. During the first three months of the year there have been 35,529 deaths, including delayed returns, a daily rate of 395, which exceeds that of the same months in 1900 by 12 deaths daily. Grippe is estimated to have caused, during March, about 1,500 deaths. the same as in February.

THE MINNESOTA MARRIAGE LAW.

THE so-called "Chilton Marriage Law," as finally passed by the Minnesota State Legislature, provides that "no woman under the age of forty-five (45) years, or man of any age, except he marry a woman over the age of forty-five (45) years, either of whom is epileptic, imbecile, feeble-minded, or afflicted with insanity, shall hereafter intermarry or marry any other person within this State. It is also hereby made unlawful for any person to marry any such feeble-minded, imbecile, or epileptic person or any one afflicted with insanity." State officials are forbidden to issue marriage licenses, and clergymen and others are forbidden to solemnize marriages in cases in which either of the parties is afflicted with any of the diseases mentioned. Violation of any of the provisions of the act is punishable by a fine of not more than $1,000, or by imprisonment in the State prison for not more than three years, or by both such fine and imprisonment.

SNAKE BITE.

McFarland (*International Medical Magazine*), *summarizes the treatment* of snake bite as follows: Stop immediately the circulation in the bitten member or part of the body, so as to prevent absorption of the poison. Incise and enlarge the fang wound freely and suck forcibly to extract the poison—the suction may be accomplished with a cupping-glass or with the mouth, the poison being harmless when swallowed. Inject hypodermically 3 to 6 drops of fresh 10 per cent. aqueous solution of calcium chloride into about a dozen areas around the wound. Gold chloride is just as effective, but it is too expensive. Potassium permanganate is of little value. Give strychnine hypodermically to stimulate the respiratory center. Whiskey should not be given at all, or only in very small doses, because an excess of alcohol still further depresses the heart, already depressed by the venom. Immediately inject 10 to 20 cc. (2½ to 5 drams) of antivenomous serum and repeat these injections frequently. People living or going into regions where there is danger of snake bites should carry a bottle of antivenomous serum with them.

THE TRAINING OF SIGHT.

"Lord Wolseley, having lately remarked upon the good sight of the Boers as one cause, at least, of their good shooting, and having ascribed this good sight to its constant exercise in the open air, Mr. Brudenell Carter has pointed out," says *The Hospital*, "that it is not merely a question of open air, but of the training of sight upon things that are far off and difficult to see. Vision, he says, like every other nerve-function, must be cultivated, for the attainment of a high degree of excellence. The visual power of city children is not cultivated by their environment. They see the other side of the street, and the carts and the omnibuses of the thoroughfares. They scarcely ever have the visual attention directed strongly to any distant object, and hence the seeing function is not exerted to anything like what should be the extent of its powers. With a country child the case is widely different."

DANGER IN GETTING "HIGH."—A DRINK-CURE SANITARIUM.

Dr. Whitmore, of Leadville, in a paper on the effects of great altitudes, in the Denver *Medical Times*, says:

"My observation leads me to believe that neither alcohol nor tobacco can be used to the same extent at great altitudes as at sea level, without more rapidly deleterious effects. At the Montezuma mine, near Taylor's Pass, at an elevation of some 13,500 feet, I met a man whom I had previously known as an excellent engineer, but who would go on frequent sprees. He informed me that working at the Montezuma was equivalent to taking the 'jag-cure'; that whiskey was not only difficult to get, but that he could not drink it. There were some thirty or forty men employed there, and they used no coffee and but little tea."

Department of Hygiene.

WITH SPECIAL REFERENCE TO STATE AND PREVENTIVE MEDICINE.

THE THERAPEUTIC VALUE OF CLIMATE.—SECOND PAPER.

COLORADO, NEW MEXICO, AND ARIZONA.

THE three climatic qualities that absorb attention and require study are heat, cold and humidity. A fourth eludes the vigilant instruments of the Weather Bureau observers and can scarcely be described. It is that nameless charm which inheres in all the genial climates, depends upon a rare combination of all the recorded qualities, refuses to be measured, and can only be experienced.

Of all the secondary influences that make or mar climatic hospitality the character and movement of air currents is beyond question the most potent. Temperature, rainfall and atmospheric humidity may be quite within the prescribed and approved limits, yet disagreeably frequent or violent winds may make the locality far from ideal, or even next to unendurable.

There are times in Colorado when high winds, eventuating in "sand-storms," try the nerves and patience of all visitors and require an unusual stock of fortitude on the part of the oldest settlers. But they are comparatively infrequent and are practically forgotten during the long intervals of delightful weather.

If one were limited to a single word with which to describe the climate of this mid-mountain region that word would be *tonic*. It is here that Nature exemplifies a ventilating system that might be profitably imitated by scientists. Volumes of air, cooled and perfectly purified by contact with snow-covered heights, are constantly sent down from the mountain summits to displace the used and impure air of the lower land, which rises to be again subjected to the process of disinfection and aseptization. This interchange is constant, day and night, and outside his own carelessness as to local surroundings or personal habits, there is no valid reason why any resident of the entire region should not at all times breathe the very best of air.

The climatic Midway Plaisance of this country includes portions of New Mexico and Arizona. It constitutes a compromise between hot and cold climates. Both these territories contain local areas that are hot enough to please a salamander, and at the same time there are altitudes where cool breezes prevail and where snow and frost are annual visitors. Between these extremes there are all gradations. The list includes lofty mountains, broad, high mesas, fertile valleys, extensive forests of pine, and stretches of arid desert. Here, climate must be spoken of in the plural, for there are many; and they cure everything but poverty and heartache! In New Mexico the Messilla Valley and Las Vegas Hot Springs rank first in popularity.

Speaking of the climate of New Mexico in general a recent writer aptly says:

"Description of the atmospheric effects of the Southwest is the most hopeless wall against which language ever butted its ineffectual head. The light that never was on sea or land spends itself on the adobe and the chaparo.

"Under that ineffable alchemy of the sky,

mud turns ethereal, and the desert is a revelation. It is Egypt, with every rock a
Sphinx, every peak a pyramid."

It is hard for one who never visited any
portion of the Great Plains or mid-conti-
nental regions to form any adequate conception of the prevailing climatic characteristics. Altitude, remoteness from any considerable bodies of water, and the peculiar,
meteorological conditions resulting from this
combination of causes make the contrast so
radical that no possible description can make
it intelligible to one who has not experienced
it. There is an average general altitude
of about a vertical mile above sea-level.
This gives at all times a rarefied atmosphere.
The remoteness of bodies of water and infrequency of springs and streams, together
with an almost total absence of rainfall,
make the absence of atmospheric humidity
a foregone and perfectly natural result. On
the plains proper and in the lower and in any
way shut-in valleys it is dry and hot. At
the greater elevations and on the mountains
it is dry and cool, that is, comparatively
cool. Between the two extremes are many
gradations, but all are dry. Physiologically considered, any considerable increase
of altitude means two things—lower temperature and increased respiratory function.
This statement is of the stereotyped order
in all ordinary localities, but when we reach
the arid regions that skirt the Rocky
Mountains we must bear in mind that we
have left all "ordinary" conditions behind us.
In the East, where the readings of the wet-
bulb and dry-bulb thermometers vary but
little, on account of the prevailing humidity, the reports of the Weather Bureau may
be consulted with some degree of satisfaction. They often lack homogenity, but
they are not universally and irreconcilably
incongruous. In Southern Colorado, New
Mexico, Arizona, and portions of California, they are little better than a jumble of
meteorological mirage. The visitor or invalid who consults the tables will soon discover that he is the victim of diurnal delusion. For example, 32° F. at Las Vegas
is quite as agreeable as 50° F. on the coast

of Maine or New Jersey, while 85° F. in
the humid atmosphere of the Atlantic coast
is far less endurable as to comfort than
95° or 100° F. in Arizona. The uninitiated
read this statement without in the least
comprehending it, if not with disdainful incredulity. Only actual experience will convince them that the sensible temperature
and not that of the air as measured by a
dry-bulb thermometer is the one with which
they have to contend, and that these often
vary as much as twenty or thirty degrees in
any arid region. In some localities in Arizona the mercury frequently marks as high
as 110° F., yet sunstroke is unknown; while
in Chicago, New Orleans or New York
plenty of cases occur with the mercury not
higher than 80° or 85° F. This proves
that there are two kinds of temperature, that
measured in degrees, by a soulless thermometer, and that realized by sentient life.
One is strictly mechanical, the other intensely vital. It is the difference between
these two that is so hard to comprehend.

In this as in all similar climates three
factors contribute to the therapeutic results,
each of the three pertaining to a condition
of the atmosphere—its tension or pressure,
its degree of humidity, and its perfect asepsis. The elevation determines its degree of
rarefaction, the absence of rainfall and remoteness from bodies of water keep it at a
uniformly low percentage of humidity, and
both these causes, in connection with the
nature of the soil, give it its aseptic character. It is a combination that is not found outside of certain topographic and meteorologic limits and can not be even approximately imitated by art.

One of the first things the novice discovers on arriving at an altitude a vertical mile
or more higher than the one he has been
accustomed to, is, that his breathing function has unconsciously assumed a new gait;
his heart is equally anxious about the new
environment, and is running a race with his
respiratory apparatus. As a mechanico-
physiologic result, air cells that may have
been dormant or collapsed for years, find
themselves suddenly pressed into service, in

order to assist in supplying the system with its due quota of oxygen from the diluted atmosphere. Every vital function soon begins to respond, in unison with the enhanced breathing function, and the whole system is soon actively involved. When invalids seek this region after organic changes have gone so far that any systemic disturbance is hazardous, it is practically too late; but at earlier stages the effects are almost invariably salutary as well as permanent. Lung capacity is increased, vital processes healthfully stimulated and the entire economy invigorated. The increased chest expansion frequently amounts to several inches in as many weeks. This is a gain that does not recede when one leaves the region. It remains as a permanent accession to the future stamina and capacity. It means added comfort and added years to any life.

All this refers to what Nature has done for the region; but this does not exhaust her resources. Sunshine predominates; it is unimpeded even by the smoky haze so common at the East, and it permeates. There are but twenty-five or twenty-eight days in any year when sunshine is not in evidence. It keeps the air and soil aseptic; it generates ozone; it dissipates malaria; it stimulates absorption and assimilation; it imparts tone to the entire system; it lifts flagging spirits, and restores waning hope

To all this potent meteorologic armamentarium Nature has added hot and cold springs that have been famed for their healing virtues from time immemorial. The principal of these are at Las Vegas, on the line of the Santa Fe Railway, where the latter skirts the Gallinas River as it debouches from the Las Vegas spur of the Rocky Mountains. The elevation at this point is nearly 7,000 feet above sea-level, that is to say, a lineal mile and a quarter nearer the sun, moon and stars than the topographically abased cities of Boston, New York and New Orleans. Now that statement is perfectly plain English, but not one reader in a hundred will stop to realize what a change of environment, atmospheric

tension, magnetic relations and general vital conditions such an elevation implies. Centuries ago the nomadic tribes that peopled this wild and wonderful country made long and frequent pilgrimages to these springs, in which they found healing for all the ills that aboriginal flesh was heir to. To this day they continue to come from far and near, camping in the vicinity and utilizing the virtues of the springs, until they have shed their physical disabilities, their damaged livers, rheumatic joints, and disgusted or rebellious stomachs, as one sheds a worn-out suit of winter underclothes. Remaining for a few weeks each season, they return to their accustomed hunting grounds, where with dance and pow wow they celebrate their recuperation and renewal of youth.

Now, the irrepressible white man is crowding the aborigine from his Mecca and turning his Fountains of Youth into a modern Bethesda. Hotels, bath houses, a scientific laboratory, a natatorium and all the addenda and equipments of a complete sanatorium have sprung into existence, and every year more and more thousands are flocking hither to do penance and regain lost vigor.

The hot springs resemble those of Carlsbad and Teplitz in chemical composition, and have a temperature of 124° F. But there are springs of cold water, and others containing sulphur and the chalybeates. The peat baths are also a notable feature.

Mud, as well as blood, is thicker than water, and if not satisfied with plainer and *thinner* baths, you can be accommodated with mud to your heart's content.

There are many other localities in New Mexico, each having its special attractions and warm advocates. In the Pecos valley they have a modern Carlsbad in name as well as nature. It has a much lower altitude—about 4,000 feet, and is surrounded by a fine farming country. It has a warmer climate, and its lower altitude adapts it to some cases which would not do well at Las Vegas. Fifty miles north of Santa Fe is Ojo Caliente, (hot lather) which was quite as famous as Las Vegas, having been visited by the early Spaniards long before it was known to any but the aborigines.

At Jemez, fifty miles north of Albuquerque, there are more hot springs, one of which is a spouter or geyser. It is a great resort for inveterate cases of rheumatism.

Twenty-five miles north of Deming are the Hudson hot springs. They are similar in character to those at Las Vegas. At both Jemez and Hudson Springs the altitude is 1,500 feet less than at Las Vegas. For those who would seek greater elevation Camp Whitcomb is 8,000 feet, and Sulphur Springs 8,250 feet above sea-level.

In Arizona, Phœnix is the center of attraction and is fast taking on metropolitan airs. It has acquired a great reputation for relieving or curing desperate cases of both asthma and bronchitis. Some of the latter are, of course, really cases of laryngeal phthisis, and the "cures" effected are fairly miraculous. Whitelaw Reid seems to consider it the only place that promptly relieves his elsewhere intractable asthma, and many others have had a similar experience.

If one is asked for a comparison, Arizona may be called the counterpart of Persia. She has the same dry air, the same hot valleys, roses, date palms, olives and fig trees, pomegranates and vineyards.

Among the pine-clad hills and high mesas of Arizona are plenty of delightful sites for health stations. Probably not a tenth part of them have yet been discovered, much less explored. Most of them are remote from settlements and lines of travel. There is the choice between valley, mesa and mountain, and any altitude from 3,000 feet to the summits of the highest mountain ranges is at command. Much of the territory consists of a hot and arid desert, and will doubtless remain a *terra incognita* until the national government or private enterprise succeeds in reclaiming its waste places by a gigantic system of irrigation. In fact this is already in process of accomplishment. One tract of 100,000 acres will be supplied with water and made ready to blossom as the rose by the end of the present season. The ultimate result of irrigating schemes

now under way can hardly be foretold. The Colorado River furnishes an ample supply of water at all seasons, and its complete diversion into this so-called desert means not only the reclaiming of wide stretches of territory now worthless and uninhabitable, it means that which is of far greater importance—*the radical modification of the climatic conditions of the entire region.* If the value of the reclaimed and fertilized acres mounts into millions, that of the reclaimed climate may be estimated in billions. The arid regions are arid simply because they are rainless. When all the melting snows of the west slope of the Rockies have been turned into the thirsty soil instead of being annually poured into the insatiate and ungrateful Pacific, rains will come in summer, dews will fall, snows will whiten the landscape in winter, and the whole face of Nature will be changed. The soil lacks nothing but water to make it the garden spot of the world. This is not a matter of theory and hyperbole; it has been practically put to the test. Ten tons of alfalfa, per annum, to the acre sounds Munchausenish to the uninitiated, but it is already an accomplished and commonplace fact, in some of the valleys where water has been made available.

As a wild camping ground for invalids, curiosity seekers and naturalists no region of the unsettled West affords a greater variety or richer promise of interesting as well as startling novelty. There are cañons and gorges too appalling in their immensity to be ventured near or looked into by any save those who feel perfectly sure of their nerves and their footing; ruins of once populous and busy cities and villages, ages ago peopled by a race of which we have little history outside of tradition and the tale told by these ruins and relics; and there are remains of forests of gigantic growth, unlike any now in existence, and which, submerged by some colossal, prehistoric cataclysm, were petrified *in situ.* They were doubtless the "Big trees" of a bygone epoch, turned by some inconceivable freak of Nature into columns of agate and chalcedony. Sections of these anomalous monoliths, that once dwarfed the most ambitious of the Egyptian obelisks, are still standing. At one point a monster trunk lies stretched unbroken, across a wide gulch or cañon, a possible footbridge for the great-great-grandfather of the Aztecs! It is a rich field for botanist, geologist and curio hunter.

It was in Arizona that an old miner, a few years ago, announced the discovery of rubies and garnets, and here that other "experts" continue to prophesy that one day diamonds and other precious gems will surely be revealed. Why not? There's Africa, Afrikander, Aztec and Arizona; Transvaal, Tugela, Tucson and Tombstone; Boer, Bloomfontein and Bowie; Cape Town and Clifton, Philippolis, Pretoria and Phœnix, Moselitkase and Maricopa—surely all these initial coincidences ought to stand for something, in a community which originated the Baconian-Shakespeare cryptography!

Phœnix, the capital, has had a phenomenal history. Within a few years its population and material prosperity have distanced even western records, which is putting it as strong as language permits.

This embryo city, which as already noted, has acquired high repute as a favorable resort for desperate cases of throat and lung diseases has all the usual and some rather extraordinary appurtenances of the typical western city. Its gambling palaces—sometimes spelled by another name!—are unique; its concert saloons—'parlors with a bar"—already rival in glittering splendor and illusive attraction the best of those in the large cities of the East. The "artists" of the dance halls and "chance" halls are constantly recruited by accessions from the traveling theaters and light opera troupes that so frequently find themselves stranded on the Pacific slope; or that have learned by previous experience to expect a spasmodic harvest on each recurring visit to this place, so that there is no lack of "first class" vaudeville in half-dress, of cowboys and acrobats in dress-as-you-please, or of gaiety girls and danseuses in little or no dress.

Thus the season is never dull, for those who "like this sort of thing," and it must be confessed that staid easterners soon get to looking on without being shocked—in fact with gusto.

HOW TO GROW BEAUTIFUL WITH THE YEARS.

Solomon says: "The hoary head is a crown of glory if it be found in the way of righteousness." In the early spring time of youth, when the soul is opening like a flower before the sun, then is the time to sow, plant, and graft, thus making ready to garner the crop in the autumn of life.

As we approach the adult life, careful preparation must still be going on—education, accomplishments, and the exercising of all the virtues that will make a life noble and great.

Strict attention must be paid to the laws of health, so that the ripe years are reached in comparative strength and vigor.

The knowledge of how to care for one's health, abstemious living, and moderate enjoyment of the good things of life tend not only to lengthen the years, but to the increase of happiness.

The possessor of a cheerful disposition is a boon to society, maintaining cheerfulness and good humor; thus cultivating a thankful, restful temperament among all with whom we come in contact.

Cheerfulness can be cultivated by habit and the law of contentment. One must accustom himself to see only the best and brightest side of everything. This creates an air of geniality and good humor which seems contagious, and its possessor is greeted with smiles and pleasant words wherever he goes. Persons who possess the happy faculty of being cheerful always have something to fall back on; and such people realize how much occupation contributes to happiness. Hence they are never without something to do.

Half of our troubles come from an idle life and an exaggerated idea of our own merits and importance; therefore the degree of happiness we would enjoy depends largely on ourselves.

Would you know an infallible secret for winning friends, and making ourselves popular, even to the concealment of our faults? Acquire these important rules in your everyday life:

Cultivate a pleasant manner, a kind thoughtfulness for doing good to others, patience and self-denial, a desire for being agreeable in all your actions, in the tones of your voice.

And, more than this, in your mind and heart mastering these simple rules, and with good self-control, you will always be amiable, and will earn and foster the respect and affection of every one whom you may meet, whether in social life, or in the outside world.

ECHOES OF THE YEARS.

One who has made the attempt to cater for the amusement and entertainment of those who have reached the shady side of life will recall their experience of the rather unsatisfactory effort to light up the beaming face of interest, the sparkling eye and listening ear, such as the modern style of song and dance arouses when caroled in sweet melodious voice and tune, in the presence of a well matured and critical audience belonging to ye olden time.

Some time ago in visiting a Home for the Aged, I had such an experience. I did not, however, take my seat at the piano with any formal announcement that I intended to entertain my "young" friends, who were promenading the room and most agreeably chatting with one another.

Striking a few chords of that old ditty, "Barbara Allen," instantly I perceived a change. The room became quiet. Then I ventured a few of Moore's melodies, so popular fifty years ago.

"Ah!" said one old lady, "my young man used to sing 'Love's Young Dream,' can you sing it?"

Fortunately I could recollect one stanza. She supplied the rest of the words, and for the time being was thrown back into youthful reminiscences of happy days. From songs we gradually drifted into old dance music, jigs and waltzes. By this time several of those who were sitting had risen to their feet, keeping time with the good old tune, "The Girl I Left Behind Me."

My audience being now aroused into a healthy condition of enthusiasm, some of them began to recite little snatches of poetry and song. I encouraged the effort by attentively listening to results of dormant faculties suddenly and feelingly awakened into life.

One dear old lady endeavored to repeat a long-forgotten poem. Much to her annoyance and chagrin she could only repeat one stanza. On retiring for the night, as I walked through the long corridor, out of a dark corner came this same old lady, approaching me with the remark, "I have thought of the rest of that poem."

"Repeat it, if you please," said I, and in that dark hall, with an impressive manner of both voice and action, that sentimental poem was recited in a way and with a spirit that would have done credit to a finished actress.

I felt for the time being that I was indebted to that cheerful evening of merriment, for it had brought me, too, a harvest of thoughts too precious for words. In the language of rollicking Gail Hamilton, "Oh the lusty luscious years!"

JEANETTE THORPE.

LIVES MORE IMPORTANT THAN MACHINERY.

WE reproduce from the *Chicago Tribune* the following sensible protest on this subject:

With the evolution of business involving vast capital and necessitating concentration of executive forces in a few heads, the wear and tear upon this directing machinery of a great corporation has been suggested as possibly of more concern to stockholders than generally has been admitted.

The question has been asked in point: Can the stockholders of a great railroad system pay a president $50,000 a year for looking after the wear and tear of its physical machinery and yet not recognize that the president himself should be looked after as of vital importance to the conduct of the road?

In the case of the president of the steel trust, would it not be a good business policy for the directorate to see that a president drawing a salary of $1,000,000 a year shall have the attention of a medical adviser in some such degree as the inanimate machinery of the mills demands of the mechanic and engineer?

Should a careless head of a great institution be allowed to wear himself out looking after the wear and tear on inanimate things that can be easily replaced?

DISAPPROVE OF SALARIES.

In general it may be said of the medical profession of Chicago that it does not look kindly upon salaried positions for doctors. Except in rare cases, it is regarded as a confession of individual weakness when a physician ties himself to a salaried position. He may go with a millionaire patient to Europe. He may put himself at the head of a great hospital or medical school. But for any position where the influence of "pull" may be exerted, there is the prejudice that belongs to the profession.

Still, as a proposition in economics, Chicago physicians say that for a great corporation to wear out its chief executive at preventing wear and tear, and at the same time to have no eye to the condition of the executive himself, could not be logical on its face.

"But the question is," said Dr. Edmund Andrews, "could a board of directors elect a competent physician to such a post? Or, having elected him, could they bring influence to bear that would lead a $10,000, $50,000, or $1,000,000 man to consult him or accept his attentions?"

"Such a man would naturally have his individuality strongly developed," said Dr. Daniel R. Brower. "If he had ever been sick he would have had his own physician. Could a corporation induce him to drop this man in favor of another?"

TO CARE FOR THE CARELESS.

As against these opinions, however, it is admitted that a man who has a family physician would not be in need of a company physician; that it would be the persistently careless man who would need to be looked after by such an official.

"I can see difficulties in the way of establishing a salaried physician for a big corporation," said Dr. Andrews, "but if a competent, conscientious man were so installed I think he would be able to earn his salary.

"In many ways the advice of a physician among the managers of a great company would be of direct benefit to the stockholders. So often a man under pressure of work that inevitably comes upon him resorts to stimulants to carry him through with it. The reaction is always certain and harmful. If, feeling the need of this stimulus, he would consult a physician, something more effective and less reactionary than alcohol could be given.

"The advantage of being under the observation of a physician, of having a record of analyses of the secretions, of the heart beats, and of respiration for comparative purposes could not be doubted. So many times such observations would save a man a spell of sickness, and, in the case of a man capable of earning $1,000,000 a year, such prevention would mean money to stockholders.

"Ordinarily, too, a man in a high executive position has certain demands made upon him as a host and entertainer. He often has to serve drinks to business acquaintances, and necessarily has to partake of them himself. Naturally he is inclined to feed well. Perhaps he is indifferent to exercise.

"The result may be a case of 'drunkard's

liver' in a man who was never intoxicated in his life, and an attack of gout in one whose ancestry showed no predisposition to the disease."

CHECK INCIPIENT DISEASE.

"The earmarks of many diseases are plain to a physician when these diseases are in their incipiency, especially if the patient has been under observation for any length of time. Capacities for work vary in individuals, but in general a physician would know if a man is overworking himself. He could see that sleep enough was taken, and, while occasionally any man in such capacity has to overexert himself, the physician could make sure that sufficient relaxation followed the effort."

Dr. Andrews says that in his experience with such men most of them suffer because of too much attention to details, and for the reason that they so grudgingly confer the power to act upon others. The one great penalty for this overwork he has found to be neurasthenia, in all its shadings, from a mere mental depression to insanity of pronounced degree.

"Bright's disease, as it is commonly called, means so many things," said he. "that it hardly can be called a millionaire's disease. They have it. but nobody can say overwork is the cause, though it may aggravate it. Insanity is a frequent penalty. Gout, while not common. is frequently met with. Its only successful treatment is to remove the cause."

As an alienist and neurologist. Dr. Brower has discovered that the millionaire manipulator of millions is not as careless of his health as he may seem. He insists that the man who sits on the side of a road and pounds stone for $1 a day is many times more careless of his health than is the man who earns $50,000 or $100,000 a year.

"Everywhere the art of prevention of disease is being considered." said Dr. Brower. "Men so often go to a doctor not because they are sick but because they don't want to get sick. There are several men in Chicago who draw big salaries who have consulted me about every three months for years. They are not sick when they come. They want a general examination, however, and to know by comparison with former records whether they are holding up under the strain."

THE GENERAL CARE OF THE SKIN CONSIDERED FROM THE POINT OF VIEW OF PROPHYLAXIS.

JAMIESON writes in the *Edinburgh Medical Journal* for December, 1900, reproduced in the *Therapeutic Gazette*, upon this important subject. He reminds us that the association of soap with ablution has come to be a fixed idea in the British mind. "What! not use soap in my bath; why, I should never feel clean," is the common answer to the suggestion that it had better be discontinued. There is reason on its side, yet when we consider that much of the soap employed for toilet purposes contains more or less free alkali, often more than less, and thereby emulsifies the protective oleaginous ingredient of the epidermis, and so in a manner does away with it, soap as usually met with is not an unmixed advantage. The introduction by Unna of neutral soaps, to which an excess of unsaponified fat has been added—superfatted soaps—is an immense stride in the right direction. There are now many superfatted soaps in the market, and among them some really reliable ones, but it has to be borne in mind what it is to be a thoroughly good soap. It is quite possible to add lanolin or some other difficultly saponifiable fat to a soap which was originally a very inferior soap, and then palm it off as a superfatted soap. Hence it is necessary to see that the soap is manufactured by a trustworthy firm, and it is well also to learn that it contains no cocoanut oil. as, if it does, it is not a proper skin soap. Neutral soaps, made from pure fats, and superfatted to the extent of from 3 to 5 per cent., should unquestionably be used in preference to any others. Medicated soaps are medicinal: they are not suited for ordinary use, but have their place, and a very restricted place it is, in the cure or amelioration of certain diseased conditions. The substitution of bags containing bran or oatmeal for soap is advisable, as by them the detersive effect is obtained while the defensive fat is left undisturbed.

Another important element in the care of the skin is the kind of water to be employed. Distilled, rain, or river water constitute perfection, but these are in many cases unattainable. We are not all in the position of Glasgow, with a practically pure water supply. Hard water, from its containing lime, acts deleteriously on the skin, and while there are chemical methods of softening such water, these are not available to the multitude. Some of the lime is deposited from water which has been boiled for a time and allowed to cool. The artificial additions to water, for the purpose of softening it, are apt to be harmful. Thus borax, soda, or ammonia render it alkaline and endow it with disadvantages similar to alkaline soaps. The sensation of softness imparted by these is deceptive. It arises from their combining with and saponifying the fat of the skin, hence they leave it harsh and dry. Bran, oatmeal, or starch lessen the injurious effect of the lime salts and are in themselves innocuous, hence such can frequently be mixed with the water with benefit. Glycerin diluted with water and the glycerite of starch are recommended as applications after the bath, to obviate the ill effects of hard water. These act through their hygroscopic power and keep the surface moist, but at the same time they swell up the epidermic cells, rendering them unduly tender. It is a method which may prevent chaps forming in cold, drying winds. Of still more consequence is to at once seal up any chance crack or slight lesion of continuity, by placing over it a film of salicylic wool, and then painting this down with flexible collodion. In so doing we carry out the principle of the famous medical maxim, "Obsta principiis," which was, as some may remember, the motto of that much-loved man and excellent physician, the late Sir Douglas Maclagan, who among many other subjects took a deep interest in skin diseases.

Some portions of the body normally bear hairs, and some are wholly destitute of them. Exposure to the weather during adolescence and early manhood increases the hirsute growth, while constant covering checks its formation or leads to its disappearance. We see the effect of the former in the hairy legs of the Highlander accustomed to wear the kilt; of the latter in the bald crown of the hat-wearing professional or city man. Though there is desquamation from the scalp surface, as there is from the rest of the body, it is slight and trivial should the scalp be thoroughly healthy. To preserve it with the natural polish is what we should aim at. This can only be done by judicious attention. It is singular that there is a prejudice among many people against washing the hair. This may be accounted for perhaps in two ways: one, that in the female sex at least it is certainly rather a troublesome procedure to wash, and still further to dry, a copious and lengthy crop; and again, when washed with ordinary toilet soap, or with solution of borax, as some do, the hair is left harsh and dry, and tends to fall more plentifully in consequence. But unwashed, effete epidermic particles in most cases accumulate around the roots of the hairs, and encourage if they do not directly cause diseased conditions. These cannot be removed by brushing, which, if at all vigorously carried out, like the small-tooth comb—an abomination now all but banished—rakes the scalp and eventually renders the plight worse than before. If a well made fluid superfatted soap, in which the alkali is potash and not soda, be sprinkled over the head, then sufficient warm, soft water be added from time to time, first to produce a lather, subsequently to wash out this lather, and with it the incorporated dust, the hair when dried will be found to be left soft and flexible, while the scalp has no sensation of tenseness. Or, in place of the soap, we may have recourse to an effusion of quillaia bark in warm water. This contains saponin, which emulsionizes the fatty matter, and floats off the dirt. Another safe and excellent shampoo is yolk of egg beaten up; this in like manner combines with the fat and renders it removable.

It may be gathered from what has been said that the proper use of a hair-brush is to polish and dress the hair, not to remove scurf. Therefore, a brush with long and fairly wide-set bristles should be used, not what is termed a hard and penetrating one. A comb with wide-set teeth should be used to arrange it, and in women it ought not to be dragged when put up. In many cases it is advisable to employ some artificial lubricant, and, as the outcome of many observations, fresh almond oil is that which has seemed to the writer to come nearest the natural unguent. Of course, it cannot quite replace it, for the hair in its growth attracts the fluid sebum from its gland, by capillary action, into its intimate fibrous structure, while we apply the oil from without. Almond oil is improved for this purpose by the addition of a little oil of eucalyptus globulus and resorcin. The former tends to keep it from rancidity, while the latter aids in maintaining the smoothness and polish of the scalp. This oil is applicable to the beard and mustache as well, and restrains the propensity to become gray. The best way to use it is to smear a little on the teeth of the dressing-comb, and thus convey it to the hair in passing it through.

THE DIAGNOSIS OF SMALLPOX.

OWING to the prevalence of smallpox at the present time, and on account of the difficulty the ordinary physician has in determing whether it be smallpox or not with which he has to deal, the Provincial Board of Health of Ontario has issued the following circuar containing the chief diagnostic featuress of the disease:

1. A prodromal period of more than twenty-four hours, with headache, pain in the back, and vomiting.

2. The rapid abatement of prodromal fever and malaise after twenty-four hours and until the appearance of the secondary eruption.

3. A primary erythematous eruption or rash, especially covering the abdomen.

4. The appearance on the third day from onset of the papular eruption with its firm, shot-like feeling, and the tendency of the eruption to appear especially on exposed surfaces, as face and wrists, notably on forehead anl about nose and lips, along with an increase of temperature.

5. The appearance early of a red areola around the vesicles, which appear first in forehead, face, and wrists, and pass gradually downward over the body, becoming mature and pustular by the fourth or fifth day, with the typical umbilication.

6. The appearance of the eruptive vesicles on the roof of the mouth and fauces— this being of special diagnostic value.

The rodent character of the pustules and the subcutaneous intercellular infiltration serve to complete a picture which, if taken with the fact that it is a disease attacking adults equally with children, along with a history of probable infection, will cause in most instances the diagnosis to become easy. But modifications of the disease have not been uncommon in the widespread outbreak of smallpox which has prevailed over the United States and Canada within the past two years. Some of these are the following:

1. Some cases have but little prodromal fever; some have pains in back, some do not; some vomit, some do not.

2. In some the eruption without shotty feeling appears altogether, and disappears with one crop; in others there is the shotty feeling with occasionally another crop of vesicles.

3. All the secondary eruptions are papular in the first stage (there being seldom any primary rash) and may become vesicles within three days; some abort at this stage and dry up, while others become semipurulent, marked at the apex with a dark spot, but with no notable umbilication.

4. In some there is no secondary fever.

CONCERNING THE TREATMENT OF RHEUMATISM.

WE find a pertinent paper on this decidedly eligible (?) subject, in one of our exchanges, from the pen of Dr. W. T. Parker, of Westborough, Mass.

Says the doctor: If there is any one subject which has received the scholarly and scientific attention of physicians, it is that of rheumatism in all its aggravating and various phases. No matter in what portion of the world we travel, whether in this country, the British Provinces, in sunny Italy, in the Alps, or in any other part of Europe, everywhere we meet people actually traveling to get rid of rheumatism. The excuses offered by these sufferers are numerous and varied. What we generally find upon close inquiry is that some feature of the sanitation of the buildings in which these patients have lived is not right.

The overshading of our homes has very much more to do with the cause than our text books suggest; and when we add poor ventilation, especially of cellar, poor food and impure water, unsuitable clothing and infrequent bathing, and last, but not least, improper footwear, it is no wonder that rheumatism in all its forms is so prevalent. It is astonishing to find the homes of well-to-do people so lacking in intelligent sanitation. Then, beside our homes, our public halls, and more especially our churches and school buildings are just the places to acquire rheumatism.

For the relief of rheumatism we must depend largely upon the hygienic measures as preliminary in the treatment. A physician may safely recommend attention to food, clothing and housing, but unless he enters into a vigorous campaign, which must thoroughly stir up or revolutionize family methods of living, he will accomplish very little good. Drug stores and even grocery stores furnish remedies for the relief of rheumatic pains, thereby entailing severe injury upon the public. Coal-tar preparations have been used to such an extent that even now a strong reaction is setting in. The New England patient suffering from rheumatism is found roaming about the world seeking for a climate cure.

We have seen many of these patients under treatment at Las Vegas, New Mexico, going through the routine of mud baths. The same method is employed at Gumunden in Ober-Austria, and in other places. In our experience we have found this method an excellent adjunct. Why cannot this mud treatment be carried on at sanitariums everywhere?

A large coffin-like box in a well lighted room, with a rain or needle bath to wash off the mud after its application is all that is required. The German bath 170° F. or the sweating-box, followed by the rain and needle spray, and winding up with the douche upon the spine, is certainly one of the most refreshing methods of treatment in rheumatic cases. With electricity we have found very unsatisfactory results, although some patients have reported decided relief.

Constipation is considered by many to be one of the most important of the exciting causes of rheumatism and in some cases is exceedingly obstinate and untractable. The regulation of diet, making use of oranges, apples, etc., and fruit in general, with massage, will be found sufficient in some cases, but the prescribing of Analeptine* is in itself a corrective of this condition even in obstinate cases. The Cascara is sufficiently well known in its action to need nothing more than to call attention to its presence in the necessary proportion in the Analeptine Cordial.

Rheumatic patients are apt to complain of suffering after midnight. From one to three o'clock is a very common time for the attack of pain. This suggests the advisability of having a wrap or blanket handy to place over the thighs at those hours of the morning. In the best regulated rooms, ventilation, although most important, is by no means properly attended to. Pure air, but not damp or cold, is what is required. A temperature below 60° F. is generally speaking injurious for the rheumatic. The use

* Reed & Carnrick, New York.

of a cold water sponge bath every morning before breakfast is almost always advisable except in acute attacks. The Saturday night hot bath can be much improved if some preparation of sea-salt be added to the water. Flannels are almost always recommended, but too often unnecessarily thick garments are worn. When this is the case, the disease is aggravated and the sour sweating so characteristic of rheumatic affections is increased.

In my experience upon the frontier and in the extreme cold of the northwest, where I have recorded a temperature upon one occasion of 57° F. (minus) I have found that the use of two moderately thin undergarments much warmer than one heavy suit of underwear. This develops the idea of an interior space so well known to arctic travelers and those subjected to low extremes of temperature. It is also important to consider how necessary it is for this class of patients, as it is indeed for all who would maintain health, to wear thick, strong shoes and light warm woolen stockings.

Here the same theory is obtainable as with underclothing. In a temperature ranging from 25° F. to 55° F. I have worn two comparatively thin pairs of woolen stockings and did not suffer from cold feet. If we can manage to keep the feet warm and the bowels regular we shall make rapid healing and cure.

For direct relief of rheumatic condition, iodide of sodium, salicylate of lithia, acetate of potash, extract of black cohosh, extract cascara; all these are contained in an admirable cordial known as Analeptine. This is an elegant preparation for the treatment of the rheumatic diathesis. These ingredients, as are well known, have proven of the greatest value in the treatment of this class of ailments. The alterative action of the iodide of sodium, the salicylate of lithia, together with the eliminative properties of acetate of potash, and the black cohosh make the most comprehensive prescription possible. The combining the saline and salicylic treatment offers the best results with the least danger from heart complica-

tions. The addition of the cascara prevents the continuance of the constipation, and favors the elimination sought for.

Rheumatism, in the ordinary sense of that term as we recognize it in daily practice, is by no means such an unmanageable disease as some would have us believe. It must be treated energetically and rationally, and without an idea that any one remedy is a specific. The "cure-alls" which have no other object than the relief of pain are worse than useless in the treatment of rheumatism. The danger from heart symptoms is not decreased by the exhibition of coal-tar products, and the heart danger is one of the most serious, although so obvious, and yet remedies known to be liable to imperil life itself are unsparingly prescribed and the older and more reliable remedies for the time being lost sight of.

✢ ✢

SCIENCE BETWEEN THE ACTS.

A REPORT comes from Paris that Dr. Hanriot, of the Academy of Medicine and the Board of Health, is creating a sensation among theatergoers, as well as consternation among theater managers in that city, by a series of experiments undertaken to prove that the air of Paris theaters is loaded with microbes. When these experiments were begun last winter, the preliminary results were so alarming that the French government interfered for fear of their injurious effects upon the approaching exposition, as well as upon the theaters. So paternal is the republic over there that it even controls the ventilation of the theaters and the distribution of bacteria. Now that the exposition is a thing of the past, Dr. Hanriot is once more at work. His method is rather sensational, as becomes the atmosphere of Paris. He arrives in the midst of a performance and settles himself in a box with his apparatus and assistants. As the apparatus makes a loud buzzing noise, he graciously sets it going only during the intervals between the acts. He and his assistants then talk in a loud tone in order to drown the noise of the machine. The immediate effect on the audience is not described, but the scientific results, as announced by Dr. Hanriot, are important. He says that the air of some of the Paris theaters is "little better than dusting." His recommendations are for better ventilation, and for the substitution of leather for plush upholstering. This latter point seems to be one of great importance, for Hanriot's observations go to show that those theaters which are upholstered in plush are the most infected.

COUGHING AS A FINE ART.

In an article on tuberculosis, contributed to the annual report of the Maine State Board of Health by Dr. A. G. Young, he treats of the above subject, and says: "There are reasons affecting both the patient and those associated with him, why cough should be suppressed by the voluntary effort of the patient so far as is practicable. How far this is possible has often been noted with surprise by visitors to properly conducted sanatoriums for consumptives. At the dinner table or anywhere else where large numbers of patients are found together, hardly a cough is heard. Unnecessary coughing is bad for the patient; loud and open-mouthed coughing subjects other persons in the same room to the possibility of infection. When obliged to cough, the patient should do so as lightly as possible, and with lips closed as much as he can. Even when the cough is hard, experiments have shown that the diffusion of particles of infectious sputum into the air can be easily prevented by holding something before the mouth. The open hand will quite effectually arrest all particles, but the rule to keep the hand as clean and as free from infection as possible, forbids the use of the hand for this purpose. A suitable object is a paper napkin or square of muslin, to be burned after it has been in use for a short time. Professor Leube, of Würzburg, has his patients, when confined to the house, keep upon their table in a suit-able dish a bunch of cotton twice as large as the fist, to be held before the mouth while coughing. A handkerchief may be used for this purpose, and for no other, but when so used it presents the same danger in a minor degree as when the handkerchief is used as a receptacle for the sputum."

HOME TREATMENT OF TUBERCULOSIS.

Dr. Lawrence F. Flick presented an admirable paper on the above subject at a recent meeting of the County Medical Society. The three ends to be attained are the restoration of the physiological functions of the body, hyper-nutrition, and the conferring of immunity. General practitioners should be more alert in making the diagnosis, an important early symptom being indigestion, persistence of which should lead to physical examination of the lungs. When the diagnosis is made three things are to be done. First, acquaint the patient with his exact condition, as this may be necessary to secure his coöperation in the treatment; second, explain to him that successful treatment means a long and persistent struggle, lasting perhaps from three to five years. Patients are often not cured when they seem to be and treatment should be kept up after symptoms subside; third, lay down a routine for governing the patient's life as to food, exercise, clothing, etc. These patients can often take large quantities of food, three to six quarts of milk and six to twelve raw eggs daily. Regarding medication, antipyretics and opium are to be avoided. The iodine compounds are first in value. Next is creosote, which is given in hot water before meals in doses reaching fifty drops three times a day. Strychnine, arsenic, phosphorus, digitalis, and iron are of value. Use any drug that will help any organ. One of the greatest difficulties in the treatment is the occurrence of complications, as colds, influenza, or pneumonia, either of which may cause a recrudescence.

STATISTICS OF GRIPPE IN NEW YORK STATE.

THE New York State Board of Health has issued a report on grippe which shows that the disease made its appearance in 1889. Every year since, in the winter season, it has recurred, the annual epidemic having various characteristics. The number of deaths which occurred each year from the disease is as follows: 1890, 5,-000; 1891, 8,000; 1892, 8,000; 1893, 6,000; 1894, 3,000; 1895, 5,000; 1896, 2,750; 1897, 3,000; 1898, 2,500; 1899, 7,000, and 1900, 11,500. The report says: "Of the distribution of the disease, it has not been found to be one of either the city or the country. It is a disease of the colder months. It has varied greatly in severity in different years; it seems likewise to have varied greatly in virulence in different localities and has shown varying types. It likewise varies in rapidity of spread. It is evidently communicable from the individual directly, and conveyable in infected clothing. Like all zymotic diseases, susceptibility to it varies; unlike some, immunity does not follow a previous attack. The State is now in the course of the twelfth recurrence of grippe. Affecting the mortality of December by about 500, it has increased the number of deaths in January by probably 3,000, and was still in progress during February.

BOILS AND CARBUNCLES AND SOME POINTS IN THEIR TREATMENT.

BIRDWOOD states in the *Indian Medical Gazette* for November, 1900, that bearing in mind the fact that the disease is probably due to a micro-organism, the following points in treatment, not generally noticed, may with advantage be considered:

1. Pay scrupulous attention to personal cleanliness of the patient. Insist, as far as possible, on frequent changes of soiled linen.

Pillow-cases may easily become infected when boils are in the neck, and may thus be the source of a crop of boils.

2. When the boil first appears, have the locality thoroughly shaved, then well washed with carbolic lotion, then dried and covered with a soft antiseptic pad. Bathe also with antiseptic lotion night and morning. These measures will tend to check the spread of boils in the neighborhood.

3. In a household, if one child gets a boil it is advisable to isolate him as far as possible from the other children till his boil is cured.

4. In a case of boils tell the patient to avoid washing the skin with irritating soaps, and do all you can to allay the irritable condition of prickly heat, which is in one way a predisposing cause.

5. When suppuration is established, the discharge should be received on absorbent antiseptic dressings. The patient should be cautioned not to squeeze the boil himself and receive the discharge on to a handkerchief or any piece of linen, which then becomes infected and is often left lying about.

6. Spraying the boil with carbolic lotion (1 in 40) twice a day for ten to fifteen minutes, as recommended by Whitla, will do much good; also small plugs of lint saturated with pure carbolic thrust into the mouths of a carbuncle seem to accelerate suppuration and to allay irritation.

7. Birdwood has found free incision across a tense boil gives considerable relief, but most will agree with Sir J. Paget that incision of a carbuncle has nothing to recommend it. Mr. Ruston Parker's treatment of excision and scraping in some cases of carbuncle seems to have much to recommend it. It is somewhat similar to the surgical treatment of malignant pustule. Under chloroform there is excision of the walls and free scraping out of the slough, and then the application of pure carbolic acid to the base. The cases in which this treatment is suitable are those cases of indolent chronic carbuncles with much pain and fever, and which, in old men especially, are a source of danger to life. Mr. Ruston Parker has

treated sixteen such cases with the best result; not only is much relief given, but the case is quickly cured, and in some instances life has been saved.

TREATMENT OF SIMPLE CHRONIC CATARRH OF THE NOSE.

BERNDT writes, in the *Columbus Medical Journal* for November, 1900, of this disease. He thinks that the first requisite to success is to keep the nasal cavities clean. This is best obtained by the use of the postnasal douche. He never uses nasal sprays, for the simple reason that the amount of medicament thus applied is so small that it is useless, and then besides, the amount or pressure required to force the spray throughout the nasal chambers is so great that the medicine could with ease be forced into the Eustachian tubes, and so cause considerable trouble.

By means of the postnasal douche a larger and sufficient quantity of medicament is applied, and the inspissated mucus and crusts thereby softened and removed, and there is absolutely no danger of any of the fluid entering the Eustachian tubes, from the fact that the direction of the force is away from and not toward their openings into the pharynx.

The solution that Berndt uses is made by dissolving one of Seiler's alkaline antiseptic tablets in an ordinary-sized glass of warm water. The amount of solution is used three times daily. This part of the treatment is carried on at home by the patient himself. Berndt usually has him call at his office every third day and makes local applications himself. After the membranes have been thoroughly cleansed, oleaginous applications are indicated to protect the surface, stimulate the absorbents, contract the blood-vessels, disinfect and render the mucosa less sensitive.

An effective treatment consists in the application of nitrate of silver water solutions, varying in strength from 1 to 10 per cent., followed by menthol in olive oil, of the strength of from 2 to 20 per cent. These remedies he applies directly to the tissues, with the aid of a head mirror and speculum, by means of the cotton swab. The whole surface of the nasal chambers is literally painted with the above named solution. This treatment is best given two or three times a week by the physician, while the patient pursues a home treatment with the postnasal syringe and solution above mentioned. By this treatment alone the writer has, with almost uniform success, treated sixty-seven cases in the past year. The few unsuccessful cases were those in which the catarrh was passing over into that variety known as atrophic catarrh, which, when it becomes offensive, is called ozena. This latter variety will resist almost every known treatment.

Berndt never uses cocaine as a therapeutic measure, because it is not of such a nature as to effect permanent results, and because of its imminent danger of converting one's patient into a cocaine fiend; he only uses cocaine as a surgical anesthetic.

Bougies and dilators of medicated gelatine, hard and soft rubber, and metal, are sometimes useful in reducing the engorgement of the turbinated bodies, and overcoming contact and pressure of the bodies on the septum. The bougies adapted in form and size to the individual cases are inserted between the turbinates and septum for a few minutes at a time at first, beginning with the smaller, and used on the same principle as sounds and dilators in other departments of surgery. When the engorgement of the vessels of the turbinated bodies produces great swelling of those structures, and consequent nasal obstruction that proves unyielding to the methods already mentioned, it has been his plan to use the cold wire snare, as in hypertrophic catarrh.

Of course, the question of proper clothing must always be considered in the treatment of all forms of catarrh.

THE NEW TONIC AND RECONSTRUCTIVE, HYPOTONE.

THE medicinal use of phosphorus and its compounds holds a place in the estimation of the medical profession which is abundantly justified. Phosphorus is one of the normal constituents of several of the tissues of the body, including those most important structures that make up the central nervous system. Hence phosphorus may properly be held to play largely the part of a reconstituent in therapeutics. The compounds of phosphorus are supposed by some investigators to act medicinally by giving up to the tissues the elementary phosphorus which they contain, but we may safely infer that it is not in this way alone that they exert a powerful therapeutic effect, for in many of the compounds of phosphorus the substances with which the phosphorus is combined have very definite and pronounced medicinal properties of their own. This is especially true of the salts of hypophosphorous acid—the hypophosphites; consequently the hyphophosphites have long been recognized as among the most valuable articles of the materia medica.

In the main, however, the indications for the hypophosphites are those for phosphorus. In *rhachitic conditions*, which are of far commoner occurrence than is generally supposed, the hypophosphites are found to be of great service while the disease is in progress, especially in its early stages, though, of course, like all other medicines, they cannot do away with the deformities due to rickets when once the disease has become confirmed. Another disease of the osseous system, but, fortunately, one of far less frequent occurrence than rickets, in which the hypophosphites are of great value, is *osteomalacia*. In these two affections phosphorus and its compounds are doubtless more efficient than all other drugs together.

In a great number of *diseases of the nervous system* the hypophosphites are of distinct benefit. Among them are *mental enfeeblement, mania, melancholia, anemia* and *malnutrition of the brain* (often mani-

fested by insomnia), *paralysis of cerebral origin, tabes dorsalis* (manifested by *locomotor ataxia*), asthenic *neuralgia*, and *nervous impotence.*

In such *skin diseases* as *lupus vulgaris, lupus erythematosus, chronic eczema, psoriasis,* and *acne* the preparations of phosphorus have been employed with success.

This new preparation—which is said to be really the revival of an old and tried formula—contains an intelligent selection of the hypophosphite salts, with nux and quinine as constitutional tonics, held in suspension in a non-saccharine menstruum.

This is a decided advance in the right direction. The syrups have long been voted inexcusable from a therapeutic standpoint. This fact alone will commend the product to many a practitioner who has become disgusted with the cloying sweet of the conventional syrup.

TO THE THERMÆ.

THE Turkish bath is always a luxury, and very many people esteem it a necessity. Without an efficient and free sewerage system a city soon becomes a pest breeder. The sewerage of the human system is even more important.

Many people appreciate this, but neglect the means on account of the expense. Really, it is the cheapest and often it is the best medicine in the market. For gentlemen who frequent the lower part of the city there is no excuse for neglecting a weekly or semi-weekly visit to the hot room, the shampooing table and the invigorating plunge at the Easton Baths—in the basement of the Bennett Building, corner of Nassau and Ann streets. Even the shorn lambs of Wall street can muster up the price of a bath—fifty cents!—which is no indication of the completeness of the appointments.

"The man who does not frequent the Turkish bath does not know what it is to rise to the moral sublimity of being clean."

EDWIN FORREST.

Department of Physical Education.

WITH SPECIAL REGARD TO THE SYMMETRICAL DEVELOPMENT OF THE BODY.

EFFECTS OF SUDDEN AND PROLONGED MUSCULAR EXERTION IN YOUNG ADOLESCENTS.

"In attempting to ascertain the effects of severe muscular exertion, we have," Collier remarks (*Brit. Med. Jour.*), "to study, first, the physiologic changes set up by moderate exertion. The effects of exercise on the two most important organs, the heart and lungs, are first noticed. The first effect of exercise is to increase the force of the heart's beat and cause an active congestion, which swells the pulmonary capillaries and diminishes the air space. As the muscular effort continues, it increases the amount of CO_2 that is thrown into the blood, stimulating the respiratory center of the brain; inspiration becomes deeper and more frequent and more air is thrown into the air cells, impeding the circulation in the pulmonary capillaries, and the heart beats more and more quickly, but each ventricular systole is less vigorous, and we have passive congestion of the lungs, which is a marked obstacle to the elimination of CO_2. This can not be done beyond a certain point, as too much CO_2 in the blood brings about the cessation of all effort. We have here, therefore, physiologic emphysema. In athletes who have been through years of athletic competitions, we often find the following signs of physiologic emphysema: (1) Absence of apex-beat, either on inspection or palpation, while at rest. (2) Absence of all superficial cardiac dulness on account of the large emphysematous lung covering the heart and separating it from the thoracic wall. (3) A hyper-resonant note above the clavicles and above the sternum. If the cause of this is repeated too often, or kept up too long, it is quite possible that it may

become converted into a pathologic condition, leading in later life to the same consequences as we have from old-standing bronchitis and chronic asthma. Another effect is to throw a great strain on the right side of the heart, since passive pulmonary congestion implies overdistention of the right ventricle." The author calls attention to a form of heart strain not uncommon among girls and young women, who do much running up and down stairs. "It is generally associated with a certain amount of anemia, and probably due to atonic conditions of the heart muscle, induced by impoverished blood. The most prominent symptom is breathlessness on exertion and great frequency and tumultuous action of the heart. Girls about the ages of rapid growth, with marked functional changes, may have minor forms of dilatation of the right side of the heart, especially liable to occur with overexertion. The effect of severe muscular exrtion on the left side of the heart is to produce a physiologic hypertrophy, and if this is overdone there is danger in it. Insomnia is not an uncommon troublesome symptom with this form of physiologic hypertrophy." Collier advises that boys in schools should be examined before being allowed to take part in athletic exercises, and especially in the adolescent periods, and when they are growing rapidly. "Cases of severe and sudden breakdown in well-fed boys and college students are rare. The danger lies in the future, some twenty years or more after." He notes the prophylaxis, advising physical examinations of school boys and students, but says that the danger is less in this class than with the lower middle classes outside of public schools. In concluding his paper he remarks on the physical standard of the army being too high. "Many men are rejected on account of insufficient weight or chest measurement. A long, narrow chest may have equal lung capacity with the broad one, but the tape only measures the horizontal diameter; it takes no cognizance of the vertical." Intermittent albuminuria is mentioned, and Collier explains it on the ground of some defect in the walls of the blood-vessels of the kidney. The condition often gives rise to no special trouble, and the treatment for it seems to do very little good.

NOTES A-SADDLE.

IT is wheel season again and although there has been some complaint on the part of manufacturers that sales have not been up to their expectations, the streets, roadways and cycle paths are everywhere alive with wheels that would be worthless if not tired and yet are never tired. (N.B. This pun is not copied from *Punch* nor from the Pirates of Penzance!) The editor of the GAZETTE has chosen his mount and is down for a season's record.

He condoles with and commiserates those who for good and sufficient reasons can not adopt the wheel, but he has no patience with those who can but will not ride, and thus cheat the doctor, the druggist, and the grave digger.

There are wheels and wheels, chain wheels and chainless, wheels with brakes and wheels that break themselves.

We haven't been bribed to mention the name of our mount, and we are so upright (when we sit in the saddle) that it would be dangerous to approach us on the subject.

Get a chainless if you can afford it, but do not grieve if you must stick to the old model. Have a coaster brake if you would know one of the luxuries of the exercise, and have also a *spring seat post*. This simple device, costing but little money, converts

any wheel into a "cushion frame," which our readers will remember we mentioned with some enthusiasm last season. There are a number of patterns. We are riding the "Berkey," and it is very satisfactory.

PHYSICAL DEVELOPMENT.

IN the popular mind the term physical development, says Dr. W. H. Kinnicutt, always means muscular development; nothing was ever more of a misapprehension; that is only one phase of its meaning. It includes the strength of the heart, the capacity of the lungs, the integrity of the digestive organs and functions, and the *balance of the entire physical system,* one part with another.

The man who is big-muscled but has not nutritive capacity to compensate, who is pale, bloodless, and slow actioned, is poorly developed.

It seems to be an easier task to start young men toward a specific impossibility than toward a common sense objective that is to be easily attained.

How many "systems of physical culture" are there to-day which claim pre-eminence as health producers, which are nothing more than muscle makers; how many appliances of wire, wood, or rubber, each possessing miraculous power to produce herculean physiques; wooden tubes to blow through or to suck, which will insure lungs like balloons; and all with an immense sale.

Getting health is no miracle; keeping it has no element of luck; just common sense living, with enough wholesome food to properly nourish the body, enough work to feel honest, enough recreation to keep the body happy, enough exercise to renovate the system, enough sleep to allow thorough repair, makes a formula which is within every one's reach.

The exercise, properly used, will cover a multitude of shortcomings in the other specified items; it is a great remedy.

BRUSH MASSAGE.

FRANK B. FRY, in the *Journal of Nervous and Mental Diseases* for January, 1901, says that dry bristle brushes have proven very effective in carrying out massage, in some instances being superior to ordinary methods. It is simple, easy, and easily· learned. As he employs the method, the brush is kept in contact with the skin and manipulated with a combined circumductory and creeping movement, and with a varying degree of rapidity and pressure. The dry brush adheres to the skin, drawing with it the superficial structures. The amplitude of the movements depends to a great extent on the length of the bristles and the spring of the brush. Specially constructed brushes are not necessary, as suitable ones can be easily selected from any good assortment of flesh brushes. Those with leather backs and well constructed are best. This method of massage is usually acceptable to patients. There is rapidly established a tolerance of the skin and muscles. A distinct advantage of the method is that there is no difficulty in obtaining operators. The procedure is effectual in the heaviest work for which massage is employed. It is an excellent means of relieving lithemic and neurasthenic pains of all descriptions.

A NEW LIGHT ON PERNICIOUS ANEMIA.

The Medical Press is very enthusiastic over what it considers a great discovery made by Dr. W. Hunter. This is that pernicious anemia is a septic affection, the poison being derived from the suppuration about the teeth or in the mouth and its dependencies. The poison passes into the stomach where it sets up a special form of gastritis, finally resulting in peripheral neuritis and blood-disturbances.

This calls for better habits of oral hygiene and antiseptic mouth washes.

TOBACCO AND BACTERIA.

"IT will be news of dubious joy to smokers," says the *London Globe*, "to learn that the flavor of their favorite brands of tobacco is not due to the excellence of the leaf, but to the bacteria which inhabit it. The bacteriologist boldly asserts that the delicate aroma, the subtle shades of flavor which affect the palate of the smoker are one and all attributable to the agency of microbes alone, and that it is to frizzled bacteria and not to any particular plant growth that the gratitude of smokers is due. A German bacteriologist, Herr S. Suchsland, was the first to draw attention to the remarkable fact that the real flavor of tobacco is not inherent in itself, but is due to the local microbes which aid in its process of fermentation. He cultivated the finest West Indian bacteria and introduced them into common German tobacco, and even connoisseurs could not tell the product from the West Indian tobacco. A patent has been applied for to manufacture high-class tobacco in Germany, and it is hoped that the bacteria may take kindly to cabbage, so that the best brands may be imitated in Germany at the lowest price. But there is, it seems, one drawback. The bacteria are local, and resent being transplanted away from their own homes. They lose their flavor away from their usual haunts, in spite of the wiles of scientific persons. Were it not so every man might grow his own microbes in his cellar, and the Custom House would have to give up taxing tobacco and levy dues on microbes."

THE SONG OF THE SWORD.

WHEN did surgery begin to be? is a question often asked and hard to answer. We know that man's first sharp-edged tools were fashioned of stone. These flint knives, axes and drills were well shaped, and we know that with them man could kill and carve the huge creatures that surrounded him. Possibly, these were the first surgical implements, but of this we have no record.

It is recorded, however, that before the first man passed away, one of his posterity, Tubal Cain, had invented and forged sharp-edged tools of both iron and brass. This was a momentous event, for it gave mankind the armed warrior, marking the beginning of slaying and wounding, giving to the primitive surgeon the first full-fashioned implements for his art. Lamach, the father of the inventor, celebrated the occasion in what is probably the first recorded poem:

Adah and Zillah, hear my voice:
Ye wives of Lamach, hearken unto my
    speech;
For I have slain a man to my wounding,
And a young man to my hurt:
If Cain shall be avenged seven-fold,
Truly, Lamach seventy and seven-fold.

MARRIED LIFE AND LONG LIFE.

SOME very encouraging statistics are gathered by the Berlin *Echo,* for benedicts, not Benedictines, i. e., if life is worth living. Dr. Prinzing states "that the experience of life insurance companies is, that the expected mortality among Evangelical pastors is 85 per thousand insured, while among Catholic pastors it is 112 per thousand insured." Yet the burdens of life to provide for, very often, large families, is against the Evangelicals. The inference is, therefore, legitimate, that married life in the same vocation is promotive of longevity.

Again, the same authority shows still greater evidences in favor of married life from the fact that the mortality of widowers who remain widowers is greater than of those who remarry.

Again, suicides and fatal accidents are far more frequent among the unmarried than among the married.

The greater mortality of the Catholic clergy is found to be owing to the frequent occurrence of diseases of the circulatory organs among them, inclusive of cerebral apoplexy. Married life is more apt to be healthy home life, and less of the tavern (saloon) life of the unmarried. The sensible conclusion of all these is, that if life is or should be made worth living, it will pay to be married, and "single blessedness" is a myth and a curse.

TALK OF MARRIAGE.

ACCORDING to the *Nineteenth Century* "A man may remark on his intention to marry at some indefinite future time, when prudeness or other considerations may make it possible or advisable, without having, as a rule, to run the gauntlet of a chorus of impertinent and stupid would-be witty remarks. But should a girl be bold enough, or, rather, natural and simple enough, to say the same thing, what would be the result? Why, every one knows that she would be promptly sneered out of countenance. And why? Is it immodest for a woman to express a determination to enter into a state which we are being continually reminded is a natural and honorable state, while it is modest and proper for a man to do so? Such a distinction would never be drawn except for the "cheapness" to which reference has been made. If a man wants to marry he can marry; if the first woman he asks refuses him, he has only to ask a second, or perhaps a third or fourth. It would be safe to guarantee that within a month any man of fairly respectable life and position and appearance who cared to make the experiment could marry in his own class, could marry probably a woman much superior to himself, But what about the girl who intends to marry "some day"? Is she not in a very different position from the man? Here is a girl of good character—much better than the man's probably—average intelligence, average good looks. Theoretically, she is free to marry whom she will; but is she? If she receives one distinct offer of marriage she has had more than her share, according to the probable average. The fact that, by an unwritten law, a woman must not take, and, indeed, does not want to take, the initiative, has very little to do with the extremely limited choice which modern conditions impose upon Englishwomen."

RHUS.

THE season for ivy poisoning will soon be at its height. Among the thousand and one remedies tried and commended the following have prominence. Those who are susceptible should be prepared. But it may be borne in mind that the poisonous (and remedial) principle in rhus is a volatile oil known as toxicodendrol. The dry herb is inert.

Chestnut, in the Bulletin of the Department of Agriculture, recommends as a remedy dilute alcohol (45 to 70 per cent.), saturated with lead acetate, well rubbed into the affected skin.

Ellingwood speaks of alnus, apocynin, hydrogen peroxide, echinacea, pilocarpus and sodium bicarbonate, as remedies. An ounce of tincture of lobelia in a pint of water, applied locally, cures rapidly.

Webster treated a case with echinacea locally and internally, and the patient was henceforth immune against rhus.

Levick found powdering with aristol useful. Van Harlingen favors lead water and laudanum, but speaks of white oak bark infusion, quinine ointment (one part to eight), sodium bisulphite (5 per cent. solution, with 1 per cent. of carbolic acid).

Hardaway praises zinc sulphate (one part to fifteen of water).

Butler adds fluid extract *hamamelis,* and that of serpentaria.

Pfaff advises the sufferer not to use oils or ointments, as they dissolve toxicodendrol and spread the eruption. Alcohol also dissolves it, and should be washed off with water.

Fluid extract *grindelia robusta* is probably more reliable than any of the forego-

ing. It is claimed that Resinol promptly allays the inflammation.

In the bulletin above quoted Chestnut enumerates poison ivy, rhus radicans; poison oak, rhus diversiloba, and poison sumac, rhus vernix. The first prevails from New England to Eastern Texas, Kansas and Minnesota, and in the moist regions of the West, except California, where the second variety replaces it, from Vancouver to Mexico. The sumac grows in damp places from Florida to Louisiana, north to Canada.

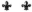

FOR FUMIGATING THE BEDROOMS OF CONSUMPTIVES.

THE following solution has been recommended to be used as a disinfectant and fumigator for the bedrooms occupied by consumptives:

Formaldehyde .... 60 parts
Creosote .... 15 parts
Oil Turpentine .... 30 parts
Menthol .... 1 part

The liquid is spread on a hot stovelid or metal plate; about 40 drops are enough for a bedroom of ordinary size.

LIME IN THE EYE.

SCHMIDT RIMPLER, in *Berliner Klinische Wochenschrift,* states that in these cases by some means the eye should be opened so that every particle of the calcium can be carefully removed from the cornea and conjunctival sac. Removal is best accomplished by the use of oil. A bit of cotton can be saturated and used to wipe out the particles. It is especially important to evert the upper lids, as particles are prone to become imbedded in them. To relieve the pain holocain is recommended, and the eye should be thoroughly flushed out with oil. If no oil can be found, water may be used, for, as a rule, the calcium has been dissolved and water causes no rise of temperature. The prevention of these accidents is highly important, and the use of protective spectacles by workers in calcium is recommended.

Stutzer, same journal, says that when an eye has been injured by lime the best method of treating the condition is to immediately cleanse the eyes with copious washings of clean water, which should be kept up for a considerable length of time. This is really a "first aid to the injured" method, as it can be readily carried out by the patient's fellow-workers. It can easily be done by one man holding the injured eye open, while another, with a clean glass and clean water, washes the eye until no particles of mortar can be seen therein.

HOME-MADE SPLINTS.

DR. THOMPSON BAIRD sends the following to the *Medical World:*

"Dissolve one pound of gum shellac in one pint and a half of 95 per cent. alcohol, with one dram of borax. Let the mixture stand until all of the shellac has been dissolved; then it is ready to be applied. Old cloth makes the best splints. I generally use an old pair of trousers. Apply the solution to one side of the woolen cloth with a brush and dry thoroughly before a hot fire. It takes about one hour to dry properly. Then apply a second coat on the same side, and dry as before. You will then have a single piece, but if you wish a stronger piece, apply the solution on one side of two pieces that have already been prepared. dry them, place them together and press with a hot iron, and they will unite and become as one piece. Always be sure to dry out all of the alcohol. To temper the cloth for use hold before a hot fire until soft, then apply. It will adapt itself to the shape of the limb at once. To make it set quickly, hold in cold atmosphere, or dip in cold water."

[Why not burn the "old clothes," and use new cloth.—ED. GAZETTE.]

NOSTRUM MANIA.

THE nostrum vendors and the newspapers and the United States copyright laws are responsible for a new type of disease. In his professional experience almost every physician must have learned of people afflicted with a genuine mania for taking so-called patent medicines. Many a man is made poor and kept so by this strange insanity. The most typical case of the disease is one cited by the *Practical Druggist,* in which a Philadelphian was arrested by his wife for failure to support his family. For several years he had followed the newspaper advertisements, and imagined himself the victim of all the diseases described by the enterprising advertisers. Apparently both poverty and pathology increased. A partial list of the takings is appended, "washed down with two gallons of lithia water each week":

48 bottles	Swamp Root
24 bottles	Celery Compound
60 bottles	Expectorant
80 bottles	Vermifuge
75 bottles	Kidney Cure
60 bottles	Peruna
36 bottles	Swayne's Specific
57 bottles	Omega Oil
75 bottles	Catarrh Remedy
30 bottles	Munyon's Remedies
50 bottles	Nervura
24 boxes	Skin Ointment
60 boxes	Magnetic Ointment
36 boxes	Cough and Catarrh Root
15 bottles	Glycerine Tonic
37 boxes	Tar Tablets
25 boxes	Cold Cure Pills

And yet—he died!—*American Medicine.*

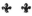

To cool water when ice can not be obtained, wrap the pitcher in cheese-cloth previously impregnated with ammonium nitrate and dried. Moisten slightly at time of use, dry and use again.—*Medical Record.*

JUDGED BY THEIR VOICES.

"THERE is a man employed in this city," according to the *New York Press*, "who employs a great number of persons in the course of a year, and yet never sees the face of one. His plan is to sit behind curtains in his office and listen to the voice of the applicant for a place as responses are made to questions put by a representative. "I believe in the human voice," said he to me. "It does not lie like the manner, the eye, the general facial expression. I do not care what a man says; indeed, I never listen. What I want to hear is the sound of his voice, its intonation, its pitch. Talk about your character being written in the palm of your hand? Rubbish! As Colonel Pierpont Milliken says, the lines in the hand are caused by hard or easy work, or by no work at all. The man who holds a plow handle ten years will have different lines from him who holds a pen. But in the voice God has written your true character infallibly. It never yet has betrayed me."

This is all rot. The poor, meek, humble, down-hearted, friendless individual who comes to-day to ask for employment has a weak little voice that a child would be ashamed of. It causes a bad impression, and our friend says: "Don't want that fellow. Let him go." But if he hires that fellow, and helps him to a good job, the chances are that in less than a month the small voice will fill the building with its rich, deep, mellow resonance, and the infallible judge of voices would imagine he heard Edouard de Reszke slinging cellar notes from "Faust" promiscuously around the corridors. Some of the biggest voices are the littlest in times of trouble and despair. Never try to judge any man by any sign when he is unnatural; and no man can be natural when looking for a job after having been out of work long enough to feel the pinch of poverty, to see the pale ghost of famine hovering over his diningroom."

DOCTOR MAY REFUSE SERVICES.

ACCORDING to an editorial in the Chicago *Record-Herald*, "Recent decisions of the higher courts in cases affecting the practice of medicine are interesting to the general public as tending to settle questions that have always been more or less controversial.

It has always been contended that a physician is morally bound to attend any patient for whom he is called. Failure to respond when called is generally regarded as a violation of medical ethics. It is well known, however, that many physicians do not assent to this view and reserve the right to refuse attendance even in cases of serious emergency. Deaths have been caused by the refusal of physicians to render medical assistance at a critical time when other physicians could not be found.

Whatever may be the moral obligation the Indiana Supreme Court has just rendered an opinion in a test case to the effect that a physician is not legally bound to attend a patient for whom he is called, no matter how urgent or desperate may be the case. An Indianapolis doctor was summoned three times to attend the wife of a prominent citizen. He refused to go, and was finally importuned by the sick woman's pastor, who offered to pay the fees in advance. The physician remained obdurate and the patient died.

In rendering his decision the judge was governed by the fact that the act regulating the practice of medicine is only a preventive and not a compulsory measure. It is plain from this that the only recourse in a case of this character is to public sentiment. A physician who would allow a woman to die in childbirth for lack of medical attendance, when no other medical aid could be summoned, is not entitled to practice medicine in any intelligent community and should not be permtted to do so.

Another important decision is that of the Circuit Court of Milwaukee in a case where two Christian Scientists were arrested for "practicing medicine without a license." It would seem to a person of ordinary intelligence that a healer who does not use drugs does not practice medicine. But it took a Circuit Court in Milwaukee several days to legally determine this fact, and it may now be definitely settled that Christian Scientists are not "practitioners of medicine."

THE SCIENCE OF SPENDING.

It is easy to spend, it is hard to keep money. Dickens illustrated the experience of millions when he called Micawber to explain: Income, twenty pounds; expenses, nineteen shillings and sixpence; result—happiness. Income, twenty pounds; expenses, twenty shillings and sixpence; result—misery." This seems to show that happiness is dependent upon the science of getting what one wants, or must have, out of what one receives, and preserving a margin, be it ever so small, to the good. For those who are secure in a regular income, such as the large number of persons can obtain, this problem is sufficiently difficult, on account of the numberless contingencies, temptations and demands over which one can exercise no foresight or control. For those who have no regular income the problem becomes one of almost impossible solution. It is said, humanity, considered as a whole, always lives within one year of starvation. Certain it is that only a very small portion of humanity is able to lay aside a whole year's income, or sufficient so that they can live through a year, spending only what they had previously earned, and laying up all their earnings for the current year. If this could be done it would be a powerful aid in learning the science of spending.

The science of spending is, in reality, the science of keeping. If one can keep, he may always have something to spend when occasion requires it. This science is learned most surely by acquiring the art of separating the essential from the non-essential objects of expenditure, satisfying the first fully and the second only so far as can be done within the inexorable limits of the fund available. If the influence of the social contact could be made as potent to assist keeping as it is to induce spending, there would hardly be a case of poverty in the land.

To spend wisely requires greater knowledge, judgment and self-control than to earn. The power to spend wisely is to the individual what the power of superior knowledge and judgment in direction is to organized labor in productive work. It is the factor of highest economic value.—*Public Policy.*

ORGANIZED IDLENESS.

"We hear much about organized labor." aptly remarks *Public Policy.* "We read many facetious stories about the efforts of tramps to avoid giving a labor equivalent for the meals they solicit, but we learn very little about the efforts of workmen to avoid giving a fair labor equivalent for the wages they receive. We are willing to believe that our lack of information on this point is due to the absence of the cause. We find confirmation for this in the fact that, while wages in America are higher than in any other country, American-made commodities are finding a wonderfully increasing sale in foreign markets. This could not be if labor cost was excessive. It also shows that the wages of labor do not affect a manufacturer or contractor so long as he receives a fair labor equivalent for the wages paid.

Organized idleness, according to two articles in this issue, "Inefficient English Labor" and "The British Workman and His Competitors," seems to be a product of English trade unionism, resulting from following the teachings of an economic fallacy. English workingmen seem to suppose that the way to make the demand for labor equal to the supply is for every man to do as little as he can. They appear to be following this idea to their own undoing. The man who does as little as he can never develops his capacity to do all that he can. By doing little and thus making his labor unprofitable to his employer, he kills instead of stimulates the demand for labor. The pressure of world competition is crowding out of the field every machine and man of inferior efficiency. Organized idleness will destroy the industrial supremacy of any country in which it is permitted."

"THE COUNTRY DOCTOR"—A NOTABLE PICTURE.

ONE of the most important and admired pictures displayed in recent years at the National Academy Exhibitions is "The Country Doctor," by Mr. W. Granville Smith.

The artistic merits of this notable picture are certified by its place of honor in the chief American exhibition, its power of appeal to human sentiment was evidenced by the persistent attention it attracted, touched by its reality, its homely humanity, its suggestion of pathos.

"The Country Doctor" is a vivid portrayal of a familiar episode—a furious winter night tempest, a long struggle through drift and storm at duty's call, an exhausted old doctor struggling wearily forward, a fatigued horse shrinking in the blinding snow-blasts, an anxious mother eagerly waiting the longed-for relief. From the porch of her humble country home she peers eagerly out into the storm. The lantern she holds above her head cuts a feeble path of light through the gloom, along which the doctor plows his way to shelter.

The artist has just issued a special art production of his painting, 16¼x24 inches, with ample margin all around, which is an absolute facsimile of the original in drawing, color and tonal spirit, on the finest of heavy plate paper, mounted with gold mat and enclosed in substantial box.

The edition is limited to 250 copies, and is sold by him at $8.00. He sends photograph on application.

Those who desire a copy should not delay, as the edition is likely to be soon exhausted.

Copies are sent subject to examination and approval, and can be had by addressing the artist, W. Granville Smith, 52 East 23d street, New York City.

IT is announced that the dates of the next meeting of the Mississippi Valley Medical Association have been changed from the 10th, 11th, and 12th of September, to the 12th, 13th, and 14th of September. This change has been made necessary because the dates first selected conflicted with another large association meeting at the same place.

The meeting is to be held at the Hotel Victory, Put-in-Bay Island, Lake Erie, O., and the low rate of one cent a mile for the round trip will be in effect for the meeting. Tickets will be on sale as late as September 12th, good returning without extension until September 15th. By depositing tickets with the Joint Agent at Cleveland, and paying 50 cents, the date can be extended until October 8th. This gives members an opportunity of visiting the Pan-American Exposition at Buffalo, to which very low rates by rail and water will be in effect from Cleveland.

Full information as to rates can be obtained by addressing the secretary, Dr. Henry E. Tuley, 111 West Kentucky street, Louisville, Ky. Members of the profession are cordially invited to attend this meeting.

Those desiring to read papers should notify the secretary at an early date.

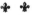

AMONG OUR EXCHANGES.

AMERICAN MEDICINE is catching up with old Father Time. There is nothing like being on time, but there are times when editors' prayers and editors' objugations are alike unavailing with the printer.

The *Philadelphia Medical Journal* makes

its appearance with the regularity of the changes of the moon's phases. The predictions of some of its contemporaries—we confess that we were ourselves agreeably disappointed—have not been able to discover any omens of fulfillment.

The *Journal* has not been devoured by any commercial ogre! We should hardly detect that it had changed management.

The *Medical Record* is as brimful as ever. In the *Boston Medical and Surgical Journal,* Dr. Robert Bell gives his experience in search of a climatic cure for asthma. We do not agree with him, as to the advantages of Southern California, for the simple reason that he did not test the real locality. The physician who ventures to Pasadena only, has seen only the northern rim of Southern California. Let him go on down to San Diego and Coronado, and then stray fifty miles eastward into the delightful Cuyamaca Mountains. His asthma and his skepticism might both be cured as a legitimate result.

The *Therapeutic Gazette* for April 15th has a suggestive editorial on "Ante-natal Therapeutics," and is as full of other good things as usual.

The *Cleveland Medical Gazette* contains four separate papers on different phases of nephritis.

* *

The following is an exact copy of an epitaph on a tombstone in a New Hampshire cemetery. It explains itself:

"Ruth Sprague, dau. of Gibson and Elizabeth Sprague. Died Jan. 11, 1816; aged 9 years, 1 mos. and 3 days.

"She was stolen from the grave by Roderick R. Clow and dissected at Dr. P. M. Armstrong's office, in Hoosick Falls, from which place her mutilated remains were obtained and deposited here.

"Her body dissected by fiendish men,
    Her bones anatomized,
Her soul we trust has risen to God,
    A place where few physicians rise."

The Brevity Club.

"MALARIA."

How long, oh Lord, how long are assumed scientists to continue to use this far-fetched and stupidly meaningless word? Even now that the guilty *Anopheles* has been brought to the bar, and although not one of the dozen new medical dictionaries has given the shadow of a sanction to its use, the term is found in common use, in formal health reports and by the most dignified authors. It was always vague and spooky; now, it is utterly absurd and without even a ghostly leg to stand on.

The word itself is well enough when in place, but it is never used in place. It would be appropriate in the noisesome tunnel of the N. Y. Central through which so many thousands of commuters daily hold their noses and swear under their breath. It would be appropriate in any of our fashionable churches after a Sunday sermon. It would fit the conditions of the Metropolitan Opera House during a popular performance. It was notoriously in evidence in the Black Hole of Calcutta. We cultivate it in our fashionable parlors and get whiffs of it in our sleeping rooms. Modern civilization and malaria are first cousins, if not Siamese twins; but *"malaria,"* in all conscience is not the name of a disease, and if we can trust the positive developments of the past year or two, it never was even a cause of the disease to which it has so long been carelessly and unwarrantedly applied. Its adoption was a popular inadvertence; its perpetuation is a stupidity. Let us have done with "malaria."

ANOTHER "IN RE."

Whether to address myself to the "God-father" or to the Editor is a conundrum, so I address neither. The spirit of the Club is antagonistic to all literary frills, and therefore the non-observance of this formality may aid my candidacy for membership.

I do not know that I am eligible, and I certainly will be ruled out on account of garrulity if I prolong this note of apology and explanation.

I take issue with some of the recommendations of the "Godfather." The publisher of the GAZETTE has not been seventeen years at his post for nothing. He has undoubtedly had his eyes and ears open and has learned many things about the conduct of a magazine of this character that Godfather has not yet dreamed of. It may be all right to drop out the "department" headings, but the publisher will probably take time to be sure he is right before he adopts the suggestion. Grouping the editorial matter under one head is a more practical suggestion. It would no doubt lead to better identification. As to reducing the number of pages of reading matter, merely to carry out this idea of condensation, I emphatically protest. Every journal is compelled to cater to numerous classes of readers. No one class reads any magazine from cover to cover. Each individual reader selects the things that interest him and leaves others unread. A certain few brief and trenchant articles are read by nearly all classes, but their number is limited. It could not be otherwise. Life is too short and too busy. We are all compelled to skim for cream. We cannot gorge ourselves with skimmed milk. For example, I do not pretend to read one in ten of the long and labored articles that regularly pad out the medical journals that come to my table. I wait till some patient editor makes a concise compend, and get my kernel of wheat from that. Hence I am quite in sympathy with the prime object of the Brevity Club.

But instead of reducing the number of pages of reading matter why not add another department, say of Recreation, either professional or literary. Doctors need dessert with their meals quite as much as any other class of mortals. Their contact with the serious side of life is too constant. It is more from want of relaxation than from overwork that physicians as a class are shorter lived than lawyers, ministers, trades-men and farmers. Some medical journals have already caught the idea and are publishing light literature, pithy stories, humorous sketches—something to rest the nerves and distract the attention from the too constant strain of serious and sordid business. Why not meet the Godfather's suggestion by devoting the fifteen or twenty pages that he would have omitted, to literature? I am confident all your readers would be delighted with the change.

But I do not consider that such a course would be a deviation from your present objects. Rest and relaxation are as essential to perfect health as dietetics and hygiene of another kind. It is the highest form of hygiene, because it is mental hygiene.

With due deference to the "Godfather" and best wishes for the future prosperity of the GAZETTE, I trust that I may be considered eligible to membership of the Club.

I want to add by way of friendly suggestion that each contributor to this department should be identified by some signature or legend so that other contributors or critics may know how to designate the particular one whom they desire to flatter or flay.

With the permission of the editor, the "Godfather" and the publisher I will inaugurate the fashion by signing myself

VIVAT.

✠ ✠

Carbonate of Creosote for pneumonia seems to be the coming fad. Prof. Andrew H. Smith, of New York, in the *Medical News*, November, 1899, after citing several writers and his own experience, goes so far as to recommend that family physicians keep their patrons provided with corbonate of creosote, or one of the salicylates, preferably the former, as being better tolerated by the patient, so that in case of indications of an attack of pneumonia (pain in the side with chill) he may take the drug at once and probably prevent the development of an attack.

A résumé of this subject in the *Medical Record* for March 30, by Dr. I. I. Van Zandt, makes a strong case for this new treatment.

Book Reviews.

A SYSTEM OF PHYSIOLOGIC THERAPEUTICS. A Practical Exposition of the Methods, Other Than Drug-giving, in the Treatment of the Sick. Edited by Solomon Solis-Cohen, A.M., M.D. To be completed in eleven compact octavo volumes, by American, English, German and French authors. Vol. I. ELECTRO-THERAPY. By George W. Jacoby. Philadelphia, P. Blakiston's Son & Co., 1901.

At first thought one would be inclined to decide that the editor had undertaken an over-ambitious, because somewhat premature, task; on second thought, we incline to the belief that the undertaking is not premature, that the new century is ready for such a work, and that, while it will not compete in the book market with "Eben Holden" or "Alice of Old Vincennes," there is a respectable audience waiting for a scientific and practical exposition of the resources of Nature and her potent agencies, physical, mechanical, vital, and mental or psychic, telluric, meteorologic, static, dynamic, and kinetic, in the alleviation of human suffering, the correction of deformities and malformations, and the cure of disease. The audience that will appreciatively greet the advent of a treatise prepared by competent hands, has already reached promising proportions and is rapidly increasing.

From the "Foreword" with which the "system" is introduced, we take the following clear-cut announcement of its origin, aims and general plans, by the editor:

"It is a work that I have long had in mind, and which, by a fortunate coincidence, had likewise been contemplated by my friend and publisher, Mr. Kenneth M. Blakiston. The system is the first of its kind to be published in America, or in the English language, and in many important aspects differs from similar works in other tongues. Among these differences are inclusion of themes, exclusion of irrelevant material, and general plan. In its planning, chiefly based on my observation of the needs and desires for information of students and practitioners, I have had the benefit of Mr. Blakiston's intimate knowledge of medical books, and in its publication the advantage of his personal supervision of the numerous minutiæ that go to make a book mechanically perfect, and thereby diminish the labor of the reader in consulting it.

"Preferring compact books by simple writers to bulky tomes of composite authorship, I have endeavored to so arrange the work that the entire field shall be covered; that nothing of moment shall be omitted, either from the general scheme or from the special articles; that theory and principles shall be sufficiently but briefly set forth, and that the descriptions of methods, indications and counterindications shall be clear, definite, full and practical, thus enabling the general practitioner to carry out for himself the important therapeutic measures recommended, and to do so understandingly and correctly.

"In the concluding volume I purpose to set forth the general principles of what, in the absence of any better word, I have ventured to term 'Physiologic Therapeutics,' and to indicate the considerations that should guide the physician in the choice and application of the remedial means discussed in the special books.

* * * *

"Health is preserved, and when disturbed by what we are all accustomed to term slight causes, is obviously restored by the automatic mechanisms of the human body.

* * * * *

"Not only must we recognize that disease and recovery are alike vital processes, in which the organism itself is the most active agent, and that neither morbific nor therapeutic influences endow the organism with new powers, but we must also keep in mind that disease and recovery are often, if not always, one continuous process. Upon the discussion of this intricate subject I shall not now enter, but will emphasize the facts that a health-preserving and health-destroying tendency exists; that it is a natural endowment, and not the gift of art, and that it is dependent upon the inherent properties of cells, tissues, organs and the organism. Some of these qualities are constantly manifested (or kinetic), and in the normal processes of recovery are merely modified—as, for instance, the thermic reaction, altered in the pyrexia of fever; while others, like the power of fibrinogenesis, manifested by blood-clotting, are latent (or potential), and are evoked only in reaction to perturbing influences. Salutary reactions, however, may be delayed, deficient, aberrant or excessive; and thus art must come to the assistance of Nature, and therapeusis finds its reason for being.

*   *   *   *   *

"The means for accomplishing these therapeutic ends fall into two great categories, which might be termed 'artificial' and 'natural,' were it not that both these terms have certain misleading connotations. * * 'Artificial' therapeutics consists in the introduction into the organism of substances ordinarily absent therefrom and, mostly, foreign to its composition, which, chemically and otherwise, provoke certain reactionary changes, and thus modify the recuperative or morbific processes. This is the great and serviceable group of therapeutic means termed 'drugs,' the use of which it is not my purpose to antagonize or decry. On the contrary, I have a robust faith in the power for good of the right drug, given in the right dose, at the right time, and equally in the power for harm of the wrong drug, the wrong dose and the wrong time of giving. Nevertheless, a more restricted use may be made of drugs, with less danger of harm-doing by reason of a mistake in the election of drug, dose, or time by the physician who familiarizes himself with the powers of the remedial agents falling into the second group—that of 'natural' or 'physiologic' means.

"But all that exists in Nature is natural—drug equally with sunlight, microbe equally with antitoxin; and under all circumstances the disordered functions of the paralytic, for example, are equally physiologic with the coördinated functions of the athlete."

"Paradoxical though it may seem, this limitation of terms leads to a broader outlook. Through it we are enabled to find a firm, scientific basis for hygienic and therapeutic traditions hitherto regarded as merely empirical.

"Nor would I be understood as decrying empiricism. Hippocrates, the empiric, was the father of scientific medicine. The dogmatists were his opponents, and dogmatism is still the enemy of medical progress."

We could profitably quote the entire 'Foreword,' which is in itself an epitome of broad-mindedness and medical progress. But we have given enough of it to make every thoughtful reader anxious to find it for himself.

In Vol. I. of this projected system Dr. Jacoby has undertaken a difficult task, and this he frankly states in his preface. He alludes to the number of volumes already extant on the subject, and cites the fact that in the light of the knowledge of the fundamental laws of electricity developed during its progress toward the industrial supremacy it has now attained, most of these statements or treatises are "replete with errors and contradictions, while they are lacking in precise statements."

The attempt to eliminate all these errors and contradictions at a stroke and within the limits of a single compact volume, and to avoid the palpable and offensive commercialism of much of the current literature on the subject requires a grasp of the subject and a degree of scientific independence which few men in the profession possess. We are not sure, and evidently Dr. Jacoby himself is not over-confident that he is the best equipped man for this work who could have been availed of; nor is he quite satisfied with his own work, for he frankly acknowledges in concluding his preface, that "No one can be more cognizant of the defects of the book than I am, but I feel certain that these defects will be least emphasized by those who have, at some time, been called upon to perform a similar work."

Chapter I. opens with a frank admission

that while we know that what we call electricity will decompose water, heat a wire through which it flows, deflect a compass needle and emit sparks under certain conditions, what it is that causes these effects we do not know.

With Meyer and Joule, our author assumes that the three great forces of Nature are heat, light and chemism, and that these are directly interchangeable as to direction and rapidity of the molecular vibrations. What utter jargon this would have been had it been uttered a century ago!

But we are lingering at the threshold, and yet we have said and quoted enough to arouse the interest of our readers, and the rest they will find in the volume itself. It is there, and it is for the most part well stated.

In a word, this is the initial volume of the most important series—and it is at all times *in series*—of Nature studies yet undertaken in the field of medical English. If carried to completion on the lines indicated, and if Vol I. can be taken as an earnest of all the rest, the finished work will be a proud monument to its industrious, audacious and talented editor and to the courage and competency of its publishers.

INFANT FEEDING IN HEALTH AND DISEASE. By Louis Fisher, M.D. Philadelphia: The F. A. Davis Co., 1901.

This work is a handsome small octavo of 359 pages, with 52 illustrations, 23 charts, and many tables, most of which are original. It undertakes to be fundamental by opening with a brief sketch of the anatomy and physiology of the infantile stomach. Then follows a very succinct statement of the chemistry of the gastric and intestinal secretions. Chapter VII. is devoted to a condensed but very lucid description of the proximate elements of food, including fat, sugar, carbohydrates, hydrocarbons (indicating the difference between these often carelessly confused names), fats, salts, salts and water, albuminous or proteid substances and proteids, to which is added a method for estimating the quantity of proteids in breastmilk.

Chapter VIII. expends itself on the bacteria found in the digestive tract and might have been compressed into two or three pages without detriment to the practical value of the work. This hunting down of harmless microbes, which abound throughout animated Nature, and without which there would be no animated Nature, is largely a waste of time.

The subject of the chemical and physical differences between human and cow's milk, and of artificial feeding, is very fully and for the most part satisfactorily treated. This is followed by an analysis of the numerous commercial foods which are too often heralded by the manufacturers with preposterous claims, and there is no evidence that Dr. Fischer was prejudiced by commercial influences—a rare thing in works of this kind. There is a chapter on infant stools and some valuable formulæ. Occasionally there is an evident effort to establish certain pet or prejudiced views assumed by the author in the face of generally accepted facts and theories. The well-read physician will not fail to detect these evidences of what may be termed the lapses of personal equation and will exercise his own judgment in estimating their value.

The illustrations are of the kind that illustrate, and, barring some careless proof-reading that occasionally amounts to faulty construction, the volume is creditable alike to author and publishers.

There is a copious index and blank pages at the end for memoranda. We advise every physician to possess the book.

TWENTY-FIRST ANNUAL REPORT OF THE STATE BOARD OF HEALTH OF THE STATE OF RHODE ISLAND, for the year ending December 31, 1898. Providence, R. I.: E. L. Freeman & Sons, State Printers, 1901.

We are at a loss to know what sort of a Rip Van Winkle has had charge of the material for the above named report. Why any State should be two years and a half in publishing its health reports is one of the conundrums of official life. If such reports are to be of value to the public they should be issued within a reasonable time after the material is in hand. Changes in matters of health are taking place so rapidly that reports have an ancient and fishy smell when detained so long in the office of publication.

Putting aside criticism, the volume in question gives a very full account of town and county sanitation, and devotes a good deal of space to the question of the disposition of sewage.

The subject of meteorology receives scant attention except in the way of statistical tables, which are apt to be rather dry reading.

The births, deaths and marriages for the year are given. The whole number of births, 10,730; males, 5,443; females, 5,287; whole number of marriages, 3,278, of which 1,522 were native born, both groom and bride; groom and bride, both foreign born, 991; native groom and foreign bride, 402; foreign groom and native bride, 363; native grooms, 1,927; foreign grooms, 1,354. Total number of deaths, 6,905; males, 3,554; females, 3,351; of these, native born, 4,957; foreign born, 1,948.

We note that of the births 4,427 were native, 6,303 foreign. At this rate the little State of Rhode Island will soon be captured by foreigners.

Of those dying, consumption claims by far the larger number, or a total of 886, heart diseases ranking next with 549 deaths; pneumonia stands third on the list with 542 deaths; 205 died of old age, and only 93 of diphtheria, which would argue that old age is a more dangerous disease than diphtheria. The birth rate as compared with the death rate for the past 12 years has been in a proportion of about 25-19. The deaths from cancer were 279 as against 234 in 1895, 226 in 1896, and 254 in 1897. The deaths from typhoid fever number 76, which is 10 more than for the previous year. The deaths from influenza number 75, or 78 less than 1897. In 1892

the total number of deaths from this disease in the State numbered 336. There were no deaths in 1898 from smallpox.

A diagram showing mortality by absolute number of deaths from 18 principal causes for 33 years—1866 to 1898—places consumption at 23, pneumonia at 14, cholera-infantum, 11; heart diseases, 10; apoplexy and paralysis, 9; diseases of the brain and accidents, 6; diseases of the kidneys, diphtheria, cancers, fevers, bronchitis, diarrhea, dysentery and scarlet fever, 5; croup, 3; childbirth and whooping-cough, 2; measles, 1½.

THE MEDICAL NEWS POCKET FORMULARY for 1901, by E. Quin Thornton, M.D. Philadelphia and New York: Lea Brothers & Co., 1901.

This is the third edition of this handy and attractive volume. The author has taken the opportunity to thoroughly revise the work, which has already become popular, by a number of new formulæ, including old drugs and new combinations, and some of the newer drugs which have been found valuable.

The work has been brought fully up to date, and will be found a present help in time of need by busy practitioners. We congratulate the compiler and the publisher on the attractive appearance of this third edition.

THE EXCURSION TO CALIFORNIA.

THE exact date of starting has not yet been fixed, but will be about the middle of June, the 18th being at present prominently mentioned.

The best rates to be had will be secured, and the object of these notices is to make the trip a pleasant one for all concerned. There will be no extra expense of any kind connected with joining the excursion. This in answer to numerous inquiries. State number to go and preferred date, addressing Editor, DIETETIC AND HYGIENIC GAZETTE, 503 Fifth avenue, New York.

Department of Notes and Queries.

FREEDOM OF DISCUSSION BETWEEN EDITOR AND READER.

Query 88. Will the editor of *Notes and Queries* give a brief explanation of the salient points of the theory of Evolution? I am often asked to do this myself, and although I have a general idea of what it implies, I confess that I stumble and hesitate when I attempt to express it.
G..R. M., North Dakota.

Answer.—The theory of evolution, first announced by Charles Darwin in his "Origin of Species," in 1859, was violently combatted by theologians and scientists, and is still denounced by narrow minds and hide-bound ecclesiastics. Since it demolished so many traditions and established theories this was to be expected. It has, however, compelled such universal acceptance, at this hour, that no sane scientist attempts to explain the laws of any of the natural phenomena of life without availing himself of its principles and phraseology.

Before Darwin's announcement various scientists had approached the theory of natural selection, among them Buffon, Lamarck, Goethe, Erasmus, Darwin and Wallace.

Herbert Spencer calls this law of natural selection or evolution the survival of the fittest. It discards the theory of special creative impulses, and traces every organization or organism as a result of natural forces. In other words, all the visible forms of Nature are accounted for through the action of forces that have always existed and are still in operation. By this theory the solar system was not the result of an instantaneous special creation, but assumed form through a slow process of the attraction of matter acting upon nebulous masses. It is the only theory that explains the observed facts of Nature, and this is the strongest possible corroboration of its truth.

To illustrate. Haeckel's statement is that we all start with the *monera*, which is the name applied to "a simple granule of protoplasm, a structureless mass of albuminous matter," the first *monera* "owing their existence to spontaneous creation out of so-called inorganic combinations, consisting of carbon, hydrogen, oxygen and nitrogen."

This had its origin early in what was formerly called the azoic or archæan, but since 1854 has been called the Laurentian period. Following the *monera*, which is not dignified by the name organic, comes the single cell, a bit of protoplasm with a nucleus. This divides by fission, forms a group of cells called a *morula*, which becomes a *blastula* or ball having cell walls and filled with a nourishing fluid. By a process of inversion or doubling in upon itself this ball becomes a *gas-trula*, or cup with double walls, its cavity forming the primitive example of an intestine. The next step is a combination of gastrulæ forming a flat worm. This worm possesses rudimentary organs, including a primitive nervous system.

Higher worm forms slowly succeed until a stage is reached in which a spinal cord and organs of respiration appear. This is technically called *prochordonia*. Next comes the *amphioxus*. Thus far no head, ribs or limbs have appeared, but in the lower Silurian epoch came the *cyclostomata* with a cranium. Then follow *fishes*, in the Devonian and Carboniferous periods; the *amphibia*; *porepilla*; the lower order of reptiles: the *protomammalia*, a new order, warm-blooded and encased in fur, with the ornythorhyncus as the exemplar; then the *marsupiatia* of the Jurassic epoch, of which there remain 150 living species. Then come the *pracentalia* of the Cretaceous period; *prosimians*, *simians*, or American long-tailed monkeys, *catarrhine monkeys*; the large *apes*, including the *gorilla, orang utan*, and *chimpanzee*; the *Pithecanthropus Erectus*, of which we find fossils in the upper Pliocene of Java;—and with something of a jump, the steps of which have not yet been accurately and satisfactorily traced—*man*.

Query 89. What form of gymnastic exercises should be resorted to, and to what extent indulged by those who desire to gain in weight?
A. H., Phœnix, Ariz.

Answer.—All forms of gymnastics that aid in promoting the nutritive processes and the general health are to be recommended. None are to be indulged to an extent that involves fatigue or exhaustion. What are termed "light gymnastics" are the proper form.

In some cases the ordinary occupation furnishes all the exercise that is desirable; but in many cases the occupation leaves certain muscles and sets of muscles almost wholly unused. In such cases some of the simple forms of mechanical exercises are of great benefit, for the reason that they call into action these unused muscles. If, however, any one will carefully study posturing, body movements and muscle-kneading for themselves, it is entirely possible to healthfully exercise every muscle in the body, without the aid of any apparatus whatever.

Your second question will be answered by letter, as being rather beyond the province of this Department.

THE
DIETETIC ᴬᴺᴰ HYGIENIC GAZETTE

A MONTHLY·JOURNAL ᵒ𝖋 PHYSIOLOGICAL·MEDICINE

Vol. XVII.　　　　NEW YORK, JULY, 1901.　　　　No. 7.

WHAT THE CENTURY HAS TAUGHT US ABOUT LIVING.

By SAMUEL S. WALLIAN, A.M., M.D.

Copyright, 1900.

IV.

WHAT SHALL WE EAT?

THIS question has been the chronic conundrum of the ages. It is still asked, notwithstanding it has been answered a thousand times and in a thousand ways. The answer is yet only partial. We know more than once we did, and we know better than we practise. We have made commendable progress in hygiene and sanitation, but have lagged in the study of the most important of the trinity, Dietetics. Paraphrasing a well-known scripture quotation, And now abideth Sanitary Faith, Hygienic Hope, and—Dietetics, but the greatest of these is Dietetics.

First breath, and then food.

This is the law of human existence. We breathe before we eat, but no sooner do we get our first breath than we expend it in a frantic cry for food. If we do not eat we soon stop breathing, and these two functions forever keep pace with each other. They are the Siamese twins of human life. Sever them and both expire.

"Who doth not work shall not eat," is but another way of saying, "Who doth not breathe shall not eat, and who doth not eat shall not breathe." Nature is inexorable; little air, less appetite. If the size of the loaf is not gauged to the size of the lungs

there will be a physiologic revolt; and if the indiscretion is repeated three times a day for a period of time beyond Nature's limit of toleration, the doctor—or the specter with the scythe—will get his inning. The vital equilibrium will be destroyed, and disease will be inevitable. Indigestion in its protean manfestations is the visible (and miserable) expression of this inharmony. Whoso ingests more than he can oxidize and assimilate becomes a victim of hypopepsia—indigestion.

Is it the nonrecognition of this fundamental law that makes us a nation of dyspeptics, and wrings from the impatient physiologist the stinging criticism that, "The average American meal is an unpunished crime?"

And do physicians temporarily forget this law when they dictate a dietary for their patients, and then wonder at the mystery of idiosyncrasy? It is not enough that the food is of unexceptionable quality. Nature is fairly indulgent, and will pardon and repair a reasonable number of derelictions; but she has her limitations, and at last her penalties follow. There has been too much teaching that if we only eat proper food all will be well. If the statistics could be accurately gathered it would be found that quantity has been at the bottom of more trouble than quality.

"For more have groaned and died from overuse
Of knives and forks, than ever fell in war
By bloody sword and bayonet and ball."

The doctor must no longer hold his peace. Let him roll up his professional sleeves and begin at the foundation.

Lord Bacon bent his mighty mind to the study of kitchen problems, and the brilliant Talleyrand, even on his busiest days, devoted an hour to companionship with his cook.

"No man is a really accomplished physician or surgeon who has not made dietetic principles and practice an important part of his professional education."—Sir Henry Thompson.

In order to answer the question proposed with any degree of intelligence it will be well to briefly consider the structure and functions of

The Digestive Organs.—In a normal and therefore healthy human organism the digestive movement begins with the mouth. The initial process is mastication and insalivation. If this process be slightingly and imperfectly performed, or if for any reason the teeth and salivary glands fail to do their proper work, the balance of the alimentary canal must perform an extra amount of labor, and in time rebels, or succumbs to the overstrain. Without this initiatory process starchy foods in particular fail of perfect digestion, and the inevitable result is amylaceous dyspepsia, acid indigestion—starch indigestion. The mouth is, then, the first stomach. To do its work well it must have its proper equipment of masticating machinery, sound teeth, well-developed masticatory muscles, and healthy secretory glands. (The salivary glands of a healthy adult secrete *from two to four pounds* of saliva in twenty-four hours.) Natural teeth, as a matter of course, as long as they can be retained and kept in good working order; but by all means artificial teeth as soon as the natural ones are lost or permanently disabled. But even the best of teeth are not all-sufficient.

The muscles employed in mastication require to be kept in training just as constantly as do the muscles of the athlete. This is another overlooked source of indigestion. Thoughtless, shiftless, and preoccupied people bolt their food, or eat soft food which requires little mastication.* The result is weakened, debilitated, and finally atrophied masticatory muscles; and when atrophied they can not if they would do justice to this primary process of digestion. The same law obtains here that applies to other parts of the muscular system. Unused muscles (in any part of the body) do not retain their strength and vigor. This fundamental law should be early and constantly impressed upon children, by precept, by example, and even if need be, by compulsion. That is, they should be supplied with food of such a nature that they cannot swallow it without due mastication; and they should be constantly impressed with the fact that they must chew their food for a long time. Children should never be hurried at their meals. They should be encouraged to spend much time over each repast, instead of being constantly goaded to "hurry up and get through when mama does." A disregard of this precaution lays the foundation of a lifelong and incurable indigestion. Too much is attributed to "pie," hot biscuit, irregular meals, and other indiscretions, and not enough to this fundamental lack of primary digestion.

The owner of the mouth that slights its duty shall surely suffer.

Unused salivary glands gradually lose their power to secrete. All these causes combine to undermine the whole alimentary process.

It follows that the saliva must be secreted in proper quantity, must be of healthy quality, and then must not be wasted on the desert air, as is practised by others than those who defile their mouths with the "filthy weed." It is from this waste of saliva that tobacco chewers almost invariably become dyspeptics.

Condiments are one of the artificial means

of stimulating the secreting glands of the mouth, but used to excess they over-stimulate and eventually debilitate. Gum chewing, if it were strictly limited to a few minutes immediately after eating, might supplement insufficient mastication; but as usually indulged is decidedly injurious. It debilitites the salivary glands by overwork and by causing them to be active when they ought to be at rest. It also throws large quantities of ptyalin and the other constituents of the saliva into the stomach at times when they are not only not needed but act in a way to neutralize and interfere with the gastric secretions. The "pepsin" gums offered in the market are delusive makeshifts, to which a certain percentage of the prevailing dyspepsias can be truthfully attributed.

The second stage of digestion is accomplished—except when it fails of accomplishment—in the stomach.

The stomach is a flexible laboratory whose walls are composed of strong, elastic muscular fibers that encircle and interlace it in all directions. These walls are motile, and this motility is the principal source of the efficiency of the organ. On account of its muscular structure the organ is amenable to the general law of the muscular system, viz.: a necessity for periodic rest, another important law that is too often lost sight of. The stomach is kept in a state of constant activity by too frequent or too liberal feeding, until it becomes utterly fatigued, and refuses to act. The practice in these cases usually is to still further burden it with "tonics" and stimulants. Its common sense treatment is simply rest. Sometimes it rejects the overload by emesis, but oftener it is over-patient and tolerates the excess until it becomes greatly distended and semi-paralyzed. If the overtasking and overdistension are continually repeated the result is chronic dilatation, which is one of the most distressing and intractable forms of indigestion or dyspepsia. It provides a constant market for oceans of "dyspepsia cures," pepsins, peptonoids, "tonics," and panaceas of all kinds, none of which

can effect anything more than temporary palliation. Ordinarily it can be cured, but the prescription sounds rather severe, since its principal ingredient is—*abstinence from food*, to a degree that to this class of overeaters savors of actual starvation.

The stomach is lined with mucous membrane and studded with countless glands and ducts, microscopic in size. These minute organs both secrete and absorb. They secrete the digestive juices which coöperate with the saliva in preparing the food elements for absorption into the circulation and their appropriation to the needs of the system. They absorb such portions of the food as require no further preparation for the needs of the system; but only certain kinds of food are suitable for absorption directly from the stomach.

The conditions for digestion are: (1) minute subdivision and insalivation of the food, by attrition or mastication in the mouth; (2) the proper temperature—about 100° F.—and, (3) a sufficient degree of hydration to convert the food into a semifluid mass—chyme. The influences which interfere with digestion in the stomach are: imperfect mastication and insalivation, too high or too low temperature, the ingestion of too little or too much fluid. The washing down of food by hot or cold drinks, as practised by a majority of people at present, is one of the most prolific dyspepsia-breeders. The use of ice water and iced drinks at meals is still more reprehensible. One prevents proper mastication and insalivation, and the other lowers the temperature below the digestive point. Slow and imperfect digestion are, in both instances, an inevitable result. If the human animal were a ruminant, and if the stomach could be safely used as a refrigerator, the case would be different.

Most dyspeptics belong to one of four classes—bolters, gormandizers, guzzlers, and those who from shiftlessness or sedentary habits take too much food and too little exercise, which means too little breathing, and involves suboxidation of both food and waste products. Those of the first class swallow without masticating; those of the second eat too much; and those of the third class drink too much with meals, or take too much soft, sloppy, and liquid food.

The aboriginal man had no soup-kettle! He ate his food as he gathered it, and afterwards slaked his natural and not excessive thirst (a thirst that was not provoked by our "civilized" condiments, salt, pepper, mustard, and the like), at some neighboring spring or running stream. His food was either so bulky or so hard that he was obliged to masticate it well before he could swallow it. Hence, although tradition has it that he was finally caught in the act of robbing an apple orchard, there is nothing in the history to show that he suffered from colic or incurred dyspepsia.

The time required for mastication varies with different varieties of food and with individuals. The rule should be rigid thoroughness regardless of the time consumed. Without worrying over the state of your teeth, see the dentist regularly, at intervals, avoid harmful dentifrices, tolerate no sensitive teeth, and whenever a molar or incisor gets beyond repair have it promptly replaced by an artificial one. Good teeth are a necessity for the maintenance of good health.

A fifth class of dyspeptics consists of smokers and chewers. Very few tobacco habitues, as already intimated, escape a final round-up from indigestion. A few are apparently iron-clad, and for years indulge with seeming impunity, but it is only a question of time.

In a sweeping sense the stomach is an elastic, expanded, irregularly pear-shaped pouch, open at both ends, or more properly at one end and one side, and holding, in the adult, all the way from two pints to two gallons, according to the degree of contraction or dilatation present. On the receipt of an invoice of food both ends or outlets are quite firmly closed, through the contraction of strong circular fibers or sphincters, the object being to retain the food during the active churning involved during the process of digestion. The lower opening or outlet, the pyloric orifice, is especially well guarded, so that no food can pass its censorship until thoroughly chymified or prepared for the subsequent processes of intestinal digestion. When from any cause, such as spasm, irritation, or disease, this orifice is so firmly closed that no food can pass, regurgitation (vomiting) occurs, or fermentation and decomposition of the contained food ensues, bringing a long train of painful and dangerous conditions.

The commonest diseases of this organ, as already indicated, are dilatation and injury to the delicate glands and ducts of the lining membrane, the resulting disturbances passing under the various names of dyspepsia, hypopepsia, indigestion, gastritis, acid fermentation, etc.

Intestinal digestion and the final absorption and assimilation of nutrient material need not be described in detail. If the materials supplied and the primary processes be efficiently performed this later process will take care of itself.

THE BUILDING OF THE BODY.

If we submit the physical body of an average man to the chemist for analysis his alembic will give, in round numbers, the following returns:

Weight of the body (average man)	154	lbs.
Oxygen (practically solidified)	97	lbs.
Carbon	48	lbs.
Hydrogen	15	lbs.
Nitrogen	4	lbs.
Calcium	3	lbs.
Phosphorus	26	ozs.
Chlorine	26	ozs.
Sulphur	3¼	ozs.
Magnesium	?	
Flourine	3¼	ozs.
Potassium	2½	ozs.
Sodium	2¼	ozs.
Iron	1¼	ozs.
Silica	?	

The gaseous elements of the body are, of course, in an extremely condensed form. If they were expanded to their ordinary gaseous condition they would occupy a space of nearly 4,000 cubic feet.

The oxygen and hydrogen elements exist chiefly in combination, in the form of water, so that about 108 pounds of our average man is water—about the same proportion as in a potato, something less than that in a cabbage.

It follows that to build, nourish, and replenish the body all the above elements must be supplied in the food. This much we have learned by means of analytic chemistry; but thus far it has been found impossible for synthetic chemistry to combine these elements in a form acceptable to the animal organism. Nature prefers her own laboratory in the preparation of pabulum from which her organized structures are to be built and nourished. They are originally evolved and elaborated through the vegetable kingdom. The lower animals appropriate them, and the higher forms then find it convenient to re-appropriate them at second hand, as supplied by the flesh of animals. Science shows, however, that all animals, even the carnivora, were originally vegetarians.

The problem of science is to determine how and where to find the necessary elements in proper proportions, and in the most economic and most readily available form. However accurately prepared in the laboratory the organism rejects the identical elements required for its sustenance and renewal. The secret of vital chemistry, as manifested in the plant, is still beyond the ken of the chemist. He is dumfounded in the presence of a growing grain of wheat or the ripening of an ear of corn. It is one of the mysteries of Nature that the scientist will never solve. It belongs to the realm of the unknowable. We have not yet given over speculating as to why the stomach does not digest itself!

Ignoring technical chemical details, the substances required for the growth and sustenance of the body are divided into four groups, viz.: proteids, fats, carbo-hydrates, and salts. To these may be added a fifth group, usually classed as accidental, but practically as essential as any other, under the head of waste products. If it were possible to isolate and concentrate the exact elements required in their proper proportions, all directly derived from organic sources, the system would not thrive under their use. The digestive organs may in time, through the law of selection, adapt themselves to aliment in this form, that is, to sheer, concentrated nutriment, but as at present constituted there is required the presence and bulk of much waste with the really nutritive portion of the food.

Proteids is a rather sweeping name applied to all the nitrogenized foods, the albumins, gluten, fibrin, casein, syntonin, etc. These were formerly called the tissue-builders, while fats and carbo-hydrates were called heat-producers. This estimate is now known to be incorrect, since the proteids are capable of heat production, and the carbo-hydrates and fats can be to some extent transformed into body-tissue. Nature's alembic recognizes no limitations, but meets emergencies in her own way, ignoring routine.

Reducing the proteids, carbo-hydrates, etc., to commoner terms, every correct and adequate dietary must contain:

1. *Water*, the quantity required by an adult in health being from 60 to 90 ounces, in some form of liquid, or contained in the food, in twenty-four hours. This seems an exaggeration, and there is no disputing the fact that many people fail to ingest even half this quantity. It is equally true that many people are not perfectly nourished for lack of simple water, which they do not take in sufficient quantity so that the various digestive and metabolic changes can be thoroughly and economically accomplished.

2. *Inorganic salts*, lime soda. potash, iron, etc.. in their various combinations, as chlorides, phosphates, etc.

3. *Albumin*, or one of its equivalents, gluten, fibrin. etc.

4. *Fat*, which is also a carbohydrate minus its oxygen element.

An adequate and balanced diet must contain all these principles, and they must be combined in such approximate proportion that a due quantity of each will be present in digestible form and free from deleterious admixtures and adulterations, in the food of every animal.

The relative proportions of nitrogenous to non-nitrogenous foods should be two of the former to seven or eight of the latter, but Nature takes care of a reasonable excess of either, through her power or fairly secernent selection, provided neither be deficient.

It has been quite generally assumed, though not satisfactorily proved, that flesh-meat is a necessary source of nitrogenous food. The vegetarian argument, though not as important as its extreme advocates contend, is unquestionably based on both logic and analogy. The vegetable kingdom supplies all the elements for perfect human sustenance, in digestible form and free from danger of degeneration or animal taint. This is not true of flesh-food.

Flesh eating is to most people an inheritance. Long custom and strong tradition endorse and perpetuate it. The food marts of the world are adapted to it, and its abolishment would entail a commercial revolution. There is, however, little danger of any such dietetic cataclysm, since with all their weight of logic and enthusiasm, the advocates of a strictly frugivorous and farinaceous diet will convert the world very slowly. Nearly all the newer "pre-digested" food products or preparations of the day are derived from the animal kingdom. Beef, blood, milk, and emulsified fats or oils are the trio from which all the nameless list of animal foods are prepared. It may be that long before the dawn of the millennium the gluten of the grains will have supplanted the albumins and fibrins of the flesh-pots. The composite and perfected man who is being slowly evolved by the advancing ages will no doubt interpret the command "Thou shalt not kill" so as to apply to the whole universe of life, and not merely to the act of homicide.

The nutritive requirements vary with the climate, the age and temperament of the individual, and also with the amount of exercise taken. The various authorities on the subject of nutrition differ as to the quantities of the several forms of food required, but they essentially agree, and an average of their estimates may be taken as practically correct.

An adult man, at rest, requires about 16 ounces of dry solids, equal to from 24 to 27 ounces of ordinary food, or that which has not been deprived of its water, per diem. The same man when at moderate work will require a daily allowance of double, and at hard or laborious work considerably more than double, this quantity.

As ordinary food contains from 50 to 60 per cent. of water this means that, according to his condition, as to labor and rest, he must daily consume from 2.5 to 7 ounces of proteids, 1 to 4.5 ounces of fats, 12 to 17 ounces of carbohydrates, and from .5 to 1.5 ounces of mineral salts. To these figures, representing water-dry food, must be added the proper proportion of liquids, which will increase the consumption to a total of from 70 to 90 ounces. In the matter of exact proportions, as between the nitrogenous and non-nitrogenous foods, Nature is indulgent within certain limits, disposing of a reasonable excess of one kind in order to avail herself of a sufficiency of another; but if from habit, ignorance, or carelessness, one or the other constituent is markedly and persistently lacking, the system is kept in a constant state of irritation, clamor and unrest, and soon falls from a state of perfect health.

The minimum amount of food necessary at the different ages is thus stated by the Munich School:

Age.	Nitrogenous.	Fat.	Carbo-hydrates.
From birth to 1½ years..........	20–36 gms.	30–45 gms.	60–90 gms.
From 6 to 15 years	70–80 "	37–50 "	25–400 "
Adult (at ordinary work).........	118 "	56 "	500 "
Elderly male.....	100 "	67 "	350 "
Elderly female...	80 "	50 "	260 "

Obviously the chemical constituents of the body are the only authoritative guide and indication as to the proper composition of food. It is possible that the traces of additional elements not found by former analysts, such as silica, silver, copper, gold, arsenic, etc., are accidental and extra-normal. With the advances in pharmaceutic chemistry nearly all the metals are being exhibited as remedies, and it is not at all strange that the liver, spleen, and some other organs and tissues should undertake to set up gold, silver, or nickel-plating establishments of their own. That most or all of these metals are extraneous is evident from the fact that they are not found in any of the principal and essential articles of food.

It is alleged that a normal or healthy appetite will instinctively select varieties of food which will afford the system all the elements required for its growth, support, and repair; but even if this is admitted it must be taken into account that habit, custom, and accident all combine to interfere with the free play of this instinct, and to make it wholly unreliable as a dietetic guide.

From its chemical composition and abundant supply it is evident that the albumin group is the most important one to be considered. This group supplies carbon, hydrogen, oxygen, nitrogen, and sulphur. The combination of these elements to form this proteid and predominating food-product, albumin, is accomplished only by plants, all animal bodies deriving their supply from the vegetable kingdom. The exact formula of the proteids is unknown, it being impossible to obtain them sufficiently pure, in quantity for elementary analysis.

Albumin is chemically the same wherever found. Its varieties are numerous, as egg-albumin, serum albumin, vegetable albumin, whey albumin, etc. Egg albumin, consisting of the white portion of the egg, is usually called *albumen*. It consists of nearly pure *albumin*, and is a representative type of all other forms. The distinction is not very radical, although the chemists now practically ignore the word *albumen*. In treating of food products a great variety of terms are used to represent the proteid group. The albumins, albumoses, albuminates, acid-albumins, alkali-albumins, peptones, protoplasm, blood-plasm, and many other substances represented by words of cognate origin, are all essentially albumins. The gluten of plants, fibrin of flesh, and casein of milk are also albumins. Less common forms are globulin, vitellin, muscle-albumin, cell-albumin, myosin, syntonin, etc. It is the coagulation of muscle-albumin or myosin that occasions *rigor mortis* in a dead body. Mucus is essentialy a proteid, and nearly all the digestive ferments, as also nuclein, keratin, gelatin, chondrin, elastin, spongin, etc., are proteids. The animal poisons, including snake poison, tox-albumins, globulins, and albumoses, are all proteids.

It will be seen that the proteids, of which albumin is the type, preponderate in the system, and must necessarily form the bulk of the food supply of every human being. It is also obvious that the leading articles of every dietary are essentially proteids in one form or other. But it should not be lost sight of that no form of the nitrogenous, albuminous, or proteid foods constitutes in itself a perfect diet.

To establish the fact that a certain article of diet is more nutritious or less nutritious than another does not by any means establish its value as a nutritive substance. Many writers on dietetics lose sight of this fact, and there is consequently a tendency to overrate and overdo the proteid group. From this cause the system realizes an oversupply of certain elements, while it is starved for others. The result is deranged functions, "clogging" of certain organs, especially the liver, and the demoralization of all the bodily functions. The individual only half lives, because even in the midst of his constant surfeit he is but half nourished. Turtle soup, *pate de foic gras*, and all the delicacies of the land may be at his beck, but he lacks the phosphates and a few other simple salts, his brain and nerves lose tone, "that tired feeling" becomes his chronic condition, and he dies a premature death, from some one of the fashionable maladies of malnutrition—diabetes, albuminuria, heart failure, or fatty degeneration of some special organ. These cases are the *bete noir* of the profession. It isn't cardiac tonics or change of climate that they so imperatively need as a change of diet.

Without quoting the mostly dry-as-dust tables of chemical proportions and food constituents from a technical standpoint, a summarized outline of the various articles of diet in common use will be instructive and helpful to those who have given the subject scant attention.

❖ ❖

THE CHEMISTRY AND DIETETIC VALUE OF EGGS.

By Dr. E. V. Parrott.

Eggs have become such a staple in all civilized dietaries that a little more careful study of their composition and nutritive qualities is quite in place. They are eaten in all the countries of the globe, and are prepared in a greater variety of ways than almost any other item of human food. There are also almost endless varieties of eggs, although the market quotations, unless otherwise specified, refer exclusively to eggs produced by domestic fowls, in common parlance, hen's eggs.

The other varieties more or less used are the eggs of ducks, geese, guinea fowls, and turkeys, in the domestic line, to which may be added a long list of the eggs of wild birds, including those of plover, gulls, terns, herons, and murres. (Mare's eggs have never been analyzed!)

Eggs other than bird's eggs have also been more or less extensively used in various countries and by various tribes, such as turtle and terrapin eggs, fish eggs, as the sturgeon, (caviar), sterlet, sevruga, beluga, shad, etc., also to some extent the eggs of alligators, lizards, serpents, and some species of insects. Fish eggs are somewhat extensively used in the preparation of artificial foods for infants and invalids.

Referring to the eggs of birds, there are two distinct varieties, and these differ materially in composition. In one variety the young resulting from the process of incubation are hatched full-fledged and ready within a few hours to hustle for themselves and scratch for a living. Ordinary domestic fowls are an example of this variety. Quails, partridges and prairie chickens also belong to this group. The other variety includes the birds, buzzards, crows, etc. The young of these are hatched in a helpless and unfledged state, and must be cared for by their parents for some time, or perish.

The eggs of the first variety should inferentially contain more nutritive elements than those of the second, and careful chemical analyses have determined that this is the case. Inferentially, the egg must contain all the elements of nutrition required for the evolution and maintenance of the young bird, and that it meets this requirement is conclusively proved by the everyday facts of natural history.

Writers on the subject of dietetics frequently refer to this fact as conclusive evidence that eggs furnish a perfect food for animal life at all stages. The same claim is made for milk, because it supplies perfect nourishment for young mammals. The inference is not warranted. The mature organism develops needs that do not exist in the embryo. This is easily proved by the history of the chick, which would suffer in later life if restricted to the eggs of its own kind as food.

The composition of the various kinds of domestic eggs, as of the hen, duck, goose, turkey, and guinea fowl, does not vary materially. Those of the hen and turkey contain a little more water and a little less fat than those of the duck, goose, and guinea fowl. Seventy-four per cent. of the substance of hen's eggs is water. In the other varieties named it is 3 to 5 per cent. less. The hen's egg contains 9 per cent. of fat, as against 12 per cent. in eggs of the duck, goose, and turkey. In the proteid element hen's eggs contain 12 per cent., duck's the same, with eggs of the goose, turkey, and guinea fowl ranging about 1½ per cent. higher. In fuel value, the variation is in accord with the proportion of fat contained. The hen's egg stands for 720 calories per pound; duck, 860; goose, 865; guinea fowl, 755.

As compared with other articles of food, eggs contain on an average 4 per cent. less protein and 6 per cent. less fat than sirloin steak, half as much protein and one-third as much fat as cream cheese, and twice as much protein, with ten times as much fat, as oysters. Their fuel value is about two-thirds that of beef, and but one-third that of good cheese. Compared with wheat flour, eggs contain an equal amount of protein, ten times as much fat, but less than half as much fuel value. Eggs contain practically no carbohydrates, while wheat flour contains 75 per cent.

Chemically speaking, therefore, eggs are rich in building and repair material, but do not furnish a proportionate percentage of energy. This is why it is now admitted that eggs do not furnish perfect nutrition for the adult body. It must, however, be remembered that Nature endows the digestive organs with a considerable degree of vital discretion, or power of transformation; so that both proteids and carbohydrates are to a certain extent commuted into energy, and vice versa. The animal or earthy elements of the egg and its fat are found in the yolk.

It is a popular notion that the eggs of different breeds of hens vary in both flavor and nutritive qualities; but the chemists do not find that this idea is based on fact. The white-shelled eggs of the Leghorns and Minorcas have practically the same composition as the brown-shelled ones of the Cochins, Brahmas, and Plymouth Rocks.

The white of eggs is generally assumed to be pure albumen. Technically speaking, it consists of two albumens—ovalbumen and conalbumen, ovomucin and ovomucoid. There is a trace of phosphorus, and the ash yields chloride of sodium.

The yolk contains a number of different bodies, including palmitin, (20 per cent.), vitellin (15 per cent.), stearin, olein, lecithin, nuclein, etc., and a small per cent. of coloring matter. The contained phosphorus amounts to 1 per cent. of phosphoric acid, in addition to which are found various chemical compounds of calcium, magnesium, potassium, and iron. Sulphur is another constituent, the formation of silver sulphide causing the discoloration of silver spoons used in connection with the cooking of eggs. The decomposition of eggs causes the liberation of hydrogen sulphide and phosphuretted hydrogen, to which gases the rank odor is attributable.

Eggs "spoil" or rot through the action of micro-organisms, which, like mold-spores, are everywhere abundant, and which gain access to the egg through the minute pores in the shell. Some of the egg-preservatives act by simply closing these pores against the organisms. Silicate of soda or soluble glass, common tallow, parafine, and various varnishes, have been used, and the process is effective if properly done and done in time. It usually fails, for the reason that it is not done before the egg has already become infected.

The flavor of eggs varies quite decidedly, first according to the kind of food supplied to the hen. The best flavored eggs result from feeding carbonaceous, and the poorest from highly nitrogenous foods.

Grains and green clover—hens requiring a considerable proportion of green food in order to do well—give the best-flavored eggs.

The digestibility of eggs is about the same whether raw, lightly cooked, or thoroughly cooked. This will seem incredible to those who have always been accustomed to insisting upon their eggs being "softboiled," or lightly cooked. Digestibility, however, does not imply so much the rapidity with which food leaves the stomach as the completeness of its absorbability and appropriation by the system. Careful experiments in this country and abroad have demonstrated that a healthy stomach digests a hard-boiled egg quite as thoroughly as a soft-boiled one; but this does not prove that the process is as quickly accomplished, or that the hard-boiled egg does not compel a somewhat greater effort on the part of the digestive organs. With healthy persons the degree of cooking may therefore be made wholly a matter of taste. In case of invalids and debilitated digestive organs the question becomes of more importance, and must be determined by the physician, or by individual peculiarities.

In case of the yolk of eggs there is no difference in the digestibility of one that is hard and one that is soft-cooked. And in case of the white of eggs, when this is hard-boiled its slowness of digestion is undoubtedly due more to the fact that it is imperfectly masticated than to the effect of heat on the albumen. There is, however, a considerable difference in the solubility and assimilability of albumen as coagulated quickly, at high temperatures, or more slowly, at moderate temperature. The white of an egg may be perfectly coagulated in water at from 160° to 185° F., if submerged in it for ten minutes or more; in which case it will not be so firm, or "tough," as when coagulated in three or four minutes, at a temperature of 212°.

Eggs are a wholesome and economic form of human food, supplying a desirable substitute for flesh. As to comparative cost, eggs are as cheap at 35 cents per dozen as beefsteak at 20 cents per pound.

❖ ❖

THE SURGEON OF THE NINE-TEENTH CENTURY.*

FREDERICK TREVES, F.R.C.S.
London, England.

THE surgeon of one hundred years ago was but a sorry element in social life. In the great towns and cities there were a few practitioners of surgery who were eminent by reason of their scientific work and successful practice. London was then the cen-

* Abstract of the Address in Surgery, delivered at the Sixty-eighth Annual Meeting of the British Medical Association.

ter of surgical activity, and the prominent exponents of the art were John Abernethy, Henry Cline, Sir William Blizard, Sir Everard Home, Sir Astley Cooper, William Lawrence and Charles Aston Key. The great John Hunter had died in 1793, having accomplished a work which marks an epoch in British surgery. In the provinces the most conspicuous surgeons were Edward Alanson, of Liverpool, and William Hey, of Leeds, while in Edinburgh the position of the leading operator was held for many years by John Bell. A little later in the century we find among the names of prominent men in England those of Sir Charles Bell, Sir Benjamin Brodie, and the ingenious and learned Benjamin Travers.

At the beginning of the century surgery on the continent was represented by such men as Sabatier, Deschamps, Boyer, and Larrey in France, Scarpa in Italy, Langenbeck, Chelius, and Diffenbach in Germany, and Warren and Physick in America.

Smollett, who was himself in turn an apprentice, an assistant, a surgeon's mate, a practitioner and a graduate in medicine, has furnished a discouraging account of the surgeon, practitioner or leech of his time. He was ignorant, illiterate, sordid, a mere retailer of physic, not above the allurements of money-grabbing, and not without suspicion of dishonest practices, and of a leaning toward the bottle. Smollett's description could not have been true of all his brethren, and there is no doubt he wrote with the bitterness of an unfortunate experience. Launcelot Crab undoubtedly represented a type not yet extinct when the century began, and he must be taken as a forerunner of the cultured and esteemed general practitioner of the present day.

The Surgeon as an Adviser.—One cannot fail to be impressed by the paramount influence which exact knowledge—or the want of exact knowledge—has had upon the attitude of the medical profession. There is no science outside of our own in which there has been during the stages of development such an extreme disproportion between the amount of knowledge professed and the amount proved ultimately to be exact and sound. The reason for all this lies more with the sick man than with the man of medicine. The sick man requires absolute and exact knowledge from his doctor. He will accept neither possibilities, doubts nor confessions of ignorance. It is no wonder that in the past the physician made good by fiction what he lacked in fact. The demands of the patient have been hopelessly beyond any power of supply, and the deficiency has been furnished by the products of invention. A good deal of the pretense and humbug with which medical practice has been associated in the past has been forced upon the practitioner by the demands of unreasoning people. With such people the surgeon, in the early part of the century, had more largely to deal than he has to do at the present day, and yet his stock of knowledge could seldom meet the demands even of the reasonable. A false attitude toward his patient was unconsciously forced upon him, and the folly of his pretense to an unattainable learning was apparent to all but the simplest. As an adviser, therefore, he spoke not as one having authority. The surgeon of the present day, as an adviser, is in a position which could hardly have been imagined by his forbears of one hundred years ago. He has to deal with a more enlightened public, with patients whose education enables them to appreciate the nature of scientific problems, and with whom it is possible to discuss difficulties, and to own to lapses of information. The additions made to surgical lore have been so substantial that in many departments surgery is an exact science. There is indeed no longer need to call upon invention to supply such gaps as still indicate the unknown.

The operator of olden times certainly possessed many qualities which are now falling into abeyance, his success depending largely on his daring, on the alertness of his eye, the steadiness of his nerve and the rapidity of his movements. He stepped into the arena of the operating theater as a matador strides into the ring. Around him was a gaping audience, and before him a conscious victim, quivering, terror-stricken and palsied with expectation. His knife was thrust through living flesh and acutely-feeling tissues, and the sole kindness of his mission was to be quick. There is less need for such qualities now. The dramatic element in surgery has gone with the men who unconsciously fostered it. The operating theater has changed from a shambles to a chamber of sleep. The surgeon's hand can move with leisurely precision, and theatrical passes of the knife are favored only by those who have not yet learned that mere brilliancy is no measure of success. It is little wonder if the older surgeon became rough and stern, if his sense of feeling became dulled, and if the sympathetic side of his nature suffered some suppression. Indeed, contemporary accounts are apt to represent the operator of preanesthetic times as rough almost to brutality, and as coarse both in his conduct and in his utterances. His language, it would appear, savored of the cockpit, and the hasty flourishing of his knife led occasionally to unintended mutilations.

MEDICAL SUPERVISION OF SCHOOLS AND SCHOOL CHILDREN.

In the *Georgia Journal of Medicine and Surgery* for May .Dr. E. J. Spretting makes some sensible and decidedly important suggestions under the above title. Our readers may not all agree with all the doctor says, but in the essentials he is right, most emphatically right.

Medical science has no higher aim, the physician could have no nobler ambition, than the prevention of disease. The heart of every true physician swells with pride when he feels within his own consciousness that he has prevented suffering, and how much greater is this when he can look his fellow-man in the face and know that that man's physical well-being since childhood has rested with him, and that he has steered him clear of the pitfalls of disease, deformity, and suffering, and from the puny child been instrumental in developing a physically perfect man. Nor is this a mere dream, but an actual possibility—an actual accomplishment in the life of every true physician.

The baby at its mother's breast, so long as it remains well and gives no trouble, comes not under our observation. And generations will have passed ere the government, State or National, will dare interfere in the management of the nursery. Then our first approach to the child as public servant and benefactor must be made in the schoolroom—preferably the kindergarten.

Is there a physician in Georgia who would not gladly give his services to the school of his neighborhood—regulate its hygiene and advise its teacher? And in return he should have the right to supervise the whole school—its building, its hours of study, and have an oversight of the individual child. The building should be warm, dry, well lighted and well ventilated. The best temperature for study has been proven to be 69 degrees F., and each hundred weight of living humanity requires for perfect health 2,000 cubic feet of air changed hourly. Floating dust must be avoided; wet clothing and draughts not allowed; seats and desks adjusted to each child to avoid curvatures and other skeletal deformities. Habit positions must be noted and corrected.

The personal cleanliness of children is one of the teacher's greatest cares. This belongs more strictly to the home, but we must remember that these children's mothers had not the advantage of medical supervision while in school, and many of them not even intelligent care at home, therefore can not be expected to know how to deal best, hygienically speaking, with children of their own; and it is by educating those now growing up that we can obtain the proper coöperation, at home, with the greatest of public benefactions.

Every school should have bathing facilities, for by personal cleanliness we avoid the great majority of skin diseases, and in the cultivation of habits of neatness we grant immunity from many infectious troubles later in life.

Boys should be questioned and examined relative to habits, smoking and masturbation being the two most baneful of all habits. It is estimated that one-tenth of male vitality is wasted in masturbation; a great deal of this could be prevented by tactful management. Both these habits are infectious—insidiously so. No boy would take up smoking were he not taught. We know that all animals masturbate, with the possible exception of the lion, but even in boys it could be limited to within harmless proportions by the right teaching of the intelligent physician.

Tuberculosis is very prevalent among children, and no tuberculous child should be allowed without precautions to mix indiscriminately with others.

The so-called children's diseases are almost always spread through the media of the school. The school physician here finds one of his most useful fields, in early detecting, isolating, and thus stamping out incipient epidemics.

No child who suffers from any cause whatever that hinders its work should be allowed to remain in the schoolroom, for that child will be an idler, and a focus of distraction from their studies for the other children.

This brings us to the branch of our subject of the highest importance, to which we should address ourselves—mental peculiarities—slight obliquities, that stamp the child as odd among its fellows. These must be noted, studied, and so far as possible corrected. It is such a crying injustice to a child to allow it to carry a mental bias through its school life—perhaps laughed at, scorned, and humiliated by its fellows to the point of half desperation, the school conditions practically destroying its future, whereas it ought to have been the means of upbuilding and straightening its mind for life's works and enjoyments. What community has not one or more men to whom friends point with rather a sneer and say, "I was in school with that fellow; he always was odd." Intelligent care would possibly have obliterated that oddness and put him on a par with his fellows.

The writer, a year or two since was invited to go through the Springfield (Mass.) public schools and assist in classifying the 10,500 children found therein. Nine and four-tenths per cent, of all the children were found unfitted for doing average work, 8 3-10 per cent. were absolutely below the standard, 1 1-10 being so-called geniuses —that is 8 out of every 100 were incapable, either mentally, morally, or physically, of competing with the children about them. Only 1 per cent. were brilliant—the restraint of the regular routine curriculum being to them a burden. Nearly 6 per cent. were found incapacitated physically, either temporarily or permanently, and one-third of these had superadded to their physical disability, mental biases. One out of three of these was tuberculous. One out of six had throat troubles, and about the same number diseases of the nose. The hearing was seriously affected in 2-10 per cent. One out of 200 had infectious eye troubles. Nearly 2 per cent. had communicable skin lesions, either parasitic or otherwise. About the same proportion were epileptic, or suffered from kindred nervous affections, such as periodic incapacitating migrain, convulsive tremors or periods of nervous excitement. One per cent. already exhibited marked symptoms of insanity. Three-tenths of 1 per cent. I found to be already strongly imbued with criminal proclivities. Only 8 out of every 100, between the ages of 6 and 18, presented anatomically perfect teeth; and it may be remarked here, that there was an apparent ratio between the teeth and the mental and physical capability. Sound teeth mean endurance and the power to accomplish by steady plodding, hard work. By way of parenthesis, let me say, that the writer carried the investigation of the teeth even further, into the colonies for the epileptic, the asylums for the insane, the schools for the feeble-

minded, and prisons for the criminal. I found that epileptics of all ages enjoy less than 13 teeth per capita, the insane 15½, the criminal slightly over 18, the feeble-minded about the same. Each class presented most striking anatomical peculiarities and abnormalities of the mouth, especially of the teeth.

Could any stronger plea than the above statements be made for the medical care of the school child?

The French government estimates that every able-bodied man is worth to the public $400 a year, every healthy woman $200 a year. Suppose of the 400,000 school children of Georgia to-day, four out of each 100 are to become public charges some time during life. That will make 16,000 to become future burdens to the State, costing the taxpayers $75 per capita, or $1,200,000 in expenses, besides losing 300 times 16,000 in the failure of these people to be self-supporting, making a grand total to the State of Georgia in the next generation of $4,400,000 a year. This is certainly an underestimate.

Suppose by the proper care of the present school children one in four, who otherwise would be lost, could be saved and made a worker instead of a drone; the State would be the gainer by $1,100,000 a year in the next generation.

Now we arrive at the question, What shall we do with the defectives? To this there could be but one answer: Correct, if possible; otherwise, segregate. Segregation may seem unfair to the defective. But we must act on the principle of the most good to the greatest number; and any teacher will tell you that more than half her time and energy will be spent on one so-called peculiar child, leaving only half for the whole rest of the class. Is this fair? Is it just to waste energies on one who is incapable of appreciation, and stint it with those upon whom the future depends?

In the country schools complete segregation is not practicable, and our only hope there is to separate as best we can, so as to get a minimum of damage from the defective and give a maximum of good to the average. Only an expert physician should be allowed to pronounce a child defective and place it under this quasi ban. On the other hand, it is not fair to hold the specially bright pupil down to the average, but his forging ahead should be regulated by the physician's thoughtful study and advice. And the peculiar bent and particular talent of each child should be noted, studied, and directed so as to make it as advantageous as possible.

In conclusion let me ask if any charity could be grander than this medical care of school children? Could any work be nobler? For do we not only help individuals, but the whole of the future generations?

And what a feeling of pride it would give the medical profession to know that each generation is better, stronger, wiser, more powerful, more God-like, because of being intelligently aided by the physician in its effort to grow and develop.

Can any other man or set of men do this task? Is it the duty of the minister? Is it possible to the lawyer? can the merchant give it his time? Would you further laden the already burdened teacher? No! Always NO! It is peculiarly within the domain of the physician. It is his fairest effort, his very crucial test. Finally, it is, par excellence the province in which disease is preventable, and we as men and physicians shall not, can not shirk.

ARTIFICIALLY PRODUCED HYPER-
EMIA AS A THERAPEUTIC MEAS-
URE.

At the recent session of the German Medical Congress at Berlin, Prof. Bier of Griefswald read a paper on the above topic of which we quote an outline:

"In the case of a diseased joint he loosely applies a tourniquet above the joint to hinder venous circulation, and tightly bandages the limb below the joint. In the case of the arm the bandage begins at the tip of the

fingers (each having a separate bandage). The inflamed area is left uncovered between tourniquet and bandage. There must be a 'hot congestion' produced. The joint must feel hot and be of a red or bluish-red color. Never should the compression be enough to produce a 'cold congestion' of bluish color. The white (lymph) congestion is dangerous. If pain is not at once diminished there has been some error in the application of the method. He advised this procedure in tuberculosis of the joints (in which case he does not claim it will render an operation unnecessary). He has obtained good results in gonorrheal joints and in acute articular rheumatism; also in pyalmic joints and in erysipelas, but no results in lues or carcinoma of the joints. The results were particularly good in subacute gonorrheal rheumatism.

"Bier ascribes the beneficial action of this treatment to several factors. (1) It raises the bactericidal power of the tissues. Animal experiments showed that of sixty-nine animals so treated, and then inoculated with otherwise fatal doses of anthrax cultures, fifty-one recovered. (2) Venus stasis is conducive to connective tissue, perforation and formation of scar tissue, which may be important by encapsulating infected areas. (3) It aids in resolving exudates, best seen in chronic articular rheumatism. Since the absorption is hindered (proven by the delay of a tuberculin reaction tested on the treated limb) Bier recommends combining the treatment with massage, the bandage being removed once or twice a day and the joint massaged. In the case of chronic rheumatism thus treated, pain and stiffness rapidly disappear.

"Active hyperemia was also recommended, produced by heat, especially hot air. The limb should be heated by as hot air as can be endured for two hours daily. In this case Bier gave reasons to show that it is not the heat but local hyperemia resulting which does the good. Like the passive hyperemia, the active aids in resolution in all chronic joint troubles, and quiets pain, but unlike the former it promotes absorption, as experiments showed, hence it is to be recommended in many cases as superior to massage where there is blood or other exudate present, and is especially good to remove edema. The bactericidal action of the active hyperemia is very doubtful. Hot air is excellent in neuralgia, and in still other conditions. Neither active nor passive hyperemia improved the nutrition of atrophic limbs.

"Müller (of Würzburg) discussing the paper reported his examinations of the blood of limbs thus treated. Hyperemia (artificial) increases the count of the red cells, even to 6,000,000 per cmm., and the Hb in proportion, while the serum diminishes, since it is pressed into the lymph spaces. Among the chemical changes are diminution of O, increase of CO_2 and an interchange of sodium and potassium salts between serum and corpuscles, probably one also of organic constituents, which may explain the beneficial results. In answer to a question Bier replied that in a case of chronic articular rheumatism he had employed the treatment steadily for four years.

"At the same meeting, Strassburger of Bonn reported the results of himself and Schmidt in connection with intestinal fermentation. They believe that on a standard light test diet there will normally be no carbohydrates in the feces. The detection of these by the fermentation test is evidence of disturbed intestinal digestion.

They described a new symptom complex to which they give the name fermentation dyspepsia (Gährung's dyspepsia), whose only objective symptom is the character of the stools, which always give the fermentation test. The feces are yellow, frothy, very acid, and smell of butyric acid; mucus is usually absent, bile often. Subjectively there are 'dyspeptic' disturbances and pain in the region of the umbilicus. In such cases the metabolism experiments showed diminished digestion and absorption of the food, especially of the carbohydrates, as their charts already showed.

"Ewald of Berlin considered the fermentation test untrustworthy. He thought the microscopic examination of the feces gave more information concerning both starch and albumen digestion. Rosenheim of Berlin doubted that the figures on the charts exhibited were striking enough to be of diagnostic importance. He thought milk should be omitted from the Schmidt standard diet since it is so poorly digested by many persons.

The Fat-splitting Ferment of the Stomach.

Vollard, of Giessen, was able to demonstrate the preesence of a fat-splitting ferment in the stomach. This may be extracted by glycerin from the finely chopped gastric mucosa of the pig's stomach. It is found only in the fundus mucosa, none in that of the pyloric region. Its independence of bacteria may be demonstrated. Its action depends more on the condition of the fat, i. e., whether emulsified or not, than on its nature. Since the acid gastric juice prevents emulsification the sphere of action of this ferment is limited to the previously emulsified fat of the food. The action of the ferment does not vary proportionally to the time allowed nor to the amount of fat present; its action is always incomplete, the maximum in the case of yolk of egg being 60-70 per cent. of the entire amount.

Discussion.—Ellinger of Königsberg confirmed Volhard's statements.

Alu of Berlin mentioned the fact that in motor disturbances of the stomach more fat acid is present after a given period of digestion of milk than in a normal stomach, and suggested that in such cases the conditions for fat-splitting were more favorable.

An industrial sanitarium for the relief of consumptives has been incorporated in Denver. It has been planned that by utilizing the labor of patients it is expected that nearly all of the work of the institution will be performed, the entire sanatorium supplied with provisions, and a great variety of remunerative industries carried on.

INTELLECTUAL WORK AND LONGEVITY.

It is told by Petrarch, when at Vaucluse, that his friend the Bishop of Cavaillon, fearing lest his too close devotion to study would wholly ruin his health, which was very much impaired, having procured of him the key of his library, immediately locked up his books and writing-desks, saying to him, "I interdict you from pen, ink, paper, and books for the space of ten days." Petrarch, though much pained in his feelings, nevertheless submitted to the mandate. The first day was passed by him in the most tedious manner, during the second he suffered under a constant headache, and on the third he became affected with fever. The bishop now, taking pity on his condition, returned him his key, and thus restored him to his previous health.

Among the moderns, Boerhaave lived to seventy, Locke to seventy-three, Galileo to seventy-eight, Sir Edward Coke to eighty-four, Newton to eighty-five, and Fontenelle to a hundred. Boyle, Leibnitz, Volney, Buffon, and a multitude of others of less note that could be named lived to quite advanced ages. And the remarkable longevity of many of the German scholars, who have devoted themselves almost exclusively to the pursuit of science and literature, must be sufficiently familiar to my readers. Professor Blumenbach, the distinguished German naturalist, died at the age of eighty-eight, and Dr. Olbers, the celebrated astronomer of Bremen, in his eighty-first year.

"I presume you carry a memento of some kind in that locket of yours?" "Precisely, it is a lock of my husband's hair." "But your husband is still alive." "Yes; but his hair is all gone."

MILES AND MEALS.

The New York State Household Economic Association proposes to discover how many steps a housewife takes in a day.

It is estimated that 2,000 steps make a mile, and the proposition is to compute how many miles are covered a day by the housewife in the preparation of her meals and washing of dishes. Considering 1,000 meals as the average for the year, the mileage involved promises to be something stupendous.

Members of the association have by no means undertaken this labor as a mere course of mental gymnastics. The purpose in view is to discover how often two steps might serve, instead of three, and to use the statistics as a basis of reform.

We shall keep an eye out for the reports of the Association, which cannot fail to be interesting and instructive.

Having arrived at the facts, we suggest that a prize be offered for the best method of reducing the number of these necessary steps on the part of busy and overworked housewives. Reversing the old saw:

The man or woman who makes two steps do where three or four have heretofore been required deserves a patent, a pension and a monument or a niche in the Hall of Fame.

CHINESE PROVERBS.

Deal with the faults of others as gently as with your own.

A man thinks he knows, but a woman knows better.

Armies are maintained for years to be used on a single day.

Oblige and you will be obliged.

If you fear that people will know, don't do it.

He who rides a tiger cannot dismount.

Has this any reference to Tammany?—Ed. Gazette.

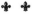

Department of Physiologic Chemistry.

WITH SPECIAL REFERENCE TO DIETETICS AND NUTRITION IN GENERAL.

THE DIETETIC DUNCE.

In his preface to "Wilhelm Meister," Carlyle makes this characteristic and mildly caustic remark: "In our wide world there is but one altogether fatal personage—the dunce, he that speaks irrationally, that sees not, yet thinks he sees."

The "Health" journal woods—rendezvous for all the prize package, pinchbeck, "and free-sample" advertising fraternity—are full of dietetic dunces. Catering to the fads of the day, "culture" and "fisical" are their catchwords. They imbibed certain notions—not from their mother's milk, but through a soft rubber nipple, for they were bottle-fed babies. Brought up on dietetic traditions, perhaps they ought not to be blamed for mental bias and ingrained obtuseness. If they ever indulged in a smattering of science it was when "respiratory foods" were in fashion, and they have never heard that the "luxus consumption" theory of Voit, and Liebig's "respiratory" hobby were both exploded a quarter of a century ago. They expatiate piously concerning "natural laws," the anatomical argument, and the Mosaic edicts, until they imagine they have made out an irrefragible case of divine design as a basis for all their sentimental pseudoscience. They harp on the command, *Thou shalt not kill*, unaware that they crush out the life of a thousand organisms every time they set foot to the ground or scald a breadpan. Some of them go so far as to denounce cooking processes of every kind on the ground that heat destroys the life of the grains and vegetables, that perhaps in a raw state they condescend to eat. They do not stop to establish premises, and have no shadow of scientific criteria on which to invoke logic or base an argument. With infinite assurance they soar and sing in the realm of assumption, half-baked science, and sentimental hyperbole, hinging all their theories of living on eccentric distortions of truth and the irresponsible vagaries of contagious lunacy. Asked concerning the requisite proportions of food elements, of metabolism, or contained calories, they are either nonplussed or indignant—perhaps both. They have no use for standards by which to compare their dietetic hobbies, and do not care to know whether their approved dishes contain 1 per cent. or 90 per cent. of nutrition, or whether nutritive elements chemically present are 10 per cent. or 70 per cent. assimilable.

The dietetic dunce has no conception of a balanced ration. To him, perhaps, bulk and value are synonymous terms, regardless as to whether bulk represents starch, woody fiber, water, or protein. The chances are that he denounces the principal proteid-bearing foods as "bilious" and unwholesome. He is several grades above the Digger Indian, and has eschewed the bark of trees, but he devours the fibrous cortex of such grains as his warped conscience approves of without knowing that he is a barkeater, all the same. To him meat is an abomination, milk robs innocent calves, and eggs blight possible chickens. Hence the use of these as food is contrary to nature, cruel and wicked. He would be shocked if told that the germ of wheat or corn is quite as much alive as the blastoderm of the egg. He feeds on bread and potatoes, with their 30 parts of carbon to one of nitrogen, and is blissfully unconscious of the palpable fact that as a consequence his brain is vapid and incapable of logical reasoning, and his nerves and muscles starved. He never tires of citing the patient endurance of the Chinese coolies, who live on rice, fish, tea, and opium, and who will never cease to be effeminate joss worshippers and whining barbarians until they are fed on a more virile diet.

But what he lacks in logic he makes up in loquacity, and hence there is a glut in the market of rump-reform, dunce-dietetic literature. Of course, we do not include legitimate workers in this field. There are health journals and health journals.

To the unthinking and casual reader much of this talk is plausible, and what isn't plausible is usually skipped, so that there are constant accessions to the ranks of the faithful, and the hundreds of self-styled "health" journals provide immensely remunerative mediums for all the pinchbeck and prize-package advertisers and freak "professors," who exploit "hygienic" cure-alls and pseudo-physiologic methods and appliances. All of these journals inculcate some wholesome ideas—mostly culled from exchanges—otherwise they would early succumb to infantile marasmus and literary hydrocephalus.

Let us cultivate charity for the dietetic dunce. His condition is congenital, and his race will either improve or become extinct.

SALERATUS AND CREAM OF TARTAR.

So common and well known are these cooking and baking requisites that the housewife scarcely gives thought to their origin or that they are likely to be adulterated and cheapened by unscrupulous manufacturers. The biscuits are soggy, cake falls flat, and the busy housewife never thinks of attributing the cause to anything but "luck" or lack of care on her part in combining the ingredients. Probably there is not one case in a thousand when a failure to secure satisfactory results is made but that it is directly due to impurities in either the saleratus or cream of tartar. In the baking powders there is the greatest opportunity for adulteration to go by undetected. An absolutely pure saleratus and cream of tartar baking powder is not obtainable. Cooks and housewives should look into these matters, not only as a means of preserving their own reputations, but from a health and sanitary point. They should inquire into the nature of the adulterations used; are they not injurious when taken into the stomach? The most common impurity or adulteration found in baking powders and cream of tartar is a compound of alum. Imagine the effect of alum on the delicate linings of the stomach. Do you wonder that people become dyspeptic? It is more wonder that their very vitals are not destroyed completely. There's danger in grocery store saleratus cream of tartar and baking powders. The grocer is not to blame; he buys the goods in good faith and sells them honestly at the prices fixed by the manufacturer. His calling is not of the character that teaches him to be careful in these things; his only guiding principle is the lowest possible price. He knows these prices carry with them no guarantee of purity. As a matter of fact, no baking powder should be used in any house, because it simply serves as a cloak under which to conceal the true character and nature of the product. Buy only saleratus and cream of tartar and bake with them. The results will be better, the general family health will be better. At the drug store you can buy saleratus and cream of tartar and feel certain that it is absolutely pure. The cost may be a few cents more, but what matters this when one's health is at stake? The druggist has uses for saleratus and cream of tartar which compel him to have only the chemically pure. He knows it is pure, he can guarantee it to be pure, and he will interest you in regard to these products if you get to talking with him about them. If you make it a point to buy cream of tartar and saleratus of your druggist you are going a long way toward perfection in cooking, as well as adopting an indirect method of establishing perfect health in the family.

SOLIDIFIED AIR.

ACCORDING to the *New York Times* Professor A. L. Metz, of Tulane University, has succeeded in making a small block of solidified air which was as substantial (for the time being) as a block of ice. It was about an inch in diameter, and lasted about fifteen minutes in a fully exposed condition. He laid it on an anvil, and as he struck it the hammer bounded off as though it had been a piece of rubber. It was so intensely cold that no one could think of touching it with his fingers. Taking a large test tube, about eighteen inches long and over an inch in diameter, Professor Metz put liquid air into it, filling it to within six inches of the top. He then corked it, and through the cork inserted a bent glass tube, which was connected with his vacuum apparatus, the full power of which was applied in order to induce the most rapid evaporation possible. The liquid air boiled and bubbled as though it had been suddenly exposed to the most intense heat. When thus exposed to extremely rapid evaporation, its temperature dropped very rapidly. The cold produced was so intense that the atmosphere in the immediate neighborhood of the test tube began actually to liquefy and drop from the lower extremity of the tube. It was caught in a Dewar test tube and found to possess all the characteristics and properties of liquid air. In the meantime the volume of air remaining in the tube was found solidified in a lump a little more than an inch deep. In order to extract this it was found necessary to break the test tube, when the lump of solid air was fully exposed to the action of the atmosphere.

THE GENUINE ST. BERNARD.

CONCERNING this remarkable strain of the race caninus we find this interesting bit of information in the *London Morning Post*: "Of late there has been a controversy between the members of the various dog societies of Switzerland apropos of the true St. Bernard dog, some declaring that the race has been altered by frequent crossing, the monks of the famous hospice, on the other hand, affirming that the type remains the same. A distinguished authority, interviewed by a Swiss correspondent of the *Figaro*, says the monks are perfectly right in stating that the St. Bernard has maintained the purity of its race. In certain cases where crossing had been tried the chief characteristics of the original breed were conserved during one or two generations, but soon these qualities became modified, and ultimately nothing remained save the defects, if the word be not too strong, of the premier couple. The particulars already published concerning the dog are, he proceeds, of a fantastic nature. The following, in his opinion, are the characteristics of the true St. Bernard: Skull raised, forehead large and hollow at base, eyes set wide apart, upper jaw protruding slightly over the under, ears big and attached low down, breast broad and deep, double claws on hind paws, loins raised, back flowing, tail carried low, the coat brown, orange, or pale gray, spotted with white, or the coat may be white with orange, brown or gray spots (pure white St. Bernards have been seen, but they are rare), and, most important, the hair should be short.'

"YOUR business is not to fight disease, but to take care of your patient.—PROF. MURPHY.

EDUCATION AND LIBERAL THOUGHT.

OUR readers will agree with this from *Public Policy*: "Education, if it is real, always tends to liberal thought. But few persons realize how much time and energy expended by them in acquiring educated minds is really used in expelling from the mind things they have learned that are not so. If they could realize this they would feel like filing a claim for substantial damages against publications or persons who imposed upon them by causing them to become the hostage of misinformation which they must get out of their minds before they can become really intelligent. The means of disseminating education is not material, but the correctness of the instruction given is everything. Organizations cannot originate thought, but are the most powerful agencies for the dissemination of thought that have ever been devised. The Norwegian inventor, Nobel, who left half a million dollars "for the promotion of liberal ideas throughout the world," has set a good example.

"It is fortunate for the cause he wished to promote that his executors have decided to publish a magazine every two weeks in France, Germany and England under the supervising editorship of Labori, who won world-wide fame by defending Dreyfus.

"Misinformation always begets suspicion and prejudice, and is the natural foe of liberal thought. Wealth has often been used to endow agencies for the promotion and dissemination of education. Bequeathers of wealth for such purposes are not always fortunate in the selection of persons to be depended upon 'for the promotion of liberal ideas throughout the world.' The attempt at sarcasm by the *Chicago American* in calling attention to this fact by applauding Rockefeller's and Carnegie's gifts to universities and libraries. while deprecating the publication of magazines under the editorship of Labori, but serves to call attention to the lamentable failure, if its purpose was to promote liberal ideas throughout the world, of the bequest that endowed such disseminators of misinformation and prejudice as the leading 'yellow journals' of New York and Chicago."

And to give the attacked a chance we append the editorial in the *Chicago American* that called out the above.

It is entitled:

MONEY CANNOT ORGANIZE THOUGHT.

THE Norwegian inventor, Nobel, has left half a million dollars in his will "for the promotion of liberal ideas throughout the world."

Three magazines, to be published every two weeks, are to be established in France, Germany and England. Labori, the able lawyer who defended Dreyfus, is to be editor-in-chief.

Mr. Nobel's bequest of half a million dollars indicates a good intention, but it cannot do much.

You can no more organize liberal thought than you can organize charity.

Charity and thought are instinctively inborn. They cannot be cultivated or organized and they cannot be suppressed. Organization applied to thought usually means ossification.

Mr. Nobel's half million dollars will probably be spent promoting the notions of some particular set of individuals and not in any way in promoting liberal thought.

The one great promoter of liberal thought and of thought of all kind is Education. Educate one man, and, if he has ability, you have one liberal thinker. Educate a thousand men and you have a thousand men with at least some capacity for liberal thought.

The real promoters of liberal thought in this world, although they do not realize it, are such men as John D. Rockefeller with his great university gifts and Andrew Carnegie with his libraries.

Henry George was a liberal thinker. It was poverty that made him think hard. It was his desperate struggle to feed his wife and children that made him sympathize with other men's wives and children.

If Henry George had been "endowed" by some one anxious to promote liberal thought he never would have done anything.

It is not comfort and ease, it is not gifts from the rich to individuals, that will promote liberal thought in the world.

No greater misfortune could befall the human race at this moment than the sudden cessation of misery, disappointment and outraged justice.

Those are the springs of progress. On them reform, higher thought, better methods, are based.

Nobel would have done better to devote his money to plain education and let the "promotion of liberal ideas" take care of itself.

FOOD ADULTERATION — ARTIFICIAL CINNAMON AND "FINEST OLIVE OIL."

A NATIVE of Ceylon, named Appo, has discovered a method of making artificial cinnamon. The adulterant which he uses for cinnamon is guava, or jungle bark, which costs about twelve cents per pound at Colombo. This bark is carefully peeled, prepared and dried like cinnamon, and resembles it very closely in appearance. The sweet odor and the still sweeter taste peculiar to cinnamon are obtained by soaking the bark in water containing a small quantity of cinnamon oil, and afterwards, when dry, by touching the end of each bundle of the "sham" cinnamon sticks with a cloth saturated with the same oil.

As the discovery of this fraud is new, no suggestions for driving Mr. Appo out of business have yet been made. But it would be interesting to know if there exists any kind of food, from coffee to carrots, which is not adulterated. It is true that many so-called "substitutes" are harmless; but if a buyer pays for a certain article, he ought to receive that article and nothing else.

Cotton-seed oil is as good an article of diet, when properly purified, as olive oil; and the difference in taste between the two must be very slight, if any exists. What is usually sold as "pure olive oil" comes from France, and is quite expensive. Italy has placed so high a tariff upon the importation of cotton-seed oil that it is virtually excluded. France, upon the other hand, last year imported from the United States as much as 10,900,000 gallons out of a total export to all countries of 44,000,000. Germany, the next largest customer, only took 3,800,000 gallons. If the French do not purify the cotton-seed oil and then export it as "the product of the finest olives," what becomes of the large quantity imported?

HOW TO BREATHE.

MOST people, when they breathe properly, says *London Herald*, do it rather by instinct, than consciously; and, on the other hand, hundreds of thousands of people do not breathe well, and are suffering from more or less severe affections of the lungs or throat, on account of this manner of incomplete respiration, or, in other words, because they breathe too much by the mouth and not enough through the nostrils. The mouth has its own proper functions, eating, drinking, and speaking; and the nostrils have theirs, smelling and breathing. It is obviously less dangerous to breathe by the mouth in summer than in winter. If you inspire through the natural tube, the nostril, the air passing over the mucous membrane lining the different chambers of the nose is warmed to the temperature of the body before entering the lungs. On the contrary, if you breathe by the mouth, the cold air comes into contact with the delicate membrane which lines the throat and lungs and gives rise to local chilling, which often culminates in inflammation. Many people in winter use respirators, which they place over the mouth on going out of doors; thus diminishing the quantity of air which passes between the lips, and compelling them to breathe through the nostrils. But they may achieve the same result by keeping the lips closed, a habit which is easily acquired and induces a natural method of breathing. We believe that if we all adopted the simple rule of shutting the mouth while breathing, there would be a noticeable diminution in lung and throat affections, which have many victims during the year. Man is the only animal who adopted the pernicious and often fatal habit of breathing by the mouth. The habit is contracted in infancy, and is strengthened in adults, thus causing consumption, bronchitis, sore throat, etc.

In conclusion, we would simply ask our readers to try the experiment. When they go out in the cold morning air, let them try the two methods of breathing, by the mouth and through the nose. In the first case, if they breathe between the open lips, the cold air rushing into the lungs creates a sensation of cold and uneasiness, often provoking a cough; but in the second they will observe that respiration is free and agreeable, for the fresh air is warmed to the temperature of the body by passing over the nasal mucous membrane and is sweet and soothing to the lungs.

[People suffering with obstructive nasal catarrh are an unfortunate exception.—ED. GAZETTE.]

NATURE AS A DOCTOR.

STRANGE as it may seem, there is nothing in the world now that was not here on the first day of creation. The difference is in form, that is all. As great or greater changes are yet to take place. Sickness and disease only come to us when we have violated some of Nature's laws. It is not always for us to trace the responsibility for disease, but in every instance it will be found to be due to failure on the part of some one to keep within the bounds prescribed by Nature. But wise, kind-hearted Nature, like a mother reluctantly punishing her child, has provided in her vast storehouse an adequate remedy for every ill. All the drugs of the drug store come from Nature, although each may be presented in different form and in combination that defies recognition. As we pluck the wild flower in the cooling woods little do we think of its power as a medicinal agent. In order to more thoroughly appreciate the mysteries and wonders in this world it is sometimes well to stop for a moment and think of these small things. Nature is the real physician in treating human ills. The druggist at the direction of the physician compounds and mixes the medicines furnished by Nature; the physician applies his knowledge of the effects of drugs on disease and sickness to the case before him; but Nature, grand Nature, impressive Nature, beautiful Nature, limitless Nature, furnishes the groundwork for all medical treatment. The "Nature" curists are well enough as far as they go, but they do not go far enough.—*Exchange.*

A WELL PRESERVED OCTOGENARIAN.

THE Catholic population of the world is estimated at about 300,000,000 souls, and the spiritual head of this vast body attained his ninety-first birthday this year. In spite of his great age, however, he is still a commanding figure in international questions and the counsels of diplomacy. He still brings an acute and balanced judgment to bear upon the multifarious matters affecting the welfare of his spiritual subjects in every quarter of the globe, and he was able to endure the fatigues of the Jubilee year without succumbing to the strain. When we remember that he was fifty-eight years of age when he ascended the Papal throne, and that of two hundred and fifty-eight Roman pontiffs only eleven have lived over seventeen years after they became popes, the twenty-three years of the pontificate of Leo XIII. becomes all the more remarkable.

And what manner of man is he who thus

seems to defy the ravages of time and of mental stress? One who saw him but a comparatively short time ago writes that as the pontiff left the chair in which he had been borne from the Vatican gardens to his apartments, "he sprang erect as if impelled by springs of steel. . . The features were fleshless. There seemed to be hardly a drop of blood beneath the dried and withered skin. The broad forehead was pale as ivory, and the lips were colorless, but the eyes lit up and vivified the living skeleton . . . there was something terrifying in their brilliancy." Of the pope's daily life we have unusually full detail. He rises about six every morning and says Mass in a small apartment adjoining his bedroom, and afterwards attends Mass said by his chaplain. His breakfast is chocolate or coffee with goats' milk. At eight o'clock Cardinal Rampolla, his Secretary of State, is admitted for a conference on current affairs. At ten he has a cup of broth after a walk if the day is fine. Thence till the dinner hour, which is two o'clock, the pontiff holds receptions. Dinner, which he usually takes alone, consists of a clear soup and eggs, very rarely meat of any kind, with a special brand of light Bordeaux wine. A short rest, with perhaps a nap, follows, and then he drives and walks in the Vatican gardens for two hours, during which he reads or talks. In the summer time he usually spends the entire day in the Leonine Tower in the gardens. At ten in the evening a light supper is eaten, after which the newspapers of the day are read to him. He seldom retires before twelve or one o'clock, working often long after all others about him have gone to rest, rarely lying in bed more than four to five hours.

Leo XIII. was born in 1810 at Carpineto, his father being Count Ludovico Pecci. He took orders in 1837, became Bishop of Perugia in 1846, cardinal in 1853, and pope in 1878.

A CASE OF SUGGESTIVE INFECTION.

WE reproduce the following illustration of the policy of suggestion, from the *N. O. Times Democrat:*

"A nervous man recently called on me," said a New Orleans physician, "and asked, 'In what part of the abdomen are the premonitory pains of appendicitis felt?' 'On the left side, exactly here,' I replied, indicatnig a spot a little above the point of the hip bone.

"He went out, and next afternoon I was summoned in hot haste to the St. Charles Hotel. I found the planter writhing on his bed, his forehead beaded with sweat, and his whole appearance indicating intense suffering. 'I have an attack of appendicitis,' he groaned, 'and I'm a dead man! I'll never survive an operation!'

" 'Where do you feel the pain?' I asked.

" 'Oh, right here,' he replied, putting his finger on the spot I had located at the office. 'I feel as if somebody had a knife in me there and was turning it around.'

" 'Well, then, it isn't appendicitis, at any rate,' I said cheerfully, 'because that is the wrong side.'

" 'The wrong side!' he exclaimed, glaring at me indignantly. 'Why, you told me yourself it was on the left!'

" 'Then I must have been abstracted,' I replied calmly; 'I should have said the right.' I prescribed something that wouldn't hurt him, and learned afterwards that he ate his dinner in the dining-room the same evening. Oh, yes; he was no doubt in real pain when I called," said the doctor, in reply to a question, "but you can make your finger ache merely by concentrating your attention on it for a few moments."

A PRIZE of $100 has been offered by a Massachusetts physician, Dr. J. B. Learned, for the best essay containing some method for inducing sleep without the use of drugs.

THE PROPORTION OF DOCTORS AMONG MEN OF GENIUS.

In the recent "Dictionary of National Biography which has been issued lately in England, and in which persons of pre-eminent intellectual ability which Great Britain has thus far produced are considered, says *American Medicine*, there are mentioned some 30,000 persons. Havelock Ellis *(Popular Science Monthly,* February, 1901), has studied the records contained in this dictionary with a view to determining the elements of intellectual ability which have entered into the success of these eminent Britons. He finds that in a large proportion of these persons there is too little recorded upon which to base a judgment, and for other reasons he eliminates from his estimates all but 859 men of a high degree of intellectual eminence. The number of doctors included in his list of names is surprisingly small, only seven being mentioned; Caius, Linacre, Mead, Pott, Sydenham, Cheselden and Cullen. It would have been possible to enlarge the group somewhat by including a certain number of medical men who are not considered by their biographers to have attained a really durable reputation. He believes that just as really able business men are not satisfied with business success, so really able doctors are not satisfied with professional success, but seek a higher success, specially in science. A number of eminent men in science, letters and philosophy have been doctors, but it has not been in medical practice that their reputations have been made. In this class he mentions such names as Harvey, Hunter and Jenner. It is questionable whether it can be truly said that these men did not make their reputations either in medical practice, or what is practically the same, in allied medical sciences, and without the experience which these men gained from their medical education and practice, it is questionable whether their intellects would have developed in such a way as to lead them to any preëminent success. Among other names which Ellis includes in his lists are those of Locke, Goldsmith, Keats, Livingstone, and others, who were educated as physicians, and some of whom practised medicine, but who cannot be said to have been deeply influenced by their medical training and practice.

This small list of names of doctors shows how little is the reward in the way of fame and public appreciation of service which can be expected even by the most successful medical men. Undoubtedly many of the men included in Ellis' lists were deeply influenced by a medical training. Without this they would never have attained their love for truly scientific study, their thorough understanding of human nature in all phases and the deeper sympathy with people of all conditions, which the doctor gains from association with the sick and afflicted of all classes; for, truly, suffering makes all men kin, and under the trying circumstances of serious illness men show their true characters as under no other circumstances. While the proportion of men who have themselves a permanent place in the archives of history among the members of the medical profession is not great, there are other rewards which are as great and in many ways more satisfactory. Ellis says that the able doctor is not satisfied with his professional success, but seeks a higher success. Can there be any higher success than the doctor's professional success? The certain knowledge that one has been able to alleviate suffering, and to cure disease, is surely worth as much as a place in the Dictionary of National Biography, and there are many unknown heroes in the medical profession who have as certainly earned a place in the hearts of their fellows as Ian MacLaren's "Doctor of the Old School."

Laborde reports that *rhythmic traction* of the tongue will keep in function the tissues of the organism for some time, even after lungs and heart cease to act. He succeeded in bringing back to life by these means individuals who had been in apparent death for three hours.

WHAT RHEUMATISM REALLY IS.

"One of the most commonly observed symptoms of a tired-out sympathetic system," says *Health,* "is disturbance of the digestive function, which is presided over by that system of nerves. The most common form of indigestion under these circumstances is the fermentative or acid. Hence the process is simple; the ingested food enters the stomach, where, owing to abnormal conditions, instead of exciting a physiological congestion of that organ and a properly increased flow of gastric juice, owing to the impaired condition of the sympathetic nerves this does not occur, and, as a consequence the food, instead of being digested, ferments, generating gas and lactic acid, the gas to be expelled and the acid to be absorbed with whatever peptones may result from the attempt at digestion, and the circulating fluid, the tissues and excretions of the body become vitiated by it, *i. e.,* the blood becomes less alkaline and the secretions less alkaline or acid, producing the state of the body most favorable for the accumulation of uric acid in its tissues. In this manner the way is paved from irritation of sympathetic nerve terminals to an excess of uric acid in the system, which constitutes, with its attendant and resulting symptoms, lythemia, and composes the necessary congeries of conditions, the next step in advance of which, the proper exciting causes being added, is acute articular rheumatism."

The late Justice Smyth, of New York, who saw about as much of the trial court as any judge of modern times, once said, "I cannot understand why it is that doctors are about the worst witnesses I know of. They are really the very worst witnesses I ever met, with one exception, and the exception is the lawyer. Doctors and lawyers are very bad witnesses. They don't know how to give a direct answer to a simple question.

Prof. A. S. Mitchell, chief chemist of the Wisconsin dairy and food commission, according to *The Sanitary Home,* appeared before the senatorial pure food investigating committee in Chicago on May 9th. The chemist told of a liquid known as "freezine." He said that the stuff had been used extensively by farmers to keep milk and butter, it being the custom to mix it with the former in small quantities and pour quarts of it into vats for the preservation of butter. "This 'freezine,'" he said, "I have found to be nothing less than a most pure formic aldhyde. This is a chemical that acts disastrously upon the tissue of the stomach, and I can only surmise the results when milk diluted with it is used constantly by a family. Where butter is placed in vats filled with this stuff the porous commodity takes up no small amount of the liquid, with a result that can only be conjectured."

HOW LEMON OIL IS MADE.

The lemons are taken to the laboratory and each is cut lengthwise into three slices. The pulp is first removed and put into a press where it is squeezed in order to obtain the lemon juice, which is sold in its natural or concentrated state to the manufacturers of citric acid. The residue of the pulp is used for animal food. The peel is put into large baskets which are stored in a cool place for some hours, when it is ready to be pressed. Each workman holds in his left hand a medium-sized sponge of superfine quality, which has been previously washed most carefully and thoroughly. Between the fingers of the same hand he has also small sponges to prevent the loss of any of the oil, which is very volatile. With the right hand the workman takes a piece of peel from the basket, which is kept within easy reach, and squeezes it against the sponge, thus forcing the oil through the pores of the rind into the sponge or sponges. When the sponge is full of essence it is squeezed into a tin-lined copper bowl having a lip, which every workman has before him. In order to make sure that the peel has yielded all the essence that can be pressed by hand, the overseer from time to time tests the rejected peel by squeezing it close to a flame. If there is any essence left it is forced through the flame and produces a flashlight. (We have seen children try the same experiment with the peel after having eaten their orange.) This hand-pressed peel is then put into brine and sold to manufacturers of candied lemon. When the tin-lined copper bowl is full it is set aside for a short time to permit the impurities to settle, after which the bowl is slowly and carefully decanted and the clear essence emptied into large tin-lined copper vessels. Before this is put into the various sized coppers for shipment, it is passed through filtering paper. This not only perfectly purifies it, but also gives it limpidity. The quantity and quality of essence yielded by the lemon varies acccording to the season. During November, December, and January most of the essence is manufactured, about 1,000 lemons being then required to make one and a half pounds of esssence. Lemons not fully ripe are preferred, as they yield a larger quantity and more fragrant quality of essence than those fully matured. While a small quantity of essence is made during spring and summer, the product lacks the delicate fragrance of that made in winter.

ANTI-CIGARETTE LAW.

Bills prohibiting the sale, presentation of, or bringing into the State, of cigarettes, cigarette paper, or any substitute therefor, have been passed by the Lower Houses in both Illinois and Michigan. In West Virginia the new law of imposing a tax of $100 on all dealers has become operative May 1. In Pottsville, Pa., cigarette smoking is so prevalent among the schoolboys that the authorities have concluded to enter suit against all dealers found selling cigarettes to boys under sixteen.

THE DEATH PENALTY.

Just so long as the law of "A life for a life" is accepted by civilized people, says, an exchange, the grim question of the means of carrying out the penalty is sure to frequently arise. Personally, we have little sympathy with those who would rob an execution of its terrors, but we do, most emphatically, protest against making public exhibitions of such, or special entertainments with which to gratify the morbid tastes of selected individuals. Already, in this country, two States have adopted electrical execution, and it is yet too early to draw any conclusions as to the effects thereof on crime *per se.*. But it has been reserved for the Japanese to suggest another method, which is perhaps more effective even than the electrical current, and at the same time more free from the reproach of inhumanity. The condemned individual is enclosed in a lethal chamber, and by means of powerful pumps the contained air is rapidly withdrawn, and death at once ensues. Experiments on animals point to the conclusions that this method is wholly painless.

It is obvious that if the principle of the lethal chamber is admitted, there are many methods of making the air within irrespirable.

DIETING TO REDUCE FLESH.

[The following rules for dieting were given by a celebrated English physician to be strictly adhered to for the purpose of reducing flesh.]

BREAKFAST.

One or two cupfuls of tea or coffee, sweetened with saccharine, no milk or cream, one ounce of dry toast, no butter, four ounces of lean broiled steak, chop or kidney, or of cold chicken, game or tongue, or four ounces of broiled or boiled sole, cod or haddock.

LUNCHEON.

FOUR ounces of lean beef, mutton or lamb, hot or cold, roast or boiled gravy to be free from fat, or of chicken, turkey or game; no bread or sauce. Four ounces of any vegetable given in the list below, plain boiled; no melted butter. Four ounces of baked or stewed apple or rhubarb, or fresh fruit, sweetened with saccharine (liquid saccharine is best for the purpose), no milk or cream. Plain salad in any quantity made without beet or oil. One graham cracker.

DINNER.

Clear soup (plain julienne or consommé), four ounces of any fish as at breakfast, and four ounces of any meat as at luncheon; vegetables, stewed fruit, salad, cracker, and liquid the same as at lunch. Later a cupful of black coffee or beef extract may be taken, in fact, a cupful of the latter may be taken at any time desired. Before retiring sip a tumbler of hot water; a squeeze of lemon may be added if desired.

The following condiments may be used: Worcester and anchovy sauces, ketchup, pepper, mustard, salt, walnut pickle, vinegar and horseradish. These salads and vegetables may be used: Watercress, radishes, lettuce, cucumber, mustard and cress, spinach, asparagus, celery, brussels sprouts, cabbage, broccoli, seakale, string beans, tomatoes, artichokes, and vegetable marrow. Lemonade may be partaken of sparingly. —*Isabel Bates Winslow, in Table Talk.*

THE following extraordinary case of fraud is reported in the *Journal of the American Medical Association:* A man aged thirty-five, described as a Dublin medical student, came to lodge in London and called on a doctor, minutely describing to him the symptoms of Bright's disease. He also brought urine for analysis, and it contained a large quantity of albumin. One day, when the doctor called, he appeared to be very drowsy and dangerously ill.

Early on the following morning a man resembling the patient called on the doctor, but he was clean shaven and in good health, while the patient had a heavy mustache. The visitor posed as the brother of the patient, who, he said, had passed away in great suffering during the night. He was given a certificate of death. In pursuance of his usual practice the doctor visited the chamber of death. In the dimly-lighted room what appeared to be a human body was perceptible on the bed, but on examination the "corpse" proved to be a dummy composed of pillows, blankets, boots, and a poker. The man who obtained the certificate, on being questioned, said: "I am the dead body," and asserted that he had committed the deception to deceive his people into the belief that he was dead. A search in his box, however, showed that he had a life policy of $1,000. For having made a false declaration for the purpose of death registration, he has been sentenced to nine months' imprisonment. It appears that the man was really ill and had a high temperature, but simulated the special symptoms of Bright's disease.

✤ ✤

TOBACCO INCONSISTENCY.

The Medical Age aptly says: "The governor of Michigan has a cabinet whose members nearly all smoke large dark cigars without reproof from his excellency. Yet there is little doubt that the governor will sign the law making it criminal to sell or give away cigarettes. This is another example of swallowing the camel. In the State of Connecticut they do somewhat the same. In the school text-books the children are taught that a drop of nicotine will kill a full-grown cat in one minute, and that the smoker shuffles in his gait and loses ambition, and at the same time the same State spends $500 a year to encourage experiments in tobacco growing."

THE MICROBES OF RHEUMATISM.

ENGLISH investigators think they have discovered them at last, according to the *New York Tribune:* "A good deal of evidence that rheumatic fever is an infectious disease has accumulated within the last ten years, and while that theory is not yet to be regarded as fully established, it has apparently gained some ground even this very spring. *The Philadelphia Medical Journal* refers to it as 'the more generally accepted view,' to which the lactic acid and nervous origin explanations have given place to some extent.

"One of the reasons for suspecting that this disorder might be infectious is that several cases will often occur in the same house, and it is peculiarly prevalent in large communities. Again, it has been asserted that the mortality and frequency of rheumatic fever fluctuate in the same way as those of erysipelas and scarlet fever.

"Now, infectious maladies are all attributed to micro-organisms, and as soon as suspicion was excited the search began for bacteria which should prove to be characteristic of the malady in question. One expert hunted in the blood; another directed his attention to the tonsils; a third examined the synovial fluid, or lubricant of the joints; a fourth tested other secretions, including exudations from the heart.

"The first definite declaration of a discovery was made in 1891, when Bonchard and Charrin believed that they had found in the joint fluid a certain well known organism hitherto associated with suppuration. This was the staphylococcus pyogenes albus. The presence of this microbe in the joint would not prove much, considered by itself; but in 1893 St. Germain succeeded in producing an inflammation of the joints by inoculating an animal with staphylococci. Of course, a single instance would not settle the question, but the experiment was highly suggestive, to say the least. Since that time several other investigators have found microbes in the blood or secretions. Sometimes these organisms were identified as the 'aureus,' or 'citrus,' instead of the 'albus,' but they were staphylococci. Occasionally, however, another microbe that is characterfistic of pus, a streptococcus, was found.

"The latest investigations which bear on this subject are those of Poynton and Paine, and are reported in the *Lancet* of May 4, 1901. The *Philadelphia Medical Journal* summarizes them without comment. These men assert that they have isolated diplococci in sixteen cases. Cultures were made of organisms found in rheumatic nodules or swellings, and were injected into the veins of rabbits. In consequence, the little creatures had pain in the joints and inflammation of the valves and covering of the heart. The fluid in their joints and some of the brain tissues revealed the presence of the diplococci. Poynton and Paine think that the nodules of rheumatism are a particularly characteristic feature of that disease.

"It will be observed that the results of this latest inquiry differ from those previously obtained. Streptococci look like chains of beads of practically uniform size. Staphylococci suggest rosaries, one organism longer than the other occurring every so often in the series. Diplococci are usually half-round objects, and come in pairs. They sometimes look like the halves of a pea, slightly separated. The pneumonia germ is diplococcus, and is pointed on one side like a raisin seed. But there are many other points of difference besides those of form. One takes a certain kind of stain which will not affect another. One must be cultivated in a manner unlike that required by another, and so on. But the most important distinction, of course, is that between the effects produced on the human system when the latter is invaded. The other characteristics are important only as means of identification.

It appears, then, that Poynton and Paine do not attribute acute inflammatory rheumatism to the same organism as do their predecesssors. Further study is essential, therefore, to ascertain which of them is right. More experiments are necessary to clear up several phases of the matter. The natural history of the newly found diplococcus should be fully worked out, so as to differentiate it distinctly from all other microbes, and if its responsibility for rheumatic fever finally be established it will then be highly desirable to try to make an antitoxin that will have a curative power.

"Meantime, it should be noted that these researches do not apply to 'muscular rheumatism,' or 'myalgia,' whose nature and cause still remain a mystery. As yet, no one can say positively whether it is a product of beer, beefsteak or the weather. Conservative physicians confess that ' its pathology is obscure.' "

THE USES OF EGGS.

THE uses to which eggs may be put are many, aside from their employment in cooking.

A mustard plaster made with the white of an egg will not leave a blister.

The white skin that lines the shell of an egg is a useful application for a boil.

White of an egg beaten with loaf sugar and lemon relieves hoarseness—a teaspoonful taken once every hour.

An egg added to the morning cup of coffee makes a good tonic.

A raw egg with the yolk unbroken taken in a glass of wine is beneficial for convalescents.

It is said that a raw egg swallowed at once when a fishbone is caught in the throat beyond the reach of the finger will dislodge the bone and carry it down.

The white of a raw egg turned over a burn or scald is most soothing and cooling. It can be applied quickly and will prevent inflammation, besides relieving the stinging pain.

One of the best remedies in case of bowel troubles is a partly beaten raw egg taken at one swallow. It is healing to the inflamed stomach and intestines, and will relieve the feeling of distress. Four eggs taken in this manner in twenty-four hours will form the best kind of nourishment as well as medicine for the patient.

A raw egg is one of the most nutritious of foods, and may be taken very easily if the yolk is not broken. A little nutmeg grated upon the egg, a few drops of lemon juice added, some chopped parsley sprinkled over it, or some salt and a dash of cayenne pepper, vary the flavor and tend to make it more palatable when not taken as a medicine.

The white of a raw egg, says the *Grocers' Monthly*, is the most satisfactory of pastes and is better than any prepared mucilage or paste one can buy. Papers intended to be put over tumblers of jelly and jam will hold very securely and be air-tight if dipped in the white of an egg.

THE PHENOMENA OF DEATH BY DROWNING.

DR. PAUL LOYE, in the *London Lancet*, has published some observations made by him, bearing on the phenomena which precede death by sudden immersion. The first stage of deep inspirations lasts about ten seconds, followed by a reaction caused by the resistance to the entrance of water into the bronchioles. This lasts for a minute, and is succeeded by arrest of respiration and loss of consciousness. Finally the scene closes with four or five respiratory efforts—the last. Immersion causes an immediate rise in the blood-pressure, with slowing of the heart-beats. The action of the heart remains slow but strong till death ensues. The pressure gradually lessens, but rises just before death, to fall to zero immediately afterward. The heart sometimes continues to beat feebly for about twenty minutes. The result is the same in animals which have been tracheotomized; the period of respiratory resistance is, therefore, due to the respiratory muscles, and not to spasm of the glottis.

THE EVOLUTION OF FOODS.

Our ancestors—if we care to trace them far enough back—no doubt lived from hand to mouth. That is to say, they dispensed with silver service, bills of fare and napkins. In their pristine state they were undoubtedly vegetarians, subsisting wholly on barks, roots, nuts and fruits. They gathered their harvests with their hands, shinning up trees for fruits and nuts, delving for roots, only as their daily needs required.

It probably took them a long time to discover that shucks, husks, and beards were Nature's *chevaux de frise* for the protection and concealment of wholesome nuts, wheat and corn. Meanwhile there was no demand for reapers, threshing machines, and roller mills. When at last they discovered the secret of the grains they no doubt munched them in their raw state. When the ripened kernels got so dry and hard as to threaten the integrity of the molars the owners of the molars discovered how to crush them with stones and soften them with water. Later they learned to roast the stuff, to make mush of it, and finally to bake it in the ashes.

From these crude beginnings has all our art culinary been evolved. The bruisers and mushmakers have developed into scientific millers and sapient chefs. Milling has become a fundamental fine art and baking the basis of all culinary processes. And now the chemist-critics are having their say. The loaf has its lacks and is not uniformly good. The crust is dietetically quite different from the heart of the loaf. It has yielded up some of its starch and replaced it with dextrin. This results from the different degrees of heat imparted by the oven, the crust receiving 500 degrees, while the heart of the loaf barely reaches boiling point. Result, the crust acquires a nutty flavor and digestibility not found in the inner portions. The former satisfies the palate and is easily assimilated; the latter often ferments, digests with more or less difficulty, and is only partially assimilated. Some of the astute bakers have learned to slice up their surface-baked loaves and rebake the slices until they are a rich, golden brown and become all crust, as in "zwieback." Some of them granulate these twice-baked slices and call the product "granola," "wheatena," "granum," and what not. Other manipulators of farinaceous products shred the wheat or flatten it into semi-transparent fish-scales, wash out a portion of its starch, dry it and call it "granose," "flaked wheat," "cream of wheat," or any one of a dozen other fancy names. But the esthetic evolution of the human stomach goes on, and the food-refining processes are compelled to keep pace. By and by we may be able to subsist on an occasional thimbleful of nectar such as the gods enjoy. Weak stomachs already rebel at the excess of cereals, and delicate stomachs are demanding further refinements. Excess of starch in the food is charged with a major part of the invalidism and prevalent indigestion. Hence the food chemists are turning their attention to other sources. Their latest triumphs are in the line of milk products. Milk was the original, and always represents the natural food of the human race. It is the first food of every infant, and chemically contains all the constituents of the human body. Acting on this theory scores of milk foods have been thrown on the market. The success of this class of foods has been phenomenal, and the traffic in them has rapidly grown into millions, and this, too, in spite of the fact that the processes of condensation and concentration have been radically faulty, deteriorating, or destroying the nutritive quality and spoiling the flavor of the product.

At last a process has been devised which claims, and seems to have obviated the defects of the former ones, in substance retaining all the nutritive properties of milk, without interfering with its flavor. The product has been not inaptly named *Plasmon*, and is a decided departure from the many forms of merely desiccated casein, which latter lacks perfect solubility and agreeable flavor. This process has been patented in all the leading countries of the world, and promises to revolutionize the manufacture of milk foods.

Dr. Hutchinson, in his admirable work on food and dietetics, has this to say of it:

"It consists of the proteids of milk rendered soluble by combination with bicarbonate of soda. It occurs as a yellowish-white powder, containing 12 per cent. of moisture, 8½ per cent. of ash and 11 per cent. of nitrogen. It is easily soluble in warm fluids, and is devoid of taste. . . . Metabolic experiments show that it is capable of replacing all the other proteids in food. It is the cheapest of all the casein preparations."

The venerable Professor Virchow testifies that a teaspoonful of Plasmon is equal in nutritive value to a quarter of a pound of the best beef. The *London Lancet* adds that the introduction of Plasmon marks an important advance in the separation of nutrient material without any deterioration of its dietetic quality, from the most natural of all foods, milk.

Chemical analysis shows what a remarkably high proportion of proteid it contains, and physiologic experiment has established that this proteid is completely available for the nourishment of the human body.

Dr. Tunnicliffe conducted an elaborate system of experiments, corroborating the previous analyses and determining that Plasmon contains 81.30 per cent. of proteids, nearly 5 per cent. of lactose, and about 3 per cent. of phosphoric acid.

What are the sweetest things of earth?
Lips that can praise a rival's worth,
A happy little child asleep;
Eyes that can smile though they may weep;
A brother's cheer, a father's praise,
The minstrelsy of summer days.
The light of love in lover's eyes,
Age that is young as well as wise;
A mother's kiss, a baby's mirth—
These are the sweetest things of earth.

EMMA C. DOWD.

TO THE POINT.

WE admire the terse aggressiveness of the short editorials in *American Medicine.* The following are examples in hand:

PHYSICIANS' STRIKES.

We have long wondered when physicians, irritated by a hundred forms of popular ingratitude, would go on strike. While laboring heroically to prevent disease and thus committing professional suicide, we are constantly maligned, the lowest kind of protection is generally denied to us by the law-makers and Government-protected quackery flourishes. But according to the proverb, even the worm will turn; and it has turned in Germany. The Sickness Bureaus (*Krankenkassen*) are the intermediaries whereby about 30,000,000 people obtain practically free medical service—of course at the expense of the profession. When the bureaus made the physicians into slaves by all sorts of demands, at about 15 cents a call, or $75 a year, most naturally there was "a strike," or what the newspapers call a recurrence of the old question of "recognizing the Union." Fifteen cent fees for cases of obstetrics, or operations, was more than human nature, even of the long-suffering bureaucratic German type, could endure. The strange thing in all these cases is that the public does not recognize that the service obtained by such methods and prices can hardly be called medical. How can therapeutics be possible under such conditions? Physicians would be more than human who could keep such ludicrous relations from vitiating into extremes of abuse and degradation. It is as poor financial policy for the patient as for the doctors. We wish that the charges of "medical monopoly" by the hate-filled antis were truer or more possible of realization among us.

THE MOST ILLOGICAL THING IN THE WORLD

Is to sacrifice life itself in the fight for the luxuries of life. The Health Department of Chicago finds that during the week of high stock speculation in Chicago there was an increase of about 25 per cent. in the normal number of deaths of people sixty years of age and over. Money, of course, represents only the means of carrying on the business of life, and when the craze for it reaches such an intensity that it hastens death, it becomes a positive disease. In all the severe symptoms of the disease exhibited in the trust-formings, stock-waterings,' and stock-speculations, our quiet professional world goes on with its beneficent work of healing, untouched, directly, we hope, by the furious greed of wealth that uses up life in the illogical chase for the means of living. It is fortunate if the gathering and analysis of vital statistics has become so accurate that the figures are able to point us to the origins of disease and the lessened death-rate. And yet there were always in our ears the warning axiomatic words, "What shall it profit a man if he shall gain the whole world and lose his own soul?" Disease and death are old teachers of morality. How slowly is the lesson learned?

PNEUMONIA MORE FATAL THAN TUBERCULOSIS.

This is the teaching of statistics. In New York, from 1890 to 1900, there were 56,092 deaths from pneumonia, and 50,490 from pulmonary tuberculosis, and in Chicago the relative figures are 25,228, and 22,957. The increased mortality from pneumonia is ascribed to influenza, which, although also increasing the fatality of tuberculosis, does so to a much greater degree in the more acute disease, pneumonia. The fact that the first death from influenza in New York was reported in December, 1889, shows how suddenly the causes of death may change, and how quickly we must be prepared to deal with new and dangerous diseases. The report of the New York State Board of Health for the month of March shows that influenza has caused about 1,500 deaths, and that 76 per cent. of the deaths from acute respiratory diseases were from pneumonia. The fundamental condition underlying the rise and continuance of an acute infectious disease, such as influenza, is probably the tremendously increased amount in travel. Re-infection from new foci constantly occurs in places in which the disease is dying out, and every city or part of the country is bound up with all others by the railroads. The problem of disease in a high state of civilization becomes more than ever one of prevention, and yet how slow is civilization to recognize and act upon the fact. Millions for tribute but not one cent for defense, is the motto of the modern "statesman."

HER RECORD FAULTY.

"Your record seems to be all right," said St. Peter to the applicant at the gate. "You were charitable, virtuous and reasonably good in other ways, I think——"

"Hold!" exclaimed the recording angel, suddenly looking up from the big book. "I find one big black mark against her. She showed an utter lack of consideration for others."

"What did she do?" said St. Peter.

"She made a regular practice of cooking onions and cabbage in a flat building."—*Chicago Post.*

HELPING A LITTLE.

(From the *American Agriculturist.*)

When the days are hot and growing hotter,
And earth is dry as a worn out blotter,
When the grass is crisp and the sky is copper,
And more than a burden is each grasshopper,
When the shrill cicada's redhot voice is
A note at which no heart rejoices,
When at every crack the dust is sifting,
And gasping hens their wings are lifting.
I like to think of the deep snow drifting,
Of frost-bound pond and icicles brittle:
      It helps a little.

Department of Hygiene.

WITH SPECIAL REFERENCE TO STATE AND PREVENTIVE MEDICINE.

DIVERSION, ETHICS AND THE DOCTOR.

ONE of our Brevity Club contributors criticizes the proverbial gravity and stern decorum of professional men; and while it must be admitted that medical men represent one of the learned and admittedly dignified and very responsible professions, an unsophisticated layman, listening to the usual medical essay, as read, with either stumbling hesitation, idiotic punctuation or absolutely no rhetorical expression, or else with a stilted pomposity that makes it sound like a schoolboy's first attempt at a funeral oration, is not astonished at the criticism. And when one considers the usual audiences before which these scientifically lugubrious dissertations are exploited it would be excusable to assume that for a medical professor to smile or to perpetrate a deliberate pun would constitute a crime worthy of capital punishment under the code.

The statement that doctors are shorter lived than the members of other professions is warranted by the facts. Is it because they seldom laugh? Victor Hugo's "L'Homme Qui Rit" certainly was not a doctor of medicine. As a class, with a few jolly exceptions, medical men are so professionally proper, and so hemmed in by a kind of stilted code of etiquette, that they can hardly be expected to enjoy good health, for lack of natural relaxation and the wholesome influences of those sweet amenities that go so far toward making human existence worth the candle!

Why should the medical, only, of all the professions, be forever done up in starched stomachers, and stuck up on stilts?

The literary man belongs to his clubs and has his carte blanche to unbend in all social circles; the judge on the bench, the advocate at the bar—even the man of God in his clerical robes—all these at times throw off their formal airs, shed their unwonted dignity, as the snake sheds its skin, and give themselves over to social relaxation. Your "Adirondack" Murrays, with their fast horses, buckboards, and beautiful women; your Beechers, Tiltons, Tallmadges, and Downs, all found a following of exculpators and apologists; but where is the clientèle to stand by the medical suspect accused by blackmailing husbands, hysterical wives, or prudish old maids?

The busy medical practitioner is practically at the mercy of every social wind that blows, the prey of every scheming man and neurotic woman, of every eccentric, monomaniac, and social crank that runs at large. He is never quite sure when an hour of the day or night is his own. If he presumes to partake of the good things of the world he must be content to receive his blessings, as it were, at the point of a hypodermic needle, or by cutaneous absorption. Even his conjugal seances—of course he must marry—are at all times subject to sudden and unseasonable interruption; and sometimes a breath of undeserved calumny, or the morbid imaginings of a hypochondriac or hystero-epileptic are sufficient to damn his reputation forever.

The truth is, medical practice is not yet on a business basis, and prevailing medical ethics are a standing illustration, in four colors, of *how not to do it*. And this statement is intended to cover the whole ground of the subject treated elsewhere in this number, as well as in previous numbers of the GAZETTE—competition, advertising, educating the public in health matters, professional intercourse and the relations of the profession to the public.

If the priest or the Levite discovers a new process or product, or learns a new application of an old principle; if the scholar, the judge on the bench, the briefless lawyer, or the theologic expounder, brings out a fresh idea, or a new way of utilizing an old one, the Patent Office or the Librarian of Congress issues him a perpetual caveat; straightway he deserts his calling and becomes a bloated patent-right monopolist, with the whole power of the State or the national government standing at his back to ward off cowans, eavesdroppers, and bandits.

How is it with the hardworked and underpaid medical discoverer and inventor? Even though he should produce a contrivance that would forever banish all pain from the universe, render manual labor a thing of the past, blot out evil and poverty from the face of the earth as sunlight banishes darkness, and that would prolong human life to the rounded period of a thousand years, yet must he publish it all without money and without price, in the next number of the *Medical Oracle*, with working drawings and every ingredient and process accurately weighed and described.

And all for what return or recompense?

To see his name spelled wrong in the next issue of the *Oracle*, and receive a dozen extra copies of that erudite publication, on which to waste postage stamps in franking them to "dear" old grannies in and out of the profession, or to jealous rivals who will take delight in consigning them to the gaping waste basket; or in cremating them to slow music, in the same batch with Patent Office reports and Hostetter's Almanacs.

The medical practitioner is unlike other professional men in that he is not allowed to choose whom he will serve. In other words, he must respond with equal alacrity at the beck of all, rich or poor, honest or dishonest, pure or impure. For him there are no lighthouse signals, no moral or commercial Bradstreets and Duns to forefend him from deadbeat shoals and confidence rocks, and no courts of equity to recoup his reputation or award him damages for abuse, heaped thickest by some of the very ones for whom he has done most. Verily he is compelled to cast his pearls before the world's swine; and when they turn and rend him the same world usually sneers or looks on with a good-enough-for-him complacency. In short, there is for him an unwritten law—usually called "moral," but is often diabolical—that compels him to squander time, brains, midnight oil, and his astutest skill, to the end that he may avoid suits for malpractice by serving and saving some very good, but too often ungrateful people, along with a good many worthless shysters, who seem to live for the sole purpose of abusing the doctor and procuring medical services under false pretences.

Again, the merchant sheds oceans of printer's ink, and finds in it his business sheet anchor; the lawyer is permitted and expected to blow his own horn, night and day, before every judge, jury, courtroom crowd, and political gathering; the judge on the bench is placarded in all the dailies and utters pettifogging decisions to gaping crowds; even the man of the cloth, the follower of the meek and lowly Nazarene, has the benefit of his Thursday sewing circles, all the periodic sociables, with house to house visiting, and full swing from his pulpit on Sunday. No one will question his goings and comings if he makes a little personal and professional capital out of public conventions, political meetings, and agricultural "hoss trots." He may even avail himself of that acme of American impudence and cheek—the repertorial interview, without losing caste.

The physician who presumes to avail himself ever so modestly of any of these avenues to acquaintance and popularity, unless he be one of the lucky few who have already acquired both fame and filthy lucre, will find himself butting his silly brains out against the outer ramparts of the sacred Code. This Magna Charta, invented for the mediocres rather than the mighty, alleges in dignified cadences that "it is derogatory to the character of the physician" to adopt business methods in announcing his wares or his qualifications to serve the public. He must resolutely hide his light under a bushel, must never mention to his nearest friend such favorable facilities as have fallen to his lot, must never advert to the extent of his experience, nor divulge the nature of any discoveries or improvements he may have made. To display any semblance of commercial enterprise or common sense businesss constitutes a professional blunder, for which he is held amenable and subjected to ostracism.

In short, for the professional medicus, bursting, perhaps, to tell the world how to do some one thing in a great deal better manner and far less time than it has ever been done, these are the only avenues.

He must become Dean of a medical college (that isn't needed!), found a hospital for green young sawbones to experiment in, invent an obstetric forceps or a lithotrite, edit a medical journal with a proprietary pull, or sell certificates to manufacturers, verifying the claims for purity, superiority, and efficacy of all the multiplying examples of lacto-pepto-pancreatized emulsions of saccharated sourkrout!

One thing more, he may say, on the lower left-hand corner of his business card, in type so punctiliously small that nobody will ever take the pains to read it: "Practice limited to diseases of the pyloric orifice of the Galenical gizzard"; or, "Specialty—Latero-posterior enucleation of the healthy appendix"; or, "X Ray illumination of congenital femurs, with press reporters as paid assistants."

All this is almost legitimate, and is quite winked at by the superannuated greatgrandmothers who still recite parrot-talk platitudes at all the association meetings.

But "Victis" has cause to thank his stars and take courage. The medical mountain is slowly but surely approaching full term. What she will bring forth no living prophet can foretell. It is, however, to be earnestly hoped that no indiscreet conduct on the part of her many and officious nurses will precipitate a calamity by causing her to abort!

ANENT THE ANOPHELES.

Mr. Newnham W. Fynn, according to *Climate*, has had an experience of twenty-four years backwards and forwards to the west coast of Africa, having been stationed there so long as two years at a time. For the last seventeen years he has been going to and from Old Calabar, where mosquitoes are very rarely seen or heard, and during that period he has never used mosquito curtains, either by day or night. There has been a lot of sickness at that place from malarial fevers, and it is his opinion, after his long experience, that these fevers are caused solely by the miasma arising at break of day from the swamps, and decaying vegetation washed down by heavy rains, the majority of fever cases having happened generally, between early morning and noon.

In Mr. Fynn's opinion, the theory that mosquitoes are the cause of fever is untrue. Mr. Fynn has nursed scores of men during the stages of malarial fever, and, although sleeping in the same room, has suffered no ill effects. It is very seldom that he has heard of a second case within a month in the same habitation. He has not suffered in any way from mosquito bites nor does he know of any one who has taken the fever owing to mosquito bites. He has had conversations with medical men and traders—friends of his—who have been for a long time on on the coast, and they one and all look upon the mosquito theory in the same light as himself.

There is more sickness from fever where there are no mosquitoes, than in parts where it is almost impossible to sleep, even with mosquito curtains, owing to those pests.

The majority of cases (in Mr. Fynn's opinion) of fever have been caused by young men not taking care of the amount of clothing they wear, especially as regards the feet and head. They neglect—after perspiring and getting their clothes damp—to change, with the result that they catch a chill. Mr. Fynn puts down his fevers, and he has had many of them, to the miasma from the swamps, etc., and from exposure to chills after being run down in health from the want of good nourishing food—vegetables and fresh milk—at times. Having to start work at 6 o'clock in the morning, before the night mists are cleared, it often happens that before 9 A. M. you are attacked by pains in the legs and back as a consequence of inhaling the miasma. Another cause of fever is taking cold baths in the heat of the day, resulting invariably in a chill. Mr. Fynn says that tepid water should always be used for bathing.

On his last day in Africa, whilst at Bakana, he was kept awake one night by mosquitoes and sandflies, but he was not laid up with malarial fever afterwards. On his first stay of three and a half years at the Rivers Bonny and New Calabar, he had two very severe fevers, but came home looking fit and well. After being at home about one month, he was suddenly taken with the African fever whilst walking in Bold street, Liverpool, where there are no mosquitoes, showing that the malaria was still in his system.

Mr. Fynn's opinion is that fair men do better in West Africa than dark men, as regards health; but every one takes the fever. Owing to the impossibility of draining the swamps on the coast, Western Africa will always be unhealthy.

The best preventatives are good dwellings, good nourishing food, but not too much of it, good protection from heat and cold, to always wear light flannel next the skin, and not cotton, be careful in the use of stimulants, and avoid night air and living in native towns as much as possible, owing to their poor sanitary conditions.

The great point when ill is good nursing and attention.

Health on the Upper Niger was bad when he was there early in the year. This surely could not be put down to mosquitos, but to bad sanitation and the use of river water.

FOOD AS A FACTOR IN THE CAUSATION OF DISEASE.

At a recent meeting of the Medical Association of the Greater City of New York, Dr. Elmer Lee read a paper with the above title, a synopsis of which we reproduce from the columns of the *Medical News:*

The science of living, he said, begins at the mouth. As a man eats and digests his food, so is he. Disease is latent in every man, and at all times. Food is both the saving and the undoing of health. Food, rightly used, means health and strength. Neglect to feed the body safely is the starting-point in pathology. The universality of sickness, suffering and premature death requires a universal cause for their explanation. The habit of letting into the system unprepared and unsafe nutriment is the only admissible solution. Theories have long been put out to explain the riddle, but have ever remained theories. In the extreme urgency to satisfy the demand for an answer to the question, plausible hypotheses have grown up. The germ theory is the one most prominent at this time, but it is incomplete and unsatisfactory, for it cannot account for the germ itself.

There is one health, and that condition which is not health is disease. Any departure from perfect health and economy of vital action is a first stage of disease. Every variation from the normal state is a degree. Sickness is composed of many degrees. The words "slight," "serious," "dangerous" and "fatal" are terms representing different states or degrees of disease. But in each instance disease is a backward process, while health is progressive. Inaction and retarded action within the body are the beginnings of disease from the misuse of food. As food enters into the substance of man, so is it his health or the opposite. All systems of medicine amount to nothing unless founded on what is carried within the human body as essential nutriment to its growth and life. The right uses of food build for health and vigor and preclude disease. Each physician should apply the test of sound and continuous health to himself as the measure of his scientific knowledge of human vital action. Sound and continuous health is the sequence of habitual living by knowledge and not by chance.

Various members discussed the paper, each from his own standpoint.

Dr. Ransford E. Van Gieson thought that all must acknowledge that the improper selection and preparation of food and imperfect mastication are undoubtedly responsible for a large amount of ill health. Man is more or less an animal, but his instincts do not always guide him correctly, as in the case of the lower animals. Doubtless the broad ground taken by Dr. Lee is measurably true, and it is a matter of observation that the physician who is most successful is he who takes the greatest pains to instruct his patients in regard to their diet and the proper manner of taking it. But, at the same time, Dr. Van Gieson said, he was not prepared to accept in its totality the theory as to the universal causation of disease set forth in the paper. He would especially take exception as regards the etiology of epidemic disease.

Other members present added suggestive comments. One urged the necessity of complete mastication.

It was urged that complete mastication was quite as essential as proper food; that every physician should be a good cook, able to give exact instructions in the culinary art to cook or nurse; and, if need be, to himself prepare the diet for the invalid. Dr. Quintard mentioned a few instances coming under his observations in which special varieties of disease were produced by particular articles of food.

Having spoken of the eczematous-like eruption caused by oatmeal, he said that he had met with three cases in which the eating of salted almonds resulted in the production of peculiar little ulcers of the tongue. He had frequently observed that the free use of sweets and pastry gave rise to a peculiar form of gastritis accompanied by hyperacidity. In subjects with a tendency to affections of the mucous membranes highly-seasoned foods were also very apt to produce gastritis. From cases he had observed he was inclined to the opinion that in chlorotic girls, much given to the use of sweets and suffering from hyperacidity, such food is sometimes the cause of gastric ulcer. There is a peculiar form of diarrhea, almost dysenteric in character and coming on almost immediately after meals, which is due to an inordinate amount of fluid taken with the meals. This had the effect of diluting the gastric juice to such an extent that it could not properly perform its function, and increased peristalsis was caused by the irritation thus set up in the intestine.

Dr. Cammac said that Dr. Lee's ideas were far from being out of accord with the results of bacteriological research. It was because of a loss of nutrition in some part of the body that the disease germs were enabled to get a foothold. Thus, pernicious anemia was caused by a gradual failure of resistance on the part of the digestive tract to the onset of micro-organisms having a destructive action upon the blood.

Dr. A. Rose thought there was a danger in generalizing too much. He had known of patients who, under a carefully-regulated diet prescribed by stomach specialists, had continued to suffer greatly, but who, when allowed to eat everything they wanted to, immediately got well. We should not forget that what is satisfactory in the case of one individual may be dangerous to another. Gerhardt had pointed out that many of the late hemorrhages in typhoid fever were due, not to typhoid ulcerations in the intestine.

but to a form of scurvy resulting from an exclusive milk diet. He therefore advised that typhoid patients should be given more or less vegetable food, such as spinach, watercress, and the like.

OBJECTIONABLE NAMES FOR INSTITUTIONS.

THE choice of a name for an institution designed primarily for the relief of suffering, or for developing arrested mentality in children," says the *Phila. Med. Journal,* "is one upon which very much depends. It is rather more than sentiment which has so often prompted objections to such titles as Home for Incurables, Home for Consumptives, Cancer Hospital, Institute for the Feeble-Minded, and even (as recently established in England) a Hospital for the Dying. There is something of pathos in the thought of a man digging the grave in which his bones will rest—there is a gross violation of the delicacy that is born of the broad spirit of humanitarianism, in the thought of tagging a man's remaining days with the stigma of the malady from which he suffers. Every physician well knows the truth of the lines:

"The wretch condemned with life to part,
    Still, still on hope relies,
And every pang that rends the heart
    Bids expectation rise."

It behooves us to champion the changing of these objectionable names of institutions. Let us select something which shall not typify so ruthlessly the blasted lives, or undeveloped faculties of the unfortunates entrusted to our care. We recognize fully the value of the element of suggestion in bettering the physical processes through the mental, and we know full well how a patient, deprived of hope, will quickly wane and die:

"Hope, dead, lives nevermore,
    No, not in Heaven."

The objects and aims of such institutions are by no means furthered by this method of designation. Rather do they become places to be dreaded and shunned. It may be urged in defense of these titles that after all a name stands for little; that the patients will know soon enough the true import of their disease and their surroundings. But how much better the late Dr. J. M. DaCosta expressed the thought in bequeathing a sum of money to the Pennsylvania Hospital for the endowment of a ward for cases "now deemed incurable." The avenue of hope is still left open. Every effort in the direction of eradicating the significance of hopelessness in these cases must be regarded in the light of removing the fetters of apparent banishment and ostracism.

THE DAY'S DEMAND.

GOD give us men! A time like this demands
Strong minds, great hearts, true faith and
    willing hands,
Men whom the lust for office does not kill;
Men whom the spoils of office cannot buy;
Men who possess opinions and a will;
Men who have honor; men who will not
    lie;
Men who can stand before a demagogue
And damn his treacherous flatteries without
    winking;
Tall men, sun-crowned, who live above the
    fog
In public duty and in private thinking.
For while the rabble, with their thumb-worn
    creeds,
Their large professions and their little
    deeds,
Mingle in selfish strife, lo! freedom weeps;
Wrong rules the land, and waiting justice
    sleeps.
                              —J. G. HOLLAND.

THE THERAPEUTIC VALUE OF CLI-
MATE, WITH A WORD CONCERN-
ING SOME AMERICAN CLIMATES.

WARMER CLIMES.

A QUARTER of a century ago the only
warm corner resorted to in this country by
invalids and frost-fearing climate-seekers
was the semi-peninsula of Florida. She was
poetically called the "Land of Flowers,"
and as such for years, both literally and fig-
uratively, bore the palm. Since other localities and claimants for popular favor have
been investigated and tested, and traveling
facilities to them have been multiplied and
improved, the fame of the older community
has been proportionately overshadowed and
diminished in brilliancy. Once the only
American Mecca toward which winter
travel regularly set in with the holidays, she
must now compete with a dozen other resorts and bear the brunt of the always exaggerated adverse criticism which invariably results from active rivalry.

The fabled Fountain of Youth and all
the cherished dreams of Sir Knight Ponce
de Leon have faded into the mists of
mythology. Nevertheless that visionary
achieved a degree of immortality for his
name, which is being perpetuated in a gor-
geous and artistic monument of brick and
stone (coquina?) at St. Augustine.

The drawbacks alleged are excessive humidity, fogs, malaria and mosquitoes. Within recent years the occasional occurrence of
severe and killing frosts must be added
to this list. Partly on account of these objections and bugaboos and partly for other
reasons, many who once spent their winters at St. Augustine, Palm Beach, Lake
Worth, or other Florida rendezvous, now
betake themselves to some of the many
competing resorts. Some cross the ocean,
go farther and fare worse, for the sake of
fad or fashion. But there are others to
take their places, and a host of those who
insist that there is no sport quite equal to
tarpon fishing, no boat ride so startlingly
picturesque as a stern-wheel chase up the

crooked, shallow and moss-fringed Okala-
waha, and positively no hotels in the world
to be mentioned in the same breath with the
sumptuous "Alcazar," the palatial "Ponce
de Leon," or the "Royal Poinciana."

Florida is, however, strictly a winter climate, and much of its winter weather is
superb. Its summers are hot, humid, and
depressing. The weather libel as to Vermont and New Hampshire might here be
very aptly reversed. There is three months
of summer and nine months of—blasted hot
weather.

THE MODERN PONCE DE LEON.

To drink from the fabled fountain is still
possible, says the modern chemico-physiolo-
gist. Hear him:

"The change from youthfulness to age is
that of increasing calcification. Youth is
gelatinous; old age is osseous. To prevent
this accumulation of earthy elements in the
tissues is to remain young. To permit and
hasten it is to grow old. It is not possible
to check it entirely, but it can be materially
delayed. The rational means are, regulation of the diet—less food that is known to
be rich in the earthy and calcifying elements, and more fruit and bland vegetables
which are not rich in calcic salts. Second,
counteraction, by promoting more rapid
and perfect elimination of any excess
of the earthy salts absorbed by the
system. This may be effected by
all the approved hygienic measures
keeping all the emunctories free, copious water drinking, plenty of open air
exercise, Turkish baths, massage, avoidance
of water that is very hard; to all of which
may be added the taking of about fifteen
drops of dilute phosphoric acid in a tumbler
of distilled water after each meal.

"Results, tissues retain their suppleness,
circulatory system remains elastic, longevity, youth in age—a practical realization of
the Fountain of Youth."

Ponce de Leon failed to definitely discover it; nevertheless, he was an unconscious prophet.

"This were to be new made when thou art
　old,
And see thy blood warm when thou feel'st
　it cold."

Thomasville, Georgia, presents some
marked contrasts. Its soil is absorbent, its
atmosphere, redolent of pines and balsams,
is drier, while fogs are less frequent and
much less overwhelming. The air-tempera-
ture is lower and much of the time enjoyable. Instead of being depressing, it is
tonic and supporting. The place and its
surroundings are acquiring a creditable and
increasing if not yet quite national reputation.

Asheville, North Carolina, and *Aiken*,
South Carolina, illustrate still further modifications, occupying a position between the
warm and cool climates. The former has
an altitude of 2,300 feet above sea-level,
while the latter is but 500 feet above tide
water. Asheville has a mean annual temperature (our first offence in the statistical
line!) of 49° F., the seasonal means being:
spring, 52°; summer 71°; autumn, 55°;
and winter 37°. The maximum for January is 60°, and the minimum for the same
month, 10°.

Aiken is some degrees warmer.

The annual precipitation amounts to 44
inches. In winter sudden changes and frequent snow squalls are a trying feature; but
when the weather is good it is very, very
good, giving opportunity to forget that
which is "horrid." The scenery about Asheville and the valley of the French Broad
River is among the finest to be found in the
United States.

WHO'LL GO TO TEXAS?

An area large enough to engulf the Republic of France, altitudes ranging all the
way from sea level at the Gulf coast to
mountain summits 9,000 feet high, in the
northwestern corner of the State, and with
climates scattered all along from downright tropic at the extreme south to decidedly chilly at the extreme north, Texas
ought to be able to furnish wealth, weather

and wildness for half a dozen full fledged
nations. And so she is.

There are local drawbacks—there was
the serpent in Eden! The principal of these
is that lurking foe that "walketh in darkness
and breeds in warmth and wetness" in many
otherwise fair corners of the United States.
It is well in evidence in the northeastern
counties, and not unknown along the Gulf
coast; but there is no need of hunting for
it. Its breeding grounds can be avoided.
The coast is subject to extremes of heat
and humidity during four months of the
year, while during the remaining eight
months this condition is appreciably and
gratefully modified by the prevalence of a
gentle Gulf breeze, corresponding to the
sea breeze of other localities.

San Antonio is the most beautiful of her
many cities, and is made the winter home
of very many fine people from further
north. It affords all the civilized and many
of the esthetic "conveniences," and is the
brightest city in the whole South.

It is, however, the middle western portion of the State that has acquired the
widest repute among invalids, especially in
the treatment of chronic throat and lung
ailments. The most favored and famous
localities are the high tablelands lying to
t'e westward of the Rio Pecos, at altitudes
varying from 2,500 to nearly 6,000 feet.
One of the principal rallying points is *Fort
Davis*, the site of an abandoned army post,
situated at the foot of the Davis Mountains,
which shelter it from the "Northers" that
are occasionally severe at other points. The
altitude at Fort Davis is 5,200 feet, soil
warm, dry, and permeable, drainage excellent, and mean annual temperature 59°
F. The annual rainfall does not exceed 20
inches; consequently, vegetation is scant,
and the average atmospheric humidity is
less than 36 per cent. at midday and but 53
per cent. night and day, for the year. Sunshine prevails during most of the day, on
an average of 328 *days of the year*, and during the entire winter there are, on an average, *but five cloudy days*, a most remarkable
record.

The place is reached by a short stage ride from Marfia, on the Southern Pacific Railroad.

El Paso, immediately on the line of the Great Southern Thoroughfare, is on the extreme western border of the State. It is both warmer and drier than Fort Davis, the mean temperature being about 65° F. The higher temperature is due chiefly to its greater longitude and lower altitude. The latter, about 3,700 feet, makes the site more favorable for certain classes of invalids. The place lacks the shelter of mountains, and is therefore a prey to some high winds that do not reach the other side.

These two localities are so nearly representative of others in this region that the latter need not be individually mentioned.

The diseases benefited are asthma, bronchitis, humid catarrh, the chronic indigestions, and consumption in its early stages. Those who have suffered from *la grippe*, but have never fully recovered, do well at either place.

THE *Medical Record* is authority for the following; On April 1st, at a sitting of the French Academy of Sciences, M. Curie, a chemist, separated a new gas from rhodium. The gas is intensely phosporescent, and will glow for months in the dark. It was also announced that M. Naudon, a scientist, had found means of producing X-rays without electricity, by exposing a metal plate to the violet end of the spectrum."

SAYS Ruskin: "Hundreds of people can talk for one who can think; but thousands can think for one who can see."

"THE greatest thing that a human soul ever does in this world is to see something and tell what it saw in a plain way."

FRUIT BREAKFASTS.

PATIENTS with thick, non-circulating blood, torpid lymphatics, and dormant secretions; patients with stiffened joints, gouty deposits, chronic neuralgias, torpid livers, uric-acid kidneys, and the irritable nerve centers that go with them, and others who suffer from errors of nutrition, can be greatly benefited, not to say cured, by the simple dietetic procedure known as the fruit breakfast.

Accordinng to *London Health*, this means just what it says. Fruit, all the patient wants, and nothing else for breakfast. No chops, bread, cereals, coffee, tea, or anything but fruit before twelve o'clock. By fruit is meant apples, oranges, and grapes. These should be of excellent quality. Preserved fruit juices do not answer as well and no other kind of fruit compares in efficacy with oranges, apples and grapes. No sugar should be used on the fruit. Cooked fruit will not do.

Just what effects these natural fruit juices have on the blood is not easy to say, but they certainly do contrive to purge, purify, and alter it for the better. Two months of the fruit breakfast will work a practical miracle in a body full of the morbid products of chronic disease. The patient feels lighter, more active and cheerful. The circulation is accomplished with less friction, and is better equalized. The glutinous quality of the blood has been overcome, and no longer paralyzes tissue cells as treacle does the wings of a fly. Assimilation and elimination are better performed. The secretions are all of a higher physiological standard.

The difficulty is to get the patient to refrain from eating all other foods in the morning. and unless he does this, he will get little or no benefit. Habit is strong, and for some days the patient may feel a craving for the usual breakfast, a gnawing sense of dissatisfaction. but if he persevere this will gradually give way. The amount of fruit is not limited. He can eat all he wants of that.

No stimulants of any kind should be used while taking this cure.

It is not necessary that the fruit breakfast should be a permanent thing. Three months will put the system in excellent order, and then the patient may return to his former habits, if he desires, making use of the fruit breakfast whenever the symptoms indicate that nutrition is again deranged.

SUNLIGHT OR SLEEP FOR CHILDREN?

A CORRESPONDENT of the *Boston Med. and Surg. Journal* writes as follows:

"I have recently passed through an experience that may prove of some value in answering the above questions. You know how prevalent the opinion is among those who have the means to enable them to take the best care of their children, that they should be put to bed in the middle of the day and sleep an hour or two. We have tried most thoroughly this system with our two children, continuing it until they arrived at the ages of two and one-half and three and three-quarters, respectively. They were very healthy children naturally, but we were constantly obliged to have medical attendance for them, and at one time they had serious difficulty with their ears, requiring surgical operations. Although they slept an hour or two, it kept them in-doors the best portion of the day. Between dressing and undressing, lunch and sleeping, there were six months in the year when they got, practically, very little sunlight, and what they did get was of very little consequence, it being so early in the morning or so late in the afternoon.

About six months ago we ceased putting them to bed, and let them play out-doors all day long, and immediately we saw an improvement. Since then they have constantly gained, until now they are as robust as any children could well be. Although one swallow does not make a summer, two swallows are twice as near to it, and our experience with these two children seems to me to go far towards proving that sunlight is one of the most effective agents for preserving the health of any living creature.

Nobody can over-estimate the value to health of sleep, but does the child get more sleep in the twenty-four hours by being put to sleep in the middle of the day? Our experience proved to us that this was not the case. For though our children slept an hour and a half during the day, they lost from one-half to three-quarters of an hour in getting to sleep in the evening, and woke an hour earlier than now in the morning."

GOLD COIN SUPPLANTING PAPER.

WE are not conducting a financial review nor coaching for the next presidential election, but we reproduce the following from the *Ft. Dodge* (Iowa) *Messenger:*

George E. Roberts, director of the mint, includes in his annual report the result of an interesting inquiry into the money supply of the world. It has been said the volume of the world's money was cut in two in 1873, and that all the ills which society has since suffered have been due to this alleged fact. Millions of well-meaning persons, not staying to discover whether the asserted thing were true or not, have accepted it and built political opinions thereon. Mr. Roberts' cold and calm figures, gathered from official sources, show that instead of the money supply having diminished since 1873, it has increased more than 150 per cent—a rate of increase much faster than the rate of increase in the world's population.

In 1873 the total stock of money in the world, gold, silver and paper, was $4,600,-000,000. The world's supply of money in 1900 was $11,600,000,000. There has been a gross increase of $7,000,000,000 in the world's stock of money since the commission of the crime of 1873. The increase in the amount of gold has been $3,600,000,-000; of silver, $2,750,000,000, and of paper, about $650,000,000. The world is using a greater proportion of metallic money and a greater proportion of gold. During the last seven years there was an increase of $950,000,000 in the world's supply of coined gold alone.

In the opinion of Mr. Roberts, the great outburst of activity in the mining of gold, which commenced four or five years ago, and which is going on with unabated vigor, promises to supply nearly the entire monetary needs of the world, without resort to any material increase in the amount of circulation. Whatever may have been true concerning the money question ten or twenty years ago, it is now obvious that there has been a complete change in conditions. The bimetallist of 1873, without the slightest inconsistency, may be the gold monometallist of 1900. The increase in the supply of gold has introduced a new element into the monetary problem which cannot logically be ignored.

With more gold alone now in monetary use than there was of both gold and silver twenty years ago, and with every indication that the stock of gold money will further increase, even students of "Coin's Financial School" must admit that something has come into the argument which the author of that plausible pamphlet did not foresee, or found it convenient to ignore. It is not true that one pile of wheat has been destroyed, thereby doubling the value of the remaining pile; the pile of monetary wheat is bigger than ever before, according to Mr. Roberts' authentic figures, 150 per cent. bigger than in 1873.

THE VITALISTIC IDEA OF LIFE.

Under this head, some one says:

"1· All organisms have in common a certain substance, that is albuminous matter.

"2· All organisms are built up by cells.

"3. All organisms are individual.

"4. All organisms have the same mode of growth.

"5· All organisms have the same mode of propagation."

ON THE "HYPURGIE" OF OBESITY.

Mendelsohn, editor of the *Zeitschrift für Krankenpflege*, has devised the term "hypurgie" to denote that special exercise of the physician and nurse which seeks to attain the comfort of the patient upon all occasions.

In the July number of his journal, according to the *Med. Review of Reviews*, Mendelsohn extracts from Van Noorden's new work on obesity various practical points which bear upon the questions of nursing and hypurgie.

The capacity for exertion on the part of the corpulent patient must first of all be determined for a given time. Those who have a normal tolerance for exertion may be made to work hard, and by following out this principle we avoid excess. The quality of the exercise must be studied. If a patient ascends an elevation 300 metres high he expends the same energy whether he takes 100 minutes or only 60 minutes for the task, but in the latter case he may overtask his heart. Both in walking on a level and in hill-climbing, the effect on the heart and voluntary muscles must be carefully supervised. The better the ventilation of the lungs, the less liability to heart strain.

The introduction of the bicycle into medicine is a great advantage in the management of obesity, but the heart is equally exposed to danger in this form of exercise. The fat bicyclist should never be allowed to bend forward, because of the prejudicial effect upon respiration. Rowing, either on the water, or with a parlor rowing machine, is strongly recommended by good authorities, and tests made after this form of exercise show that the pulse and heart are not overtasked. Vigorous obese individuals may play active outdoor games—tennis, football, golf, etc. The principal value of gymnasium exercise lies in the development of certain groups of muscles, and the general strengthening of the entire muscular system.

On the other hand, horseback exercise is not recommended. It is good to reduce the horse's weight, but not so good in this respect for the rider.

Baths, both for the sake of cleanliness and as hydrotherapy, are of the greatest benefit to the obese.

With regard to diet Van Noorden believes in the expediency of small and somewhat frequent meals. In this way we avoid the profound weakness which comes from an empty stomach (often causing fat women to swoon), as well as the danger of overeating.

Wine should never be taken with meals, but between meals it is often grateful. Mineral waters, weak tea, lemonade, etc., may be taken either with or between meals.

A SPECIAL PROCESS FOR PRODUC- ING ARTIFICIAL SLEEP.

P. HARTENBERG, in the *Journal de Neurologie:*

IT often happens in the experience of every physician that hypnotic sleep is indicated, but for various reasons cannot be employed. The practitioner is thus obliged to relinquish a method of treatment from which good results would be obtained. Under these circumstances the possibility of indirect suggestion occurred to the writer. Might not the therapeutic measure be applied without the patient being aware either of the name or the manner of the procedure? The difficulties would be avoided while preserving all the advantages of the direct method. To accomplish this the word "sleep" must not be mentioned, being in this respect exactly contrary to the usual method of hypnotic suggestion, where the word is constantly repeated and the subject knows that sleep is the end and aim of the maneuver.

The principle of procedure employed by Dr. Hartenberg is the influence of forced respiration upon the circulation and the cerebral activities. It is well known that forced respiration produces a flow of blood toward the thorax and at the same time a certain degree of cerebral anemia, followed by less- ened mental activity, dulness of consciousness and psychic rest. A series of inspirations, sufficiently deep and rapid, will even produce short anesthesia sufficient for slight surgical operations. A simple experiment demonstrates this fact. Seat yourself comfortably and breathe rapidly and deeply, so as to expand the chest to its utmost. Almost immediately there occurs a feeling of lassitude, a heaviness of the limbs and eyelids, a cerebral torpor. If continued, the eyes close involuntarily, and you are seized by an almost irresistible desire to sleep.

In practice, however, some excuse is necessary to the patient for these respiratory exercises; for this purpose Dr. Hartenberg employs electricity. He makes a pretense of electrical application and uses a faradic battery, which is a valuable auxiliary; in a word, he attributes his curative results to the use of electricity.

He seats the patient in an easy chair, directing complete relaxation of all the muscles; with his hands he holds over the forehead and thorax two large electrodes; these are connected by cords to a small faradic battery placed near by, the vibrator of which is set in motion, but from which no current passes to the patient. He then directs the patient to breathe deeply and regularly, inflating the chest as much as possible, and to concentrate the entire attention upon this exercise. He assures him that scrupulous compliance with these directions will increase the good effect of the treatment he is about to give. These instructions he repeats to the monotonous and continued accompaniment of the faradic interrupter for some little time. As a result the patient rapidly fatigues himself and little by little the inspirations decrease in amplitude and frequency, the eyelids gradually droop and close. The operator then lightly presses the eyeballs with one hand, and lowering his voice, directs the subject to breathe quietly and make no further effort. The restful position, muscular relaxation, pressure on the eyeballs, monotonous and continued sound, go far to reenforce the hypogenic action of the respiratory exercises.

This is the moment for the therapeutic suggestion, although in certain cases it may be necessary to repeat the breathing procedure two or three times before doing so. The operator closes with a general assurance of bien-être and satisfaction, removes his hand from the other electrode, stops his machine and leaves the patient to himself. In some cases the patient gradually awakens, in others he continues to sleep until forcibly aroused.

If the patient be questioned, he describes the condition as a very agreeable and comfortable one. He remembers what has occurred, although sometimes these recollections become confused at a certain point, and he forgets what has been said to him, or he believes it to have been a dream. This condition is absolutely the same as that obtained by verbal suggestion of sleep. The subject passes through every stage from light sleep to profound unconsciousness. The therapeutic advantages are the same obtained by verbal suggestion, viz.: repose, passivity, absence of control, and a receptivity favorable to curative suggestions. Furthermore, the concentration of attention upon the respiration is favorable to a monoidism in which the idea of a cure may be directly substituted for the respiratory idea.

Dr. Hartenberg does not, however, make any curative suggestions until the second or third séance. It is first necessary to accustom the patient to the treatment and teach him how to breathe.

The treatment has had no bad effects whatever, the only counter-indication being some cardiac trouble which may be easily discovered. In the three years during which the writer has employed this method his results have been invariably excellent. It has all the advantages and none of the disadvantages of a direct suggestion of sleep, and equally with it leads to the realization of curative suggestion. It can be employed where a thousand obstacles (prejudice, fear, amour-propre, religious belief) render hypnotism impossible. More than all, showing how dear to the mind is the illusion of free will, when the subject goes to sleep during the séance it does not disturb him. '' was

so comfortable I went to sleep.'' There lies the difference! He went to sleep but was not put to sleep!

Dr. Hartenberg believes this simple and easy procedure will be likely to render good service in nervous therapy.

THE "PAPYROS-EBERS."

BELIEVING that physicians, of all men, are most interested in the history of their art, the makers of Hemaboloids are now prepared to present to their friends in the medical profession a fac-simile reproduction of the beginning of the earliest medical treatise extant, together with transcription into hieroglyphics and translation of a portion of the text.

The famous "Papyros-Ebers," which was written during the reign of the Egyptian king Bicheres, 3,500 years ago, was discovered by the celebrated archeologist, George Ebers, in 1872, when an Arab brought him a metallic case containing a papyrus roll enveloped in mummy cloths, which he claimed had been discovered between the bones of a mummy in a tomb of the Theban Necropolis. A complete description of the papyros and its history is included in the reproduction and is certainly extremely interesting to physicians and antiquarians generally. A copy will be forwarded by The Palisade Mfg. Co., Yonkers, N. Y., to any physician who may have failed to receive one.

Do not worry, eat three square meals a day, say your prayers, be courteous to your creditors, keep your digestion good, steer clear of biliousness, exercise, go slow and go easy. Maybe there are other things that your special case requires to make you happy, but, my friend, these I reckon will give you a good lift.

ABRAHAM LINCOLN.

INFANT FEEDING.

A LITTLE treatise on "The Feeding of Infants," by Joseph E. Winters, M.D., Cornell University Medical College, published by E. P. Dutton & Co., New York, contains the following summary of the several preceding chapters devoted to modification, sterilization, etc. We quote first from the author's prefatory remarks:

"Two facts should be ever present in the mind when considering the feeding of infants.

"First—Of children born healthy and exclusively breast-fed, very few die during the first year of life, even in institutions or among the poor in tenements. A breast-fed infant is seldom ill, rarely coming under a physician's care until after the period of weaning.

"Second—Of children artificially fed, in institutions and in tenements, very few survive the first year.

"In these two immutable facts we have consummate proof that mother's milk is the ideal food for infants.

"When this is impracticable, the only method by which we can establish the value of an artificial substitute is to compare it with woman's milk.

"A substitute for human milk must resemble that perfect model as closely as possible in chemical composition and physiological properties."

*   *   *   *   *

RECAPITULATION.

"We have seen, then, that for the successful substitution of cow's milk for human milk the following conditions are essential:

"First—Pure, fresh milk.

"Second—It must be so modified that the proportions of the different constituents are made the same as in human milk.

"Third—Scrupulous cleanliness.

"Fourth—Quantity at each feeding, as indicated by the tables.

"Fifth—Semi-erect position during feeding.

"Sixth—Feeding slowly.

"Seventh—Regularity, as given in schedule.

"Eighth—Temperature of food 99° to 102° F.

"Ninth—After the first few weeks, six or eight hours of rest at night for the digestive organs."

SMALLPOX IS A PREVENTABLE DISEASE.

No intelligent person need have smallpox. It is a fact of common knowledge that vaccination destroys the susceptibility to the contagion. The experience of an hundred years throughout the civilized world has proved the absolute protection against smallpox, afforded by *thorough* vaccination, with *reliable* lymph, and repeated with *sufficient frequency.* The protection afforded by vaccination is not perpetual in all persons. Therefore revaccination should be practised after a few years, especially if the disease is prevalent.

A genuine vaccination in infancy and revaccination at the age of twelve or fourteen, will protect through life. The exceptions to this rule are exceedingly rare. There is no objection, however, to a subsequent vaccination as a means of additional safety, if one has been specially exposed or is liable to be.

Observe, the statement is made of "genuine vaccination." There are many spurious vaccinations. They are worse than none, because they give a false sense of security, and when they fail to afford the protection expected of them, they not only imperil the lives of the subjects, but bring an unjust odium upon the practice.

Trivial and simple as the operation appears, it nevertheless is one requiring skill and special knowledge to secure successful results. It is not only a foolish but a dangerous economy to entrust this responsible duty to nurses and midwives, or even to school teachers or ministers of the gospel. A person is usually capable of being vaccinated fully and successfully only *once in a* lifetime. The revaccinations are almost always more or less modified, if the first was genuine. Hence, it is of great importance that the first vaccination should be performed by a competent person, well acquainted with the phenomena of the vaccine pustule and the responsibilities of the act. The vaccine inflammation should always be inspected once or twice during its progress.

It is a well established fact, that if the operation is properly performed, under right conditions, it is not followed by any bad results other than a temporary inconvenience.

Every infant should be vaccinated about three months after its birth, unless an educated and intelligent physician advises against it, temporarily.

No parent or guardian should permit a child to go to school until it has been successfully vaccinated.—*Circular on Smallpox of the Connecticut Board of Health.*

THE *New York Times* aptly says: "When Surgeon General Sternberg, in his recent formal order, informed his subordinates that hereafter the existence of malaria at any army post would be regarded as proof that a previous order in relation to the destruction of mosquitoes had not been obeyed ill-informed critics may have thought that he was accepting a new theory somewhat hastily. As a matter of fact, however, the relation between mosquitoes and malaria is now thoroughly established, and public sentiment everywhere should hold local Health Boards to the same responsibility that General Sternberg has imposed upon the post surgeons. In Italy, where the ravages of malaria have long been greater than anywhere out of the tropics, action suggested by the recent discoveries has been taken by municipalities, corporations, and individuals, and always with excellent results. A consular report from Naples illustrates what has been accomplished in regions formerly of the very worst reputation for fevers. It says that the Mediterranean Railway Company has spent a large sum of money in equipping all stations and employees' houses in the malarial districts with mosquito proof wire screens. Switchmen and others who must be out of doors at night have been provided with clothing through which the insects cannot bite, and to make places of family resort after sunset, the porches of the houses have been inclosed with gauze. The result is described as marvelous. Formerly, to be appointed to these districts meant for the railway employee little less than a death sentence, and no man could have his family with him in the summer with any prospect of escaping the scourge, which affects one-third of the communes in Italy with more or less severity. Now the railway company has secured absolute immunity for its servants and their families, and even in such poisonous localities as Battipaglia and San Nicola the families in protected houses have this summer been perfectly healthy. Of course what can be done in Italy can be done elsewhere, and Gen. Sternberg's position is fully justified."

A PARADISE OF SPINSTERS.

THE celibate tendency of the modern woman is becoming to worry the vital statistician. The decadence of marriage is threatened, and the gradual extinction of the race. Mr. Carroll D. Wright has been investigating the subject, and finds that of 17.427 representative workingwomen, living in 22 cities, 75 per cent. of them being under 25 years of age, 15,337 were single women. These figures are simply appalling. In the good old times, it is claimed, one-half of these young women would already have been married from three to five years. The fact seems to be that there is a tendency to the postponement of marriages on the part of both sexes. In the case of women this postponement is too often fatal, and in the case of men it gets to be a bad habit. But the evil being recognized, and reduced to figures, the next natural thing to do is to seek for the causes of it.

Several theories have been advanced to account for this increasing unpopularity of marriage. The statement that young men have become more shy and embarrassed in the presence of the modern go-ahead girl, may have some truth in it. The present tendency is undoubtedly to cultivate self-assurance and independence in young women, and to encourage them to become self-supporting. Many avenues are open to them; they can make a comfortable living and enjoy life. Many a woman, in fact, can make a better living for one than the majority of young men can make for two (with prospects of more). This situation tends to check marriage in two ways: First, it makes the women more independent of men, and therefore, in the second place, perhaps a trifle less attractive to them. Marriage is an odd affair, anyhow. It is largely a psychical business at the start, based upon a delicate emotional instinct; and all the logic and reason of a progressive age cannot alter that fact. The pushing and business-like modern woman is not conducive to it.

The competition and the stress of modern life are deterrent to matrimony. Every one can see this in his daily observation. How few men are able properly to marry before they are 35 or 40. But by this time the girl companions of their youth are almost fitted to become grandmothers. We would suggest to Mr. Wright that he should write up the statistics of bachelors—both young and old (if any of the latter can be found). In France a law has been introduced into the Senate to tax all celibates over the age of 30, and all married couples who remain childless after five years. We heartily approve of this plan. Let these people contribute to the support of other people's families if they persist in not having any of their own.

MEN are born to be serviceable to one another, therefore either reform the world or bear with it.—*Marcus Aurelius.*

A NEW FRUIT.

THERE is every reason to suppose, says the *Detroit Medical Journal,* that before long a most delicious fruit, new to America, will dominate our markets; already a few specimens have found their way to the seaboard cities. This is the mangosteen—native to the Moluccas and extensively cultivated in Ceylon and Java, and latterly introduced to Jamaica and other portions of British West Indies. It is about the size of a small orange, spherical in form, and when the rind is removed a juicy pulp, "white and soluble as snow" is revealed, possessing a most delicious flavor—something like a nectarine with a dash of strawberry and pineapple combined. It promises, in a few years, to supersede the orange in popular favor, and attempts are already being made to introduce it into the Southern United States.

"To apply a plaster-of-Paris bandage in fractures below the knee," says Dr. J. S. Dodds, "have a stocking put on. This gives a clean, smooth inside surface. Apply circularly, then up and down, finishing with the circular application. Apply so as to leave a thin streak in front, to be more easily cut. A bandage so applied fits like a glove, and leaves nothing to be desired to hold the fragments in place."

"IN order to relieve the pain and irritation caused by the removal of dressings adhering to a wound," says the *Canadian Practitioner and Review,* "pour some peroxid of hydrogen over the adherent part of the dressing. This will rapidly soften the coagulated discharges and the dressing will come off readily. This method saves the time employed in prolonged soaking with ordinary solutions, and relieves the apprehension so usually shown by patients at each fresh dressing."

Department of Physical Education.

WITH SPECIAL REGARD TO THE SYMMETRICAL DEVELOPMENT OF THE BODY.

TIMELY BUSINESS HINTS FOR PROFESSIONAL MEN.

By H. W. Perkins, M.D.

Professional men have acquired the reputation of being poor business managers. The reputation fits a majority of its owners.

Every doctor needs to be a fairly good business man, otherwise he can not be a thoroughly successful doctor. Many of the best-read physicians are hustled aside and distanced in the professional race simply because their competitors happen to be better business managers.

What are some of the more common of the doctor's faults from a purely business standpoint?

He lacks method.

Method and system will hide a multitude of professional shortcomings. Method has untold value all the way through, from his pocket visiting list to his writing desk, his woodpile and the arrangement of bank notes in his wallet.

He tells his patients too much about their maladies.

His responses to inquiries should be at all times guarded, sententious, and, if not ambiguous, a shade mysterious.

He should avoid expressing an opinion except when he can assume it with the utmost positiveness and assurance. Hesitant opinions are a sign of weakness and worse than none.

He degrades his business by treating medical science as if it were a trade. If it is a trade it is because he makes it such. It is the noblest science that has ever been given a name.

He practically lets the druggist and pharmaceutic manufacturer dictate his prescriptions, when he should be compelling them to sue for his approval.

He tells his patient what remedies are being used in his case.

This is a fatal mistake, and is rapidly developing a most disastrous form of practice—self-treatment.

He disparages, if he does not condemn, his competitors.

He tattles from one patient to another.

He falls into a rut, and is content with what he knows.

Instead of this, every week of his professional life should be a post-graduate course.

He lies awake over his patient's condition, but goes to sleep over his own health. Hence his clients, the preacher, the lawyer, and the baker, outlive him by ten years.

He weakly yields to indulgences that his judgment condemns.

Alcohol, opium, and tobacco have wrecked more medical intellects than all other causes combined.

He buys too many cheap aids from a sense of mistaken economy.

On the contrary, he is parsimonious in his purchases of the best.

Ten dollars expended for the best is worth ten times as much to his business as twenty dollars frittered away in catchy but only half-made gimcracks that will be thrown aside in a month.

He suffers addlepates and idiots to monopolize too much of his time with idle talk on indifferent subjects, and thus abridges his time for study, reading, and rest.

He pays too little attention to social life, neglects his wife and children, and subjects himself to the charge of indifference or inconstancy.

Sometimes he is indifferent as to his personal appearance.

He wears ill-fitting or ill-fashioned garments, an inappropriate hat, soiled linen, or torn gloves. Or he neglects the bath and lavatory.

He should never appear before a patient in any other condition than that of immaculate cleanliness, from headgear to boots.

He permits obstacles and opposition to depress and frighten him, instead of crushing them by force of faith, will, and perseverance.

He gives up his patients too easily. He should never admit that any patient is going to die until after he has been dead fifteen minutes.

Finally, he is not prompt and business-like in presenting and collecting his bills.

In relation to all these items he can reform.

ENLIGHTENING THE LAITY.

WE are glad to note that the medical press is taking this subject seriously. The GAZETTE has been an advocate and exemplar of the idea from the date of its initial number. Dr. Smith's paper, the substance of which we reproduced, has aroused more than passing interest, and we hope it means the inauguration of a new era in national medical literature.

The *Post Graduate,* in a recent issue comments as follows:

Now, in the light of what has been lately read in various quarters, and at one of the recent meetings of the Academy of Medicine, in the discussion of the subject of the "Relations of the Public to the Medical Profession," in a paper by Dr. Andrew H. Smith, let us inform the public as to just what can be done by the medical profession and what has been done. Scientific men of other cults have not failed to let the public know what can be done in their science, and why should our profession fear a proper publicity? How are people to know what the medical profession has accomplished and can accomplish unless our exponents tell them? It is easy to distinguish between the personal advertisers, who allow accounts of their great operations to be heralded in the newspapers, and who grant interviews on subjects in which they are personally interested, and whose airing will consequently benefit them personally—it is easy to distinguish between this kind of publicity and the instruction of the public that we advocate. There ought, at various intervals, to appear in the monthly and quarterly magazines, interesting and clearly written articles on certain points in medical science. For example, the mosquito and malaria, the revelations of the X-ray, the value of serum injections for diphtheria, the necessity of the continued prevention of the spread of smallpox by vaccination, the nature of the bubonic plague. Such a list as this may be multiplied tenfold. If the magazines do not care to publish these things, the profession ought to establish a magazine of its own, devoted to the education of the public at large. We could soon make our superiority over all the pretenders and miracle workers so apparent that the position of the profession in this country would be markedly changed for the better. We are perfectly well aware of the prejudice existing in certain quarters against the appearance of a physician's name anywhere than on a prescription or in a medical magazine, but if the distinction named above. which is so clear that no truly scientific and humane member of the profession can misunderstand it, there need be no fear of any violation of a written or unwritten code of ethics in informing the public of the things that are and may actually be done, for the mitigation of disease by the regular profession. Crusades against Christian Scientists, except in the way of legal prosecution, when they undertake to take charge of the cases, are of no avail, and will simply increase the number of those who adhere to these dangerous beliefs.

IT is only the optimist who extends the frontier of civilization.—*Wm. E. Smythe, in Sunset.*

THE EMPLOYMENT OF HEAT AS A THERAPEUTIC AND DIAGNOSTIC MEASURE.

MANY pages have been written of the therapeutic value of the local application of dry heat or moist heat in the treatment of various painful and inflammatory processes. It is a familiar fact to many practitioners that soaking a sprained ankle in very hot water will often do much toward relieving the pain and allaying inflammation and swelling, and that the use of repeated very hot vaginal douches will often relieve pelvic pain due to congestion or spasm. So, too, irrigation of the external auditory canal with very hot water is not only a pain relieving but a curative measure in cases of inflammation of the middle ear. The other external and internal uses of hot water are exceedingly numerous.

The object here, however, says the editor of the *Therapeutic Gazette,* is to call attention to a proposition recently advanced by Lewin, of Berlin. He claims that by the use of the local application of heat we can make a diagnosis as to whether an acute inflammatory process has gone on to suppuration—as, for example, in a case of appendicitis. He asserts that if pus has not yet formed, the application of heat will be a comfort to the patient, whereas, on the other hand, if pus is present, it will so increase and exacerbate the pain that a diagnosis of the presence of this material can be made with assurance. He states as an example that in cases of swelling of the knee associated with rheumatism or otherwise we not infrequently are able to give great relief if the knee is put at rest with a fixation splint, and heat is actively employed. If by any chance pus is present the pain is augmented and becomes intolerable. Lewin states that he has employed heat for this purpose in a sufficient number of cases to make him feel confident that he cannot be mistaken in regard to this point, and he cites ten cases of appendicitis in which the heat was applied for two hours by means of hot compresses and without the use of internal pain relievers. Eight of these received this treatment with a good deal of relief, but the remaining two showed marked increase in pain. Of the eight cases all went on to cure in the space of from five days to three weeks, while, on the contrary, the two which suffered an increase in pain after the application of heat required the administration of opium for the relief of pain, and both of them died.

The experience of Sphor, of Frankfort-on-the-Main, is also quoted. In fifteen cases of appendicitis which had hot applications without internal treatment very similar results were obtained. So, too, in three cases of perimetritis two were relieved by the application of heat and recovery promptly took place; while in the third patient the pain was greatly increased, and later on a large quantity of pus was discharged by the vagina.

If further investigations show that this method of diagnosis is at all accurate, it is so simple in its application that it cannot fail to prove of value.

BETTERING THE QUALITY OF LABOR.

WILLIAM C. REDFIELD, of J. H. Williams & Co., Brooklyn, a concern that employs machinists on a large scale, says concerning this subject:

"The nine-hour day has been a gain, and not a loss.

"A man is more than a machine. The policy which treats him as a machine ignores one of the greatest factors in production—namely, human nature.

"A clean man produces more in the long run than a dirty man. A well-informed man produces more than an ignorant man. A justly treated man produces more than an unjustly treated man. A contented man is a better and cheaper producer than a discontented man. A well-paid man is a more economic producer than an ill-paid man.

"It would be well, when seeking to economize, to give less attention to the pay roll and more in other directions."

MERE MENTION.

UNDER the guise of medicine-selling and bitters-traffic there is a deal of the worst sort of whiskey-shop business done by apothecaries and by country stores. Many if not all of these pernicious "bitters" are sorry mixtures of cheap alcohols, wines, etc., with various disguising drugs, which quickly and surely destroy both body and soul of the unfortunate habitué. We are glad to see that the law of Maine prevents shipment into the State of these "medicines."

The United States Senate Committee have reported the results of their investigation as to the relative merits of the slow sand filtration of water and the rapid or mechanical filtration for the supply of Washington. The committee find that either system removes the bacteria, and that the slow method is the better for clear water, while the rapid method, with a coagulant, is preferable for turbid water.

An examination of the brains of two great mathematicians by Professor Retzius and Professor Möbius, leads to no definite location of the mathematical centrum. There was in both cases a shortening of the Sylvian fissure. Whether this will finally be placed in the lateral parts of the frontal lobes, or in the parietal region, remains for future researches to determine.

There is a very general feeling that the repeal of the army canteen law was a bitter mistake. The repeal seems to be increasing drunkenness and insubordination and disease among the soldiers. A total abstainer writes: "All the good the women wanted to do they undid, and all the good that was being done without them they have utterly ruined."

Chicago thinks of flushing the streets to keep them clean, while Milwaukee is about to abandon the method for a dry sweeping patent process which draws the dust and dirt by an air blast into a chamber so that it is not blown or scattered about. If it works, the patentee of the machine should have his million dollar reward.

Dr. A. P. Grinnell, of Burlington, Vt., says that there are more than 3,300,000 doses of opium annually sold in Vermont by the general stores. This does not include that dispensed by physicians or sold in patent nostrums. This equals a half dose daily for every inhabitant. Is this an indirect result of prohibition?

Some bacteriologist should investigate the trailing skirt of city ladies and tell us how many cases of tuberculosis and how many deaths are probably due to this disgusting fashion.

The *London Post-Magazine Almanach* has compiled a table with estimated losses of all the great fires of the last century. No fire loss of less than $500,000 is included. The two greatest fires, characteristically, were in the United States—that of Chicago, $165,000,000, and that of Boston, $70,000,000. The table foots up $440,000,000, and if the small fires could have been included the entire loss would have been at least $1,000,000,000. Has there been made any estimate of the number of lives lost by these fires?

WHY THE BLIND SELDOM SMOKE.

ACCORDING to the *Family Doctor,* a peculiarity about blind people is that there is seldom one of them who smokes. Soldiers and sailors accustomed to smoking, and who have lost their sight in action, continue to smoke for a short time, but soon give up the habit. They say it gives them no pleasure when they cannot see the smoke, and some have said that they cannot taste the smoke unless they see it.

VALUE OF HEALTHY EMOTIONS.

It is difficult to define the emotions, but it seems to us they grow out of our feelings; the feelings are simple. Prick your hand with a pin, it is a feeling, but out of it may arise emotions of many kinds. Or the emotions may be called complex feelings; they are pleasing and painful. Love is a pleasing emotion; hate, a painful one. If one makes a long or even a short journey with friends and enjoys it to the fullest extent, the mind is filled with a series of complex and pleasant emotions. If one does not enjoy the journey, the emotions will be unpleasant; but in either case they arise out of the multitude of feeling or sensations which come to the brain through sight, hearing, and the other senses. In all our recreations and in our work, a prolonged flow of pleasing emotions does a great deal to brace up the body and fit it for work. The nervous system is refreshed by them; the energies of the brain accumulate. On the other hand, painful emotions act just the opposite. They exhaust the nervous energies, take away the appetite and reduce the sleep, and help to break down the constitution. Whether life is worth living or not depends largely upon whether we can keep up a surplus of happy emotions. Can one control his emotions so as to keep a constant stream of pleasant ones and keep away those which are painful? They are, no doubt, to some extent controllable by the will, and, by training the will, may become more so. Few ever try to control themselves and do this, but those who do, and who persevere, are sure to be repaid many fold. It is not so much the keeping out of painful emotions as in bringing in pleasing ones that this is to be accomplished.— *Health.*

Love gives itself, and if not given,
  No genius, beauty, worth nor wit,
No gold of earth, no gem of heaven,
  Is rich enough to purchase it.

ELECTRICITY AND NERVE FORCE.

The statement is not infrequently made that nerve force is identical with electricity, but there is little scientific ground for such a claim. The two forces are distinguished in a variety of ways. Thus, the speed at which they travel is very unequal; the nerve impulse travels at the rate of only about 100 to 120 feet per second, while the rate of electricity is vastly greater. But while the two forces are apparently not identical, it is true that the generation of nerve force seems to be accompanied by electrical phenomena. This may be merely in accord with the fact that all chemical changes are thus accompanied; as, for instance, the reactions between the elements in a Leclanché jar. Vito-chemical reactions in a neuron-body probably in the same way generate electrical force, but this is not necessarily the same thing as the nerve force itself. Another, and still more potent argument is based on the fact that nerve force is variously differentiated until in its psychic manifestations it reaches its highest display. This would be quite inconceivable of such a force as electricity, for certainly no one would say that thought and consciousness are merely electrical phenomena.

M. August Charpentiere has recently made observations which tend still further to prove that the two forces are distinct. He found that an electric stimulation of the nerve trunk causes a double transmission. (1) An almost instantaneous transmission just as in an ordinary conductor. This is evidently the electric current. (2) A current, also with electrical phenomena, transmitted at the very moderate speed of the nerve impulse (65 to 100 feet). That this true nerve impulse is accompanied, however, by electrical energy, is proved by the fact that it can send a stimulus over a wire to a nerve in another animal and thus cause a response. But Charpentiere found that a second, third and even fourth impulse or wave is carried over this wire, the inference being that the nerve impulses are "oscillatory." This latter display is probably simply in accord with the idea of Schaefer and Horsley, that neurons have a rhythmical discharge. M. Charpentiere's observations are discussed in the *Revue Scientifique*.

THE KARNICE.

Dr. Garrigues, in a letter to the *Medical News*, describes this unique invention. "The Karnice" is the name of an apparatus destined to bring help to persons buried alive.

It is the invention of the Russian Count Michel de Karnice Karnichi, who was impelled to his researches by being witness to the narrow escape of a young lady who was thought to be dead and was about to be buried.

The apparatus consists of an iron tube, 10 centimeters in diameter, one end of which is screwed to the circumference of an opening made in the lid of the coffin, while the other end is connected with the small quadrangular metal box containing signals. This box is the only part visible over the grave; the tube is buried in the ground.

Through the whole length of the tube passes a metal rod which enters the coffin below and is connected with the signals above. At the lower end it has a metal ball which is placed four or five centimeters above the chest of the supposed dead. Whether this ball be pushed or pulled it causes a sliding movement in the mechanism contained in the box, in consequence of which the box opens, a metal ball is displayed above it, and a loud bell is made to ring for a considerable length of time. The person enclosed in the coffin receives immediately all air necessary for comfortable breathing. A lamp throws light down to him, and the tube serves as a powerful speaking trumpet to make his voice audible at a great distance.

All joints being hermetically closed, no emanation of gases due to decomposition can escape.

When the tube is removed a thick metal plate lined with rubber and moved by a strong spring closes the opening in the coffin.

The box cannot be opened from without. The construction of the apparatus is of the simplest. There is no complicated machinery to get out of order, nor is that unreliable factor, electricity, used at all.

THE OLD WAY OF TREATING HYSTERIA AND THE NEW.

Our grandfathers in medicine laid the foundations of therapeutics, and in many ways their work is worthy of them. When, indeed, shall the world ever see the equal of Watson, or when again shall there appear such a resplendent genius as John Hunter? The great need of the present time is for a great genius like Sydenham to arise and bring all of the scattered facts of medicine together and make of it a work which will bring out in an orderly system all the truth which the patient workers have laid on the altars of medical science.

In nothing has the profession made greater advances in recent years than in the treatment of nervous affections, and particularly is this true of hysteria. Formerly a patient with hysteria was treated with derision. She was looked upon as one who was pretending to be diseased, and who was in fact a vicious or lazy person.

The present day physician is altogether out of such loose unscientific methods. He carefully goes into the merits of a case and adjusts his treatment accordingly. Hysteria is now fully recognized as a disease which merits not only the sympathy of the patient's friends, but also the sincere efforts of the physician to cure.

Hysteria is generally evidence of neurasthenia, or impaired nervous system, and its treatment should comprehend the exhibition of those remedies which will bring about an improvement or removal of these conditions.

These patients should have open air exercise, and should have such remedies as will build up the system. The hypophosphites is one of the best general remedies at the disposal of the profession. The physician will find the greatest source of benefit to his patient in such a remedy as will give his patient a sufficiency of sleep and rest. In fact many physicians now place their sole reliance upon Daniel's Conc. Tinct. Passiflora Incarnata. This remedy is an anodyne and nerve sedative of power and as a hypnotic it has no equal. Given in doses of a teaspoonful every two or three hours these patients get a sufficient sleep, the nerve tension and hyperasthenia are relieved, the patient ceases to be restless and weary of herself, and in a short while all the elements in the case rapidly disappear and the progress toward recovery is often so marked and quick that it is noticeable by all with whom the patient comes in contact.

Another excellent quality of this remedy consists in its mild laxative action. As is well known, in hysteria there is generally more or less fecal autoinfection and fecal anemia associated with these cases, and the laxative influence of the remedy makes it indeed an ideal remedy.

Some physicians give certain remedies supposed to be nerve "foods" or nerve tonics. To say nothing for or against any remedy let us ask the physicians if a remedy which brings about a quiescent state of the nerves, and which brings about normal sleep, is not in the truest sense of the word a nerve tonic?

Daniel's Conc. Tinct. Passiflora Incarnata is not a remedy which is attended with evil results from continued employment. It does not set up drug addiction, or any other condition which is unpleasant or dangerous. Another point in favor of the remedy too is that it is entirely non-toxic, and can be given in large doses without producing any evil result whatever.

In prescribing this remedy I am frank to confess that I am partial to Daniel's Conc. Tinct. Passiflora Incarnata, as I consider it the only reliable preparation of the drug that has come to my notice.—DAVID L. STOCKING, M.D., Ponce, Porto Rico.

WOMAN.

HE is a fool who thinks, by force or skill, to turn the current of a woman's will.—*Samuel Tuke.*

A perfect woman, nobly planned, to warn, to comfort and command.—*Wordsworth.*

The most beautiful object in the world, it will be allowed is a beautiful woman.—*Macaulay.*

If the heart of a man is depressed with cares, the mist is dispelled when a woman appears.—*Gay.*

Oh, woman! lovely woman! . . . Angels are painted fair, to look like you. —*Otway.*

Lovely woman, that caused our cares, can every care beguile.—*Beresford.*

Raptured man quits each dozing sage, Oh, woman, for thy lovelier page.—*Moore.*

Kindness in woman, not their beauteous looks, shall win my love.—*Shakespeare.*

He that would have fine guests, let him have a fine wife.—*Ben Jonson.*

A woman's strength is most potent when robed in gentleness.—*Lamartine.*

All I am or can be I owe to my angel mother.—*Abraham Lincoln.*

Disguise our bondage as we will, 'tis woman, woman, rules us still.—*Moore.*

Heaven will be no heaven to me if I do not meet my wife there.—*Andrew Jackson.*

Women need not look at those dear to them to know their moods.—*Howells.*

Oil and water—woman and a secret—are hostile properties.—*Bulwer Lytton.*

Remember, woman is most perfect when most womanly.—*Gladstone.*

Earth has nothing more tender than a pious woman's heart.—*Luther.*

AMERICAN WOMAN'S PHYSIQUE.

DR. CHARLES A. L. REED, in his new text-book of Gynecology, published by D. Appleton & Co., makes the following observations in the opening paragraph of Chapter II., devoted to the general etiology of diseases of women:

"There is a prevailing impression that the diseases peculiar to women are increasing relatively to the population. There exist no data upon which such an affirmation can be based. The impression probably depends for its existence upon the fact that such diseases are now better understood and more generally treated than formerly. Evidence is not wanting to indicate that the Anglo-Saxon woman is not degenerating. Bowditch has made some interesting observations on the physique of women, as follows: Of over 1,100, he found that the average height was 158.76 centimeters (five feet three and one-half inches). Sargent, in nearly 1,900 observations, the ages of the women ranging from sixteen to twenty-six, found the average slightly higher. Galton, in 770 measurements of English women from twenty-three to fifty-one years of age, also found a higher average—a difference due in part, no doubt, to the younger age of a number of American subjects. In 1,105 subjects in ordinary indoor clothing, Bowditch found the average weight to be 56.56 kilogrammes (125 pounds). These observations, compared with 276 by Galton, show that the average weight is a little greater among Americans. It would seem that while the tallest English women surpassed the tallest American women in height, the heaviest American women exceeded the heaviest English women in weight. Specific observation of this systematic character, however, is not necessary to impress the intelligent traveler with the generally satisfactory physique of the women of England and America. It is true that many defective specimens are found, and these come with relatively greater proportion under the observation of the physician. But no one can fail to be impressed with the fact that they comprise a distinct minority of the masses. The improvement in the physique of women has been very noticeable since the sentiment for athletics has supplanted that for the cloister, and since outdoor exercises have taken the place of those sedentary habits which but a few decades ago were considered the proper affectations of refinement."

SPOON LORE.

ONE of our English exchanges thus discourses about spoons:

Spoons have been in use for many centuries. In early times it was the fashion for ladies and gentlemen to have their own spoons and spoon cases, which they carried with them wherever they went. Two hundred years ago we find frequent mention in the newspapers of a "lost case containing a knife, fork, and silver spoon." The spoon was usually described as bearing the crest of the owner, upon its handle; or a picture of the Blessed Virgin. The "apostle spoons" were a dozen of these silver implements, each containing an image of one of the apostles in relief upon its handle, sometimes with and sometimes without his name. If the name was omitted, there was usually some emblem of the worthy supposed to be represented on the spoon. In case emblems were used instead of names, St. James would be attired as a pilgrim; St. Jude was usually pictured with a club, the emblem of his martyrdom, or with a boat, to show his occupation; St. Simon, with a saw, because he was sawn asunder, and generally with an added oar, to show his earlier tastes. The use of these spoons as gifts from godparents to godchildren dates back nearly 500 years. When the giver was too poor to present the whole twelve, he gave one spoon with the image of the patron saint after whom the child was named, or to whom he was dedicated, or who was the patron saint of the donor, not always in such cases an apostle. The images of the four

Evangelists were often thus used, the spoons being called "apostle spoons," although all were not apostles in the usual meaning of the word. Shakespeare, in "Henry VIII.," when Cranmer declares himself unworthy of being sponsor to the young princess, makes the king reply: "Come, come, my lord, you'd spare your spoons," in plain allusion to the gift expected on such occasions. The earliest notice we find in print of this form of spoon is an entry on the book of the Stationers' Company, made in the year 1500. It is this entry: "A spoyne of the gyfte of Master Riginold Wolfe, all gylte, with the pycture of St. John," showing that "apostle spoons" were well known at that early day.

FORCED FEEDING FOLLIES.

THE physician who undertakes to give a patient the "Rest Cure," says the *Northwestern Lancet*, should be endowed with a fair amount of common sense and judgment. He must study the individual as well as the technique of his treatment, and keep in mind the fact that not all of his patients can be subjected to the same routine. * * *
A patient who has spent three months under mismanagement, discharged with a two or ten-pound gain, perhaps, who suffers from indigestion and autoinfection, and is still a broken-down neurotic, is an unprofitable advertising agent who might have done the physician much credit, and saved the reputation of the "Rest Cure," if a more careful study had been made of individual requirements. * * *
There is much folly in forced feeding.

A SIMPLE METHOD OF WRITING PRESCRIPTIONS FOR CHILDREN.

MAX HUHNER, in the *Medical Record*, gives a simple dose method for prescribing for children. It is based on Cowling's rule

that the dose suitable for a child is obtained by dividing the age of the child at the next birthday by twenty-four. The simple method of writing the prescription is to have it contain twenty-four doses; hence for a child one year of age the amount in the prescription would be exactly the adult dose; if the child is three years old, three times the adult dose; if ten years, ten times. The method is simple and avoids a complicated calculation. It holds good for all those remedies to which Cowling's rule is applicable. In the case of opiates the amount must be diminished one-half.

IS ALCOHOL A FOOD?

ACCORDING to *La Tribune Medicale*, R. Romme declares that our knowledge of the physiological action of alcohol and the alcoholic beverages is very limited. In medicine, alcohol passes as an excitant or stimulant—a very vague term. But it really appears from its effects, according to many authors, to be a paralyzant. It alters rather than stimulates the functions of the organism. It presents the action of a toxic substance whose effect is more paralyzing than stimulating. Alcohol is not a food, properly speaking. It should be considered a condiment. But in order to play this rôle, which is one of considerable importance, it should be sufficiently diluted, and natural, as it is found in a drink naturally fermented, such as wine, cider, or beer. In any other form it is a poison.

"THE moving finger writes, and having writ,
Moves on; nor all your piety nor wit
    Shall lure it back to cancel half a line,
Nor all your tears wash out a word of it."

"And some loquacious vessels were; and some
I istened perhaps, but never talked at all."
                        —*The Rubaiyat.*

SOME MEDICAL APHORISMS.

THE following more or less sensible aphorisms are going the rounds of the medical press: (1) Life is short, patients fastidious, and the brethren deceptive. (2) Practice is a field of which tact is the manure. (3) Patients are comparable to flannel—neither can be quitted without danger. (4) The physician who absents himself runs the same risk as the lover who leaves his mistress; he is pretty sure to find himself supplanted. (5) Would you rid yourself of a tiresome patient, present your bill. (6) The patient who pays his attendant is but exacting; he who does not is a despot. (7) The physician who depends upon the gratitude of his patient for his fee is like the traveler who waited upon the bank of a river until it would finish flowing that he might cross to the other side. (8) Modesty, simplicity, truthfulness!—cleansing virtues everywhere but at the bedside; there simplicity is construed as hesitation, modesty as want of confidence, truth as impoliteness. (9) To keep within the limits of a dignified assurance without falling into the ridiculous vauntings of the boaster, constitutes the supreme talent of the physician. (10) Remember always to appear to do something—above all when you are doing nothing. (11) With equal, and even inferior, talent, the cleanly and genteely-dressed physician has a great advantage over the untidy one.

HIS UNCERTAINTY.

FARMER HONK—Say, Lem!

Farmer Stackrider—Har?

Farmer Honk—Is that 'ere solemn, spectacled young nephew of your'n that's bein' called "Doctor," and goes around lookin' as wise as a treeful of owls, a dentist, a hoss-physician, a corn-curer, a layer-on-of-hands, a presidin' elder, or just a common doctor that saws bones and kills folks?— *Puck.*

The Brevity Club.

A NEW MEMBER'S MAIDEN EFFORT.

"THEREFORE since brevity is the soul of wit,
And tediousness the limbs and outward
   flourishes,
I will be brief."

All's well that ends well, therefore, The best part of a story and the only part of most jokes that is tolerable is the end of them.

If you want a recipe for being wretched, take the following:

Marry some one who has more money than you have and is not overmodest about reminding you of it. If this fails try again by marrying some one who does not love you through and through and for all you are, good, bad, and indifferent; or whom you fail to dote on in the same unquestioning and unselfish way.

People who call this a dreary and wicked world and life not worth living generally do about as much as they can to make it so.

With the beautiful heavens overhead, the teeming and glorious earth underfoot, and the best thoughts of the best minds so easily at command, no one has any logical or moral right to call himself or herself "poor." To be really "poor" one must be poor in thought, poor in spirit, poor in feeling and appreciation, and poor in the consciousness of personal rectitude.

The only real riches are of thought and feeling, of appreciative capacity of enjoyment. Riches never consist of gold and silver, houses and lands, government coupons and railway bonds.

We surely all know these to be facts, but very few of us are living as though we believed them!

Nothing is more evident than that the Millennium will not materialize during the reign of the materialistic and money-worshiping age.

New version: Brevity is the soul of— quit! I quit!

HOW TO "GET THERE."

I AM going to state right here, for the benefit of humanity at large, that there is not a soul in the world who cannot make the leading inclination of his life a success by being *faithful* to it; by centering every faculty he possesses upon it; by never wavering in his fidelity to it. The idea must be strongly defined by the man's intelligence and endorsed by his conscience. It must be endorsed by his conscience, because there must be no pulling back from it by any part of him. The whole man must be centered on it—on the idea; not on the money necessary to bring out the idea, but on the idea itself; and the money will follow as the waves follow the moon. For brain potency, will power, undaunted resolution, courage, faith, and patience, these things are the real gods, before whose throne principalities and all external powers, including gold—the great power of all—doff their beggarly caps and prostrate themselves in the dust.— *Helen Wilmans.*

A FEW OF THE CLINICAL USES OF LIQUID AIR.

PEARCE (*Cincinnati Lancet-Clinic.*) As a local anesthetic it has been most satisfactory, minor operations being done with no pain at all, and no injury to surrounding tissues. In neuralgias, and pain of herpes zoster, it has given prompt relief. A case of erythematous lupus, in which it was used, healed nicely, without the deep seaming attended by other forms of treatment. A case of epithelioma of the face yielded easily. In cases of small tumors of the face, nævi, etc., it can be used, and leaves a scar which is hardly perceptible. Cases of boils, carbuncles and bubos show marked modification in their course. A case of facial erysipelas was subjected to the spray until the infected surface felt very cold, and three days later the patient returned, having had no other

treatment, and the inflammation had completely subsided. Sluggish ulcers seem to take on a new growth when they have been subjected to the spray of liquid air, which appears to have all the effects of a caustic, without its attendant inflammation.

TRANSLATING THE MENU.

A NOTED satirically-minded epicure one day dropped into a *café* for dinner. The obsequious waiter had just flicked a bit of lint from his customer's coat collar when this gentleman opened out on him.

"Yes," he said, glancing at the menu, "you may bring me some eggs blushing like Aurora."

"Beg pardon, sir," explained the waiter, "it's not on the bill."

"Isn't, eh? What's this, *œufs à l'aurore?*"

"Oh, yes," replied the young man, blushing and shifting somewhat uneasily.

"And I feel like having some breeches in the royal fashion, with velvet sauce."

The waiter turned red, white, and blue.

"Got you again," chuckled the epicure. "Well, I suppose you call it *culottes à la royale, sauce velouté.*"

"Oh, that! Yes, sir; yes, sir;" and the waiter briskly rattled the cutlery around the plate as though he would fain drown the epicure's voice.

"Be sure you bring a stew of good Christians."

"Now you are joking," mildly expostulated the waiter, with a sickly smile.

"Not a bit of it, man. See here on your bill. *Compote de bons chrétiens.*"

"Oh—ah—ugh," gulped the waiter.

"And a mouthful of ladies."

"Eh?"

"*Bouchée de dames*—quick, help—a glass of water—dash it in his face!"

But the epicure was too late. The waiter was in a dead swoon, from which he never recovered until later in the afternoon.

Book Reviews.

FOOD AND THE PRINCIPLES OF DIETETICS.
By Robert Hutchison, M.D. Edin.,
M.R.C.P., with plates and diagrams; oc-
tavo, 548 pages. New York: William
Wood & Company, 1901.

There is no dearth in the mart of books
on diet, books on food and feeding, books
on the chemistry of catering, books with a
feeding fad, books crammed and padded
with chemical chestnuts and nutritive nonsense. All this is so patent and notorious.
that it would seem that a new volume must
necessarily thresh old straw and find little
grain.

This is a hint of the mental attitude in
which we read the unassuming and rather
overmodest title page to Dr. Hutchison's
work. We are frank to say that the most
critical reading of a dozen pages of the
book, selected at random, will effectually
cure any such preconception.

At a time when so many authors, especially medical authors, have fallen into the
habit of dawdling through a dozen lines,
after the fashion of the big-type headlines
of a yellow journal aping sensations that
do not exist in the text—to tell what it is
they are going to talk about, the very brevity and directness of the title is a suggestive object lesson to ambitious medical scribblers. When we read these abstrusely pre-
tentious and interminably long titles we are
quite inclined to accept them as abstracts
or briefs of what is to come, and to skip
the voluminously padded body of the work
entirely. No doubt this is an indignity and
injustice to some writers who discourse
well and really have something to say; but
it is their own fault. It is the busiest age
since time began, and there is no kind of
doubt as to the fact that many an able paper
goes unread, dammed by its pointless and
long-winded title.

We often feel like imitating the "Philistine" that flourishes at East Aurora, by becoming "A Magazine of Protest."

The contents of Dr. Hutchison's work

were first addressed to the students of London Hospital, as a course of lectures, in
1899-1900. Quoting from the preface: "In
recasting the lectures for publication a
large amount of additional matter has been
used, and no pains have been spared to make
the book fully representative of the present
state of our knowledge on the subject of
which it treats."

The author adds that "a considerable
amount of space has been devoted to the
patent and proprietary foods, and an effort
has been made to deal fairly and honestly
with their merits. The great number and
variety of these now offered for sale makes
this specially necessary."

For this the author is to be commended.
In this country we have fallen into the idiotic habit of branding every effort in this
direction as a literary commodity purchas-
able at a definitely understood price. Dr.
Hutchison's frankness and conspicuous
want of bias in this direction is refreshing.

There isn't a dull chapter in the book nor
one that is not full of facts so freshly and
aptly stated that they fairly seem new.

No matter how many works you have
in your library on the engrossing subject
of dietetics and nutrition, the subject which
underlies all successful medical practice,
don't hesitate for a moment to possess yourself of this volume. The physician who
will study it and keep it at hand for daily
reference may safely relegate all the other
works of the kind to an unused shelf.

The price, $5, is apparently high; but
it will prove the best investment of a lifetime. It is not so technically worded but
that the intelligent layman will find it full
of the practical facts of which he can not
know too much.

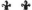

PRACTICAL HYPNOTISM, by Comte C. de
Saint-Germain. Laird & Lee, publishers,
Chicago.

As a rule works on hypnotism have
been either too deep and scientifically technical to be easy and pleasant reading for

the non-professional, or they have proved of such a flimsy and weak character as to lack any value, even as the mere recreation of an idle hour. The question of the production and nature of this strange state of trance which by the curious variety of its manifestations still puzzles the masters of psychological and physiological research, is so important on account of the power it seems to give certain human beings over others, that it ought to be treated, not by irresponsible and ignorant stage performers or dangerous quacks, but exclusively by authorized savants of well-known disinterestedness and honesty. It is to this class of authorities that Comte de Saint-Germain has applied for the information herein classified and presented in most readable form. The French, German, English, American, Italian, Swedish, Russian and Belgian specialists have all contributed to make "Practical Hypnotism" a systematic and reliable work on Hypnotism, Magnetism and Suggestion—three different names for really the same series of phenomena. Concerning Suggestion, we are glad to see that the Comte energetically combats the idea so dangerously insisted upon by the "Professors" of hypnotism, that any one can be taught to place hypnotizable subjects under his or her control. As a matter of fact, out of the comparatively few persons who can be placed under the influence of the hypnotic sleep a very small minority are made to obey, or simply to understand the orders of the hypnotizers. This is a first safeguard against the misuse of the power of Suggestion; the second protection against scoundrelly attempts to abuse with impunity these spells of submissiveness, resides in the fact that the subject who has been induced by Suggestion to commit certain acts of a detrimental and even criminal character, of which he has no remembrance in the waking state, can be made to tell everything about them when thrown again into hypnosis by some other operator in quest of the truth. These two points must not be lost sight of, as they place Comte de Saint-Germain's book among the

few respectable and safe manuals on hypnotic matters. The work is divided into three parts: Historical, Theoretical and Practical, the latter containing methods to induce hypnosis, and to apply it to the relief of sundry diseases. A vocabulary of all medical words used in the work and a number of most interesting foot-notes help to make "Practical Hypnotism" a guide for all those who are attracted to this fascinating study. Some of the illustrations might have been improved.

[Large 12mo, 264 pages. Cloth, unique cover design, 50 engravings, 20 half-tone cuts, 75c. Paper, lithographed cover, 30 illustrations, 25c.]

ON THE EDITOR'S TABLE.

HYGIENE and Humor are first cousins, if not more nearly related.

This will absolve us for all time for not apologizing when we introduce snatches of humor, curt sayings and witty selections, into our columns.

Here are the TRIBUNE PRIMER and NONSENSE FOR OLD AND YOUNG, by Eugene Field, published by Henry A. Dickerman & Son, of Boston.

They are trifles in the book line, but trifles that talk. Copies of the original edition, a wee 24mo, bound in pink paper covers, bring $125.00 each. This quaint edition costs but fifty cents. Buy it, read it, and stave off biliousness, the blues, and the undertaker.

From the SELF AND SEX SERIES, issued by the Vir Publishing Co., Philadelphia, we have: *"What a Young Boy Ought to Know; What a Young Man Ought to Know; What a Young Husband Ought to Know; What a Man of Forty-Five Ought to Know."*

These four volumes comprise the essentials of what should be known by boys, youths, and men, told in a convincing and attractive style, with no leaning toward either prudery or pruriency.

They are safe volumes to be placed in the

hands of those for whom they were written.

The Delineator for July is already on our table. It is a superb edition of this popular publication.

Its special feature is the three-color printing in the illustrated article on the Pan-American Exposition.

The publishers seem to have been fortunate in securing the advantage of working directly from the original water color sketches of C. Y. Turner, Director of Color to the Exposition.

Some of the effects are simply wonderful.

Modern Culture for June appears with a new cover design, the work of Sarah Noble-Ives, of New York. It is a clever drawing of a modern girl in unconventional pose against a poster effect of hollyhocks and summer greenth, and is an advance upon previous work by this gifted artist. It adds greatly to the general attractiveness of the most notable number of *Modern Culture* which has been issued. The perfect balance of the June table of contents and the superior excellence of all the articles presented are the especial features of a magazine which in this number, if never before, has fairly earned its title.

Among the many pseudo-hygienic and health journals that ape the name "Culture" it gives us pleasure to note this ambitious aspirant for literary honors and popularity, which anon was called *Self Culture*. It is published at Cleveland, and need not hesitate to be critically compared with the best of the dollar magazines. The table of contents for June is specially attractive.

The Philistine.

We often wonder if our readers are but few of them familiar with the character, aims and quaintness of this unique little magazine, published by a little band of uncommoners calling themselves "Roycrofters," at East Aurora, New York. The moving spirit is Fra Elbertus Hubbard, who is quite as much in earnest in his work as was the Apostle Paul.

These Roycrofters are a band of coöperative, socialistic, and humanitarian brothers and sisters, who seem to have attuned themselves artistically, commercially, socially, and spiritually, which is saying a good deal for the moral and humanitarian progress the members must have made. They issue the quaintest and daintiest of volumes in the quaintest and daintiest of typography and bindings, and are doing their utmost to disseminate the most advanced ideas of genuine progress and philanthropy as they see them. They inculcate the strictest straightforwardness in every field of human effort, and assume to despise all the literary and commercial tricks and subterfuges in vogue.

Here is a sample of the way Fra Elbertus talks:

"All the money I make by my pen, all I get for lectures, all I make from my books, goes into the common fund of the Roycrofters—the benefit is for all. I want no better clothing, no better food, no more comforts and conveniences than my helpers and fellow workers have. I would be ashamed to monopolize a luxury—to take a beautiful work of art, say a painting or a marble statue, and keep it for my own pleasures and for the select few I might invite to see my beautiful things. Art is for all—beauty is for all. Harmony in all of its manifold forms should be like sunset—free to all who can absorb and drink it in. The Roycroft shop is for the Roycrofters, and each is limited only by his capacity to absorb and assimilate."

WHAT do we live for, if it is not to make life less difficult to each other?—*George Eliot.*

Department of Notes and Queries.

FREEDOM OF DISCUSSION BETWEEN EDITOR AND READER.

Query 90. You will remember that sometime last year I wrote asking for practical information concerning the selection of a typewriter for the use of physicians. After a considerable delay you were kind enough to reply by personal letter, which was not what I desired, since I know there are many others equally anxious for suggestions. As I wrote you before, I had indulged in one of the cheap "one-hand" machines. I had trusted the advertisement (in your own journal) and had invested an X in a "one-hand" toy machine. It has made my little daughter a most interesting plaything!

I have not repeated the experiment, and now venture to repeat my inquiry of last year. The market is full of typewriters and they all claim everything in sight. I have procured catalogues from a number of them and am more puzzled than ever. The so-styled "standard" machines all insist that none of the cheaper kinds are reliable or economical. I do not care to waste any more money and therefore hope you will excuse me for again pressing my question. As you no longer advertise the toy machine, and probably do not hold any "trust" stock, I see no ethical or professional reason to bar your frankest advice.

I have the catalogue of a machine advertised in Chicago, but it does not answer to the description of the one advised in your letter, the name of which you did not see fit to give.

E. C. S., Minn.

Answer.—In replying to your former inquiry we followed an established precedent, under which we refrain as far as possible from mentioning the names of competing manufacturers. Like all other set rules this one is often absurd and useless. Your second inquiry deserves a frank reply, which we will undertake to give.

No class of business men is more benefited by the use of the typewriter than the busy physician who writes for his medical journal or conducts a considerable correspondence. Proverbially careless about his penmanship, the active practitioner soon finds it irksome to take sufficient pains with it to make it readable. Those whose business is so extensive as to require the employment of a stenographer are interested in the particular make of the machine used only as far as regards its cost and the quality of its work. A majority of doctors who need a typewriting machine want one that is not extravagant in price, that does good work, is thoroughly durable, not likely to get out of order, and that is easily learned so that they can manipulate it themselves. Portability is another feature of considerable importance to the doctor. The so-called "standard" machines, costing on an average, $100, obviously lack some of these qualifications. They are expensive and they are too heavy for ready portability. Of the lower priced machines some are quite as cumbersome, others are inferior in material and construction, made to sell, while others are restricted or inefficient in their working capacity. In this office we are using two varieties, a "standard" machine and a light, portable style which is not listed with those that have entered into a "trust" and which we have no hesitation in recommending to physicians as the best one by odds for their personal use. It is thoroughly well made, weighs only one-fifth as much as the heavier machines, does all kinds of work done by any machine, and does it better than most of them, it has the scientific keyboard, which is easiest of all to learn, and the fact that it is composed of but about 250 parts as against the something like 2,000 of other makes is prima facie evidence that it is proportionately less likely to get out of order. It is called the *Blickensderfer*, and is made at Stamford, Conn., by the Blickensderfer Manufacturing Company, in two styles, the most portable size being No. 5, which without its case weighs about six pounds, No. 7 having a little greater range and weighing a few pounds more. We prefer this machine to any other yet offered. The prices are $35 and $50, and while these companies do not as a rule advertise in medical journals we shall modestly but unhesitatingly suggest to the proprietors of the Blickensderfer the propriety and advisability of advertising their ingenious and every way desirable apparatus to the readers of the GAZETTE.

Among the good points that distinguish this machine from most others we will mention a few.

The line you are writing is in plain sight as you write it. It does away with the use of ribbons entirely, substituting a small ink-roller which can be removed in a jiffy, without soiling the fingers, and costing but 4 cents. There are no long type-bars to get out of alignment, and one can have half a dozen styles of type, instantly interchangeable, extra type-wheels costing but a dollar. The spacing can be varied from the width of a line to half an inch or more at will. It manifolds well, the printed line never "wabbles," that is, it cannot get out of alignment, and it stands all sorts of abuse without kicking. The writer has used one of these machines for nearly eight years at a cost of less than two dollars for repairs. This is one of the most important items in connection with the use of any machine, and fully warrants any seeming enthusiasm we may have expressed.

Dear Editor:

Query 91. I am frequently encountering the word *Kinetic*, but no dictionary to which I have access gives me a satisfactory definition. In fact, to be quite frank, the word does not occur in my dictionary, only some of its derivatives being mentioned, as *Kinetoscope*, the definition of which is "An instrument for illustrating the results of combinations of arcs, arcs of different radii in making curves." Evidently this does not explain its medical meaning. Can you lift the clouds?

E. L. A., Arkansas.

Answer.—The word is from the Greek *Kineo*, to move. Hence *Kinetic* is defined as "causing motion; motory; pertaining to or causing motion, as *Kinetic Energy.*"—*Century.*

"That which produces motion. Pertaining to those forces which produce motion."—*Gould.*

"Pertaining to, manifested by or causing motion."—*Foster.*

The derivative, *Kinesitherapy,* although ignored by Foster, is coming into use as a scientific appellation for a system of cure based on Swedish Movement and Gymnastics. The *Century* thus defines it.

Gould spells it both *Kinesotherapy* and *Kinesitherapy,* while Foster gives *Kinesipathy,* and refers the reader to *Cinessonosus,* and also to *Cinesitherapy.* If the original "Osteopath" had been a better linguist and devoid of ambition to straddle a fad, he would have adopted the word *Kinesitherapy* instead of the other awkward term to describe his system.

The word is now much used by the "Physical Culturists" in lieu of the straight-from-the-shoulder English, *Movement-cure.*

THE GRAND MEDICINE MAN.

ACCORDING to the *Open Court,* the ceremony of the Grand Medicine is an elaborate ritual, covering several days, the endless number of gods and spirits being called upon to minister to the sick man and to lengthen his life. The several degrees of the Grand Medicine teach the use of incantations, of medicines and poisons, and the requirements necessary to constitute a brave. "When a young man seeks admission to the Grand Medicine Lodge, he first fasts until he sees in his dream some animal (the mink, beaver, otter, and fisher being most common), which he hunts and kills. The skin is then ornamented with beads or porcupine quills, and the spirit of the animal becomes the friend and companion of the man." The medicine men have only a limited knowledge of herbs, but they are expert

in dressing wounds, and the art of extracting barbed arrows from the flesh can be learned from them.

In olden times—yes, to within the memory of living Ojibways—the medicine man at the funeral ceremony thus addressed the departed: "Dear friend, you will not feel lonely while pursuing your journey toward the setting sun. I have killed for you a Sioux (hated enemy of the Ojibways) and I have scalped him. He will accompany you and provide for you, hunting your food as you need it. The scalp I have taken, use it for your moccasins."

OLD PROVERBS IN NEW DRESS.

Quacks are stubborn things.

It's a wise girl who knows her own mind.

Society's the mother of 'convention.

Home was not built in a day.

Modesty is the best policy.

Circumstances alter faces.

A rolling gait gathers no remorse.

All's not old that titters.

Let us eat, drink, and be married, for tomorrow we dye.

Charity uncovers a multitude of sins.— CAROLINE WELLS, in *The Smart Set.*

THE ratio of physicians to population is 1 to less than 600 in our country, while in Great Britain it is 1 to 1,100, and in Russia, 1 to 8,500. Proportionately, we have four times as many physicians as France, five times as many as Germany, six times as many as Italy, and six times as many medical schools as any of these countries.

✦ ✦

"UNCLE JOHN," said little Emily, "do you know that a baby that was fed on elephant's milk gained twenty pounds in a week?" "Nonsense!" exclaimed Uncle John, and then asked: "Whose baby was it?" "It was the elephant's baby," replied little Emily.

THE
DIETETIC AND HYGIENIC GAZETTE

A·MONTHLY·JOURNAL ᴏꜰ PHYSIOLOGICAL·MEDICINE

Vol. XVII.	NEW YORK, AUGUST, 1901.	No. 8.

WHAT THE CENTURY HAS TAUGHT US ABOUT LIVING.

By SAMUEL S. WALLIAN, A.M., M.D.

V.

SOURCES AND SELECTIONS OF FOOD.

In a general and sweeping sense food must supply the wants and waste of the body. No dietary is complete that does not accomplish both these objects.

America is the land of abundance, the granary and grazing-ground of the world. Every form of food-supply either exists or is produced in lavish quantities. The very profusion of Nature's gifts is here a source of actual embarrassment. It leads to surfeit and to waste. We indulge in too great variety and too many luxuries. True, the race is steadily advancing in many directions, but there is plenty of room for improvement in our methods of living which would add to our span of life, and to our progress as a nation, as representatives of the human race.

In the matter of how we shall live we substitute fashion for frugality, elaborateness for economy, and whims of appetite for wholesomeness of aliment. Earth and air and ocean teem with food-supplies that are unapproachable in quality and unlimited in quantity. It is our own fault that we blunder in our adaptations, make indiscreet selections and combinations, and are stupidly careless and negligent in our manipulations and methods of preparation. The generous earth germinates the seeds and grows the roots and tubers; the sun, air and rain mature and ripen the grains, fruits and nuts; beasts, birds and fowls feed on these and fatten; and the sea yields up its generous store of crustaceans and finny food, so that our tables groan with their loads of luxuries and their burden of bounties. Scientists insist that the quadruped is a four-footed man, the bird a flying man, and the fish a swimming man; and that the tree and grain and grass are but vegetating men. If we accept this version of creation, then the biped man is at best nothing less than a cannibal. He dominates the whole and subsists on his own kind! He levies tribute on every species, from gastropod to Graham bread, from mollusk to moose-deer, and from the oyster to the ox. The very affluence of his inheritance confuses his judgment and tempts him to riotous living.

From whence shall we draw our supply of the proteids, the nitrogenous or albuminous foods, which must compose at least one part in four, or four and a half, of all we eat? Shall it be from the gluten of grains, the albumen of eggs, or from the blood, fibrin and gelatin of flesh, from beef and bluefish, or from bread and beans? This question has already been broached. The radical vegetarians are confident and enthusiastic, basing their arguments on the logic of esthetics and the history of various races. A few of these may be cited:

The Japanese are a race of great physical and mental development. This is evidenced by their political progress and acumen. Physically they have strength, hardness and suppleness of muscle, such as astonishes the world. Intellectually they are giving evidence of similar virility; they have conquered China and are holding Russia and all other nations at a respectful distance; and they have forged ahead in the arts and sciences until America is not ashamed to imitate their manufacturing processes and purchase their art products. Her people subsist almost entirely on grains, vegetables and fish, and the quantity of food they consume is "astonishingly small," when compared with that devoured by the flesh-eating nations of the Western world. The Japanese peasantry, living wholly without flesh-meats, perform the most wonderful feats of manual labor, actually taking the places usually filled by horses and oxen, and they possess an endurance of both heat, cold, and severe muscular strain that is simply marvelous. All those races which have ranked high as to their civilization, and as to their beauty of form, feature and complexion, as witness the Circassians, have invariably been an agricultural people, subsisting almost exclusively on the direct products of the soil. On the other hand, the most brutal and disgusting forms yet described as belonging to the human race, for example the Calmucks and Cannibals, have been those who subsisted chiefly or wholly on animal food, and that of the most depraved and disgusting type. The strongest men of the three manliest races of the present world, the Schleswig-Holstein *Bauern*, who furnish the heaviest curassiers for the Prussian army and ablest men of the Hamburg navy, the Mandingo tribes of Senegambia, and the Turanian mountaineers of Dahgestan and Lesghia, are said to be non-carnivorous. There is no question but that the advocates of a direct grain, fruit and vegetable diet

for man have history, logic and esthetics all on their side; but as society is at present organized and established by habit, custom and strong prejudice, they must be content to make slow but steady progress toward popularizing their arguments and principles. Each succeeding generation will add to their numbers; but a century, and it may be several centuries, will be required to inaugurate the dietetic millennium of which they dream and bring about that

"one far off, divine event
Toward which the whole creation moves."

Meanwhile, works on dietetics, to be practical, must be adapted to conditions and society as they are, and not as they should be.

PERCENTAGE OF PROTEIDS IN VARIOUS FOOD PRODUCTS.

Long tables of chemical details are the driest of dry reading. They would be drier but for the fact that they are seldom read. If scientific writers realized that not one in ten of their readers—perhaps this estimate is ten times too liberal—ever follows to the end a single one of their labored and elaborate tables of minutiæ and infinitesimals, they would either omit them entirely or skin and skim them until only the essentials were left. Let this protest and counterblast be a sufficient explanation of the absence of most of these scientific space-fillers and cemeteries of chemical coefficients.

At best, tables are lame guides. Like the tables of the Weather Bureau, they all need interpreting before they can be understood and their value estimated. For example, the physiologic chemists tell us that one ounce of protein represents a fuel value of 129 calories, which is equal to 198 foot tons; an ounce of carbohydrates exactly the same, while an ounce of fats represents a fuel value of 143 calories, or nearly 220 foot tons; and this fuel value is called potential energy. Practically a man derives more real strength and vital endurance from 1 ounce of protein than from half a pound of fats. Again, a pound of beef and a quart of un-skimmed milk represent about the same quantities of nutritive material; but for or-dinary use the nutrients of the beef differ in proportion as well as kind, and can be turned to more practical account in certain ways. In all the analyses of foods two im-portant items are ignored—the contained water, which is reckoned as a non-nutrient, and that indefinable mystery that yet eludes our art, the vital principle of plants, the secret of vito-chemical combinations. To grasp these would be to pierce the eternal secret through and to find the Philosopher's Stone. The hard and fast lines of separation between the several proximate principles of food are both artificial and arbitrary. Na-ture ignores them, since proteids serve their purpose as body-builders and are then, as occasion requires, broken up by cleav-age and oxidation into "fuel," and the car-bohydrates, though in a much more limited degree, may replace the proteids when the latter are temporarily absent in the dietary. Furthermore, since the fasting cranks have proved it, the water constituent of foods can no longer be termed "non-nutrient."

The practical question is to determine as nearly as possible what articles of the cur-rent food-supply will furnish the nutrients required by the body, in the kinds and the proportions adapted to the perfect nutri-tion of every organ and tissue, and at a minimum cost. This covers the whole ques-tion of food economy.

The confusion in the use of terms may be summarily disposed of by the broad and comprehensive statement that "proteids," "nitrogeneous products," "gelatinoids," "albuminoids," "amids," etc., which include the glutens or vegetable albumins, myosin, the base of lean meat or muscle, gelatin, col-lagen and ossein, all come under the head of nitrogeneous bodies and are principally tis-sue builders.

This confusion is not surprising, since what we know of the real or vital chem-istry of foods is still rudimentary, tenta-tive and inaccurate. Works on dietetics in-dulge in a good many ambitious terms, con-cerning "potential energy," fuel value, and transformations into mechanical power, of a given food substance; and of how carbo-hydrates and fats act in a conservative way by preventing the consumption of proteids. Much of this science is more lucid than logical.

This table contains the salient facts, all that is really practical, from nearly 100 pages of analytical statistics, as tabulated in the bulletins of the Experiment Stations conducted by the United States Department of Agriculture. As an example of the ex-tent to which condensation has been prac-tised, the one line covering the item of beef, in the above table, occupied nearly 1,000 lines or entries in the tables referred to. The 1,000 entries are not, however, repe-titions, but referred in detail to all the vari-ous portions of the animal and fancy prepa-rations from which analyses were made, varying all the way from horns to heels, and from soup and shin bone to sirloin steak. The figures quoted above give the extremes.

It is charged that of all the various forms of lying now current in the world, statis-tical lying, which technically is not lying at all, is the most mischievous. Ordinary lying has ceased to do harm, since it deceives no one; but your scientific lying consists in presenting essential facts in such a blind, diffuse or confused form as to deceive the very elect. These facts assume such an air and attitude of dignity that, however mis-leading, they always appear in the livery of exact mathematical truth.

It must be confessed that, unless it be the delusive tables of the Weather Bureau, there is no department of inquiry and inves-tigation in which figures can be made to say so much and mean so little as in the do-main of food statistics and food analyses. This may be chiefly because the exact for-mula for protein, the most important proxi-mate principle of food, is not yet, and may never be, known.

There are few reliable analyses of the nut family at command, but nut foods are at-

COMPARATIVE COMPOSITION OF FOOD MATERIALS.

(BY PERCENTAGES.)

Condensed Essentials of a Hundred Tables.

Articles.	Water.	Total Nutrients.	Protein.	Fats.	Carbo-hydrates.	Mineral Salts.	Fuel Value, in Calories.
Vegetables :							
Irish potatoes	78.9	21.1	2.1	.1	17.9	1	375
Sweet potatoes	71.1	28.9	1.5	.4	26	1	536
Beets	88	11.5	1.5	.1	8.8	1.1	195
Turnips	89.6	10.6	1.2	.2	8.2	1	185
Carrots	88.6	11.4	1.1	.4	8.9	1	205
Onions	87.6	12.4	1.4	.3	10.1	.6	225
Squash	88.1	11.9	.9	.2	10.1	.7	215
Pumpkin	93.4	6.6	.9	1	4.9	.7	110
Cabbage	90.5	9.5	2.4	.4	5.3	1.4	155
Cauliflower	90.8	9.2	1.6	.8	5	.8	155
Spinach	92.4	7.6	2.1	.8	3.1	1.9	120
Asparagus	94	3	1.8	.2	3.3	.7	105
Tomatoes	96	4	.8	.4	2.5	.3	80
Green peas	78.1	21.9	4.4	.5	16.1	.9	400
String beans	87.2	12.8	2.2	.4	9.5	.7	235
Green sweet corn	81.2	18.8	2.8	1.1	14.2	.7	360
Baked beans	67.2	32.8	7.1	3.2	20.3	2.2	615
Fruits :							
Apples	83.2	16.8	.3	.4	15.9	.2	320
Cherries	86.1	13.9	1.1	.8	11.4	.6	265
Strawberries	90.8	9.2	1	.7	6.9	.6	175
Blackberries	88.9	11.1	.9	2.1	7.5	.6	245
Whortleberries	82.4	17.6	.7	3	13.5	.4	390
Cranberries	87.6	12.4	.4	.9	10.9	.2	350
Grapes, Catawba	74.8	25.2	1.6	1.7	21.3	.6	500
Lemons	79.3	10.7	1	.9	7.3	.5	210
Banana	63.3	33.7	1.4	1.4	29.8	1.1	640
Pineapple	89.3	10.7	.4	.3	9.7	.3	200
Watermelon	91.9	8.1	.9	.7	6.2	.3	160
Nutmeg melon	76.4	23.6	1.4	.2	20.5	1.5	415
Flesh Meats, Fresh :							
Beef, various cuts	24-60	10-60	8-19	2-53	....	.6-1.2	235-2435
Veal	50-64	25-26	15-18	5-10	....	.9-1	570-717
Mutton	32-51	31-60	12-15	16-44	....	.5-.9	925-2145
Lamb	41-53	29-40	14-17	12-24	....	.8-.8	820-1255
Pork	31-49	40-46	13-14	25-70	....	.8-.9	1325-1425
Chicken	69-92	27-31	21-25	1-5	....	1-2	330-633
Turkey	63-66	25-37	17-24	5-14	1	.9-2	550-1015
Corned beef	71	24	17	5	....	2.4	525
Smoked ham	37	52	15	35	....	2.4	1735
Fresh Fish :							
Averages	27-62	15-39	14-24	5-19	....	.7-2	250-1130
Shell Fish :							
Oysters	87	13	6	1.6	4	.9	260
Clams	86	14	9	1	2	2.6	240
Scallops	80	20	15	.2	3.4	1.4	345
Lobsters	31	18	15	1.9	....	1.7	350
Crabs	77	23	18	2	....	3	415
Shrimps	71	29	26	1	....	2.6	520
Terrapin	75	26	21	3.5	....	1	540
Green turtle	80	20	19	5	....	1.2	365
Dairy Products :							
Milk, cow's	87	13	4	1	4.7	.7	325
Butter	10	89	1	85	.5	5	3615
Cheese	30	70	28	36	1.8	4.2	2070
Oleomargarine	11	89	.6	85	.4	5	3605
Miscellaneous :							
Sugar, granulated	2	98	....	....	97.8	.2	1820
Starch	2	98	....	....	97.5	.2	1820
Wheat bread	32.3	67.7	8.8	1.7	56.3	.9	1280
Graham bread	34.2	65.8	9.5	1.4	53.3	1.6	1225
Rye bread	30	70	8.4	.5	59.7	1.4	1285
Pilot bread	7.9	92.1	12.4	4.4	74.2	1.1	1795
Eggs, hen's	63.1	23.2	12.1	10.2	....	.9	655

COMPARATIVE COMPOSITION OF FOOD MATERIALS.—(Continued.)

Breadstuffs :						
Wheat flour, ordinary	12.5	87.5	11	1.1	74.9	.5	1645
" " roller process	14.8	93.5	13.8	1.9	78.1	.5	1715
G aham flour	13.1	86.9	11.7	1.7	71.7	1.5	1625
Whole wheat flour	13	87	13.6	2	70	1.4	1640
Cornmeal	15	85	9.2	8.8	70.6	1.4	1645
Buckwheat flour	14.6	85.4	6.9	1.4	75.1	1	1605
Rye flour	13.1	86.9	6.8	.8	78.7	.7	1625
Oatmeal	7.8	92.2	11.7	7.1	68.4	2	1845
Rice	12.4	87.6	7.4	.4	79.4	.4	1630
Nuts :						
Almonds	4.8	52.3	21	54.9	17.3	2.5	3030
Beechnuts	4.1	21.9	57.4	13.2	....	3.9	1655
Brazil nuts	5.3	17	66.8	7	....	3.8	3265
Butternuts	4.4	27.9	61.2	3.5	....	2.9	3165
Chestnuts, fresh	45	6.2	5.4	42.1	....	1.3	1125
" dried	5.9	10.7	7	74.2	....	2.2	1875
Cocoanuts	14.1	5.7	50.6	27.9	....	1.7	2760
Filberts	3.7	15.6	65.3	13	....	2.4	3290
Hickory nuts	3.7	15.4	67.4	11.4	....	2.1	3345
Lichi nuts	17.9	2.9	.2	77.5	....	1.5	1505
Peanuts	9.2	25.8	38.6	24.4	....	2	2560
Pecans	3	11	71.2	13.3	....	1.5	3455
Pistachio nuts	4.2	22.3	54	16.3	....	3.2	2995
Walnuts, Calif., soft shell	2.5	16.6	63.4	16.1	....	1.1	3285
Peanut butter	2.1	29.3	46.5	17.1	....	5	2825
" Malted nuts "	2.6	23.7	27.6	43.9	....	2.2	2240

tracting much more attention than ever before, except, perhaps, in the primitive day, when our ancestors subsisted upon nuts, fruits, barks and roots. At least one large company in this country is extensively engaged in preparing various forms of palatable, wholesome and nutritious nut products for the table. The success of this movement has aroused fresh interest in this promising class of nutritives, and the nut oils bid fair to supersede the use of some of the less desirable varieties of the animal oils. The esthetic sanitarian can feel no regret at the prospective banishment of lard, oleomargarine and cottolene from the cuisine catalogue, and if even Elgin creamery, with its remote suspicion of tubercular taint, should eventually follow, it would be in keeping with some other hygienic reforms that are more or less agitated.

There are two classes of edible nuts, those which are comparatively free from, and those which contain, a considerable percentage of, starch. All of them yield more or less oil, bland in quality and both palatable and digestible. To this statement there are a few exceptions. All contain a considerable quantity of the proteids, and hence are very markedly nutritious. Sweet almonds head the list of non-starchy, chestnuts and peanuts representing the starchy varieties.

It is a popular fallacy that all nuts are hard to digest, and predispose to "biliousness." Manna from heaven would disturb the digestion and rattle the liver if eaten between meals, and after a hearty and sufficient meal of other food, which is the usual way of eating nuts.

Glancing at the table, those who have not already made similar comparisons will be surprised at the apparent anomalies. Thus the figures make Irish potatoes and apples each contain two and a half times as much "total nutrients" as the poorest cuts of beef, quite as much as the best cuts of veal or corned beef, twice as much as oysters or milk, more than either lobsters, scallops, crabs or green turtle, and nearly as much as turkey or terrapin. In fuel value sweet potatoes, peas and beans rank with corned beef and chicken, while apples, bananas, grapes and cranberries are nearly equal in nutritious value to the poorer cuts of beef and other flesh meats. The three items which rank highest in nutritive value are sugar, starch and pilot bread, and in fuel value butter and oleomargarine leave all the rest far in the shade.

Of course these values are theoretical and

comparative. No man can subsist for any length of time on either sugar, starch, butter or oleomargarine, and an exclusive diet of pilot bread would soon become unendurably monotonous. Buckwheat flour, which, according to the musty traditions, is very "heating," not to mention many other alleged perversities, has less fuel value than that blandest of all foods for invalids and Celestials—rice. Wheat bread, it will be seen, exceeds in nutritive value the best cuts of beef, and is in itself an almost complete food. One dietetic authority asserts that the two items, wheat and apples, are capable of supplying all the elements of nutrition.

Butter stands credited with 89 per cent. of nutritive value, while a juicy sirloin steak has but 27 per cent.; whereas, practically, a pound of steak will nourish a man far better than twice that quantity of butter. It is the so-called "fuel value" of the butter which makes it rank so high in the tables. Of real tissue-builders it possesses a bare trace. So, too, flank beef and flank mutton are rated far above the best loin cuts of the same animal, simply because they are one-half fat, and fat ranks high in "calories." No man could live on cheese, and yet cheese possesses a stunning amount of nutritive equivalents. The tables are full of similar inconsistencies.

In the condensed table given the variations in the quoted values of beef, as already indicated, depend upon the "cuts." To separate the proximate principles which go to make up a rational dietary and say that one of these is more important or valuable than another is out of the question. It may be assumed that protein is most important as a single item, but protein alone will not sustain life. Each principle is valuable only as it is found combined with the others in due and proper proportions.

For the most part the butchers of to-day are nothing more than meat carvers, the refrigerator car having revolutionized this business. The actual "butchering" is done a thousand miles from the market shops.

A cut to illustrate the various "cuts," as

named by standard marketmen in New York City, will not be out of place.

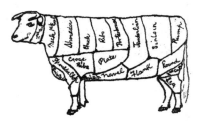

This sample of the geography of the *corpus bovis* corresponds as nearly as any in use to the current designations and practice of New York marketmen. Esthetic Boston has a bovine topography of its own. Here is the map issued by the "Boston Cook Book" (Mrs. Lincoln).

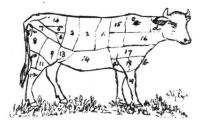

(This diagram needs a key, just as the animal that posed for its picture needed corn. But then, it is more intellectual, and has larger ears than its New York competitor!)

1. Top of sirloin.
2. Middle of sirloin.
3. First cut of sirloin.
4. Back of rump.
5. Middle of rump.
6. Face of rump.
7. Aitch bone.
8. Lower part of round.
8½. Top of round.
9. Vein.
10. Poorer part of round.
11. Poorer part of vein.

12. Shin.
13. Boneless flank.
14. Thick flank, with bone.
15. First cut of ribs.
(c) Chuck ribs.
(d) Neck.
16. Rattle rand.
17. Second cut of rattle rand.
18. Brisket (a, navel; b, butt end).
19. Fore shin.

✣ ✣

SOME SUGGESTIONS ON SEA-SICK-NESS.

By Daniel R. Brower, M.D., LL.D.

More than the ordinary amount of ocean travel has fallen to my lot, and I am more than usually susceptible to mal de mer; hence, I have been compelled to give some special consideration to the subject. While it is a disorder of the brain, yet inasmuch as the principal sensory nerve of the brain is also the sensory nerve of the stomach, a disturbance of this will intensify and precipitate an attack.

There is no infallible cure, yet very much can be done in the way of prevention and mitigation. The two days before sailing should be as restful as possible; the foundation of many a bad voyage is laid two or three days before the ship sails, by overfatigue and over-eating. Persons go aboard tired and "bilious," and the slightest thing then will bring on an attack of nausea, vomiting and headache. The second day before sailing, at bedtime, a dose of blue mass, 3 to 5 grains, should be taken, and followed the next morning by a saline; this may be a Seidlitz powder, a glass of Hunyadi water or a moderate dose of Rochelle salts. After the evacuation of the bowels the bromide of sodium should be taken in 20-grain doses every four hours, until the ship is out of port. If relief has not been obtained he should stretch out in his steamer chair, with his back to the ocean, apply a capsicum plaster over the stomach, and take 20 grains of the bromide, with 15 grains of chloralamid keep the eyes closed and rest quietly, go to sleep and when he awakens he will, in all probability, have his "sea legs" on. If not the dosage must be repeated.

The bromide of sodium and chloralamid should be dispensed in separate *waxed* papers.

The sea-sickness sometimes lingers around because the person does not eat judiciously, exercise freely, secure daily evacuations of the bowels and keep on deck.

✣ ✣

CHLOROSIS.

Says *the London Hospital:* The point of view from which many of the phenomena of chlorosis are regarded has altered considerably during recent years, so that now again, as in that long ago when by giving the disorder such names as *febris amatoria, icterus amantium,* and so forth, physicians expressed their belief in its sexual origin, the tendency is to regard the disorder as associated in some way with the function of reproduction, perhaps, in fact, as but an exaggeration of certain changes which normally occur in woman preparatory to her great function of childbearing. Time was when attention was principally fixed upon the changes in this blood in disease. Poverty of blood was looked upon as the central fact to be regarded. Anemia and debility being considered as almost of necessity coincident, and chlorosis being evidently a condition of anemia, every effort was made to "build up" new blood.

Perhaps the microscope was responsible. At any rate, we can have no doubt that by depending too much upon the counting of blood corpuscles both in diagnosis and in estimating progress physicians have for many years past hovered on the verge of error.

Of late, however, with more accurate

clinical methods at our disposal, doubt has been thrown upon much that was not so long ago considered certain. Speaking at a recent meeting of the British Balneological and Climatological Association Professor Clifford Allbutt pointed out that some of the tests on which we have relied can no longer be trusted. "For many years," he says, "we, or our clinical clerks for us, have been industriously engaged in making blood counts. Now of the value of blood counts in the more eccentric deviations of the blood from the standard of health I am at present not called upon to speak; we leave such perversions out of account. But even if we regard for the moment the red corpuscles only, as in chlorosis, for instance, the value of blood counts, if not depreciated beyond all usefulness, proves to be far less directly interpretive than we had supposed." He goes on to show that a drop of blood taken in the usual way is not by any means representative of the mass of the blood in the body, varying as it does according to the condition of the cutaneous circulation, according to the exercise taken or of mental work done, according to the time in relation to sleep, and in other ways.

Not only do we thus have it that the blood counts, on which so much has been made to hinge, are useless or misleading, but by new methods of research new factors are being introduced into the problem. More especially do we now have to consider the total quantity of blood present in the body. We are now told that the impoverished condition of the blood in chlorosis, which to some observers has appeared to be the main departure from health and sufficient to account for all the symptoms of the disease, is after all only apparent, that there are corpuscles enough and hemoglobin enough, only that they are scattered through far too large a quantity of plasma—plasma which, useful as it may be for purposes of nutrition, is obviously of but small service in carrying oxygen to the tissues and in thus maintaining the functional activity of the body.

Taking this more recent view of chlorosis it would appear that the dyspnea, the palpitation, and the not infrequent dilatation of the heart in chlorosis are to be explained, not by lack of blood, but by the fact that in this disease the bulk of the blood is increased without proportionate increase in the corpuscular element. Thus the therapeutical problem is not so much how to multiply the red corpuscles as how to diminish the plasma in which they are extended. "Pull the blood together and there will be corpuscles enough, the heart will not have to deliver excessive parcels of blood to the lungs and elsewhere, and its dilatation will recede in so far as it may have been due, not to malnutrition, but to need of greater temporary capacity." On this hypothesis many of the symptoms of chlorosis appear easy of explanation, and the somewhat mixed ideas which have long prevailed as to the therapeutics seem to receive some degree of clarification. We cannot admit, however, that we are any nearer the prime cause and origin of the disease. Probably the old physicians were right, and certainly a considerable number of modern physicians are inclined to agree with them in thinking that sexuality has much to do with the matter, that this excessively rich blood plasma is in a sense a preparation for maternity, and that many of the symptoms which accompany the condition are but the organic expression of that deeply-rooted desire for maternity which, however little it may be shown, or even felt so far as the ordinary consciousness is concerned, is the motive power in the life of normal woman. This raises at once the ticklish question of marriage as a cure for chlorosis, about which we will only say that "it is a wasteful thing to use a steam hammer to crack nuts. Still, the nuts do generally crack."

THERE is no arguing with the inevitable. The only argument available with an east wind is to put on your overcoat.—*Lowell.*

DIETS FOR EVERY DAY USE.

By J. WARREN ACHORN, M.D.,
Boston.

THE treatment of eczema should properly begin in childhood. Children, either of whose parents have developed hay fever, asthma, salt rheum or eczema, should never be allowed to eat foods that produce these disorders or invite them, if latent.

These dyscrasias are certainly related; the children of parents who have suffered from either are liable to an outcropping of eczema, especially if fed at random.

We often see children educated by unthinking parents to eat the very food that, later on, will cause them to suffer the disorders from which their betters are begging relief and paying the doctor prescription fees in vain.

All cases of eczema do not call for specific dietetic treatment; in some instances the condition seems to be due to nervous or neurotic causes associated with a delicate skin, the food and digestion being all right. It is a good plan, however, in obstinate cases, to test the digestive apparatus for hidden help or negative influences that unconsciously protract the disease. Surprisingly beneficial results will often follow independent exploration of the digestive tract.

Washing out the stomach, for instance, is a source of benefit in cases where liver torpor or uterine disorders are suspected, especially in immature girls or unmarried women; and when no cause is made an excuse for the trial it works well; probably by freeing the system of acids that induce intestinal fermentation and act as irritants inside and out.

Uterine pains before or during menstruation that light up periodical eczema and acne or aggravate an existing dyscrasia, often disappear, and with them the skin trouble, after stomach washing is begun, showing plainly the effect of stimulation of the pelvic organs through gastric channels.

Percolation or stimulation of a lazy liver with water, when no recognized disorder of the stomach or intestines is present, works unthought of results sometimes. The eczema begins to dry up or improve at once; if not, one has the satisfaction of knowing that neither the stomach, liver nor intestines are at fault.

Many cases of eczema are due, in part, to dilatation of the stomach, where lavage goes far toward a cure.

Seborrheic eczema due to acid fermentation in the stomach has been made to disappear in this way. A *red nose* will fade for the same reason if allowed to.

The water for washing should be tepid, fairly hot or moderately cold, according to the patient's general condition, and whether the stomach, liver, uterus or circulation is the thing aimed at in particular. It is best, perhaps, to wash with tepid water until experience has been gained as to the effect in a given case, when a change, if indicated, may be made.

The stomach should be empty when washed, and half an hour, at least, should elapse after each flushing before food is eaten. Bilious looking subjects may be treated the first thing in the morning, when considerable bile will often be found in the stomach. This soon disappears if treatment is continued. Five o'clock in the afternoon, or an hour before the principal meal of the day, are good times for washing if the patient is hard worked and too tired to digest a substantial meal. The stomach does better work in these cases after it has been flushed out.

The sessions should not be too protracted. Two and a half gallons of water are usually sufficient for a sitting. Not more than two pints should be introduced at one time, better less than more, to be immediately syphoned out.

Some patients undergo this form of treatment daily and thrive on it. Three times a week is a good practice. Flooding the colon is not a patch on the procedure outlined here, for effectiveness, and the same may be said of hot water drinking between meals.

A healthy nose, throat and digestive

tract—in a word, healthy mucous membranes and lively eliminative organs, that are not aggravated, irritated and impoverished by all sorts of indigestible stuff—go far towards preserving a normal outside skin.

Lack of oxidation, lack of air, lack of exercise, are certainly factors in causing and maintaining this disorder. Lovers of ease and eating are most subject to it.

Inside washing is of benefit in diseases of the skin, while outside washing in eczema is often harmful.

The local treatment of eczema is very important.

DIET IN ECZEMA.
(Copyright.)

As soon as awake, or while dressing, take a glass of hot or cold water, sipped slowly, or of hot skimmed milk or of plain milk, cut one-third with Saratoga Vichy, etc.

BREAKFAST: *Cereals*—"Cooked gluten," wheaten grits, whole wheat, Ralston Breakfast Food, shredded wheat, hominy, with cream and a dash of sugar, or with butter and salt; rye mush thoroughly cooked, cornmeal mush with skimmed milk or cream.

Meats (red)—Rump steak, round steak, sirloin; mutton chops, lamb chops; thin bacon with dry toast; broiled fresh tripe. Pepper and salt.

Fish—Chicken halibut, cod, haddock, flounder, scup, butterfish, smelts, the lean of shad, any lake or brook fish, boiled or broiled; salted herring occasionally.

Eggs—Soft boiled, poached or scrambled. The yolks.

Breads—Whole wheat bread, gluten bread, rye or French bread, Cestus brown bread, pilot bread. Butter, jam, marmalade.

Fruits—Orange juice, pineapple juice, cantaloupe, melons; stewed prunes, stewed figs, French prepared prunes, Turkey figs, prepared peaches.

Drinks—Clear coffee, cereal coffee, Phillip's Digestible Cocoa, one glass of hot or cold milk, or of hot or cold water; buttermilk.

A.M. BETWEEN MEALS: Hot or cold water, hot or cold milk cut with French or Saratoga Vichy, skimmed milk, buttermilk. Phosphated crackers, Turkey figs, prunes, etc.

NOTES.

In acute eczema the diet should be chiefly bread and milk, or other non-irritating liquid food—no stimulants. This form of treatment for two or three weeks in chronic eczema often makes a good beginning.

The dyspepsia of eczema is usually a chronic gastric catarrh, associated with dilation perhaps or a sluggish liver.

Eczema is also due to acid fermentation, more often intestinal than otherwise.

Eczema in children is usually due to indigestible food.

Deficient fat is a cause of eczema in children; this is true no matter how plump the child is in appearance. It is a causative factor in the eczema of grown people.

Ichthalbin (oil of fishes) is an excellent remedy for children with this disorder. Mixed with Vigor Chocolate it is readily taken. The yolks of eggs are sometimes beneficial.

German Seltzer and milk (half and half), served hot, make a good morning drink.

Water, hot or cold, may be flavored by holding a checkerberry lozenge between the teeth.

Coffee should not be drunk with any meal where milk or cream have been used in quantity. Avoid the after-dinner-cup. On account of the uric acid in tea and coffee both may prove injurious.

Wines or liquors that disturb the circulation of the skin, such as beer, ale and red wines must be avoided. Shinnecock whiskey goes best or some white wine, such as Moselle. These must be taken by measurement with meals—never more better less, except in old burned-out subjects.

Cane sugar is the least harmful of the sweets, but all sweets are objectionable.

Starch and sugar must be greatly restricted in an eczematous patient with gouty diathesis.

Only fresh foods should be eaten; the few things specified may be made the exception, if they are desired and are found to agree.

Fresh fruit may be eaten in moderation in most cases. Cooked or prepared fruits are safer than raw ripe fruits. Apples, pears, grapes and bananas are generally denied. Do not eat fruit and vegetables at the same meal. Fruits, if they agree equally well, were better eaten at the close of a meal.

Prepared peaches constipate. Potatoes by irritating the stomach and alimentary canal disturb the action of the skin. Sweet potatoes should not be eaten at all.

Oatmeal and buckwheat are injurious in this disorder.

Certain shell fish disagree with some. This is a matter of idiosyncrasy.

Vegetables, cereals, bread and milk (nitrogenous) should constitute the basis for a diet in eczema; albuminous foods are to be used only to

LUNCH: *Meats* (red)—Roast beef, roast lamb; boiled ham, cut thin and served cold; (white) chicken, capon, breast of turkey, squab, partridge, quail, any game bird (except as mentioned in notes), boiled or roasted.

Any fresh fish mentioned.

Any vegetable mentioned, if desired.

Any bread mentioned. Cestus phosphated crackers, soup sticks, rusk, zwieback, somatose biscuit, bread and milk.

Any fruit mentioned.

Any drink mentioned.

Any dessert mentioned, if desired.

P.M. BETWEEN MEALS: Same as A.M. Weak lemonade, root beer carrying sarsaparilla.

DINNER: *Soups*—Any clear vegetable soups, with rice, sago, bisbak, vermicelli, or okra; veal broth, lamb broth, chicken broth; croutons.

Any fish mentioned. Oysters (raw), with horseradish or lemon juice, if known to agree; shredded codfish.

Any meat mentioned.

---

the extent of the needs of the system, as determined by the general health of the patient. Vegetables are especially indicated on account of the alkaline salts they contain, care being taken not to use rhubarb, tomatoes, etc., too freely, as they yield acids also.

Avoid solid food between meals unless constipated or in need of nourishment.

Red meats should be eaten but once a day; the top of the round is best. Eat only lean meat pulp, avoid connective tissue.

Avoid cold meats and cold meals as a rule. Avoid duck and goose, domestic or wild. Ham that has been boiled until it is as tender as stewed chicken may be eaten. Eggs may be eaten three times a week if known to agree.

Gluten (30 per cent.) is an admirable substitute for meat.

Soups must be eaten sparingly, if at all.

All breads should be at least one day old, and eaten cold. Gluten and breads carrying phosphates in excess are best.

Salines taken regularly for a time, especially magnesia, helps eczema. Constipation must not be tolerated.

Tobacco is especiallly injurious.

Sea-bathing aggravates eczema.

Soft water to bathe in is indispensable; distilled or rain water is to be preferred.

Strained gruel should be used in place of soap, or corn bran if the eczema is moist.

Soft linen or cotton should be worn next the skin. Soft moist air is beneficial. Harsh winds are irritating.

Vegetables—Lettuce, beet greens, dandelion greens, with pepper and salt, lemon juice, horseradish or oil; new string beans, new peas, new corn, if it agrees; squash, pumpkin, minced carrots, celery (stewed or raw). Spinach, asparagus, onions, watercress, tomatoes—of either twice a week. Rice, with platter gravy in place of potatoes. One baked potato, daily, baked with jacket on; macaroni, plain or with tomato.

Any bread mentioned. Cæstus bisbak and milk, toast and milk, pilot bread and milk.

Any fruit mentioned.

Any drink mentioned. Cocoa nibs, weak tea, Vigor Chocolate.

Desserts—Cup custards, blancmange, orange jelly, rice pudding, coffee jelly, calf's foot jelly, clear jellies, not too sweet; strained cranberry, cottage cheese.

9 P.M.: Hot or cold water, hot or cold milk, Turkey figs, bisbak.

THE PHYSICIAN WHO ADVERTISES.

THE *Medical Examiner and Practitioner* gives us the following: A matter came before us a few days ago which seemed particularly unfortunate. A party said he knew an individual who had a cancer, said to be a sarcoma, who wished to have it "removed." He had seen the advertisement of a cancer doctor whose splendid announcements are spread all over the land by public prints and circular letters, embellished with woodcuts of magnificent buildings and grounds where crowds of patients seemed to glory in the fact that they had a disease which granted them the privileges of the sanitarium which none others could enjoy. This doctor, it is said, had made an examination, and alleged that he could remove the growth by a remedy which only "himself and his God knew of," but the price which he demanded was what was in the way. The patient was not able to pay it, and yet the doctor insisted upon an enormous fee. We looked the "doctor" up in a medical directory, and sure enough his name appeared in the list of other doctors—whose names are well known—and apparently carrying as much weight professionally as the best of them. But he advertises in the most brazen manner possible to be at certain hotels certain days and cure dyspepsia, fistula, Bright's disease, cancer, consumption, and the Lord knows what.

We were under the impression that physicians of this class were not entitled to the privileges of the medical directories. This particular individual has no distinctive note opposite his name, neither is there any means of knowing that he is not altogether regular in his practice. If this sort of thing is permitted, what guarantee is there that we will not be dragged down in the unprofessional mire, on the principle that a man is known by the company which he keeps, or, as in this case, is compelled to keep? Isn't there some remedy for this sort of thing? Or is it the correct thing for such a "physician" to advertise as he does? If not, why not? If yes, why is it not proper for any other doctor to advertise in the same way, receive the sheltering arms of these publications and scoop in the shekels? Why should an honest physician go through life poor and hungry, while the brazen-faced doctor rides in his automobile, dresses in purple and fine linen, and lives on the fat of the land? We advised the party to go to the proper hospital, but the objection was, and probably with truth, that the hospital physicians would advise against the advertiser and his secret nostrum, and would suggest the knife which these patients fear so much. There is always that delusive hope in desperate cases which leads one on and on to one knows not where.

FAIRLY EAT QUININE.

THE New Orleans *Times-Democrat* seems to have a rare faculty of gathering out-of-the-way items of news, literature and science. It is one of the most quotable and quoted of all the journals in the country.

From its columns we reproduce the following:

"The quantity of quinine taken by foreigners on the southeast coast of Mexico is something simply incredible," said a resident of this city, who is interested in coffee culture in the sister republic. "There is a general belief among the Americans and English all through that region that the drug is necessary for the preservation of life, and they keep full of it from one year's end to another. The first time I visited the coast I stopped at Frontera, the first port east of Vera Cruz, and as soon as our ship tied up it was boarded by a tall, sallow man, who turned out to be an American engineer, in charge of a big sugar plant up the country. He made a bee line for the purser. 'Hello! Billy!' he said; 'did you bring that quinine?' 'Sure,' replied the purser, and diving into his cabin he came out with an armful of tin boxes, about the size of tea cannisters, and japanned green. Each of them held a pound of quinine. I never saw it put up that way before and, naturally, I was surprised.

"I soon scraped an acquaintance with the engineer and made bold to inquire what in the world he wanted with such a supply. 'Are you getting it on a speculation?' I asked, with a vague idea that it might be intended for some Mexican army contractor. He laughed heartily. 'Speculation nothing!' said he; 'this all goes to our little colony of Americans back in the interior, and it won't last very long. either.' With that he drew a pen-knife from his pocket, opened a blade that had been ground off round, like a spatula, and thrust it into one of the cans. He brought out a flaky, white mass—enough to heap a teaspoon—put it on his tongue and swallowed it like so much sugar. 'Have you any idea how many grains you are taking?' I asked in amazement. 'Only approximately,' he replied carelessly; 'a man quits weighing quinine after he has been down here a few months.' That was my first encounter with a *bona fide* quinine-eater," the coffee-planter went on, "but I met plenty of them afterward. They generally keep the stuff in rubber tobacco pouches, to protect it from perspiration, and when they feel like taking a dose they dig in with one of those spatulated knives that they all carry and swallow as much as they see fit. As they go entirely by guess, it is hard to say how much will be taken in the course of a day, but I have weighed the amount that can be lifted on the ordinary knife blade and found it to range between 25 and 50 grains. You see, quinine is as compressible as cotton, and two wads of it that look about the same size will vary a hundred per cent. in weight. One would suppose, as a matter of course, that such enormous quantities of the drug would produce an intolerable ringing in the head; but, strange to say, they do nothing of the kind. The average white man down there who keeps under the influence all the time experiences nothing except a slight feeling of exhilaration—at least so I was assured by dozens of habitues. Whether the use of the stuff is of any real benefit is something I am sceptical about. I never took a grain of it myself, and I was the only man on our plantation who didn't have a touch of fever."

THE ASSOCIATION OF AMERICAN MEDICAL EDITORS.

THE annual meeting of the editors' association, was held at St. Paul, June 3-5, 1901, the sessions being convened in the library hall of the Ramsey County Medical Society. This was the most successful meeting held for fifteen years, both from point of attendance and the high standard of excellence of the papers presented. Of especial moment was the paper presented by Dr. Burnside Foster, of St. Paul, entitled "Some Thoughts on the Ethics of Medical Journalism," which was discussed by Drs. Lancaster, Gould, Love and others. At the instance of Dr. Foster, a committee consisting of Drs. Simmons, editor of the *Journal of the A. M. A.*; Gould, of *American Medicine,* and Foster, of the *St. Paul Medical Journal,* was appointed to amend the constitution and by-laws of the association by adding certain rules concerning the nature of the advertising which is to be admitted to the pages of the journals in affiliation with the association. These rules are to be binding on all members, the committee also being advised to suggest such revision of the constitution and by-laws as may be deemed advisable.

Among other papers read were those of Dr. John Punton, entitled "The Relative Value of Medical Advertising"; that of Dr. Dudley S. Reynolds, entitled "Improvements in Medical Education"; Dr. Harold N. Moyer, "Relation of the Medical Editor to Original Articles."

The association adopted resolutions favoring the establishment of a psychophysiological laboratory in the Department of the Interior, at Washington, D. C. It also appointed a committee to draft a resolution requesting the Board of Directors of the Louisiana Purchase Exposition Co., in charge of the St. Louis World's Fair, to recognize and commemorate in a suitable manner the great work done in medicine and surgery. *The American Medical Journalist* was selected as the official journal for publication of papers and proceedings.

The annual dinner of the association was held at the Metropolitan Hotel, on the evening of June 3d, President Stone acting as toastmaster. The speakers of the evening were Drs. Love, Stone, Moyer, Matthews, Marcy, Fassett, and Hall. They confined their remarks to subjects of interest to medical editors, and contributed not a little towards the scientific features of the meeting.

At the session of June 5th the officers for the ensuing year were elected as follows: President, Dr. Alex. J. Stone, of St. Paul; vice-president, Dr. Burnside Foster, of St. Paul; secretary and treasurer, Dr. O. F. Ball, of St. Louis.

The executive committee appointed for the ensuing year consisted of Drs. Gould, Matthews, Lillie, Fassett and Marcy.

The next meeting will be held at Saratoga Springs, N. Y., in June, 1902.

A WELL-EARNED PROMOTION.

MISS MINNIE A. STONER, Dean of the Woman's Department and Professor of Domestic Science in the Kansas State Agricultural College, has been elected Professor of Domestic Science in the Ohio State University.

Professor Stoner's preparation consists of six years of collegiate training and eight years as a teacher. Her collegiate training includes a four-year course in Domestic Science, a year's professional normal course in Dakota and a year's course in the Boston Normal School of Household Arts. To this, she has added a year's advanced work in both psychology and chemistry.

Her experience as a teacher comprehends work in both Domestic Science and Domestic Art in high school, manual training school, college, and university. During the past three years, she has been at the Kansas State Agricultural College, where she has had a very successful career. She is spoken of as a woman of unusual ability as an organizer, of pleasing and commanding personality, and an excellent teacher. She has been further characterized as one who "Will always surpass expectation and never disappoint the highest confidence or fail in the greatest demand upon ability, power, and efficiency."

The work in Domestic Science and Art at the Ohio State University has taken such a high position under the leadership of Miss Bowman, whose marriage to Professor Gibbs of the Ohio State University occasions her withdrawal, that the Board of Trustees are exceedingly anxious that no backward steps should be taken. Professor Stoner's qualifications are such that the Board of Trustees materially increased the compensation that it has been customary to pay in order to secure her services. Miss Stoner's work in Domestic Art was also recognized by a substantial increase in compensation.

ERRONEOUS NOTIONS ABOUT THE TOAD.

IF one reads in old books and listens to the fairy tales and other stories common everywhere, he will hear many wonderful things about the toad, but most of the things are wholly untrue.

One of the erroneous notions is that the toad is deadly poison. Another, that it is possessed of marvelous healing virtues, and still another, that hidden away in the heads of some of the oldest ones, are the priceless toad-stones, jewels of inestimable value.

Giving Warts.—Probably every boy and girl living in the country has heard that if one takes a toad in his hands, or if a toad touches him anywhere he will "catch the warts." This is not so at all, as has been proved over and over again. If a toad is handled gently and petted a little, it soon learns not to be afraid, and seems to enjoy the kindness of attention. If a toad is hurt or roughly handled, a whitish, acrid substance is poured out of the largest warts. This might smart a little if it got into the mouth, as dogs find out when they try biting a toad. It cannot be very bad, however, or the hawks, owls, crows and snakes that eat the toad would give up the practice. The toad is really one of the most harmless creatures in the world, and has never been known to hurt a man or a child.

A boy might possibly have some warts on his hands after handling a toad; so might he after handling a jack-knife or looking at a steam engine; but the toad does not give the warts any more than the knife or the engine.

Living without Air and Food.—Occasionally one reads or hears a story about a toad found in a cavity in a solid rock. When the rock is broken open, it is said that the toad wakes up and hops around as if it had been asleep only half an hour. Just think for a moment what it would mean to find a live toad within a cavity in a solid rock. It must have been there for the thousands, if not for millions of years without food or air. The toad does not like a long fast, but can stand it for a year or so without food if it is in a moist place and supplied with air. It regularly sleeps four or five months every winter, but never in a place devoid of air. If the air were cut off the toad would soon die. Some careful experiments were made by French scientific men, and the stories told about toads living indefinitely without air or food were utterly disproved.

It is not difficult to see that one working in a quarry might honestly think that he had found a toad in a rock. Toads are not very uncommon in quarries. If a stone were broken open and a cavity found in it, and then a toad were seen hopping away, one might jump at the conclusion that the toad came out of the cavity in the rock. Is not this something like the belief that the little toads rain down from the clouds because they are most commonly seen after a shower?

FLIES AS DISSEMINATORS OF DISEASE.

According to *American Medicine* a number of investigators recently have called attention to the important rôle played by insects in disseminating disease. Because of their great numbers and active habits, flies are no doubt the most dangerous insects in this respect. After feeding on the expectoration of the tuberculous, on the feces of typhoid patients or other infective material, they carry disease germs into innumerable places and deposit them not only by direct contact with their filthy little bodies, but by their excreta and the dust formed by the crumbling of their dead bodies. Restaurants infested with flies are special abominations. The danger from this source is not small and as the summer is now up on us in good earnest with hordes of these pests, it seems desirable that everything possible shall be done to limit the amount of mischief done by them. More effective measures are needed for destroying flies and preventing their multiplication. The war on mosquitos by our sanitary department in Cuba has shown what can be done in exterminating insects, and the preparations which are already being made in several different places in our country to carry out the Cuban methods show that the people are willing to act if they are shown the best ways. Until some successful method has been devised for exterminating flies special care should be taken to prevent their access to sputum, pus, or other infectious material; fruits and foodstuffs should be thoroughly cooked or washed if flies have been allowed to come in contact with them, and should be protected from flies after preparation for use.

THE SACROSANCT TUB-BATH.

The typical Englishman, says *American Medicine*, has been pictured as refusing to enter heaven when he found that he would not be allowed to carry in his bath-tub with him. We have never been able to determine whether this gentleman flattered himself more by his pronunciation of the word *baahth* or by his reputation for cleanliness by means of it. Both the bath and the cleanliness are excellent things, far superior indeed either to the assumption of superiority, the pronunciation or the immersion. There is only one Lodge of Perfection above that of the tubber—the unexpressed contempt of the clean man for the tubbing egotist who advertises that there is no cleanliness without the tub. The simple truth is, of course, that perfect cleanliness of the body is far more easily secured by means of the sponge or a wet towel with a pitcher of water than by a huge tub full of water. We have no doubt that the rage for tubbing has not only harmed or (mercifully), killed thousands of tubbers, but has in a general way made the world a dirtier one. By everlasting inculcation of the untruth that there is no (sanitary) salvation except by immersion, millions of people go to another extreme and do not bathe at all or use an insufficient amount of water. Do half the people in the world wash their bodies once a year? Bathing in such water as we have in many cities may be considered dangerous or disgusting, according to the amount of water used. In order to have pure water for bathing or anything else it must be filtered. This will inevitably bring the water meter. Then the financial argument will reinforce the sanitary one, that perfect cleanliness is as attainable with two gallons of water as with 200 gallons.

THE muscles of the human jaw exert a force of 534 lbs. The quantity of pure water which blood contains in its natural state is very great; it amounts to almost seven-eighths. Kiel estimates the surface of the lungs at 150 square feet, or ten times that of the external. The blood is a fifth the weight of the body. A man is taller in the morning than at night to the extent of half an inch or more, owing to the relaxation of the cartilages. There is iron enough in the blood of forty-two men to make a ploughshare of twenty-four pounds or thereabouts. The human brain is the twenty-eighth part of the body, but in the horse the brain is not more than the four-hundreth.

Infallibility in diagnosis is a sign of medical dilettanteism.—*R. von Jaksch* (Prag).

Surgery depends upon knowledge and skill. A development of the one with a neglect of the other will conduce to the injury of surgery. It is only by the uniform use of both that the whole will develop harmoniously into full bloom.—*Otmar v. Angerer* (Munich).

Department of Physiologic Chemistry.

WITH SPECIAL REFERENCE TO DIETETICS AND NUTRITION IN GENERAL.

GLEANINGS FROM RECENT PHYSIOLOGIC-CHEMIC LITERATURE.

Arsenic in Animal Organisms.—It has been quite currently stated, but not satisfactorily proved, that arsenic is a normal constituent of all animal organisms. This assertion has not passed without being questioned, and has instigated further and more exhaustive analyses. These latter tests seem to show that those organs which are usually examined, in cases of suspected poisoning, the liver, spleen, kidney, pancreas, etc., and the blood, urine, etc., do not normally contain any trace of arsenic. On the other hand, traces of arsenic are so uniformly found in the thyroid, thymus, and mammary glands, in milk, brain, bone, hair, and skin, that the presence of this element is now assumed to be normal in these organs and substances.

In order to be normally present in the body it must of necessity be present in the food. No trace of it appears in such leading articles of diet as bread, eggs, and fish, but minute quantities are found in potatoes and some other vegetables. Since the practice of using arsenical compounds in destroying the potato beetle has become so universal, it may be well to make further tests before positively assuming that arsenic is a normal constituent of any vegetable.

Iodine in the System.—Iodine is found in the thyroids and parathyroids of even new-born children, except when the mothers have been suffering from some abnormal condition.

Digestibility of Casein.—For a long time it has been currently asserted that the casein of cow's milk is much more difficult of digestion than that of human milk. Recent experiments go to prove that this is one of those scientific inaccuracies that passes for truth, simply because no one takes the pains to refute it.

A similar case of acquiescence in a current error is found in the belief that children digest casein much more perfectly than do adults. This assumption has given rise to the plausible inference that milk is not a natural food for adults. Both these errors have now been exploded. It is found that there is practically no difference in the digestibility of the casein of cow's milk and that of human milk; and careful experiments prove that adults digest and absorb casein quite as readily and completely as infants.

Absorption of Inorganic Iron.—For a number of years the German chemists have been teaching that inorganic iron is never absorbed in the slightest degree by the human system. Abderhalder and some other authorities now claim, and seem to have conclusively demonstrated, that ferric chloride is absorbed to some extent, chiefly in the duodeum. It has also been shown that animals fed on their normal diet absorb more of the inorganic iron administered to them than others fed on a diet poor in iron, but to which inorganic iron salts have been added.

The inference is plain that the exhibition of organic mineral salts of any kind is much more likely to prove efficient than the use of the same salts in an inorganic form.

Phosphorus Absorption.—It is found that the feeding of phosphorus-bearing proteids is followed by much better results than when phosphorus-free proteids to which phosphorus has been added are exhibited. This is quite in accord with the foregoing deductions regarding iron.

Goat's milk is found to be rich in phosphorus, but it is a rather curious fact in animal chemistry that less of this element exists in the form of organic compounds in goat's milk than in case of human or of cow's milk.

The administration of phosphorus in the form of glycerophosphate of calcium does not increase the phosphorus in the milk of the goat. This does not prove that this salt is not utilized in other portions of the animal economy.

Effects of Boric Acid.—Boric acid in the form of boroglyceride is extensively used as a preservative of various perishable food products, especially of milk. This fact has led to some careful experiments to determine the general effect of this drug when used for some time. In the proportion of forty grains of boric acid to the gallon, the usual strength resorted to to prevent milk from souring, the mixture proves fatal to kittens fed upon it. The animals die within four weeks, at the longest.

The danger of feeding infants on milk thus treated is obvious.

As it is claimed that much of the milk supplied to all our large cities is thus treated, the question becomes one of decided importance. Unless a given brand of milk is known to be free from either boric acid, formalin, or any other artificial preservative, it would be better to rely on a good brand of condensed milk, properly reduced and modified.

Effects of Alcohol on the Blood and Milk of the Mother.—Experiments conducted by Nicloux show that alcohol administered to the prospective mother is found in the blood of the fetus.

In case of nursing mothers even small quantities of alcohol are quickly found in the milk. The birth of children with an appetite for alcoholics, that develops in later life, is thus easily accounted for. The mother who is in any degree addicted to her cups, or who is plied with stimulants at any period of either gestation or lactation, under medical direction, may readily lay the foundation for an incurable and unfortunate habit in her progeny.

FOOD BEFORE SLEEP.

WE quote the following by Dr. Cathell, but decidedly take issue as to some of his positions: "Many persons, though not actually sick, keep below par in strength and general tone, and I am of the opinion that fasting during the long interval between supper and breakfast, and especially the complete emptiness of the stomach during sleep, adds greatly to the amount of emaciation, sleeplessness, and general weakness we so often meet.

Physiology teaches that in the body there is a perpetual disintegration of tissue, sleeping or waking; it is, therefore, logical to believe that the supply of nourishment should be somewhat continuous, especially in those who are below par, if we would counteract their emaciation and lowered degree of vitality; and as bodily exercise is suspended during sleep, with wear and tear correspondingly diminished, while digestion, assimilation, and nutritive activity continue as usual, the food furnished during this period adds more than is destroyed, and increased weight and improved general vigor is the result.

All beings, except man, are governed by natural instinct, and every being with a stomach, except man, eats before sleep, and even the human infant, guided by the same instinct, sucks frequently day and night, and if its stomach is empty for any prolonged period it cries long and loud.

Digestion requires no interval of rest; and if the amount of food during the twenty-four hours is in quantity and quality not beyond the physiological limit, it makes no hurtful difference to the stomach how few or how short are the intervals between eating, but it does make a vast difference in the weak and emaciated one's welfare to have a modicum of food in the stomach during the time of sleep, that, instead of being consumed by bodily action, it may, during the interval, improve the lowered system; and I am fully satisfied that were the weakly, the emaciated, and the sleepless to nightly take a light lunch or meal of simple, nutritious food before going to bed, for a prolonged period.

nine in ten of them would be thereby lifted into a better standard of health.

In my specialty (nose and throat) I encounter cases that, in addition to local and constitutional treatment, need an increase of nutritious food, and I find that by directing a bowl of bread and milk, or a mug of beer and a few biscuits, or a saucer of oatmeal and cream, before going to bed, for a few months, a surprising increase in weight, strength, and general tone results; on the contrary, persons who are too stout or plethoric should follow an opposite course."

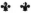

EAT ALL YOU CAN, MOTHER.

AN old man whose hair and beard were cut in a chaste, rural design appeared in one of the table d'hote restaurants the other day. He had his wife with him. That was more than the old lady could say of her hearing. She was almost stone deaf, which gave everybody a chance to find out what splendid lungs her husband had.

The meal was luncheon. The price which the old man was asked after he had ordered two meals was 75 cents.

"Seventy-five cents!" he exclaimed. "You don't mean apiece?"

"Yes, sir."

"Gracious!"

He thought it over a minute or two. Then he looked at his wife, as if considering whether he should try to get the dreaded news past the old lady's tympanum. Evidently he gave it up. But he did what he could. When the first course came on, he leaned over and shouted in her ear:

"Eat all you can, mother! I'll tell you why after awhile!"—*New York Sun.*

"TELL you what I like the best
'Long about knee-deep in June,
'Bout the time strawberries melts
On the vines—some afternoon
Like to jes' sit out and rest,
And not work at nothin' else!"
JAMES WHITCOMB RILEY.

OLEAGINOUS SCIENCE.

THERE have been many reported "strikes" in oils, and now it is asserted by some scientist that petroleum is really a distilled and fossil fish oil! Is it possible that Norway cod were really at the bottom of the Standard Oil Company? Who can say? If science says so, one may go on downing the oil, but there is no downing science.

Hagee evidently believes in science and in oil in the same breath. In any event Hagee's *Ol. Morrhuæ Comp.* is the outcome of scientific combination and adaptation. Its formula makes it a food of the greatest value in all wasting diseases and low states.

If there is anything better in the market we shall be glad to herald its virtues.

REDEEMING THE COLORADO DESERT.

IN the absorbing interest of great mergers with capitalizations which a few years ago would have been deemed impossible, we are apt to overlook the fact that a great deal is going on in the world which makes for good in very much larger degree than do the operations of the Wall Street financiers. For example, a work is now in progress which will redeem for cultivation and occupation 400,000 acres of waste land in Colorado and 500,000 in Mexico, and before the close of the present year one of the most desolate and forbidding of the American deserts will be redeemed and prepared to become one of the garden spots of this continent. Artesian wells which have been drilled near Indio are flowing copiously, and these are to be supplemented by an irrigation canal sixty miles long, which will bring the water of the Colorado River into the heart of the desert. This will furnish the water to abundantly irrigate nearly 1,-500 square miles of land, which will become wonderfully fertile when thus treated. Great climatic changes may be expected to follow, diverting the waters of the Colorado into this arid waste, where the heat is intolerable and the distance between springs is greater than in Sahara. A similar work is in progress on the Arizona side of the rvier, and before winter, at least, another 100,000 acres of now uninhabitable land will be made desirable by irrigation.

Such enterprises do more for the progress of civilization than all the banking deals which can be evolved in the board rooms of the Napoleons of finance. They not only make blades of grass grow where none grew before, but they make homes for the homeless and add something tangible to the National wealth. This is better territorial expansion than can be effected by colonization or conquest.

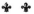

HER DEBT OF GRATITUDE.

WHEN she entered the pharmacy the proprietor was too busy stacking almanacs to hear her footsteps. She tapped on the brass scales and he came out smiling.

"What can I do for you?" he asked, with a courteous bow.

"Ah, monsieur," she replied, "you can do nozing now; you have done much in ze pazt. I come to say zanks."

"I am afraid I don't recall the circumstances," he said, shaking his head.

"Ah, monsieur's memory is weak. Two years. I come one night. Ze wind. How ze wind blew zat one night two years ago! Ah, monsieur, and ze sleet. Horrible ze thought! I come and ask for ze poison. I was ze one miserable singer. My voice fail. No longer ze audience call for Marie. Ze audience hiss ze song. I no longer want life. I come for ze poison. Monsieur sell ze belladonna without ze prescription or ze question."

"Did you take it?" gasped the pharmacist.

"Monsieur will listen. I stand in ze dressing-room. I would take ze poison in ze moment. While I wait I have one idea. I put ze belladonna in my eyes. Zey shine like stars of ze North. Glorious! I run

out on ze stage. In ze box sit ze rich man. He fell madly in love with my bright eyes. He beg me to marry him. He worth many millions. I am his wife to-day. Suppose monsieur had refused ze poison on zat wild night two years ago?"

"It would have been bad for you."

"Horrible! And now I will buy somezing of monsieur. Give me two stamps and one postal, please."

The pharmacist sighed and opened the stamp drawer. When the visitor was at the door smiling a farewell he beckoned her to return.

"Was ze change right?" she queried.

"Yes, but you forgot to take an almanac."

He forced a collection of variegated pamphlets in her hand.

"Here is a good selection. Calendars, recipes, jokes and pictures of great men who take preparations."

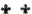

WHAT "V" MEANT.

"MANY years ago," says the *Youth's Companion*, "a young fellow entered the freshman class at Amherst College—a lad with a square jaw, a steady eye, a pleasant smile, and a capacity for hard and persistent work. One day, after he had been in college about a week, he took a chair from his room to the hall, mounted it and nailed over the door a large square of cardboard, on which was painted a big black letter V, and nothing else.

College boys do not like mysteries, and the young man's neighbors tried to make him tell what the big V meant. Was it "for luck?" Was it a joke? What was it? The sophomores took it up, and treated the freshman to some hazing, but he would make no answer to the question they put. At last he was let alone, and his V remained over the door, merely a mark of the eccentricity of the occupant.

Four years passed. On commencement day Horace Maynard delivered the valedictory of his class, the highest honor the college bestowed. After he had left the platform, amid the applause of his fellow students and of the audience, one of his classmates accosted him:

"Was that what your 'V' meant? Were you after the valedictory when you tacked up that card?"

"Of course," Maynard replied. "What else could it have been? How else could I have got it?"

Maynard needed to tack no other letters over his door. The impetus he had gained carried him through life. He became a member of Congress, attorney-general of Tennessee, minister to Turkey, and post-master-general, and adorned every position to which he was called.

NERVOUS DISORDERS.

London Hospital contains some good advice as follows:

Nowadays, when every one seems to be suffering from nerves, it is more than ever necessary to try to cultivate reposeful habits. When you sit down to rest, be still, and do not start at every noise. A long-continued noise might have a wearing effect upon the nerves, but the little noises, which are over in a moment, hurt no one, and it is quite absurd to jump and start as some people do, at them. Control of nervous movements acts beneficially on the nerves themselves; whereas, if the nerves are allowed to run riot, bodily health is imposssible. Uncontrolled nerves are responsible for terrible disasters caused by panics in fires and other accidents, which often result in the loss of hundreds of lives. Giving way to nerves without a strugggle for mastery over them is, therefore, not only very bad for one's self, but exceedingly selfish to one's neighbors. Every one should strive to attain a quiet, even manner under all circumstances, and then when an emergency comes the chances are that they will be able to act with cool courage.

HEALTHY SLEEP.

HE who has no sleep, says the *Kneipp Water Cure Monthly*, is just as sick as the one who always feels sleepy. A healthy human being only feels sleepy during those hours which are designated by Nature for rest. The sleep of the healthy will always last for the same length of time.

How long should one sleep? Children are growing sleep a good deal of the time; old people very little. For grown-up people a sleep of seven or eight hours should be sufficient.

How could one produce healthy sleep?

Fresh air is a fundamental rule for the production of sound and healthy sleep. He who wants to sleep well must not take a late supper, the stomach cannot rest while digesting such a late meal. The activity of the stomach will influence other parts of the body and disturb their rest. Food hard to digest should not be partaken of in the evening.

Rest a little before you go to bed. He who works mentally or physically up to the last moment before retiring will not get a healthy and sound sleep.

The sleep before midnight counts double, says an old proverb. Nine or ten P.M. ought to be the hour for retiring. He who goes to bed later hurts his health. This ought to be the rule. Exceptions may be taken, but not too often.

When out on the path the step is ringing,
And keen as a whip the sleet is stinging,
When buffalo robes are heaped to the
   shoulder,
And the cold moon makes the night seem
   colder,
When a few thin leaves on the beeches
   shiver,
And dead and buried and gone is the river,
And out of the north the flakes are flying,
I like to think of the new hay lying,
Of summer airs in the branches sighing,
Of the hammock at noon where I lounge or
   whittle:
       It helps a little.

THE HOT AIR CURE.

A WRITER in the *London Chronicle* says: "In all cases the Tallerman treatment is applied under the direction of medical men and of a nursing staff, but it is an open secret that Mr. Tallerman (whose headquarters are at No. 50 Welbeck street, London, W.), has had an uphill fight for the recognition of his system. I have been going through the reports on the work of the free institutes, and have also perused a series of hospital reports of cases treated at home and abroad, and I have no hesitation in saying that there is no other mode of treatment known to science which can effect the cure of stiff and deformed joints in the fashion accomplished by the Tallerman system. It is a very simple affair, so simple that, as usual, one is given to wonder that medicine did not think of it ages ago. Mr. Tallerman in cases the affected limb or joints in a special case or copper chamber. Hot air is then laid on, as it were, by means of gas or oil, so that a temperature of from 250 to 300 degrees or more can be generated without any discomfort. The effect of the application of this hot, dry air is literally marvelous. Joints which were practically immovable become useful, and patients, from being cripples, have the use of their limbs restored to them. It is not claimed that the Tallerman treatment will cure every case. Some are beyond its aid, but, from what I have seen of its effects, I have no hesitation in saying that it should be made widely known, and especially among the poor, to whom the loss of a useful limb is a calamity of no mean order. Nothing, to my mind, has been more disgraceful than the tacit boycotting of Mr. Tallerman's treatment in certain medical quarters. Against this, of course, he has the satisfaction of seeing his treatment applied in certain of our big hospitals, but I have thought that if Mr. Tallerman had been animated with the desire to make money he could by this time have acquired a considerable fortune had he regarded his own pocket more decidedly than the relief of the sick poor."

The treatment is now gaining headway in this country, and America bids fair to excel Europe in the matter of improved apparatus.

OH, FORTUNATE WORLD.

(From the Chicago Times-Herald.)

HE dropped from Jupiter one day,
A stranger from the starry way.
He sought our world intent to find
A solace for a wearied mind.
For, though from Jupiter's fair zone,
Our guest had troubles of his own.
We took him joyfully in tow
And gladly hauled him to and fro.
We showed our architectural freaks;
The furrows deepened in his cheeks.
We boasted our electricity;
"Our system has no wires," said he,
"We launch a thunderbolt to move
A little world like yours, by Jove!"
He saw an automobile drive,
And asked them was the toy alive.
Then yawned and looked another way
As if too tired and bored to stay.
But one place was unvisited—
The marble mansions of the dead.
"Dead?" "Who are they?" with interest new,
His wonder and attention grew.
We told him what we knew of death
And what we hoped. He caught his breath.
Then shouted with a wild, weird cry:
"Oh, fortunate world, where people die!"
And vanished, leaving no excuse,
As if in haste to tell the news.

L'ENVOI.

This may be true or may not be,
I tell the tale as 'twas told to me.

The diagnosis is and will remain the foundation of every rational proceeding of the physician. Examine again and again. For it is only uncertainty that leads to completeness of truth.—*Wilhelm Erb* (Heidelberg).

And this from *Our Dumb Animals:*

A BRAINLESS ASS.

In our January paper we published the remark of a prominent Boston gentleman that a man who voluntarily rides or drives a horse mutilated for life by docking proves that he is a brainless and heartless ass.

On this January 30th we receive a letter from a California editor, in which he says:

"Alameda, California.

"I protest on behalf of the ass. It has been my fortune to become more or less intimately acquainted with various and sundry specimens of the *genus asinus,* and never have I seen one that did not possess more brains than any of these fool humans who mutilate horses. No, sir; on behalf of the ass I protest. He is a gentleman and a scholar as compared with the idiots who dock horses' tails."

"Yours for humanity,
"G. F. Weeks."

✢ ✢

"IF I SHOULD DIE TO-NIGHT."

By Ben King.

"If I should die to-night—
And you should come to my cold corpse and say,
Weeping and heart sick, o'er my lifeless clay,
If I should die to-night—
And you should come in deep grief and woe,
And say, 'Here's that $10 I owe,'
I might rise up in my great white cravat
And say, 'What's that?'

"If I should die to-night—
And you should come to my corpse and kneel,
Clasping my bier to show the grief you feel,
I say, if I should die to-night,
And you should come to me, and here and then
Just even hint about paying me that ten,
I might arise awhile—but I'd drop dead again."

SIR HENRY THOMPSON'S METHOD OF COOKING A HAM.

Recipe for cooking a ham at a low temperature long continued: I prefer a thick, plump ham—say from 10 to 12 pounds—for a moderate-sized party (12 to 16), York or Cumberland by choice. It must first lie some hours in cold water; if a highly smoked one, and you desire to retain the flavor, 8 or 10 hours will suffice; if it is not much smoked, but has been fully salted, it should remain 12 hours or more. This process should be concluded at least 36 hours before the hour fixed for dinner.

As soon as it is removed from the cold water, scour with a softish scrubbing brush, so as to remove all dirt from the surface.

You will have already prepared the day before a good meat stock, well flavored with vegetables, carrots, turnips, parsnips, onions, and a faggot of kitchen herbs.

The ham is to be placed in an oval cooking pot just adapted to its size; sufficient of the above stock to cover the ham is to be added, allowing room for a few slices of the fresh vegetables just named to be put in also. Place the pot on the fire, and bring the stock soon to the boiling point, maintaining this for five minutes only, no more. Then withdraw the pot from the fire so that the stock may gradually cool to a temperature about 170 degrees, but not exceeding that. Keep it thus 12 hours. For this purpose it is best to place it over a gas ring, which is easily regulated, and to have a thermometer which ranges up to 212 degrees, the boiling point, precisely like a bath thermometer, that is, with a tin receptacle at the lower end guarding the bulb, only that the bottom of the receptacle should be cut away for kitchen use; otherwise organic matter would lodge there, soon decompose, and become noxious.

Suppose at the end of this time that by means of the thermometer and by adjustment of the gas, that the temperature has been steadily maintained, preparation must be made for leaving it for the night, so that the temperature shall not henceforth exceed 150 degrees Fah.; on the other hand, it shall not fall below 130 degrees. With a little observation, it is easy to ascertain how much gas suffices to do this during the night; and a small quantity of fresh stock to fully cover the ham is added the last thing. The cover of the pot being always on, the loss by evaporation is very small; but towards the close of the process the stock may be allowed to diminish one-third or so of the original quantity.

Supposing you have arrived at about four hours before the time for serving; the ham is now taken out and skimmed in the usual manner, then returned to the pot, together with a bottle of good wine emptied into it, which of course reduces the temperature. Raise this gradually to 140 degrees, as before. If a red wine, let it be a good mid-quality Burgundy; or a good red Italian wine may suffice. If white be preferred, a bottle of fair Sauterne or Graves.

THE SAUCE.

The temperature last named is to be continued until the ham is served. The remaining contents of the pot are now to be carefully skimmed to remove fat, a portion strained through a tammy without addition, reduced to a glaze in a small saucepan, and served in a sauceboat apart. Or, if preferred, a cherry or other acid-sweet sauce may be substituted. I strongly recommend the former for a ham which is served hot.

It is very easy to over-cook a ham in 36 hours, so that the flesh falls from the bones, and can scarcely be cut. It is equally certain that it will not be so, although it will be deliciously tender, provided that the rules above given respecting the temperature are followed.

✣ ✣

PASTEUR TREATMENT OF RABIES.

In connection with recent discussions of the subject of rabies, pro and con, in the columns of THE GAZETTE, the following summary is interesting:

THE Department for the Preventive Treatment of Rabies of the Baltimore Col- of Physicians and Surgeons report 209 cases successfully treated, of which 85 per cent. were from the rural districts. Of those treated 159 were males, 50 females, 70 children, none of whom were over 10 years of age. The wounds were inflicted by dogs in 188 cases, in 13 cases by cats, in 1 by a calf, and in 1 by a pig. Those who came to receive treatment during the first week after being bitten numbered 147, those in the second week 27, those in the third week 11, those in the fourth week 7, those in the fifth week 11, and 4 and 2 came in the sixth and eighth week respectively. There were 5 abscesses in 6,270 injections. There was but 1 death from any cause. This death was caused by rabies. A lad, 8 years old, bitten February 2, 1900, was admitted February 4. He received only 1 treatment, consisting of 2 hypodermic injections. He was removed from the institution and treatment discontinued on February 5th against the advice of the physicians. After the inoculated rabbits and a cow bitten by the same dog developed rabies, the child was brought back on February 25. He developed rabies March 14 and died March 17. A case of this character cannot be attributed to failure of the treatment, but to delay in resorting to treatment.

✣ ✣

DOG DEFENDS THE LOST CHILD.

GEORGE FINDLAY, candidate for United States internal revenue collector for Kansas, has returned from a trip through the Indian Territory, and he vouches for the following story of the devotion to his little mistress of a dog owned by Jim Hay, a quarter-blood Quapaw Indian.

Hay's four-year-old girl Nellie wandered into the woods near his place last week and became lost. She was accompanied by her dog, a gigantic yellow staghound. After wandering a mile and a half from home she became tired and fell asleep.

Her father was searching for her at midnight, when he heard the baying of the hound out in the woods. He found his daughter, with the big hound standing guard close to her, and in the underbrush near her were *the bodies of two big gray wolves.* The child was unable to give a very intelligent account of what had happened, but she said she was awakened by hearing Nero fighting with the wolves. The hound is badly scratched and cut.

A CHILD OF THE WOODS.

He knew the first sweet wood notes of the
    thrush,
The first wind-flower, hidden in the grass;
The little shrines where fire-flies, saying
    mass,
Swing low their censers through the marsh-
    land's bush;
The quickened sound before the poignant
    hush
Which preludes charges at the old earth's
    cuirass—
That magic moment, when the seasons pass
And all live things to newer promise rush.
He loved the bob-o-link's familiar call,
The friendly clover nodding to the bees;
The tiger-lilies flaunting, gay and tall,
Their motley coats of spotted harmonies;
And when the night lay on the forest grim,
He heard the tree-tops croon a song for
    him.—*Charlotte Becker, in Outing.*

PURIFICATION OF WATER BY CHEMICALS.

Prof. Dobralsanée, of St. Petersburg, recommends the following to precipitate the impurities of water:

To 12 quarts of water he adds 7½ grains of perchloride of iron, and 10½ grains of crystalline sodium carbonate; in forty-five minutes the water was perfectly pure.

AMERICAN CHILDREN.

According to *The Literary Digest,* Julius Szavay, an Hungarian editor and poet, and secretary of the board of trade of Raab, has been sojourning in this country and publishing in book-form his observations. This is what he has to say about American children, as quoted in the *Neue Pester Journal:* "The education of the children is only another name for extreme liberalism, the children being regarded as exceptional creatures, almost as saints, who may demand anything and are superior to all others. After the women, the children receive the greatest protection from the laws, and everywhere there are societies for the prevention of cruelty to children. . . . This comprehensive protection naturally has its dark side also. The American children are the worst in the world. It is they who chase the Spanish ambassador because they believe his gala costume does not become him; it is they who throw stones at the Catholic priest when they see him in his official vestments; it is they who steal the boxes and barrels they find piled before the stores and burn them in the middle of the street (Americans, by the way, incline very strongly to pyromania); and it is they who steal the wooden steps before the doors of residences, a business in which they are assisted by the policemen, who complacently turn their backs to their mischief, for they tell themselves that they themselves were children once and that they have children of their own. On the other hand, these incomparable American scalawags are perfect marvels of adroitness and easily excel all their brothers on this side of the Atlantic in the art of making money. They are adepts in all the lighter kinds of business; not only in selling newspapers and blacking shoes do they find profit, but there are many other sources of income with which they are familiar and to which they devote themselves body and soul. One would have to smile at them if they did not know, in spite of their finicalness, how to turn to profit the zeal with which the attend to business. From these embryonic men, educated in utter freedom, and entrusted to accident and the natural development of instinct, comes the average American who is every inch an individuality, not content with the leveled and uniform compendium of scholastic wisdom, but who is swayed by a bold and original habit of thought that is prolific of tricks and stratagems, and which bewilders with its record of keen successes."

MATHEMATICS IN MEDICINE.

A DOCTOR WHO FIGURES OUT JUST WHAT YOU NEED TO TAKE.

HE was a doctor of the advanced school. He laid his fingers on my pulse, and, with his watch in his hand, gave it a fair start and observed it carefully all of the way around, says *Harper's Bazar*.

"Strong, seventy-four," he said, in a moment. Then he consulted a card that was covered with figures and continued: "That equals sixty-three," and he placed that number on a slate. "Put out your tongue. Good! That is fourteen," he said.

"Inches?" I asked.

"How is your appetite?" he inquired, ignoring my question.

"Equal to the supply."

"That makes 204," he replied.

"Can't you reduce it a little?" I asked, but failed to get his attention.

"Cold feet?"

"Yes," I answered.

"Three," he said.

"No, two," I replied, to correct him.

He set the three under the other figures. He then placed a thermometer in my mouth, which he afterward consulted in connection with the card.

"A good 198," he said.

"Impossible," I suggested, mildly.

He wrote down the 198 and asked if I had headaches.

"Sometimes in the morning, after being kept late at the office," I answered.

"Four," he said.

"Isn't that rather low," I asked.

"Do you smoke," he inquired.

"Yes."

"Ten," he replied.

"No, two for ten," I said.

He put down the ten.

"Do you sleep well?" he asked.

"That depends upon the baby," I answered.

"We won't consider that," he said.

"You had better call it 980." I suggested.

"He added together the figures that he had placed on the slate.

"That makes 496," he said.

"Is that the amount of the bill?" I asked.

"Bill?" he replied. "That is the number of the prescription. I want you to know that medicine with me is no longer an experiment, for I have reduced it to a mathematical certainty. Every symptom has its number, and the sum of these numbers indicate the medicine that is needed. I have worked for fifteen years in formulating my prescriptions and perfecting the treatment, but I have it now. Your bill is $10."

I understood that number, and left the office feeling relieved and deeply impressed by the doctor's learning.

CARIES RARE IN HINDU TEETH.

THE *British Med. Journal* is responsible for the following:

Pessimistic prophets declare that future generations of humanity will be toothless. Civilization has certainly brought with it, from one cause or another, a great increase in dental troubles, and the number of people nowadays whose teeth are either lost or diseased at an early age is very large. To a great extent this must be ascribed to neglect. Some observations on the teeth of the Hindus, by Dr. Egbert, were recently quoted in the.*British Jour. D. Sc.* In his experience, natives of all castes, from the Brahmin to the pariah, have uniformly large, strong, and exceptionally well-developed teeth, with the third molars and lateral incisors developed proportionately to the other teeth. In the hundreds of dentures which he has examined among Indian natives, he has never seen a single malformed molar or lateral incisor, and these teeth were always present. The Indian people are remarkably exempt from caries, and do not often lose their teeth from this cause. There can be little doubt that this immunity is largely due to the fact that careful and regular cleaning of the teeth is a universal habit in India. It is strictly observed, because it is laid down as an important part of religious ritual. Very exact rules for its performance are given in the great book of Brahmin ritual, called "Nitia-Karma." To clean his teeth the Hindu uses a small twig, one end of which he softens out into the form of a painter's brush. Squatting on his heels, and always facing either east or north, he scrubs all his teeth well with this brush, after which he rinses his mouth out with fresh water. There is, indeed, much in the personal habits of the Indian races which might with advantage be imitated by Western peoples. All Hindus, for instance, strictly observe the custom of washing with water after answering a call of Nature, and the European habit of using paper is looked upon by them as an utter abomination, of which they never speak except with horror. They object just as strongly, also, to our use of a handkerchief, which is afterwards put in the pocket. The general neglect of the teeth in this country is certainly deplorable. Even among the richer classes, it is quite uncommon to meet with people who make a regular practice of cleaning the teeth after each meal—a most desirable habit on hygienic grounds—and large numbers of the lower orders never use a tooth brush at all. The vegetable nature of the Hindu's food probably has its influence in rendering him less prone to caries than the meat eater, but there can be no doubt that he owes immunity from much pain and ill-health to the salutary habit his religion has wisely enjoined.

AN ANESTHETIC FOR AN ELEPHANT.

An elephant in the zoological gardens at Hanover, Germany, was recently found to be suffering from a growth upon the lower part of one of its hind feet, and it was decided to remove this malformation. In order to make the animal insensible a dose of 600 grains of morphia in six bottles of rum was administered. About an hour after the elephant had consumed this combination narcosis was complete, and the operation was performed without any trouble.

MASQUERADING AS A MAN.

The *London Lancet* records these curious histories:

On March 2d a person described on the charge sheet as "Catherine Coome, aged sixty-six, house decorator, of no fixed home," appeared in connection with a case of alleged fraud. She appeared in court dressed as a man, and, according to her own story, she was married at fifteen years of age. Having served as a schoolmistress she went to Birmingham, where she determined to personate a man, as she thought she would get on better. She served for two years on board of a Peninsular and Oriental liner as ship's cook, and became acquainted with the maid of a lady who lived at Hampton Court. This maid she "married" and they lived together for fourteen years. The "husband" then returned to London, where, on account of meeting with severe injuries, she had to enter the workhouse, where her sex was discovered. The story is strange enough, but there is nothing particularly new about it. Besides such heroes of romance as Billy Taylor, the immortal Rosalind, and the lovesick crew who (according to Mr. Gilbert) shipped with Lieutenant Belay, there are historical instances of women who have passed their lives as men. Such a one was Christina Davis, who died in July, 1739, after having served many years in the Second Dragoons, afterwards the Scots Greys. She was born in 1667, and when quite a young woman married a man named Welsh. One day Welsh was forcibly recruited and sent to serve in Holland in Lord Orrey's regiment. Christina thereupon dressed herself as a man and enlisted as a foot soldier so as to find her husband. After many adventures, during which she served in the battle of Landen, was wounded, taken prisoner, exchanged, and fallen in love with, on account of which last affair she had to fight a duel, she enlisted in the cavalry and was present at the siege of Namur. After the peace of Ryswick she returned to Ireland without having found her husband, but on war being again declared she took up service again. After the battle of Blenheim she was on prisoners' guard, and there met her husband, who had long thought her to be dead. They decided to pass as brothers, and continued to serve. At Ramillies she was severely wounded and her sex was discovered. Her husband was killed at Malplaquet, but she was twice married afterwards. At her death she was buried in the grounds of Chelsea Hospital with military honors. Two other remarkable women were Anne Bonney and Mary Read, who lived about 200 years ago and carried on a successful career as pirates, but the classical instance of a woman passing as a man is that of James Barry, M.D., of the Army Medical Staff, a full account of whose remarkable career was incorporated into a novel, "A Modern Sphinx," by Lieutenant Colonel Rogers. The sexual problems involved in such cases form a curious chapter in medical psychology. Our readers will recall the case of a woman passing as a man and wielding a considerable influence as a Tammany politician, who recently died in this city.

⚹ ⚹

The greatest progress in my opinion that modern medicine has made is that it has taught not only to diagnosticate and to cure diseases, but also to prevent them.—*H. Chiari* (Prag).

PINE-NEEDLE OIL.

IN OREGON THE INDUSTRY IS OF SOME IMPORTANCE.

THE utilization of the pine needles of the yellow Oregon pine, botanically *Pinus ponderosa,* is becoming an industry of considerable importance on the Pacific Coast. Fifty years ago it was discovered that the extracts and products of the long, slender leaves of the pine possessed real efficacy in complaints of a pulmonary character. It is claimed that insomnia yields to the influence of the pungent odor, and asthmatics have found a real relief in partaking of the oil and in sleeping upon pillows stuffed with the elastic and fragrant fiber manufactured from the interior substance of the pine leaves. The illimitable forests of yellow pine abounding in the State of Oregon, with their accessibility to through lines of transportation, suggested to a German from the forests of Turingia the transfer of a lucrative business to the Pacific Coast. In Germany the leaves never exceed two inches in length, while in Oregon they often exceed thirty inches, and average twenty. In the former country the forest laws are extremely strict and often prohibitive, obliging the maker of the product to use the dried leaves, that have fallen to the ground, and thus insuring an inferior and less effective quality of goods. In the Western States denuding the yellow pine of its leaves has been encouraged, the expert of the Forestry Commission having pronounced the process as beneficial. A tally kept of the weight gathered from a certain number of trees indicated that the crop taken in April weighed 650 pounds, while that of the same trees in October yielded 775 pounds. Two crops are gathered yearly, the later one being always the largest. The leaves of the young trees are preferred, yielding a better quality of oil, it is said., though this fact is doubted. The leaves are stripped from the trees by women and men, who are hired for the purpose, and are paid 25 cents a 100 pounds for the needles: 500 pounds is considered an average day's work. The leaves are packed into sacks and hurriedly sent to the factory. Exposure to the sun causes the leaves to wilt and impairs the quality of the product. In picking, the thickest bunches of leaves are selected, and the scanty ones are neglected. The vast quantity available, so far beyond any present demand, permits the picker to thus discriminate. The factory at which the essences and extracts of the needles are manufactured has a capacity for handling 2,000 pounds of leaves per day, but it is soon to be enlarged to about four times its present size.

In the extraction of pine oil, 2,000 pounds of green leaves are required to produce ten pounds of oil. The process is the ordinary one of distillation. In the manufacture of fiber the leaves pass through a process of steaming, washing, drying, etc., twelve in all, occupying four days. Two qualities are produced, first and second. The first, from which no oil has been distilled, is worth, upon the market, about 10 cents per pound. The fiber is elastic, and the staple only little shorter than the green leaf from which it was made, and with strength sufficient to enable it to be spun and woven into fabrics. Mixed with hair, the fiber makes an excellent material for mattresses or pillows, and repose comes quickly when resting upon them. It is also used as a partial filling for cigars, imparting a flavor not the least disagreeable, and calming to the nerves. The oil extracted gives an agreeable flavor to candies. Toilet soaps are made, strongly impregnated with essential oil of pine needles.

The fiber itself, after curing, looks like a slender shaving of some dark wood, retaining its odor indefinitely. Insects abhor it on that account. It is said that the Oregon factory is the only one in the world outside of Germany.—*Enos Brown, in the Scientific American.*

✠ ✠

INTESTINAL ANTISEPSIS.

CONSERVATIVE men of the older school of therapeutics still look upon the modern claims as to the efficacy of the various antiseptics in sterilizing the digestive tract with pronounced incredulity. The Woodbury method in typhoid is based on this theory, and has now so many reputable and competent advocates that its practical success can hardly be longer called in question.

Undoubtedly it will be further improved by other observers and experimenters; but it certainly is itself a great improvement on the usual practice, which so often proves unavailing. On this topic Dr. Chas. F. Hope has this to say:

"Every physician knows that the intestines can be affected by calomel, salol, thymol, sulpho-carbolate of zinc and sodium, bismuth, turpentine, beta naphthol, and a large number of other drugs. But that these drugs should be able to affect intestines which are the seat of typhoid ulceration seems strangely incredible to those physicians who are wedded to the older doctrines of therapeutics. Every physician knows, or should know, that acute enterocolitis in infants and children can be benefited if not entirely cured by small broken doses of calomel, especially in connection with some of the other reliable intestinal antiseptics, and that the same drugs are equally valuable in the enteritis of adults; but that these drugs should be employed in typhoid fever to influence the condition of the intestines and the intestinal contents is a view to be met by the haughtiest skepticism! For my part, so long as I am engaged in the practice of medicine, I propose to be steadfast and loyal to the advocacy and use of this modern treatment. I shall do what little I can to popularize the antiseptic treatment of typhoid fever.

"Starting from the positive observations that the intestinal antiseptics will cure enteritis in children and adults, it will be found that they also possess remarkable value in combating typhoid fever. Under their use the intestines can be practically sterilized and the contents rendered harmless for the organism. After the continuous employment of these antiseptics for several days absorption of poisonous substances from the bowels is greatly modified, and in many instances wholly stopped. In this manner ptomain-intoxication is forestalled. The effect is shown by the disappearance of the symptoms of toxemia, the stools lose their offensive character, and the formation of gases in the bowels ceases."

The future of medicine depends on prophylaxis.

JAM, MARMALADE AND GLUCOSE.

COMMENTING on a recent legal decision in England in a case in which a manufacturer was accused of adulterating marmalade with 13 per cent. of glucose, William Murrell has undertaken a series of observations to see whether the amount of glucose sold in the ordinary jams and similar preparations is injurious or not. He comes to the conclusion that its alleged injurious properties are greatly overestimated. In fact, he says that he often orders commercial glucose as a food, in two dram doses three times daily. He has never known it to disagree with the patient. He declares that it may be safely affirmed that there is no valid objection to the use of glucose as a substitute for cane sugar or beet sugar in jams or marmalade, and that prosecutions for employing it for this purpose are vexatious, and serve no useful purpose; but, on the contrary, are prejudicial both to the consumer and the maker, inasmuch as they tend to restrict the production of the best and most palatable form of an article of everyday consumption.—*Medical Press and Circular.*

Mistakes we make in scientific articles, which are called to our attention by others, we should honestly acknowledge, and should endeavor to keep free from a feeling of personal injury.—*Isidor Hernheiser* (Prag).

DIGESTION AND THE DIGESTIVE FERMENTS.

BY C. W. CANAN, M.D., B.S., PH.D.,
Orkney Springs, Va.

FROM a physiologic and dietetic standpoint, the relations existing between the food from the time that it first enters the mouth until it passes the ileo-cecal valve, and the glandular tissues of the intestinal tract are of the greatest importance in their bearing upon digestion and assimilation, and consequently upon the general nutrition of the body. That the modification and digestion of the food is dependent upon the action of specific enzyms, manufactured by the glandular tissues of the digestive tract, has long been appreciated by physiologists.

Our present knowledge of digestive ferments is very far in advance of that of a decade past, and constant research is bringing out additional facts with regard to the action, source and chemical constitution of the primary zymogens and their resultant enzyms.

One point which affects not only the physician in his practice, but his patient in its results, has been constantly reiterated. That is, the practical necessity of *all* of the individual ferments of the digestive tract to achieve a *complete* digestion of the food. It is this which renders pepsin unsatisfactory when taken alone, and the lack of the various pepsin preparations to perform the entire duties of complete digestion arises from the impossibility of a single enzym performing the work ordinarily executed by the ptyalin of the salivary glands, the pepsin and rennin of the glands of the stomach, the trypsin, pancreatic rennin, amyolytic and fat-splitting enzyms of the pancreas, the enzyms of the succus entericus (produced by Brunner's and Liberkuhn's glands), and, lastly, by the action of the specific principles secreted by the spleen and liver, which exert such an important action in regard to the regulation of the general metabolism of the body.

This can be easily demonstrated to the student by a comparison of the effects of the various digestive preparations, with the combined extracts of all of the above glands, and the fact will be quickly noticeable that the combined enzyms exert a more rapid and complete digestive action upon the food.

Peptenzyme* has thus demonstrated its efficiency as a digestive agent, since it corresponds in every proportion and effect to the combined normal secretions of the alimentary tract. It contains all of the enzyms of the various glands mentioned above, and also the extracts of the spleen and liver.

This product not only aids Nature to digest the various foods, either in health or disease, but it furnished the different glands, through the blood, the essential protoplasmic elements from which they can produce the necessary digestive ferments. Peptenzyme is compatible with most of our best drugs and enhances their action by promoting digestion, absorption and assimilation. As a product, I have found it of extreme value in organic diseases of the stomach, pancreas and liver, since it rehabilitates disordered digestion and thus sustains the vitality of the patient. The elixir makes an excellent vehicle in which to administer bromides, iodides, salicylates, etc., and can be combined to great advantage with fluid extract cascara. The powdered form of peptenzyme can be combined with codeine, bismuth, salts, muriate of caffeine, strychnine, acetanilid and many other drugs, when such combinations are indicated.

The clinical results obtained by the use of this preparation coincide with the researches of the leading physiologists, in that they go to substantiate the statement that *all* of the enzyms of the alimentary tract are necessary in the process of a *complete* digestion, and thus serve to emphasize the conclusion that in treating cases of impaired digestion and nutrition it is always advisable to use that preparation which most nearly resembles the natural physiologic conditions of the alimentary tract.

✣ ✣

The result proves the right.—*Prof. E. Behring* (Marburgh).

*Reed & Carnrick.

THE DYNAMIC VALUE OF CARBO-HYDRATES.

According to the *Georgia Journal of Medicine and Surgery*, Abel summarizes the value of carbohydrates for muscular work as follows:

1. When the organism is adapted to the digestion of starch, and there is sufficient time for its utilization, sugar has no advantage over starch, as a food for muscular work, except as a preventive of fatigue.

2. In small quantities, and in not too concentrated a form, sugar will take the place, practically speaking, weight for weight, of starch, as a food for muscular work, barring the difference in energy and in time required to digest them, sugar having here the advantage.

3. It furnishes the needed carbohydrate material to organisms that have as yet little or no power to digest starch. Thus milk sugar is part of the natural food of the infant.

4. In times of great exertion or exhausting labor, the rapidity with which it is assimilated gives it certain advantages over starch.

✣ ✣

MORE ADVICE FOR THE OVER-FAT.

Dr. Strebel, in addition to the well-known dietary prescriptions, contributes some interesting details to the treatment of this obstinate condition. He adds the electric light to the usual procedures. Hot-air baths constitute one of the best means of keeping the condition in check, but it is only too frequent that precordial distress, palpitations, syncope, and vomiting are induced by this means; certain patients with heart trouble can not take such baths. For such especially are the electric-light baths available. Among the gymnastic exercises advised by the author is the familiar one of resting on one's back and coming to the sitting posture. This should be done regularly ten to twenty times at a séance, once or twice a day, on rising and retiring. As a cardiac tonic he recommends camphor, preferably in oil, used hypodermically. The electric-light séances are to be carried out twice a week. After an exposure of twenty minutes to an arc light, the neck is enveloped in cold compresses, and after the séance a bathing at a temperature of 86° F., followed by five minutes at 64° F., then massage and friction.

An *Atlantic* contributor points out what he believes to be a parallel between the autobiographies of Benjamin Franklin and Booker Washington:

"Their autobiographies are admirably written; Franklin's with a superior ease, fluency, unction; Washington's with more naïveté, candor, warmth. Franklin's has long been a classic. We think it not unlikely that the story of Booker Washington's life will also become a classic; but whether it does or not, it has always proved itself something better than another classic, namely, an inspiration to an unfortunate race—a book that by an irresistible compulsion teaches youth to live cleanly, to work honestly, to love one's neighbor, and to have that long patience which is another name for faith."

During the summer the Abbott Alkaloidal Company is advertising its remedies for cholera infantum and other summer diseases with the bold assertion that with these agents properly applied there is no need for a solitary infant's death from these maladies. Is it not worth while to look into the matter, and see what is the foundation for such faith?

GOOD-BYE.

"We say it for an hour or for years,
    We say it smiling, say it choked with
        tears;
We say it coldly, say it with a kiss,
And yet we have no other word than
        this—
        Good-bye.

"We have no dearer word for our heart's
        friend,
For him who journeys to the world's far
        end,
And scars our soul with going—thus we
        say,
As unto him who steps but o'er the way—
        Good-bye.

"Alike to those we love and those we hate,
We say no more in parting. At life's gate,
To whom who passes out beyond earth's
        sight,
We cry, as to the wanderer for a night—
        Good-bye."

THE FARMER AND PATENT MEDICINES.

It is believed that the farmer is the greatest consumer of patent medicines, and no doubt it is a serious source of harm to him. Under a notion that it is necessary to purify the blood, pounds of iodide of potash are taken under the false name of sarsaparilla, saltpetre under the name of kidney cures, and alcohol under the names of celery compounds, nervura, and so on.—*Health.*

Department of Hygiene.

WITH SPECIAL REFERENCE TO STATE AND PREVENTIVE MEDICINE.

THE THERAPEUTIC VALUE OF CLIMATE—FOURTH PAPER.

SOME PRUDENTIAL PRECAUTIONS.

AFTER deciding upon a change of climate, invalids and their friends are quite inclined to be rash in their movements, and before resuming the study of the climatic characteristics of the remaining portions of our country a few timely suggestions will not be out of place. A degree of precaution is especially appropriate to those who contemplate a removal from a low to a comparatively high altitude.

It is well for an invalid, through his medical adviser, to study his own case and the nature of the locality for which he is about to set out, before starting. If he has a "weak heart," or is much "run down" he should not make the trip in a "lightning express," without sundry halts *en route*. To start from an elevation not much above sea-level and land at a point a vertical mile or more "up in the air," as if shot out of a dynamite gun, may prove a fatal, or at least harmful, experiment. It is better to take weeks, and in some rare cases even months, for the journey. In this way one can gradually accustom himself to the marked influences of the changing altitude, and thus avoid doing himself irreparable damage.

For example, if starting for the mountain heights of Colorado, New Mexico or Arizona, plan in advance to pause for a week or more at several intermediate points —say Omaha or Julesburg, Kansas City or Hutchinson, according to route chosen. If inclined to hemorrhages, stop another fortnight at a second point that about evenly

divides the altitude of these places with that of Denver. At the latter place bear in mind that you are a lineal mile higher than when you left the Atlantic Coast. Pueblo is lower by nearly a thousand feet, Colorado Springs nearly a thousand feet higher.

Test each tarrying point by very gradually increased exercise until it is found that no serious disturbance of the circulation results from a brisk walk. It will then be prudent to advance to the next elevation decided upon.

On reaching the final destination be circumspect as to any severe exertion until well accustomed to the diminished air-pressure. Do no mountain climbing, and even walk with "dignified deliberation" for a month or two, until the breathing capacity has thoroughly adapted itself to the new requirements.

But do not interpret these suggestions to mean that you shall mope, be afraid of shadows and stay indoors. On the contrary, make it a point to live out of doors at once, and most of the time, and to begin the process of augmenting the lung capacity and the tone of the heart from the first. Every day will give you increased assurance, unless you are bound to nurse an overweening and unwarranted timidity. In reality these precautions are wholly unnecessary except for those with damaged hearts or those who have already suffered from pulmonary hemorrhages. Excessive timidity and over-apprehensiveness are ten times as dangerous as high altitudes, if the latter be not too recklessly or suddenly approached. For all other classes of patients the transition to higher altitudes will prove immediately beneficial in nearly every case. It will compel them to breathe as they have never breathed before, and every accession of breathing function will prove a positive and permanent benefit.

Of a hundred invalids resorting to any fairly good climate perhaps not more than fifty will realize any appreciable benefit, for the reason that they will be afraid to take a full breath in the oper air, and so will insist on housing themselves in stuffy, ill-ventilated rooms, where they will breathe an atmosphere no better than the one they left behind them in the East.

Such unfortunates would do well to commit to memory the following rules, or similar ones, dictated by their medical advisers:

1. Break your last fever thermometer, or hire a boy to drive it into the sands of the sea at low tide.

2. Throw all your cares, fears and chronic worriments to the winds.

3. See that your trunk contains seasonable wraps, to meet the exigencies of weather changes, but do not carry this precaution to the extreme. There is more danger of over-coddling than of hurtful exposure. Porous linen underwear is actually safer than the heaviest woolen. The cuticle needs to help you breathe. Gradually accustom it to the wholesome tonic of the air.

4. Make the best selection of locality possible from information at hand, and then make the most of your selection. In other words, second the climate in every possible way.

5. Take a solemn oath in advance not to chafe or grumble at the inevitable. There will be surprises and annoyances everywhere. The Garden of Eden has never been restored!

6. Leave behind you as many of your bad ways of living as possible. In this respect seek the careful advice of the medical man in whom you have most faith, and then promptly ignore the meddlesome counter advice of bores and grannies. Reform your cranky diet, discard hurtful beverages, uncomfortable dress, shiftless habits of exercise, despondent moods and mental mullygrubs.

7. Co-operate with the *vis medicatrix naturæ*, of which the world is full. Don't coddle yourself. Live out of doors. Death lurks in the shadows, crouches in the parlors and revels in the easy-chairs. Don't sit motionless for hours, reading morbid and exciting literature. Read but little, and always let that little be wholesome, entertaining or amusing, the more of the latter character the better.

8. Don't be a recluse; and don't be over-suspicious. Get acquainted with somebody in your vicinity, and induce them to join you in the cultivation of hope and confidence in the outcome. Other people are just as human, and may be quite as decent and honest as you are. There are some social sneaks and boors, but don't be always on the lookout for such. There are lots of good people in this wicked world. Find some of them, and make the most of them; but shun the croakers and pessimists as you would the bubonic plague.

9. Open your mental and spiritual eyes; get into the sunshine; climb the hills; get interested—really enthusiastic over something or somebody; laugh; eat sensibly, and all you want; breathe generously, and sleep a full ten hours of the twenty-four.

10. Finally, don't blurt out your final verdict concerning the climate selected within forty-eight hours after reaching it! Your opinion will be more valuable after three or six months.

If you heed these hints, and do all these things for yourself, you will probably have no occasion to find fault with what the climate will do for you.

All climates help those who help themselves!

CLIMATES OF THE PACIFIC COAST.

The climates of the Pacific Coast remain

to be considered. This region has recently acquired fresh interest and new significance. As evidence of this we have but to refer to the recent battle royal between rival capitalists for the control of transcontinental lines of travel. It was an exhibition of far-seeing financiering such as the world had never before witnessed. It involved more capital than it cost to build Solomon's Temple or the Suez canal. The geography of this hemisphere has been readjusted. The nation has expanded, regardless of the whining of the "anti-imperialists." As a nation we no longer rank as merely continental; henceforth we are cosmopolitan. All the strained rhetoric and sounding rhodomontade was wasted breath. There never was a shadow of either statesmanship or policy—not even respectable politics—in it. The discussion is closed; the Gates of Progress are wide open before us, with all the bridges burned behind; and we cannot retreat if we would. It is one of the inevitable results of the progress of events. Granted that we have assumed grave and great responsibilities, we have at the same time fallen heir to brilliant possibilities. "Our Pacific Coast" must now be written in the plural. It is no longer our continental Ultima Thule, but has become the *entrepot* to the Orient, its permanence and supremacy guaranteed by a protective tariff three thousand miles long, as wide as the continent and as irrepealable as the everlasting mountains that stretch from Canada to Mexico.

History is being made with electric rapidity; only the most alert and astute can keep pace with the changing phases in the evolution. The new West greets the new East as a near neighbor. Henceforth the oldest civilizations must pay tribute to the newest. The opulent Orient must find its Open Door to the model republic of the world through the hospitable harbors of Seattle, San Francisco and San Diego.

Said an eminent financier, recently, when asked concerning the significance of the late struggle of the railway barons:

"My friend, bear in mind that during the nineteenth century the development of this country was east of the Mississippi, and chiefly along the Atlantic coast. In the twentieth century it will be along the Pacific coast. Seattle and San Francisco are destined to become great cities and great ports. An immense commerce with Asia is springing up, and then, too, consider that over 100,000 troops have been transported to the Hawaiian Islands and the Philippines, with equipment and army stores, and that that special business will continue, and you will see why a new era has started for all the transcontinental railways. The Pacific slope will repeat the history of the Atlantic coast."

THE NEW NORTHWEST.

It is but a few years since Nebraska, Minnesota and the Dakotas constituted the far-famed and only "Great Northwest."

The march of empire has transformed these broad stretches of eminent domain into plain and matter-of-fact Northern Central States.

They have become the granary of the nation, not by the Midas touch of the Man with the Hoe, but by the irresistible sweep of the soil-civilizing gang-plow, the traction engine and the locomobile threshing machine.

Once not without fame as a retreat for coughing consumptives and starving dyspeptics, it has been transformed into an acknowledged purveyor to the cookrooms of two continents.

A generation back the pioneers of this region were largely composed of wheezing asthmatics, hacking and hawking bronchitics and distressed dyspeptics, who ran away from the harsh, humid and inhospitable coasts of New England and New Jersey to the bracing air and bright sunshine of Minnesota; or to the welcoming hills and broad plateaus of one of the Dakotas. There, by roaming the flower-fringed prairies, rusticating among the lakes and forests, or tilling the generous acres of this realm of restoration, many a weary, disease-smitten and hope-hunting pilgrim lost his heavy burden, pulled safely through the slough of despond and secured a new lease of life. Whether he chose his abiding place on the bosom of one of the great valley plains, beside some gurgling spring or hill-embanked lake, or in the wilds of the unfrequented forest, everywhere Nature became his willing handmaid, and in good time led him into green pastures, beside clear, rippling waters and into broad fields of waving grain.

It is true Minnesota no longer lures the sick and starving to her borders, but she sends them "Pillsbury's Best" or "Washburn's Gold Medal" brands, both high-water mark standards of the miller's art, in sacks and barrels, and feeds them back to health at their own fireside.

The Dakotas boast of mineral springs as sparkling and refreshing and restorative as any in the world. They cure rheumatics, dyspeptics and diabetics to order; and there are—pardon the coinage of the word—*antogamous* springs for the healing of matrimoniacs. The latch-string is always on the outside, and non-residents are welcome at all hours of the day or night, regardless of the state of the weather, age, sex or previous condition of marital infelicity. (Cures warranted to wash after six months' exposure to the northwest wind, —fees always in advance!) Special tourist trains, with free staterooms in vestibuled sleepers, to accommodate the relieved and released, leave for the East on the adjournment of court, stopping twenty minutes in Chicago—ample time for the disconnected to re-connect, and thus complete the one-act opera bouffé of "How to Get Out of the Fryingpan Into the Fire."

Testimonials and genuine certificates on file in the offices of the county recorders.

"Knew that we ventured on such dangerous
          seas,
That if we wrought our life, 'twas ten to
          one;
And yet we venture for the" . . .
          (man) proposed.
     —*"Henry IV." slightly altered.*

THE NORTHWEST OF TO-DAY.

Including Idaho, Montana, Washington and Oregon—a quartet large enough in area, rich enough in rare natural resources, and commanding geographic and topographic features in more than ample variety from which to build an empire—this is an outline of the new Northwest!

Much as they have been harped upon in the exaggerated yet only half appreciative language of irresponsible boomers, the climatic, commercial and industrial wealth, the illimitable possibilities of this intensely interesting region are yet only superficially conjectured.

The pioneers of this new realm have thus far been too much absorbed in the preliminary battle of subjugation, settlement and the sale of city lots to fully investigate or half realize its matchless material and developmental advantages.

With plenty of scenery grander than any in Switzerland, mountain peaks that have never been scaled, cataracts and waterfalls that are yet unknown to any but trappers and Indians, there are rushing rivers and gushing springs as full of healing as any of the most renowned spas of Europe.

There are climates to order; warm and cold, wet and dry, high and low, mountain and valley, coast and inland, forest and plain, with miniature examples of intermontane, and even purely insular climates.

As to weather, it is the cream of New England when on her good behavior, transported across a continent, immensely improved by the journey, and with all the disagreeableness and cantankerous moodiness left out. In short, the climatic invitation is so cordial and full of promise and assurance that chronic invalids who are slowly but surely dying at the East, need not hesitate or delay. Whether they must have coolness or warmth, moist air or dry, sea-level, sunny plains or shady mountain heights—all are here at their command.

For those who are not invalids the region affords practically incalculable and unlimited opportunities. In mining wealth, in particular, it is a Klondike right at home. Prospectors who have resisted the Klondike craze and have been spared the forlorn hope and imminent risks of the icebound realm, from which a thousand disappointed to one fortune-striker have been lucky to escape with their lives, have been rewarded with rich finds in nearby and accessible fastnesses.

Its agricultural, horticultural and pastoral possibilities and its stored-up mineral wealth are simply untellable. Its mountains are seamed with veins of gold that coming ages will fail to exhaust, and there are limitless deposits of all the other valuable metals, silver, zinc, antimony, lead, iron and copper, while the supply of coal is ample for her own needs and for all the contiguous States, for ages to come. Her stately forests are the marvel of the world, supplying exhaustless quantities of timber such as can be found nowhere else on this continent. Add to this valleys of matchless loveliness, broad plateaus that bask in as glorious sunshine as ever streamed from heaven; a soil of unparalleled productiveness, majestic rivers freighted with fish, that find a market in every corner, hamlet and mart in the civilized globe; coast lines, inlets, bays and sounds nowhere else duplicated, and landlocked harbors that would furnish safe anchorage and commodious havens for the shipping of all the seas and nations of the world.

When one attempts to describe such a rare and comprehensive combination of natural advantages and material resources language has its limitations, and the most glowing and extravagant terms seem tame, because they fail to depict the simple truth. For example, no pen, pencil or camera can do justice to the giant forests of the State of Washington by giving more than a faint and inadequate impression of their marvelous extent, the monstrous size of their trees or their magnificent grandeur. In their presence the lumberman of other famous regions stands aghast and mute with awe. What! Half a million feet of lumber from a single giant of the forest? Well, hardly.

As a background and guaranty to the permanency of all this greatness is that *sine qua non* of supremacy in any nation—a soil so fertile that fruits, grains and every form of soil-product all are equally marvelous as to size, quality and yield. And underlying this generous soil are hidden deposits of silver and gold, and other precious metals, that have never been scratched, and the extent of which can scarcely be imagined.

The salmon fisheries of this realm are without a counterpart or competitor, its commercial possibilities can only be measured by the wants and tonnage of the world, and its climatic hospitality is comprehensive.

In view of these facilities, possessions and advantages it is not surprising that the region has attracted a population of progressives who hesitate at no obstacle or undertaking, commercial, financial or political, no matter what its magnitude or difficulty.

This new Northwest is a very giant in its youth. It is the gateway to the Klondike, outfitting its adventurous miners and receiving its treasure.

It supplies and safeguards Alaska, neighbors with British America, hob-nobs with Hawaii, and holds a commercial balance of power over China and Japan.

It is, as stated, the nation's *entrepot*, through which must come the commerce of all the opulent Orient.

Already five trunk lines of transcontinental railways have grappled the realm with hooks of steel, linking it with the populous East, and organized lines of monster steamers regularly ply between her ports and those of the Old World.

What a revelation and astonishment for an Easterner to be suddenly dropped into the midst of the restless, ambitious and irrepressible throng that surges from early dawn till dewy darkness in all the business streets of the many young communities—communities that are fast merging into cities, with blocks and blocks of solidly-built business structures and public edifices that would do credit to Boston, Chicago or New York.

Here is a palpable refutation of the trite saying that the days of miracles have passed, for this is a land of miracles. They are daily and hourly wrought by the magic wands of the tillers of the soil, by the monitions of the mariner's compass, the revelations of the miner's pick, the rejuvenation of chronic invalids, and the architectural evolutions of the mason's trowel. Except that they are performed in the broad light of day they would be recorded as miracles.

O sun-land, sea-land, thou mine own!
Have I not turned to thee and thine,
And sung thy scenes, surpassing skies,
Till Europe lifted up her face
And marveled at thy matchless grace,
With eager and inquiring eyes?
Be my reward some little place
To pitch my tent, some tree and vine,
Where I may sit above the sea,
And dream, or sing some songs of thee;
Or days to climb to Shasta's dome
Again, and be with gods at home,
Salute my mountains—clouded Hood,
Saint Helens in its sea of wood—
Where sweeps the Oregon, and where
White storms are in the feathered fir.

Joaquin Miller.

✠ ✠

COLD AIR FOR CONSUMPTION.

Good results are claimed for the treatment of consumption by the practice of sleeping in the pure, cold air out doors. With plenty of covering dampness will do no harm, and the patient at once shows gain in strength and weight. The colder the air the better, since cold air seems to have a retarding effect on the growth of the tubercle. Something like this has got to be done, for the London *Lancet* says, "tuberculosis is still progressing in spite of the incessant anti-microbic warfare during the last ten years."

AN AUGEAN STABLE.

Do the missionaries to China, the Committees of Fifteen, and the "Settlement" promoters realize what a prolific source of moral filth, debauchery, and crime exists openly and constantly in the advertising columns of the daily and weekly press? With a few, alas how few honorable exceptions, the daily papers are crammed with adroitly worded advertisements that stimulate, pander to and instigate a variety of crimes that are too indecent to be named, too vile to be tolerated.

It seems impossible that the civilization of the twentieth century, whose progress has been so brilliantly inaugurated in regard to nearly all other reforms, should have made almost no progress toward abating such a notorious and almost universal nuisance. Most nuisances have some more or less plausible excuse for being. This has absolutely none. The average newspaper of the day is unfit to be read or seen in the family circle. Of course, doctors are not more to blame for this state of affairs than other members of a community; but if the 125,000 doctors of this country should resolutely and absolutely throw out the dirty sheets, their example would soon be imitated by other thousands, and the combined influence would soon begin to tell.

It is true that a goodly number of our citizens are aware that New York publishes at least one daily paper that steadfastly refuses to resort to large display type, glaring red ink, and bogus or freak sensations of every kind. We also know that it contains no advertisements concerning "lost manhood," "female irregularities," "private masseuses," "guaranteed cures," or of other like indecencies. It rigidly excludes all advertisements that promise something for nothing, prizes for solving puzzles that are solved in the ad. itself, and all the hundred other ways of dishonestly luring money from credulous dupes.

Its standing promise, thoroughly kept, is, "All the news that's fit to print." Lest some country reader may be in doubt as to the name of this courageous sheet we print it in capitals; it is THE NEW YORK TIMES.

If the pessimists were within several centuries of being right in their estimate of the drift of affairs this epitome of journalistic exclusiveness would be a financial failure of the first magnitude; but it is nothing of the kind. On the contrary, it is a decided success, and its patronage has become so substantial that the other day its leading spirit went over to Philadelphia as a journalistic missionary. He bought in the stock of the *Philadelphia Times,* called in its staff of editors, reporters, and advertising managers, and read the riot act to them in tones that they all comprehended. In substance the new rules amount to this:

No more flare-heads, fake advertisements nor filth.

The result is that two cities, at least, have each a clean newspaper, that no father need hesitate to put into the hands of his young and innocent daughter.

If physicians everywhere would take the initiative and form Hercules clubs for the purpose of ridding communities of this incubus of foul stables, decent people would soon join their ranks, and in time the evil could be abated.

The GAZETTE is willing to act as Corresponding Committee on organization.

THE Hellespont or Dardanelles is a narrow strait betwen Europe and Asiatic Turkey, which connects the Sea of Marmora and the Ægean Sea. The legend describes Leander as nightly swimming across the Hellespont to visit Hero, his sweetheart. It was really swam by Lord Byron. The actual distance betwen Abydos and Sestos is about a mile and a quarter, but the current is so strong that about four miles is made by a swimmer, because of his drifting, ere he has touched from point to point. The first attempt of Byron to swim the Hellespont was a failure, but on a second venture he performed the feat in one hour and ten minutes.

NOVEL CLASS REUNION.

THERE was a reunion of the class of 1891 of Jefferson Medical College, at Philadelphia, on the 28th and 29th of June.

The president of the class issued the call and suggested the following rules to guide the members during the reunion:

1. Each member of the class will be sworn before being permitted to relate the amount of business he has done since graduation, or the amount of money collected annually.

2. Benedict members whose families do not attend will be allowed to exhibit pictures of the same, at a time fixed by the committee on rules.

3. All unmarried members must render their excuses for being single in writing, and no verbal explanations will be accepted.

4. Every member whose facial expression has been changed by hirsute appendages will be required to wear his name and residence in a conspicuous place.

5. No member will be allowed to sit higher than the third gallery while in attendance upon the theatres of the city.

6. All anatomical and pathological jokes must be thoroughly sterilized and wear the badge of originality before demonstration at this reunion.

7. Any member of the class caught wearing a downcast expression during this period of jollification will be at once "corralled" and initiated into the Buffaloes.

We have no doubt there was a jolly time for the classmates.

TOO CHANGEABLE.

"HERE, young man," said the old lady, with fire in her eye; "I've brung back this thermometer you sold me."

"What's the matter with it?" asked the clerk.

"It ain't reliable. One time ye look at it it says one thing, and the next time it says another."

PHYSICIANS HAVE THE RIGHT OF WAY.

Over eight hundred physicians in Chicago, says *The Chicago Chronicle*, have already taken advantage of an ordinance passed by the Council a few weeks ago, giving them the right of way on the streets and over bridges ahead of processions, parades, fire lines, and other obstructions that usually stop their ordinary traffic. Each of the physicians applying has been furnished with a badge and a special permit, which entitle him to the privileges of the ordinance and demonstrate his authority.

The badge is a very pretty affair, about the size of a quarter, and is made of German silver in the form of a circle 3-16 of an inch wide, around a red cross in the center. The cross is of red enamel, and the circle of white.

The ordinance also applies to ambulances, and is made to include all physicians driving in answer to professional calls, to fires or accidents. It is designed to afford relief as quickly as possible to people who require the services of a physician. The permits are signed by the Mayor and City Clerk, and the badges are issued from the City Clerk's office on the payment of a 50-cent fee. The ordinance has been effective about one month, and the number of doctors using the privileges granted them will soon reach 1,000, demonstrating the popularity of the ordinance and its provisions.

The *Chicago Clinic* has the following "suggestive" illustration of human nature: "A gentleman came into Dr. A.'s office and requested a diagnosis. The doctor looked at the man's tongue, placed his hand on his pulse, and handed him a prescription, with the remark, 'Two dollars, please.' The man passed down stairs and entering a drug store, asked to be directed to a good physician. He was referred to a Dr. B., up the street. He at once called upon the new man and asked him the same question he had just propounded to the eminent physician adding that the other doctor did not examine him at all, hardly. The doctor last consulted required him to strip and put him through all kinds of gymnastics, and pounded and thumped him for an hour, and finally told him there was nothing the matter with him. When he asked what the charges were he was told 'one hundred dollars,' which was paid very gladly by 'the happiest man in the city, who had feared he was gradually going down and would soon reach the end of his existence.' "

We venture to add that the mortgage on Dr. A.'s "humble cottage in the suburbs" is about the size of the sum of Dr. B.'s quarterly coupons as he clips them from his Spanish war bonds.—Ed. GAZETTE.

ANOTHER BACTERIA BUGABOO.

According to a Russian savant, M. Lakherbekoff, who carried out an elaborate inquiry into the bacterial quality of the milk supplied to St. Petersburg, the condition of affairs in that city is appalling. Milk described as the purest obtainable, was found to contain a minimum of over 10,000,000 and a maximum of over 83,000,000 bacteria in from 20 to 25 drops; while in other samples a minimum of 20,000,000 and a maximum of 114,000,000 were found. Such pollution as this is unnecessary, for milk under normal, healthy conditions contains very few bacteria as it issues from the cow. Indeed, some authorities consider that it is absolutely devoid of microbic life. If due precautions are taken in keeping the cows and their stable clean, if the milker is made to keep himself and his clothes in a thoroughly cleanly condition, milk can be placed upon the table which is practically free from all micro-organisms. Of course, the milk-cans require proper attention, and the cows ought to be under the supervision of a veterinary surgeon.

NUISANCES.

IN the fifteenth annual report of the State Board of Health of Pennsylvania this definition is given of nuisances:

"Whatever is dangerous to human life or health, whatever renders the air or food or water or other drink unwholesome, and whatever building, erection, or part or cellar thereof, is overcrowded, or not provided with adequate means of ingress and egress, or is not sufficiently supported, ventilated, sewered, drained, cleaned or lighted, are declared to be nuisances, and to be illegal; and every person having aided in creating or contributing to the same, or who may support, continue or retain any of them, shall be deemed guilty of a violation of these regulations, and also be liable for the expense of the abatement and remedy therefor."

DISHWASHING.

DISHWASHING, by the general consensus of opinion, would seem to be the most unimportant task in the whole realm of housework. An inexperienced girl or a very young girl may be considered good in so far as being able at least to wash the dishes, and sometimes she is allowed to wash them her own way without let or hindrance. But even about dishwashing there is a right way and several wrong ways. One of the latter consists in putting everything, from teacups and silverware to cooking utensils, through the same water, which grows more and more mixed as the process goes on, and then drying these same dishes without putting them through hot rinsing water. Common sense should show the necessity of changing the washing water frequently, because it grows cold as well as dirty. Common sense should also dictate that a good hot rinsing water is a necessity that will free the dishes from soapiness. Without plenty of hot water

and plenty of clean towels, clean sweet dishes are an impossibility, and no one who has ever had experience with rough dishes need be told of their disagreeable suggestiveness. A bottle or pitcher that is to hold milk or water needs great care. You may boil every drop of your drinking water and yet your trouble will count for nothing if the water is stored in bottles that have not been properly washed. Such details are not to be left too confidently to the average kitchen girl. She may mean to do all that is necessary, but microbes are not in her reckonings, and she is likely to slight their claims to recognition. Soap suds is a prime necessity with greasy dishes; in washing silverware, however, it is a good plan to substitute borax for soap, using hot water. The silver is not so likely to need polishing after it has been washed in borax water. All glassware that has contained milk must be rinsed out in cold water as a first step. Hot water cooks the particles of milk and renders the glass cloudy. Jars which have become stale should be filled with hot soda water and left to soak until clean. Even stale butter or lard jars may be rendered sweet and fresh if they are filled with hot lime-water and left while the water gradually cools. Remember in cleaning out an ordinary bottle or cruet that, good as are crumbled eggshells or shot for the purpose, a cut up raw potato is far better. Cut the potato into very small bits and put it into the bottle, with some warm water, shaking it about rapidly until the bottle is clean.—*Exchange.*

DIETARY (THOMAS).

BARLEY WATER.—Wash two ounces (wineglassful) pearl barley with cold water. Boil five minutes in fresh water; throw both waters away. Pour on two quarts boiling water; boil down to a quart. Flavor with thinly cut lemon rind; add sugar to taste. Do not strain unless at the patient's request.

Flaxseed Tea.—Flaxseed, whole, one

ounce; white sugar, one ounce (heaping tablespoon); liquorice root, half ounce (two small sticks); lemon juice, four tablespoons. Pour on these materials two pints boiling water; let stand in hot place four hours; strain off the liquor.

Sterilized Milk.—Put the required amount of milk in clean bottles. (If for infants, each bottle holding enough for one feeding.) Plug mouths lightly with rubber stoppers; immerse to shoulders in kettle of cold water; boil twenty minutes; or, better, steam thirty minutes in ordinary steamer; push stoppers in firmly, cool bottles rapidly and keep in refrigerator. Warm each bottle just before using.

Junket.—Heat one pint fresh milk just lukewarm; add one teaspoonful essence of pepsin or one-half a rennet tablet; stir just enough to mix. Flavor, if desired, with sugar, grated nutmeg, and brandy. Pour into custard cups; let stand in cool place till firmly curded.

Egg Lemonade.—Beat one egg with one tablespoonful sugar until very light; stir in three tablespoons cold water and juice of small lemon; fill glass with pounded ice, and drink through straw.

Peptonized Milk Toast.—Over two slices of toast pour gill of peptonized milk (cold process); let stand on the hob for thirty minutes. Serve warm, or strain and serve fluid portion alone. Plain light sponge cake may be similarly digested.

Wine Whey.—Put two pints of new milk in saucepan, and stir over a clear fire until nearly boiling; then add gill (two wineglassfuls) of sherry, and simmer a quarter of an hour, skimming off curd as it rises. Add a tablespoon more sherry, and skim again for a few minutes; strain through coarse muslin. May use two tablespoons lemon juice instead of wine.

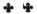

FRENCH METHODS TO INCREASE BIRTH-RATE.

THE proposed tax on bachelors and old maids and upon childless couples in France, says the *Journal of the American Medical Association*, will, if carried out, be an interesting experiment. If it succeeds in arresting the decrease of the birth-rate it will show the possibility of the more economic method. In any case it is the pecuniary consideration that is involved; if the thrifty French peasant, who, under the bounties for children is a regular proletarian in Canada, can be made such in France by the reversed inducement of fines, the problem is solved. The question is essentially an economic one, but it has some medical interest also, and the experiment, if tried, will be worth watching.

MENINGITIS AND THE OVERDRAW CHECK.

IN a recent issue of the Wilmington, Del., *Republican*, the writer of the New Castle Items states that many of their horses were dying of spinal meningitis. Just so long as a man is fool enough to torture his horse with the overdraw check, which we are informed by the highest authority in the land especially brings on that disease, he deserves to lose his horse. The same authority states that the overdraw check should be prohibited by law, that it is a great evil, a constant torment, causing paralysis and making horses liable to stumble and fall, as it cramps the heavy muscles of the neck with which he balances himself. Such a glaring breach of Nature's laws brings its own punishment.—[But the man ought to suffer in the neck as well as in his purse.—Ed. GAZETTE.]

BLINDNESS REMOVED BY REMOVAL OF BRAIN TUMOR.

DR. C. PRUYN STRINGFIELD, assisted by others of the Chicago Hospital staff, succeeded, February 24th, in relieving Mrs. F. G. Parker of blindness, which had been increasing for seven years and had lately become complete. She had met with no accident; there had been no unusual strain on the optic nerves, neither was there any physical condition that could be considered in any way associated with the affliction. For years no relief could be given her, and Dr. Stringfield could determine no reason for the condition unless there were an obstruction of the blood-vessels supplying the optic nerve.

The X-ray was employed and a skiograph was obtained, faintly outlining what seemed to be a tumor in the upper portion of the occipital lobe. By trephining the tumor was exposed to view. By the removal of the tumor the blood supplying the optic nerve is again permitted to flow freely, tissues for many years in disuse were rehabilitated, and the woman's sight will be restored in a short time.

THE patient's mental condition, says *American Medicine*, is often quite as important a matter in the proper treatment of disease as is his physical status. Failure to realize this fact has doubtless been in the past a professional sin, for which we are duly and justly punished by Un-Christian, Unscience Faith-cure, and the rest. Our text-books on therapeutics and materia medica tell us about hundreds of drugs; some of them will allude with too vague indifference to hygienic methods of treatment, but how many of them recognize and advise as to the highly important conditions of the patient's will, disposition, etc.? Every physician of discernment knows that the mental attitude of the patient governs, often entirely, always to some extent, the morbid processes and the nutritional reactions. The cheerfulness and friendliness of the old-time general practitioner was perhaps needed to neutralize his bad medicines, and they were certainly powerful therapeutic agents. Choate found the dying Lowell reading "Rob Roy," whereby, the poet said, he forgot his bodily pains. Two items universally omitted from the books on therapeutics and treatment should be henceforth

important constituent parts—music and books. Above all things nurses should be good readers, and, if possible, good musicians. Physicians should advise about what books to be read, as much as about what drugs to be given and what food to be eaten. The best nurses' training schools should have teachers of music and of literature, as well as professors of surgery, obstetrics, etc., etc.

SOME CONSIDERATIONS REGARDING THE HYGIENE OF EARLY SCHOOL LIFE.

J. STOER says children work too much, too soon and badly; that is to say, under unfavorable hygienic surroundings. We are reminded of the long list of studies, the rushing through of courses, the long duration of hours and the useless studies, the method of teaching unscientific, and the disregard of the laws of physiology and purely in favor of psychology, the evil of home tasks which rob the children of their short periods of recreation. The fact that mental and physical abnormalities exist in school children must be realized, and also that these abnormalities are always aggravated, if not, indeed, produced by pedantic and pseudo educational methods of teaching. It is eminently proper for the physician to interfere in matters relating to school hygiene. The protests of medical men may be summarized as follows. There is no evidence by which educational values may be determined except through the study of material manifestations transmitted through the nervous system. Education produces nothing new in the child. It simply unfolds and brings into intelligible activity the latent forces in the nervous system. One of the most important prerequisites for good education is good nutrition. Vigorous intellectual activity is possible only through the medium of brain-cells that are well nourished and physiologically active. All methods, therefore, which ignore the physical development are faulty and open to criticism. There is such a variance in individuals that it becomes absurd to attempt to lay out a uniform system of training and education applicable to all alike. The early discovery of the dull and the backward and the defective child, and their segregation for special training, is one of the problems of public importance in school life. The child is an exceedingly immature and delicate animal, undergoing important developmental changes. His delicate tissues and plastic nerve cells are easily warped and injured by long continued mental and physical efforts, and for this reason children are often injured by injudicious school work. Cases of this sort are of common occurrence. These abnormal consequences can, and must, be prevented, and the child's intellectual development must be allowed to proceed without detriment or hindrance.

Discussion.—Dr. Work thought that the cry that came up from all parts of the country proved that there was something radically wrong with the school system, and it was not confined to any one locality. The classification of scholars should be according to their intellect, and schools should be selected for children which were fitted to their needs. He was particularly impressed with some of the facts brought out in Dr. Darnall's paper with regard to the close fitting and often unhygienic dress of the girl. The two important factors in all dress are equal pressure and equal warmth. Another most important factor is the food of the child, which often is badly and carelessly prepared. Regular habits should be taught the child with regard to baths, elimination, eating, etc. Every child should be taught what the organs of the body are, and for what purpose they are intended, and how they should be taken care of, and how they may be injured. If a child goes to school without a proper evacuation of the bowels or bladder, he cannot study properly. His intellect is dull and clouded. If a child does not have plenty of water to drink his mind will be more or less affected from the lack of it. The greatest trouble in most of the schools is not so much with

the school or with the child. It is because we have not got trained mothers who understand these things themselves to teach the child at home. The duty of the profession is to educate the mothers of the community how to take care of the health of their school children.

Dr. A. W. Wilmarth referred to the importance of special training for the backward child, and the work that might be done by schools set apart especially for this purpose. Such a school has been provided in Philadelphia and in a few other localities.

Dr. Learned thought that the highest ideals of development might be reached by plenty of outdoor exercise, and good air and plenty of sleep. It is a mistake to start the child to school so early, and begin to burden its little mind, pushing it always to an extreme and keeping it on a tension. The child would learn faster and more thoroughly, and really make more progress in the long run, if he were not started to school until he were eight or nine years of age, at least. The child's brain is fatigued and stunted by overwork when he is started so early.

THE ETIOLOGY OF YELLOW FEVER.

FROM the long and exhaustive paper of Surgeons Reed and Agramonte, of the United States Army, on this subject, we extract for our readers the kernel, in the following conclusions:

1. The mosquito (*C. fasciatus*) serves as the intermediate host for the parasite of yellow fever.

2. Yellow fever is transmitted to the non-immune individual by means of the bite of the mosquito that has previously fed on the blood of those sick with this disease.

3. An interval of about twelve days or more after contamination appears to be necessary before the mosquito is capable of conveying the infection.

4. The bite of the mosquito at an earlier

period after contamination does not appear to confer any immunity against a subsequent attack.

5. Yellow fever can also be experimentally produced by the subcutaneous injection of blood taken from the general circulation during the first and second days of this disease.

6. An attack of yellow fever, produced by the bite of the mosquito, confers immunity against the subsequent injection of the blood of an individual suffering from the non-experimental form of this disease.

7. The period of incubation in thirteen cases of experimental yellow fever has varied from forty-one hours to five days and seventeen hours.

8. Yellow fever is not conveyed by fomites, and hence disinfection of articles of clothing, bedding, or merchandise, supposedly contaminated by contact with those sick with this disease, is unnecessary. ·

9. A house may be said to be infected with yellow fever only when there are present within its walls contaminated mosquitoes capable of conveying the parasite of this disease.

10. The spread of yellow fever can be most effectually controlled by measures directed to the destruction of mosquitoes and the protection of the sick against the bites of these insects.

11. While the mode of propagation of yellow fever has now been definitely determined, the specific cause of this disease remains to be discovered.

CLEAN MILK.

Cow's milk, according to *Archives of Pediatrics*, is practically the universal food of early life and hence its production and handling are most important considerations for the physician. That the profession is becoming alive to this question is evidenced in a number of ways. The hygienic condition of the dairy farm, the care of the cows, the personal habits of the milkers, the utensils used in collection and transportation of the milk, the proper temperature to be maintained and various other factors in the problem have all been subjected to the closest study. The question practically reduces itself to one of strictest cleanliness and a constant application of cold in the care of the milk. The test of uncleanliness consists in an increase in the proportion of lactic acid generated in the milk and in a large increase in the number of bacteria per cubic centimeter. Lactic acid is an expression of bacterial growth.

In a recent work by Farrington and Woll is found the following paragraph, which well epitomizes present knowledge on the subject: "Bacteriological examinations of milk from different sources and of the same milk at different times have shown that there is a direct relation between the bacteria found in normal milk and its acidity; the larger the number of bacteria per unit of milk, the higher the acidity of milk. The increase in the acidity of milk on standing is caused by the breaking down of milk-sugar into lactic acid through the influence of acid-forming bacteria. Since the bacteria get into the milk through lack of cleanliness during the milking, and careless handling of the milk after milking, this being kept under conditions that favor the multiplication of bacteria contained therein, it follows that an acidity test of fresh milk will give a good clue to the care bestowed in handling the milk. Such a test will show which patrons take good care of their milk and those who do not wash their cans clean, or their hands and the udders of the cows before milking, and have dirty ways generally in milking and caring for the milk." These facts should be brought to the attention of farmers and milk-dealers generally, as a very simple test will show the proportion of lactic acid present in a given sample of milk, and, hence, indirectly of its cleanliness. Over 200 species of bacteria have been found in milk, about 20 of which produce lactic acid. Some species of bacteria produce peculiar effects in milk that may embarrass the dealer. These effects may show as ropy, slimy, blue and red milk. The way to keep the bacteria out of milk is to collect and keep it under conditions of the strictest cleanliness. With such precautions milk will keep sweet and wholesome for a long time. Chapin, in a recent article, makes the statement that properly handled and cooled milk shipped from Illinois, New York and New Jersey to the Paris Exposition last summer, was used when it arrived, and was then better than the average daily milk supply of Paris. This shows the possibilities in the problem of clean milk.

The certifying of clean milk by medical commissioners, as inaugurated by Coit, is now carried on in Boston, New York, Philadelphia, Newark and Buffalo. These commissions deal usually with one dairyman, who must follow the rules of the commission and subject his milk to frequent examinations. The New York County Medical Society has recently appointed a commission that stands ready to certify the milk of any dealer that comes up to the required standard. Directions concerning the care of the stable, the cows and the milk are furnished as a guide.

The circular containing the directions closes as follows:

"The Milk Commission of the New York County Medical Society agrees to guarantee or certify the milk of all dealers desiring such certificate. A special label will be furnished for this purpose. The standard required to obtain this indorsement will be that the acidity must not be higher than .2 per cent., and that the milk must not contain more than 30,000 germs, or bacteria of any kind, to the cubic centimeter. This will be tentatively adopted as a standard of clean milk, as bacteria get into the milk through lack of cleanliness during the milking and careless handling of the milk after the milking, and, hence, is a good clue to the care bestowed in the production and general handling of milk. The milk, before testing, must be in its natural state, not having been heated, and without the addition of coloring matter or preservatives. The butter fat must reach 3.5 per cent. Examinations must be made by the experts re-

tained by the commission, with a frequency at its option, according to the season and the general condition of the milk under inspection, and at least once a month. The commission reserves the right to change its standard, in any reasonable manner, upon due notice being given to the dealer. The expense of the examination will be met by the dealer. All reports of examinations will be strictly confidential between the commission and the individual dealer."

It is to be hoped that this movement in the direction of better and cleaner milk will be successful, and extend wherever milk is used for infant feeding.

UGLINESS THAT COSTS MONEY.

"By tradition rather than necessity, the modern factory is a paragon of ugliness. The owner appears to think that he has fulfilled his duty to his employees if he has provided running water and fire escapes. It is not so greatly to his discredit that he does no more, because he has accepted custom in such matters, and if, now and then, he hears of improvements in other mills or in the way of running them, he dismisses the subject as the whim of sentimentalists, as of no practical consequence, and as a probable drag on business. Experience has proved this view to be a wrong one. The best protection against labor troubles is interest in the laborer. This interest need not and should not take the form of condescension and charity, which are demeaning and humiliating to their object, but should be a practical service which is no more called in question than is the workman's right to air, water and protection against danger from the explosion of chemicals or the escape of noxious vapors.

"The things to be done need not involve great labor or expense. To keep the floors and windows clean does not appear to be a difficult undertaking; yet in a majority of factories in this country the floors are covered with oil and dirt, and the windows are so grimy as to make a sort of twilight, which is not only trying to the eyes but is depressing to health and spirits; and a dispirited man never works as does one who is cheerful. Soap and sunshine, therefore, are prime agents in the creation of comfort and content. But it is possible to do more than this. . . . It is sometimes argued that pleasant surroundings detract from the attention that should be given to work—as if a person ever worked the worse for being clean and warm, and having plenty of air and light!

"There is yet another reason for concessions to the mill hands, and it is based on the present public interest in all schemes of betterment. The destruction of city slums, the increase of kindergartens, the establishment of free lectures, the appearance of the university settlement and of such institutions as Hull House, in Chicago, the substitution in reformatory cases of the interminate sentence for fixed terms of imprisonment, the legislation that enforces safety in mines and sweatshops, are tokens of the widening of a Christian spirit, and the improvement of factories is but in line with these reforms."—CHARLES M. SKINNER, in the *Saturday Evening Post.*

HYGIENE AND SANITARY SCIENCE.

COMMENTING on the address of Dr. Geo. M. Kober on "The Problem and Tendency of Hygiene, and Sanitary Science in the Nineteenth Century," the *Philadelphia Medical Journal* has this to say:

"In view of the fact, as Dr. Kober has pointed out, that hygiene is not an independent science, but a correlation of the teachings of physiology, chemistry, physics, meteorology, pathology, sociology, epidemiology and bacteriology, it is not surprising that the progress of this branch has been phenomenal. To emphasize that this science is not of modern origin, he alludes to the hygiene of the Greeks and Romans—the care they paid to their water supplies and

bathing facilities, and the special attention paid to the physical culture of their youth.

The greater portion of his address is confined to the discussion of the progress of sanitation in the United States, referring to the duties of health boards, quarantine regulations, the results derived from improved water supplies, the value of pure food and drug legislation, industrial, rural, and school hygiene, and the management and control of infectious diseases. The enactment of proper sanitary legislation, and the education of the public in regard to the nature and causation of infectious diseases, will be important advances in the solution of the problem of prevention. In this connection of special interest is the statement that enteric fever, a so-called preventable disease, causes an annual loss in the United States of $185,000,000. Dr. Evans has estimated that the annual loss sustained from tuberculosis in the United States is $574,-000,000. However, the mortality statistics of 1890 and 1900 show a marked decrease in the death rate from typhoid fever and consumption, and the American medical profession has much to be proud of in the century's progress in preventive medicine.

In this important contribution to medical literature we cannot fail to be struck with the development of modern hygiene, especially when we reflect upon the ignorance and superstition that prevailed in former times. With the ever-increasing means of observation and the more intimate co-operation of the profession throughout the civilized world, further progress and perfection in hygiene are to be expected with confidence."

A CHEAP, HOMEMADE FILTER.

A VERY good filter can be made out of a common earthenware flowerpot. To make it, proceed as follows: Get a new flower pot with a hole in the bottom; line it with a piece of new cotton flannel; put into the bottom of this, to the depth of two inches, some clean sand; over this put a layer of pounded charcoal, and fill up with fine gravel. This domestic filter will answer the purpose of the most elaborate, and it is very easily made. After several weeks' use it should be renewed. —[Better than none, but not germ-proof.—Ed. GAZETTE.]

FORESTRY AND ITS RELATION TO HEALTH.

FROM *American Medicine* we reproduce the following sensible remarks on this important topic:

"Until quite recently few people have given much thought to the rapid destruction of our magnificent North American forests. The necessity for limiting this destruction from the purely economic standpoint has been recognized only within the past ten years, and since the act of March 3, 1891, the President has been given power to segregate forest reservations from the public lands. Professor J. W. Toumey (*Popular Science Monthly*, June, 1901), in discussing the subject of our forest reservations states that no less than thirty-nine national forest reservations have been established, containing in the aggregate more than 46,800,000 acres, an area more than fifteen times as large as the State of Connecticut, and about one-fortieth of the total area of the country exclusive of Alaska. As the legislative act provides that the reservations are to be taken from public lands, they are for the most part in the Rocky Mountain region and in the Pacific Coast States, where large areas of public forests and land are available. Much controversy has arisen as to the wisdom of withdrawing such large areas from sale or other disposition under the laws of the land office. This opposition has become less during the past few years and public sentiment in favor of forest reservations is rapidly increasing. In fact, this change in sentiment has been so rapid that a movement is now on foot, with the prospect of success, to establish a national forest reservation in the Southern Appalachian Mountains, where it will be necessary for the government to purchase the land at an expense of several millions of dollars. A few State reservations have been established, the most splendid example being the State forests in the Adirondacks of New York. Similar reservations have been established in Pennsylvania and it is likely that others will be set aside in Michigan during the present year. Unfortunately, the lumber interests in Northern Minnesota are likely to prevent the establishment of a national reservation at the head of the Mississippi River.

Professor Toumey considers the importance of forests more from the standpoint of value in producing lumber and in maintaining the water-supply of the country. However, there is another side to the question which is quite as important and which should not be overlooked. The value of forest reservations as great national parks for recreation and sport is very great. In such reservations those so inclined can get in touch with Nature at her best, where the streams abound in trout, where wild animals are not confined behind iron bars and where there are no signs "Keep off the grass." There a man can reinforce his physical strength with wholesome mountain air, pure water, vigorous exercise, and plain food. It is a pity that the present state of development of our country makes such reservations impossible in the vicinity of most of our large cities. The park systems are of great importance as breathing places for the poorer people, but most of the real forest is too far distant to offer possible aid in gaining health for the masses. In certain foreign countries, notably Germany, there are forests of considerable size within a short distance of some of the largest cities and these are constantly frequented by picnicking parties from the poorer classes during the summer season. Even now the reservation of such areas of land would not be impossible in the neighborhood of some of our large American cities, and they would prove a good investment if the health, comfort and pleasure of the masses were considered.

Department of Physical Education.

WITH SPECIAL REGARD TO SYMMETRICAL DEVELOPMENT OF THE BODY.

GYMNASTIC TRAINING IN THE NEW JERSEY STATE NORMAL COLLEGE.

BY H. B. BOICE, M.D.,

Trenton.

IN the February number of the GAZETTE there was a somewhat extended notice of the starting of a department of physical training in the Institution of Technology, of Boston, to take equal rank with other departments in that institution, and recently in the daily press there appeared an article on the same line of work as conducted at Brown University.

It is cause for congratulation that physical training, the building of a firm foundation for mental training, is being more and more accepted as a *sine qua non* in general education by our higher institutions of learning, but it is also a cause of surprise as well as of regret that the work in that line of the normal schools throughout the country, from far-away Texas to Maine, is passed over without notice.

Yet there are, and have been for years, normal schools where a course in physical training is part of the regular curriculum, which must be passed satisfactorily in order to obtain a license to teach in the public schools of the State, the point being thoroughly understood by the directors of these institutions that to obtain the best results in physical training it is necessary, as our German friends have always urged, to begin with the child.

To reach the children of our public schools the teachers should know the *why* and the *how;* they needs must have a knowl-edge of hygiene as well as of physical exercises, the objects to be obtained and the method of obtaining them.

As an illustration of what has been said, and in the hope that it may be of interest to the readers of the GAZETTE who have at heart the education of the child, the course is given as pursued at the State Normal School at Trenton, N. J.

As a preliminary, the following excerpts from the principal's annual report will give an idea as to what is required from the standpoint of physical education:

"Applicants must be at least sixteen years of age. They must be in good health and able to sustain a good examination in physiology and hygiene.

"The work in the Normal is professional, so far as the qualifications of the pupil will permit. . . . In physical training the basis is special work and instruction in hygiene for the individual, depending on the student's physical history and on such a physical examination as is necessary to prescribe for individual needs. (See note.) In general, the work is hygienic, educative and technical.

"The primary object is, by regular general exercises, to promote, as far as may be, the student's own health, that mental power may be at the maximum.

"The exercises are, secondly, of a nature to improve the carriage and physique, and to make the 'body the servant of the will.' The agents relied upon are school tactics, exercises including free hand work (including the Swedish exercises) with light apparatus and chest weights.

"Finally, the intention is to give the student a certain amount of drill in exercises which can be used in schools where appliances are not at hand, the bearing of these exercises upon the health, physique and bodily control being brought out during the course in Theory of Physical Training."

A post-graduate, or fourth year course, includes physical training in the list of subjects pursued.

The following is an outline, in brief, of the course in the *theory* of physical training, which seems best adapted to the requirements of this institution:

I.—THE SKELETON AND MUSCLES.

The necessity of considering them together.

A—Muscles.

1. Function.

2. Arrangement.

3. Elasticity, as affecting relative position of bones, as in spine, shoulder-blades and chest, etc.

4. Changes in muscle due to work.

B—Skeleton.

1. Spine.

(*a*) Correct position of body; its bearing on physiological curves and abnormalities of the same.

(*b*) Spinal curvature; recognition, frequency, desirability of early recognition and correction.

(*c*) The spine as the foundation of all body building. Straight back and strength of back, frequent assumption of correct standing position; free exercises for, etc.

2. Boxes of the skeleton.

(*a*) Skull and pelvis; shape, strength, attached muscles.

(*b*) Thorax; arrangement of bony wall; deformities, depressed ribs and sternum, flat chest, etc.

(*c*) Action of attached muscles in movement of ribs in breathing, with importance of large mobile thorax in relation to contents, and hence to general health and vigor.

Effect on thoracic wall of action of attached muscles in various defined exercises.

3. Limbs.

(*a*) Shoulder blades; correct position on thorax; "round shoulders," uneven shoulders, bottle neck; causes, effects and exercises for correction.

(*b*) Lower limbs; curvature of leg bones, breaking down of arch of instep; causes and exercises when applicable.

II.—NERVOUS SYSTEM.

A—Inter-relation of nervous and muscular systems.

B—General effect of muscular exercise on nervous system.

C—Special effect of various forms of exercise; defining and illustrating the strict meaning of muscular training.

III.—CIRCULATORY SYSTEM.

A—Forces of the circulation.

1. Heart; brief anatomy, work of, dangers of overstraining, desirability of strong heart; exercises.

2. Suction action of movements of thorax. Mechanism of breathing. Importance of diaphragm, and necessity of freedom of action. Light clothing.

3. Muscular action, general and local, on circulation of blood and lymph.

B—Purification of the blood.

1. Lungs.

(*a*) Brief anatomy, function.

(*b*) Effect of muscular exertion on breathing.

(*c*) Bearing of lung capacity and rib mobility on expression of energy, either physical or mental.

(*d*) Deterioration of atmosphere by lights, stoves and human beings.

(*e*) Exercises.

2. Other excretory organs. (See skin.)

IV.—SKIN.

A—Effect of general exercise.

B—Baths and bathing.

C—*Clothing.*
1. Color.
2. Material.

V.—DIGESTION.

A—*Foods.*
B—*Tight and heavy clothing around waist.*
C—(1) *General exercise; effect.* (2) *Special exercises.*

VI.—GAMES AND GYMNASTICS.

Discussion based on the preceding points, as to relative value from physical, mental and moral standpoint.

VII.—SCHOOL HYGIENE.

Ventilation; heat, light, situation of pupil in room (sight and hearing); height of seats and desks; deformities incident to school life.

VIII.—THE PHYSIQUE.

1. Common defects.
2. Harmony of parts.
3. Relation of function to beauty of physique.

In considering the course here presented it should be borne in mind that the pressure of subjects which seem to be essential in the training of a teacher is ever on the increase, and that the time given to any one is necessarily limited. It may be criticized, perhaps, as to its depth and breadth, but, to twist Mercutio's meaning somewhat, " 'Tis not so deep as a well, nor so wide as a church door, but . . . 'twill serve."

The department of physical training is housed in a building which includes a gymnasium having a clear floor space of 45 feet by 90 feet, 26 feet to the ceiling, a running track, and fitted with German apparatus after the American method, offices for the director and assistant, locker rooms and shower baths, and in the basement a pair of bowling alleys.

MINISTER WU ON DRESS REFORM.

AN amusing as well as suggestive interview between a reporter and Wu Ting Fang, Chinese minister to the United States, was published some time ago in the Washington *Times,* from which paper we quote:

"It is but fair to say that Minister Wu did not express uninvited, his opinion on this somewhat delicate subject. He was asked to do so. The way in which he did it was characteristic.

"Instead of allowing himself to be questioned, he turned the tables and catechized the interviewer. Before he told what he thought of the evening dress of American ladies, he addressed a small volley of questions to the reporter. He said:—

" 'Will you tell me the reason for the American ladies dressing this way? What is the history of the evening dress? Where did it originate? Who first introduced this style? Is the evening dress worn for beauty of effect, for coolness, for convenience, or from a sense of feminine modesty?'

"The reporter's breath was almost taken away, and he was also somewhat nonplussed. He finally suggested that the reason for the present style of dress probably was that it was considered becoming. Minister Wu responded with the tactful remark, that in all matters of taste, of course, one must follow the custom of the country. Then he came out with another conundrum:

" 'But the long skirt that trails along the street—what is your reason for that?'

"The interviewer suggested modesty as a possible reason for the long street skirt— it was all the explanation he could think of. It did not satisfy Minister Wu. He protested:—

" 'But it drags in the dirt . It is so inconvenient. I never see a lady walking on the street that she does not have to use one hand to hold up her skirt. Would you consider it immodest for ladies to wear garments that would not drag in the dirt?'

"That was too much for the reporter, and in self-defense he asked the Chinese minister if he could suggest any improvement for the evening dress and the long skirt. His answer was an epigram:

" 'Use less cloth at the bottom and more at the top of the dress!'

"Then he went on:

" 'I have often wondered at the reason for the American custom. Your people, who are progressive in everything, have, I believe, started a dress reform. What has become of it? The way you accomplish things here is by calling together a great convention and deciding what is to be done. Why do you not call a great convention, and have your experts decide wnat is the best thing in dress for women, and for men as well? Surely there are improvements which could be made, even in American dress.

" 'For instance, if the corset is harmful, if it cramps the body and impedes the free circulation of the blood, it could be loosened. To me a woman is beautiful when she dresses to her natural figure. If she is fat, let her dress becomingly and naturally for a fat woman, and not try to appear thin. If she is thin there is no use of her putting on more than Nature has given her, in order that she may appear well rounded. She is pretty when her natural self, if she is pretty at all.'

"The spectacle of a Chinese gentleman lecturing the wide-awake and progressive American on common sense, propriety, and the laws of beauty and hygiene, appeals to one's sense of humor, especially as his remarks are so very wise and truthful. It suggests that America did not do everything that could be done in the cause of progress when it evolved a Constitution, and a Declaration of Independence, and a World's Fair. There is still room for improvement in some of our fundamental ideas and customs.

"The subject of dress reform has been agitated, off and on for many years. The view which the Chinese Minister takes of the European style of dress for woman is the only sensible one possible. The spectacle of a richly dressed lady trailing along the streets a gown at least a foot longer than it ought to be, gathering in course of her progress all the filth of the pavement and crossings, to be afterward shed on the carpet of her house, is absolutely ridiculous. Sometimes the long skirt is not only absurd, but an actual source of danger. The average woman, if she is obliged to walk any distance in bad weather, finds herself at the end of the walk with her skirts wet all around the bottom, and she is often obliged to sit for hours with them in this condition. There is no earthly reason for this state of things. The only sensible style of skirt for walking is one short enough to need no holding up."

MEASURE OF SENSIBILITY TO PAIN.

A CHICAGO correspondent says the "temporal algometer" is to be tried on public school children there. It was invented by Arthur McDowell, of Washington, D. C., psychologist of the United States Bureau of Education. It is designed to test pupils' sensibility to pain. By this device pressure is applied to a child's temples, and gradually increased until the child cries out from the pain. The quicker the cry comes the greater the child's sensibility, and, by the theory, the greater its cleverness. The storm of opposition is rising. A "temporal algometer" has been offered to the Board of Education. Every suggestion of cruelty is said to have been removed from the test. One of the objects of making the test is to establish the relation between the keenness of the senses and the intellect. It is shown that the more sensitive children are to pain the brighter pupils they make. This is explained by the fact that knowledge is obtained through the senses, and the keener the senses the better opportunity for knowledge. The pain test is not entirely new. It has been tried with adults, and several interesting theories have been formed. It was shown by tests that washerwomen are less sensitive to pain than women clerks in stores.—*The Sanitarian.*

THE HYGIENIC TREATMENT OF SUMMER DIARRHEA OF INFANTS.

By Henry C. Hazen, M.D.,

WE lay before our readers a condensation of this seasonable paper from the *Medical News:*

Summer diarrhea has been proved to be of bacterial origin, and it is through the agency of these bacteria and their products, toxins, the growth of which is favored by improper food supply, impure air, and insanitary environments, that so many little ones succumb to it. But, first we must appreciate the fact that many children are rendered susceptible to an acute attack of enteritis by a pre-existing condition of indigestion or of intestinal catarrh. The stools should be examined, and, if necessary, the food modified as indicated. The child should not be given an execssive proportion of fats or proteids, nor should it be fed too often or too abundantly. This latter condition commonly occurs through the anxiety of the mother that the child should thrive. The first indication of rachitis should be noted. In other words, as warm weather approaches, special care should be given to the feeding of the child; thus we may avoid predisposing causes, and should the child be attacked by the disease, the prognosis will naturally be better.

In regard to the food supply, if the child is nursing, and digestion is impaired, the mother's health may demand attention. If the child is bottle-fed, the milk supply should be of the best quality possible. The control and regulation of the sale of milk by the Board of Health has saved many thousands of infants' lives, by giving a fresher and a better milk. Nevertheless, the distant source of the milk supply and the resulting delay in forwarding it necessitate an elapse of from twelve to twenty-four hours before the consumers receive it. With milk at this age, the danger of lactic acid, the multiplication of bacteria, and other fermentative changes may be considerably lessened if the mothers are shown—I mean shown by actual demonstration—how to sterilize it and how to keep it sterile.

The purchase of bottled milk rather than of milk kept in bulk in grocery stores is most desirable, and I never fail to insist upon this among the poorer families, where it is the rule rather than the exception to patronize the corner grocery.

The food should be given at regular intervals. It is well for the child to be allowed to drink frequently of cool water that has been boiled. Often a child cries when it is thirsty, and the mother, believing it to be hungry, gives it food and thus overfeeds it. If the child does not vomit the surplus food, it may collect in the intestines, cause irritation, and produce the diarrhea.

The potency of unhygienic conditions as a joint factor in producing this summer diarrhea, is also entitled to our careful consideration in the treatment of each patient. Many suggestions can be made as to the sanitary environments, which will contribute to the welfare of the child. The room should be selected so that at some period during the day it is exposed to the beneficent effects of the sun, and we must see that it is kept perfectly clean and well aired, and its furnishings as well.

Only those who are in attendance on the child should be permitted to remain in the room. Often in visiting among the poorer classes, we will find the sick room filled with neighbors and friends, and it will be close and foul smelling from the overcrowding. Absolute quet is essential. We know how often a loud or startling noise will cause a convulsion in a weakened child.

All garbage and refuse should be immediately disposed of, and it should not be allowed to collect in heaps out-of-doors, where it so readily decomposes in hot weather. The effluvia from this alone not infrequently causes diarrhea in young children. Should we notice noxious odors for which we can not account, we should have the plumbing inspected and active search instituted.

The little patient should be placed on a comfortable mattress— not, as often seen, on a hot pillow in its carriage. The clothing should consist only of a light, *white*, loosely woven woolen [we prefer linen.—Ed. GAZETTE] shirt, a loose, light robe and diaper. Socks are not advisable. The lower extremities and feet, in severe cases, may demand artificial heat. The napkins must be immediately changed when soiled, and washed, boiled, and thoroughly dried before used again. All superfluous clothing must be removed from the vicinity of the child. The sheets and bed coverings should be changed and aired frequently.

I believe that the use of water internally and externally is far too often neglected. A bath by tub or sponge, with use of a good soap, given daily, is essential not for cleanliness alone, but to aid diaphoresis. Bathing, by sponge, at intervals during the day, refreshes the child and may supply to a slight degree the great loss of water caused by the evacuations.

The facilities that New York and some other cities offer for various long and short trips upon the water afford great assistance to the physician in his treatment. Many cases that have seemed desperate have recovered by removal from the city by water. The daily excursions of St. John's Guild have saved and prolonged many lives. The recreation piers recently built by the city offer advantages that are not to be neglected. We should also utilize the many parks, where the child may be carried for a portion of the day, and given a substitute, though perhaps a poor one, for the country.

CLINICAL EXPERIENCE WITH ADRENALIN.*

By Emil Mayer, M.D.,

Surgeon, New York Eye and Ear Infirmary,Throat Department, Fellow, American Laryngological Association and of the New York Academy of Medicine, New York.

The aqueous extract of suprarenal gland is, perhaps, the best culture medium known.

* Abstract from original paper, in the *Philadelphia Medical Journal*, April 21, 1901.

Its instability, the involved method of preparation, its unsightliness, and the inexactitude of its various strengths tend to make us welcome a preparation that is exact, stable, and, above all, clean. Dr. Jokichi Takamine undertook the task of isolating the active principle of the suprarenal gland. He obtained a substance in stable and pure crystalline form, which raises the blood pressure, and which he named "Adrenalin."

The author has used solutions of Adrenalin chloride, 1 to 1,000, 1 to 5,000, and 1 to 10,000: his cases were all rhinological. Blanching of tissues followed the application of the strongest of these solutions in a few seconds, and was very thorough. In no instance was there any constitutional disturbance. He has employed no suprarenal extract since, for any purpose whatever.

The effect of the solutions was not altered by their change to a pink color; they were used for six weeks. Subsequently a small amount of chloretone was added to the fresh solutions and now there is but slight change of color and no floccules appear.

Thirty-five cases are reported in tabulated form, showing that the usual effect of the aqueous extract of the suprarenal gland was obtained. A few operative cases bled freely, but in every instance the hemorrhage was promptly checked by a second application of Adrenalin. The Adrenalin was used not only as a hemostatic, but for the relief of nasal congestion, as a diagnostic aid, and for the continuous treatment of acute inflammatory affections of the accessory sinus.

The author arrives at the following conclusions: 1. Adrenalin solutions supply every indication for which the aqueous extract has been used.

2. They are sterile.

3. They keep indefinitely.

4. Solutions 1:1,000 are strong enough for operative work; and 1:5,000 and 1:10,000 for local medication.

5. They may be used with safety.

In this connection it is interesting to note that E. Fletcher Ingals, M.D., of Chicago, also has had a very satisfactory experience with Adrenalin. In a paper entitled "Notes on Adrenalin and Adrenalin Chloride,"* he reports that he experimented with solutions, varying from 1 to 1,000 to 1 to 10,000, of the chloride of Adrenalin in distilled water or normal salt solution, and kept careful records until satisfied of its activity. In nine cases a very small quantity of a spray, of one part of chloride of Adrenalin to 10,000 parts of water was applied to the nasal cavities, with the effect of blanching the mucous membrane quickly, and in most cases causing contraction of the swollen tissues similar to that caused by cocaine. The first solution used was made with distilled water and caused smarting; normal salt solution was then used as a solvent with perfect satisfaction. The smarting may have been due to the presence of a small quantity of formalin in which the atomizer had been washed just before use.

Experiments were also made with insufflations of a dry powder consisting of 1.5 per cent. (75 parts) each of biborate of sodium and bicarbonate of sodium; 3 per cent. (150 parts) light carbonate of magnesium; one part of Adrenalin, to 5,000 parts sugar of milk. This powder cleared the nasal cavities when obstructed by swelling of the turbinated bodies, and diminished the secretions decidedly. A case of daily epistaxis was relieved by sprays of a 1 to 10,000 solution. Another of conjunctival congestion from overwork was entirely relieved by the instillation of a similar solution. The author has had equally satisfactory results in cases of conjunctivitis; laryngitis, acute and chronic; acute laryngitis with edema glottidis; acute coryza; chronic laryngo-tracheitis with acute exacerbation; and in preparation for operations upon the nose.

In conclusion the following results are presented: This remedy will be of great value in the treatment of acute inflammatory affections of the nasal cavities, either in sprays of 1 to 5,000, or in powders of 1 to 5,000 or 1 to 2,500, sugar of milk. In acute coryza and in hay fever, in epistaxis from various causes, in acute inflammation of the fauces,

solutions of 1 to 1,000 will have good effects. In acute or subacute laryngitis, solutions of 1 to 1,000, applied with moderate force, will give very great relief. It appears probable that vocalists may obtain sufficient relief from congested cords, for at least two or three hours, to obtain normal efficiency in the use of the voice.

In a paper read before the Chicago Laryngological and Climatological Association, W. E. Casselberry, M.D., called attention to the fact that Adrenalin chloride solution is clear, colorless, odorless, sterile, and stable, if protected from heat, light and oxidation. It is non-irritating to mucous membranes. When applied locally it exerts identically the same vaso-constrictor influence as the aqueous adrenal extract. Sprayed into the nostrils in the strength of 1 to 10,000 it produces a visible change from turgidity to compactness of the turbinated tissues, and a decided pallor of the mucous surfaces. In the strength of 1 to 1,000, or even 1 to 5,000, it has the power to limit hemorrhage during operations and is an aid in the treatment of epistaxis. It may be substituted for cocaine in all cases in which an ischemic effect is desired, e.g., to facilitate inspection of the deeper recesses of the nasal cavities and to make them more accessible. Adrenalin has little or no cerebral stimulant effect, exciting no desire for more of the drug; hence there is little risk of habit-formation.

The author expresses the opinion that Adrenalin should afford relief in asthma associated with bronchitis and vaso-motor paralysis, although he would expect little benefit from its use in asthma characterized by bronchial spasm. It may be formed into an ointment with vaseline, or mixed with stearate of zinc, powdered starch, or sugar of milk to make powders for nasal or laryngeal insufflation. The bibliography is very comprehensive, covering the literature of the subject down to the present date.

* Journal of the American Medical Association, April 27, 1901.

FEEDING ACCORDING TO CLIMATE.

In the May number of the GAZETTE we quoted the essential points of a paper on "Meat Ration in the Tropics," by Dr. Egan of the U. S. Army, and ventured to criticise the conclusions of the author.

We are glad to find our strictures amply corroborated in an address by Major L. L. Seaman, late Surgeon First U. S. Volunteer Engineers, made before the annual meeting of military surgeons of the United States.

Dr. Seaman adds to his own conclusions a letter on the same subject, written by the U. S. Consul at Formosa, James W. Davidson, F.R.C.S.

We append the two reports. Dr. Seaman says:

"If any vindication were necessary for the theory for regulating the ration of an army to suit climatic conditions, unanswerable proof can be found in Peking in the study of the statistics of every company serving in the Chinese Expedition. At my earnest solicitation, Captain Anderson, commanding Company A, Ninth U. S. Infantry, obtained the following figures for me. His command, now numbering eighty-five, came from Manila to China with the first American troops landing at Taku last June. At that time, twenty-nine (or 33 per cent.) of the men were suffering from chronic diarrhea contracted in the Philippines. On their arrival in China the combined weight of the company was 12,304 pounds. (I have the individual figures.) On February 15, 1901, these same men weighed 13,284, or an average gain of about thirteen and one-half pounds. There was not a case of so-called 'digestive disease' in the company, nor a man in the hospital. On the contrary, to illustrate the state of the men's digestive ability, the captain adds:

"'During the month of January, 1901, the following extra commissary supplies were used by my company 3 bbls. (78 gals.) pickles, 240 cans cream, 240 lbs. oatmeal, 75 lbs. maccaroni, 60 lbs. cheese, 75 lbs. onions, 12 lbs. baking powder, 2 gals. syrup, 117 rations of bread, 127 lbs. beef. Total cost of extras $93.30, and paid from the company fund.'

"The reason for this remarkable difference lies in the changed climatic conditions, the extreme winter temperature of Pekin being fully 100° F. lower than that of Manila; in Pekin this rich ration was requisite for the proper nourishment of the system.

"As further bearing upon this point, let me submit the testimony of a witness, our American Consul at Formosa, whose opportunities for personal observation on this most important subject have rarely if ever ben surpassed. His letter is better reading than medical statistics.

"The letter from Consul Davidson is in substance as follows:

"I have perused your very interesting pamphlet on the Army Ration, and the following personal observations may be of some interest to you. As you are aware, I have had rather an unusual opportunity of confirming your statements on the subject of diet. The years 1893 and 1894, as a member of the Peary Arctic Expedition, I spent in North Greenland, within the Arctic Circle. On returning from this trip I departed almost immediately for Formosa, which is within the tropics, and called the most deadly climate in Asia, and the last six years have been spent in this island.

"In North Greenland our supplies were naturally limited to most portable foods; delicacies were left at home and we did not always have as much in quantity as we wished. It is not strange, therefore, that we, as young men, sometimes turned from our dry pemmican and biscuits to discuss the probable joys, from a culinary standpoint, awaiting us on our return to the States. You will doubtless surmise that oyster stews, roast turkeys, or pies 'like mother used to make' were the subject of our discussion. These we could give warm welcome, still they were far from that glorious dish for which we all yearned and, I might say, almost prayed—it was nothing more than a *side of bacon.* Not the streaky article marked 'prime,' but the kind that is practically solid fat, and which the butcher in the temperate zone usually throws in the lard pot. We wished no side dishes, and even the cooking did not worry us much; in fact, I believe we would have preferred it merely warmed. On an occasional trip to the southern headquarters we were sometimes the recipients of a thin slice or so, dealt out from our slender stock. And how good it was! There was nothing that could approach it. On one occasion I was fortunate—at least I looked upon it in that light, then—to obtain out of meal hours from the cook the outer skin, or end piece, of a side of bacon. I immediately sought the seclusion of my room, warmed it slightly over the flame of my candle, and then ate it with all the pleasure that a young boy obtains from his favorite confectionery.

"Before our return from Greenland I arranged with my roommate that, on our arrival at St. Johns, the first port on our downward journey we should go together to the leading grocery, which we had visited on our upward journey, and purchase a side of bacon. This we would take quietly to the hotel, and for once have simply all the bacon we wished. Of course, on our actual arrival at St. Johns, the subject of bacon never entered our heads. We had entered the temperate zone, our systems ceased to call for fat, and we were prepared to give warm welcome to dishes of quite a different nature. This appetite for fat and fatty meats, so keen in the far North, is merely Nature's call for help in repelling the almost overpowering cold, and if it is answered there is but little fear of disease. There is probably not a healthier race on earth than the Eskimo of these regions, and our party suffered not the slightest indisposition while there. Yet the same diet in the tropics would be absolutely fatal.

"In tropical Formosa, the idea of fat bacon was as repulsive as it was entrancing in the North. There did I think of home delicacies; it was the splendid fruits, the strawberries, the luscious peaches that in-terested me. Nature had given me new tastes, new fancies, an appetite for something that would induce energy, without heat. If we were wise and obeyed her, and left aside intoxicants and heavy, fatty meats, we found our life a pleasant and not unhealthy one. And, although Formosa has the reputation of being the unhealthiest spot in Asia, I am convinced from my own experience of six years that one who is careful in one's diet, selecting only the foods which will tend to assist Nature rather than oppose it, will find life quite as healthy in Formosa as they will out of it, assuming, of course, that they live in suitable quarters raised above the ground, and protect themselves against the midday sun when in the open.

"In 1892, on my departure for Greenland, I weighed 148 pounds; after six weeks of Arctic life, on a suitable diet, my weight increased to 190 pounds. During several months' confinement with a frozen foot I lost heavily, and on my arrival in Formosa in 1894, weighed 155 pounds. After a six years' stay in the island, during which I had not had a single sick day, I am now returning to my home land weighing 194 pounds. The practical diet for a tropical country should, as you suggest, be light meats, chicken, fish, fruits, sugar, tea and rice, which are to be found there in abundance. This is what I lived upon. During the two years I was attached to the Imperial Japanese Army, in its campaign against the Chinese rebels in the island, I suffered as severe physical hardships as the average soldier finds in any military campaign in the tropics. By carefully obeying the dictates of Nature in the selection of foods, I have not—either in Greenland or Formosa—suffered *a single day from sickness.*"

A good physician must not only be a true and exact observer of Nature, but also a deep student of mankind and self-sacrificing friend of his fellowmen.—*Herman Eichhorst* (Zurich).

Brevity Club.

PITH AND POINT.

THE FIGHT FOR LIFE.

PRACTICALLY we are all fighting for Life, Liberty, and the Pursuit of Happiness. We adopt divers methods of warfare and use an endless variety of weapons. Nobody is exempt from military service, desertion is out of the question, and neither potentate nor millionaire has ever been able to decree or purchase an armistice. The battle is to the death.

We choose weapons according to individual whim, or rely on those handed down by tradition. Most of us fight strictly on the defensive, and our weapons vary all the way from peppermint, paregoric, and patent medicines, to ice-trusts, tennis, and the Turkish bath; from blood bitters to bicycles, faith cure and the phosphites, and some of us have a leaning toward myths, miracles, and madstones. Latterly we have been banking rather heavily on antiseptics, antitoxins, and horse serums. When our superannuated equines lose all their pull, instead of being pensioned with green pastures and a peaceful old age they are turned over to the sanatory laboratories, where they heroically shed the last drop of their toxintainted blood in behalf of diphtheritic babes and the victims of the tetanus-bacilli.

The rules of warfare are as variable as the weapons employed. There are no statutes against gullibility, and only those who ostentatiously throw away all their weapons are held amenable to the law.

We average to surrender at thirty-five, whereas we ought to live to a hundred.

The heated season is again upon us, and with every upward hitch of the mercury the battle waxes fiercer and the death rate increases.

Most of us fight blindly. Every professional pretender has a system of tactics of his own and practises a manual of arms chiefly inherited, but partly devised within his own empirical and prejudiced consciousness.

There is no doubt but that we know much better than we practise, and hence need to be frequently reminded of the simplest first principles. Hence the pertinency of a few seasonable

HEALTH HINTS.

Eat less.

If this precaution were universally observed it would overcome a multitude of other dietetic sins.

Drink less at meals and more between meals; sparingly of iced drinks. Avoid all stimulants, and drink no water of questionable quality.

There are the effective and inexpensive water stills in the market, and there are safe and effective filters; but fake filters are plentiful and immeasurably worse than none.

Tea is a mocker and strong coffee is raging.

In the end they are both sappers and miners. This isn't fashionable, but it is a fact. They are slow, but they are sure.

The best hot weather foods are cereals, fresh vegetables, ripe fruits, eggs, and milk. For variety, nuts, fresh fish (extremely fresh), and now and then for relish a slice or two of canned bacon, nicely broiled. (Armour's is exceptionally fine. Other brands may be equally good.) Avoid salted fish, cheese, fine crackers, and all other constipating foods.

Bathe more.

Keep the emunctories one and all free, open and active. It is in hot weather that the ptomains and toxins are so rapidly engendered. Keep them washed out. When you take your weekly Turkish omit the "alcohol rub," but have the attendant treat you to an inunction of an ounce or two of olive-cottonseed oil or white vaseline. If he (or she) rubs it in long enough there will be little of it outside to be wiped off before dressing.

Wear porous clothing, linen open-mesh underwear, if you can afford it. Change and air it as often as possible when perspiring freely.

Let narcotics alone.

The cigar is a slow fuse, but in time it explodes the best heart that ever beat.

Take needed, but not excessive, exercise in the open air.

Don't rush!

The next train will carry you at the same price, and may be a great deal safer than the one you will lose by not hurrying.

Keep your temper well in hand.

This will make ten degrees difference in the temperature.

Finally, the water-still and the filter cost a little care and cash; but it is better to pay ten dollars for one of these preventives than risk typhoid, pay the doctor a hundred, or the undertaker twice as much!

A REMINISCENCE OF ARTEMUS WARD.

THERE has never been another just like him. His humor was unique and irresistible. But his amiability and what the French call "camaraderie" hurried him out of the world. He never could say "No" to the boys, and whenever he lectured, whether in New York, New England, California, or London, there was sure to be a knot of young fellows to gather round him, go home with him to his hotel, order supper, and spend the balance of the night in telling stories. feasting, and having a "good time." They toasted him early and late, compelled him to keep them in a roar over their wine, and to join them in singing humorous or sentimental songs. This kind of life will kill any man, in time, even the most robust, whereas Ward, whose real name, as many readers will recall, was Charles F. Browne, was quite delicate. He was not like Poe and some other erratic geniuses who might be mentioned, a heavy drinker. In fact, he had no strong appetites or bad habits; but to yield to his "friends," the thoughtless and rollicking convivials, deny himself of needed rest after an exhaustive evening's entertainment, catch only a wink of sleep before he must hurry to the train, in order to keep his next engagement—this was what sent him to his grave at thirty-three. He died of consumption, in Southampton, in 1867, forty years too soon, his unnecessarily premature death a loss to the world in general and to the world of philosophic and wholesome humor in particular.

Among his works, of which the present generation knows little, were: "Artemus Ward, His Book," (1862); Artemus Ward, His Travels Among the Mormons," "On the Rampage," "Artemus Ward, His Book of Goaks," and Artemus Ward Among the Fenians," (1865); "Artemus Ward in London," (1867), and contributions to *Punch*, 1866-7.

His lecture at the Egyptian Hall, London, with pictures from his panorama, was edited in 1869, by Robertson and Hotten.

Much of our present-day humor seems flat and superficial beside the "Goaks" of Ward, which never lacked pith, point, or pertinency.

SLEEP INDUCED THROUGH MUSCLE FATIGUE WITHOUT DRUGS.

BREATHE slowly, with deep, full, regular inspiration and expiration, and at the same time, while in the recumbent position, raise one foot slightly and hold it motionless until the muscles are weary; then the other foot. Extend one arm to its fullest extent, as though reaching for the footboard; then the other. Elongate the body to its fullest, as though trying to touch both headboard and footboard at once. Remove the pillow and raise the head slightly until the muscles are weary. Other similar muscular efforts will suggest themselves adapted to the recumbent position. With the tired feeling sleep will come.

Book Reviews.

A SYSTEM OF PHYSIOLOGIC THERAPEUTICS. A Practical Exposition of the Methods, Other than Drug-Giving, Useful in the Treatment of the Sick. Edited by Solomon Solis Cohen, A.M., M.D., Professor of Medicine and Therapeutics in the Philadelphia Polytechnic; Lecturer on Clinical Medicine at Jefferson Medical College, etc. Volume II., Electrotherapy, by George W. Jacoby, M.D., Consulting Neurologist to the German Hospital, New York City; to the Infirmary for Women and Children, etc. In two books: Book II., Diagnosis; Therapeutics. Illustrated. Published by P. Blakiston's Son & Co., 1012 Walnut street, Philadelphia, Pa. Price, eleven volumes, $22.00, net.

We noticed at length in these columns the initial volume of·this series. Volume II. is a continuation of Dr. Jacoby's work on Electrotherapy. It is made up of Part III., Electrophysiology and Electropathology; Part IV., Electrodiagnosis and Electroprognosis; Part V., Electrotherapeutics, and an Addendum of about a hundred pages, for which we can see no valid reason. It is quite as important as anything between the covers and should have been spared this apparent mark of disrespect. This Addenda includes The Surgical Uses of Electricity, by Dr. Da Costa; Electricity in Diseases of the Eye, by Dr. Jackson; The Applications of Electricity in Diseases of the Nose, Throat, and Ear, by Dr. Scheppegrell; Electricity in Gynecology, by Dr. Martin, and The Electric Therapeutics of Skin Diseases, by Dr. Ohmmann-Dumesnil.

It is sufficient to say that there has been no lapse from the high standard set up in the production of the first volume of the series. The paper and presswork are both superb.

How TO COOK FOR THE SICK AND CONVALESCENT. By Helena V. Sachse. Philadelphia, Pa.: J. B. Lippincott Co., 1901.

The Philadelphia Cooking School has turned out Miss (or Mrs.) Sachse and Miss (or Mrs.) Sachse has turned out materials for a clear cut, concise, and well-arranged volume under the above title.

Doctors are criminally careless when they prescribe a given diet for a patient, in that they have no notion as to how it will be cooked and served, and most of them, it must be confessed, are incompetent to give direction for its preparation, or to prepare it themselves.

This little work might, therefore, be conned by every practicing physician to the advantage of himself, and with unquestioned benefit to his patients.

The author wastes no words in circumlocution or theory, but drives straight at the thought in hand.

THE DISEASES OF THE RESPIRATORY ORGANS, ACUTE AND CHRONIC. By William F. Waugh, A.M., M.D. Chicago: The Clinic Publishing Co. 1901.

Dr. Waugh has a way of plunging directly into his subject, without any pause for preliminaries or flourish of exordium. We verily believe that if he were about to offer a prayer in church he would purposely forget to mention to whom it was addressed! This incisive directness is in such vivid contrast with the long-winded prefatories to which we are all accustomed, that it is decidedly refreshing. Why don't we stop dawdling and apologizing, and obey the semaphore that is always at right angles on the literary main line—"Go ahead!"

The general preface to this rather unique and decidedly practical little handbook is condensed into twenty lines, yet it says all that need be said. Conciseness and directness are the dominant characteristics of the body of the work.

For example, hay fever is disposed of in two pages; acute laryngeal catarrh in less space, and acute coryza in four—and they are small pages, set in type of easily readable size, at that.

Probably no reader of this volume will agree with its author in some opinions advanced with a good deal of emphasis and assurance; but if there is a practising physician in the country who can peruse it without gaining valuable aids in the treatment of his patients, we pity him for his obtuseness or his obstinacy!

In the light of personal experience and observation in a number of "climate" resorts, including the Adirondacks, Florida, Colorado, and California, we cannot fully agree with Dr. Waugh as to the imminent danger of infection in all these climatic resorts. The tubercle bacilli can not survive the dry, aseptic soil and atmosphere of New Mexico, Arizona, and Southern California. Some sections of Colorado, at least at certain seasons, are favored in the same way.

The volume is interleaved for notes, and can not fail to prove a valuable aid in the treatment of all respiratory diseases.

PROGRESSIVE MEDICINE. A Quarterly Digest of Advances, Discoveries, and Improvements in the Medical and Surgical Sciences. Edited by Hobart Amory Hare, M.D., Vol. II., June, 1901. Philadelphia: Lea Brothers & Co., 1901.

What we have said in general of the character and scope of this valuable work may be unhesitatingly repeated of this latest issue of the series. The topics treated in this volume comprise "Surgery of the Abdomen, Including Hernia," by William B. Coley, M.D.; "Gynecology," by John G. Clark, M.D.; "Diseases of the Blood and Ductless Glands"; "The Hemorrhagic Diseases," "Metabolic Diseases," by Alfred Stengel, M.D.; "Ophthalmology," by Edward Jackson, M.D.

The opening article on "The Radical Cure of Inguinal Hernia," is alone worth many times the cost of the volume; while the pages devoted to the "Surgery of the Intestines," "Surgery of the Stomach," and "Surgery of the Appendix" are scarcely less complete and comprehensive.

In connection with the subject of the Surgery of the Liver" some curious, if not even startling, statistics are given. In

1,150 autopsies Schroeder found that under 30 years of age gall stones are found in from 2 to 3 per cent. From 30 to 50 this percentage rises to over 11; and above 60 amounts to 25.3 per 100.

The illustrations, paper, presswork and binding are quite equal to that used in previous volumes, leaving nothing to be desired.

FACTS AND FIGURES, MEDICAL AND OTHERWISE, FROM THE CENSUS OF 1900, AND OTHER RELIABLE SOURCES.

UNDER this title our enterprising friends of the Arlington Chemical Company have issued a quite unique and instructive 12mo. volume of 64 pages. Of course, this firm always has an eye to business and couples an advertisement with each of its literary and scientific contributions; but even the advertising matter is so deftly and artistically put that it is not obnoxiously dominant, and the science, statistics, or other information imparted is always apt and acceptable.

A series of diminutive but well executed maps in colors gives the distribution of population by States, increase and decrease of population, 1890-1900, and Cuban and Puerto Rican populations. These are followed by a chart, also in colors, showing the rank of each State and Territory, at each census from 1790 to 1900. Then follow maps giving respectively the altitudes of the various States and Territories, average yearly rainfall, and percentage of normal sunshine. Another chart groups the elevation, average annual temperature and average annual rainfall of the principal health resorts of the country. In this chart are some palpable inaccuracies. Example, the average annual rainfall of Los Angeles is stated at five inches, whereas it is nearly thirteen. That of Santa Barbara is given at eighteen inches, which, if we are not mistaken, is too high, the two places being in the same general range and receiving about the same amount of precipitation.

A more instructive set of charts indicate

the number of deaths by specific infectious diseases in the ten principal cities of the country for the year ending June 3, 1900. Familiar as we all are with the fact, it is fairly startling to be reminded that *tuberculosis claims more victims than all the other infectious diseases combined.*

Of the ten cities named, San Francisco shows the greatest percentage of death from this fatal death scourge—1,049, against 229 from all other infectious diseases. St. Louis stands second, with 1,067 deaths from tuberculosis, as against 545 from all other infectious diseases. Then comes Baltimore, New York, Boston, Buffalo, Philadelphia, and Chicago, in the order named, each with a considerably greater percentage of deaths from tuberculosis than from all the other infectious diseases. In the two cities, Cleveland and Pittsburg, the fatalities from typhoid exceed those from tuberculosis. In Cleveland deaths from typhoid numbered 167, and those from diphtheria 80, as against 120 from tuberculosis. In Pittsburg, 457 from typhoid, 385 from tuberculosis and 114 from diphtheria. The combined statistics of these ten cities show as follows:

Deaths from tuberculosis, 18,763; from diphtheria, 5,117; from typhoid, 2,716; from measles, 1,709; scarlet fever, 1,456, and whooping cough, 1,273.

There are numerous other tables of statistics that every physician and professional man should always have at hand.

As the book can be had for the asking we will not quote further from its instructive collection of practical information.

Despite the presence of their advertising rider, the publishers of such valuable compilations deserve "honorable mention."

DR. JOSEPHINE. By Willis Barnes.

The same old story, ever new, of love and adventure. The heart is touched with memories which we, who have passed the meridian of life, would feign keep green. To the youths and maidens "Dr. Josephine" points the way to many charming love pictures. But more than this, "Dr. Josephine" tells the old yet ever new story of the brotherhood of man, by exploiting the economy of profit-sharing, showing how labor strikes may be avoided. "Dr. Josephine" is a book for the home, the capitalist and the laborer, each of whom will find in the reading of this story much to his liking. The author, Willis Barnes, of New York, is a charming writer, and knows what he is writing about.

Cloth, 12mo, daintily produced, $1.00. Will be sent on receipt of price by the DIETETIC AND HYGIENIC GAZETTE.

Editor's Table.

Lippincott's Magazine greets us with its usual store of interesting and instructive reading matter. Its contributors are sensible rather than sensational. It is always readable whether at home, at the seaside or among the everlasting hills.

Success has a taking name, but its history is not all in mere name. Every month we marvel at the scope and variety of practical and helpful matter served up by its enterprising publishers.

The Ladies' Home Journal maintains the high standard to which it has attained both as to character of contents and excellence of mechanical execution. Its illustrations, paper and press work are simply incomparable.

The Literary Digest occupies a field in American literature unoccupied by any other publication. If one could have no other magazine of art, science, music, theology or political economy, he need not grow rusty if he reads *The Literary Digest*.

A FOOLISH consistency is the hobgoblin of little minds, adored by little statesmen and philosophers and divines.—*Emerson.*

Notes and Queries.

Query 92. The medical journals mention cases of appendicitis occurring in very young children. Are there any well authenticated cases on record in which the diagnosis has been verified by an autopsy?   C. L. K., Pa.

Answer.—Yes. The *Archives of Pediatrics* for March, 1900, copies a report by Goyens, published in the *Gas. Méd. Belge*, Vol. 12, No. 14. The child was six weeks old, and the autopsy showed the existence of general peritonitis with perforating appendicitis. This condition supervened upon infectious gastro-enteritis, in a bottle-fed infant.

Other cases have been reported, but without the exact verification supplied in this case.

Query 93. It seems to be authoritatively settled that mosquitoes are the principal if not the only means of disseminating "malarial" fevers. (I quite agree with your strictures on the misuse of the word "malaria.") Stagnant pools and lack of drainage, it is now claimed; do not breed "malaria," except as they breed the diabolical kind of mosquitoes. I do not feel quite sure that the mosquito is the only source of intermittent fever; but it behooves every citizen living in a district that is subject to this disease to use every possible means to destroy this prolific source of infection. Will the editor suggest the most practical and inexpensive of the methods now recommended?
          C. E. N., New Jersey.

Answer.—Kerosene, fresh tar, anilin dyes, Dalmatian crysanthemum flowers and permanganate of potassium are all recommended. Kerosene is the easiest of application. It is to be floated over the surface of all the pools that can be reached, and the application should be repeated every four weeks during the season. Fresh tar is said to be equally effective and to last longer, since it does not evaporate so readily. Permanganate crystals are to be sprinkled in small quantities into the pools and over the wet places where the insect breeds. This chemical is not expensive in the quantities required.

As a matter of course, the radical cure of the evil lies in perfect drainage and the filling in of pools and low places as fast as this is feasible.

The best time to destroy mosquitoes is in winter and spring. This does not at first sight seem feasible, but it really is. The entomologists assure us that every female *anopheles* destroyed in the spring prevents the hatching of all the way from 200,000,000 to 20,000,000,000 larvæ.

This sounds rather Munchausenish, but the bug-sharps insist that figures will not lie, and refuse to cut off a single cipher.

Query 94. The question of how best to combat chills and fever will now be uppermost in all "malarial" districts, for months to come. I have grown tired of the prevailing method of giving large and repeated doses of quinin sulph. to my patients, but our best authorities do not seem to have discovered any better way. Some of the more susceptible patients find the quinin treatment almost as bad as the disease.

Warburg's Tincture is again coming in vogue, and thousands are doctoring themselves with it; but it is the rankest kind of a shotgun prescription, and even more demoralizing to human constitutions than the overuse of quinin alone. It certainly breaks up "chills" and it certainly undermines the blood of those who patronize it. They all have a washed-out look, and are always "tired."

Can you or any of your readers suggest a better treatment for uncomplicated intermittent fever?
          T. S. M., Conn.

Answer.—We sympathize with our correspondent. Large sections of our country are subject to annual outbreaks of chills and fever. There is, too, no doubt as to the almost universal prevalency of the peculiar type of fever caused by the plasmodium malariæ in connection with very many other diseases occurring in paludal districts. We also share our correspondent's objections to the lavish use and abuse of ordinary quinin. It may not have slain its thousands, but it has undoubtedly shattered the nerves, injured the sight and hearing and confirmed many painful conditions of joints and muscles in uncounted myriads of people. Its popular use has increased to an extent that few can realize. It might be not inappropriately termed a species of cinchono-mania. When the writer was in San Francisco a few years ago he was much amused as well as astonished to see business men to whom he was casually introduced treat each other to quinin pills, just as Easterners offer a cigar or a glass of something at the bar.

Preventing the occasion for the wholesale and indiscriminate use of this drug—some of it now being prepared from the coal tar series—is, of course, always preferable when it is feasible. This is to be sought by all available means, first, by a strict attention to hygienic laws, a careful but thoroughly supporting dietary, attention to all the emunctories, especially the skin. Frequent hot and occasional Turkish baths should be practised, and in many instances the semi-occasional use of some drug known to be prophylactic to the infection.

For this purpose, as well as for the treatment of the disease after it has been incurred, we have found the salt of quinin, known as the hydro-ferro-cyanate, administered in frequent but decidedly small doses, much more efficient than even large doses of ordinary quinin sulph. We have never noted any disastrous after effects from its use in this manner. It proves effective in doses so small that they might fairly be called homeopathic.

We have also used a tablet composed of the arsenates of quinin, strychnin and iron, as prepared by the Abbott Alkaloidal Company, as a prophylactic and general tonic, and always with good results.

The radical method of prevention, of course, includes the renovation of the breeding grounds and culture beds. On this point see the reply to Query 93.

MOVING TIME AND DISINFECTANTS.

THIS is the natural moving time. Some people change their place of residence regularly the first of every May. Moving is one of the institutions peculiar to this free land of ours. It makes no difference how careful and cleanly a housewife may be, there is urgent need every spring and often during the summer for a liberal use of disinfectants. Warmth and decaying refuse matter are a combination that is responsible for a great deal of sickness, mostly typhoid fever. A house that has been shut up all winter needs a pretty thorough airing in the spring time. Sunlight and pure air are very good disinfectants, but they are not enough. Regular spring house cleaning time is another period when disinfectants should be used freely. The small cost of effective disinfectants places them within the reach of every one, and if every one used them there would be less sickness. There are different kinds of disinfectants, each best adapted for some particular purpose. Talk disinfectants over with your druggist; he is informed on these matters, and can interest you with details about the

different disinfectants, and why one is better for one purpose and another for another, and so on.

Platt's chlorides are applicable almost everywhere.

"REST."

MORTAL doest thou look for rest?
Dost thy nature's stern behest
Wish to silence or oppose
All for thine own sweet repose?
Foolish is thine effort—vain;
Senseless, hopeless is thine pain,
With the march of motion keep,—
In thy walk and in thy sleep!
O'er us in the evening sky
Whirling planets pass us by
Resting never, always spinning
Countless years without beginning,
Worlds are moving on their way;
Always night moves on the day.
The stern yoke of constant motion
Binds the planets, land and ocean,
All the world is by it held;
None escape it, all must yield,
Rest is nowhere to be found,—
Each to all in motion bound,
No might can deliver thee,
Mortal, from activity.
In thy life as in thy death,
In thy heart as in thy breath,
In the heavens, as in the earth,
Whirling motion finds its birth;
Always raging, always spinning,
Endless, and without beginning,
And from death and dying break
Forth new growth, for Nature's sake;
On, then, sluggard, on with zest!
Mother Nature has no rest,
Not for e'en thy weary soul.
On! the part obeys the whole;
Even Death's most grewsome portal
Gives no Rest, O selfish mortal.
From thy coffin blossoms spring;
From thy flesh new life takes wing.

—M. T. AYEEZ.

THE
DIETETIC AND HYGIENIC GAZETTE

A·MONTHLY·JOURNAL·of·PHYSIOLOGICAL·MEDICINE

| Vol. XVII. | NEW YORK, SEPTEMBER, 1901. | No. 9. |

WHAT THE CENTURY HAS TAUGHT US ABOUT LIVING.

By Samuel S. Wallian, A.M., M.D.

VI.

THE LOST ART OF BREATHING.

As a prelude to further discussion of dietetic questions it will be a mark of good seamanship to cast an anchor to windward and take fresh bearings.

The process of digestion is fundamentally based on oxidation. The action of all the digestive ferments is essentially a form of oxidation. At every step in the digestive process oxygen is in immediate and incessant demand.

The Lord breathed into his nostrils the breath of life and man became a living soul.

Through the chemic necromancy of a puff of oxygen a lump of clay was transmuted into a thinking being.

From that initial impulse Aeration has never ceased to be the sine qua non of every vital process.

Philologists acknowledge the supremacy of the function in the wealth of terms allotted to its description. Thus, Aspiration, Inspiration, Respiration, Inhalation, Exhalation, Asphyxiation and so on.

Nor is this function monopolized by the animal kingdom. Plants breathe; and the transformation of inorganic into organic material, of mineral and earthly matter into structural and sentient tissue, is never accomplished except by direct contact with this control agent, *oxygen*.

The intervention of a transformer makes the current evolved by the dynamo safe and manageable; without its natural transformer,—oxygen, food is never perfectly utilized. Mastication, insalivation, and hydration are important; but they are auxiliaries to the process of oxidation.

Air and water are the bread and wine of life.

Modern customs and carelessness, the fads and fashions of civilized life, the very architectural arrangements we imitate, all tend to inhibit the normal use of both these elements. We breathe, because no genius has yet invented a breathing machine; but we breathe under protest, and would farm out this function entirely if we could hire it done by proxy.

Our ancestors were admittedly more virile, retained their hair, teeth and eyesight until each of these had earned the right to be placed on the retired list; and they lived to be centenarians, on a daily regimen simple even to crudity, and prepared in the most primitive manner imaginable. But they practically lived in the open, housed themselves in rustic huts and within walls through which the winds of heaven entered freely, day and night, in winter as in summer. Parlor, dining-room and kitchen were all in one, and communicated with the outside world through the throat of a fireplace, as wide as a modern hall, and with a draft like a miniature Trade Wind. Through this open airshaft ventilation was never interrupted, and it furnished ready exit for all the lurk-demons of disease borne in the "infectious dust" constantly present in our modern parlors.

If that shadowy bugbear of pseudo politicians, a "grasping monopoly," should actually materialize, and could manage to "corner" the atmosphere we should hereafter receive our breath of life through a meter, paying for it by the thousand cubic feet, as we now pay for legalized dilutions of it called illuminating gas.

We spleen against cast-off clothing, the remains of another's dinner, and the baby's bath-water; but we voluntarily immerse ourselves in second-hand air, and breathe it day and night, with only now and then a sigh of regret or a spasm of remonstrance. We have so long schooled our olfactory nerves and respiratory apparatus to the use of admixtures of air, ammoniacal emanations, smoke, carbonic oxid, nicotin and sulphuretted hydrogen that we now tolerate if we do not even prefer them.

The inconsistency is that we should be surprised at the inevitable results,—semiorganized tissues, flabby fibers, useles adipose, all these instead of normal and alert nerves, brain and muscles, self-poise and self-reliance.

Deprivation and depravation, this a sequence of that, go hand in hand. They readily account for the fact that so many of us drag out a handicapped existence, strewn with failures, saddened with shadows, and punctuated with moral surrenders; or that so many flag at the first serious strain and collapse entirely before they have reached their prime. They make the pessimism and protest of Schopenhauer plausible;—so many lives spent in the shadows of a veritable hell, so many homes a perpetual hospital!

The cheated vital mechanism struggles valiantly and sounds alarm after alarm to no purpose; and when finally the tired central pump stops short the survivors excuse themselves for cheating the doctor, with the plausible plea that he cheated them, by failing to fashion a beaded silk purse from a sickly sow's ear!

If causes were self-recording at the Bureaus of Vital Statistics many entries of "tabes mesenterica," "phthisis," "neurasthenia," "heart-failure," and the like would be changed to "unintentional asphyxiation." Against this form of *felo de se* no penal statutes have been enacted.

There is no lack of advice on the subject. All the libraries groan with their loads of works on hygiene,—most of them standing on undusted shelves and with uncut leaves, and "health" journals are thick as leaves in Vallombrosa. But the myriad victims do not learn to *breathe*. They helplessly go on coddling themselves, hunting for panaceas, enriching the nostrum vendors, and suffocating by inches. A few profit by the advice, ride a little, take occasional walks "on an empty stomach," flourish a tennis racket, go golfing by spurts and to excess; or invest in somebody's "exerciser," with which they enthuse for a fortnight and then discard, sine die. Other few patronize dusty gymnasiums, spasmodically swing clubs, hang on a trapese, or punch dummies, a la pugilists. A majority do nothing of the kind. They maintain the even tenor of the conventionalities, exercise as little as possible, wear clothing dictated by fashion rather than physiology—impediments that restrict muscle movement and debilitate the integument, by excluding that all-potent ally, the air. They live shut-in lives, work or sit long and late hours in cramping positions, and are chronically too "tired" and too much bored to indulge in any of the made-to-order contortions called "physical culture," or to care a rap whether zoologists classify them as monads, mollusks, or mammals.

Meanwhile the papmongers and proprietors of placebos wax plethoric of purse and swell at Newport, Saratoga or Aix-la-Chapelle. We go on smiling incredulously at the health-warnings, much as we formerly read the weather prognostications of the cheap almanacs. In short, we go on breathing second-hand air, day and night, impatiently anathematizing the doctor-druggist and druggist-doctor because their complexion wafers, cassia buds and cachou pellets do not clear up a turbid skin and correct a fetid breath.

It is of no avail to charge the results to climate, "malaria," environment, polluted water, tainted soils, or much libelled heredity. Nor can we migrate en masse to Colorado, New Mexico, or California, nor put to sea in houseboats, to escape an alleged unfavorable environment. Criminating Nature or Fate will not absolve us. It isn't so much the surroundings as it is the respiratory functions that are demoralized. If the environment has become insalubrious it is because we are all suffering for want of breath. To elevate, it is only necessary to aerate it.

To begin with, we must no longer accept the bungling work of builders who persist in giving us air-tight death-traps, in the shape of dwellings, offices, halls, churches, and public buildings, insisting that they are "up-to-date" structures, with "all modern improvements." As we can not be born again, so most of us cannot build again. But we can call in—if he can be found—some sane "sanitary" architect, one who has the fear of God and the gallows in his heart, and who knows how to healthfully warm and permanently ventilate every room, hall, nook and closet in the building. But his work will not be effective unless we call in the carpenters and plasterers and give them carte blanche to tear off and cremate whatever the plumber and ventilator leave of the walls and ceilings—"old churchyards stuffed with buried crimes,"—and to replace them with new ones, clean, aseptic and absorption-proof. Follow this with a raid on the carpets and upholstery, all the fluffy, dust and germ-harboring draperies, —tear them all up or down, and ship them to Siberia or Sheol; after which processes one can hope to keep the air of the rooms respirable.

Outside the premises there may be occasion for a similar exhibition of "muscular Christianity." Do away with excessive shade; fasten the blinds or shutters wide open and never allow them to be closed except during a hailstorm, a cyclone or a funeral. Aerate, levigate, and give t he antitoxic rays of the midday sun a chance to flood the entire premises with their unimpeded potency of revivification.

Only thus will ventilation be made all that it should be made, and without perfect ventilation the breathing function will never be adequately performed.

Sometimes it seems a mortal pity that the present generation can not be born again, with its present knowledge and facilities; or that it cannot at least circumvent the results of pre-natal coddling. Its culmination is evidenced by the universal over-sensitiveness.

Our mothers and nurses should have sung, with the Sage of Concord;

"Cast the bantling on the rocks,
    Suckle him with the she-wolf's teat,
Wintered with the hawk and fox,
    Power and speed be hands and feet."

But regrets aside, if we now realized all that the free air of heaven can do for the human bantling, we might assure him of a reasonably fair start in the vital race. We could bar the heredity bugaboo, teach him to breathe, tear his suffocating swaddling clothes into paper rags, and make him forget how to "take cold." With that haunting hobgoblin forever laid what an army of nameless but deadly ills would be effectually jugulated!

For the present generation it is perhaps too late to do more than modify the immediate environment and mitigate susceptibilities. Many of us were taught to breathe through a rubber nipple, were coddled and suffocated in wool and linen, and fur and feathers, until we have come to think it is necessary.

So, we spend half our leisure hours in "taking cold," and a goodly portion of the other half in making the nostrum-vendors rich and ourselves more susceptible to the next "exposure." by self-doctoring with quinin, coal-tar derivatives and something prefixed "bromo"; or we invoke the vapid gibberish of some latter-day juggler who practices his confidence game under a pseudo-sacred name.

Goodness knows there is room enough and sore need for reform in the feeding habit:

"For more have groaned and died from
    overuse
Of knives and forks, than ever fell in war
By bloody sword and bayonet and ball."

A majority of us are confessed gourmands, gluttons, nibblers, and so, dyspeptics; but the gastric apparatus successfully copes with almost any form of dietetic abomination, from rice to raw beef, and from pine-bark puddings to pancakes of infusorial earth,—if only this apparatus be kept generously supplied with the transforming element, *oxygen.*

Possibly many of us "dig our graves with our teeth"—shop-made teeth at that— but the funeral usually waits until the victim has cheated himself of a few stingy last gasps of the adulterated air about him.

The man at the sawbuck eats with impunity a diet that would send his sedentary brother to his long home, or to a Home for Incurables. It is because while the sawyer eats he aerates. Exercise compels him to breathe, and his food digests and invigorates. The other semi-suffocates in his tainted atmosphere, mincingly munches his food without zest or appetite, and it ferments and generates putrefactive poisons. Hence that other stupid old saw that even the unthinking doctors quote and requote, as if it were gospel, instead of a dietetic bugbear.

While *aeration* is the dominant, subdominant and diapason of the new doxology of deliverance from dietetic evil, it is of little use to perfunctorily reiterate the same old ding-dong of physiology,—"Get out of doors, exercise, breathe!" The advice has lost its significance, because it falls on leaden ears. It has become an old saw that sadly needs filing and resetting. It is time

to retire it on a pension, and to write on the walls of our domestic temples in letters of fire, as a shibboleth—not a new gospel of health, but the old basic factor restated:

Who doth not aerate shall not assimilate.
. *Whoso skimps his lungs and his skin skimps his life.*
Who only half breathes only half lives.

In the sweat of thy brow shalt thou find thy breath, and so, be able to eat bread, and beef and beans. Nature cares not a rap except for the result; whether it is work with a grim purpose and market value, or idle roving and silly skittles; whether bobbing in the wake of a tennis racket, cavorting over the landscape and swinging a putter or leaning against a tired hoe. To her, exercise is exercise; but it must be embraced with a vim. Nature hates a flunkey.

The rich and indolent would cheat her by affecting massage, which is better than nothing when nothing better can be had; but it is a makeshift, that may temporarily delay muscular atrophy, without inducing a single gasp of increased respiratory effort.

Cycling, the golf links, mountain climbing and various other forms of robust recreation are having an inning, and, until turned down by inexorable fashion, will give good account of themselves; because they compel their devotees to breathe. But what a beggarly few care to or can engage in them; whereas the overwhelming majority they do not reach are the ones who need them most.

In the sweat of thy brow shalt thou win thy breath, and the breath is the life. There are no substitutes, and Nature is the only pharmacist.

To harmoniously develop, fortify and inure the body can not be accomplished except by enhancing the facilities and increasing the capacity for *aeration.* The lungs and the skin are the laboratory and outer guard. To develop one and reenforce the other is to permanently enhance the vigor of every vital function, and strengthen the defences against all exposures and infections.

Every health crank has his particular fad.

One attributes the national malady to inefficient mastication; another performs all his oblations before a bathtub; a third ascribes everything to mentality, the domination of mind, faith "suggestion," superstition. A fourth is hysterical at the sight of blood, and morally shocked at the odor of roast beef or lamb stew; while a fifth finds his chief delight in lampooning the medical profession. All these continually harp on half-truths, giving credit where little is due; yet all of them, consciously or unconsciously profit by indirectly invoking this magic spirit of the air, the spirit that instigates all remedial effort.

In what direction lies the remedy?

It is a case in which no measure can be made to take the place of *Inflation*. Most of us possess twice as much lung capacity as we ordinarily utilize. The first thing in order is the recovery of collapsed and unused lung tissue. This is to be supplemented by systematic movements which tend to increase this normal lung capacity. Every increment of the respiratory function will be responded to by every other function, and by every fiber of the entire organism.

Then comes the integument, with its multi-million hungry mouths. It, too, is a breather and powerful auxiliary to the process of aeration, if given half a chance at the atmosphere into which it was originally born.

The naked Indian and New Zealander do not shiver and absorb influenza and rheumatism every time the wind shifts or the mercury fluctuates. The exposed and inured integument is their birthright and bodyguard. It repels cold, and wards off distempers, because its owners breathe and live in a perpetual air-bath, and bask in sunshine that is unimpeded by the civilized disguises we call clothes. Of course, Nature is not to blame for the "fatal invention," as Du Maurier put it. But we modern guardians of esthetic art and the proprieties are barred from anything more bold than a faint approximation of the privilege of the aborigine. We can not hunt the wild boar, nor climb trees, in search of our morning meal, clad only in our glove-fitting inauguration suits, as our remote ancestors undoubtedly did; but we might devote a little time, night and morning, to the cause of external and internal aeration. Thus we could emerge from the couch like Venus from the sea, clad only in smiles and resolution, and pacing the room for fifteen minutes or half an hour, like so many dancing dervishes.

For the next ordeal, improvise a cat-o'-three-tails, of manila rope, covered with haircloth or worsted plush; and with this formidable scourge briskly flagellate, and then spank, knead and percuss every inch of the exposed integument until it blushes with astonishment and tingles with delight. All this while inflate the lungs to their utmost, repeating the effort fifty times or more, and each time retaining the breath in the lungs as long as convenient. Conclude this gymnastic demonstration with a few special motions of another kind. Twist, gyrate, bend the body as far as possible in all directions, guard, thrust, parry, as if handling the foils with an imaginary foe, or as if on the verge of chorea; the final touches to consist of a brisk grooming with a hair mitten, or with bare-hand friction, if an assistant is available. Twice a week this last touch may be varied to advantage by an inunction with olive, almond or cotton-seed oil or white vaseline, to be well rubbed in.

Thus honored, the surface vellum will acquire such a vigorous glow that the accustomed weight of conventional coverings will seem a burden, and every one of thirty million epidermal mouths will be rosy with thanks, and wide open to say, in its dumb way, "Do it again!"

As a legitimate and assured result of all this combination of ærotherapy, gymnastics and kinesitherapy—begging pardon for such a string of jawbreaking names—the whilom flabby, blanched, debilitated and over-perspiring skin will gratefully and rapidly respond to its tonic treatment, burdensome adipose tissue, if present, will melt, thaw and dissolve, and the hypersensitive organism will become assured, self-protective and hygienically defiant.

And as for the baby, bless the innocent little heart that flutters on in utter unconsciousness of the dreadful "failures" that lurk in its future path!—We can make him a Spartan, by inuring every inch of his body to the constantly recurring vicissitudes of the airworld into which he has made his involuntary début. Spare him the paps, namby-pambyism, coddling and semi-asphyxiation to which our over-fond parents and ignorant nurses subjected us; and thus forefend him from the over-susceptibility and vital effeminacy that have made so many millions of human lives only half worth living!

It will compel us to face custom and defy tradition, but the end will amply justify the effort.

SPECIAL INSURANCE FOR TOTAL ABSTAINERS.

THE *Medical Record* has the following: In answer to a numerously signed petition, the Equitable Life Insurance Society of this city has agreed to put in a special class any successful applicant for insurance who declares that he has been a total abstainer from the use as a beverage of alcoholic liquors, including wine, beer, and fermented cider, and as a condition of membership in this class agrees to remain a total abstainer as long as his policy is in force. Any surplus apportioned to the policy will be based on the experience of the society on policies belonging to the total-abstinence class. It is believed by the petitioners that the number of the total-abstinence class will receive the benefit of largely increased dividends. A number of British life insurance companies have for many years segregated their total-abstinent policy holders.

POLYPHARMACY WITH A VENGEANCE.

BY GEORGE T. WELCH, M.D.,
Passaic, N·J·

AN aphorism by Prof. Murphy, in the July number of this GAZETTE, that "It is the physician's business not to fight disease, but to take care of his patient," causes me to relate how this matter is differently regarded at a fashionable watering place when business is booming.

A client of mine, of his own volition, as a species of recreation, after passing a dull winter, went to the Hot Springs, Ark., the last of February. He found a lively town, a hotel fairly reeking with gaiety, and a medical contingent at sword's points, but in the art of keeping a patient in chancery, fully *fin de siècle.*

My client being of a progressive turn, felt that he ought to drink the waters, and take the baths, and not be a mere looker-on in Venice. Prompted by a newly-found friend, he consulted a physician, who looked him over with the eye of an enthusiast, and who assured him that he was really in a bad way, and that he must take the baths at 98°, and return to him daily, for further advice. This he accordingly did, and was much debilitated, but on his return to the doctor he was greeted with much satisfaction, and a complication of drugs was incontinently ordered, as a preliminary to further proceedings.

The patient was accompanied by his wife and she prudently prompted him to ask for his bill. The doctor told him it was thirty-five dollars, and obligingly itemized it as follows: For advising a bath at 98°, twenty-five dollars; for noting its effect, ten dollars. The patient was stunned, and began to pay the bill without a murmur. His wife, however, was of an ardent temperament, and she characterized the whole proceeding as a swindle. The doctor gave her a condescending smile, and then in a burst of confidence he added, "If you were in a hell-hole like this, wouldn't you pull yourself out by tugging at other men's pockets?"

My client having paid thirty-five dollars as initiation fee, did not want to lose all that he had invested, so again returned to the baths, and again was debilitated, and finally an acute articular rheumatism set in. To add to the distress he was unable to get properly accommodated in the dining-room, the headwaiter being a *grand seigneur*, whom it was necessary to fee every day, and the lesser flunkeys had to be bribed as often, and if the least neglect was shown dinners became short commons indeed.

Barely able to crawl about, my friend sat in the lobby one day gloomily ruminating, when a gentleman came to him, saying, "I have been watching you, and I think I know just what is the matter. You look just like I felt four years ago, when I went to Dr. Fake, who is simply the smartest physician this side of the Atlantic Ocean. I may have his card about me, but if I have not, I will take you right to his office."

My friend demurred, and even said, "I have already been to one who was recommended to me as the smartest doctor in America, and you see where I have been landed." But the other would not hear a word of protest, he vigorously denouncing the first physician; in fact, had had the same experience with him himself, when at the threshold of four years ago, nearly lost his life on account of his blunders, was just as incredulous about the ability of Dr. Fake, but was persuaded to see him at the last gasp, and, lo! he had done miracles, saved a valuable life, and he, the speaker, was going to sound his praises as long as he had a tongue to sing. Well, what could a pain-tormented mortal do when beset by such a plausible mascot? He went to see Dr. Fake.

The doctor treated him with much hateur —gave a supercilious smile when he heard of his first experiences, remarked that none but an ass would recommend a bath at 98° to an unseasoned man. It was not his custom to parboil his clients in the beginning. "Then, doctor, what do you propose to do?" asked the sufferer. "Sir," returned the great man, "I propose to do nothing—at least until I find out what is the matter. First, I will have an analysis made of your urine, and to-morrow I will advise you." And here he waived him haughtily away. On the morrow he presented to the effete Eastern man the result of the urinalysis, for which he afterward paid twenty-five dollars. "I have discovered," said the doctor, "that you have rheumatism." "I knew it all along,"ventured the invalid. "Sir," thundered the autocrat, "I do not permit my patients to talk back at me. You go at once to your hotel and to your bed, and I will follow you presently, and after I have examined you thoroughly I will prescribe for you. Go at once, sir."

After a prolonged examination, which began at the occiput and ended at the last phalanx of the pedal extremities, the doctor once more declared that the man had rheumatism. He thereupon wrote the following:

For Acute Rheumatism:

℞ Tr. Aconite............ ℈ i
" Belladonna
" Bryonia alb. } aa.... ℈ ii
" Conium mac.
" Colchicum. } aa.... ℈ v
" Rhus tox.
" Cimicifuga Rac....... ℈ x

M. Sig: Thirty (30) Minims, in water, every hour, until better, then every 3 hours. —*Fake.*

On the following day, the patient being no better, was roundly scolded by Fake, and after being taunted with his baths at 98° he was ordered:

For the Liver and Bowels:

℞ Laxative tablets, Frasier & Co., No. XXV.

Sig: One at bed-time.—*Fake.*

Daily, the sick man grew worse. The old prescriptions were continued, and the new ones grew apace. He was, at length, using, besides the former:

℞ Thialion .... 1 bottle

Sig: Teaspoonful in glassful of hot water every morning, on waking.—*Fake.*

℞ Tr. Cactus Grand...... ʒ iv,
Spts. Ammon. Aromat... ʒ xx.

M. Sig: 30 Minims, in cool water, as a stimulant.

Repeat the dose every hour, or oftener, if needed.—*Fake.*

Tonic Digestive, Stimulanti, etc.:

℞ Strych. Nitrat. Mercks. } aa grns. ii
Acid. Arsenit:

Tr. Berbis Vulg.
" Cactus Grand. } aa.... ʒ iv
" Pulsatillac
' Squills

" Apocynum Can......... ʒ viii,
" Fairchild's essence peps. q. s. ʒ iv

M. Sig: Sixty minims in half a glassful of water, half an hour before each meal.—*Fake.*

℞ Pl. Digitalis. } aa. gr. i. No. 100
Squills.

M. Sig: One every 3 hours.—*Fake.*

℞ Merck's Guaiacol. } aa. ʒ ii.
Glycerin.

M. Sig: Apply 60 drops with camel-hair pencil to each inflamed joint. Then apply raw cotton and oiled silk.—*Fake.*

Not much time was wasted now. The first prescription was being given every hour; the second was due constantly, as it was bed time all the while, with him, after that first day. The thialion came every morning; the cactus and aromatic spirits of ammonia followed hard on the rheumatism medicine; the digitalis and squills came punctually eight times in the twenty-four hours. And while the stomach was being fired within, the joints were being basted without. Only one prescription bided its time, and that was the tonic, digestive and stimulant, for there was no longer an interval for meals.

While the deadly notation went on, the patient fell into a frenzied nightmare, only broken momently by the click of spoons on his teeth, or the passage of ordinance in the shape of pills. Before his window stalked the gamblers, masquerading in shiny silk hats and with dyed mustaches. Over-dressed women from St. Louis and New Orleans lolled in their hired carriages; the oblivious police seemed to be spotless in Spotless Town; while the highwaymen held up their victims in broad daylight. The arrogant doctor was coming and going, hectoring the worse and writing additional prescriptions, and the harsh discord of the Hotel Directors at a meeting in a back room could be heard, as they, like our army in Flanders, swore terribly if a proper division of spoils was not coming in from every one who practiced his art in the big hostelry.

It was at this juncture, when the patient was drifting between shadowy banks to the unknown sea, "the helm of reason lost," that a clever physician from Paterson, N. J., looking over the hotel register, came across the signatures of this family from Passaic. A fellow feeling made him wondrous kind, and following his card to the sick man's room, he made himself known. When he had heard the story, and had viewed the bristling array of bottles, and realized that the man was taking about thirty different drugs daily, he broke out into impious admiration, but ended with urgent advice to leave Hot Springs at once and forever.

Dr. Fake was furious next morning when he found his victim had the temerity to announce that he wanted his bill and that he was going home. "You can't go too quick for me!" he sneeringly ejaculated. "I don't want any such patients as you. You are no man at all if you quit before I am half through with you. Go." And go he did, minus thirty-one pounds of flesh, twenty-five dollars to Fake for the urinalysis, ten dollars for having his rheumatism given the stamp of authority, and ten dollars apiece for fifteen visits.

The experience was bizarre, and the whilom patient is now at the other extreme of the compass, endeavoring in Nova Scotia to regain the flesh he lost.

✣ ✣

DIETS FOR EVERY-DAY USE.

By J. Warren Achorn, M.D., Boston.

THE question of water drinking is not an idle one. Generally speaking, people do not drink water enough, or if they do, it is at the wrong time. Water goes best on an empty stomach an hour and a half before meals, and it were better sipped. Large quantities in this way leave the stomach readily. Ordinarily a glass of water may be taken at the close of any meal; if taken, however, in large draughts or at improper times without regard to the condition of the stomach, it is apt to produce disorders of digestion. Three or four glasses gulped down during a meal or used to wash down half masticated food is sure in the long run to bring on the whole chain of dyspepsias that begin with catarrh or loss of motor power in the stomach.

In myasthenia (loss of motor power), the use of water should be restricted to the needs of the system—enough to quench normal thirst and promote the healthy action of the skin and kidneys. This condition can be diagnosed by a glass of hot water on an empty stomach; if, at the end of an hour, with the patient on his back and abdomen relaxed, the stomach can be made to splash, myasthenia exists as evidenced by slow absorption. Care should be used not to confound splashing here with water or gas in the big bowel. If the papillæ of the tongue show red, the stomach is irritated, when a glass of hot water taken at the close of a meal should prove beneficial. In myasthenia with lack of secretion, cold water does better. Hot water is soothing and quickly absorbed; it stimulates the secretion of bile, especially if the liver is repeatedly signalled by the water taken in sips; it is a solvent of retained products in the system.

In chronic rheumatic states, where there is no disorder of the stomach, hot water is obviously beneficial. The same holds true in auto-intoxication. In hyperacidity hot water affords relief taken half an hour before meals. The free use of hot water taken on an empty stomach tends to reduce weight in some cases; in others it increases adipose by water logging the tissues. Water starvation certainly reduces weight, the food problem being also satisfied. An actual trial is the only way for determining the action of water in a given case.

Cold water is an intense stimulant of gastric secretions, if taken on an empty stomach. Its use would be contraindicated then, in chronic gastric catarrh. A glass of hot water on the other hand, an hour before meals should prove helpful, because it washes out the mucous.

Chronic gastric catarrh can only be demonstrated accurately by the introduction and use of the stomach tube. Cold water benefits constipation, if not associated or dependent on some other disorder, where water in excess would do harm. Ice water, unless sipped, retards digestion; if freely used it may cause acute gastritis or aggravate an existing catarrh. Its use in chronic heart disease is dangerous. Water does harm in dilitation of the stomach, especially if coupled with retention and fermentation. Water that is refreshingly cool should be taken at *all* times, when there are no indications for the use of hot water or it cannot be procured. The protracted use of hot water is debilitating to the alimentary tract, and the same is true of its too free use externally.

A healthy condition of the skin, bronchial tubes, kidneys and intestines, and their full activity as eliminators, can best be secured and maintained by exercise and the proper use of water. We see "dessicated" nerves, tongues like parchment, skins as dry as sand paper, urine as red as wine, and faces filled with grease and blackheads from the lack or misuse of this grateful solvent.

DIET IN RHEUMATISM.

(Copyright.)

Take a glass of hot water on rising, sip slowly. Hot milk is a good drink, cut one half with vichy.

BREAKFAST: *Cereals*—Gluten (30 per

cent.), mush 5; rice, cornmeal mush, rye mush with prune or pineapple juice; oatmeal, cracked wheat, coarse hominy, with cream, milk, or grape juice; w h e a t e n porridge (from groats); popped corn for a separator.

Fish—(Fresh only), cod, haddock, butter-fish, smelts, flounder, chicken halibut, shad, shad roe, perch, pickerel, trout, or other lake or brook fish, boiled or broiled.

Eggs—(Fresh only), soft boiled, poached or scrambled, twice a week.

Breads—Cestus gluten bread Nos. 1 or 2; gluten cakes, gluten biscuit, other glutens. Whole wheat, rye or French bread; Cestus brown bread. Butter, orange or prune marmalade, unsweetened jam.

Fruits—Baked or stewed sour apples, orange juice, pineapple juice, cantaloupe, watermelon, melons; stewed prunes, unsweetened; other stewed or prepared fruit in moderation.

Drinks—Hot skimmed milk, hot or cold water, grain coffee, water with lime or lemon juice; one cup or glass of either.

A.M. BETWEEN MEALS: Water, hot skimmed milk, buttermilk, French or Saratoga vichy, clam water. Pure fruit juice in water.

LUNCH: *Meats* (white)—Stewed or roasted chicken, breast of turkey; capon, squab, partridge, quail or other game bird; breast of duck (dry.)

Any *fish* mentioned.

Any *vegetable* mentioned.

Any *bread* mentioned. Cestus phosphated crackers, soup sticks, rusk, zwieback; crackers and milk, pilot bread and milk.

Any *fruit* mentioned. Grapefruit, white grapes, ripe olives; berries, except strawberries.

Any *drink* mentioned. Imported ginger ale.

Any *dessert* mentioned. Nut food with fruit or crackers.

NOTES.

In acute rheumatism the diet should be entirely fluid, milk cut with distilled water; whey, barley water, thin oatmeal gruel, arrowroot, rice or bread in milk. Or the oatmeal gruel, barley water or arrowroot, may be stirred into the milk. If the latter constipates, use bi-carbonate of soda instead of lime juice or lime water to alkalinize. Vegetable broths are a substitute for milk, if the latter is not well borne. Weak lemonade.

Twenty-drop doses of the oil of wintergreen in milk, every two hours, will relieve the pain of acute rheumatism. The heart should be examined daily during an attack. If it becomes involved the diet and medicines should be regulated to satisfy this complication. After the fever has subsided, clear soups and broths are suitable, flavored with vegetables. Stale bread goes with these. Fresh fish and the white meat of chicken are among the first solid foods admitted. Stewed celery, mashed potato, spinach and the pulp of stewed fruit are among the foods for convalescence. Pounded meat sandwiches may be required if the patient is very anæmic. Later comes cauliflower, bean omelette, Parmesan cheese, macaroni, cayenne, vermicelli, mushrooms, white cabbage and apples. Only a strong digestion can dispose of mushrooms.

A diet of cheese, milk, potatoes and fruit will keep the urine free from "red sand."

In both chronic and acute rheumatism a highly nutritious diet must be maintained.

Mush of any kind should be eaten with bread crumbs or other discreet food, as a separator; this practice helps digestion. Toast made of zwieback, with fruit makes a good breakfast.

Plain milk, diluted, is to be preferred to skimmed milk in chronic rheumatism. If fleshy, skimmed milk or milk that has been largely diluted would meet the requirements better, perhaps. If fleshy, constipated or bilious, gluten is the best bread or cereal for regular use. Meat in any form should not be eaten oftener than once a day, white meat or fish having the preference. Elderly persons, whose nutrition is poor, may require meat once a day aside from some fibred fish.

Sugar with vegetables and fruit, if meat is withheld, does no harm. With meat in the diet it increases the acidity and the uric acid in the system (Haig).

Sugar and sweets of all sorts must be practically let alone if this diet is liberally used.

Peas and beans are substitutes for meat, if they agree; beans should be avoided by the obese, constipated or bilious. Peas and beans are relatively poor in fat; they contain much albumen, however. Their action tends to inhibit the free elimination of uric acid by upholding the acidity of the urine; on this account they should not be eaten too often. All vegetables and cereals tend to maintain a highly acid urine. Peas are to be preferred to beans, and are best stewed; they are best served mixed with barley or rice.

Gluten (30 per cent.) is a substitute for meat; the flavor for some is improved by adding a little

P.M. BETWEEN MEALS: Same as A.M. Lime juice in water, with a lithia tablet added; sweeten slightly.

DINNER: *Soups*—Any clear vegetable soup with bisbak, sago, pearl barley or ground rice; chicken broth. Pea or bean soup with milk, best made from pea or bean flour.

Purees of—Potatoes, young peas, corn, squash or celery, adding milk, when possible; milk soups thickened with discreet cereals and flavored.

Any *fish* mentioned. Oysters (raw) with lemon juice, little neck clams, plain lobster.

Any *meat* mentioned. Baked or stewed peas or beans.

Cheese—American (fat 31); Single Gloucester (24); Dutch (17); Suffolk ( ); Camenbert (21); Parmesan (16); skimmed milk cheese, (8½); cottage cheese, buttermilk cheese. Cream (35); Neuchatel (43); Edam and Roquefort.

Vegetables—New peas, new string beans, new corn in moderation; celery, dandelion greens, beet tops, beet root, cucumbers, cauliflower, lettuce, with oil or lemon juice; squash, turnips, artichokes, carrots. Spinach, tomatoes, asparagus, watercress, onions, of either twice a week. Baked potatoes with butter, potatoes with milk or cream, macaroni plain.

Any *bread* mentioned. Water, milk or dry toast.

Any *fruit* mentioned. Apricots, peaches, and ripe bananas.

Any *drink* mentioned.

Dessert—Milk pudding, plain custard, floating island; rice, apple tapioca or bread pudding; apple charlotte; clear jellies not sweet; blanc mange, junket. Puddings of milk, egg and grated cheese. ·

9 P.M.: Hot milk, weak lemonade, an orange with Vichy, and apple with milk.

---

rice or other light cereal that has been previously cooked.

Cheese is the equal of meat in force production; like milk, it contains no uric acid. It must be thoroughly dissolved in the mouth before swallowing. Grating helps the digestibility: or it may be cooked into the various dishes served. Parmesan, Edam and Roquefort cheeses are hard and likely to be better chewed, and consequently better digested. than the softer cheeses. A pinch of bicarbonate of potash should be taken with each ounce of cheese eaten to negative the fatty acids sometimes present in it that interfere with digestion. The proportion of nitrogen in cheese, generally speaking, equals that of meat with the exception of cream cheese, where the nitrogen falls to 8½ per cent. Cheese should be eaten early in the meal. Cottage cheese is laxative.

Cestus phosphated crackers are especially indicated in chronic rheumatism. Phosphates in some form in excess are highly beneficial. The phosphates in bread can be readily multiplied by increasing the proportion of bran present, by adding the phosphates of milk secu.ed by evaporation. They diminish acidity.

Almonds. pecans or filberts with crackers or fruit go well for lunch; masticat: thoroughly. If found to be indigestible. some of the Sanitas Nut Food products should be trie..

Oily fish. such as salmon, mackerel, bluefish, swordfish and eels may be eaten by those having a strong digestion and for whom their use is not denied. Avoid in acid stomach. furred tongue, biliousness or loss of appetite. The free use of potato by the fleshy, flatulent or constipated is denied. Green olives are very indigestible, ripe olives much less so; they contain considerable fat.

Milk and vegetables do not go well together. Bread and milk with some light dessert makes a good supper.

Hot milk and bisbak or phosphated crackers and a glass of milk, may be tried on retiring, if there is any tendency to insomnia, or if one is faint or in need of nourishment.

If the splitting up of medicine into constantly narrowing specialties continues as it has during the past few decades, scientific medicine will soon be a thing of the past. Even more dangerous is the complete division between the theoretical branches, anatomy and physiology on the one hand, and the practical branches on the other. Medicine without anatomy and physiology is not knowledge.—*Karl v. Bardelben* (Jena).

THE TOXIC ORIGIN OF NEURAS-
THENIA AND MELANCHOLIA.

SHAKESPEARE was incredulous as to the ability of the physician to minister to a mind diseased; but in these days it is the commonest thing in the world. A Turkish bath, a few granules of calomel and soda, or podophyllin, and a saline often transforms a hypochondriac into a cheerful citizen.

Under the above title Dr. M. Allen Starr, in the *Med. Record* of May 11, advances some novel ideas as to the origin and rational treatment of a quite common and very distressing malady. Says the doctor:

"While the interest of the physician is commonly excited by rare and unusual cases rather than by the common run of disease, it is after all the ordinary light type of case which comes most frequently under his attention and demands his effort. There is no need to affirm the frequency of mild cases of neurasthenia and of melancholia, inasmuch as every practitioner sees such cases constantly. The complaints of a neurasthenic are so numerous and the general frame of mind of these patients is so depressing, that the disease fails to elicit very much interest on the part of the practitioner, or of the neurologist to whom in despair he often refers these cases. Yet it is my experience that a little care in their examination often enables one to classify them into a variety of different types, not only cerebral, spinal, and vasomotor types, but also into different classes according to the origin of the disease. Thus one can recognize clearly cases that are due to anxiety and worry; cases that are due to overexertion, mental and physical; cases that are due to beginning degeneration of the neurons, destined to go on to organic disease; and lastly, cases that are distinctly toxic in their origin. It is to the latter class that I wish to direct attention at the present time.

I do not wish to delay you by any long study of the symptomatology of this variety of neurasthenia. It usually occurs either in poorly nourished women, or in men about the age of forty-five who have lived rather freely, have taken little care of their diet and have indulged in the use of alcohol and tobacco, and who have neglected exercise.

The chief symptoms in this form of neurasthenia are headache, dull pressure in the head and back of the neck, sensations of fulness in the head with inability to concentrate the attention, irritability of temper, manifest irregularities of the circulation shown by cold extremities, and by frequent flushings and burnings in different parts of the body, and general disorders of the digestion either of the nature of acid dyspepsia, or of considerable evolution of gas in the stomach and intestines, with irregular and very offensive stools. In these cases the urine is irrregular in quantity, at times scanty, of high color and of high specific gravity; at other times profuse, light, and of low specific gravity, and at all times it contains large quantities of indican or indoxyl. In this condition a mild state of melancholia is very frequently associated with the neurasthenia, and in almost all cases of mild beginning melancholia the same symptoms are present.

The chief characteristeric of this type is the alternation of feelings and symptoms at different times of the day. One can draw a curve representing the intensity of symptoms in these patients with remarkable accuracy, a depression in the curve representing the depression of spirits and intensity of suffering. From noon such a curve rises gradually toward the normal level. At 9 A. M. it begins to descend; during the night falls to its lowest level, so that at 4 A. M., when these patients commonly awake, they are in the deepest distress of mind and are .suffering the greatest discomfort of body. For a period of three or four hours the curve is then at its lowest point, but by breakfast time it begins to rise and continues to rise slowly until the normal level is almost reached at noon. This cycle of misery and well-being is so constant and so uniform that patients themselves readily recognize it. It is perfectly evident that a variable condition of this character must be produced by a varying intensity of cause, and the fact that the maximum of distress occurs in these patients after the sleep of the night, is an indication that it is not the wear and tear of exhaustion which produces their chief symptoms. It must be some toxic agent which accumulates in the blood during the period of sleep, which reaches the point of irritation early in the morning, which is counteracted by the activity of the day, and hence is less intense in its action toward afternoon. That this toxic agent is manufactured either in the intestines on in the stomach seems to be the most natural theory, inasmuch as activity in the digestive process appears to aid in the elimination of the poison. Exactly what this toxic agent is I do not know. As already stated, I find that indican or indoxyl is the one particular thing found in the urine in varying quantities, according to the general condition of these patients, and yet I do not suppose that indican is the active poison. It would be as foolish to affirm this as it would be to judge of the results of heat and power produced in a steam furnace by analyzing the character of the slag in the ash pan. Very much more exhaustive studies in the chemistry of digestion are necessary before we begin to approach any true knowledge of the active agents producing these effects.

But it is not necessary for us always to wait in medicine for scientific facts before attempting treatment. Some of the most valuable remedies that we have at our disposal are purely empirical in their origin. When a patient presents these evidences of toxæmia, he can be materially helped by a certain regimen and treatment, no one particular element of which is necessarily curative, but all of which combine to give relief.

First: Diet. This cannot be laid down in a uniform manner for all patients. The majority of them, I believe, do not digest milk well, and eggs as a rule do not agree with them, though occasionally raw eggs will be digested when cooked eggs will not. Meat of all kinds seems to me to agree very well with this t ype of patient, but meat soups are not well digested and therefore cream soups are preferable. Fish in all forms and oysters usually agree with such patients and also certain types of vegetables; but potatoes, turnips, beets, and tomatoes are liable to give more trouble than other vegetables. Rice, macaroni, and hominy are usually well borne, but should not be cooked with cheese, and cheese as a rule is not well digested. Patients differ entirely from each other in their capability to assimilate breads and sweets, and it will not do to lay down any rule for the use of these articles; in fact in these cases various forms of diet and various articles of diet should be tried until the articles which disagree are ascertained.

Fluids: Tea almost uniformly disagrees with these patients, making them nervous and increasing their indigestion. In many of the patients, coffee acts as a desirable and pleasant stimulant, both in the morning for breakfast and after dinner, and does not in any way interfere with sleeep. In others it acts as a poison and should be excluded. I believe that in all these cases alcohol should be avoided in every form, especially the sour wines and champagne. In about one-half of the cases whiskey can be taken without ill effects, but the stronger wines, like port and sherry and all liquers are to be avoided. Occasionallly a patient can take Rhine wine diluted, or the Austrian Vöslauer, without ill effects. Water should be taken very freely, and a good alkaline or lithia water is often of much benefit.

Drugs: The digestion must be aided in these patients by two classes of remedies: one which stimulates the liver to activity, the other which counteracts the evolution of toxic agents in the intestines. First, it is my habit to give these patients small doses of calomel (gr. $^1/_{10}$ every half hour till one grain is taken) every ten days and to give them a dose of podophyllin (gr. $\frac{1}{4}$) every ten days alternately with the calomel. It is also well to stimulate the liver by the use daily in the morning of either Carlsbad salt or a salt made by mixing gr. x. of salicylate of sodium with ℨi. of phosphate of sodum and ℨ ss. of chloride of sodium. If this mixed salt is put in a large tumbler of sparkling water of any kind, and taken during the act of dressing in the morning, it will usually be beneficial. In this manner the liver is stimulated to action.

The second object—the counteracting of the toxic agent—is attained by one of three different remedies, and it is never possible to determine exactly which of these three in any one case will prove of service. The first is a combination of gr. v. of the sulphocarbolate of sodium with gr. i. of permanganate of potassium put up in a capsule, which is coated with shellac so as to be insoluble in the stomach, and hence dissolve only in the intestine. Such capsules are given after each meal and on retiring. The second remedy that I use is a capsule of salol and castor oil—gr. v. of salol and Mx of castor oil. This also is rendered insoluble in the stomach by a coating of shellac. The third remedy is given in the same manner, in capsule after eating, and consists of benzoate of sodium gr. ii., sulphocarbolate of zinc gr. i., and beta-naphthol gr. i. It is my experience that by the administration of these remedies continuously for a considerable period a steady amelioration in the symptom of intestinal indigestion will ensue, and, what is much more noticeable, an entire cessation in the periodicity of the alternations of the symptoms; the first evidence of relief being a quieter rest during the night without any early awakening and a relief from the depression that occurs early in the morning.

Baths: The use of a hot bath on rising, at a temperature of 104° F. for three minutes, followed by cool sponging for one-quarter of minute, is of importance, as nothing stimulates the general nutrition of the body better than such a measure, but in this type of patient the cold bath in the morning usually produces distress and is followed by a feeling of exhaustion, cold extremities, and discomfort.

Exercise and rest: In all cases an increased amount of exercise should be insisted upon, yet in many cases any long-continued exercise is most exhausting and is followed by a rapid action of the heart; hence it is far better for these patients to swing clubs briskly or to play a game of tennis for twenty minutes, thus getting into a pleasant perspiration, than it is to take an hour's horseback exercise or to play a game of golf which requires tramping two miles, though both of these measures occasionally can be endured and are beneficial. One very important element in the treatment is regularity in the amount of rest. These patients should be urged to lie down and relax all the muscles, the clothing being properly loosened, for one-half hour after each meal, and after any active exercise rest of the same duration should be enforced. One of the essential elements of successful treatment in these patients is a pleasant occupation for the mind, as their depression leads them to intensify their nervousness by introspection and self-observation. A variety of occupation should be sought and every means should be employed to keep them interested and diverted. An outdoor life is far better for them than a life indoors, and therefore if an occupation can be found which involves some activity in the open air it is desirable: the study of botany, the study of forestry, the running of a farm, the care of chickens the occupation of an engineer or surveyor, the study of landscape gardening—all of these are pleasing occupations for men and women, and it is on this principle that travel and change of scene may be urged upon these patients. But whatever means are employed in their treatment, it seems to me that the essential element in their success is the counteracting of the toxic product within the body and the prevention of its formation.

Without pathological anatomy practical medicine is a patch work.—*Hans Eppinger* (Graz).

MEDICAL PROSPECTS

UNDER this title Dr. George E. Francis of Worcester, Mass., read a very thoughtful paper before the Massachusetts Medical Society.

His concluding remarks are decidedly pertinent.

We should like to produce the entire address as it appears in the *Boston Med. and Surg. Journal:*

"EVERY physician, without exception, helps his patients by the expectation of relief which his very presence brings; and most of us go further, and consciously or unconsciously use the very helpful power of direct suggestion, of a partially hypnotic character. It is curious to note that this faculty and habit of suggestion is the only feature which is common to all who attempt to heal the sick. When the last veil of mystery shall have been torn from our art by the advance of science, I fear that little will be left of our special power of suggestion, and that humanity will be much the poorer thereby.

"We observe that the Syrian's leprosy was cured without the use of any drug. We may not all agree as to whether there is any visible tendency toward the disuse of medication; and certainly it would appear that the number of drugs in use or recommended for use, was never so great as now. On the other hand, we have learned that the virtues of much of the old materia-medica were purely imaginary; while as to the value of the new synthetical compounds so pertinaceously thrust upon us, there appears to be widespread doubt. They are formidable weapons, indeed, but many of them have more than one cutting edge.

"The growth of another doubt, of a more radical sort, is also to be noted—as to whether chronic organic disease is ever cured by drugs, if by cure we mean restoration to the normal state. Some form of compensation seems to be the extent of the benefit which is to be hoped in such conditions. This, at least, can be confidently affirmed: That in the chronic diseases which figure most largely in the bills of mortality, the use of drugs is decidedly on the wane.

If we are asked to name the specific whose power is most generally granted and least questioned, we should probably at once point to the control which quinine exercises against malaria; yet it seems exceedingly likely that the next century will see less and less use of this great remedy, simply because there will be less need of it—malaria is going to be prevented. Prevention is a watchword of great promise in the years which are before us; but the promise is to the community in general, and not to those whose incomes depend on the abundance of disease. Our profession prides itself on its constant and eager search for methods of preventing and diminishing disease, and we gain some public credit for our aims and achievements in that direction; but few seem to appreciate the full extent of our unselfishness, and that complete success means professional suicide. This sad result is not yet in sight, even of the prophetic eye we are using to-day.

"Returning to the text from which we have wandered so far, we are struck by the statement that it was the little maid waiting on Naaman's wife who called attention to the skill or power of the healer. This little detail has a very modern and familiar sound.

"We further read that the grateful Syrian attempted to reward his benefactor with gifts of value, but that the offer was refused. There is nothing modern about this statement. Even that new sect which boasts of its reversion to ancient modes of healing does not carry its reverence for antiquity to such an extreme; it demands the regular fees. Yet to find a modern analogue to the refusal of Elisha, we need only view some of our public and semipublic establishments for medical and surgical treatment. This very day, in almost any city in this State, any person, rich or poor, who is coming down with a fever, or needs a surgical operation, will be received into a city hospital, where he will get first-rate care and treatment. At his departure he will be asked to pay a proper price for his room, board and nursing, but for the professional services not a cent will be charged. What lesson is this likely to teach him and his friends, if not that the municipal supply of medical skill is an excellent and most economical idea, which might be carried further to great advantage.

"This practice seems to me altogether wrong, not simply because it diverts much money from the pockets of doctors who deserve and need it, but because it so forcibly teaches a lesson in applied socialism which is very dangerous to the financial future of our guild.

Our text might easily guide us into many other lines of thought, but I mercifully refrain from further turning of the hourglass, and will simply ask you to observe that this old story of the healing of the leper has long been known to the whole civilized world. Once, and not so long ago, this was a distinction almost unique; to-day every important medical case or discovery is promptly carried to the remotest regions of our globe. On this opening year of the twentieth century let us not withhold the tribute of gratitude and admiration due to the medical press, and particularly to medical journalism. Not all of these journals are admirable, and not all are truely scientific; perhaps in some might be suspected a slight bias from commercialism; but as a whole they are doing wonderfully good and useful work, and are to be ranked among the great improvements of modern times. Not all of us are called upon to write papers for them, but every one of us should look upon it as a duty, as well as a privilege, to subscribe to at least one good medical journal.

After all our searching and discussing, the summing up shows but a brief list of plausible predictions. That specialism will increase, and competition become more fierce, we may feel as confident as of any future event. That medical treatment will become more scientific in its basis and methods; that disease will be more effectively prevented; that hygiene agents will largely supplant drugs—all these seem to be among the strong probabilities. Very probably the family doctor is about to be eclipsed for a time; perhaps to reappear later in a more glorified aspect.

The darkest cloud which rests upon our future seems to arise from the combined forces of greatly increased competition and the growth of socialistic and co-operative ideas.

We must not forget that the past is the only test by which we judge the future. In his great vision, Dante observed that all the prophets had their heads turned backward. The most accurate inferences we can draw from experience are liable, indeed are almost certain, to be deranged by the entrance of new and unexpected factors. Let us therefore face the future with the hope and confidence which befit men who believe that creation is not without a plan, and that the grand trend of evolution is toward better things.

"New times demand new measures and new
    men;

The world advances, and in time outgrows
The laws that in our fathers' days were
    best."

Department of Physiologic Chemistry.

WITH SPECIAL REFERENCE TO DIETETICS AND NUTRITION IN GENERAL.

A WAITING OPPORTUNITY.

AN OPEN LETTER TO MONEYED AMERICANS.

To-DAY wealth is increasing more rapidly than ever before in the world's history.

Once it was a distinction to be known as a millionaire. Now it is too common to elicit a passing remark. It now implies nothing beyond financial mediocrity. There are hundreds of millionaires whose names have never been mentioned in the catalogues of the wealthy, and but for the revelations of the Surrogate's Court would never be made public.

Coincident with the increase in the general wealth of this nation, and the unprecedented massing of individual holdings, the practice of distributing, generally but incorrectly called "giving," has proportionately and by no means always grudgingly increased. The word Charity is rapidly losing all its old signification. It is even acquiring a sinister sense. One of these days it will be written, EQUITY.

In line with the other changed and changing conditions the forms of distributing and selection of fields of distribution have also materially changed. Money and material assistance are not now doled out indiscriminately, and direct to mendicants, beggars and unfortunates as it once was.

Charitable organizations have gradually but positively demonstrated that the old-time impulsive giving is subversive of its primary object and perpetuates the evil it is designed to cure. They have shown that poverty too often degenerates into a profession, and that when genuine it is often the deserved and inevitable result of cultivated shiftlessness and inexcusable faults. This is why benefactions are being diverted into other and new channels.

Hence, the last decade has witnessed a veritable mania for the endowment of colleges and universities, and the founding of hospitals and public libraries.

Carnegie, Rockefeller, Morgan, Gould, Astor, Vanderbilt—these are a few of the successors and eclipsers of Crœsus, whose discretion or whose consciences—an attribute not accredited to him of old—are prompting them to give some account of their stewardship while yet among the living.

It is perhaps natural that their first thought should be of institutions of learning, of literary boards, retreats for invalids, cripples and the injured, and for immense hostelries and homes for the helpless and homeless.

But colleges, universities and even libraries are not and never can be made available to the masses; they are all for the Minority. They are not for the poor but for the rich and the comparatively well-to-do All of them combined fail to reach and remedy the condition of those who most sorely need, elevation, enlightenment and succor. They are above the heads of a large element of that substratum majority, many of whom do not know one letter from another, and would consequently prefer a loaf of bread, a lump of sugar or a pair of shoes to all the volumes in the Astor-Tilden library.

The primary bane, the original and unrelenting handicap of large numbers of the baseborn masses is not so much Illiteracy as Disease. They need Physical Recuperation, Vital Regeneration, rather than financial assistance; Medicine rather than Money. Give them better health, an immunity from the prevalent infections and contagions, and they will become self-helping, will outgrow their need of charity and be less inclined to criminal ways. They must have better physical environment before they can cultivate an ambition to learn. Facilities for enlightenment are second in order.

A man whose wife is slowly dying of consumption, and who is compelled to leave her every morning, to strugggle through the day with the care of a houseful of scrofulous, putty faced, and tubercle-doomed children, while he wields a shovel, pushes a barrow or carries a hod, ten hours for a dollar and a quarter, has little appreciation for free scholarships and the classics.

As society and business are now organized and administered even the moderately well-to-do, when stricken with pulmonary or other wasting disease, have no other recourse but to remain in their own communities and in the midst of their anxious but helpless families, thus further disseminating the seeds of their fatal malady, as it slowly and distressfully saps their existence. By the nature of their maladies the stricken fathers are even debarred from leaving to their dependants an ameliorating pittance in the form of life-insurance.

Pasteur and his confreres, with their microscopes, test-tubes, culture-media, and proving animals,—in a word, Science, has now placed in our hands the necessary knowledge by which nearly all the suffering, physical degeneracy and premature deaths occuring in the world, with most of the prevailing diseases can be either prevented, mitigated or cured. The methods are at last unquestionably within our reach, and neither the Age nor our own consciences will absolve us if we knowingly continue to withold the means, and thereby doom other thousands and expose ourselves to infection and premature death.

The infection can be prevented; the lives can be saved!

Twenty of every hundred human beings, one-fifth of the race, are, to-day, victims of a preventable scourge—Consumption; a plague that can be warded off in advance,

and when incurred can be cured, by proper measures promptly invoked. This "Great White Plague" annually claims *more than three millions of victims.*

These statements are not the haphazard exaggerations of an alarmist; they are statistically demonstrated facts.

And yet, in the face of these facts *the menace of infection is permitted to remain in every community.*

The modern physician girds himself as best he can for the lifelong and unequal combat with suffering and disease; but he is constantly and almost hopelessly hampered and his best efforts wholly balked or seriously restricted by lack of conditions, and lack of ability to command equipment and environment.

Not that all medical men would be philanthropists on a large scale, if it were in their power, for not all are thus endowed; and all have their own private and personal obligations to be met and discharged. Leaving out of consideration the, let us say, comparatively few narrow, selfish, and instinctively mercenary members who misrepresent the profession, of that unenumerated and unobtrusive army of practitioners who patiently devote themselves to an incessant and often poorly paid effort to fittingly respond to the never absent and always pressing demands for help in their immediate vicinity, none succeed in accumulating a sufficiency of the world's material wealth with which to undertake a materialization of their humanitarian ideals. They clearly realize what could be done, but can only dream on while they drudge on, waiting for future workers and dreamers to devise methods and induce means to shape their dreams into realizations.

Much has been essayed and something accomplished in the way of "Health Resorts, "Invalid Retreats," and Sanatoriums;" and much is being written of "Climate-Cures."

But thus far all the efforts have necessarily been rudimentary and subject to limitations. None of them have compassed breadth, scope and breathing room. Besides, all of them have been compelled to shift sail to the unconstant breezes of popular favor and material success.

This is fast merging into a standing reproach to the sagacity and foresight, let alone the magnanimity and benevolence of the age.

The necessary facts concerning the prevention and cure of diseases heretofore intractable are no longer wanting; but as yet no adequate and comprehensive effort has been made toward the realization of a System of either prophylaxis or cure, based on these later and sweeping advances in Physiology, Sanitation, the laws of Contagion, and the possibilities of antiseptic and antitoxic therapy. Scientific and sanitary possibilities have been sacrificed to commercial success.

No sane man will question the motives or criticise the judgment of those who have with such unstinted liberality endowed institutions of learning, libraries, hospitals and laboratories for research. The race can never be made too wise in matters of health. Ignorance is a constant bar to every form of progress and prosperity.

But while we accord all honor to those who have thus munificently founded Homes of Learning, let us not longer fail to remind them that the grandest field of all yet remains untrodden.

Its longer neglect is a constant menace to every citizen of every populous community, regardless of his rank or station, and regardless of his most punctilious precaution. It maintains in a condition of constant jeopardy the inmates alike of hovel and palace. It plants an invisible but deadly viper in every susceptible bosom. It fastens the fangs of an insatiable vampire at the throats of millions of helpless victims by propagating, distributing and perpetuating the seeds of the deadliest contagion known to man. It invites the annual and hourly visitation of the Destroying Angel into the heart of uncounted thousands of homes; and against its uninvited and insidious entrance the costliest time locks of the most favored multi-millionaire are powerless to protect.

It is not content with common sacrifices, but demands the fairest and sweetest lives. It pauses at no threshold. Neither blooming youth, prime manhood nor maturest age is immune. It is unerring and insatiate, so long as its victims are harbored and its sources of incubation and infection continue to be nursed by neglect.

But it is becoming evident that this neglect and omission have been unconscious and not deliberate or premeditated. The attention of those who are in position to cope with the problem of all problems, in its relation to human happiness, has not yet been aptly and definitely engaged.

This is the most obvious shortcoming of the profession.

It can hardly be questioned but that the means to execute has awaited the inspiration to suggest, the brain to plan.

The medical profession will not be blameless if this needed admonition be longer withheld. Recent occurrences that need not be cited furnish abundant evidence that *willing millions await the needed suggestion.*

The leading inheritors and accumulators of wealth have demonstrated by their deeds a profound and intelligent appreciation of the fact that they are but temporary custodians; that unuseful millions are but a bar-sinister on the escutcheon of manhood, a stigma on the face of honor that no distribution of posthumous charity can possibly erase; that they can carry with them no jot of their hoarded possessions when they go out of life; that life is short, and that whatever good they can do for themselves and humanity must be done soon if they themselves would have any hand in selecting its objects or directing its methods.

Of this class, more numerous to-day than at any former period in the world's history, each will contribute toward the particular object that to him or her seems most worthy or more immediately in need; or to that cause to which his or her attention has been most incisively and impressively directed. Some feel constrained to build churches and inaugurate missions; some fit out scientific exploring expeditions; others found colleges, endow professorships or establish whole systems of libraries, such as no age or nation has ever known. Still others erect commodious hospitals for the alleviation of human suffering in our large cities, or provide costly laboratories for the scientific study of health problems.

All these are worthy objects, and it is not at all probable that any one of them will be overdone.

But not one of them is radical and fundamental; all are secondary and palliative. They are reparative, but neither constructive nor preventive.

For example, the hospital: it binds up wounds, alleviates present suffering, looks after the unfortunate victims of accidents and criminal assaults, and subdues or supersedes deformities. All these mitigate; they wipe up the floor, but do not mend the leak in the roof.

Generations, ages, all the centuries have waited for the Opportunity that now presents itself.

Moreover, contradictory as it may seem, in embracing it the broadest philanthropy can go hand in hand with the supremest selfishness; because it is a case in which *he who saves others saves himself.*

To longer neglect the peril of the masses is to partake of their peril. No one is wholly immune until all are immune. A selfishness that binds itself to this phase of the situation is simply suicidal.

This is the unmistakable attitude of science, and it is daily and hourly becoming more clearly defined. It amounts to an ultimatum promulgated from the inner temple by the Goddess of Health. Ancient Greece and Rome ignorantly or wilfully ignored it, and went to swift ruin. The Children of Israel trampled it under their feet and soon had no soil of their own on which to plant their feet.

It remains to be seen whether a nation that has never had a compeer, whose wealth is boundless, and whose enterprise knows no restrictions, will heedlessly invite the same fate.

The object and necessity being fully realized, it need not take long to decide as to means and working methods.

The first requisite is *environment.*

This involves everything that is afforded by climate, soil, altitude and all terrestrial influences.

The second is *isolation.*

But this must not be made to mean banishment to some forlorn desert, where loneliness and desolation will add their depressing influence to the destruction already begun by disease.

It is now the privilege and duty of free America to inaugurate a history-marking epoch in the progress of sanatory science.

What more fitting or more in accordance with her aggressive enterprise than that the New World should take the initiative in this forward step. It is here that human thought becomes impatient of the restraints of precedent. It is here that the champions of human freedom first dared to freely breathe the unmeasured air and bask in the unclouded sunlight of heaven; here that the human soul first sundered its inherited bonds and learned to use its stifled voice; and here that the human intellect first dared to think, act, invent and advance, unhampered by the iron laws of despotism. Here innovation had its birthplace and here it maintains its nurtured ground.

Not for a moment relaxing her vigilance nor losing her prestige, America must remain in the forefront and give to the world the needed impulse which will finally culminate in the establishment of a mental and physical freedom, and a standard of physical perfection and immunity as far in advance of all existing models as the principles of true democracy and the law of equal rights are in advance of the unjust and arbitrary canons of monarchism.

This does not call for a multiplication of "sanatoria," on the plan of existing models; nor for massive hospitals and "health" hostelries, each sheltering a thousand invalids, who inhale each others' breath and imbibe each others' infection.

The unmistakable demand of sense, science and the hour is for *sanatory reservations, invalid preserves, recuperative retreats*—call them by whatever name you will, so that they are broadly based, favorably located and intelligently arranged and administered in the light that now shines, and in the light that is sure to be evolved by the coming years.

The sanatorium system has had its mission; has been a pioneer in demonstrating the value of the numerous localities and of systematized effort; but it lacks scope, and has its definite limitations and fatal drawbacks. Because of these it can never rise above the sphere of patchwork and palliation. It is based on *congregation,* whereas *segregation* is the primal and indispensable necessity.

The waiting opportunity calls for the sequestration of a large tract of land in each of the more favored and convenient localities of the country, each of which is to be transformed into a colony of convalescents, a salutary retreat for physical degenerates.

Abandoning the fatal practice of concentration, each site should include thousands of acres, whole townships or even a fair-sized county. Nothing short of this will give science full swing and secure the needed breathing space, so that sanitation and segregation can be made complete and effective.

The first step is to acquire the sites, while lands appropriate for the purpose and in the proper localities can be had at nominal cost. The various States and the nation may need to be invoked in order to secure all the lands required. Sites should be secured, not singly but in series, including every variety, from seashore to mountain heights, and from the Adirondacks and the mountains of North Carolina to Montana, Colorado and Southern California. Then, every class of chronic invalids can be favorably located, and every climatic condition made available.

Evolved strictly in accordance with our advanced knowledge of sanitary requirements, each of these reservations or retreats can be developed into a co-operative colony and in time may be made partly, if not wholly, self-supporting. Resort to it will involve virtual banishment, since, when that seems desirable entire families can be entertained and kept intact. Not technically ideal; there are many cases in which any other course would be impracticable and inadvisable. It would reduce the number of the exposed to a minimum, and would supply facilities so adequate that henceforth no case of tubercular disease need be compelled to remain at the site of its inception to slowly but irresistibly proceed on its downward course, while at the same time insidiously distributing the fatally infective germs of its malady to all within the circle of its contact. Every case, as soon as diagnosed, could be placed in surroundings most favorable for its arrest and cure, and thus be withdrawn from contact with the general community and from those who might at any moment become susceptible to the infection.

This is what science-to-date demands, and nothing short of this will satisfy her or absolve those who have it in their power to inaugurate this all-important and waiting movement.

It is neither necessary nor opportune to suggest details as to locations and general plans. Nor should the undertaking offer any encouragement for individual aggrandizement. The country is rich in the possession of inviting and unobjectionable sites, and the plans can be safely referred to competent sanitary engineers, under the surveillance of those who have made climate-cure a feature of their therapeutic investigations. An undiscovered Waring is sure to appear when his hour arrives!

SIR WILLIAM LONG tells a story of an old Scotch lady who could not abide long sermons. She was hobbling out of kirk one Sunday, when a coachman, who was waiting for his people, asked her:

"Is the minister dune wi' his sermon?"

"He was dune lang syne," said the old lady, impatiently, "but he winna stop."

COOKING OATMEAL.

A FEW medical men may still be found who will neither use oatmeal themselves nor advise it for their patients. They perhaps admit that it is the most nutritious and dietetically desirable of all the cereals, but for the fact that it is not always well borne by weak stomachs. They admit that the Scotch yeomen were noted for physical vigor and as athletes, but they assert that even the Scotch who lived on oatmeal porridge were subject to waterbrash and sour stomach, from eating so much "horse fodder."

They haven't taken the trouble to discover that the trouble has all been with the cook. Even the Highlanders who lived on groats only about half cooked them; but they had stomachs that were almost as competent as that of a horse, which does not require that its oats shall even be hulled, to say nothing of cooking. Those who in any way acquired a dyspeptic habit no doubt suffered from waterbrash and other stomach troubles. The average civilized stomach requires that all starch-bearing cereals shall be thoroughly cooked. To such stomachs half-cooked oatmeal is about as indigestible as corn husks. Every doctor knows this in a theoretical way, but the "few" referred to seem to overlook the fact.

There are two ways of cooking oatmeal, and a dozen ways of half-cooking it. Too many people adopt one of the latter and never know the luxury of one of the finest dishes that is ever brought to the table.

First of all, there are oatmeals, and oatmeals, and oatmeals. The different brands in the market are counted not merely by scores but by hundreds. This shows the popularity of the food. There is but one tone of advice to be given, and that is to *get the best in the market.* There are several good brands, and connoiseurs in cereals are inclined to have their preferences. A few manufacturers rigidly maintain the grade of their product. Too many of them put out excellent samples, advertise extensively, and when they have acquired a name, at once begin to flood the market with in-ferior goods, for the sake of temporary gains. Some patrons are silly enough to continue the use of the deteriorated article, thinking it is the best in the market, because it was once so.

The American Cereal Company puts out no less than seventeen distinct preparations from the oat. It is no doubt an effort to cater to the varying tastes and prejudices of the public. At the head of their list— we mention this company because it is the largest manufacturer of cereals in the world —stands Quaker Oats. Whatever merits other brands may claim this one has strictly adhered to its original standard of quality. With discriminating housewives and cooks it has become a standard, for the reason that as yet no inferior goods have been offered under this label. If Quaker Oats as brought to the breakfast table are not both toothsome and digestible it is the fault of the cook and not of the product.

The first method of cooking this food may be called the primitive way. The meal is slowly stirred into rapidly boiling water until a thick porridge is made, and this is kept over a hot fire and constantly stirred until thoroughly done. The time required is a full half hour. If not thick enough it will be sloppy and too much on the order of "spoon victuals." If made too thick it will not be thoroughly cooked. The good cook acquires a "knack" of getting it just right, a knack for which no rules can ever be put into words. The stirring required is really an objection to the method, since it changes the consistency of the mush and injures its flavor.

The second method and the one to be universally recommended is to stir the meal into rapidly boiling water as before, but to use a double boiler, and to do no more stirring than is absolutely necessary at the outset, to prevent the formation of lumps. The water in the outer vessel is then to be kept actively boiling until the process is complete, which will vary with the size of the vessel, the quality of the oatmeal, and with *the altitude above sea-level.* For most people this latter point has no significance, since the boiling point of water varies but little except in high altitudes. Those who have tried to cook white beans in mountain camps will appreciate the remark. Half an hour will suffice for ordinary stomachs, but the dish will be much improved by giving it more time. For invalids and weak stomachs it will be the better if kept at the boiling or simmering point for three or four hours.

Few cooks have the time or patience to thoroughly cook oatmeal by the first method described. Not one in a hundred gives it time enough, and the hundredth burns it on the bottom of the kettle. Frequently the entire mass is injured in flavor by the burning process.

Theoretically pre-roasted oats would seem to be ideal, but in practice they do not seem to have been made a success. In case of wheat the "Parched Farinose" is much preferable to other preparations of this grain. Perhaps the same manufacturers will finally give us Parched Groats or Parched Avinose, answering to Parched Farinose. It ought to be an ideal preparation, and would simplify the process of cooking oatmeal.

We have dwelt thus at length on this subject in response to numerous and repeated requests.

We shall be glad to hear from any of our subscribers who can add to our advice or who are in the least inclined to criticize it.

ALUM IN FOOD.

THE following very sensible remarks on this topic are from the columns of the *New York Tribune*s

There is before the Legislature of the State of New York a bill prohibiting the sale of baking-powders containing alum. There are similar bills before several other State Legislatures. One State at least, Missouri, already has a law prohibiting the manufacture or sale of alum baking-powder. A recent attempt to repeal this law failed.

Dr. William H. Thomson, President of the Academy of Medicine, said: "The use of alum baking-powders is very injurious. I am positive of this. It has a tendency especially to produce rickets."

Dr. Abraham Jacobi said: "Alum baking-powders are harmful. There is no doubt about it."

Dr. George F. Shrady said: "Alum used in food in any way is deleterious. This is the opinion of the medical profession."

Dr. Louis F. Bishop, Secretary of the Academy of Medicine, said: "Bread made with alum baking-powder is almost certain to have alum in it, often considerable quantities. All admit that alum in food is injurious, and the best authorities state that bread made with alum is harmful, even if there is no alum left in the bread after baking, the residue of alum being itself injurious, or being reconstituted into alum in the stomach. Consequently, physicians generally believe that the manufacture and sale of alum baking-powder should be prohibited by law."

Dr. Ralph Waldo, the noted surgeon, said: "I think that alum baking-powder ought not to be used at all."

Dr. J. E. Winters, one of the foremost authorities in the country on children's diseases and Professor of Children's Diseases in Cornell University, said: "If Professor Vaughan, of Ann Arbor, says that alum baking-powders are injurious, and I understand that he does, you need go no further. What he says is practically certain to be correct. He would not make such a statement unless he was sure of his ground. Alum is a powerful astringent. It is simply impossible to introduce it into the system by means of a staple article of food without doing harm. It would be sure to cause serious injury to the digestive organs, which in turn brings on various other diseases."

Prof. Charles F. Chandler, of the Columbia School of Mines, the great chemist, said: "This is a subject that has been much investigated and written about by chemists and hygienists. It is the general impression among chemists and hygienists that alum baking-powder should not be used. While a person in a 'brutal' state of health might eat bread made with alum baking-powder and experience no ill effect, yet those not in perfect health might be seriously injured by it. In doubtful cases the stomach should always have the benefit of the doubt. There is no object in using alum baking-powder. There are others cheap enough and entirely free from any suspicion of being harmful. For that reason I would never allow alum baking-powder used in my house.

Dr. Cyrus Edson, formerly of the Board of Health, said: "Alum has two effects. First, it renders the flour more difficult to digest, and, second, it has an injurious effect upon the stomach, as it diminishes the flow of gastric juice, the fluid which digests the food. There is no question that taking alum in bread, frequently and for a long time, even in very minute quantities, would prove very injurious."

A mass of testimony has appeared before the public recently going to show that adulteration, including the use in food of injurious drugs, and the sale of injurious articles to be used in food have assumed vast proportions, and there is not the slightest doubt that as a result millions of people suffer injury to their health, many of whom die in consequence. In many cases the government can furnish the best protection, and in some cases the only adequate protection, against these impositions. Unless each family employs a chemist and his each separate can, bottle, or package of food material tested, it is impossible for them to know whether the food or articles they buy to use in food, are wholesome or injurious, except in those cases where the brand or name of the manufacturer is a guarantee of purity.

That there is nothing more important to people than their health goes without saying; consequently, to prevent the sale of things injurious to health is among the most important duties of legislators as well as of judicial and executive officers.

The people should demand that efficient laws for the suppression of this evil be passed and that they be stringently enforced. It is to be hoped that the various State Legislatures will put upon the statute books effective laws to this end.

VEGETARIANISM.

THAT epitome of dignified and astute conservatism, the *British Med. Journal*, puts the case after this fashion.

In an interesting paper recently published, Professor Ferdinand Hueppe discussed the question whether vegetarianism can be supported on scientific grounds. He considers that geological evidence proves that the cradle of primitive man was in a northern land, and fixes his evolution in the tertiary period when Asia was still partly separated from Europe, but connected with Africa and united with America by a land bridge. The human-growing anthropoid, owing to hard times, left the forests and became a beast of prey, probably the most cunning and ferocious that has ever stalked on the face of the earth. In the interglacial period man was a mammoth hunter. The Danish kitchen middens show that the primitive Europeans were fish and flesh eaters. The Asiatic stock, meanwhile, evolved into shepherds and began to cultivate cereals in the alluvial plains of the great rivers. The irruption of Asiatics into Europe brought about the introduction of cereals and domesticated animals, and a mixed diet became usual. With the overgrowth of population in the East vegetarianism arose, and man took to rice eating, not from desire, but through the scarcity of animal food. The Eskimo remains to this day an example of a pure flesh-eater. The anthropoid stock from which man evolved fed on nuts, fruit, eggs, small birds and insects. Such is still the mixed diet of the ape, as well as of the Arabs of this age. Owing to the struggle for existence man has evolved into a flesh-eater, a mixed feeder, and lastly into a vegetarian, but vegetarianism became possible to him only by the introduction of fire and cooking. He has neither the teeth nor the gut of a herbivorous animal; otherwise he would naturally graze the fields, and in winter chew oats in a manger. It has been abundantly proved by breeders of pigs and other animals that the best proportion of albumen to carbohydrates in the diet is 1:5. Among the Eskimo it is found to be 1:29, among Europeans on a mixed diet 1:5.3. The Irish peasant, on the other hand, consumes, or used to consume, a diet containing ten times as much carbohydrate as albumen (1:10.6), and in a Munich vegetarian Voit found the proportion to be 1:11. A diet such as that of the Irish peasant increases the death-rate in the young and the old; that is to say among those in whom the excess of carbohydrate cannot be burnt off by hard bodily labor. Such a diet can be consistently borne only by a man bred to it from infancy, and accustomed to the doing of hard work. There is no advantage in vegetarianism as a working diet. The same amount of potential energy (33 per cent.) consumed as food appears as work in the carnivorous dog, the herbivorous horse, and the omnivorous man. No vegetarian animal, not even the horse, ox, camel, or elephant, can carry the weight of his own body. The carnivorous lion, on the other hand, gripping a calf equal to himself in weight, can jump a hurdle 6 feet high. The lifting power of man, the mixed feeder, exceeds that of any other mammal. Louis Cyr is recorded to have lifted 1,669 kg., Little carried 600 kg. fifteen steps, a Tyrolese in six hours carried 110 kg. to an altitude of 1,500 m. A man of 75 kg., working in the docks will, many times in the course of one day's work, carry sacs weighing 100 kg. The diet of the vegetarian. reckoned in calories, is found to value 86 calories per kg. of body weight, and the proteid is worth only 6 per cent. of this. The man on a mixed diet, on the other hand, eats only 39 calories per kg. of body weight, and the proteid equals 14 per cent. of this. The vegetarian is like an overheated steam engine which is in danger of explosion owing to the use of a wrong kind of

fuel. His digestive system is forced to deal with a far greater bulk of food and energy which might be used for the higher purposes of mental activity is wasted. Only in the condition of hard manual labor in the open air can a purely vegetarian diet be borne. Of course, he who consumes milk, eggs, butter and cheese cannot be considered a vegetarian. Vegetarianism does not, as is sometimes suggested, lead to a mild and gentle spirit, for the wild buffalo, the rhinosceros, and the rice-eating Chinese pirate are alike remarkable for ferocity and cunning. Finally the vegetarian is exposed to as many chances of poisoning as the flesh eater. The vegetarians of our time, Professor Hueppe tells us, belong to the class of neurotic men who, failing to meet the strain of town life, ever seek for a "heal-all" in one or other crank. Their doctrines, pushed with fanatic zeal, make no impression on the healthy, and only tend to overthrow the balance of others who, like themselves, are the victims of an unnatural mode of existence.

CARELESSNESS IN THE INTERDICTION OF STAPLE FOODS.

On this important topic *American Medicine* has this to say:

"Of all the advice which the physician has to give his patient, in many cases, the most valuable is his advice as to diet. Instances not infrequently occur, however, of specialists, who in their endeavor to *"reconstitutionalize"* their patients, as the elder Jackson of Dansville fame was wont to put it, broadly condemn in a most unwarranted way some one or more of the most healthful of foods.

"Sweeping generalizations as to the harmfulness of widely used foods and beverages, such as wheat flour, milk, and coffee, are too often made by physicians and as a result there have arisen numberless attempts to replace these great staples with substitutes more or less inferior to the article condemned, and in many cases actually harmful through active ingredients,or from the omission of valuable constituents found in the natural product.

"The time is nigh when the fad for substitutes and modifications of natural foods will pass, and the effort of the physician will be largely confined to the securing of purity and conformity of standard. The harmfulness of the great universal food stuffs lies rather in the methods of use than in constitution.

"Notwithstanding the astounding increase in the consumption of wheat among the nations of the earth, and in face of the fact that the dominant races are wheat eaters, we constantly find persons of more than ordinary intelligence in most things who have been needlessly frightened into the disuse of this prince of foods. To account for the taboo placed upon wheat, the most specious and contradictory reasons are given.

"In a recent case a specialist of prominence, in one of our great medical centers, forbade his patient the use of wheaten bread on the ground 'that wheat contains such a large amount of silica that it hardens the arterial walls.' There are many cases in which the use of wheat or other starchy foods might be wisely forbidden and for valid reasons intelligible to anyone conversant with the rudiments of the physiology and chemistry of digestion; but, if reasons must be given the patient for such interdicton, what excuse can there be for an attempt to satisfy his inquiring mind with this sort of twaddle. In the case noted, the sand was surely in the possession of the learned exponent of well-living rather than in the wheat flour. Silicic acid, the solluble colloid form of silica, though present in minute proportions in wheat, is not likely to be absorbed to the extent of warranting any fear of silicious arterial sclerosis. Adverse opinions regarding common articles of food soon become widespread and serve as the basis for foisting upon the confiding public all sorts of 'green-gourd substitutes' for those foods which most nearly represent the staff of life. There is room for the dietist, but he should handle the taboo with discretion

and with reference to the individual case, and beware how he imposes on the public misleading notions as to the general injurious nature of common foodstuffs."

THE ENZYMS.

THE term enzym according to an editorial in the *Medical Times* has been given to the unorganized or chemical compounds of vegetable or animal origin which cause fermentation, as pepsin or rennet.

The enzyms have rightly been called soluble ferments, but what they are and how this work is accomplished is an enigma which has never been fully solved, notwithstanding the vast amount of study which has been bestowed upon them.

Professor Kestle, of the Texas Academy of Science, expresses the idea that they are the residuum of the vital force of the living cell. It is demonstrated that they are albumenous and contain phosphorous, and probably iron, in addition to carbon, hydrogen, oxygen and nitrogen, and occur in every living animal or vegetable cell.

Without undergoing any chemical change themselves, they seem to have the power of breaking down complex chemical substances to an extraordinary extent.

Thus far over fifty varieties of enzyms have been named, some of them of great physiological importance, such as pepsin, found in the gastric juice; ptyalin, found in the saliva, and trypsin, found in the pancreatic secretions. Trypsin occurs not only in the digestive fluid of the intestines, but is found also in the pine-apple, as pepsin, found in the stomach, is also obtained from the papaya, and, as papoid of vegetable pepsin, is used in indigestion with even greater benefit than the pepsin. Wherever the enzym is found, either in the vegetable or animal world, its action upon complex chemical substances seems to be the same, and is one of the principal elements of what is called digestion.

Professor Harper, in a paper read before

the Cincinnati section of the American Chemical Society, advances the theory that the enzym action is to be accounted for, not by the chemical interaction of molecule with molecule, but by the molecular vibration of the enzym molecule itself. If we grant the existence of molecules we must grant the existence of molecular vibrations, and from this the existence of ether waves spreading out from these vibrating molecules. If these ether vibrations correspond in period with the vibrations of the molecules of the fermentable substances, then fermentation ensues by sympathetic vibration, and, of course, the enzym is not destroyed in the process.

According to this theory, and we must remember it is a theory only, the enzym action is not due to the enzym substance, but to the energy radiating from the substance, and it is therefore comparable to light or electricity.

VIEWS ON VEGETARIANISM.

THE GAZETTE invites views from all sides. Here is another view of vegetarianism, being an editorial from the *Medical Age*.

The advocates of exclusively vegetarian diet are not so numerous as they used to be, and it is interesting to note the change of opinions which has resulted from more extended knowledge of the effects produced by restricted dietaries. This change of opinion was well reflected in a recent discussion of the matter before the Berlin Medical Society, in which many leading clinicians and investigators participated.

Rosenheim declared an exclusively vegetarian diet harmful because it contained an insufficient amount of albumen, and led to diminished resistance in infections, besides which the persons who strictly observed it could not do the normal amount of work. He had renounced the strictly vegetable for a lacto-vegetable regimen, one which included milk, butter, and eggs. This diet he

employed with advantage in gastric ulcer and in patients who exhibited a distaste for meat. In constipation it was not unwise to recur to an exclusively vegetable diet with plenty of fruit and nuts.

Gravitz thought that exclusively vegetable alimentation was of much use in neurasthenia, diminishing fermentation in the digestive tract.

Schonstadt regarded a vegetarian diet as in the nature of a graduated fast, and ending in an ultimate loss of strength. In order to maintain nutrition it would be necessary to take 1,740 grammes of bread, while it was difficult to obtain consumption of more than 800 grammes. He recorded how in 1854 a bad epidemic of scurvy occurred in a prison in Waltenburg, in which the prisoners had an exclusively vegetarian diet; the epidemic disappeared on the resumption of a mixed diet.

Furbringer thought many of the good effects of vegetarianism were due to suggestion. He employed exclusive diets in obesity, sexual neurasthenia, and in alcoholism. For nephritis a lacto-vegetable dietary was the best.

Meyer, who had experimented on himself thought that exclusive vegetarianism exalted the gastric acidity.

Ewald did not deny that certain individuals could exist on an exclusive diet, but claimed that for these a special digestive apparatus was a necessity.

Hanchecorn pointed out that in all zoological groups the carniverous animals are superior in force and intelligence to the herbivorous.

Exclusive vegetarianism will therefore in all probability in the near future be relegated to the limbo of defunct theories, mankind being nevertheless the wiser if not the happier for having tried it.

Upon the development of a scientific biology depends the future of medicine.—*Otto Bergmeister* (Vienna).

OUGHT THE STARCHES TO BE ELIMINATED FROM THE NOURISHMENT OF VERY YOUNG CHILDREN?

Borde, although admitting that mother's milk ought normally to form the nourishment of the infant, still, when this is impossible to procure, believes that aqueous solutions of starches should be combined with cow's milk for feeding. These decoctions are soothing to the intestine. They are also nutritious. In the starches he includes the starch of the potato, tapioca, starch of wheat, arrow-root, etc., also the decoctions of rice, barley, oatmeal, etc. He emphasizes the advisability of making these decoctions with water, not believing in their efficacy when cooked with milk. But milk can be mixed with the prepared decoctions with benefit. He concludes that: Aqueous decoctions of starch are digested by very young infants; they do not irritate the intestines, but exert a soothing influence, preventing the acute infectious gastro-enteritis of s u m m e r; they also aid in curing these affections by replacing advantageously cow's milk and even mother's milk during the acute stage of these maladies. These foods are very nutritious, preventing rachitis and chronic digestive troubles in the babe brought up on cow's milk; the best of these is oats coarsely ground, which contain, besides the starches, albumen and assimilable vegetable phosphates, very useful in the dietary of the child. These starches should first be cooked in water and the resulting product mixed with milk.—*Gazette Hebdomadaire des Sciences Médicales de Bordeaux*, April 28, 1901.

THE HEN AND HER EGGS.

The common hen lays about 500 or 600 eggs in ten years. In the first year the number is only 10 to 20; in the second, third and fourth 100 to 135 each, whence it again diminishes to 10 in the last year.

INFANT FEEDING.

John J. Hanley, in the *Medical Council*, makes a plea for the baby. The article is addressed to mothers who can and will not nurse, and to physicians who can restore an ancient and commendable practice by preaching it.

He says that mothers should suckle their young:

Because it is a natural obligation.

Because it is a moral (religious) one.

Because it is a pleasure.

Because it is the most beautiful living picture in the world.

Because it charms a man to see it.

Because it is a sermon in tableau.

Because of its refining and softening influence on the higher emotions.

Because the child wants to.

Because it has a right to.

Because it is "open day and night".

Because it is "always ready."

Because it doesn't need to be sweetened or heated.

Because it is the only ideal infant food.

Because it is not a perfect substitute, but the "real thing."

Because there is no perfect substitute.

Because the baby likes it (not important).

Because it doesn't make him "tired."

Because it doesn't have to be sterilized.

Because you don't have to cudgel your brains about the proportion of milk-sugar and lime water and other confusing things.

Because you serve the State better.

Because it is cheaper (you get it for nothing).

Because you don't have to read chemical analysis of various celebrities on the containers, declaring the extraordinary skill and knowledge in producing such wonderful rubbish as some milks are.

Because you don't have to get out of bed at night to get "the other" ready.

Because you can "modify" it by your diet and hygiene.

Because Nature is a better chemist than you are.

Because you don't have "to run" a chemical laboratory in the house.

Because you will feel better yourself.

Because the mutual love will be greater.

Because your husband will prefer it (or ought to).

Because all true mothers do it.

Because you will show good example to other women.

Because the baby will be physically stronger to fight for its existence both in health and sickness.

Because it is the same as mother and grandma "used to make," a strong recommendation daily observed.

WHAT TO EAT IN SUMMER.

BY MRS. MOSES P. HANDY.

THE selection of the daily bill of fare, always a more or less difficult duty for housekeepers, becomes doubly so during the heated term. Appetites are capricious; dishes devoured one day may be sent away untasted the next, and the conscientious mistress of a household stands perplexed between the Scylla of wastefulness on one side, and the Charybdis of niggardliness on the other. The praiseworthy economy practiced at King Arthur's court, where

"What they could not eat that day
The Queen next morning fried";

becomes an impossible virtue; things will not keep, and the most capacious of ice-chests will scarcely avail to preserve cooked food from one day to another. Warmed-over summer vegetables are almost invariably flat, stale, and unprofitable; while fruit kept upon ice quickly loses its freshness, and ergo its wholesomeness. To eat is a weariness to the flesh, and yet there is a prevailing sense of emptiness which clamors to be filled.

Nature is in most cases a law unto herself, and for every season she provides convenient food. In winter, when the fires of the system need keeping up, game is abundant, fat, and easily tracked; in summer, on the contrary, fruits and vegetables abound, and point to the expediency of a vegetable diet.

The school of medicine, of which Dio Lewis was the first apostle, which reduces the science of health to a system of diet and exercise, with abundant bathing, declares that no meats, excepting lamb and chicken, should be eaten in hot weather; to which list however they add fresh fish. Certain it is that much meat is unnecessary for even laboring men with the mercury among the nineties. The lazy West-Indian negro grows fat on conchs and bananas; the East-Indian coolie toils all day long on his rations of rice. The hardy Arab conquered the world on a diet of dates and barley-bread, and ceased to be the terror of Europe only when he found such fare too simple for his taste. Oatmeal and milk for breakfast; bread and eggs with fruit, for luncheon; soup and vegetables, with little or no meat, for dinner; this is the diet on which one is able to work best, and keep in best condition, during hot weather.

The Philadelphia Board of Health, in its instructions how best to avoid disease in summer, condemns the use of stimulants in any form, and emphasizes the fact that temperance is the best insurance against fevers of all sorts, besides aiding the chances of recovery in case of attack. A glass of cold milk or lemonade will be found much more refreshing in mid-summer, than one of beer, or a mint julep, and leave no disagreeable after-effects.

While fresh fruit may, in most cases, be freely indulged in, much of the mortality arising from summer diseases is due, more or less directly to the use of unripe, or still worse, stale fruit. This is especially the case with children, both because they are more sensitive to disease, and because they lack judgment as to the quantity and quality of the fruit they eat. Green apples are a stock subject with the humorous newspaper paragrapher; they are also a source of anxiety to every careful country mother. The old-fashioned rule is not to eat an apple until the seeds are black; but children are apt to be color-blind where apple seeds are concerned. Cooked apples are, however, among the most useful articles in the summer store of the housewife, the tart, green apple being far superior to the ripe for baking, as well as for pies and sauce.

Fresh tomatoes are anti-bilious, and thus not only wholesome for healthy people, but may be used with advantage in many cases of fever. Dio Lewis used to say that he expected to see the day when tomatoes would take their place in the pharmacopœia, among established remedies for fever. Fresh tomatoes, gathered from the vine before the sun is on them, are excellent for dyspeptics. They should be eaten without seasoning, or at most with a little salt.

When in doubt as to the freshness of any food, throw it away, the waste may be deplorable, but it is much worse to attempt to prevent it by running the risk of sickness, not to say death, from the use of unwholesome food.

The ice chest is well nigh a necessity in hot weather, yet unless it is carefully attended to, will prove a source of danger. Anything, however little, which is allowed to spoil in the refrigerator will develop into a very nest of germs. The Jewish law which forbids that milk and butter shall be kept in the same place with meat, is like most of their dietetic rules, a wise one; milk especially, absorbs impurities readily, and should always be kept covered. The ice should be wrapped in a blanket, unless kept in a compartment to itself, and never allowed to touch the meat it is used to preserve. When ice is scarce, butter may be kept firm by means of evaporation. Set the bowl or crock containing it in a dish, with cold water, to the depth of an inch, and cover with a linen cloth (cheese-cloth is next best to linen, letting the ends of the cloth come down, and tuck in the water, under the bowl. Capillary attraction keeps the cloth wet, and the evaporation keeps the butter firm. The water should be changed twice a day, and the cloth kept clean and sweet.—*What to Eat.*

LEARNED ROT.

HERE is a sample of some of the scientific twaddle that gets started by some learned pundit, goes the rounds of the medical journals, and finally crops out in the daily press to frighten people who never think—far worse than nothing. It is from the *Munchiner Medinische Wochenschrift;* the author must have suffered from water on the brain!

"*Pure Water Harmful.*—Distilled water, or chemically pure water, is harmful, even poisonous, when introduced into the digestive tract. The addition of salt to enemas, and water used for lavage of the stomach, has become a general practice because of the knowledge that otherwise the delicate cells of the epithelial lining are apt to break down, as do the blood corpuscles, in pure water: For the same reason, 'physiologic' salt solution is employed in nasal irrigation. The destruction of these cells is due to the abnormal endosmotic entrance of watery fluid, and consequent gorging and rupture, because of the unequal specific gravities of the interior and exterior fluids. Hence, when distilled,-ice-, or boiled water are used as beverages, under a mistaken idea of their greater purity and wholesomeness, the unavoidable consequence is peptic disturbances eventuating in gastro-intestinal catarrh. A spring at Gastein, Germany, has from time immemorial borne the name of *giftbrunnen, i. e.,* 'poison spring.' the only successful charge brought against its waters being that they are unusally free from mineral constituents."

FOOD VALUE AND DIGESTIBILITY OF THE BANANA.

IN a communication to *Domestic Science Monthly,* Aug. F. Knudson contradicts certain statements that have been going the rounds of the medical journals for some months past. He says: "All I know about the banana is mostly my own personal experience. I know that Von Humboldt calls it the most nutritious of all foods, and the most productive, area for area, of all man's foodstuffs. I know by experience that one can live on ripe, uncooked bananas for an indefinite period. I have lived on them for weeks at a time and was perfectly nourished.

"In India the banana is looked upon as one of the best foods that can be wished; and in the Hawaiian Islands it used to be considered the most nourishing and the best food for women in delicate health. My own experience is that it is a very easily assimilated food.

"One strange feature is that any alcohol in the stomach causes a very rapid fermentation, and almost poisons the unfortunate drinker. This accounts for the universal bad name the banana has in India. Singapore, and other tropical countries where there is so much liquor consumed.

"The chemical reason for the change I do not know, but I think it is a universal fact."

WASTE IN THE KITCHEN.

In cooking meats the water is thrown away without removing the grease, or the grease from the dripping pan is thrown away.

Scraps of meat are thrown away.

Cold potatoes are left to sour and spoil.

Dried fruits are not looked after and become wormy.

Vinegar and sauce are left standing in tin.

Apples are left to decay for want of sorting over.

The tea canister and coffee box are left open.

Bones of meat and the carcass of turkey are thrown away, when they could be used in making good soups.

Sugar, tea, coffee and rice are carelessly spilled in handling.

Soap is left to dissolve and waste in water.

Dish towels are used for dish cloths, napkins for dish towels and towels for holders.

Brooms and mops are not hung up.

More coal is burned than necessary by not closing dampers when the fire is not used.

Lights are left burning when not in use.

Tin dishes are not properly cleaned and dried.

Good new brooms are used to scrub kitchen floors.

Silver spoons are used in scraping kettles.

Mustard is left to spoil in the cruse.

Vinegar is left to stand until the tin vessel becomes corroded and spoiled.

Pickles become spoiled by the leaking out or evaporation of the vinegar.

Pork spoils for want of salt, and beef because the brine needs scalding.

Cheese is allowed to mould or be nibbled by mice.

Woodenware is left unscalded and left to warp and crack.

These may seem small leaks, but in the aggregate the loss is considerable.

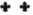

SUCRAMINE, A NEW SWEETENING AGENT.

This substance has been placed on the market by a chemical firm under the name of *sucramine* or *"sucre de Lyon."* It is easily soluble in water, insoluble in alcohol, ether, etc., neutral in reaction, leaves no residue on combustion in air, and is supposed to be 700 times as sweet as sugar. The author found that sucramine presents all the chemical characteristics of saccharine, except as regards solubility. This indicates that sucramine is a salt of saccharine. Yet, as it leaves no residue on calcination, the base is not a fixed one. On boiling an aqueous solution of sucramine with magnesia a great deal of ammonia is given off, and sucramine is, therefore, probably the ammonia salt of saccharine. The manufacturers also offer what they call *"sucre double sucramine"* (double sucramined sugar) in pieces of 1 gm. each, equivalent to a lump of sugar weighing 5 gms., and whose power of sweetening is ten times that of sugar. The author found this compound to be ordinary sugar, with the addition of 2 per cent. of the ammonium salt of saccharine.—*M. J. Bellier.*

THE DREARY MONOTONY OF HOTEL AND RESTAURANT COOKING.

THE editor of *American Medicine* voices the plaint of uncounted thousands who manage to exist without realizing the comforts of home and the gastronomic luxury of home cooking. (This does not refer to husbands who are in the habit of being domestically basted).

This is the plaint:

There is no country in which the menus of hotels, dining cars, and restaurants, contain so many items, and yet there is none in which there is such a monotonous and tiresome sameness. From Maine to California, from Florida to Wisconsin, the same choice of foods is offered, all cooked and served in the same way. But a few years ago one found some variety the "spice of life" and of cookery, in the old-fashioned dishes of New England, the baked beans and brown bread, the hulled corn, the baked Indian pudding, etc., but now these things are not to be had anywhere, or if the names greet one, the things themselves are disappointing travesties of the olden toothsome delights. It is the same with the indigenous dishes of all other parts of the country. The refrigerator car makes possible the dull uniformity of the menu, and fashion stupidly demands that the palatable things of one part of the country shall be perhaps ignored where they are fresh, and transported 1,000 or 2,000 miles where they are out of season and stale. It has been said that whether one smoke good or bad tobacco, or indeed whether one's cigar be lit or not, is a matter of indifference to the smoker sitting in the darkness. To the blind man it must be "all one" wherever he dines. Is it useless to appeal to chefs, cooks and caterers for the native dishes of the country, cooked as the natives cook them? Individualism is as good for health in the culinary as in the sociologic art.

TALK HEALTH.

Talk happiness. The world is sad enough
Without your woes. No path is wholly
   rough;
Look for the places that are smooth and
   clear,
And speak of those to rest the weary ear
Of earth, so hurt by one continuous strain
Or human discontent and grief and pain.
Talk faith. The world is better off without
Your uttered ignorance and morbid doubt.
If you have faith in God, or man, or self,
Say so; if not, push back upon the shelf
Of silence all your thoughts till faith shall
   come;
No one will grieve because your lips are
   dumb.
Talk health. The dreary, never changing
   tale
Of mortal maladies is worn and stale.
You cannot charm, or interest, or please,
By harping on that minor chord, disease.
Say you are well, or all is well with you.
And God shall hear your words and make
   them true.—Ella Wheeler Wilcox.

SEARCHLIGHT FISH.

MANY deep-sea fish carry searchlights. One species, called the chiasmodon, emits a strong, white light. Another glows with a rich, golden light, like a small incandescent lamp, while yet another carries a lantern on its head that emits bright green rays.

Department of Ibygiene.

WHAT ARE REMEDIES?

THE one department of the healing art hopelessly behind all others, in the degree of progress attained, is that of materia medica. There is no dearth of experimental and commercial laboratories to give us annual grists of "original researches," "exhaustive studies," and plausible, if not quite reliable "provings" of new and far-fetched barks, roots and extracts from the vegetable kingdom, and new and unnamable chemical compounds and derivatives from the inorganic and mineral kingdoms. The current medical literature is full of reports, speculations and clinical investigations of the claims of the newer aspirants for professional favor, and volume after volume of ponderous compends on the subject appeal to us from the publisher's catalogues. But if we could for a moment go back to first principles, invoke the aid of Bacon and Euclid, and fortify ourselves with a clear comprehension of the rigid laws of logic, we should be compelled to admit that all these painstaking labors and compilings are based on the same old assumptions which have been accepted without question from time immemorial, and which have as yet scarcely been questioned by the proverbially incredulous investigators of the present day. These assumptions cannot be traced to any particular age, nation or individual, but like all traditions have had a universal origin, every age, nation and tribe having inherited its own version.

That "This cures That" is as old a faith as any other folk-lore philosophy that has come to us from the most recent as well as from the remotest ages, and from all peoples. Like all folk-lore learning, it has its origin in, first, vague and unreasoning tradition; second, in blind superstition, which is but another name for distorted imagination; and third, in a kind of consensus of intuition. None of these sources is either scientific or reliable. All are quite unscientific, unreliable and misleading. Yet out of them springs nearly all the prevailing and decidedly heterogeneous faiths as to the "curative" potency of drugs proper as applied to the treatment of physical ailments.

Remedial measures may be divided into two primary classes—the so-called "remedies of Nature" and artificial remedies. The means and measures embraced under class one are many in number, of almost universal utility and applicability, and are more or less relied on by all schools and sects in medicine. Progress in adapting this class of agencies to the multiform pathological conditions which are constantly presenting has not been as marked and rapid as in the manipulation of articles classed under the head of materia medica proper, of which they usually form an unimposing part.

The list of substances used and recommended as artificial remedies, from time to time, as history gives us its details, is an incongruous and almost interminable one. The hell-broth brewed by Macbeth's witches was mild and innocent in comparison with some of the brews, concoctions and grewsome messes of which we read in the history of medicine.

The word *Remedy*, from the Latin *remedium*, is defined by Swift, Worcester and others as *"That which cures a disease; a medicine that cures."* The Century Dictionary's primary definition is the same. Stormonth defines the word as *"That which cures a disease or restores health."* The Latin root is formed of the prefix *re*, and *medior*, "I heal." Lexicographers are thus in accord as to the signification of the term. Taking this definition as a guide, it will occur to every inquirer that in the indiscriminate use of this word a great degree of laxness has crept into medical literature. Thus, it is made to include all measures, substances and agencies, no matter how rational or irrational, which are intended by the prescriber to prevent, cure or alleviate disease, and to materials and measures designed merely to mitigate suffering when cure is out of the question. Perhaps in time lexicographers will recognize this greater latitude of signification now so generally accorded to the word.

Artificial remedies may be sub-divided into two general classes, determined by their mode of exhibition, namely, internal and external, a further and natural subdivision classing them as direct and indirect. Direct remedies are such as are intended to act directly upon and antagonize the disease itself, or its causes. Indirect remedies are such as are relied on to provide conditions, supply materials, remove obstructions and permit or render feasible the access of more direct agencies. Innumerable further subdivisions, pertaining to the nature, particular effects and assumed action of different substances, are included in all treatises on the subject of materia medica, but they are not germane to the present inquiry.

Some substances called medicines properly belong with nutritives, since they supply in minute quantities some one or more of the proximate principles which are essential to the perfect growth, maintenance or renewal of some portion or tissue of the body, which element or principle may be lacking in the usual dietary.

To intelligently analyze the nature and scope of remedies or substances resorted to in inharmonious or pathological conditions, we must first consider the functions of the animal body in health, a condition which may be defined as an expression of harmonious normal or undisturbed physiological action.

Setting aside the instinctive function of reproduction, which is limited to the perpetuation of the species and need not be considered at this time, the two primary and fundamental objects of all physiologic processes and functions are nutrition and deobstruction.

Nutrition is accomplished through the action of the digestive and assimilative organs, beginning with the mouth and teeth, and including the stomach, bowels and numerous auxiliary glands and secreting organs and surfaces. In the complete process of digestion, excretion of excessive, unusable and injurious material is quite as essential to the correct result as any other item of the somewhat complex succession. To a very limited extent nutrition may be accomplished without the interposition of all these organs, as by cutaneous absorption, intravenous injection and some other unimportant methods, but in a general sense the alimentary tract is the only intermedium of normal and prolonged nutritive processes.

The rejection and ejection of waste and noxious material—deobstruction—is as essential to the integrity and maintenance of the health and status of the organism as the preliminary process of maceration and selection. The organs of digestion and assimilation are constantly called upon to act as inspectors of materials, to decide what elements are safe and useful, and what must be promptly condemned and ejected. It therefore becomes a logical truism that every material substance, whether fluid, solid or aeriform, mineral, vegetable or animal, when taken into the human system, is received and dealt with as either food, rubbish or poison, its office and attitude toward the organism being either nutritive, nil, or noxious. This estimate and classification does not ignore that principle of selection and combination which, through a happy conjunction of instinct and reason secures a due variety of the essential elements of nutrition. This covers the field of correctives—the use of alkalies, acids, diluents, absorbents, ferments and antiferments, as also the exhibition of a considerable list of saline, earthy and other salts, which, although generally considered as coming under the head of remedial measures are, for the most part, and quite properly, included in any really comprehensive study of nutrition.

To every substance ingested certain attributes, which are common to all matter, inhere, such as gravity, momentum, inertia, extension, penetration, and the like. Each also possesses a limited range or province of direct and indirect chemical reactions, which are, however, materially modified in the presence of the vital chemistry inherent in every living organism. As matter cannot be said to possess either instinct or intelligence, consciousness or volition; and since even its chemical relations are either abrogated, modified or inhibited in the presence of vital energy it can hardly be said to "act" in such presence except in a passive, limited and figurative way. In other words, under ordinary circumstances, and with few exceptions, when brought in contact with living organisms and vital chemistry, matter of every kind is as passive as clay in the hands of the potter. Food, therefore, cannot be said to possess any active attributes. It is as passive as the flax and wool that pass from the cards, over the spindles and through the shuttles to the loom. It is triturated, macerated, dissolved, assorted and, finally, either appropriated or rejected and ejected, according to the use or non-use that can be made of it by the vital laboratory into which it is introduced. Food is the building material; the living forces the constructors, and the resultant structure is the complex system of tissues, varying from crudest rudimentary cell, through all the coarses gradations of bone, muscle and cartilage, up to the most exquisitely delicate fibers that lend enchant-

ment to the vibrations of the *chordæ vocales*, and culminate in the composition of those inexplicable organs through which is manifested cerebration and those physiopsychic miracles we call audience and vision. Throughout the entire series of complicated processes, from original bioplasm and cellformation to the perfected retinal image, the living forces—that mystery of mysteries—organic energy, the secret of which is as far off as the wand of Midas, the perpetual motion or the Philosopher's Stone—these, by whatever name designated or guessed at, with their instinctive and inerrant power of selecting and rejecting, of transformation, assimilation and expulsion, and their incessant, but as yet imperfectly understood actions, reactions and transmutations, are the only real factors, and, using the term in its technical and logical signification, the only active or actual *agents*.

To this law apparent exceptions are numerous, but they are only apparent, and arise from the occurrence of another law, which may be termed the law of vital limitations. Thus, animal organisms are naturaly endowed and fortified to repel, resist and countercheck inimical influences and contact up to a certain limit, beyond which they succumb and are themselves destroyed, overwhelmed and disintegrated. But this fact does not contravene the law already laid down; it is simply exterior to its jurisdiction, beyond its fixed limitations. When chemical affinity becomes stronger than the inherent law of organic cohesion, the organism is no longer capable of maintaining its individual integrity. It dies, and is resolved into its original elements, or into new compounds. This is the direct result in case of the contact of caustics and corrosives, indirectly but none the less definitely, and certainly the result in the presence of noncorrosive and non-caustic, but so-called toxic substances and elements. There is no known law for determining the limit of toleration, as regards the contact of organic structures with organic or inorganic incompatibles or inimical chemic elements. A recent authority asserts that "The intensity of the action of different substances upon organisms increases with their atomic weight." But evidently any such law is merely approximate, and by no means universal in its application, the element of uncertainty being the same as is encountered in the study of psycho-biology when it is attempted to establish a fixed law of personal equations.

The term "action of remedies" is, therefore, a misnomer—a species of medical metonmy—and must be understood as relative rather than real. Within its limitations living force dominates chemic as well as mechanic force. Up to that limitation what is usually termed action on the part of the non-vital material or agency exhibited is really the reaction, antagonism or revulsion of the living organism into which it has been introduced, or to which it has been applied. While physiologists do not admit that "vital force" is "a special force of a peculiar kind," they demonstrate beyond question that, while they are composed of material atoms and are, therefore, subject to the general laws pertaining to all matter, living organisms, and especially that highest and most complex type of organized matter, the human body, is at once a generator and a reservoir of both potential and kinetic energy. In other words, organisms possess the power and discretion, if the word be allowable, to transform the elements of matter into compounds, forms and structures peculiar to themselves, and as much superior to the most complex chemical combinations as living cells are above the unorganized and amorphous elements of which they are composed. Therefore, while the ultra-materialists may claim that all matter is at all times subject to all the laws of matter, it is sufficiently evident that organized matter or living organisms to a certain extent defy the laws of chemical affinity, set at naught material laws and interrelations, which under all other conditions are unerring and irresistible. In other words, the chemistry of unorganized matter is quite distinct from the province of vital chemistry, finding itself distinctly modified and restricted when brought to bear upon elements and materials which have been erected into living structures. Furthermore, it is found that living organisms are fortified with a certain degree of inherent immunity from the operation of physical laws, and with unique powers of resistance and self-preservation which are wholly wanting in unorganized matter. Thus, irritants, revulsives, escharotics and the like are followed by no results if applied to the cutaneous surface of the cadaver, although the chemical elements which go to make up the living organism are the same in the cadaver. This subject calls for much more extended treatment.

CONCERNING BOVINE TUBERCULOSIS.

THE discussion of this subject will no doubt be in evidence for some time to come. Dr. Koch's announcement is not generally accepted, and various authorities are marshaling clinical facts to contradict it.

Dr. G. Murray Edwards, of Denver, contributes the following to the *Denver Republican*:

I desire to offer briefly the history of two cases which came under my observation in the East.

A gentleman living in Philadelphia consulted me in June, 1898, about his father and brother living in Morristown, Pa. As I considered the cases interesting, at my request the father called at my office a few days following, with a history as follows:

Mr. R., age 63. Quarryman (proprietor.) Family history negative. Family consisting of wife, two sons and two daughters, adults, were all well except one son. Father was well until about five months previous, when he developed a cough, attended with general languor and loss in weight. Could not attribute the decline to any special cause. History of having drunk freely of milk from a pet cow which had been used exclusively in the family for two years. Father and son each drank about two quarts daily, while mother and two daughters took none. Will say here, that this cow, showed signs of disease a year before, but was pronounced free from disease by a veterinarian. She died, however, about six weeks previous to this consultation, and upon investigation by a competent vegetarian was found tuberculous. Using the language of the patient, "she was rotten throughout."

Physical examination showed cavity in right lung with rapid breaking down of left. Emaciation marked. Temperature of 102 degrees. Gave him not to exceed six months to live. At a subsequent examination of the son, aged 25 years, a clear case of phthisis was in evidence with all the symptoms of an advanced stage. Sputum showed bacilli. Patient was unable to continue at work.

Now, while of course one or many cases similar will not prove or disprove the validity of the point in question, we cannot ignore the fact of two previously healthy individuals suddenly stricken, while other members of the family, with identical environments remain exempt, as being very significant.

I have great respect for Professor Koch, and would there were more such devotees to medical science, but none are too great to err, and much harm might result from lack of prevention were such teachings practiced by boards of health, etc. We should be slow to accept any dogmatic theories, although emanating from apparently reliable sources, lest the very purpose for which medical science is laboring be worse than defeated.

We would suggest that Professor Koch apply the maxim, "Be sure you're right, then go ahead."

Bronardel, at the head of the Paris faculty, rejects Koch's theory in toto, and holds the cow to strict responsibility. He is, however, in accord with other authorities as to the principal sources of propagation of tuberculosis, viz., by the careless distribution of the sputum of the patient.

Professor B. compliments this country on its prompt legislation on this subject, and predicts that when this source is suppressed tuberculosis will rapidly disappear.

BATHING AND CIVILIZATION.

SOME writer with more zeal than common sense undertakes to prove by analogy that man was not intended to bathe, that it is unnatural and therefore to be avoided. He argues that the human cuticle is simply a layer of scales that are constantly maturing and being exfoliated, and that to rub them off, as they die, with the hand or a dry cloth is all that the laws of health require.

As a counterblast to this sort of sophistry, we subjoin the following from Dr. C. W. Lyman in the *New Voice*. "A learned German professor has said that in a state of absolutely wild nature a man would require no bathing. That is to say, the skin, exposed constantly to sun and wind and rain, brushed by dewy branches and grasses of mornings, and inured to periods of chill and cold, would keep itself clean enough. The skin, when exposed to all the vicissitudes of the weather, develops a vastly more extensive circulation than is seen in the clothed man of civilization. Lay a hand on the thigh of a Nez Perces Indian in winter-time. It is covered only by flaps of buckskin fastened roughly at the side edges with two or three thongs. Even in zero weather it feels hot. That means circulation of blood. But a savage pays for this by having most of his nervous force taken up in adjustments to the various inclemencies. In civilization we want this force for other things. So we dress, and heat our houses, and always shade the body (except hands and faces) from the sun-rays, and get quiet and equable conditions for the skin and its thousands of nerve endings. The brain can work better thus than when the skin-nerves are in excitement. But incidentally to this almost incessant shielding of the skin, its circulation falls off vastly more than we ordinarily realize. Its glands become less active by far than in the savage. It becomes thinner in its working elements; or, worse, becomes a sort of shelving-place for half-vitalized fat and water—this especially in women of leisure lives or men in sedentary occupations. And its nerves from lack of employment become relatively inert. Finally the constant exertions, so necessary to the general well-being, tend to accumulate in the top layers of the skin, on its surface, and in the clothing, and impede the escape of other excretions that should be having right of way.

"This brief history is necessary to bring the mind to the point where it realizes that baths are the compromise made by civilization to savagery. We need constantly to work back toward the superb skin circulation of the savage and his completer glandular activity, and to this end can gladly devote from a quarter to half an hour out of each day, taking all the rest for other things. It is not otherwise with a horse or a cow. Turned out in a brushy pasture, and (for horses especially) free to roll in the dirt, and getting betimes showers and sun and wind, their hides keep clean. The bushes curry them the whole day through. But if horse or cow or calf or bull is kept in a barn, and there are enough reasons for doing so in winter,—then it becomes imperative, for the best results, to curry the creature thoroughly every day. We take extra work from the horse or more milk from the cow, and give in exchange currying—along with hay, grain, and shelter."

In this connection *Good Health* suggests some timely precautions, and, these, too, are a sequence of our own civilized and artificial habits. The original man enjoyed a bath every time it rained and every time he had occasion to cross a stream.

It is highly probable that he made his daily frolic in the water one of his regular pastimes.

We append the *Good Health* precautions referred to:

1. When fatigued, as the result of the loss of sleep or severe muscular exercise, a cold application should be preceded by a hot douche or immersion bath for three to seven minutes.

2. If but slightly fatigued, a short cool or tepid douche, or cold friction may be substituted for the cold bath.

3. A very cold bath should always be short, and should never be administered when the body surface is cold or chilly. The hot bath carried to the point of gentle perspiration is an excellent preparation for a cold application.

4. The temperature of the air of the room in which a cold bath is taken should always be higher than that of the bath.

5. Avoid frequent hot baths at all seasons, and especially in winter, as they are depressing, and lessen the vital resistance to cold and other disturbing influences. The best time for a hot or warm bath in cold weather is just before retiring.

AFTER TREATMENT OF SUMMER DIARRHEA OF INFANTS AND CHILDREN.

By William M. Taylor, B.S. M.D.

As supplementary to the foregoing, we condense from this paper by Dr. Taylor, found also in the *Medical News:*

The after-treatment of this condition is essentially hygienic and dietetic. Even after all immediate symptoms have subsided, it becomes a serious question as to what food shall be used. Of the various kinds of prepared foods, I think the most satisfactory is the pure modified cow's milk, using as a diluent barley-water previously dextrinized by a diastase or maltine. By beginning with a percentage milk, a food that will agree with the child is almost invariably attainable. The tendency is to begin with too high a percentage, for it is noticeable in changing the diet of any child that its digestion will be disturbed at the first feedings by an amount which will later be taken without the slightest ill effects. A good plan is as follows: Decide upon the number of feedings, amount of milk, sugar, cream and diluent to be taken by the child. As, for example, we would take three ounces of whole milk, one dram each of sugar and cream and three ounces of barley-gruel. Seven feedings of this amount and proportion may be given in twenty-four hours. To prepare the barley-gruel, add two full tablespoonfuls of barley-flour to one quart of water and boil for fifteen or twenty minutes; to this is then added two teaspoonfuls of Cereo, or dextrinize the barley-water with any other reliable preparation on the market. The diastase partially digests the starch of the barley-water, causing it to form with the milk a much looser and softer coagulum. This is shown by actual experiment in the laboratory and also in the curdled vomitus of children taking milk thus modified, the curds being softer and less tenacious than the firm, ropy curds which are almost invariably present when such diluents are used without diastase. Wheat or oatmeal flour may be used instead of the barley flour in making the gruel, though from my experience I favor the latter. This is a simple method of preparation and one in which the proportions may be easily modified. Any mother may be instructed in its preparation so that there will be little chance for error.

If the above treatment fails, kumyss in my estimation stands next. The dislike for kumyss manifested by some is usually overcome after the first few feedings, though it is sometimes more readily taken if one part of water be added to four parts of kumyss. I have seen patients with whom it seemed that all else had failed, begin to improve immediately when put on this. It is especially well taken during the summer months, having a cool, pleasant taste and a fondness for it is soon developed. Beef-juice given three times daily is a most valuable aid in the condition under consideration, seldom, if ever, causing intestinal disturbance and being easily assimilated. This should be expressed from fresh, lean beef daily, thus having it perfectly sweet and fresh. A good method for giving it is one dram to an ounce of barley-water.

In the dietetic treatment during this stage, milk, of course, should form the principal factor, but children of two or three years of age will not always submit to a milk diet, nor is it best to keep them on it. They may have in addition beef, mutton, or chicken broth from which the fat has been carefully removed. Finely chopped or scraped rare roast beef is also a valuable addition. However, we should not rely on these broths to take the place of milk for any length of time, since upon them alone the child invariably loses ground, but they are unquestionably of value in supplementing the milk diet. Dry toast or zweiback seems the safest and best form of farinacious food to begin with in children who are accustomed to a mixed diet, but at first a liquid diastase should be administered to aid the digestion of starch. Some form of pepsin, as the wine or cordial, is of undoubted service in the management of these cases when a mixed diet is begun.

The general condition may be favorably influenced by inunctions of cod-liver oil and they are especially indicated in children whose circulation seems sluggish, with blue skin, cold feet and hands. A most marked improvement is often seen in a short time from this treatment. The cod-liver oil should be warmed and rubbed in by the hand from the head to the feet. This should be continued for half an hour, repeated twice daily, and followed by a warm sponge bath. By the sponging the unpleasant odor is done away with and the comfort of the child enhanced. Aside from the absorption of the fats, the massage has a decidedly stimulating influence.

Cleanliness is the best prophylactic measure.

A kilogram of soap is a better prophylactic than ten kilograms of carbolic acid.

The final aim of the practice of medicine is to *keep* the organism healthy, not to *make* it healthy.

WHY DO WE SLEEP? WHAT ARE DREAMS?

WE reproduce from the *Mass. Med Jour.* the following interesting paper from the pen of James D. Ferguson, M.D., of Manchester, N. H.:

Some one recently said that notwithstanding the almost universal dread of dying, everyone, once in each twenty-four hours, yields gladly, or at all events without shrinking, to sleep, which in all respects resembles death except that the latter knows no waking.

The immediate cause of sleep, as likewise its object, is still an unsolved problem, and will, I think, ever remain an open question for thought and discussion. It is contended by some authorities that "in the invasion of sleep, the senses first experience its inroads; the sight is dimmed, and the eyelids close; the taste, smell, and hearing are suspended; and lastly, touch ceases to be exercised. The internal senses, as hunger, thirst and pain are in like manner suspended. The intellectual and moral faculties suffer the same oppressive lassitude, their exercise becomes languid and painful; the ideas, dull and confused, are formed with difficulty, and without connection; thought is at an end; a species of reverie, or rather delirium, succeeds, and, finally, every act of the mind is suspended; perception and consciousness, the internal evidences of existence, cease; organic life alone is manifest; animal life for a time has terminated. The act of sleeping resembles, and is in reality, a rehearsal of the act of dying." Now, as I do not endorse the above in all the fullness of its meaning, I shall further on advance and express my belief and opinion.

Dreams "are an intermediate state between sleeping and waking; imperfect consciousness continues, but the faculties are sluggish, and attention is dull; complete suspension of all the psychological operations does not exist, some continue in activity, or awake; ideas are formed and consciousness is not entirely absent. From this state of imperfect sleep and partial repose of the intellectual and moral faculties, proceed dreams."

Dunglison defines sleep: "A temporary interruption of our relations with external objects, a repose of the organs of sense, intellectual faculties, and voluntary motion;" and dreams, "A confused assemblage, or accidental and involuntary combination of ideas and images, which present themselves to the mind during sleep."

In that great, grand Book of all books, the following passages are found: "And my sleep was sweet unto me;" "Yea, thou shalt lie down and thy sleep shall be sweet;" "In thoughts from the visions of the night, when deep sleep falleth on men;" "For in the multitude of dreams and many words, there are also divers vanities;" "Your old men shall dream dreams, your young men shall see visions," etc.

It is a well-established law of nature that sleep is absolutely essential to the existence of all mankind; the loss of it seriously impairs health, and existence is often shortened; but to enjoy the blessings of "tired nature's restorer," no one should attempt to get to sleep immediately after a full meal nor with an excited and disturbed mind, for to sleep well and enjoy perfect repose, all gloomy or depressing thoughts should be banished. The duration of sleep is not uniformly the same with all persons; some require more than others. The time requisite for the reparation of the functions of relation is said to be from six to eight hours. Thus sleep occupies nearly a third of life, and he who has reached sixty years, as it respects the operations of the psychological faculties, and including the time of infancy, has not lived more than twenty years. Infancy and old age demand longer periods of sleep, and females sleep more than men. Napoleon slept but little, and Caligula, it is said, but three hours out of the twenty-four. The celebrated John Wesley says that for a period of more than sixty years, he was in the habit of going to bed at ten and rising at four, and that he had six hours of uninterrupted sleep, which he considered to be sufficient for his own health; he, however, very properly remarks that invalids and persons of delicate constitution, and those accustomed to much bodily fatigue, may require from seven to eight hours. Of abnormal somnolence, the following is from the pen of M. Lasègue:

"A barkeeper was often taken with an irresistable desire to sleep while serving his customers, and putting his glasses on the table slept for a few minutes. A porter, in a glass merchant's, would stop in the street, lean against the wall with his basket on his shoulder and sleep, then, waking in a few minutes, would rub his eyes and go on his way. A young farmer was out hunting, when he sat down in a field and went to sleep, his companions being unable to awake him. He awoke in five or six hours, but the next day he went to sleep at the same time, and ever since has done so every day. This was a hypnotic sleep, which could be brought to an end by blowing on the face. A young girl went to sleep always at eight o'clock, day and night, with or without a clock. A Belgian countess went to sleep regularly at nine o'clock, whatever she might be doing, and remained until the following day in the position she then occupied. Her catalepsy was joined to hypnotism. She recovered after two years."

Dr. Gibbons Hunt, on one occasion said, that he thought "sleep was only a lazy habit we had got into"; but I think that even if we leave out altogether the evidences from the lower animals, the phenomena of plant life would be sufficient to convince us that organized nature requires rest. Nevertheless sleep is certainly much under the control of habit. Many of the readers of the *Journal* doubtless have heard the story of the miller who was very sick, and for whose comfort the mill was stopped. But he was unable to rest quietly except under the influence of the noise to which he was accustomed, and the mill was again started. It is in fact a matter of common observation and experience, that the most violent motions or sounds will not wake up a sleeper if he is accustomed to

them and for this reason, some sleepers do not wake up during a thunder-storm, the ringing of bells, a passing train of cars, or by the conversation of members of the family, but will awake quickly at a change of noises.

There is a funny story related of an Irishman, and many good stories are peculiar to that class, who, on being told that a severe storm had occurred during the night, said to his companion, "Why did you not wake me up, for you know I can't sleep while it thunders."

It is asserted that the sensitive plant, so-called from its motions imitating the sensibility of animal life, if carried in a railroad car or any other kind of vehicle, will at first close up under the influence of the jolting motion, but will eventually get accustomed to it, will open, and then close when the motion is sudddenly stopped.

But the momentous question, What is Sleep? I come now to that point where I beg leave to differ somewhat from the quotation in the commencement of this article. Sleep, in my opinion, does seem to be merely an interruption of the relation between consciousness and sensation, and is not an entire suspension of either of these functions, for I believe that to some extent we smell, taste, hear, and feel when asleep, and the reason that we do not see is simply due to the fact that our eyes are closed, and not to any positive suspension of their powers. Vision is the only sense which we are able to fully interrupt by special mechanism; we cannot shut our ears, our noses, our tastes or feelings, against unpleasant sensations, and it has often been the expressed wish of many, "Oh, if I could only shut my ears as easily and completely as I can shut my eyes, what a satisfaction it would be."

But to return to the subject, we know that consciousness is not wanting in sleep, because dreams are evidences of its power; it must then appear that there is simply an interruption of the relation between these two functions, and the act of waking is simply the restoration of the normal relation between them. In true anæthesia, the influence is more profound; the activity of both sensation and consciousness is diminished; as under the influence of anæsthetics the sensations experienced are, so far as impressions go, very different from those of naturally going to sleep or awakening.

As a general rule persons do not sleep well in a change of beds or in new places; this may be due to an unconscious influence of the instinct of self-preservation, the mind being in a temporary alarmed state. There may also be something in the position of the sleeper in reference to the points of the compass; some persons think they can sleep best with their head to the north, and others to some other point. If the view that sleep is a break between sensation and consciousness is correct, then we should expect that as we awake, this relation is gradually restored, and we may have a confused or mistaken interpretation of consciousness, which we call a dream. It is doubted by some, and I incline to the opinion, that dreams do not occur during a profound sleep; many think that they only do occur at the moment of transition from sleep to waking, or vice versa, circumstances that may cause dreams. If, for instance, by some accident, one's foot should get uncovered during a cold night, the sensation of cold would be finally sufficient to push its way through the dormant brain cells until the consciousness was reached, and then might come an imperfect perception, which the mind would refer to some cause known to be capable of producing it; thus the person might dream he was walking on ice. I lean to the view that dreams are never out of the sphere of our experience, that nothing is ever revealed to us through them, and I am sure that often they do not represent the most important topics upon which the mind may be engaged. Sometimes we dream (though somewhat disconnected) of our daily duties, and very often of secondary matters. Dreams present some features which seem to be common to all persons. It is not an uncommon thing, especially with women, to dream of being naked in the street. This is obviously the result of circum-

stances under which they retire. If they went to bed fully dressed, such dreams would be rare. It is not an uncommon thing to dream that one tries to run and cannot. This I believe is due to the recumbent position, the usual stimulus to the soles of the feet is missing and the pressure of the bedclothes upon the lower limbs gives a sensation of restraint, which makes us think we cannot run. Such dreams, I think, always occur when we are nearly awake. Sometimes we hear persons say that a dream occurred long after they got asleep or long before they got awake, but I doubt whether they can tell anything about it. If dreams do ever occur during a profound sleep, they are purely subjective, that is, they arise from influences entirely within the body. Such are the dreams produced by indigestion, disordered blood, etc., and are not the result of impressions on the senses proper, though even in such dreams it is not improbable that for the first effect of the subjective influence to partially wake the sleeper and then produce the dream.

Some interesting experiments on this subject were made by Delaunay. According to psychologists, dreams are generally illogical and absurb. Delaunay, however, by covering his forehead with a layer of cotton wool, rendered at will his dreams healthy and intelligent. According to his experience, the dreams which people have when lying on their backs are sensuous, agitated and erotic. Those which occur when the dreamer is lying on the right side are changeable, full of exaggeration, absurb, and relate to old recollections. Those which occur when lying on the left side are intelligent, reasonable, and relate to recent occurrences. People often talk during the last mentioned dreams. The author considers that dreams, intelligent or otherwise, erotic or sober, can be induced by causing variations in the cerebral circulation, and by the nutrition of the various regions of the brain, either by the elevations of the cranial temperature or by decubitus. They, therefore, form an interesting field for psychological research. Much of the above, in my opinion, is dubious. Atkinson, after describing the nervous manifestations of sleep, and especially "night terrors" in children, says:

"The treatment must be directed to the avoidance of the causes, as fright, silly-shines, sleeping without a light, injudicious feeding, the relief of constipation, the use of abundance of fresh air and exercise; the latter even to the point of approaching fatigue, so that the child may sleep soundly without dreaming; and the employment of nervines and tonics, preferably those containing phosphorus and iron."

The further consideration of the subject of sleep and dreams, recall the words of the poet Armstrong. He says:

"Great Nature droops
Through all her works. Now happy he
        whose toil
Has o'er his languid powerless limbs diffused
A pleasing lassitude; he not in vain
Invokes the gentle Deity of Dreams,
His powers the most voluptously dissolve
In soft repose; on him the balmy dews
Of sleep, with double nutriment descend."

Hence, I may well add to the foregoing sentiment, that "tired nature's sweet restorer, balmy sleep," under no circumstances can be dispensed with. Both the body and mind enjoy (as we would say in our school days) a glorious vacation, by which the thoughts of the mind, the labors of the hand and our weary limbs, would secure the needful rest for a few hours, to prepare and fit us for life's duties on the following day.

But in the night through which we have passed we had dreams, producing impressions on the memory. They are a kind of vision in sleep, an idle fancy, a groundless suspicion; to which I may add that dreams are not of Divine origin, but are self-formed. Do you ask what share you have had in a pleasant sensation of dreaming? I reply, precisely the same that it has had in the coursing of your blood through your arteries and veins, in the pulsation of your heart, or of your brain.

As I am now treating of things which take place during the night, hence let me suggest a few thoughts. Do not uneasy and horrible dreams denote pain either of body or mind? or, in other words, a body overcome with food, or a mind occupied with melancholy ideas when awake? If this doctrine is true, based upon the principles of sound philosophy, then we must arrive at the irresistible conclusion that dreams are produced by some excess either in the passions of the soul or the nourishment of the body. Hence we conclude that nature very properly punishes us by suggesting ideas and making us think how derelict we have been in not living a more acceptable life.

This question necessarily opens up for contemplation the subject of spectres and manes, of prophecy and prediction, but which I have no inclination to enter upon.

Petronius, a writer of antiquity, says that dreams are not of divine origin, but self-formed; and I will only add, that whatever view we take of the question, whether the memory impels the brain, and the brain acts upon the soul, I think we must admit that our ideas come in sleep independently of our will.

Before concluding this subject, I desire to allude to one other topic, which, I think, is worth considering. Our ancestors of the Middle Ages slept naked. We surely have improved on that habit, but there is still room for more improvement to insure our personal comfort and good health. It is my opinion that when the time arrives to prepare for our night's rest, we should, if circumstances will allow it, have a complete night sleeping suit, of warm shirt, drawers, and stockings, which should fit us as well as our day's clothes. The recent custom of men wearing pajamas at night, seems a step in this direction. In our houses a room should be provided which could be warmed during the early evening, and in this room every member of the family could dress for bed, and to it they could come in the morning and change the dress. When all were up and dressed, the room could be opened, and the night clothes thus aired. Such a system would give great encouragement to the ventilation of sleeping rooms, the want of which is fertile of disease.

THE SELECTION OF SUMMER CLOTHING

Is a matter of considerable importance not only from the influence it may have in comfort, but also in promoting health. Yet this is a mater to which most people give comparatively little attention, and the question of style and appearance is certainly more considered than the effect on health. From the hygiene standpoint we are concerned with the questions of what form and quality of clothing will maintain the proper body-temperature, protect from changes of temperature and absorb the sweat with the excretory products contained in it. In both summer and winter, as a general rule, too much, too heavy, and irrational clothing is worn by most people. This keeps the body overwarm, and promotes free sweating, thus the skin is most of the time kept covered with moisture, in a condition in which it reacts most readily to changes of temperature and is likely to become suddenly chilled. The frequent summer coughs and colds, most of them, arise in this way. Besides weight of clothing, the ventilation, if we may use that term in this sense, is important. Goods of loose texture, loosely fitting and without constricting collars or bands allow free circulation of air and escape of perspiration vapor. Clothing which is not properly ventilated retains a layer of steam-like perspiration which gives a feeling of oppression. The sweater is an example of a properly ventilated garment, and every athlete knows how warm and comfortable a sweater is. Its loose mesh permits of free escape of perspiration, the skin dries rapidly, but without becoming cold. Very little clothing is needed to maintain the bodily temperature

in summer, but it is necessary to protect against sudden changes in our changeable climate. Wool, cotton, linen and silk each have their enthusiastic advocates. Experience has very certainly shown that woolen garments are better adapted to protect those whose occupation subject them to very sudden and considerable changes of temperature, especially if accompanied with much exertion. But it is unfortunate that practically no light loose mesh woolen undergarments are to be had that have any durability; and thus for persons engaged in sedentary occupations the lighter cotton and linen mesh are better adapted. For both cleanliness and health very frequent changes of underwear are needed, thus keeping the skin in the very best condition to eliminate as much waste matter as possible, and this is fully as important as the material of the garment worn.

Less clothing, looser mesh garments, fewer stiff collars and constricting bands are needed reforms in summer clothing for our hot cities. If sensible people will demand such clothing, the demand will not long remain unsupplied and what sensible people wear soon becomes, to a certain degree at least, the fashion.—*Am. Medicine.*

THE SANITATION OF HEALTH RESORTS AND COUNTRY HOUSES.

It is a duty which dare not be neglected to call public attention to the fact that many so-called health resorts are more insanitary than our crowded, smoke-grimed, steam-sodden factory towns. It is not the large popular seaside or "spa" town which is so much to blame in this connection, as the newly-born and pretty little seaside village, which had been discovered and had had greatness thrust upon it by railway companies and excursion agents before it was really prepared to start housekeeping on its own account, and has no such thing as a sewerage system or a water supply, and perhaps no engineer to prepare either. The man with a large family is easily lured into sending the said family to such a place, or perhaps to one of the many advertised country farmhouses or cottages, with never a thought of inquiring into anything but the rental. It is not too much to say that the average "small country-house to let during the summer months" is a danger trap, which should be most carefully examined before it is entered. Adults do not suffer from the bad conditions of such houses or "health resorts" to such an extent as children, for they can wander abroad more and their constitutions are firmer; but what a common experience it is for parents on returning home from such places to exclaim with amazement that they cannot understand their child being ill, because it has come back from the seaside or the country only a few days ago! The preventive remedy for such things at present is for parents to get their medical man to make inquiries from the local medical officer of health as to the sanitary state of the place in which they propose to spend their holidays, and to be guided by his advice. But surely it is a matter in which the government might interfere by prohibiting the letting of houses for holiday purposes, unless such houses have previously been certified by the local sanitary authority to be free from all conditions dangerous to health.—*Medical Magazine.*

STAR DUST.

MAN, at least the female part of him, takes more trouble in looking earthward for pins and dirt than for stars. From recent researches and investigation, it would seem that cosmic, or star, dust has an important bearing and influence upon things terrestrial. Our earth, according to some scientists, received its first cell life from star dust. If the assertion of these scientists be true, all the life which goes on here on earth is the result of moss-grown fragments dropping upon this earth from the ruins of a celestial world. Star dust is a regular visitant to this mundane sphere, for it is not unusual for various portions of the earth to be caught in the throes of cosmic dust, during which time rich and rare metastatic elements flood the atmosphere. Ships at sea under a cloudless sky have been known to accumulate quite a quantity of star dust, its composition being totally unlike that of volcanic or flue dust, and is of meteoric origin. Here is a field of investigation for some eager student to benefit humanity who can tell since we know that the mosses may undergo immensely low temperatures and yet, under proper conditions, germinate into life. May not this star dust convey some form of microbic life and be the occasion of terrestrial disease? Anyhow, the study of star dust is open for future investigators. Perhaps the bacteriologists may find some new form of germ life existing in star dust. It is sad but true, even with medical investigation, that the terrestrial is studied more than the heavenly. But then what the heavens shower down the earth must take, even the dirt from the stars.

THE OPEN WINDOW.

UNDER this heading the *Medical Press and Circular* adds its voice to what we have long and constantly been urging on the subject of "drafts" and air-cure:

" 'It is only since the introduction of glass for use in windows that such a disease as consumption has become a scourge; before that time life had generally to be lived in window-open, ventilated houses.' So pregnantly remarks, in a modest foot-note, the author of a very able and suggestive article in the *Westminster Review.* We are doubtful whether this statement can be verified statistically, but we have no doubt whatever as to the truth of the lesson it teaches. As to the value of the Nordrach treatment there can no longer be any doubt whatever. It, however, labors under the disadvantages inherent to all 'systems' of treatment. It has been vigorously taken up in England, but still as a 'system,' and the author of the articles in question will have performed a real service if he succeeds in making the public understand that the virtues of treatment reside in the *raison d' etre* of the system, and not in the particular institution or physician charged with its administration. The point, too, must be emphasized that the open-air treatment is no specific treatment for tuberculosis; it is of far wider application. Briefly, the method is an amplification of the old-fashioned treatment—put the patient in the most healthy condition available and trust to Nature. This can be and should be the object of every one, not only in the treatment of disease, but in everyday life. The policy of the open window is capable of universal application, but it will not, we fear, be generally admitted without much insistence, for the prejudices which exist against draughts are very deep-rooted, and invested with all the hereditary awe of our grandmothers' teaching. The germ theory of disease has done much towards giving us an intelligent appreciation of many of the mysteries of infection and contagion, and is in a fair way towards giving us the master key to treatment, but at best it is only half the matter. A seed cannot grow without suitable soil, nor can a patient harbor a bacillus to his own detriment unless he is in a fit condition to do so. Typical diphtheria bacilli exist in perfectly healthy throats without causing any pathological condition, and virulent tubercle bacilli are ubiquitous, yet we are not all tuberculous. In other words, for disease two factors are necessary. the infecting organism and a soil capable of supporting its growth. The distribution of the organisms in our habitations has been to a certain extent controlled by modern sanitary methods, but sufficient attention is not paid by the public to control the condition of the soil. A rich man will spend his money in making his sanitary service resplendent with glazed bricks, lined and jointed pipes and polished copper tubing, but will give no attention to procuring

sunlight and fresh air—that is, he will guard against infection, but will take no trouble about safeguarding the condition of the soil the infection is to grow upon. For health both are necessary and equally important."

✦ ✦

THE PRESERVATION OF THE TEETH OF SCHOOL CHILDREN.

RULES recommended by the School Children's Committee of the British Dental Association and circulated for the information of managers and teachers of the national schools in Ireland:

"Without good teeth there cannot be good mastication.

Without thorough mastication there cannot be perfect digestion, and poor health results.

Hence the paramount importance of sound teeth .

Clean teeth do not decay.

The importance of a sound first set of teeth is as great to the child as a sound second set is to the adult.

Children should be taught to use the tooth brush early.

Food left on the teeth ferments, and the acid formed produces decay.

Decay leads in time to pain and the total destruction of the tooth.

The substance of the following rules should therefore be impressed constantly upon all children:

1. The teeth should be cleansed at least once daily.

2. The best time to cleanse the teeth is after the last meal.

3. A small tooth brush, with stiff bristles, should be used. brushing up and down and across, and inside and outside, and in between the teeth.

4. A simple tooth powder or a little soap and some precipitated chalk taken up on the brush may be used if the teeth are dirty or stained.

5. It is a good practice to rinse the mouth out after every meal.

6. All rough usage of the teeth, such as cracking nuts, biting thread, etc., should be avoided, but the proper use of the teeth in chewing is good for them.

When decay occurs it should be attended to long before any pain results. It is stopping of a small cavity that is of the greatest service.

In 10,000 children's mouths examined, 86 of every 100 required skilled operative treatment."—*Journal of the British Dental Association.*

THE FUTURE MAN.

PROFESSOR McGEE, chief of the United States Bureau of Ethnology, has been formulating an estimate of the man that is to be in the good time coming.

He does not prophesy that the present specimen of the genus homo will gradually evolve into a new being, but will essentially remain a man. The changes that will take place will be modifying and complementary rather than revolutionary.

The future man will have a better brain than the present, and his brain will more thoroughly communicate its expertness to his hand. In other words his handicraft will become more exact and intelligent.

He will develop the spiritual side of his nature, gradually becoming more conscious that he has a soul, and that it can readily intercommune with disembodied souls, thus doing away with all the present questionings as to the reality of a future existence. In other words, immortality will become a scientific demonstration instead of a dream.

While some of his hypersensitiveness will be gradually lost he will acquire a more general perceptivity. He will feel some things less acutely than now, but will feel more things.

The man of the future will be taller, more symmetrically developed, will live longer, suffer less from disease, enjoy more, do more effective work, and will attain to a moral standard and degree of social equality at present only dreamed of.

The professor predicts much more in the same general vein, his conclusions being summed up as follows:

HE WILL—

Develop a better brain.
Transfer more brain power to his hand.
Become more inventive.
Speak more logical and economical language.
Remember more.
Have greater range of vision.
Perceive more odors.
Have more delicate sense of feeling.
Have a more expressive face.
Have better teeth and hair.
Be stronger physically.
Live longer.
Grow taller.
Have power to predetermine sex.
Be more beautiful.
Suffer less pain.
Have thought-saving machines.

HE WILL NOT—

Change his general characteristics.
Develop wings.
Develop into a hairy creature.
Have as acute perceptions.
Talk or write as fast as he can think.
Expend energy on mathematical drudgery.
See as far.
Hear sound as far off.
Perceive odors as far off.
Be as much the victim of climate.
Have any new sense.
Betray his feelings as plainly.
Lose control of vocal organs.
Retain either blond or brunette characteristics.
Be bald.
Suffer as greatly from disease.
Be pursued by germs and insects.

DANGERS OF ALCOHOLISM.

IT is needless to enter into details, says *The Westminster Review*, as to the consequences entailed by overindulgence in the use of alcohol. Most of us are familiar with cases of ruined lives and wretched homes as the result of the fatal habit, and in these days of high pressure living it is becoming more and more common. Mental worry, overwork, ill-health, want of sufficient nourishment and clothing, tend to swell the numbers of chronic alcoholists, and the habit so easily acquired is extremely difficult to relinquish.

The real danger to the race, however, lies in the fact that the great majority of inebriates need no incentive to acquire the habit; they are born with the tendency, and it is to this cause chiefly that we must ascribe the increase in the number of deaths from chronic alcoholism during the last twenty-three years. A reference to the table of statistics shows that in 1875 27 persons in 1,000,000 died as the result of chronic alcoholism; in 1898 these figures had more than doubled themselves, the number then being returned as 65 per 1,000,000 of population.

The following quotations point to the conclusion arrived at by some of the most eminent men of the day.

"Heredity as a causation is estimated to be present in nearly 60 per cent. of all cases of chronic alcoholism."

"Sur 97 enfants nés de parents alcooliques 14 seulement etaient sains."

"There are not a few human beings so saturated with the taint of alcoholic heredity that they could as soon 'turn back a flowing river from the sea' as arrest the march of an attack of alcoholism."

Much that has been said respecting insanity applies equally to inebriety. Both belong to the group of diseases of the nervous system, showing a marked tendency to degeneration, and both are liable to be transmitted hereditarily.

DEVICES FOR COOLING THE AIR— WET WINDOW SCREENS AND BOWLS OF QUICKLIME SUGGESTED FOR USE DURING THE DOG-DAYS.

"THERE are several devices that may be used to cool the air during the dog-days," writes Maria Parloa, in the *Ladies' Home Journal* for August. A modified form of the *Tattie* employed in India for this purpose could be made in any country house. On frames like those used for window screens tack enough narrow tapes to make a support for a thick bed of grass. Now cover with long grass fastened to the frame by sewing with twine. These screens should be placed in the windows and kept wet. The air passing through them is cooled. A garden syringe may be used to spray them with water. Three or four of these screens will do a great deal toward keeping the air in the house cool and fresh. A simpler screen may be made by covering a frame with coarse flannel, which should be kept wet. It is not so effective as the grass screen, and the flannel dries more quickly than the grass. A still simpler device is to have wet flannel over the ordinary screen, wetting the flannel from time to time. Some of the moisture may be removed from the atmosphere by placing large lumps of quicklime in earthen bowls about the rooms."

JUDGE LINDLEY, of the St. Louis Circuit Court, like many another good judge, is fond of a quiet joke. A raw German, who had been summoned for jury duty, desired to be relieved.

"Schudge," he said, "I can nicht understand English goot."

Looking over the crowded bar, his eyes filled with humor, the judge replied.

"Oh, you can serve! You won't have to understand good English. You won't hear any here."

Department of Physical Education.

WITH SPECIAL REGARD TO SYMMETRICAL DEVELOPMENT OF THE BODY.

ADVANCING THE STANDARDS.

In the course of his Valedictory Address to the graduating class of Cooper Medical College of San Francisco, Prof. Geo. D. Somers pointed out the high degree to which modern medical ideas have attained. He said:

"The conditions to-day are greatly changed. We are no longer compelled to grope about in the dark. Rays of light shine from many different directions. We have to guide us well-known laws, scientific methods, many instruments of precision, and the accumulated experience of the past. It is the custom nowadays for nearly every physician to establish a laboratory in connection with his office, in order that he may have the aid of science constantly at hand. We are conscious that our present knowledge gives us immense power over disease. In the great realm of surgery we are masters of the situation. In contagious diseases our methods of treatment are based on scientific principles, and we attack them with the greatest confidence. Smallpox and diphtheria are practically under control, and it remains for you to overcome in similar fashion the next two diseases on the list—tuberculosis and typhoid fever. How have you prepared yourself for the task?—You have acquired the necessary knowledge and experience entitling you to enter the ranks. Your training has developed certain qualifications of mind necessary to impartial judgments in estimating the various factors that influence disease. Compare yourselves now with yourselves as you were when you took up the study of medicine. You will find that your powers of observation, your methods of thinking, your ideas, your associations, your interests have all changed. These points distinguish you from your neighbors and mark your professional character. They do not make you better than others, but make you different—necessarily so—because henceforth you are to become observers and advisers rather than companions of men.

Grant that you have all the knowledge that science can give. Is this sufficient to insure your success? You will find that there are other qualifications, partly natural, partly acquired, which must go hand in hand with science. Let me quote you something from Dr. Oliver Wendell Holmes. He says, 'Science is a first-rate piece of furniture for a man's upper chamber, if he has common sense on the ground floor; but if a man has not got plenty of common sense, the more science he has the worse for his patients.' This is no reflection on science, but means that a physician must temper his knowledge with sympathy and a kindly spirit. As an example, take any simple case of sickness to which you may be called. Science will tell you that you can find out a great deal about the man's condition if you examine him systematically. Therefore you thump his chest, run a tube down his throat to examine the stomach contents, and stick pins into his skin in order to examine his blood. On the other hand, judgment may tell you that the man is not very sick, and that all he wants is to be assured of the fact and made comfortable."

IDEALS IN PHYSICAL EDUCATION.

BY D. A. SARGENT, M.D.,

Of Cambridge, Mass.

FROM Dr. Sargent's very instructive paper in the *Medical News* we condense the following:

In considering the present status of physical training in the United States we find it established in some form or other in 270 colleges and universities. 98 are doing organized work, 72 require physical exercise, and 24 give credit for it in the course which counts for a diploma. About 300 cities have introduced physical exercises into the public schools, and 100 of them have special teachers. There are about 500 Y. M. C. A. gymnasiums in different parts of the country, with a corps of some 300 physical directors and 80,000 members. The North American Turnerbund has some 300 gymnasiums and about 200 instructors, and some 45,000 members. There are perhaps 100 athletic club gymnasiums of one description or another and a few out-of-door and public city gymnasiums. There are many gymnasiums in private houses, churches, hospitals, sanitariums, army and navy depots, police quarters, engine-house stations, mission houses, industrial schools, and many other institutions to the number of several hundred. In addition to this form of physical training there are a great variety of special athletic clubs for boxing, fencing, bowling, boating, canoeing, swimming, bicycling, etc. Then there is golf, tennis, baseball, football, with their ardent devotees and numerous following, together with the more passive forms of exercise, such as riding, sailing, driving, etc., which have many admirers.

Taking all the sports, games and well-established forms of exercise into consideration, it is safe to affirm that they represent millions in capital invested and affect the lives of millions of our people. The amount of money which a people are willing to spend in the furtherance of a movement is a pretty good indication of its value in their estimation, though if judged from an educational point of view this value would probably be considerably discounted. If we were to estimate the value of the century's efforts in physical training by the effects produced, the problem would be a difficult one on account of the many factors involved, and the increasing number of influences that tend to neutralize all the good that might be derived from systematic physical exercise. Bicycling, lawn tennis, and golf have been especially valuable to our women, inducing many to exercise who never exercised before. These three sports have probably done more to overcome the evils of tight clothing than a whole century of preaching and lecturing on this subject. Boxing, football, basketball and other antagonistic games have done a great deal to lessen the evils of over refinement and excessive sentimentality, and they may be conducted in such a way as to develop a firm character and a manly spirit. But there are certain inclinations connected with the development of competitive sports and antagonistic games that are not only detrimental to physical training in its best sense, but are also demoralizing to our youth and to the public in general.

Let us consider some of these drifts and tendencies. Thirty years ago amateur baseball was at its height in America, and there were well-organized clubs in nearly every city in the Union. To-day there are a very few amateur baseball clubs outside of the colleges, and the interest in this once popular sport is declining in our institutions of learning. Professional baseball has superseded amateur baseball in popular interest, and although the game is just as beneficial from a physical and recreative point of view as ever, it does not have anything like the following it once had. The interest in college boating culminated in 1875, when thirteen crews were represented at Saratoga. In some colleges this sport has been abandoned altogether. In a few institutions it has been re-established, and in some, especially at

Harvard, there is a great revival of interest in boating, as many as twenty eight-oared crews being on the river at one time. The practice of archery was quite generally established in this country in the early seventies, and there were numerous clubs of both sexes that rallied around this form of recreative exercise. The interest culminated in 1879, and at the present time there are few archery clubs in existence. The so-called higher gymnastics attained their greatest prominence in the colleges and city gymnasiums in the early seventies. Boxing and wrestling contests attained their greatest popularity at Harvard in 1883, '84, and '85, and are now practically abandoned, although there are two instructors in boxing regularly employed at the gymnasium. The interest in lacrosse and cricket has waxed and waned, but the games have never been entirely abandoned. Field and track athletes have a strong following in the vicinity of New York, Boston and Philadelphia, but attract small audiences and little attention in the colleges and other communities compared to what they did a few years ago. The great city athletic clubs, which once fostered track and field athletics, now seldom have any representatives from their own membership in the public contests, and confine their attention to exploiting the athletic abilities of outsiders for the entertainment of their regular members. Some of these athletic clubs, notably the Boston, act as patrons for school and college athletes, and do a great deal to encourage the practice of out-of-door sports and systematic exercise among their junior members. Many of these city athletic clubs, like the Orange of New Jersey, Washington, Detroit, St. Louis, Providence, Pastime in Brooklyn, Manhattan in New York, Staten Island, Fitchburg, Nationals, Louisville, Philadelphia, etc., have been given up entirely or turned into social clubs.

Now, the important question is, what are the factors which cause some sports to decline and others to be perpetuated in popular favor? In answer to this question we are forced to admit that fashion plays a very prominent part, bringing into vogue at one time sports which have but few valuable features, and sweeping away at another time exercises of the greatest importance. Some of the special forms of exercise like archery, fencing, Delsarte, etc., may be taken up as society fads, and be rushed for a few seasons and then become obselete. Even the more serious forms of exercise are sometimes taken up by society because they are thought to be the "proper thing," without regard to their hygienic or educational value. In fact, I should be rather loth to admit to this semi-scientific association how much of our work is without scientific or artistic value, because it is governed so largely by fashion and caprice. Again the spirit of emulation and competition which we try so hard to foster and cultivate has its limitations, and it is a serious question just how far it can be carried without detriment to the cause we are striving to advance. A high spirit of emulation breeds rivalries and enmities and often stirs up bad blood and leads to the establishment of more or less permanent factions which may work great harm to a school or club. This is especially likely to be the case where competitions are confined to members of the club or to the different classes of a school or college. The hardest struggles on the athletic field are frequently between classes or members of the same institution for positions on class or university teams. The feelings of bitterness and enmity often engendered by these hard contests in schools and colleges are softened and assuaged by the thought that knocks, strains and bruises must be endured in practice in order to enable the chosen school, college, or university team to vanquish its rival from some other school, college or university.

Another disrupting influence is the establishment of too high a standard. This is one of the evils of professionalism, and really marks the underlying difficulty of settling who is and who is not an amateur. The poorest professional must be a better performer than the best amateur in order to constitute himself a professional and be able to receive money for his services. But the receiving of money is a secondary consideration which follows the presumption of superior merit. This results from long and persistent practice or training such as a person is obliged to undergo in preparing for a life's profession or occupation. When therefore students, clerks and young men who work with their brains rather than with their muscles are urged to practise certain exercises or sports as a means of improving their health and physique, and are offered prizes or trophies of victory as incentive for them to train and compete, one of the first essentials of a fair contest is to see that those who entered the competition are of the same class or on somewhere near the same footing. Now, if the contest is in rowing and those who make a business of rowing are allowed to enter, the conditions would be unfair, as students who are engaged in their studies, or clerks with their bookkeeping through the working hours of the day, and who only take up rowing as a recreation or pastime, cannot compete on anything like equal terms with professional oarsmen. It would be just as absurd to expect the professional oarsman to compete on equal terms with the student in solving mathematical problems or with the clerk in bookkeeping or penmanship.

When, however, sports and pastimes are pursued with so much intensity as ends in themselves, rather than as means to an end, and the devotees give so much time to practising them that they haven't time or energy enough left to give to other pursuits, these persons are just as much professionals in the true meaning of that term as they would be if they received money for their services. These are the type of athletes that have been supported and exploited in the past by some of the large city and university athletic clubs. Although they have won prizes for their clubs, I can hardly believe that they have won honors, indeed I am sure that this style of athleticism has done great injury to the cause of physical training. First, by placing all the records so high that bona-fide amateurs will find great difficulty in surpassing them; second, by discouraging and literally driving out of existence the smaller clubs that could not afford to follow the same tactics; third, by causing a decline in active interest among the members of these clubs who cannot give the time and attention from their business that will enable them to compete with the performances of star athletes and who, therefore, do not compete at all. As long as the public is content to see the best performances without regard to the status of the competitors, there will always be a tendency towards professionalism which will have to be guarded against by very stringent rules. One of the best ways of meeting this objectionable tendency in school and college athletics is for the authorities to insist that all contestants must not only attend to all of their school and college exercises, but they must give evidence of having done a certain amount of work and attained a certain rank therein. If the school curriculum is what it ought to be, this will insure that the students will not give too much time to their athletics and that the work that they do engage in will tend to give them a sound mind as well as a strong body.

I have dwelt at some length upon this tendency of antagonistic sports and highly competitive games to exterminate themselves, when not properly managed, because I deem it of the greatest importance that this fact should be thoroughly understood. There is no use denying the fact that athletic contests afford a stimulus to effort to a great many boys and young men, and even to girls and young women, which no other forms of exercise can give. The problem is how to control these sports and yet keep up the interest, or to eliminate the evil and yet preserve the good. When we ask a friend to assume to be an enemy in order that we may arouse our fighting spirit and practise our animal instincts upon him, it is not a little strange that the imaginary attributes which we repeatedly give to him, are after a while difficult to efface. This is especially so if the fancied realism adds so much to our fierceness of attack and defence as to enable us to win a victory. A man instinctively shrinks from falling upon another man's head under the ordinary circumstances of life, but a man so considerate of an opponent's head or person would not make a successful football player. When the papers were filled with denunciations of the West Point cadets for their rough and cruel practices upon under class men, it did not occur to the general public that these are qualities that must necessarily be bred into the man who would become a professional soldier. A much more agreeable way for us to become reconciled to the stern qualities in our young men, especially if we wish to raise an army, is to attribute these rough, cruel and even fiendish qualities to those who happen to be for the time being our enemies. We have all read about the inhuman cruelties of our Southern brethren during the Civil War, the barbarous cruelties of the Spanish soldiers, and the fiendish conduct of the Chinese Boxers and the Filipinos. By attributing diabolical qualities to an opponent we may excuse ourselves for trying "to do him up" or "put him out of the game." These are simply the remnants of primitive characteristics, possessed by our early ancestors, when those who were not members of the tribe were enemies of the tribe, whom it was one's first duty to wound or kill. When rival boxers deliberately try to "knock each other out," and friendly baseball players "spike" a runner, or throw dirt in a baseman's eyes; when the fair devotees of basketball hiss every attempt of the visiting team to make a goal; when grave and dignified professors rush up and down the side lines of the football field shouting, "down him," "kill him," and delicate ladies who but a moment before shrunk from witnessing the "brutal" game, with flushed cheeks and staring eyes wildly shriek their approval, one might reasonably ask if this, also, is not an exhibition of some of the recurrent traits of our barbaric ancestry.

Of course these are exceptional occurrences, but if you have any real doubt as to the passions which are swaying the minds of most of the spectators, as well as the participants, during an exciting football game or boxing match, just watch the faces of the audience during these antagonistic exercises. To be sure there is the joy of victory to the side that wins, there is also the chagrin of defeat to the side that loses, and it is a question if the prolonged depression that follows defeat does not more than offset the temporary pleasure of victory. As this movement, which has now been in operation for twenty or thirty years in some of our colleges, is beginning to breed the inevitable bitterness of feeling that sometimes finds expression in a phrase that consigns a whole institution to the infernal regions, the question arises whether these rival colleges cannot unite against some common enemy or institution and thus work together in harmony. The union of Harvard and Yale against Oxford and Cambridge in their athletic games in England, and the American team at Paris and at Athens, are illustrations to the point.

At the present day every alumnus rejoices in the athletic victory of his school or college team because he thinks the public will consider the achievements of this team a fair representation of what his institution is doing for the physical training of its youth. How seldom this is true! In intellectual training all school men are required to come up to a certain minimum standard of excellence before they can enter college, and again before they can receive their diplomas. There is no such incentive to keep the mass of students up to a required physical standard, and the gulf between the lowest and the highest is great indeed. A few years ago the college gymnasium directors, believing that a moderate degree of physical strength was the fundamental basis, not only for all forms of athletics, but for health itself, decided upon a uniform system of strength tests by which to gauge certain functional powers in their respective pupils. The test consisted of an all-round trial of strength of back, legs, arms and chest, in which the sum total of the several trials was to represent the total strength of the individual. After the candidates for all the athletic teams have been chosen, a great many men who desire to have something definite to compete for, are left without any incentive.

The great objection to all forms of athletic competitions and strength contests is that after a while, as the standard rises, they are likely to be pursued as ends in themselves, as I have stated before, rather than as a means to an end, which is the betterment of the whole organism. But unfortunately this objection is not inseparable from mental contests, and in both instances those men come to the front whose constitutions are best adapted to stand the strain to which they are subjected. By this method of selection our higher schools and colleges are fostering two distinct types. One type devotes itself to the supreme development of the mind, and the other type to the supreme development of the body. The latter type is best calculated to survive, because it has to meet certain mental requirements of the faculty. But neither type represents the average student, and yet it is the condition of the average student who shows what our schools and colleges are doing for the country.

The more experience I have in teaching physical training and the more I observe its results, the more I am convinced that the highest ideal for which we should strive is the improvement of the individual man in structure and in function. This was the conclusion that I came to some twenty-five years ago, and time and experience have given it confirmation. With this ideal in mind, all the diverse forms of exercise and games, all fads and specialties, all methods and systems may be weighed in the balance and credited for what they are really worth. For it is not a runner, a jumper, a boxer, a ball-player, an oarsman or a gymnast that we are trying to produce, but the highest type of a physically perfect man. This forbids excessive development in any one direction, which specialists are constantly striving to attain. It also makes overexercise and overtraining inconsistent with the object in view. It furnishes a constant incentive to well-directed efforts and right methods of living. It is not necessary to hunt for a competitor, for one is always in competition with himself, endeavoring to make his condition to-day better than it was yesterday, and so on from week to week and from month to month. If one wants an opponent, he accepts him as a friend. For, as Burke says: "He that wrestles with us strengthens our nerves and sharpens our skill. Our antagonist is our helper." The great thing to be desired and attained is that prime physical condition called fitness—fitness for work, fitness for play, fitness for anything a man may be called upon to do. Is not this a condition worth striving for? How few of us realize the dignity and importance of the work in which we are engaged. Trying to assist Nature in developing and perfecting her handiwork, not simply mending bones, patching wounds and relieving functional disturbances, but trying to lift man on to a higher plane of living, by improving the structure of his bones, muscles, nerves, and tissues, and increasing the functional capacity of his whole organism. This is the highest kind of constructive work, in which the building of all other material structures sinks into utter insignificance. If there are those among you who sometimes get disheartened and discouraged because you think your particular branch of service is not appreciated, I trust you will let this ideal take possession of you.

Free exercises, dancing steps, plays, games and "sleights of art and feats of strength," even the schoolboy's "stunts," all will be brought under tribute and made to aid you in getting hold of some indifferent soul, and inducing him to make efforts for himself. All criticism against childish sports, trivial plays and undignified movements and exercises will be simply laughed to scorn, for what dignity has any movement or exercise except the dignity of the mind that directs it? Something of this spirit must have possessed the minds of Agesilaus and Socrates of old, who did not disdain to practice the child's play of "riding a stick" for exercise.

It is the same spirit that induces many over-brain-worked business and professional men, many closely confined clerks and shop girls, to take regular systematic exercise at their homes or boarding places, when golf, tennis, the bicycle and gymnasium are inaccessible. And I regret to say that it is a lack of this spirit that puts so many of our college athletes out of condition after they have entered upon their life's work. Finding no opportunity to practise their favorite sport, they find no incentive for exercise of any kind, and frequently break down in health for the want of it. There are scores of such men in New York to-day, and their early breakdown is not unfrequently attributed to overindulgence in college athletics. In some instances this may be true, but the fundamental weakness in the whole athletic movement at the present time is a failure to recognize the primary objects for which athletic exercises are fostered and encouraged—in other words, a failure to recognize proper standards and high ideals.

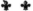

THE HYGIENE OF THE WHEEL.

ACCORDING to London *Health*, it is doubtful if health culture ever had a more helpful agency than is found in the bicycle. To many a house and office-tied man and woman this has proved the first incentive to seeking outdoor life. The healthful, exhilarating exercise which comes to them from the proper use of the bicycle might never have come from any other source. The wheel takes those living and working in the close city atmosphere out into the open fields and woods, where there is a chance to breathe the pure undefiled air, and to come into contact with and study nature. There are some who from choice of force of circumstances, have maintained the riding habit throughout the winter months, either for business or for health and pleasure, but with a large majority, and especially those who are most in need of the exercise, at the appearance of cold weather the wheel was stored away for the winter, waiting for the return of spring with its balmy days, birds and flowers. Now that the time has come the cycle paths, park roads, and highways are filled with those who are riding the wheel for pleasure or from the standpoint of health. Notwithstanding the craze for bicycling, as it may have been called at one time, has in a measure passed, there is no question but that it will always maintain its place; still we can but wish there were even more who were seeking this form of outdoor life.

MARY SARGENT HOPKINS,

in her chapter on Bicycling and Beauty in "Womanly Beauty of Form and Feature," says: "It is difficult to induce the home woman to go out and take sufficient exercise in the open air. She will always find some excuse for putting it off until to-morrow. If she goes out she will not stay long enough to do much good unless she has some object in view. She must have something to divert her mind to gather any degree of enthusiasm; this she can find in bicycling.

"The wheel stands to-day the greatest emancipator for woman extant—women who long to be free from nervousness, headache, and the train of other ills. The wheel stimulates the circulation and regulates the action of the bowels, thus driving away headache, and is a cure for insomnia which stands unequalled. In every motion which the rider makes the muscles are brought into play and gently exercised. With head and shoulders erect those of the chest and arms are given a chance, while the pedal motion gives ample play to those of the legs."

Many riders have come to know something of the hygiene of the wheel, and still words of caution may not be considered untimely or out of place. Like all other good things this can be abused. One of the dangers in cycling comes from the tendency to overdo in the way of speed, of distance or time given to continuous rides.

AN HOUR'S RIDE

at a leisurely pace, giving abundance of opportunity for taking in deep breaths of the life-giving, morning air, taking note of the scenery and attractive surroundings, listening to the birds or enjoying the company of congenial companions and covering a limited distance, is far more beneficial than the strained ride in an effort to go a specified number of miles in a given time. Remember when going that you must return, and that the distance back is never shorter.

Another point for consideration is the proper adjustment of your wheel. Study this and see that it is right; give attention to the saddle; do not be satised with whatever you happpen to have, but experiment and get that best adapted to yourself; some find one and some another make the most desirable. See that the handle-bar is so adjusted to obviate the necessity for the stoop. This unhealthful and ungraceful position cannot be too strongly condemned. It is always injurious, giving the lungs no chance for expansion, and is very likely to lead to a permanent stooping of the shoulders; especially should young people be careful of this.

In a general way the morning is the best time for this form of exercise, as the atmosphere is new and less contaminated. Remember never to ride beyond the point of fatigue, and this with proper food, sleep, and rest, and taken at the right time, will do much to promote a healthful condition, physically, mentally, and morally.

THE law that holds this universe together is the law of affinities; like will seek like. Make your choice now for the good things of that time that go into eternity with you. —August *Ladies' Home Journal.*

THE TREATMENT OF INTERMITTENT AND REMITTENT FEVER— WITH CLINICAL REPORTS.

By CHARLES W. MCINTYRE, M.D.
New Albany, Ind.

IN the spring, summer, and fall of each year these two most prevalent types of malarial fever usually prevail in this section of the country to an extensive degree. These affections are not only in themselves most prevalent, but they tincture, as it were, all other diseases that we encounter. In other words, it is very rare to see a case of pneumonia, dysentery, or typhoid fever in which there is not some well marked malarial complication.

The practical physician has now come to realize this clinical fact and directs his medication acordingly.

The treatment that has been most successful in combating these fevers will be considered singly.

Intermittent fever, commonly spoken of by people as chills and fever, is a disease which demands prompt and effectual treatment. This clinical fact stands out boldly, when we remember that the second chill may be one of pernicious intermittent. When a simple intermittent may develop into a "congestive chill" no one can tell. I, therefore, look upon all cases of chills seriously, and try to cure them at once.

My way of treating chills, whether the type is quotidian, tertian, or quartan, is to give to an adult patient twenty grains of quinin six hours before the paroxysm is due. In other words, if the chill comes at 10 o'clock in the morning I have the patient takes twenty grains of quinin, so that all is taken two hours before the expected chill.

I employ this drug in the form of Dad's Quinin Pills. Each of these pills contains two grains of a salt of quinin which does not cause congestion, head noises and the great depression which is so distressing to some patients. Two of these pills can be taken every four hours till ten of them have been taken.

It is best to give these pills every other day for a week after the paroxysms have been interrupted.

Remittent fever is a disease which is in fact, curable only by quinin. I have not employed any other drug that ensures anything like as good results as quinin. Here Dad's pills serve us admirably, since they do not produce any disturbance in the brain.

The headache and congestion of the brain in some cases is often fairly dreadful, and ordinary sulphate of quinin will often make the symptoms worse and in some cases death will follow the depressing action of the drug. Dad's pills are not open to these objections.

One of Dad's pills is to be taken every two hours, and to be continued until the fever has ceased, and for a day or two after it has ceased.

REPORTS OF CASES.

1. Mrs. S., age twenty-two, had had chills for two weeks. The chill appeared every other day at 9 o'clock. She was given two of Dad's quinin pills at four, five, six, seven, and eight, and missed the intermittent fever paroxysm. I gave her this number every other morning for a week to overcome the malarial plasmodia that might yet develop. I had her move her sleeping apartment to the second floor. This patient got on well and has had no further recurrence of the fever.

2. Mr. B. F., called me and I found him with a temperature of 106° F. He had a severe headache and his fever had not left him for two days and nights. The case was one of remittent fever, and I began by giving him a Dad's pill every two hours. In twenty-four hours the fever had ceased and he continued without fever. He took no other medicine except the pills. He took a pill, however, after each meal for several weeks as a plasmodicide.

3. C. W. B., age eighteen. This young fellow has been a sufferer with chills for two months—one appearing every other day. Quinine caused him to have nausea, head

noises, and vertigo, so he could not take it.

I put him on Dad's quinin pills, as in the other case of intermittent fever already detailed, and had none of the symptoms which annoyed him before. He made a complete recovery.

Mrs. A. I. L., aged sixty-nine. This old lady was quite feeble and I feared that the quinin sulphate would prove too much for her. But as she had remittent fever quinin was the only thing I could use. I put her on Dad's quinin pills and they had the desired results without producing any head symptoms or depression.

4. A. Y. F., age twenty-one, of extreme nervous type, in whom I could only expect trouble when I exhibited the sulphate of qninin, was treated with the pills and made a speedy recovery.

THE MOST IMPORTANT THING IN LIFE.

Says J. H. Kellogg, M.D., in *Good Health:*

"To live and to live uprightly and well, is the sum total of everything important in life.

"Education, as Colonel Parker of Chicago well says, is simply life. If we go to the right kind of school, we shall be taught how to live—how to live righteously, happily, and comfortably. Many people never learn how to live. They blunder through life as one floats down stream, taking things as they come. They give no heed to the morrow, but live like squirrels. However, they are not so provident as squirrels, for the squirrels lay up something for a rainy day, or at least for a wintry day.

"The man who comprehends life—what it really is—thinks of the future, and husbands his resources. Nearly all of us do that in relation to financial matters. Everybody is, if possible, laying up something for a rainy day, for the hour of trouble, for the time when an emergency will force some extra burden upon him. But how many are laying up energy, vitality, and health in preparation for a sick day?

"The reason so many people fall at their post—congressmen, judges, lawyers, clergymen, doctors—doctors even more than anybody else—is because they have been squandering their resources. A leak has been going on for years. Their vitality has been slipping away. Their strength has been dissipated, so that when the emergency comes, they go down. Some time ago I was crossing a bridge; it shook and trembled. Soon a dog came over, and it shook and trembled still more, because the dog went over on a rhythmical trot. A week afterward that bridge went down when a horse passed over it. Now there had been great loads of hay, heavy yokes of oxen, and ponderous loads of vegetables carried across that bridge, but it held up. A single week afterward it broke down. Why?—Because there were timbers in it that had become rotten. They had been growing rotten for a long time until simply the weight of a horse caused the bridge to collapse.

"It is exactly so with the human constitution. It is not the last thing a man does that makes him sick, but the things that he did years before. I once asked a gentleman who was in a very bad physical state what brought him into that condition. 'Oh,' he said, 'overwork. I have not been well since I was engaged in my winding-up work, looking over my books of accounts, and straightening things up. The first night afterward I did not sleep well, the next night it was worse, and for several nights I did not get a wink of sleep. I have never been so well since.' But it was not the overwork that made him sick. A year before he had been through the same work, and it did not make him sick, and he did not consider it a strain. Five years before he had probably enjoyed that amount of work. He had had no ill success, and no losses. It was not his business that broke him down. It was his big dinners, his sedentary life and neglect of exercise, his lack of sweating.

"The lack of sweating breaks down the business man a great deal more than the actual work he does. I never heard of a man's breaking down in business who was in the habit of taking a good sweat every day. It is because business men sweat their brains instead of their muscles that they break down. It is because they neglect their proper exercise so that poisons and waste materials accumulate in the body until by and by the brain is paralyzed; and not only the brain, but every other part of the body also. The accumulation of these poisons causes apoplexy, degeneration of the heart, the kidneys, the liver.

"The business man gets very little benefit from the sunshine. Yet there is great virtue in the sunshine. By our indoor life and our black clothes we shut out a great deal of its wonderful health-giving power.

"One of our greatest faults is that while we should cultivate life, we cultivate death. We do it at our dinner-tables and in our sleeping-rooms, which we shut up so tight that the life-giving oxygen can not come in. We stop up the keyholes and put listing around the windows, until the oxygen, the most essential thing to life, is driven to moaning and sighing to get in. But we keep it barricaded away. Then we sit down at our dinner-tables and cultivate death. We swallow things that ought to be buried in the ground and carried to the bone-yard and soap-factory, instead of being put into the human stomach.

"If we want life, and health, the most important thing in life, we must cultivate life. We must eat the things that have the most life in them. All the life in the world comes from the sun. Living things go to sleep at night, and in the morning the sun shines on them and wakes them up to life again. All energy comes from the sun. The tree receives its energy in the form of chlorophyl, from the air, the sunlight, and the earth. It is the energy of the sun stored in the tree that we find in coal. Electric light is simply resuscitated sunlight, which shone upon the earth centuries ago. The energy came into the tree through the sunlight. The tree became coal under ground. The coal was converted into steam, and then in the dynamo the energy is converted into electric light. Grain, wheat, corn, barley, nuts, fruits, and vegetables—all these things which are wholesome foods, are simply stored-up energy. The energy taken into our bodies through them becomes mental energy and digestive energy, and also moral power.

"All our energy comes from our food. When we take food in the form of vegetables, the energy is all ready to be transformed into life. The vegetables store the life, and the animals eat it and transform it into animal life. But suppose we eat the animal instead of the vegetable. The animal was made, not to impart energy, but to use energy—to consume it. An animal is a machine, like a locomotive. We eat to supply the energy that we are consuming. So when one animal eats another animal, it is like a locomotive eating a stove, or like feeding a stove with kerosene lamps. It is like one large machine being fed upon a number of small machines. The kerosene lamp has fuel in it, and by throwing the kerosene lamps into the stove, the stove receives a small amount of fuel. So the animal consuming another animal receives a little food, but he gets also along with it a great deal of that which is not nutrient material.

"In eating animals we have to eat death as well as life. The reason man dies is because death gains the ascendency over life. If we took nothing but life into our bodies, it would be a very long time before death could gain the ascendency; but if we eat things with death in them, death will finally preponderate."

THE late William M. Evarts had a farm in Vermont where swine were bred with especial care. He once sent a barrel of pickled pork to the historian, George Bancroft, with this letter:

"I am glad to send you two products of my pen to-day, a barrel of pickled pork and my eulogy on Chief Justice Chase."

Brevity Club.

PITH AND POINT.

A WORD ABOUT CLUBS.

BY ANOTHER NEW MEMBER

CLUBS are very old institutions. They date clear back to the Garden, where Cain's club proved a stunner for Abel, otherwise. the history of the race might have been written in ink of a more cheerful color. Had the result of that primeval battle been reversed, had the amiable Abel successfully ducked or landed heavily on Cain's solar plexus, or below the line where his belt ought to have been, we might have had to revise all our genealogical trees, and the outcome would have been racially radical. There would have been no need for that historic "Mark of Cain" which so many modern men continue to wear.

Cain's motive does not appear in the record, and no Delia Bacon, or Delia Ignatius Donnelly has appeared to champion the cause of Cain or bring to light his lost cryptogram. Perhaps it was a case of emotional insanity, in which case he should have been acquitted, and the experts in "Higher Criticism" owe it to the world to clear up his smutty memory.

Of course the brothers might have been rivals for the hand and heart of one of their hirsute and half-naked sisters, and this is a plausible theory, since it brings out the inevitable woman in the case. This sounds rather funny; but we must remember that there were no chic actresses nor fly grass widows to distract their attention; and if not in love with their own sisters pray whose sisters or other men's wives could they elope with?

Abel must have been a non-combatant, or an anti-imperialist, or a "goody-goody." Had he lived to people the other half of the world his descendants might have been a great improvement over the "Heathen Chinee," and perhaps that would have forefended all this long-winded international muddle.

The next club of which we have any authentic record was the Antediluvian Yacht Club, of which Noah the First was chief navigator. That was before the grades of commodore, rear admiral and vice-admiral had been invented. This ancientist of ancient mariners should have sent for Lieutenant Hobson to take charge of his bureau of construction, for then his floating hippodrome could have advertised all the sailing qualities and "superior appointments" of our modern liners. Not being up in maritime lore, and Herreshoff being just then otherwise engaged, Noah devoted his attention to capacity rather than speed. The Ark must have been all hold; that is, it accommodated such an extensive menagerie as to beat the "Deutschland" about a hundred per cent. in tonnage, and of course it was all gross tonnage.

How fortunate it was for the race, the ritualists and the ringmasters that he succeeded! There would have been no descendants of Ham. Had he foundered at sea, Barnum's Greatest Show on Earth would have never materialized, the allegory of the theologasters would have lacked plausibility, and zoology would have been set down as a lost science.

It has always been a conundrum as to how the Noah family managed to take on their incongruous cargo. Did they back the bronchos and zebras and Berkshire pigs up the gangplank? And did Mrs. Noah chuck the clucking, contrary sitting hens into a gunny sack, and carry them aboard? Surely none of these animals ever went in head first! Imagine the angel Gabriel trying to persuade a balky jackass that delay was dangerous!

But then some men, even to this day, always go about their business backwards, and a good many join the church in the same way. Their heels are with the saints, but their faces are dead set after the shekels of the wicked world!

Had it not been for clubs the race would have surely perished during the very first generation, from the ferocity of wild beasts. Clubs and claws were the original and aboriginal weapons of offense and defense. Our forefathers, the orang, the chimpanzee and the gorilla, all wore clubs; and perhaps if mother Eve could have swung an Indian club to some purpose she might have worsted the snake, and what then! The theologasters would have had to invent something to take the place of the "Original Sin!" And what is more, we poor, deluded, blundering mortals might now be howling ourselves hoarse over some other real or imaginary set of trusts or monopolizing corporations than the ones just now flourishing; or we might be railing about some other climate, some other administration or some other government! *Quien sabe?*

A good deal can be said about clubs that is not set down in the cyclopedias. When giants walked the earth and frightened naughty children into terrified but temporary goodness and shaking palsy, clubs were trumps; and ever since that time more battles have been fought with clubs than with cannon. In modern warfare the crisis frequently comes only when the combatants club their muskets and wade in for all they are worth. Some of the most successful hunters, when they get within clinching distance of a bear prefer a stout club to their rifles, because the club is always loaded.

All modern cities are proud of their multitude of clubs, and when a noted or notorious man dies it takes half a column in the daily press to enumerate his club affiliations, while half a dozen lines sum up all he has done for his country, for charity or the church. For an equally prominent man who has not divorced three wives, wrecked a bank or committed a felony or a murder, three lines are considered superfluous for his obituary. To this rule there are a few exceptions, such as millionaire misers and wife-poisoners. The latter, in particular, are loaded with wreaths and buttonhole bouquets on their way to the electric chair!

But your regular city club does not entirely fill the bill. When the city fellows become ambitious to take the thirty-third degree in club rituals they shake the city dust from their patent-leather bals and organize a country club. This is an example of true avatism, a reversion to original types. In fact, the word club could not have originated in the city. It is strictly a country product, and had its origin before cities had an existence.

In his celebrated battle with the Philistines, Sampson—not the Admiral!—is supposed to have seized the first club within reach. Had it proved to be a regular Irish shillalah no doubt his victory would have been swifter and more brilliant. But then, his ordinance department hadn't yet been placed on a war-footing.

But for the modern policeman's club civilization would never have attained to its present high state of advancement. With his night stick argument—by no means a "Brevity Club"—the bluecoat can persuade almost any pugnacious and pertinacious culprit to keep the pace and keep step to the station house.

That clubs are a permanent institution is evidenced by the fact that in our later lexicons the members are known as "clubbists."

In cities a man's social standing is quite apt to be measured by the number and character of his club affiliations. Since it is assumed that a respectable club lends some of its respectability to each of its members, "good standing" in such a club acts as a passport to "good society." Clubs are sometimes more discriminating and exclusive in admitting new members than is the church, the latter actuated no doubt by an overweening sense of Christian charity.

In these latter days not to belong to a club or two is not to be anybody in particular. Even the women are numerously and proudly wearing club buttons, hence there is no reason • why any enterprising man need be without membership in a club or two! When both the members of these limited clubs are amiable and a trifle forbearing, there is a chance for them to be highly entertaining.

This dual club business is the most momentous as well as the most maligned of all. If men and women could only manage to keep their heads when they lose their hearts, and could be persuaded to keep in mind the old Latin maxim, *festinat in lente,* many of the saddest catastrophes of human experience might be averted. You can withdraw at will from the ordinary club, but this domestic club business may become— well, here I am on dangerous ground, and in a field where every soured critic has pranced and cavorted with free rein and high toe-and-heel calks. When the naked facts get to the surface it generally turns out that the chronic carpers who have drawn blanks in the lottery of matrimonial life generally realize all they deserve and deserve about what they get.

There are several methods of withdrawing from such a club. The sneaking and cowardly one is suicide. Another is to go to the courts and ask to have your charter or your character annulled, which may take you to the salubrious climate of Dakota, and rid you of phthisis and a termangent at the same time. A thousand times better divorce than diurnal, nocturnal and eternal discord!

But whatever the condition, there is another way. Don't suicide! Don't get desperate and go to the devil or the Klondike or South Africa or the Philippines. Brace up, dissolve the club and go it alone, or try again. Next time you may draw a capital prize and forever after wonder how you happened to be a fool the first time!

Meanwhile, join the "Brevity," or some wide-awake social club, where you can possibly pick up some of the crumbs that fall from happier tables than your own!

Much might be said about clubs, but in this somewhat restricted organization patience and forbearance have definite limits; and lest an avenging club may be already hanging over my head, I desist.

"EF the left hind foot of a rabbit wards off danger so sartin, like some folks says it does, why don't it keep the dog frum ketchin' the rabbit? That's what I'd like to know."

Book Reviews.

ANNUAL AND ANALYTICAL CYCLOPEDIA OF
PRACTICAL MEDICINE. By Charles de
M. Sajous, M.D., and One Hundred Associate Editors. Illustrated with chromo-
lithographs, engravings, and maps. Vol.
VI. Philadelphia: F. A. Davis Company, 1901.

This sixth volume is the last of the first
series of this present work. The mass of
medical literature brought together in these
volumes has probably never before been
condensed into the space of six volumes.
It is a medical library in itself.

The aim of the talented editors has been
"to furnish the general practitioner with a
clear outline of the entire field of practical
medicine."

This volume comprises 1043 pages, beautifully printed on extra paper, bound with
a taste that is unusual with medical publishers, and illustrated with cuts that illustrate, and that are a credit to both designer
and printer. Although arranged alphabet-
ically, the work is supplemented by an index that will greatly aid the searcher for
particular topics or special facts. The binding is of the same general style as the last
volume, but the artists who designed and
the artisans who have executed it, seem to
acquire new skill with each succeeding effort, so that each new volume is a little
better and more attractive than its predecessors.

The editor and his corps of accomplished
assistants have acquitted themselves of this
latest effort in such a manner as to add to
his and their already enviable fame.

"A YEARNIN' to learn things an' keep
posted is somethin' to be commended, but a
man that'll stop on the railroad crossin'
to ask what they've got the danger signal
up an' the bell a-ringin' fer, is carryin' the
idee a little too far, accordin' to my way o'
thinkin'."

Modern Culture. The table of contents
for August, 1901, has reached us and is very
attractive. The reading papers are: "The
Morning Walk" (illus.), Irving R. Wiles;
"Some Minor Painters and Their Work"
(illus.), N. Hudson Moore; "A Camera-
Girl on the Midway" (illus.), Miliccent
Olmstead; "The Bicentennial City" (illus.),
Webster Sterling; "In Our County—VI.
The Lethe Mystery—II.," Marion Har-
land; "Subordinate Territory and the Su-
preme Court," Prof. Albert Bushnell Hart;
"Wood-Notes—II. Midsummer," Nora
Archibald Smith; "Church Music in Colo-
nial Days," Mercia Abbott Keith.

EVIDENTLY no effort has been spared to
make the *Ladies' Home Journal* for August
a positive boon to its readers during these
warm midsummer days. Its light, readable articles, bright stories, clever poems,
charming music, and numerous beautiful
illustrations afford the easiest and pleasant-
est kind of entertainment for leisure hours.
Enchanting views of the lovely scenery in
the Engadine Valley and among the Swiss
and Italian lakes, as well as such delightful
articles as "The Singing Village of Germany" and "What Girl-Life in Italy
Means," allure the thoughts to foreign lands
while there are timely suggestions about
"The Picnic-Basket," "Keeping a House
Cool in the Dog-Days," and "Sea-Side
Toys and How to make Them." Other
thoroughly interesting contributions are
"The First White Baby Born in the North
west," "My Boarding School for Girls,"
and the usual serial and department articles. By the Curtis Publishing Company,
Philadelphia. One dollar a year; ten cents
a copy.

Notes and Queries.

Query 95. In a recent number of the GAZETTE there was an editorial on the subject of bread. You made out the ordinary grades of baker's bread a rather sorry substitute for the traditional staff of life.

It is much easier to tear down than to build up, and you did not tell your readers how to correct the particular faults of the baker's loaf. For one I would be glad of some more practical directions for making good bread from "the best wheat in the world." In a future article please point out the shortcomings of the baker, the much abused baker, and tell us how to avoid his dietetic faults.

For my part I think he supplies the kind of loaf that a majority of the breadbuyers appreciate, or else he would not be so universally patronized.

A. D. R., Ohio.

Answer.—In the article referred to we indicated the general faults encountered in the ordinary baker's loaf:

1. He begins by utilizing as great a proportion of low grade flours as can be made to answer his purpose, in order to save something in the matter of cost.

2. To overcome the defects of second or third grade flour he doctors it with alum, ammonia salt, and the Lord knows what else.

3. He uses brewer's instead of baker's yeast, which gives his product a harsh, yeasty taste and as a rule overferments it.

4. He makes his loaves too large and bakes them too rapidly. The result is a loaf with a thin crust and a large center "crumb" that is only half baked—its starch left in a semi-raw state that is well adapted to the work of dyspepsia-breeding. Weak stomachs cannot digest it. Many of them wear themselves out in the attempt.

In a future number of the GAZETTE we will undertake to discuss this question more thoroughly.

Query 96. Does the Editor of *Notes and Queries* credit the announcement by Dr. Koch that human beings cannot be inoculated with bovine tuberculosis? J. C. M., Penna.

Answer.—Judged by his former announcement of tuberculin and his surrender to the commercial spirit of the time, one is inclined to take a fresh announcement from the German professor with liberal grains of allowance. Some palpable facts may be cited to corroborate his announced theory. We all know that tubercular cows are by no means scarce. We also know that milk from these cows finds it way into city markets in spite of the efforts of the inspectors. Now, while it is quite the fashion for medical journals to reiterate the dangers from feeding tuberculous milk, it is not certain that a single case of infection has been directly and unmistakably traced to milk as its source. Perhaps it can only be assumed that no such cases of infection have occurred, but it is evident that if tuberculous milk is a prolific or even occasional source of infection, the race would soon become extinct from the ravages of tuberculosis. One may therefore credit the plausibility of the announcement without admitting any degree of over-confidence in the word of Koch.

IN the May number of the *International Monthly* appears an article on "Dietetics," by Professor Karl von Noorden, of Frankfort-on-the-Main. It is in the line of what *The Post-Graduate* discussed last month, on the theme of informing the public on medical matters. This article will do a great deal of good among the educated men who read it. Perhaps they will reflect—although we are not certain of that—that all this knowledge comes not from Faith Curists, and Christian Scientists, but only from members of the Medical Profession, who have gathered together all the available knowledge that there is in the world in regard to dietetics. We hail the entrance of Professor von Noorden into the field of medical science for the laity.

HUSBAND of Novelist.—Is your novel finished?

She.—No, my dear. The hero must die, you know.

H. of N.—Well, after you have killed him, will you sew this button on for me?——*Public Policy.*

DEACON BLIMBEN'S WISDOM.

"If you want your child brung up in the way he should go, you want to travel that way yourself, now an' then."

"The kitten that gets drownded ain't so bad off, after all, fer she won't live to have her tail pinched in the woodshed door."

"An' I want to tell you this. It ain't always the man what builds a sky-scrapin' buildin' that's goin' to have a mansion in the skies, an' you mind what I tell you!"

"There ain't nothin' truer than that the race ain't always to the swift; but, all the same, if I was a bettin' man, I'd put my money on the fastest hoss."

"Don't never git down-hearted 'cause you hain't got somethin' good that somebody else has got. A hen hain't got no teeth, but jes' see the luck she strikes by it. She don't have to have no gum biles."

"There ain't no rose without its thorn. Jest look at new cider. If there's a luxury on 'arth sweeter an' fuller o' satisfaction than a tin dipper o' new cider I'd like to know it; but the achin' an' doublin' up it kin interduce into your system is a caution to wildcats!"

"It's awful to read in the papers about them unpardonable fellers that eats pie with their knife an' tucks their napkins under their chin, but sence I come to think on it, them ain't never the fellers that gits pulled up to be examined in supplement'ry proceedin's, so I've noticed."

"Goodness ain't always rewarded jest accordin' to the way the books has it sot down. Now I never sold my mother's three-dollar brass kittle fer two shillin' when I was a boy, to git money to go to the circus, an' I never played hooky to see a ball game, an' I never robbed birds' nests, nor tied tin pans to dogs' tails, an' yit, by Josh, I hain't never got to be President yit!"

After a man has learned enough to instruct others he knows too much to try to do it.

Ice cream is buttery when it is churned before the cream is icy cold. Turn slowly at first until the mixture begins to freeze, then rapidly for a few moments until it is frozen.—August *Ladies' Home Journal*.

Trying goes above studying.—*P. Greitzner* (Tübingen).

The physician can receive no higher honor than the confidence of his colleagues, but only the knowledge that he has earned it can make him happy.

❧ ❧

APHORISMS.

Stone monuments are rarely erected in honor of the neurologist by his fellow-men. But so many stones are thrown at him by his patients that he can build a pyramid for himself.—*L. von Frankl-Hochwart* (Vienna).

Antisepsis is the triumph of modern surgery, but perhaps also the ruin of the old surgical skill, for to-day, under its protecting wing, children and fools operate unpunished.—*Anton v. Frisch* (Vienna).

❧ ❧

AN EFFECTIVE PRESCRIPTION.

Two Deacons of the same church were of different political faiths. Politics waxed warm in the little town where both made their home, and so, although they spoke when they met, as Christian brothers should, they never had much to do with each other. One day Deacon Smith's horse fell ill, and hearing that Deacon Brown's horse was troubled with a like malady, Smith approached Brown, and, after the customary short "Good morning," remarked: "My horse is sick; what shall I do for him?"

Deacon Brown responded: "Give him a pint of turpentine."

They passed on, and the next morning Deacon Smith on meeting Deacon Brown remarked:

"My horse died last night."

"So did mine," said Deacon Brown. "Good morning!"

THE
DIETETIC AND HYGIENIC GAZETTE

A·MONTHLY·JOURNAL·of·PHYSIOLOGICAL·MEDICINE

| Vol. XVII. | NEW YORK, OCTOBER, 1901. | No. 10. |

DOES PERSPIRATION INCREASE ELIMINATION?

By G. H. PATCHEN, M.D., NEW YORK.

IT has been aptly remarked by some one who possessed a mind well trained in the art of observation, that "when a lie once gets into the world it travels so fast that the truth can never overtake and correct it." While, of course, this saying is not literally true, it is a humorous exaggeration of the well-known fact that the exact truth in regard to any matter is very difficult to find. No wonder the ancients claimed that truth lay at the bottom of a well!

Even in our own time, with all the assistance science and experience can give to aid us in our search for truth, we meet with so many fallacies, specious probabilities and even half-truths, all masquerading in its garb, that we are often led to accept as the truth statements and conclusions which, later, are discovered to be egregious errors —errors the very belief in which is harmful and which, when adopted as a rule of practice, are positively injurious.

Although man, in his present stage of development, is denied the possession of the whole truth concerning any subject, he is created to know it, and his restless mind will not be satisfied until by searching he has found it out. Hence, the zest in the quest of it which will, undoubtedly, be continued, with added interest, upon the infinite plane of his existence.

Much to our discredit and even shame, must it be said that in no department of knowledge does there exist such a dearth of essential, demonstrated facts as in that which pertains to the needs and welfare of our own bodies. We invent the most ingenious and wonderful machinery and learn how to use it to the best advantage, and what kind of care is necessary to protect and preserve it; we engage in the largest and most complicated business enterprises, and, by reason of thorough knowledge of every detail, favorable or unfavorable, connected with it, conduct it to a successful issue; we have gained such complete and practical knowledge concerning the vegetable kingdom that we know the nature and habitat of each different species and what particular environment of soil and temperature is best adapted for its perfect development; we have studied the habits and needs of domesticated animals until we know how to raise them and care for them in such a way as to promote their health and longevity, and, yet, after thousands of years of experience, we possess so little accurate knowledge of the action, powers and requirements of our bodies that, even among those occupying places which entitle them to speak with authority, there exists no concord of opinion as to what we shall eat and drink, when and how we shall exercise, when and how we shall bathe, how we shall breathe or what we shall wear. There are even the most divergent expressions of opinion, by the same authorities, in regard to what is the proper method of walking, sitting and standing.

In shorter phrases, man, the most gifted

of all earthly creatures, is obliged to confess that, after unknown years of existence, he knows really less about the proper care of himself and his family than he does of his dogs or his horses—a sad reflection upon his wisdom, if not upon his intelligence.

The only redeeming feature about this humiliating admission is that, racially considered, man is still in his infancy—a period in which knowledge and wisdom is acquired very slowly. But the fact that he has already learned what are the needs of such of his animal associates as minister to his comforts and necessities, and willingly provides for them, is ample proof of his ability to acquire and apply physiological knowledge, and leads to the hope that, when he has arrived at the stage of maturity and discretion he will have a thorough comprehension of the beneficent laws which regulate and control his own physical and mental powers, and will be wise enough to live in harmony with them.

Already there are encouraging signs of a desire both to know and do what these laws require. The most tangible evidence of this character is the interest manifested by nearly every one in all matters relating to the subject of hygiene. Besides the increasing number of books and magazines published, for the purpose of promoting a general knowledge of the principles and facts of this science, new sects and schools, devoted to the study and practice of some special branch of it, are constantly appearing. As might naturally be expected, the information disseminated by these numerous centers of instruction, although unlimited in quantity, is not always of the most reliable character. Much careful winnowing is often necessary to separate the few grains of truth from the bulky chaff of error with which they are surrounded. But the most serious hindrance to this method of obtaining correct hygienic knowledge is not the unavoidable winnowing process itself, however tedious and expensive it may be, for truth is always worth its price. It is the lamentable fact that the great majority are unable to recognize the precious grains of truth after their

separation has been effected, unless they bear the stamp of some professed authority. But, as there is no authority for truth save that of itself, the difficulties attending its pursuit are not materially lessened by unreservedly accepting as the truth every statement which bears the trade-mark of an illustrious name. The consequence of it all is that, strive to prevent it as we may, error, to a greater or lesser extent, becomes an integral part of much of the knowledge we possess, and its elimination is as necessary a factor of scientific advancement as the acquisition of new facts and ideas.

The history of the development of the science of hygiene is a pertinent illustration both of the slowness of scientific progress and the difficulty of detecting and eliminating error when once it has been accepted as truth.

Although the facts and principles upon which the science of hygiene rests are necessarily few and simple, such as any ordinary mind can easily understand, and, although they have been studied with more or less interest since the birth of the race, it possesses, as yet, only a modicum of truths which have been universally recognized and accepted. It still harbors many erroneous and even superstitious ideas, which are not only believed but lived by thousands to their undoubted detriment.

The accuracy of the above statements is proved by the fact that there is hardly a single important matter relating to practical hygiene which meets with unanimous approval. A subject as simple as the object and uses of the bath is debated with as much zeal and diversity of opinion as the most abstruse problems of mental philosophy. There is, at once, expressed such a difference of opinion as to the proper time and proper temperature for taking it, its immediate and remote effects upon the skin, nerves, kidneys and other organs—questions which one would think should have been definitely settled generations ago—that the enquiring student of hygiene begins to have serious doubts about the propriety of bathing at all.

Upon nearly every other hygienic topic of practical interest similar differences of opinion are found to exist, and as but one of them, if indeed any, can be right, the amount of error which must be eliminated before this noble science can lay any claim to perfection is sure to be very great.

There being no absolute, isolated standard by which the accuracy of statements and conclusions can be determined, the work of elimination must proceed slowly. The method employed must be that of comparison. One truth never conflicts with another, whether in the same or an entirely different department of knowledge. Hence, any statement, belief or even alleged fact which conflicts with any definitely known and previously established fact cannot be accepted as the truth, no matter how plausible it may appear, or how completely it may seem to explain or harmonize certain phenomena.

The object of this article is to show that what for generations has been almost universally taught and believed to be a specific functional effect of one of the simplest and most familiar organs of the body is physiologically impossible, and, therefore, does not occur. The organ referred to is the skin, and the functional effect, the elaboration and elimination of physiological waste in exact proportion to the amount and activity of the perspiration induced.

To avoid any possible misunderstanding, it must be stated that by physiological waste is meant those residual, chemical products which are both the result and evidence that the successive processes of nutrition have been completed in an orderly and normal manner.

Physiological waste should not be confounded with adventitious waste which includes all substances, irrespective of their manner of introduction, which are foreign to the system, or which, like the insoluble portions of food, are dismissed from the body without being subjected to chemical change.

The alleged fact that the chief function of perspiration is to promote depuration has taken possession of the minds of both physicians and laymen to such an extent that a "good sweat" is quite universally believed to be the best possible remedy for any diseased condition of which faulty elimination is the cause. As a consequence of this belief, various devices for the artificial production of perspiration are abundantly provided. While it is undoubtedly true that many beneficial effects—some mental, some physical—occur as a result of copious perspiration, it is evident, from the following considerations, that the elaboration and elimination of waste to an extent which always corresponds to the amount of perspiration induced, is not one of them.

Physiological waste arises from only one source. It is a product of oxidation resulting from the final union of oxygen with the nutritive elements of food. It consists principally of carbonic acid, water and urea, forms of matter from which all vital energy has been extracted, and for which the system has no further use.

Unlike nutritive residuals, which, for some reason, have failed to reach a completed stage of reduction, whose prolonged retention in the system in an intermediate form is injurious and whose elimination is so difficult that it becomes a pathological process, perfected waste is not only not harmful, but its elimination cannot be prevented. As soon as formed each of its several ingredients finds immediate and ready exit from the body through channels provided for this purpose.

Physiological oxidation, although a chemical process, is subject to the laws of vitality, and, for this reason, can neither be inaugurated or maintained in the absence of organic activity. It is not enough that oxygen be abundantly supplied. The oxygen bearers of the blood may be filled to repletion with their precious freight, but none will be released until a legitimate demand for its use has been created by the functional, atomic activity of some tissue or organ.

As the muscles exceed all other organs both in size and activity, they are, at once, both the principal seat and instruments of oxidation. This important function of the muscles—that of supplying the system with the chemical power required for all purposes—is one which is too little appreciated and understood. It is not only the means by which health is normally maintained, but, when deficient, its augmentation becomes a most effective remedy for the successful removal of many serious forms of disease.

Again, under normal conditions all vital action is automatically regulated. There always exists an exact ratio, in degree, between the amount of work done by any function or organ and the incitation which leads to its doing. There are three prominent incentives to oxidation: muscular and nervous activity and the loss of vital heat. Of these incentives, the latter is undoubtedly the greatest, for, while each of the others occasions, at most, only a fitful and irregular action of oxidizing processes, the constant necessity for replenishment of vital heat allows no cessation of them.

It is the explicit of teaching physiology that the amount of oxidation taking place in the system at any given time is greatly influenced by the state of the external temperature. It is at its maximum when the temperature is 40 or 50 degrees below that of the body, so that the heat interiorly produced radiates freely and rapidly into the surrounding air. When the external temperature equals or excels that normal to the body, a powerful incentive to oxidation is lacking. The result is not only a diminished amount of vital heat, but a notable deficiency of other necessary forms of chemical energy inseparably associated with heat production. Hence, to subject the body to a degree of heat sufficient, in any form, to induce free perspiration, instead of increasing the production of eliminative matter, positively lessens it.

Cold, on the contrary, promotes oxidation by inciting muscular action, thereby making an increased demand for the chemical union of oxygen for the double purpose of supplying the heat, constantly lost by evaporation, and of preparing new, nutritive material to take the place of that destroyed by the muscular effort it has induced.

Furthermore, although the skin performs several useful functions it is not an elabora-tive organ like the liver and kidneys, nor the seat of chemical activity like the muscles. Therefore, beyond the preparation of the perspiratory fluid and its own products of waste, it does not participate in the general processes of oxidation. The channels of perspiration, it is true, afford egress for some of the products of perfected waste, but, like the lungs and bladder only for such as are conveyed to them already prepared for exclusion.

Moreover, the proportion of physiological waste which finds exit through the skin is very small, whether compared with the total amount, from all sources, or with that from each source singly. No urea is discharged, and the carbonic acid which escapes is only about one one-fiftieth part of the amount furnished by the lungs, while the quantity of water eliminated is less by far than that which appears from any other source.

Lastly, the main object and use of perspiration is to cool the blood. Over 99 per cent. of its composition is water. This water is not depurative; it is only regulative of the temperature. Its production is more the result of a mechanical than of a vital process. After passing through numerous minute coils of tubes in close proximity to the overheated blood of the capillaries upon which it exerts a perceptibly cooling influence, it reaches the surface of the skin to add to its cooling effect by more or less rapid evaporation.

From the foregoing brief presentation of the fundamental facts concerning the origin, composition and manner of elimination of physiological waste, it is evident that nothing can be more erroneous or further from the truth than the idea, still widely spread and popular, that perspiration is, of itself, a purifying process. The error, undoubtedly, arose long before the functions of the skin, or any of the vital organs became known, from ignorantly believing that the relief and sense of good-feeling which follows copious perspiration is due to the escape of pent-up waste matter, and that perspiration is both the cause and means of its expulsion.

Such a conception, in the absence of better knowledge, was natural and excusable. Modern methods of scientific investigation, however, have proved that this assumption is far from correct. Elimination of waste matter consists of two distinct processes—its preparation, or elaboration, and its dismissal. The first of these processes is the all-important one, for, contrary to another erroneous opinion, perfectly elaborated products of waste require no assistance of any kind to aid them in their escape from the body. The pores of the skin are never so tightly closed that carbonic acid and water with the few organic salts it contains —forms of perfected waste normal to these channels—cannot pass through them, in any amount, without any hindrance or disturbance; the lungs afford egress with equal facility to all the water and carbonic acid presented to them, and the kidneys, never, for an instant, refuse passage to urea, however rapidly and abundantly it may be formed.

But, it may be asked, do not the pores of the skin sometimes become clogged with waste matter seeking an outlet, and does not free perspiration, even if artificially induced, assist in removing these substances and in keeping the pores open? The answer is that if the pores become clogged it is with other forms of matter which do not find ready exit, there or elsewhere, because the oxidizing forces are too weak to change it into elements prepared for dismissal. Its presence, wherever found, is a menace to healthful interests, and its lodgment in the skin is a wise provision, because, there, it cannot interfere with the necessary work of more vital organs. Its presence in the pores of the skin does not indicate that the system is trying to get rid of it. Its physical composition precludes such an idea; for, besides the fact that it contains elements of nutrition and power which, by such a procedure, would be wholly lost, its passage would be both unnatural and unnecessary; unnatural, because difficult, and, therefore, irritating, and unnecessary because a better way has been provided. Faulty chemical action is the only cause of its existence in its present form and location.

Restore, therefore, the defective oxidizing functions and processes to a normal degree of vigor and efficiency, and this offending material obstructing the eliminative pathways of the skin will be quickly removed through the agency of the circulation, and resubmitted to the powerful chemistry of the organism which will extract its nutritive portions and insure the rapid and easy dismissal of the residuals.

Elimination depends upon, and is measured by, oxidation, a process which is quickened and intensified by activity and cold, and retarded and repressed by repose and heat. Perspiration bears only an incidental relation to oxidation; its function is to modify the heat to which the body is subjected by oxidation from within and that of the temperature from without.

Such, logically stated, are the truths of physiology regarding the depurative influence of perspiration. That they are squarely antagonistic to prevailing belief and practice does not lessen their value or importance.

20 West Fifty-ninth street.

DR. SPRATLING writes: "It would be well if epileptics could be made to understand that in taking patent nostrums they are consuming quantities of poison that is destined in time to injure them physically and mentally. These patent nostrums have the superficial and false virtue of *suppressing* the attacks for the time; but that is all, they simply *suppress*, they do not cure. In doing this they do infinitely more harm than they do good, for when the drug is withdrawn the attacks always recur with greater violence than ever. In the meantime the patient has suffered great damage, both to his mind and to his digestive organs, the one set of organs above all others that the epileptic should keep free from disease, and unhampered in healthful activity. I have seen numbers of epileptics made insane by patent nostrums, and so far have wholly failed to observe any case that has ever been cured or benefited in the slightest degree by these poisons."

WHAT THE CENTURY HAS
TAUGHT US ABOUT LIVING......

By Samuel S. Wallian, A.M., M.D.

(*Copyright*, 1901.)

VII.

The Ethics and Evolution of Cooking.

Without doing violence to the established laws of evolution, it may be assumed that before he had reached a stage of development entitling him to the generic name *homo,* man possessed several stomachs, or at least gastric dilatations and subdivisions that might be said to correspond with the several stomachs of the ruminants. Possibly there was originally a septum at about the cardiac flexure, separating the organ into two sections or stomachs. Perhaps the duodenum is an atrophied, constricted but not yet wholly obliterated third food receptaculum. Further on are the cæcum and vermiform appendix, both now practically functionless. Are they, too, rudimentary, having once performed their respective functions in connection with the transformation or assimilation of nutrient material?

It is evident that if the professional biologists finally answer this question in the affirmative the human race has at last emerged from the ruminant or semi-ruminant stage and can no longer call upon the digestive tract to grapple with the cruder forms of nutrient material. Uncooked starch and woody fiber prove obnoxious to the modern stomach.

It is therefore rational to insist that in his stage of physical development the food of mankind requires to be modified and in a sense partially predigested by either thermic or chemic processes.

Cooking is an art. It has become a necessity. But for the existence of a sprinkling of nondescript philosophers who loudly advocate the use of raw food and denounce cooking as subversive of the laws of nutri-

tion and hygiene it would not be necessary to emphasize this assertion. There are certain enthusiasts who plead for a return to the primitive habits and practices of the race, to the time when our ancestors wore hair all over their bodies, "shinned up" trees for "shack," and fought their duels and battles with teeth, claws and clubs.

Cooking is the principal process by which alimentary products are modified for human use. Heat transforms starch, woody fiber and cellular structures of all kinds into much more digestible and assimilable forms. The same agency disintegrates the tough fibers and cells of fleshmeats and thus puts them in condition to be promptly and thoroughly acted upon by the gastric secretions.

The various methods of cooking include baking, broiling, and frying, boiling and steaming. To these might be added a modified form of boiling called simmering, and a modification of roasting which is accomplished by submitting, especially meats, to prolonged heat of moderate degree, as in the Aladdin oven invented by Professor Atkinson.

Baking and roasting are susceptible of almost unlimited modification as to degree or thoroughness as exemplified in the pale semi-cooked "crumb" or inner mass of the ordinary white loaf and the well-browned outer crust of the same. Zwieback, bisbak and sundry forms of "sticks" and crisps are other examples of twice-baked and hard baked breadstuffs. Still other forms are being introduced in the form of granose flakes and biscuit, shredded wheat, granola, rusks, etc. The multiplication of these products is an apt illustration of the persistence of the law of selection and evolution. Even the better grades of the ordinary baker's loaves are beginning to show more crust and less crumb; and the bread of the future will undoubtedly show further modification in this direction. The loaf will be made thinner and the baking process prolonged.

The cooking process, if carried to a sufficient degree and if sufficiently prolonged, converts starch and gluten into dextrin and glucose, which tax the digestive organs much less than the original forms.

For generations the sturdy Scotch yeomanry successfully grappled with semi-raw starch, living, and developing into men of great stature and unparalleled endurance, on their diet of under-done oatmeal porridge. Now, the same regimen gives them waterbrash and painful hypopepsia, and they are entering into a stage that may be called one of dietetic transition. No doubt they have deteriorated somewhat in the matter of brawn, but by and by they will give more attention to cooks and the cuisine, and perhaps will resume their former reputation as athletes and men of physical sturdiness and endurance.

The opinions and practices in relation to the cooking of fleshmeats have not made the same progress. Authorities, both numerous and prominent, still insist that raw or rare-cooked flesh is more digestible than when thoroughly cooked. Other authorities are beginning to assert that this is only the persistence of a primitive instinct, and that it is closely related to the raw cereal delusion.

Heat does not induce changes in the fiber of flesh analogous to those produced in case of starch and the cereals. The carnivora do not need that their food be cooked, and the raw food advocates revert to this fact as an argument in support of their theories; while the advocates of thorough cooking intimate that this is nothing more than a partial reversion to animal instincts.

The law of evolution is progressive, not retrogressive. In the order of creation art is not an alien and an interloper; it is a legitimate expression of Nature. The two are always in close sympathy, never in contrast or antagonistic. Fire is a resultant of chemical combinations that are constantly taking place. It has never been and never will be quenched. It is as natural as freezing. Cooking is, therefore, by no means an unnatural process.

The first European treatise on cookery of which we have any account emanated from the Romans, and its authorship is rather uncertainly accredited to Cælius Apicius. This supposed author flourished under the reign of Trajan, early in the second century. Samples of his recipes sound queerly enough to modern ears:

"First, for a sauce to be eaten with boiled fowl, put the following ingredients into a mortar: Aniseed, dried mint, and lazar root, cover them with vinegar, add dates, and pour in liquamen (a distilled liquor made from the large fish which were salted and allowed to turn putrid in the sun), oil, and a small quantity of mustard seeds. Reduce all to a proper thickness with sweet wine, warmed, and then pour this same over your chicken, which should previously be boiled in aniseed water."

"Take a wheelbarrow of rose leaves and pound in a mortar, add to it brains of two pigs and two thrushes, boiled and mixed with the chopped-up yolk of egg, oil, vinegar, pepper, and wine. Mix and pour these together, and stew them steadily and slowly till the perfume is developed."

Other examples might be cited, such as pigs stuffed with live thrushes, peacocks, killed by suffocation, skinned, stuffed with the flesh of other birds, the whole sewn together, roasted (presumably, affixed to a small branch as if alive), and served as a prelude to dinner.

As recently as during the reign of Charles the Second, these recipes were imitated and made even more atrocious. Thus, two pies to be served jointly were made as follows:

One contained live frogs and the other live birds. "When the pies were opened. the frogs skipped, and the birds flew directly at the lights, of course putting them out, which made the ladies to shriek and fly from the room in a panic."

The discovery or invention of cooking was undoubtedly an accident. Some animal, caught in a forest fire or in some other way was partially cremated. A hungry hunter sniffed the savory carcass, was curious enough to taste it, and instantly became a convert to the new cooking school.

Or, the same fire roasted some nuts, browned some edible tubers, or parched some of the primitive grains. The modern French *chef* is only a lineal descendant evolved from such an unpromising ancestry.

A few general principles may be formulated:

In a general way, baking, roasting and broiling are more effective processes than boiling, since the heat can be carried to a higher degree. The limit in boiling is 212° F., and this extreme is attainable only at sea-level, since as one ascends to higher altitudes the boiling point of water falls, until at great elevations it is so low that it will not cook either flesh or vegetables. Even at the moderately high elevations at which mining and other vocations are carried on, it is found impossible to thoroughly cook beans and other leguminous edibles, as any Rocky Mountain miner or prospector will attest. It is a common remark that boiled meats are not as digestible as roasts, and the old-fashioned boiled pudding has never stood high as a diet for delicate stomachs. It is because the starch granules are but partially converted by the degree of heat attained. The sogginess complained of is due to this lack of cooking rather than to the presence of water.

The prolonged exposure to even a moderate degree of heat, in boiling, induces the thorough changes in flesh and in some forms of vegetable fiber that are required to make them easy of digestion, as in the various stews; but this rule is not applicable to substances containing a preponderance of starch.

Broiled and roasted meats are more appetizing and more digestible than either boiled or fried meats. In frying some portions are sure to be over-done or scorched, and certain chemical changes occur in the fatty portions thus overheated which render the meat obnoxious to the digestive organs. In the language of Dr. Rainsford:

"The frying-pan is the enemy of civilization; it drives women to despair and men to drink."

Another eminent authority says: "If the frying-pan is a terror to the well it is death to the sick."

This is a rather exaggerated estimate, but there is no question as to the desirability of substituting the broiler for the frying-pan. There are, however, two methods of frying, the first of which is by cooking things in hot fat, the other by cooking them rapidly, in a dry frying-pan or on a hot griddle. This latter may be called superficial roasting. It can be done so as to be unobjectionable from a dietetic standpoint.

As man is at present constituted, raw starch is not digested until it reaches the small intestine, and its digestion there is slow and imperfect. Much of it is not digested at all. For this reason, if for no other, as already intimated, it is not an economic form of food. Since the principal portion of all human food belongs to the starch group, it is possible to devolve much of the labor of the digestive organs upon the range and oven. Proteids and fats can be digested with little or no cooking, but a large share of the process of starch digestion must now be accomplished in advance by the application of heat. Slightly cooked starch is not much more digestible than when raw, and it is largely due to its presence that starch indigestion and "dyspepsia" are so prevalent.

Thus, in the preparation of food, vital or digestive energy may be conserved by a systematic resort to heat. One reason that green fruit is so obnoxious to weak stomachs is that it contains a certain percentage of starch which, through the ripening process, is converted into sugar. For the same reason cooking green fruit partially or wholly overcomes the principal objection to its use.

It seems to be admitted that cooking will be further studied and better methods of applying it devised as the age progresses.

Perhaps, in the near future, the grains will all be roasted or parched before grinding, and it may be that radically new processes for turning them into nutritious and economic bread will follow.

THE PROBLEM OF HAPPINESS.

Stanton Kirkham Davies,
In the July number of *Mind*.

WE are born into the consciousness of material things and are brought under the dominion of the senses when first we open our eyes, and so it is that men fall naturally into the belief that to eat and be clothed, to marry and beget sons and accumulate property, are the paramount considerations —nor ever question it. Only now and then is one born into the consciousness of the Spirit; only now and again one who sees these things to be secondary and not in themselves sufficient ends in life. What wonder, then, that as men grow older they grow disheartened and become cynics? What wonder, indeed, that the problem of happiness finds so seldom a solution in terms of actual life; for, considering the neglect of essential factors, how else can it be?

Many factors, of a truth, enter into our problem. There is courage, for instance, which were it a man's sole possession would in itself confer a considerable degree. There is perception, will, habit—education, which has reference to all of these. Are we being educated, that is, or stimulated, in the direction peculiarly our own, that we may come to express that something which is in us? It is obvious that education without reference to this will not contribute to happiness. If capital lie unused, if character be unformed, there must be unrest. In such case we cannot too soon have done with book learning and begin the culture of the will and the affections. Does our mode of living tend to educate us, above all, away from our false and negative tendencies, in the direction of aspirations and real aims—out of the Adam into the Christ? And this is the education that is never ended, and it is never too late to begin. Nor let us neglect the sense of humor—a brave virtue, a practical virtue, a friend indeed. "To sit on a stile and continue to smile" is a better philosophy than many another, and is vexed with no dogma. We cannot laugh too much so long as our mirth is kindly. True humor need create no false occasions, and it brings no heartaches. It begets good will and is a mental and moral buffer. The man of coarse habit and coarse thinking needs it not so much as the gentle soul—to him it is indispensable. Out of the flux of things it everywhere extracts some gold. Its possessor carries his own sunshine—gilds the dreariest circumstance and enlivens what else would be monotony. So is it recuperative and wholesome, and, being cultivable, it, no less than the love of the beautiful, comes within the scope of a liberal self-education.

* * * * *

It has thus been the chief office of any true philosophy of living to show that happiness is something apart from pleasure, which is but a fool's paradise; that it reverts to an inner state, is the outcome of an inward poise and serenity, and therefore not greatly dependent upon externals. We may be unhappy—uneasy—in spite of ease of circumstance and the most favorable surroundings. Again, we may be sick and happy, poor and happy, alone and happy. But, thanks be to the genius of the hour, we need no longer state our doctrine so narrowly as did the Stoics, who placed such things as health and environment beyond the will.

* * * * *

If you have no revolution in your life, and are as yet in your period of feudalism, you shall experience anarchy and the overthrow of a whole line of degenerate kings before you emerge from despotism and evolve at last a stable self-government. Alas, if when the time is ripe we leap not to our feet and don the red cap in the name of Liberty!

* * * * *

It is a thankless task to read philosophy if we can live none. What does it concern us what Kant said, what Hegel, or Fichte, or Schelling, if we have no convictions of our own? Some little philosophy for this daily life is the crying need. But it is alone a spontaneous and inspired utterance that can aid us. Who has not felt the futility of all "systems" of philosophy? They fall cold on our ears—do not warm in us any new life nor hope: just as a treatise on morals is a bore, and rules of conduct an impertinence, while the shining example of a free and noble life is refreshing and uplifting. Because life and love are one we must live from our hearts, write from our hearts, speak from our hearts.

* * * * *

Much reading, much listening, much wrestling with the angel, and yet wisdom comes slowly. But it is realization only that we lack. We have capital enough for the enterprise of life in our being; the question is to render it available. So need it be no discouragement that wisdom conditions happiness. *Still* the mind and the Soul will make itself known. It is thus the main purpose of concentration to hold the mind in check, to render it passive that self-illumination may take place. More often than not we are oblivious of the soul through the over-activity of the mind. Concentration, in fact, should always be in the direction of repose. But in our revolt from mental tyranny let us not disparage the mind as an unworthy agent of the Soul's divine estate. In this connection Emerson says: "Everything has two handles; beware of the wrong one." There's no faculty of the mind but its use is beneficent, but it needs be taken by the right handle.

* * * * *

Any stable condition of happiness must be the outcome of balanced forces—a rounded character. It is not genius which is happiest, nor is great attainment essential—unless it be the genius to find one's self, which is, to be sure, a very considerable attainment. Life is not so hard as we make it. But we cannot enough see the divine in it. Our living is perfunctory; we live because we must. So in our daily life, if we occasionally pray for heaven, we as often invite the reverse in the character of our thought. Living is too dear thus. We are more than sheep. He alone who begins life anew each morning is truly living. It is ever morning to the Soul, and it would seem a constitutional

defect of the mind that measures life by days and months and years, as if the world were a huge clock and mankind the minute hand, and the main business to count the minutes. Let us count cycles rather, and aim to live epochs and eras. For we may crowd a cycle into a day if we live to the Universal.

What matters it that we are dead to custom, dead to society, if only we are alive to Beauty? 'Tis the stream in which we bathe and forget our cares, and are renewed. So does the Spirit contrive that here on this dear green earth we are beset with beauty. The very sod is packed with it, so that it must continually overflow, now in green fields and buttercups, now in golden rod and asters. It lies over the moonlit ocean and purples the distant hills. It skims with the martin and floats with the cloud—is showered upon us in October leaves and winter snows. All the days of my life it knocks at my door. Let us not be unheeding, lest we become withered and sere in the desert wind of the commonplace; lest we become infected with the pessimism of church and society—parched and shriveled with the dulness of men's thinking, and so succumb at last to the Prosaic. Keep, then, the lamp burning at sacred Beauty's shrine, and may it be constant as the Greek fire; for, give me in my heart the love of Beauty and naught shall keep from me the World Beautiful. In view of this it is only the frivolous, or the melancholy and half insane, who can talk of "killing time." A healthy mind does not know the meaning of *ennui*.

* * * * *

To have kept the house or tended the baby —managed the farm or financiered the nation—one is as insignificant as another; for house and baby and all are destined for mortality's speedy end. But if in so doing we have acquired love, patience, insight—these are ours for evermore, and make the task noble and the game worth the candle. Neither is it much to give happiness that we ourselves may be happy, nor to love for the sake of being loved. Our problem will not admit of so easy a solution. No conscience money! No robbing Peter to pay Paul! But motive—always motive, and this alone.

In the pursuit of happiness we travel the world over—we forever seek new conditions. Now it is money will give it, and now it is marriage. But happiness lies not in new conditions: it is the outcome of a superiority to all conditions. Once married we find it is to impose strange and unlooked for circumstances to which in turn we must rise superior. When men say marriage is a failure, they mean that selfishness is a failure—that egotism is not a success. Marriage is indeed the true state of man, and true marriage can never be a failure. But we play at marriage; we are but half married at best. Unselfishness is that basis alone on which marriage can rest secure. Here, above all, is it required. True marriage requires a gradual self-renunciation. It grows beautiful as it becomes impersonal: two living and acting together to the ends of the Universal; two in one, and that the Soul; two going out to humanity in each other—that is marriage. But two living to their own ends will bring up like the monkey and the parrot. Nature resents a too personal and restricted love and finds a way to turn the tables. From the hearth our love must go out to the world, else it will grow stale. It is the same with property. Whatever is hedged in has lost its best value. The exclusive exclude themselves. We are only here for a day; let us hold a feast, then, and celebrate the event. What is love for but to express? Lavish it, then, on the cat, if no other outlet presents itself. But there is occasion enough—never fear; the aged and neglected need it, the unwelcome children need it, the downtrodden animals need it. Ah, but they are a sorry lot of specters, these austere men and women who have bottled up their natural affections until they have turned to vinegar. We can be as miserly with love as with dollars.

*　　*　　*　　*　　*

Marriage exacts a purification as well as a renunciation. Every happy marriage implies evolution: an evolution from the personal man or woman of selfish ends, to broader views and nobler aims and a deeper love, a sanctified love. It demands there should be a community of such interests as these—that man and wife should hold the Ideal in common. For merely to hold the flesh in common is to seek a common grave; to have nothing in common is an affliction. And yet even this is not hopeless but capable in noble natures of bearing fine fruit. All experience goes to corroborate what wisdom reveals to rarer natures, that there can be no perfect union on personal grounds—so unreliable and fluctuating is personality. But where two are joined in the Spirit nothing indeed can put asunder.

*　　*　　*　　*　　*

Oh, happy day for him who gives up striving to be richer, wiser, more clever than his fellows, and settles down content to be himself! And when abates the fever of possession and he perceives that the riches of the rich, the joy of the happy, and the strength of the strong are his as well—then indeed for him has the millennium dawned. Then shines the sun for him; for him blooms the rose; for him the waters murmur and the wind sighs in the forest, or croons to the rustling corn. He shares the speed of the trout and the song of the wren. He welcomes the souls that are coming and bids God-speed to the souls that are parting. Alone on the mountain or one of the crowd, everywhere is he in touch with the heart of humanity. All joys are his joys; all sorrows are his to assuage. Child is he with childhood everywhere. To him flow the love and heroism of the world; for he has no longer a private and particular life. His bark has sunk to another sea—sails now on the serene and smiling waters of the Universal.

A LIBERAL EDUCATION AND THE STUDY OF MEDICINE.

THE *Outlook* has recently published, says the *Philadelphia Medical Journal*, a laudatory notice of the utterances of Dr. Edmund W. Holmes, of this city, in respect to a liberal education for professional men, especially medical men. Dr. Holmes has analyzed the figures supplied by a number of American universities, and finds in some of them, especially those which are noted for their medical curriculum, a distinct tendency away from what is usually called a "liberal education." He attributes this tendency to three principal causes. First, the desire to begin professional work early. Second, the encouragement of the belief, held by some professional men, that a college education. is a waste of time. Third, the popular error that a professional or technical education is of itself a liberal education. Dr. Holmes does not agree with these views, and we agree with Dr. Holmes. We have never sympathized with the opinions of those medical teachers who are constantly declaiming against a liberal education for the medical student. We understand fully the grounds upon which they base their objections. It is, if we mistake not, the utilitarian objection that a liberal education is not necessary to success in the practice of medicine. We do not attempt to combat this statement. We know that it is in large part true. It is easy to point to very many men who have been eminent in our profession without the assistance of a liberal education. We grant this without dispute, and we honor these men not the less, but rather the more. We think, however, that the argument is doubly fallacious and unreliable, and that in fact it has nothing whatever to do with the real question. A liberal education is not intended for mere utilitarian advantages. One might as well speak against the fine arts, or literature, or ethics, or even against religion itself, because these are not absolutely essential to a technical training, as to decry a liberal education. Such an education is not intended to be a mere aid in the winning of bread and butter, neither is it intended to be a mere accessory to a technical training, although we believe the time is coming when it will be more and more a necessity for success in some of the purely technical pursuits. But, laying that aside, it can be broadly stated that a liberal education has

an entirely different object, and that that object is the cultivation of the mind, the broadening of the intellect, the endowment of the moral sense, the acquaintance with the best attainments, history, cultivation, literature, and development of the race, and that it is far above all considerations of mere utilitarianism.

The case of Huxley is well in point. This eminent man suffered from the deficiencies of his early education, but he realized this so fully, and devoted himself so assiduously and so successfully to the remedy of these defects, that he became a man of wide cultivation, not only in science, but in literature, languages, philosophy, metaphysics, history, and even theology, to all of which he added the advantages of a fine literary style. Was this liberal education of no advantage to Huxley?

With respect to medicine, which is a profession that brings a man most intimately into contact with his fellows, we believe that from a mere personal standpoint, a liberal education is a desirable and appropriate thing for a physician to have. We do not contend for a moment, however, that it is a necessity for his success or profit. We think it should be apparent, nevertheless, to most thoughtful observers that the argument that a young man cannot spare the time to be liberally educated is a most unconvincing one. It makes practically little difference to his success whether a young man receives his medical degree at twenty-two or twenty-three, on the one hand, or twenty-five or twenty-six years of age, on the other. If there is any advantage it is on the side of his not taking his degree too early. Few men succeed in the practice of medicine until they are well past thirty, and the years before thirty can be well devoted to education in the widest sense of that word. A young man has lost nothing who has given a few additional years to the cultivation of his mind. Such a curriculum certainly does not disable him for anything, while as a rule, it not only makes him more readily efficient as a student of the intricate sciences of medicine, but it gives him a personal endowment which is of inestimable advantage to him as an individual and a citizen. The claim that a young man wastes three or four years of his life in the cultivation of his mind in attaining a liberal education can only be based upon an erroneous view of what constitutes one of the highest aims in life.

THE FIGHT AGAINST MOSQUI-TOES.

THIS is a decidedly engrossing topic at this particular season, and will remain such until the frosts of winter have annihilated the last of the *anopheles.*

The *Medical News* has this to say: "The average young person probably harbors a hazy notion that whatever is good for his health is disagreeable. There are many instances, however, in which health and comfort are promoted by the same means. One of them, as we have only lately learned, is the prevention of mosquito-bites, and,in our opinion, the Division of Entomology of the United States Department of Agriculture has done the people a distinct benefit by issuing a circular (No. 13, second series) concerning mosquitoes and fleas. While the entomologist whose signature is appended to the circular, Mr. L. O. Howard, recognizes that the thorough screening of windows and the use of the bed net are the best means to employ against the access of mosquitoes in dwellings, he makes some very practical and useful suggestions as to the destruction of those mosquitoes which, in spite of these measures, do inflict their bites even in the best-regulated families. As some of the defensive means suggested may not be generally known,we will mention them briefly. The slow burning of cones made of miostened pyrethrum powder gives great relief from the attacks of mosquitoes in a room, but does not kill the insects, and is only a palliative. Mosquitoes found on the ceiling of a bedroom may be killed easily and quickly by placing under them a shallow tin vessel nailed to the end of a stick and moistened on the inside with kerosene. But the most satisfactory means of fighting mosquitoes is to destroy their larvæ or abolish their breeding-places by draining ponds and marshes, by stocking pools with fish, and by the use of kerosene on the surface of the water. Approximately, an ounce of the oil to every fifteen square feet of surface is sufficient, and generally the application need be made only once a month. Mr. Howard doubts, however, if it will prove feasible to treat extensive salt marshes in this way. Cesspools, cisterns, etc., should be treated in the same manner. If drinking-water is drawn from the bottom of a tank, as is commonly the case, there is no objection to coating the surface of the water with kerosene. In the matter of tanks, cisterns, cesspools, etc., there should be concerted action in a district, for a family may suffer from their neighbor's mosquitoes."

Assuming that the guilty *anopheles,*—the female only, for the males are all pious members of the anti-imperial society, and never harm anybody!—are strictly and solely chargeable with all the annual devastation ascribed to "malaria." Dr. G. N. Lawson has an article in the *Yale Medical Journal* of which we summarize:

1. There are three varieties of malaria, (1) the tertian, (2) the quartan and (3) the estivo-autumnal, each produced by its special plasmodium.

2. The female mosquito of the genus anopheles is the extra-corporeal host of the plasmodium of human malaria.

3. The mosquito must first bite a malarial patient in order to become infected.

4. Malaria is only produced clinically as far as our experimental knowledge goes, by the bite of infected anopheles, (and hence, granting this.)

5. Malaria can be entirely avoided by avoiding the bites of the anopheles.

6. Anopheles can be easily distinguished from culex in all its stages.

7. Anopheles bite mostly by night.

8. The three most effective ways of avoiding bites of anopheles are, (1) by

draining the breeding pools; (2) by applying petroleum once a month to such pools as cannot be drained; (3) by protecting sleeping rooms by mosquito netting and avoiding bites during the evening.

9. Malarial patients should be protected from mosquito bites, especially early in the season.

In the old days it was deemed necessary that every physician should be something of a botanist. He has always needed to be a chemist. During the last decade, all students of medicine have been made to some degree bacteriologists, and now unrelenting Science has decreed that we all become entomologists.

Let us cheerfully shoulder our new duty, pick up our magnifying glassses and kerosene cans, and fight the bugs.

A HANDY DEVICE IN THE TREATMENT OF OPIUM NARCOSIS.

Dr. Lyne, in the *Vir. Med. Semi-Monthly,* has the following pertinent remarks concerning this frequent and fatal accident:

"I wish to call attention of the medical profession to a means always 'at hand' in the treatment of coma incident to poisonous doses of opium or morphine, which enables the attendant physician, at least from the standpoint of the laity, to appear less brutal, and often save a patient from any marks of violence, as bruising, arising from flagellation with the often used wet towel.

"All text-books condemn flagellation, which I most heartily endorse; but it often becomes necessary to use it in a modified way, particularly in the absence of the sanctioned electric battery, which every physician does not possess, or if so, in many instances, is either out of fix or out of place. I have never seen in print this method advocated nor have I heard of its being used prior to my suggestion, in 1896, while in the Richmond City Ambulance Service.

"To enter into a discussion of the "rationale," I would first say that if one is observant of a hypodermatic injection of morphine or dose per orem, he notices an itching or tickling sensation about the nose and mouth; the same being manifested by the drowsy or asleep patient rubbing his face now and then. This, as we all know, is a physiologic action of the drug. Tickling or itching are both nervous manifestations, and though not the same, for all intents and purposes, when either is present to a marked degree, sleep is more or less disturbed, if not entirely abandoned.

"Take, for instance, how, when pesky flies promenade during sleep, the realm of infant smiles, or if more mature life, the wince, the fidget, the movement to shoo fly, a semi-conscious act.

"Look at the constant irritation produced by scratching, when asleep, in eczema, scabies, etc. How impossible sleep, in exaggerated pruritus ani, vulvæ vel scroti!

"We all know the efficacy, much to our discomfort and annoyance, when in the bliss of our second or third morning nap to have our helpmeet or room-mate interrupt abruptly the possibility of realizing or enjoying the sensation of a millionaire (alas! only in sleep), when she or he throws the cover off and digs into our sides with both hands, in anything but mirth-inspiring tickling. Have you noticed or experienced how mad or angered one gets under these circumstances?

"My friends, I have practiced *tickling* during the sleep of opium in poisonous doses. It acts like a charm, not only awakening, but angering nearly to the point of fighting. My advice, however, is to stop short just this side and give it in broken doses *pro re nata.* If it be a woman, so much the better, because of their delicate nervous poise making them better subjects; and I care not how degraded her morals, if she think her person threatened or any liberties taken, defence will come in the supreme effort of resistance.

"Of course, I do not claim that tickling is Gabriel's trumpet, which awakes the dead, or even those in which reflexes are entirely lost. I do not refer to the abolition of pain reflex, for we must ever remember that opium is the 'pain killer.'

"Further, I claim that this method of tickling has a very wide range of application, on account of the big percentage of ticklish persons. I do not dwell on the recognized methods of treating opium poisoning, which are well known to junior students of medicine; but always *treat the patient*.

"To summarize the advantages of tickling:

"1. The doctor has it handy.
"2. Wide range of application.
"3. Simplicity.
"4. Leaves no marks of violence.
"5. Efficacy."

CONCERNING THE ANTIPHLOGISTIC ACTION OF COLD APPLIED TO POINTS DISTANT FROM THE SEAT OF INFLAMMATION.

EMMERT (*Fortschritte der Medicin*, 1901, xix., p. 161), in Goldscheider's clinic, has repeated some experiments which were made by Samuel in 1892, with regard to the antiphlogistic action of cold applied at points distant from the seat of the inflammation. Samuel noted that if croton oil were applied to one ear of the rabbit, while the other was immersed in water, the inflammation was materially delayed. In control rabbits the process came on in five hours, while in those in which the opposite ear was immersed, no signs of inflammation were to be noted throughout the experiments, which lasted up to twelve hours. On removing the ear from the water, however, the inflammation began. Samuel's explanation of this antiphlogistic action was, that owing to cooling of an extensive vascular area, the leucocytes which passed through the vessels were, for a certain length of time, deprived of their active motility. In repeating Samuel's experiments, Emmert adopted a somewhat different plan, as he found it

difficult to keep the rabbit's ear under water for long periods of time without bringing about conditions which interfered with the experiment. An arrangement was made by which, without much distress to the animal, one leg could be kept under water. It was found that under normal circumstances the time at which the evidences of inflammation set in, varied so greatly that it was necessary to retain the leg under water for at least twelve hours, by which time, in the control animals, the inflammation invariably came on. The experiments showed that, by immersion of the lower half of the left hind leg in water at a temperature of from 12° to 15° C., the croton oil inflammations were delayed as long as the leg remained in the water. Some of the experiments were continued as long as thirty hours. Another series of experiments, in which the leg was immersed after the inflammation had begun, showed distinctly that the inflammatory process stopped at the point which it had reached at the beginning of the bath.

With regard to the explanations of this phenomenon, Emmert differs from Samuel. He noted, contrary to the observations of the latter, that the temperature of the animal always fell several degrees, and that this fall in temperature always preceded the disappearance of the inflammatory process. It was found, further, that if, while the leg was still in the bath, the animal was warmed so as to prevent this fall of temperature, the inflammation occurred exactly as in the control animals. In another animal exposed simply to cold air there was also a marked fall of temperature and a material delay in the onset of the inflammation. He concludes that the observation of Samuel, that the immersion of one extremity of a rabbit in a cool fluid is sufficient to hinder the development of a croton oil inflammation in another part, is true; that, indeed, the antiphlogistic action of this procedure is even greater than Samuel suspected. Emmert's experiments, however, appear to show that the delay and prevention of the croton oil inflammation depends not upon any special action of the cold on the leucocytes in the exposed area, but upon the marked fall of temperature throughout the animal's whole body.

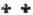

TRANSMISSION OF SOUND.

A striking example of the magical effects capable of being produced by any one conversant with the laws of sound, says *Chamber's Journal*, was shown by the late Prof. Tyndall, in one of his lectures. He placed on the floor of the room an ordinary guitar. No one was near, and yet some unseen hand drew sweet music from it, so that all could hear. The guitar was replaced by a harp, with the same result. A wooden tray was then substituted, and even from that issued mysterious harmonies. The marvelous effect was simply due to the sound-conducting quality of wood. In a room beneath, and separated by two floors, was a piano, and connecting the rooms was a tin tube containing a deal rod, the end of which emerged from the floor. The rod was clasped by rubber bands so as to close the tube, and the lower end of the rod then rested on the sound-board of the piano. As the guitar rested upon the upper end of the rod, the sounds were reproduced from the piano, and when the sound-board of the harp was placed on the rod it seemed as though the actual notes of the harp were heard, the notes of the piano being so like those of the harp. As the professor said: "An uneducated person might well believe that witchcraft was used in the production of this music," and

it is certainly more than probable that if he had done the same thing publicly in an earlier age, he would either have been reverenced as possessing supernatural powers or have been burned as a sorcerer!

HUXLEY ON PHYSIOLOGY.

In the recently published Life and Letters of Huxley, the subject of the biography in one of his letters says: "I would urge that a thorough study of Human Physiology is in itself an education broader and more comprehensive than much that passes under that name. There is no side of the intellect which it does not call into play, no region of human knowledge into which either its roots or its branches do not extend; like the Atlantic between the Old and the New Worlds, its waves wash the shores of the two worlds of matter and of mind; its tributary streams flow from both; through its waters, as yet unfurrowed by the keel of any Columbus, lies the road, if such there be, from the one to the other; far away from that Northwest Passage of mere speculation, in which so many brave souls have been hopelessly frozen up."

Dr. Anchorn's "diet list" in obesity will be published in November GAZETTE.

Department of Physiologic Chemistry.

WITH SPECIAL REFERENCE TO DIETETICS AND NUTRITION IN GENERAL.

A WORD TO THE OVERFAT.

OBESITY is apparently becoming more and more common, so common, in fact, that it is a drug in the market. Furthermore, it is the impression of those who have traveled much in foreign lands that a greater proportion of the population of the United States have the appearance of being stall-fed or overfed than in any other country. The daily papers and the illustrated monthly advertisers with storiette accompaniments, abound with cuts of "before and after taking." According to these "genuine" attestants whole mountains of too, too solid flesh melt, thaw and dissipate, in the presence of somebody's magic obesity belt, pills, salts or antifat—and what oceans of them are being sold!

At regular intervals the medical journals, and after them the newspapers, discuss the subject of reducing diets and "systems" of semi-starvation recommended by this or that celebrity, or spread broadcast some eminent nobody's prescription for shedding one's flesh and keeping down the bodily avoirdupois, their advertising pages full of guaranteed "antifats."

In spite of all this the unfortunate inheritors of the tendency to adipose tissue go on accumulating, or go off with suffocation or fatty heart. Many of them avoid severe exertion and resort to heart tonics, and thus manage to live on for many uncomfortable, apprehensive and out-of-breath years.

The trouble with all the vaunted obesity "cures" is that they are lame in theory and lacking in a physiologic basis: hence they lack horse sense and fail to get at the bottom of the matter.

Of course, overfeeding is one of the prolific sources of obesity, but many people grow "stout," as they modestly call it, without being chargeable with gluttony. Some very fat people are very sparing feeders, and some of the heartiest eaters are lean as Cassius. No matter how little the former indulge in the good things at table, they steadily pile up flesh, and no matter how much the latter eat they are always thin— all muscle, tendon and nerve fiber. They have not enough fat to round out their arms, cheeks or calves. Many of them are positively cadaverous. They are the "lankeys" so often lampooned and caricatured.

Most of the advertised panaceas for obesity are mere tricks to inveigle dollars from the pockets of gullable victims. Some of them reduce flesh and ruin lives at the same time since they rely upon measures or drugs that ought to be placed on the poison list and prohibited by law. Aside from the Vichy and Kissengen salines the alternate and systematic use of which has been urged by physicians of eminence and honorable repute, all of the so-called obesity or "antifat" salts depend upon iodide of potassium, and any prolonged use of this drug is destructive to the red corpuscles, and hence destructive to vitality.

In a general sense, obesity is a disease. It depends, first, upon slow and imperfect metamorphosis of food products, and, second, on imperfect oxidation and elimination. Those who have a tendency to it—usually this is inherited—should observe three fundamental rules:

1. Never to eat a mouthful more food than the system actually requires.

2. To use every effort to accelerate the nutritive changes required to transform food into normal, living tissues.

3. To maintain the function of elimination at the highest possible point.

Under rule 1, the selection of a nourishing but not naturally fat-forming dietary is essential. Those who have a marked tendency to obesity will, to a certain extent, transform almost any form of food into fat; but they should rigidly exclude all the decidedly fat-forming items from their daily regimen.

Under Rule 2, they should persistently cultivate the art of *breathing*. Most of them have small lungs. Practice will enlarge them, and systematic exercise will make them doubly efficient. Every form of vigorous exercise, especially one that calls for the continuous and active use of the arms, abdominal and chest muscles, will enhance the breathing function and enlarge its capacity. Every increment in this direction will fortify them against their distressful infirmity and help them to overcome it.

We are collecting data for a symposium on the rational prevention and cure of obesity, and will be glad of experiences and suggestions from all our readers.

COLDS.

EVERYBODY suffers more or less from "colds," and everybody ascribes these troublesome afflictions to exposure and the total depravity of the weather. This is an ancient and popular mistake. If common sense were a little more common, colds would be less common. For example, "drafts" are considered the chief causes of taking cold. Drafts are bad things to have in a family, but often the most fatal draft is the one that takes its direction from the turn of the table fork, begins with soup and ends with salads and dessert. Eating is a very necessary habit. Too many people unthinkingly let the habit dominate. Habitual overindulgence at table is responsible for more "colds" than we are aware of. Another prolific source is close rooms, not always overheated, but underventilated. Air

that is too impure (the system can cope with an ordinary degree of contamination) is much more dangerous than air that is too warm.

Other causes are excessive wrapping and coddling of the throat and chest, sleeping in poorly ventilated bedrooms, wearing the same underclothing night and day, neglect of the cleansing bath, want of reasonable physical exercise, and general inattention to the important bodily functions.

If one precaution, however, is more important than another, it is to keep the feet warm and dry, at whatever cost. No mortal who tolerates habitual cold feet can long remain well. It is the first grip of the icy fingers of the final foe. Influenza is no longer ranked among the trivial inconveniences. It is the foundation of nearly all the serious maladies. It is far easier to prevent it than to recover from its often deep-seated effects.

A single precaution is worth a hundred prescriptions.

THE NATURE OF VITAL FORCE.

FROM a very thoughtful and temperate paper by Dr. M. A. Blanton in the *Wisconsin Med. Recorder* we extract the following:

This vital force which we call life and with which we are constantly battling—of what does it consist?

Take your microscope, graduate your chemicals, search it out as you may you cannot find it.

It is not in the brain, it is not in the spinal cord.

Electricity is one of the subtlest known forces in Nature.

Is that the vital force? Perhaps so.

Or does not this mysterious element which courses through all our systems dwell in the fact that the constant movement of particles of matter one upon the other produces warmth, warmth nervous energy, nervous energy vital force?

"God breathed into the first man the

breath of life and he became a living being"
—set the heart in motion sending its life-
giving current throughout our entire bodies
and thus inter-dependence sprang into being, one particle catching energy from another till the whole organism moved in one
grand cycle of living pulsating life. When
death comes motion ceases.

We approach that form so recently throbbing with the thrill of existence and how
cold and still it lies in its abrupt conclusion.

That form so lately touched at birth with
the warmth-giving power of life, death has
stilled so soon, sooner than the great possibilities of so grand a being as man would
seem to merit.

The casket of life is there, but its vital
energy has fled and no mysterious power
of physician, necromancer or magician can
bring it back to its former habitation and
we turn away—impotent in the face of this
dull, unanswering silence.

LAUGHTER AND LONG LIFE.

FROM the *London Lancet* we get the following bit of good sense: "It may be that
some enthusiastic and laborious German
statistician has already accumulated figures
bearing upon the question of length of life
and its relation to the enjoyment thereof;
if so, we are unacquainted with his results,
and yet have a very decided notion that people who enjoy life, cheerful people, are also
those to whom longest life is given. Commonplace though this sounds, there is no
truth more commonly ignored in actual
every-day existence. 'Oh, yes, of course,
worry shortens life and the contented people
live to be old,' we are all ready to say, and
yet how many people recognize the duty of
cheerfulness? Most persons will declare
that if a man is not naturally cheerful he
cannot make himself so. Yet this is far
from being the case, and there is many a
man who is at present a weary burden to his
relatives, miserable through the carking care

of some bodily ailment, perhaps, or some
worldly misfortune, who, if he had grown
up into the idea that to be cheerful under all
circumstances was one of the first duties
of life, might still see a pleasant enough
world around him. Thackeray truly remarked that the world is for each of us
much as we show ourselves to the world.
If we face it with a cheery acceptance we
find the world fairly full of cheerful people
glad to see us. If we snarl at it and abuse
it we may be sure of abuse in return. The
discontented worries of a morose person
may very likely shorten his days, and the
general justice of Nature's arrangement
provides that his early departure should entail no long regrets. On the other hand,
the man who can laugh keeps his health and
his friends are glad to keep him. To the
perfectly healthy laughter comes often.
Too commonly, though, as childhood is left
behind the habit fails, and a half-smile is
the best that visits the thought-lined mouth
of a modern man or woman. People become more and more burdened with the accumulations of knowledge and with the
weighing responsibilities of life, but they
should still spare time to laugh. Let them
never forget, moreover, and let it be a medical man's practice to remind them that 'a
smile sits ever serene upon the face of Wisdom.'"

SHOULD COUSINS MARRY?

FROM A MEDICAL POINT OF VIEW.

CONSANGUINITY in marriage is still a
much debated topic. A great number of
physicians are opposed to unions of this
kind. Yet, consanguinity being only a special case of heredity, it is generally held
nowadays that if a husband and wife as
well as their ascendants are of a healthy
mind and body, the result will be good; in
the opposite case it will be bad. Regnault is
of opinion that not only the descent of husband and wife produce consanguinity, but
also their sojourn under the same condi-

tions, while, on the other hand, it may happen that relatives living separated by space should cease to be regarded as consanguineous, being able to intermarry without the character of consanguinity. It has been pointed out that in most nations several laws have been enacted against marriage between relatives .Regnault, on the strength of his investigations, thinks that the nations have endeavored with at least equal energy to prevent intermarriage between individuals living in the same place without being relatives, *i.e.*, topographic commingling. As instances the author quotes the Indians of North America and the Australians, who used to get their wives far away from their own tribal district. In France, and probably elsewhere, it has been noticed that the strict observance of the religious prohibition of marriage between relatives decreases in the same proportion as the number of marriges between individuals of the same locality. The latter decrease is connected with the increasing facility of transportation. In the Middle Ages marriages were prohibited between relatives even in the seventh degree, and kings themselves obeyed this law.

In the last century the Church limited her prohibition down to the fourth degree, and in the present century cousin-germans are allowed to contract matrimony, although with special dispensation. The author explains this disappearance of the laws against marriages between consanguineous persons by the fact that by the progressive and unceasing commingling of individuals topographic consanguinity came to an end by itself. In France there are some localities constituting an exception to the rule, such as Pollel, Boury de Batz, Fort Modyk, where marriages are strictly limited to people of the same place. At Orthez, where this rule existed among the Protestants, epilepsy had become endemic and inevitable to such a degree that each house contained a special room provided for it. After the railways have led to intermarriage with Protestants of other localities, espilepsy has decreased in a surprising manner. Observations of the same kind have been made in

animals long ago, and Cornevin quotes a striking instance of this fact. Darwin points to the habit of agriculturists, who, for the purpose of improving the quality of crops, will always employ seeds from other localities. The fact that consanguinity in a marriage between two persons having lived in different localities is of minor importance. A physician consulted about the opportunity of a marriage between relatives should consider not only the blood relation, but also the topographical circumstances. Provided both parties are strong, healthy, and without taint, any possible objection to their union will be lessened by their not having been raised in the same locality under the same conditions.

OLD HOUSEKEEPER ON COOKING.

THE New York *Sun* is responsible for the following apt comments of an Old Housekeeper:

"Not every one makes a good cook," said the old housekeeper, "in spite of all you hear about exactness and attention to detail. It is quite possible to be a careful cook and an exact cook, and yet be a very poor cook just as it is also possible to simply go by judgment and show good results day in and day out. One of the best cooks I have ever known is unable to give an exact account of how she makes bread or anything else. She will make a brave start with exact proportions, but very soon she will be found switching off and saying 'well, you have to use your judgment about that.' Her cake is mostly judgment cake; her pies are judgment pies; and her waffles are judgment waffles. I made up my mind a long while ago that the person who isn't endowed with the right kind of judgment need never try to cook very well. It doesn't come from experience; it is a gift or a knack, as some folks call it, and if you were born without it you can do no better than to cling to exactness and leave inspiration alone. What started me talking about this is a recent experience with a recipe. A recipe that reads one cup of this and a teaspoonful of that and a tablespoonful of something else ought to assure an unvariable quality, you would think, and it may if the same cook always has the work in charge. Otherwise, it is hardly to be recognized.

"It is a fact that one may be a first-rate cook in most lines and never be able to conquer a certain sort of dish. Sometimes you will run across cooks who will make the kind of pie crust that melts in your mouth and puddings that are dreams, who know how to get up a perfect dinner, and yet who never conquer cake baking. Bread is really a much more difficult thing to build than cake is, but nevertheless it is impossible for some persons to become good cake makers. Of course there are the rules to remember, such as that which says that the butter and sugar must first be creamed together and then the yolks of the eggs, previously well beaten, added, and that the well-beaten whites of the eggs should go in last. But even closely following the directions the woman who isn't a good cake maker may be rewarded by a failure. Perhaps she lacks the judgment about how much stirring the cake will take after the eggs are added. Everything ought to be as light as possible, but too prolonged effort to make it so may produce a soggy cake. Remember, too, when you wish cake to be light and airy that it is better to sift the flour three or four times.

"Again, the cook may be successful in every line except pie-making. If that is the case, she may get her supplies all ready, sift the flour and the salt together and use a knife for cutting the butter into the flour. She may add the water a little bit at a time and mix it in ever so lightly. She may know theoretically just how to roll that crust out and how to fold it over and roll it out again. She may have everything as cold as possible and may use the hands as little as possible. Nevertheless, ten to one, if she is a good cake maker she will not be especially good at pastry. As for the theory, I can't tell you why it is—it is simply true.

"Good bread-makers are rare, and yet it is possible to give the most explicit directions about what to do and how to do it. From the flour, which should be of a yellowish white tinge and rather granulated, up to the dough, which should be strong and elastic, yet easily kneaded, every step in the bread-making can be put into words and yet one may become lost, all because she has not the proper kind of judgment. Judgment must come in about the shortening. Bread made with unskimmed milk needs no butter or lard, and instead of being improved, it is really harmed when shortening is added because too much clogs the glutinous cell walls and checks the rising. Most good bread-makers put all the flour in when mixing the dough.

"Another thing I have noticed is that the same cook who is successful with bread knows how and has the knack of making delicious pastry. I can't explain why the two go together.

"Some persons have a special dish that they are unable to manage. One woman I know owns up to complete defeat in making crullers. She knows the way they should be made and can teach any one else what to do but her own crullers never come up to the standard.

"Yes, I have an enemy in hot biscuits, the kind you call baking-powder biscuit or tea biscuit. Any inexperienced housekeeper can make them and make them well after a few trials, and there is nothing about which I could give better advice if you want to learn. But I'll tell you right here and now that I cannot make them myself."

POPULATION AND BREAD SUPPLY.

ONE of our Western contemporaries discusses this question with fairly prophetic intelligence:

"There is a good deal to be said on each side of the proposition that the population of the world will increase so fast that the wheat supply will not be adequate to furnish bread for all the people. Sir William Crookes, of England, expressed that fear some three years ago, and during the recent session of the American Science Association Mr. Edward Peters, of the Department of Agriculture, made a similar prediction, but in a greatly modified form.

"There are two great factors in this problem, and neither is definitely known—the increase in population, and the amount of land available for successful wheat production. It is by no means sure that during the twentieth century the population of the world will increase as rapidly as it did in the nineteenth. The population of France is nearly stationary, and the recent census of England shows that the situation in that country is no better, even if it be no worse. Statistics in certain parts of this country and also in Europe indicate that Nature makes provision against too rapid an increase in population after a certain stage of growth has been reached.

"Unless the population of the world increases rapidly, instead of there being danger of a shortage in the wheat supply, there may be a lack of civilized people to occupy and improve the comparatively new and undeveloped parts of the earth.

"The wheat supply may be increased in two ways—by increasing the yield per acre, and by bringing new lands under cultivation. There is ground for hope in both these directions. Improvements in seed and better methods of cultivation will in all probability greatly increase the yield per acre. The Department of Agriculture in Washington is doing good work along these lines, and there is excellent reason to believe that much will be accomplished.

"It is a matter of conjecture, and yet it is probable that a large area in both South America and Africa, of land now uncultivated, will ultimately be brought under cultivation, and that each country will make large contributions to the world's wheat supply in addition to that now made. In this connection one should not forget the possibilities of the arid part of the United States. Through irrigation and probably other means a large part of the country west of the 100th meridian may be added to the

wheat producing area; and there is furthermore a vast expanse of land in Western Canada which will add more or less to the wheat product when it is brought under cultivation.

"The danger that the inhabitants of the world will have to cut short their bread supply because of a lack of wheat is rather remote. The world will be much older than it is to-day when that time comes, even if there shall continue to be a large increase in population."

✤ ✤

BAD FOOD VERSUS LONGEVITY.

WE find the following in the *New York Times:*

From a leading article in the *Times* in relation to the influence of muscular exercise upon health and longevity, some readers may draw conclusions not strictly in agreement with facts. Of all the animals the deer is one of the most active and one of the most healthy, always dying of old age if not killed by accident or by the hand of an enemy. On the other hand, the farmer's hog is one of the most inactive and shortest lived of animals. This illustration is, of course, not a fair one, but is given to show how facts without explanation may mislead those not very well acquainted with a subject that is being discussed. If the shorter life of the farmer goes to show that the amount of physical labor he performs is not favorable to longevity, then why should saloon keepers, whose labor is light and who are not out in all kinds of weather like the farmers, be still shorter lived than the latter?

There are several conditions that have more or less to do with health and a continuance of life, but there is one upon which more depends than on any other one, or, perhaps, on all the others combined, and this most important factor is the use of good food. Life and health are maintained and labor performed by a continual generation and expenditure of strength, and this involves a continual supply of suitable food. If a baby, a puppy, or a kitten be fed on milk that has been deprived of its cream it will for a time appear not to thrive, but after a while it will be healthy and vigorous, and will continue so until the food is discontinued. Now, on the other hand, if the baby or the young animal be fed on cream only, it will die of starvation as certainly, though not as quickly, as if fed nothing at all. If the milk be deprived of half the normal percentage of any one of its most important mineral constituents, there will be partial starvation, or a lessening of vitality, which is a condition favorable to the development of disease.

If any reader of this article will inquire of a dog-breeder as to the best food for a puppy just weaned, he will very likely be told "bread and milk." If further inquiry is made about a bit of meat now and then, the reply will be quick and emphatic, "No meat till he is a year old." The breeder may explain that the puppy will not thrive on a meat diet, that he will get sick and perhaps die, and that any way he will not make a good dog. For a long while after I learned this I was puzzled to know why food that was good for a grown dog was not good for one only half grown, but one day the problem was solved when I saw a puppy trying to eat a bone and not able to do it for want of strength in his teeth and jaws.

Then the important fact was revealed that meat alone, while containing all the nutritive elements, does not supply a sufficient amount of the minerals that are needed for health, and which the grown dog gets from his bone.

The increased consumption of meat during the last fifty years in this country is out of all proportion to the increase of population, and there is a corresponding increase in the number of doctors, druggists and dentists; and we may judge by the advertisements, there is an unparalleled boom in the sale of quack nostrums, all of which indicates a steady physical degeneration on the part of the people. If the use of less meat is the ounce of prevention and a saving of expense as well as a saving of life, there

should be no delay in reducing the amount of our meat rations.

We Americans take pride in our being a practical people. In our ordinary business transactions we look sharply to the "main chance." If we contract for the building of a house we employ a man to stand, specifications in hand, to see that no rotten lumber or badly burned bricks are used in its construction. Our clothing and boots must be made of strong and durable materials, but when it comes to supplying to our bodies the elements that will enable them to endure the strain and labor of life, we proceed with a reckless disregard of results that is sublimely idiotic. We spend fabulous sums in establishing and maintaining universities in which our young men are taught to "skilfully rattle the skeletons of dead languages" while they remain so densely ignorant of the conditions upon which life depends that a large proportion die before attaining the age of greatest usefulness and enjoyment. Is human life worth preserving? Am I mistaken in saying that the preservation of life depends mainly on the use of good food?

WILLIAM PORTER PECK.

TABLE DRINKING.

GEORGE E. WALSH, in *Table Talk*, discusses this topic as follows:

"Scientific experiments help to establish more clearly each year our knowledge concerning dietary matters so that we can the better judge how to eat, what to eat, and what not to eat. No question has caused greater diversity of opinion than that of drinking at meals, and all sorts of recommendations are given by those who may or may not know. The great trouble with all this free advice is that no two people are alike, and what suits one does not necessarily agree with another. Another common error is that we are apt to draw conclusions from insufficient premises. Thus, if a thing disagrees with us once, we are inclined to conclude that it will always produce the same evil results. Now, it is a fact well known to science, that the condition of the system at the time any food is taken makes all the difference in the world as to its chemical action. We may be in a state where any food might cause trouble, and it is not right to blame the food for causing it any more than we would say that a change caused an attack of typhoid or malarial fever, when the germs were in our system, ready to develop at any moment. What we need to establish a rule of living and of hygiene is to make several careful tests of any one thing, and if the results are all practically the same, we are safe in saying that we know what effect such a thing has upon us.

"If people would apply this in their drinking and diet we would have few cases of indigestion, dyspepsia, nervous disorders and headaches. We cannot get this knowledge in all cases from even the physician. He must make general rules, but after all he must make allowances for individual constitutional peculiarities. On these depend to a large extent the condition of our future health.

"In the matter of drinking at meals, it is safe to say that this practice has directly contrary effects in different individuals. Some people have to refrain from drinking at the meals to keep from getting too fat Where there is one such person there are scores of others who refrain from it because they are afraid of inducing indigestion and getting too thin. Is there any safe rule then for any one to follow in regard to drinking at meals?

"It is not possible to lay down any absolute rule, but a few general hints about a common-sense way of looking at the matter can be stated, which should enable every one to make a modified rule for his own living. There is first the general condemnation of ice water, either with the meals or between them. This practice is detrimental to the health of nine-tenths of those who indulge in it, and yet a few are blessed with such vigorous constitutions that the ice water does not appear to hurt them. For most of us, however, the less ice water we drink, the better for our health. The next point is that of the relative purity and temperature of the drinking water. If there is any question of taint to the water, have it boiled and filtered. Pure water washes out the system and leaves no sediment behind, but impure water causes trouble through the lodgment of germs in the system.

"A little water taken with meals is not injurious to any, except those with very delicate stomachs, where the juices are supplied in very small quantities. The injury then comes through the dilution of the gastric and pancreatic juices, and may in time prove serious. A certain amount of liquid is needed in our stomachs. It is possible to prepare a meal of dry bread, dry mush, and similar articles, so that half a pint of water is needed to digest it well. Of course we overcome this difficulty usually by eating the mush with milk, or drinking tea or other warm beverage. Whatever it is, the liquid is needed. Another prepared meal might contain so much liquid in the food that even a small amount of water would be injurious.

"Consequently water may be either a poison or a medicine. It is common to say water, and not include tea and coffee. in condemning this practice. Either tea or coffee will produce just as evil results if taken in excess as water. The only virtue in these drinks is that they warm the stomach when taken. We drink cold water, usually, but there is no reason why we should not drink warm water with our meals. It is merely a question of habit. Many who do not dare drink tea or coffee, or water, can compromise by warming the water, and putting a teaspoonful of tea or coffee in it. This will take away any nauseating flavor that is experienced sometimes in drinking hot water, and the amount of tea or coffee taken into the system in this way will hurt no one's nerves. The exercise of a little common sense will in most cases show to each one the most desirable course to pursue."

COLDS.

THE editor of the *Pacific Health Journal* submits a very apt paper on this important topic. He arranges his advice under several sub-captions:

HOW TO AVOID THEM.

1. *Have confidence in the power of your body to resist disease.* Faith and hope are wonderful curative agents. Fear is a depressant. In every epidemic there are many who succumb to the disease as a result of fear, who might otherwise recover.

2. *Determine not to yield to disease.* Men have gotten up from sick-beds, after being given up by their physicians, by mere force of the will. The writer recalls a case, a number of years ago, where a patient was so low with lung trouble that a consultation was called, the result being that the patient was told that he could not live. "I'll fool you," he said, and he did. He is still living.

3. *Let tonics and drugs alone.* Nothing will so effectually weaken the system and render it an easy prey to disease.

4. *Breathe through your nose.* It was placed there to warm and moisten the air before it reaches the delicate tissues of the throat and lungs. Breathing through the mouth is an excellent way to invite sore throat.

5. *Do not overeat or abuse your digestive organs.* A large proportion of colds originate with some dietary indiscretion.

6. *Do not wear too much clothing.* Extra wraps tend to produce perspiration and weaken the reactionary powers of the body.

7. *Do not live in close, ill-ventilated rooms.* Plants raised in a hothouse are never so hardy as those grown outside. Animals in their native haunts are not subject to lung difficulties, as they are in confinement. When savages exchange their outdoor life for the dwellings of civilization, they become the victims of a decimating scourge in the form of pulmonary diseases. Living rooms should be supplied with thermometers.

8. *Take a daily hand bath in as cold water as will be followed by a good reaction.* This, followed by a vigorous rubbing, will greatly increase the power of the body to resist disease.

9. *Keep warm, if possible, by exercise, and place little dependence on artificial heat.* Not that one is to live without fire in the cold weather, but that the room should only be heated to a point, say sixty-five degrees, where the body will have its part of the work to do.

2.   WHAT TO DO FOR A COLD.

The first and most important advice is, "Don't get it." But for those to whom this injunction comes too late, the following directions will be of value, *provided they are carried out.*

Colds beginning at the back of the throat may often be broken up *at the start*, by swabbing the throat or gargling with some antiseptic solution. Peroxide of hydrogen diluted with four parts of water is excellent, and is harmless if swallowed. Carbolic acid in one per cent. solution* is also valuable, but care should be taken not to swallow it, as it is poisonous.

SORE THROAT.

One of the best remedies for sore throat is a compress worn over the throat at night. A piece of muslin or light cloth about half the size of an ordinary handkerchief should be folded so as to cover a space about three by four inches, wrung lightly out of cold water, and placed over the throat. This should be covered by a piece of rubber cloth, oiled silk, or oiled muslin. obtainable at any druggist's, or a piece of flexible table oilcloth may be made to do service. A long narrow strip of dry cloth should now be wrapped around the neck in such a way as to hold the compress firmly in place. If this compress is so put on as to retain its place, prevent evaporation, and exclude the

* This may be obtained at the druggist's; or the ninety-five per cent. solution can be obtained, and one dram of this to twelve ounces of water will make a one per cent. solution. Shake well, and see that no drops of the strong carbolic acid remain

air, it is a sovereign remedy for cold in the throat. It should be put on when retiring at night and taken off on arising in the morning, the neck being washed in cold water and rubbed until the skin glows.

"SNIFFLES."

For cold in the head the nasal passages should be thoroughly cleansed. This is best accomplished by sniffing from the palm of the hand water as hot as can be borne comfortably, containing a teaspoonful of baking soda or borax to the pint. The head should be held at different inclinations (tipped forward, vertical, tipped backward) during this process, in order that the cleansing fluid may reach all parts of the nasal cavities.

It is well to follow this treatment with an oily spray, from one of the excellent oil atomizers now on the market, which should contain some mineral oil, as albolene, or liquid vaseline, in which is dissolved one dram of menthol, or one dram each of camphor and menthol to two ounces of the oil. Spraying this solution into the nose at intervals of half an hour will often break up a cold in the head, *if taken in time*, without any other treatment. This spray is often useful, also, in cutting short an attack of sore throat affecting the larynx and vocal cords.

STEAM INHALATIONS.

An excellent remedy when the cold is farther down, is the inhalation of steam. The effectiveness of this is increased by adding to the boiling water a teaspoonful of compound tincture of benzoin. Many forms of apparatus have been devised for the administration of medicated vapor; but an old teakettle or other vessel from which steam can be inhaled will answer every purpose. In order to keep the water hot it should be on the stove or over a spirit lamp. A funnel can be made of paper and held over the vessel in such a way that the steam enters the large end of the funnel below,

and the patient inhales from a hole at the small end of the funnel.

GENERAL TREATMENT.

So much for the local treatment of cold. For general treatment nothing is superior to a full hot treatment to produce vigorous perspiration. This is best accomplished in home treatment by giving a hot leg bath at the bedside. The bath should come well up to the knees, and hot water should be added as fast as the patient can bear it. The patient should be well wrapped in blankets; and as soon as he is perspiring freely, he should be put into bed, still wrapped in the same blankets, and the other clothing tucked snugly around him. He may now be given a pitcher of hot water, or, better, hot lemonade to drink. If he now sleeps several hours, he will probably awake free from his cold. On arising, he should be sponged in cool water and rubbed with a coarse towel until a good reaction is induced.

All these treatments are efficacious in proportion to the promptness and vigor with which they are given. During a cold one should eat lightly, of simple food. Indeed, it is not a bad plan to skip a meal or so.

THE CLERGY AND THE DOCTORS.

ON this topic the *Phila. Med. Journal* has this to say: The absolute inability of some religious writers to appreciate the real force and trend of the modern science of pathology, is curiously shown in their methods of criticising so-called Christian Science. They naturally fear this new cult for its effects on existing religious systems rather than for its menace to the public health and the public intelligence. In a recent contribution to the *Churchman,* a prominent Anglican divine discusses the relation of the early church to the treatment of disease. He thinks he finds evidence that the clergy in those remote times exercised the functions of the physician, but he adduces no adequate proof whatever in support of this claim, for it is not the function of the physician to cure by miracles and wonder-working. Lecky ("History of European Morals," Vol. I.) has shown that the early church relied upon thaumaturgy, just as Christian Science is doing, whereas legitimate medicine does nothing of the sort. The *Churchman,* commenting on this paper, makes the astonishing statement that "many a clergyman is already a consulting physician." It seems to think that the two offices—that of the priest and that of the physician—should be combined in one and the same person. All this is evidently suggested by the progress of Christian Science, but the point of the whole matter is curiously missed.

These writers should at least understand that the whole therapeutic power of any religious system lies simply in the domain of mental impression or suggestive therapeutics; that this power is not, and never has been, confined to any one religion or sect, but has been exerted by all of them in every period of history and in every region of the globe in which they have prevailed; that this suggestive therapeutics is potent for good in only a limited domain of medical practice; and, finally, that suggestive therapeutics can just as well, if not better and more rationally, be used by extra-theological methods. The Hindoos and the Chinese, as well as the ancient Greeks and Romans, have not been unfamiliar with the therapeutic value of religious emotion. This is shown by Regnier in his work on hypnotism in the ancient religions, ("Hypnotisme et Croyances Anciennes," Paris, 1891)' and by Nevius in his book on demon possessions in China, ("Demon Possession and Allied Themes," 1896).

To see in all this any evidence that the enormous fabric of modern medical science will be, or even can be, entrusted to the hands of the clergy (as seems to be the idea of a writer in the *Literary Digest*) is an evidence of a critical insight that would have done credit to a medieval monk.

ALCOHOL NUTRITION AND INEBRIETY.

An eminent writer on the diseases following the use and abuse of alcoholic beverages sums up his conclusions in this wise:

"The appearance of inebriety is usually sudden and without any exciting causes, and the change in conduct and manner of living is unexplainable. The same methods of using spirits and the same food impulses and tastes, and the same surroundings as far as possible, appearing after a lapse of a lifetime, show that early defects are not affected by time. I conclude at this point with a summary of what I have intended to make clear in this study:

"1. Inebriety is a most complex neurosis. The causes are equally complex, and include all the various states of degeneration which influence and disturb nutrition.

"2. Obscure indigestion begins, and for this drugs and bitters containing alcohol are used. The narcotism which follows is so grateful that it is continued.

"3. Dietetic delusions are fostered in the minds of parents and children, and from this many different forms of inebriety begin.

"4. Often the most maniacal and chronic inebriates are from these delusional dyspeptics.

"5. Starvation is present in many of these cases. The quality and variety of foods are deficient, and defective nourishment follows.

"6. The uniformity of taking foods and the quality and variety are essential. This and nutritional rest and mental anxiety are important factors.

"7. The inebriety following these conditions is successfully treated by elimination of the toxins and special correction of the nutrition.

"8. Nutrition is a very active cause in the production of inebriety, and should receive a careful study in all cases."

✤ ✤

THE RECREATIONS OF SCIENTISTS.

WITH men in our profession all seasons are times of work; therefore, all seasons for them are likely to be times also for play. How else can your poor overworked doctor (who is so apt to condole with himself) even things up? He must snatch his moments of sport even from the grasping hours of toil and duty. Who shall blame him for this? If he hurries from the sick room to a game of cards, he is not to be charged with cynicism and indifference. The season, for the meetings of the numerous medical associations is the great recreation time for the doctors. There is no use in denying the fact; many a good man goes to the yearly meeting of his association with his mind bent on pleasure as well as on science. And we are not going to berate him for this in these columns. If we were a self-constituted reformer of the medical profession (which we are not), we might find occasion here for some labored editorial rhetoric. But a fellow-feeling makes us wondrous kind, and we confess that the humorous side of this whole picture appeals strongly to us. That doctors should travel many hundreds of miles to attend a grave assemblage of their colleagues, and then should rush off from the meeting at a moment's notice to attend a horse-race or to take a ride on a river, strikes us as being peculiarly man-like. We recently saw a big base-ball match deplete an afternoon session of an association of specialists, many of whom are well known to fame. One unfortunate member confessed aloud that he would like to go with the sport-loving delegation, but could not, because he had to stay and read a paper. He was in the position of the small boy who would like to play truant but dares not. The man who would propose on such an occasion that the society adjourn in favor of the ball match would be frowned down. He would be judged guilty of levity and would be voted a Philistine. But the man who deliberately gets up, takes his hat, and leads off a coterie of his weaker brethren to the neighboring ball field, is en-

vied rather than scorned. And when one thinks that the bold man has come hundreds of miles and spent much money, one must at heart have a little sympathy with his desire to get some fun out of it all. And then, after all, the papers can be read just as well when they are published in the journals.—*Exchange.*

✤ ✤

TESLA ON VEGETARIANISM.

How to provide good and plentiful food is a most important question of the day. On general principles the raising of cattle as a means of providing food is objectionable. It is certainly preferable to raise vegetables, and I think, therefore, that vegetarianism is a commendable departure from the established barbarous habit. That we can subsist on plant food, and perform our work even to advantage, is not a theory, but a well-demonstrated fact. Many races living almost exclusively on vegetables are of superior physique and strength. There is no doubt that some plant food, such as oatmeal, is more economical than meat, and superior to it in regard to both mechanical and mental performance. Such food, moreover, taxes our digestive organs decidedly less, and, in making us more contented and sociable, produces an amount of good difficult to estimate. In view of these facts, every effort should be made to stop the wanton and cruel slaughter of animals, which must be destructive to our morals. To free ourselves from animal instincts and appetites, which keeps us down, we should begin at the very root from which they spring: we should effect a radical reform in the character of the food.—*Nicola Tesla,, in Century Magazine.*

✤ ✤

"A HOUSE is no home, unless it contains food and fire for the mind as well as the body."—Margaret Fuller.

SNATCHES OF THOUGHT.

"Elegies, and quoted odes, and jewels five
words long,
That on the stretched forefinger of all time
sparkle forever."

The ancient Theologs held that "The face of the wicked man is a map of the Empire of Sin."

Dumas said of the gourmand, "He is a Sanctuary of Gluttony."

Every effort that finally fails was either a mistake or an abortion. Every undertaking that finally succeeds is simply another item in the Records of Destiny.

The average annual product of each cow in the country, as figured by the department of agriculture, is milk, 380 gallons; cheese, 300 pounds; butter, 130 pounds.

Snakes, it is said, appear to delight in being shocked by electricity. Several thousand volts passing through their bodies merely induce a pleasant sleep with these curious reptiles.

VEGETABLE BUTTER.

Is the cow to be altogether eliminated from the dairy? The British Consul General at Marseilles hears that "a new fatty substance, for consumption in the United Kingdom, to take the place of butter, is being put on the British market. It is called vegetaline, and is nothing else than the oil extracted from copra (dried cocoanut), refined, and with all smell and taste neutralized by a patented process. It becomes like sweet lard, and is intended to compete with margarine on the breakfast table as a substitute for butter." A Liverpool firm, we are told, will this year help in an effort to popularize the stuff.

ONE HUNDRED AND FIVE YEARS OLD.

A remarkably interesting man is Goddard Ezekiel Dodge Diamond, of San Francisco, Cal., who claims to have been born May 1, 1796. He is a wonder of all who see him. A photographer who made a portrait of him on his hundreth birthday, gave this testimony as to his appearance:

"Naturally expecting so old a gentleman to be very feeble, on the day appointed for the sitting, I made preparations accordingly. I covered my skylight with cloth, thinking that eyes at that age would not be able to stand the light. I remember also, placing an easy chair ready for the sitting. Presently my friend came in, with another gentleman, and announced the arrival of Mr. Diamond. I asked them to have the old gentleman's carriage driven around into the court, when, to my great astonishment, my friend introduced the gentleman with him as Captain Diamond, himself. I was dumfounded! Here was a man standing straight as a young prince, moving with an elastic, sprightly step, with a bright, youthful twinkle shining in his eye! I could see at once that I had gone to much unnecessary trouble in my preparations. Photographers are often obliged to refuse direct sittings for large portraits, and instead enlarge from small pictures, because of the inability of the subject to remain perfectly quiet for the requisite length of time. In spite of his great age, there was not the slightest difficulty of this kind with Mr. Diamond. He certainly is the best sitter I ever had. During the long exposure necessary to insure the quality in a direct life-sized portrait, he never moved a particle. Every hair of head and beard came out as sharp as in any other sitting I ever made of a man of thirty, no matter how much I braced the latter up with back and head rest."

A San Francisco physician who made a clinical examination of Mr. Diamond at the age of one hundred and two, reported in part as follows:

"Height, 5 feet, 6¼ inches. Present weight 141 pounds. Nine years ago he weighed 225 pounds. Reduced himself by diet. Appetite always good; digestion excellent. Diet plain; no sweets, no meats since 1852. Never used a stimulant of any kind; never used tobacco. Drinks hot water thrice daily; no tea, no coffee. Temperament passive. Uses olive oil externally and internally. Never been married. Keeps the same weight. No difficulty in breathing. Can lie in any position, preferring an abdominal one. No palpitation. Pulse regular in rhythm, tension slight, easily compressible, irregularly intermittent. Pulse rate, 76. Respiration regular, full 18. Vision good; reaction of pupils normal; range of vision somewhat shortened, reading a 10-foot chart, short at 8 feet. Physical appearance good, resembling a well-preserved man of 78. Absence of wrinkles, face slightly flushed; condition of the skin in all parts of the body excellent, except over the abdomen, which shows the loss of tissue, owing to the great reduction in weight. Hair gray, not bald. Chest well formed with exception of a deep depression in the lower sternal region, which has persisted since youth.

"The physical examination of Captain Diamond reveals a remarkable preservation of tissue integrity and functional activity. There is no factor or combination of factors which would suggest any approach to dissolution; and if the same vegetative routine of life is maintained, and no intercurrent complication supervenes, it would be purely speculative to hazard an opinion as to the probable future span of life."

Mr. Diamond, in describing the methods by which he has preserved his health and vigor so far beyond the ordinary term of human life, says that he gave no especial attention to the matter until he was sixty-five years old, although he had always lived a temperate life. At this time, however, he began a systematic study of the measures necessary to promote comfort and longevity. He came to the following conclusion, as expressed in his own words:

"The two things, as it appeared to me, required to attain the results which I desired, were diet and oil. To carry out my plan I knew that self-mastery was the chief obstacle to overcome. By this I mean that personal attention must be given the body, and that the palate must be educated to self-denial and correct taste."

At this time Mr. Diamond began the practice of rubbing himself daily with olive oil after a cool sponge bath—a practice which he has continued, sometimes using the bath and the oil both morning and evening, for forty years. As to what he eats and drinks he says:

"Long life and good health are not sustained alone by external applications. That which enters within a man, tells the story of building up and pulling down.

"Breathing, eating, drinking, are the three processes of taking into the body the vital forces of Nature. These forces work outward, and afford something to be washed, rubbed, and oiled. Three things I have faithfully practiced in the last half century, jointly. The first is that of breathing the freshest air possible—long, deep draughts. The second is the selection and eating of the best bone and blood food at my command. The third is the use of pure water at proper time and temperature. When I began to prepare the body for long and healthy life, I left out of my diet slaughtered meats. Strong meat, often taken, is the source of all kinds of disease, laying the foundation for untold suffering."

Upon the philosophy of the subject, he declares himself as follows:

"The selection of food and drink is of vast importance in youth, but it does not become of first importance in the estimation of men until they have reached the meridian of life. By this time the machinery of the physical man has been running several decades with but little attention, and there is rheumatism, chronic headache, liver pains, kidney trouble, stomach rebellions, dyspepsia, which means chronic constipation. It is generally known and admitted by the most thoughtful people, that by far the greater amount of physical suffering is the result of eating too much or eating the wrong kind of food. A man will be systematic in allowing to his horse two quarts of oats, and is careful to confine him so that he can not get to the oat bin and eat all he wants, lest he 'founder,' and swell his body and feet, undermining his constitution, knowing that ever after, the chances are that the horse will 'founder' on every little provocation. The same man will go from the stable to the table, and sit down to eat of at least ten varieties of food, the most of it cooked in poor oil fats, and during the meal drink freely of water, wine, and coffee, capping it off with a cigar.

"That man will get into his road wagon, behind that scientifically fed horse, and reel off ten miles at a two-forty clip; and when he gets there, his horse is in good condition, but he walks up the lawn slope of two hundred yards, winded, holding his stomach with both hands, and panting like a fat ox. He is a crank on horse-feeding and a fool about feeding himself. . . .

"There are better uses to which to put cash, food, and raiment, than to overfeed and clothe the body, cut short the life, and fail to enjoy this world. The man who sins against his own body, sins against his neighbor, against Nature, and against his Maker.

"My rule is to avoid ice water, and not to drink unboiled water unless it be distilled. Nature intended that man should live on the products of the earth. To provide for his thirst, Nature draws up the water from the rivers and the rills, distills it, sends it down into the earth, and up through the roots of vegetation into the leaves and bark, fruit and nuts, and in such proportions as to provide for hunger and thirst in Nature's own gifts. Even dried fruits can be restored to their original quality by the free use of distilled water. But men tell me that they thirst, and must take large quantities of water to satisfy that thirst. Certainly! But they are large meat eaters, hot because of the meat they have taken; or perhaps they are accustomed to the use of stimulants and narcotics, introducing foreign elements into the body, thus reversing Nature. As the

jaded horse submits to the lash, so the exhausted energies of man resort to stimulants. The body seeks to obey Nature in rest, but the ambitious man urges it on by the use of strong coffee, wine, beer, or liquid, until Nature is exhausted.

"The man who thinks well of his body will study how much Nature can endure, as the architect studies the weight of the superstructure before he selects the size and material for supports. The thin man can put on flesh, and the fat man can put it off. At the age of ninety-three years I weighed 225 pounds, with but 5 feet, 7 inches height; for two successive summers I went into the hot climate of California, lived mainly on fruits, nuts, and melons, and dropped to 142½ pounds, since which time I have not gone above 160 pounds. The thin man can fatten his cattle and hogs, why can not he put flesh upon his own skeleton? I have never used the pipe, cigar, or cigarette; never indulged in wine, liquors, nor any stimulants, omitting entirely the use of tea and coffee. None of these things contain food, and Nature rebels at their use until, through custom or social life, the taste is educated to indulge in them, after which Nature receives them because too weak to resist an encroaching enemy.

"My practice and advice is not attractive to the man who has 'money to burn,' and passions to serve as a master. The after-dinner man, the banquet man, the rich clubman, and the high-tea ladies may not be interested in these simple methods of living long and living happily, because they prefer the good things of to-day, and let the morrow come with its heavy bills, in the shape of pains, aches, and early death. The rich man who fares sumptuously is ill, peevish, goutish, and miserable; but his valet nurses, cares for, and ministers unto him, feeding himself upon the crumbs from the rich man's table.

"My practice is such as comes within the reach of the common people. The working man and woman can ward off disease, suffering, and premature death by the use of these means, and enjoy life to a ripe old age."

LONG HAIR AND NERVOUSNESS.

THE man who runs the bath house at Sharon Springs, N. Y., is full of theories about difficult diseases, and some of his theories are at least interesting. Speaking to a patron, who had very thick hair, he said:

"I see you are one of those nervous people. You had better take pine needle baths."

"What made you conclude I was nervous?" inquired the gentleman.

"I knew it from your hair," was the reply.

"How so?"

"Because all thick, coarse-haired people are nervous."

"Why?"

"Well, it stands to reason, don't it, that if you overplant a small patch of ground you will deplete the soil. It's the same way with a man's head. When a man has a big crop of coarse hair his nerves pay the penalty. Bald-headed men are seldom nervous."

DESIRABLE FOODS FOR SUMMER.

LEAN meats, eggs, milk and cheese are, in proper proportions and when taken with succulent vegetables and fruits, desirable foods for summer. But the fats of meats, and fat meat such as pork, large quantites of cream and butter, as well as olive oil, should be avoided. The latter, however, is preferable, as it does not contribute so rapidly to the bodily heat as do the animal fats. Avoid hot and heavy deserts. Use fruits in season in abundance.—*Mrs. S. T. Rorer, in the Ladies' Home Journal for August.*

CLEANLINESS IN COOKING.

SAYS a Chinese writer of the eighteenth century: "Don't cut bamboo shoots (the Chinese equivalent of asparagus) with an oniony knife. A good cook frequently wipes his knife, frequently changes his cloth, frequently scrapes his board and frequently washes his hands. If smoke or ashes from his pipe, perspiration drops from his head, insects from the wall or smut from the saucepan gets mixed up with the food, though he were a very chef among chefs, yet would men hold their noses and decline."

LACTIC ACID AS A REMEDY FOR BALDNESS.

BALZER practises friction of the bald part daily with a 30-per-cent. solution of lactic acid until the skin becomes inflamed. Then the treatment is suspended for a few days, and resumed when the inflammation has subsided. He reports that he has often observed a new growth of hair in the course of three or four weeks.—*Medical Times.—*

HOPES.

"Do you think that the trusts are capable of serving any philanthropic purposes?"

"I have hopes in that direction," answered the optimist. "I understand that a peanut trust has been organized, and I am waiting to see whether it won't put up the price so that you can't get enough for five cents to make you sick."—*Washington Star.*

Department of Hygiene.

WITH SPECIAL REFERENCE TO STATE AND PREVENTIVE MEDICINE.

THE THERAPEUTIC VALUE OF CLIMATE.

(*Fifth Paper.*)

THE LAND OF THE LATTER-DAY SAINTS.

IF this recentest recruit to the Sisterhood of States, in which sisterhood and citizenship had wellnigh become synonymous while she was yet in her swaddling clothes, has not established a world-wide reputation as a desirable site for health stations and invalid retreats, it is more herself than her climate that is to blame. She possesses a really genial climate; is interspersed with rugged and ragged mountain ranges, and has numerous valleys than which no lovelier or more delectable can be found on the western slope of the continent. Beautiful lakes nestle among her rugged hills and innumerable springs gush from her mountain sides. All to herself she has an inland ocean that is practically the only one of its kind on the American continent.

This was a wise provision of Providence, to the end that when a Mormon patriarch is translated his numerous widow can moan her moan by the sad sea-waves and add her tears to the brackish waters of the Great Salt Lake! And as they bear his sacred and silent remains to the crypt of the Temple, the numerous widow might chant in chorus:

"After life's misfit fever, he sleeps well!"

Utah winters are mild and her summers enjoyable. Her natural resources are rich in variety and abundance—fertile valleys that could furnish a site for Eden Restored, mineral deposits that have never acknowledged any competitors and that show no diminution in their annual yield of treasure.

Her one handicap in the social, commercial and political race is this shadow of religious fanaticism, which in the light of the present day ought not to become a perpetuity. Time slowly cures all great evils; the Millennium is a perennial anticipation; and so, Truth crushed to earth will rise again even though a hundred false prophets sit on her prostrate stomach!

The day seems rapidly approaching when all this incubus of socio-religious insanity will have been dropped behind. There is nothing else to hinder Utah from making material, social and political strides that will be the envy of her elder sisters.

CLIMATES THAT BORDER THE SILVER SEA.

The climates that border the placid Pacific are in many respects unique. Other countries furnish some semblance but no exact counterparts. Unique causes combine to produce them. Topographic limitations, meteorologic precedents, hydrographic maxims—all these are set at naught. She wrenches isothermal lines from their normal and traditional bearings and sends them wandering at right angles to precedent, tradition and parallels of latitude. The older meteorologists were astounded when they discovered that their law of the trend of these lines had been rudely and radically dislocated. To them the change meant climatic chaos and an infraction of the laws of the universe.

To say that this phenomenon is a scientific anomaly and wholly unique is to repeat a platitude. The word unique has come to be so common and so much abused that it has lost its significancy. So many things are called unique when they are scarcely less than humdrum.

So, also, the glossary of expletives and enthusiastic adjectives concerning the climate, contour, physical features and meteorological anomalies of the west coast of America has been exhausted and made meaningless. The painter, the poet and the photographer have exhausted their arts in a vain attempt to reproduce the strange scenes and sensations they have encountered in their wanderings through Wonderland. They can carry away and reproduce neither the landscapes nor the largesses of the region.

There is and can be but one Kuroshiwo or Great Japan Stream. Another would render it necessary to write a new system of hydrography and revolutionize the climatology of the world. Hot at its outset and seven hundred miles wide, this Arbiter of the Climates of the World, ceaselessly sweeps over the beds of all the oceans, from Orient to Occident. It kisses to life the frozen shores of Alaska, cools itself as it dallies with the Arctic icebergs, and then swerves southward to do its work of climate-building along this favored coast ere it again loses itself in the illimitable bosom of the wide Pacific.

But for the influence of this monster current, Alaska would have remained a frozen zone, her glacial epoch a perpetuity, and the incredible stores of gold hidden away in the sands and seams of Nome and the Klondike would have forever remained ice-locked and unknown. But for this current British Columbia would be inhabitable only by the fur-hunter and the fisherman, the walrus and the polar bear. It was this current that unlocked the frost-portals of Alaska and invited the ingress of humanity and the hummingbird. But for this current there would have been no American Eldorado, no onrush of the forty-niners, no monster trees in the forests of the Oregon, no *sequoia gigantea,* no San Francisco, with its Nob Hill, Cliff House and Chinatown; no Pacific railways spanning the continent; no Stanford University, no sand-lot philosopher, nor Lick Observatory. In truth, there would have been no settlements or sojourn of human beings from Behring's Sea to Southern Mexico.

And yet the effects of this current, at certain points, are at first sight inexplicable and apparently contradictory. Thus, the isothermal line that touches New York, lat. 41°, reaches the west coast at Vancouver Island, lat. 52°, and the mean temperature of San Diego is 9° below that of Charleston, which is in the same latitude.

But for the impinging of that stream on the Pacific coast of the American continent, there would have been no settlements by human beings north of the Gulf of California; the gold fields of Eldorado would have remain undiscovered; the iron horse would never have climbed the Rocky Mountains, and no New Empire of the West would have blossomed into existence.

The forty-niners have nearly all passed off the stage. The few survivors have forgotten the stress and fierceness of the ordeal through which they passed. The obstacles they had to face would have appaled the most daring spirits of any other race. Savages occupied all the desirable localities and stubbornly disputed every inch of the coveted ground. Water famine stared them in the face, along all the trails, and the victims of thirst planted their bones in the scorching sands of treeless deserts. Scorpions, the deadly crotalus and the dreaded Gila monster lurked in wait in the vicinity of every water source. Starvation, heat and the scalping knives of the treacherous Apaches decimated their ranks; and yet the undaunted few neither faltered nor turned back. Although gold was their immediate allurement, they well knew that no amount of the coveted treasure could repay them for their sufferings and struggles, and that though they might walk on gold, only brawn, bravery and sheer endurance could be made to win. Murder stalked in open day. Human life was held of little value; and many who won, robbed of their winnings, went booted and spurred to dishonored graves, scooped in the inhospitable sands, or were left where they fell to be devoured by · hungry wolves or birds of prey. They lived on cactus, roots and mesquit-beans, drank the rankest alkali water, and slept on pistols. Hundreds who soon realized that they could not win and live willingly threw away their lives, that their comrades might win. Not many won for themselves, even though they survived, but won for their children or their successors.

Withal, they builded better than they knew, and the irrepressible Empire of the Pacific stands as a proud and exultant monument to their tragic heroism and defiance of Fate. If laws interfered with them they were promptly repealed at the muzzles of loaded revolvers. Of precedent they made no account, and once they had put the dreadful deserts behind them, the elements became their allies. They recuperated and grew virile, as a result of the new climate and the new environment. They learned to meet and outwit the wily Apache on his own ground and at his own methods of warfare.

And they won—not merely the gold they sought, but an empire. That empire lies before us—California!

Restoring the word *unique* to its legitimate signification, it means, when applied to California, that no other State in the Union extends through ten degrees of latitude and half as many of longitude. It means that she has a longer coast line, more mountain ranges and the richest educational institution of any country or state in the world. It means that among all the States she ranks second in size, and first in the production of gold, honey, fruit and grain. There is but one Yosemite, and there are no trees on the face of the globe to be spoken of in the same breath with her *sequoia gigantea*. She has contributed more than $2,000,000,000 to the world's stock of the yellow metal. It

means that she is the only raisin-producing State, and that she produces more sugar beets than any other. She has the largest horse-breeding establishments in the world; has half a million horses, a hundred thousand milch cows, and supplies the markets with $50,000,000 worth of beef annually. She has six millions of sheep, clipping $35,-000,000 worth of wool every year. It means that the State and her largest city are practically out of debt; that the United States mint at San Francisco is the largest mint in the world; that her State University has an endowment of $7,000,000, and the Leland Stanford, *over twenty millions*, while the school revenues of the State are nearly eight millions. She produces 30,-000,000 gallons of wines annually and ships more "genuine" French wine from France to New York in a year than all France can produce on her lousy vines in ten.

California has had her days of trial; she is entering upon those of triumph. And why not.? All her natural and acquired resources, mineral, agricultural, horticultural, pastoral, and even political, comport with her area in square miles.

But further, her commercial position with relation to the rest of the Republic and with the new realms that destiny has brought under our tutelage is unlike that of any of her sister States. In addition to her extensive coast line she has two of the safest and roomiest natural harbors on the continent. The national Government is constructing a third at an expense of millions. She measures her grain, fruit and nut crops by centals and carloads instead of by baskets and bushels. Her common school system is a decided advance over the famous Eastern models, and her universities, colleges, normal and technical schools and kindergartens are not content to imitate those of older and more conservative communities. Visiting professors from New England and New York are genuinely surprised and go home with a very large flea of disillusionment in their ears, just a little ashamed of their slowness and want of enterprise.

These features and developments might be attributed to the fact that the settlers of this new realm were from among the most enterprising spirits of the older sections of the country, and no doubt this is correct to a certain extent; but it is climatic superiority that underlies it all. Her atmosphere is full of ozone and her soil is rich in iron. Both put brilliancy into the eyes and intellects of her citizens. The combination begets a temperament that transforms opportunity into accomplishment, success into sequence, and fortune into fatality. Here the aboriginal races and pioneer settlers were noted for their fine physical development, their virile health and powers of endurance. Per consequence, the white race that has supplanted barbarism and turned savagery into civilization, is already showing unmistakable evidences of physical gains.

Looking at the animal kingdom, the studs of Leland Sanford, J. B. Haggin and "Lucky" Baldwin have turned out more winning horses to the turf than any three other States—perhaps, as is claimed, than all the other States.

In the human line, it was a Californian who won the championship from the slugger Sullivan. A Californian rescued it from the iron-sinewed Australian, and still another Californian now holds the belt against the onslaughts of the world's athletes.

Nor is this superior development confined to muscle, physical brawn and endurance. Gray matter is quickened, brains teem with inventive enterprise, and special talents develop and shine. Music and the arts are more commonly cultivated than in any of the older communities. Nowhere else have so many exceptionally fine singing voices appeared. Not merely a duet or two, but scores of them could be named, all of which are winning laurels on the concert stage and in the operatic world.

These are significant facts, not fancies born of enthusiasm, and they are not merely accidental. They are largely and legitimately the results of a tonic and inspiring climate.

Take a sanitary example. San Francisco is in many respects badly situated from the standpoint of the sanitarian. The lower portions of the city were originally veritable sloughs of despond, the drainage of which is next to impossible. Her summers are really her winters, furs, overcoats and winter wraps being regularly kept at hand throughout July and August. Heavy fogs rush in from the ocean at frequent intervals in all seasons, drenching the city and vicinity as thoroughly as an ordinary summer rain. Grate fires are grateful in dogdays, and dog-day weather may occur in February.

In spite of all these contradictory conditions and other serious drawbacks, and of the criminally negligent and unsanitary habits and practices of the thousands of Mongolians who swarm and burrow like rats in their various "quarters," San Francisco shows the cleanest health record of any city of its size in the country. The disciples of Esculapius have no health saws by which to acount for such anomalous results, results that seem to set at naught all precedents. The apparent sanitary conditions and climatic factors are contradictory. Isotherms march by the right flank; there are mountains with snow on their summits and ripening oranges at their bases; there is summer in winter, cooler weather inside the houses than out of doors; streams running two-thirds of the year bottom-side up, and cloudy weather at a premium.

This aggressive city, watching the sun as it dips its day colors in the waters of the silver sea that laves the western rim of a continent through the open portals of the Golden Gate, is free from the endemics and epidemics that periodically decimate other cities of the land. Cholera has never put in its appearance; puerperal fever is practically unknown, and the eruptive fevers run a mild course; while neither bronchitis, consumption nor catarrh is indigenous.

Northern California is full of interest to the traveler, the student of nature and the climate-seeker. Shasta, most impressive of isolated mountain peaks, stands as a silent and eternal sentinel at the boundary line.

A thousand crystal rivulets dash from her dizzy heights; natural soda fountains burst and bubble from rock crevices at her base, and the fertile valleys on which she frowns and smiles, according to her ever-changing moods, are the orchard and vineyard of the world.

The climates of Northern California, like those of all other sections of the State, are always to be spoken of in the plural and are ranged in terraces. Climatic terrace No. 1 lies between the Coast Range and the ocean. Terrace No. 2 is the valley behind the Coast Range, and No. 3 is the westerly slope of the Sierras. The sea terrace is perhaps the most interesting of the three, but there are sequestered nooks and favored slopes here and there in both the others that are delightful beyond the power of description. There are mountain lakes where ice forms in summer nights, rushing rivulets and springs innumerable, hot, cold and mineral, and sites for health stations that would make Eastern proprietors green with envy.

But the culmination of climatic quaintness and excellence is attained in Southern California. This includes that portion of the State lying south of the Tehachapi Divide. Monterey, with her luxurious Hotel del Monte, Santa Cruz and Pacific Grove are delightful halfway breathing places to which San Francisco, Oakland and Stockton society can periodically retire to do meet repentance for dissipations and indiscretions that, if indulged with equal abandon in any other climate or country, would inevitably end in early physical collapse; but when a thorough change is desired these social penitents must go farther south. It is only south of the Tehachapi that all the climatic factors get in their perfect work.

On the statute books of the State there is an almost forgotten act looking toward the division of the northern and southern portions into two States. Nature has already made the division, and her hint will no doubt some day become a political realization. There will be two States and each will be larger in area than the average Eastern State.

Let there be a prize contest over the name of the commonwealth-to-be, the Sunland and Zephyrland of the South.

This new realm, no longer new except to those who have not found and enjoyed it, lies between the 32d and 34th parallels, and its more desirable portions are embraced within a triangle, of which San Diego, Santa Barbara and San Bernardino represent the vertices. There are patches, nooks, favored valleys and timbered heights outside these limits that compare fairly well, but their number and area is limited.

Tourists rushing through the country, seeking for novelties, visitors and paragraphers have essayed to describe the climate of this region; but they generally fail to make the story intelligible to others, because so much of it and the pith of it are untellable. The most enthusiastic admirer is impatient with his attempt at description. His would-be rose turns out a vulgar hollyhock; and when he would photograph the delightful touch of a sea breeze that is never heavy with humidity, his negative develops only an unprintable blank. The climatic cynic glances at the region through his colored-to-order glasses and reports only chromatic distortions.

Southern California is climatically ideal just as certain fortunate mortals who were born with a sixteen-to-one spoon in their mouths are rich—she can't help it! She lies on the shores of an ocean which has earned its name by its behavior. Its temperature is regulated and equalized by that monster of all the great ocean currents, the Kuroshiwo, already described. Originating in torrid regions and embracing in its volume a dozen degrees of latitude, this moving sea does not acquire its perfect thermal equipoise until it reaches Santa Barbara and Santa Catalina. Lack of this perfect blending of its cold and warm streams, further north, rationally accounts for its less uniform and less benignant effects along the coasts of Washington, Oregon and Northern California.

The special features of this climate, as to its therapeutic inducements, will be presented in a future paper.

THE LESSON OF THE PAN-AMERICAN.

WE do not know what farseeing genius is responsible for the legends and prophecies emblazoned on the principal buildings of the great Fair at Buffalo; but he has certainly condensed its objects, its lesson, and its history into a few pregnant and eloquent sentences that deserve the immortality they will surely win.

The GAZETTE will not vie with the daily press and the illustrated monthlies in detailed description of the commercial, mechanical, and ethical features of the Exposition, but takes pride and satisfaction in reproducing such of the inscriptions as sharply arrested the attention of the Editor as he elbowed his way through the maze of buildings and the throng of eager and awe-inspired beholders.

On the Railway Terminal Building:

"Here, by the great waters of the North are brought together the peoples of two Americas; in exposition of their Resources, Industries, Products, Inventions and Ideas."

Beginning with the more material subjects, Machinery Hall bears these dedicatory legends:

"To the Great Inventors and Farseeing Projectors, to the Engineers, Manufacturers, Agriculturalists and Merchants who have developed the resources of the New World and multiplied the homes of freemen."

"To those who in the deadly mine, on stormy seas, in the fierce breath of the furnace, and in all perilous places working ceaselessly, bring to their fellowmen comfort, sustenance and the grace of life."

On the buildings devoted to Manufactures and Liberal Arts:

"To the Explorers and Pioneers who blazed the westward path of Civilization; to the Soldiers and Sailors who fought for Freedom and for Peace, and to the Civic Heroes who save a priceless heritage."

"To the Prophets and Heroes, to the Mighty Poets and Divine Artists of the Ancient World, who inspired our forefathers and shall lead and enlighten our children's children."

On the United States Government building are the following:

"To those Painters, Sculptors and Architects, Tellers of Tales, Poets and Creators of Music; to those Actors and Musicians who, in the New World, have cherished and increased the love of beauty."

..*"To the Statesmen, Philosophers, Teachers and Preachers, and to all those who, in the New World, have upheld the ideals of Liberty and Justice, and have been faithful to the things that are Eternal."*

On the building devoted to Ethnology:

"Knowledge begins in wonder."

"Speak to the Earth and it shall teach thee."

"Nothing that is human is alien to me."

"The weakest among us has a gift."

"All are needed by Each one."

"And hath made of one blood all Nations of the Earth."

"No se gano Zamora en una hora."

"O rich and various man, thou palace of sight and sound, carrying in thy senses the morning and the evening, and in the unfathomable galaxy of thy brain the geometry of the City of God, in thy heart the Bower of Love and the Realms of Right and Wrong."—EMERSON.

On the Agricultural Building:

"To the Ancient Races of America, for whom the New World was the Old, that their love of Freedom and of Nature, their hardy courage, their Monuments, Arts, Legends, may not perish from the Earth."

"To the Scholars and Laborious Investigators who, in the Old World and the New, guard the Lamp of Knowledge, and, Century by Century, increase the Safety of Life and enlarge the Spirit of Man."

On the entrance gateway to the Stadium:

"Who shuns the dust and sweat of the contest, on his brow falls not the cool shade of the olive."

"He who fails bravely has not truly failed, but is himself also a conqueror."

"Not ignoble are the Days of Peace, not without courage and laurelled victories."

THE VALUE OF EXAGGERATION.

MOST ably has the subject of the doctor's fee been treated by Roberts (*Philadelphia Med. Journal*, May 11, 1901) and most thoroughly has he exposed many of the unethical and dishonest methods by which it is increased. He scathingly denounces the system adopted by some consultants of offering commissions for patients and dividing fees received from them with the sender. The furnishing of testimonials to manufacturers of drugs for pecuniary or other recompense is justly condemned. The overcharging of the wealthy on the ground that they can afford to pay and of the estates of deceased patients, because the dead cannot complain, comes in for a share of denunciation, while the surgeon who will wait with the patient anesthetized and upon the table until his fee is forthcoming, is given the notoriety which he deserves.

The subject is decidedly unpleasant. Far more agreeable is it to discuss the effects of the abuse of alcohol by others, and to point out the resemblance between the so-called Christian Scientist and the guinea pig on the ground that the latter is not a pig and that it did not come from Guinea. It is hard for a member of that profession which is composed of men whose relations to others most demand justice and a high moral sense to acknowledge the shortcomings of the fraternity. The family skeleton in the closet is not a congenial companion and the one exposed to view by Roberts is not the only one which the medical profession possesses. Advertising is one which has been given considerable notoriety. But what of exaggeration for the sake of impressing an actual or prospective patient? It is certainly one of the most common and most successful methods of enlarging a practice, but he must be careful indeed who escapes detection by others of the profession. We do not refer to self-glorification at society meetings, references to the extent of one's practice, or to others as the younger men; not to the publication of articles describing unique methods of palpating the impossible, of performing a whole series of operations through a microscopic incision of stated dimensions; nor to seeking notoriety by receptions given to persons of note, or by newspaper interviews in which the speaker is more emphasized than the subject. These are merely phases of the advertising skeleton, showing various degrees of taste.

The form of exaggeration which is an indication not merely of lack of taste, but of dishonesty, appears in many shades. One of its best known examples is that of the physician who is invariably called just in time to prevent a threatened pneumonia or to save the patient's life; the man who diagnoses every case of bronchitis as pneumonia and claims that he has never had a death from the latter disease. Closely allied is the surgeon who with equal frequency dwells upon the seriousness of every case and every operation, however trivial, and lives upon the reputation acquired by the brilliant results he attains in spite of his dark prognoses. He is usually not one who is diffident in regard to mentioning such results or the number of his operations. The patient is usually pleased by the idea that he is a most unusual or serious case and is the last to suspect exaggeration. A well-known surgeon called to treat a case, apparently a limited cellulitis of the ankle, pronounces it "blood poisoning" and evacuates a small amount of pus. At a second visit a similar spot appears upon the anterior aspect of the ankle and is also relieved by a slight incision. The patient is surprised that he feels well with so serious a difficulty, but is assured that it is nevertheless an ominous malady. After three weeks of treatment he is cured; he then publishes to his friends, lay and medical, the wonders of his case. His professional friends say nothing, but has their opinion of the well-known surgeon been improved, and are they the more likely to call him in consultation? Again a patient with chronic appendicitis, recovering from an exacerbation, is advised to wait until the interval and then be operated upon by his own surgeon in Boston. A surgeon who is as well known as he can make himself is called as consultant. Without a word to the attending physician he informs the patient and his family that his condition is serious and immediate operation is necessary. He is removed to the hospital where the surgeon operates, is kept in bed for twelve days and then operated upon after the attack has subsided. Incidentally suppuration of a clean case occurs, but this point is not exaggerated and is referred to as a slight oozing from the abdominal fat. Will he be called in consultation by those who know his name?

And concerning those whose statistics are manipulated; if such liberties with strict truth are not evident upon the face of their articles there are almost invariably enough witnesses to compare the published accounts with what they have seen. And of what advantage is it to minimize the dangers of a procedure which one advocates? Suppose that an operator publishes a long series of operations under lumbar anesthesia and claims that the inconveniences are insignificant, the headache following so slight as to be negligible. Investigation will undoubtedly show that morphine has failed to relieve the suffering which the injection of cocaine caused, and the reporter's reputation has suffered by inaccuracy.

The tendency to specialize has become so strong that it has been said that diseases of the umbilicus is the only field that has not been filled. Convalescence is evidently the specialty of some physicians, for it is well known that there are those whose daily visits rarely terminate until the patient, in self-defense, is obliged to assume the responsibility of deciding that a cure has been accomplished for some time.

Where competition is so keen as in New York and exaggeration is so common a bait for the patient, the fact that such procedures are not ethical will have little weight with those most concerned. But after all, honesty is the best policy. Murder will out, and eventually many a dishonest act will work untold harm to its performer.

LEPROSY IN THE UNITED STATES.

According to a Washington dispatch in the *New York Tribune,* the surgeon-general of the Marine-Hospital Service is not ready to publish the results thus far obtained under his direction in the attempt to enumerate the known cases of leprosy in the United States, as the returns are far from complete. But sufficient material has already been secured by the experts who have been diligently investigating for the last two years to indicate that there are at least one thousand lepers in this country, most of them immigrants from abroad, and to warrant strong recommendations to Congress for their segregation. The commission, consisting of Surgeon J. H. White, Chairman, and Passed Assistant Surgeons

G. T. Vaughan and M. J. Rosenau, have been working under Congressional authority since 1899, making a scientific investigation of the extent of the disease in America. They sent circular letters to physicians, health officers, hospital superintendents, and others in 600 localities, covering the entire country, asking for reports and information regarding leprosy patients. Eight thousand circulars have been sent out, and only 2,000 replies have been received. From these, 277 lepers have been located and their names and addresses obtained. About one hundred are known to live in New Orleans, many of whom are well-to-do persons of good families. In Minnesota about twenty cases have been reported, the disease there being found mostly among the Scandinavians living in the rural districts. In New York seven cases have been reported, while in Chicago only three have been found so far. In San Francisco fifteen cases are known, twelve of which are confined in the pesthouse. There are fifteen in North Dakota, and only two in South Dakota. In New Mexico there are at least a dozen, and Baltimore reports three cases. The remainder are scattered throughout the country. Owing to the fact that three-fourths of the circulars have brought no replies, especially from suspicious districts, the authorities estimate that only about one-fourth of the cases of leprosy have been reported. The commission will almost certainly recommend to Congress in its forthcoming preliminary report in December that national lazarettos be established in several parts of the country—one, herhaps, at New Orleans, one in New Mexico and another in Minnesota or Montana. A generous appropriation will be asked, large enough to cover the erection of fine isolated buildings, attractively equipped with every imaginable convenience for the comfort and pleasure of the sufferers. By this means it is hoped to overcome the general antipathy to isolation of the diseased, and thus remove the greatest obstacle in the way of preventing the disease from spreading. Not the least interesting result accomplished by the investigation is the conviction of the experts that, notwithstanding the widespread distribution of leprous patients in the United States and the increase in the last decade, there is little ground for alarm.

ON THE PROPER USE OF HYDROGEN DIOXID.

DR. MORRIS, of New York, says of the use and misuse of hydrogen dioxid, now called *dioxogen:*

I emphasize the fact that I am now more than ever convinced of its indispensableness to the best surgical practice. I am also satisfied that some excellent surgeons have been inclined to drop the use of it because of apparent failures in results attained. These untoward reports, I am sure, arise from inadvertence in the methods and periods of using the remedy. It is my firm conviction, after more than ten years of continuous use, that nothing yet discovered can take its place in cleansing and rendering aseptic blind cavities, sinuses, and fistulæ; but at the same time my experience and observation have taught me that in certain cases its use can be continued too long, after the prime object of complete asepsis has been fully attained. The explanation is perfectly rational and logical, viz., that as soon as all pus, pus germs, detritus, and culture fluids have been decomposed, broken up and driven out of the hidden recesses of a wound or fistula, the continued use of hydrogen dioxid (dioxogen), with its incessant avidity and affinity for the albumins, undoubtedly tends to destroy the incipient exudations of plastic lymph, which are the beginning of and absolutely essential to the healing process. When this occurs, the efforts of nature are constantly thwarted, and the process of repair greatly delayed.

To illustrate, he cited the case of a young man operated upon for appendicitis, in whom the fistulous opening left for drainage remained open for a year or more, simply because the attending surgeon overlooked or did not suspect the action above referred to, and continued to syringe out the wound or cavity with the dioxid. On consultation, it became evident that this was the condition: the young man was directed to omit further treatment and to go about his ordinary business, and not even to avoid any active field sports to which he had formerly been accustomed. The fistula promptly healed.

The indications for stopping the use of dioxid are the *vital signs.* In other words, when the patient's condition reaches the turning point between retrogression and improvement, when he ceases to grow worse, or to exhibit signs of degenerative processes and begins to improve, the dioxid should be promptly discontinued. No mistake can be made if this *vital sign* be carefully noted and adopted as a guide.

CORPOREAL SPECIFIC GRAVITY.

ALTHOUGH the absolute weight of the body is a valuable sign in determining the physical condition of a patient, yet it does not always reflect the true state of health, for a very heavy man need not be obese, nor need a light man be emaciated. Much more definite and valuable assistance can be had from the determination of the specific gravity. H. Stern (*Med. Rec.,* February 9, 1901), after considerable expense, suggests that the simplest method of ascertaining this point is by the archimedean principle, by which the density is obtained by dividing the absolute weight of the body by the loss of weight which it sustains when suspended in water. He believes that if the specific gravity is below 1,063 or above 1,073, unsoundness of the organism is denoted. Low density means satiation with water or preponderance of adipose; the high figure means disturbed metabolism, general atrophic state, or senility. There is also a greater predisposition to infectious diseases when the density is low, and increased sus-

ceptibility to eliminative disorders when it is high. Strength and endurance are deficient among those at either extreme, and the duration of life depends so much upon corporeal density that this physical sign should become a valuable one to life insurance examiners.

A NEW USE FOR VASELINE.

WHEN sterilized vaseline is introduced within the tissues it undergoes no change and appears to be retained for an unlimited period. This property, says the *Int'l Jour. of Surgery,* has been made use of for plastic purposes by Gersuny, of Vienna. In an individual upon whom a double castration had been done for tubercular orchitis, several injections of white vaseline were made, finally resulting in the formation of two deposits, which were a fair representation of the original contents of the scrotum. An individual suffering from a difficulty of speech after an operation for harelip received an injection of vaseline under the pendulous fold of the upper lip, and was thus given the amount of labial resistance needed for proper articulation. It is therefore evident that the ingenuity of surgeons will find new and original uses for this procedure.

FOREIGN BODIES IN THE HUMAN SYSTEM.

Two or three months ago we published an item about *"la dame aux aiguilles"* or the "needle woman"—a young woman who was then mystifying Parisian physicians and surgeons with the needles which she claimed to remove from all parts of her body. She proved to be a hysterical fraud, but the publication of the item in a French medical journal elicited from a correspondent the following curious facts:

"M. D. Antonio Marcus y Cabot cites, among others one noted also by Brodie in which a demented person passed by the rectum, some twenty-four hours after he had swallowed it, a pair of carpenters' compasses of iron or steel, and quite large and bulky. Legendre tells of a case where an iron fork, of ordinary size, swallowed by a drunken man, worked its way through the system in fifteen months, and was finally extracted entire. The case of Block is also referred to—a young subject who passed at various times 429 articles, among which were iron keys, bits of iron and of lead, etc., and all were passed without accident.

Marcus y Cabot relates the case of an old man of sixty-seven years, who suffered from an abscess in the anal region. An incision was made, and catheterism discovered, at the depth of 2½ inches, a hard substance, which proved to be the stem of his pipe, made of horn, which had disappeared one evening some two and a half months previously. He was in the habit of taking a nap every afternoon, with his pipe in his mouth, and it is supposed that he swallowed the stem on one of these occasions.

Tactron removed a partridge bone from near the prostate in one of his cases. Merlin removed a fish bone, encysted in the shoulder, and other bones in the thigh of a fetus. Morris tells of a fecal abscess in the cecal region, which he opened and which had been caused by a calculus of cholesterine as big as a nutmeg.

It is wonderful how foreign bodies, sometimes of large dimensions, can traverse the intestines, apparently without causing any damage, when some little insignificant thing will cause the gravest of accidents."

❧ ❧

It is said that automobiles have so cheapened the cost of harvesting grain in the immense California fields that wheat can be raised there at less actual cost than in the Argentine Republic.

❧ ❧

CLEANLINESS WITHOUT SOAP.

From the *London Truth*.

Surely too much importance is attached to the scarcity of soap in the Boers' farmhouses. People may be very clean and use very little soap. The Russians and Japanese cleanse themselves with vapour baths, rarely using soap when they do so. A really healthy skin cleanses itself. Rough inside clothing, which, I presume, the Boers wear, is a great skin cleanser. I have known of doctors curing skin diseases by insisting on linguerie de luxe being cast aside and coarse undergarments worn instead. The late Emperor of the French hardly ever soaped his hands until he went to England. I have come across a paper found in his desk at the Tuileries. It contained the instructions of the King of Holland to the Governor of his two elder sons. Among the things forbidden was for the young princes' hands to be washed with soap. They were to use bran and a slice of lemon. The lemon was to remove ink stains, and in summer to keep off gnats and mosquitoes. Napoleon, whose hands were good to model and beautifully white, also used bran but no soap, unless to shave. I never use soap of any kind without a sense of skin discomfort which not even a deluge of quite pure water will wholly remove. In England, on account of coal, smoke and smut, soap is more needed than in countries with clear air. The Boers enjoy, perhaps, the purest atmosphere in the world except when there are dust storms. I know French ladies who have discarded soap for vaseline. They smear themselves with the latter, and then rub it off well with a soft cotton towel. A doctor tells me that nothing is more cleansing, but that he prefers, as more tonic, plain cold water, followed by the same sort of rubbing. Dr. Leyds really should not take to heart what Sir Henry Stanley said about the Boers being badly off for soap.

❧ ❧

FEAR LITTLENESS OF SOUL MORE THAN LITTLENESS OF FORTUNE.

THIS commercial age is not the inferior of any preceding age in morality. Never before have the principles of justice been more intelligently understood or applied. The machinery of commerce, like the machinery of industry, is being continuously developed in the directions of accuracy and power. Instruments of precision do not vary their measurements or movements to accommodate the instability of any man's views or movements. He must comply with their requirements or they will not serve him. Only small minds regard such compliance as servitude. Weaklings are the slaves of conditions which master minds command to serve them. Punctual attention to every business requirement is as necessary for the employer as for the employed. Few employees realize that, were the employer to shirk his duties as they do theirs, were he to limit his work, his thought and care for the business as they limit their work, the business which furnishes occupation to both would soon dissolve for lack of cohesive force, and the money for the payroll would not be forthcoming. Littleness of soul always limits endeavor and dwarfs accomplishment. The gains of life are property and character. The poorest man on earth is he who has gained wealth at the expense of character. When the day for his departure comes he must go forth empty-handed, a beggar. Mr. Forgan well says: "It is better to die a pauper in purse than a pauper in soul."

METALS NEED REST.

METALS get tired as well as human beings. Telegraph wires are better conductors on Monday than on Saturday on account of their Sunday rest, and a rest of three weeks adds 10 per cent. to the conductivity of a wire.—*Med. Age.*

ANTIQUITY OF MAN.

THIS problem receives an interesting answer in the latest edition of De Mortillet's "Origin and Antiquity of Man." The total number of years elapsed since, according to geological evidence, man first appeared upon the earth is placed at 238,000. Of this 78,000 years belong to the Pre-Glacial epoch; 100,000 to the Glacial; 44,000 to the interval between the Glacial and Proto-Historic; 10,000 to the latter and the Neolithic, and 6,000 years to the time elapsed since the beginning of the Historic period in Egypt.

THINGS WORTH REMEMBERING.

CHRISTIAN SCIENTISTS say that as an evidence of the necessary faith the fee must invariably be paid in advance.

Nine per cent. solutions of essence of cinnamon, 11 and 12 per cent. of essence of thyme, and 18 per cent. of essence of geranium assure complete disinfection of the hands.

When a child complains of pain in the knee for any length of time, without any evidence of local disease, invariably be on your guard. Nine times out of ten it means that the child has hip-joint disease.

"Here, young man," said the old lady with fire in her eye; "I've brung back this thermometer you sold me."
"What's the matter with it?" asked the clerk.
"It ain't reliable. One time ye look at it it says one thing, and the next time it says another."

Rigg—Yes, Jigg and I are good friends now; but when we were boys he gave it to me in the neck.
Tigg—That so?
Rigg—Yes; I caught the mumps from him.

CONCENTRATION IN SCIENTIFIC WORK.

WE are not advocates of specialism where the term is used as, too often, a synonym for narrowness. "The man of one idea" is neither a safe physician nor a wise counselor. Deliver us and our patients from the man who is always ringing in his pet hobby and peculiar theory. Such a man looks only through glasses with a limited field, and sees but the organ in which he is specially interested. He ignores all else, and magnifies the importance of this.

Although this danger attaches to all special work, yet it is true that most men should have a lifework in some definite direction. This need not lead him to neglect general acquisition—rather it should stimulate him to become familiar with all that enters into the building of the wall, in order that the key-stone in his efforts may be securely laid.

It is not needed that the physician should abandon general practice to become expert in some chosen line of investigation, but let him at least be, if he can, well grounded in the advanced thought and progress of that special department. Such a man in even a small village may become an authority and be the consultant for the whole district. A physician living in a small mining town in Illinois is deservedly looked upon as the best posted practitioner on cardiac diseases in all that country, and his advice is sought from far and near. Another, in a still smaller town, is one of the best microscopists in the West.

Where it can be done, we believe that practice should be limited to the class of diseases that the practitioner is best fitted to treat. It is a reproach to our profession that in our Western cities a surgeon who claims distinction as an operator will attend a case of measles in the morning, operate for appendicitis at noon (funeral three days later), and preside at the delivery of a pickaninny after supper. Such surgeons would criticise harshly an oculist who would set a broken leg or an aurist who would "cut for stone;" yet they will treat anything from fever to fibroids, and prescribe for all things between hemicrania and hemorrhoids.

Of course, each man must judge for himself how far he can specialize; but we are sure that in so far as he does limit himself to one line of work (not study), he will be more successful and more honored.

CREMATION AND CRIME.

THE increase in popularity of cremation as a means of disposing of the bodies of the dead, and the thoroughness of the process in destroying any evidence of crime about the body, should such evidence exist, must needs interest any municipality where cremation is permitted and encouraged.

The only precaution practiced is to have a burial certificate signed by some physician in good standing, together with a request from some friends or relatives that they desire the body cremated.

The body is thereupon cremated, and should any suspicious circumstances arise after the death of the individual, but very little room for investigation would be found.

THE NORMAL SALT SOLUTION.

THERE is some variation in the formulæ given by different writers. Dr. Charles A. L. Reed, in his new "Text-Book of Gynecology," remarks that Locke has suggested the following formula and reported favorably upon it:

℞ Calcium chloride ......gr. iij 3-4
 Potassium chloride ...... gr. iss
 Sodium chloride .... ʒ iiss
 Sterilized, distilled or tap
 water .... q. s. ad 1 quart

M. The solution may be injected subcutaneously, into the intestine, or into a vein.
—*N. Y. Med. Journal.*

TO BANISH MOSQUITOES.

THE following generally proves effective in banishing these pests from a room into which they have found their way and from which it is often difficult to expel them:

Mix formaldehyd of 40 per cent. strength with four times its volume of alcohol. Wood alcohol is probably better than ordinary spirit. Saturate small bunches or tufts of absorbent cotton with this mixture, place in a saucer, soup plate, or some metallic dish and apply a lighted match. Do this two or three times during the afternoon and half an hour before retiring.

NAPOLEON'S TOMB AT PARIS.

A LITTLE while ago I stood by the grave of the old Napoleon—a magnificent tomb of gilt and gold, fit almost for a deity dead—and gazed upon the sarcophagus of rare and nameless marble, where rest at last the ashes of that restless man. I leaned over the balustrade and thought about the career of the greatest soldier of the modern world. I saw him walking upon the banks of the Seine contemplating suicide. I saw him at Toulon. I saw him putting down the mob in the strets of Paris. I saw him at the head of the army in Italy. I saw him crossing the bridge at Lodi with the tricolor in his hand. I saw him in Egypt in the shadows of the pyramids. I saw him conquer the Alps and mingle the eagles of France with the eagles of the crags. I saw him at Marengo, at Ulm, and at Austerlitz. I saw him in Russia when the infantry of the snow and the cavalry of the wild blast scattered his legions like winter's withered leaves. I saw him at Leipsic in defeat and disaster—driven by a million bayonets back upon Paris—clutched like a wild beast—banished to Elba. I saw him escape and retake an empire by the force of his genius. I saw him upon the frightful field of Waterloo, where chance and fate combined to wreck the fortunes of the former king. And I saw him at St. Helena, with his hands crossed behind him, gazing out upon the sad and solemn sea.

I thought of the orphans and widows he had made—of the tears that had been shed for his glory, and of the only woman who ever loved him pushed from his heart by the cold hand of ambition. And I said I would rather have been a French peasant and worn wooden shoes. I would rather have lived in a hut with a vine growing over the door, and the grapes growing purple in the kiss of the autumn sun. I would rather have been that poor peasant, with my loving wife by my side knitting as the day died out of the sky—with my children upon my knees and their arms about me. *I would rather have been that man* than to have been Napoleon the Great.

TO IMPROVE THE HYGIENIC AND PHYSICAL CONDITION OF THE SLUMS.

BY L. I. BOGEN, M.D.,
of Omaha, Neb.

From *American Medicine.*

IN the first number of your valuable journal in an editorial on "Heredity and Human Progress," the writer strikes the keynote to the situation, when he says: "It cannot be doubted that modern city life, with its unhygienic, underfed slum population, must inevitably produce some such horrors as Dr. McKim outlines." After reaching such conclusions the remedy would naturally suggest itself, viz.: to improve the hygienic and physical conditions of this underfed slum population, and the cause once removed, the effects will themselves disappear. Instead of it the writer suggests "for those classes who are unquestionably hopelessly depraved," etc., the unsexing of these classes and thus preventing them from producing others of their kind.

The writer's remedy would be consistent and logical if. like Dr. McKim, he would contend that the world's degeneracy is due solely to the survival of bad and weakly people. If, however, modern city life, etc., be the cause of it, then degenerates must always be produced as long as this modern city life with the unhygienic surroundings will continue in existence.

It may not be amiss to remind the writer, as well as Dr. McKim, that about a hundred years ago Robert Owen was confronted with the same problem and he solved it very effectively and in a very much more humane way than Dr. McKim and the writer suggest.

Robert Owen was manager of a large mill in Scotland employing 2,000 people; 500 were children, and nearly all of them had been taken at the age of five or six years from charity institutions. He found his workingmen in a most deplorable condition, many of them being hopelessly depraved. Most of the families were living in single rooms, and theft, drunkenness, and other immoralities, together with long hours of factory work, kept respectable people from working in the mill.

Robert Owen reduced the hours of labor, established schools for children and adults, improved their dwellings, sanitarily and otherwise, and he put the sale of intoxicating liquors under the strictest surveillance. In a short time this once demoralized village became the most civilized, industrious, intelligent, happy and prosperous community in Great Britain.

FORMALDEHYD AS A DISINFECTANT.

As a result of a review of French literature on disinfecting by formaldehyd, by Assistant Surgeon S. P. Gruble, it appears to be a recognized fact that formaldehyd gas is a surface disinfectant only and will not penetrate deeply into the bedding and the like. The lack of penetrating power of this gas seems to be that when it comes into contact with any fibrous or porous body it changes its form and polymerizes into an inert solid.

USEFUL HINTS.

WE are indebted to the *National Druggist* for the following recipes:

FLOOR POLISHES.

The following are all good and cheap:

Stearin .... 100 parts.
Beeswax, yellow .... 25 parts.
Potassium hydrate .... 60 parts.
Yellow laundry soap ...... 10 parts.

Water and coloring matter to suit—ochre is usually employed. Heat together until saponification takes place. Another, which is said to be most excellent, is as follows:

Beeswax, yellow .... 25 parts.
Yellow laundry soap .... 6 parts.
Glue .... 12 parts.
Soda ash (80° B.) .... 25 parts.
Water and ochre, sufficient.

Dissolve the soda in 400 parts of water, add the wax, and boil down to 250 parts, then add the soap. Dissolve the glue in 100 parts of hot water, stir in the ochre, and mix the whole with the saponified wax.

For light, unstained parquettes, the following is recommended:

White wax .... 75 parts.
Bleached shellac .... 75 parts.
Clear rosin (transparent) ... 6 parts.
Oil of turpentine .... 100 parts.
Alcohol, wood .... 400 parts.

Melt the wax, shellac and rosin together, remove from the fire, let cool down somewhat, and add the turpentine, under active and constant stirring. Warm the alcohol, carefully, to a point near boiling, then add, under rapid and constant stirring. This preparation should be slightly warmed before applying (except in summer time), and afterwards polished with woollen cloths.

LEMON JUICE—TO PRESERVE.

There are several more or less reliable processes. The following has given satisfaction in our hands:

Express the juice and filter *at once*, through two thicknesses of best white

Swedish paper, into a container that has been sterilized immediately before letting the juice run into it, by boiling water. The better plan is to take out of water in active ebullition at the moment you desire to use it. Have ready some long-necked 8-ounce vials, which should also be kept in boiling water until needed. Pour the juice into these, leaving room in the upper part of the body of the vial to receive a teaspoonful of the best olive oil. Pour the latter in so that it will trickle down the neck and form a layer on the top of the juice, and close the neck with a wad of antiseptic cotton thrust into it in such manner that it does not touch the oil, and leaves room for the cork to be put in without touching it. Now cork, and cap or seal the vial, and put in a cool, dark place, and keep standing upright. If carried out faithfully, with due attention to cleanliness, this process will keep the juice in a perfectly natural condition for a very long time. The two essentials are the careful and *rapid* filtration, and the complete aseptization of the containers. Another process, in use in the French Navy depends upon the rapid and careful filtering of the juice, and the addition of from 8 per cent. to 10 per cent. of alcohol.

LASTING OFFICE PASTE.

(SUBSCRIBER, Kansas City, Mo.)—We find the following in our files: Dissolve a teaspoonful of alum in a quart of warm water. When cold, stir in as much flour as will give it the consistency of thick cream, being particular to break up the lumps; stir in as much powdered resin as will lay on a sixpence, and half a dozen cloves to give a flavor. Have on the fire a saucepan with a teacup of boiling water, pour the flour mixture into it, stirring well all the time. In a few minutes it will be of the consistency of porridge. Pour it into a jar. Let it cool, tie a cloth over the jar and set in a cool place. When wanted for use take out a portion and soften with warm water. It will keep twelve months.

SAUSAGE POISONING (BOTULISM).

LAUK, in the *Munchener Medicinische Wochenschrift*, says that this form of poisoning is due to a special bacillus which produces a specific toxin. The poison may be developed in ham or bacon, but is by far most frequent in liver or sausage. The striking characteristic in this form of intoxication is that the symptoms are slow to appear, twelve or thirty-six hours often elapsing from the time the tainted food is eaten. The first to show themselves are a general malaise, with pain in the epigastrium, nausea, or actual vomiting. Later there is a sense of suffocation and great prostration. All the secretions are diminished, and the skin and mucous membranes are very dry. Ulcerated patches appear in the mouth and larynx, and certain cerebral nerves are generally paralyzed. Ptosis is common, the pupils being commonly dilated and reacting slowly to light. Difficulty in swallowing may be so marked as to necessitate the employment of the stomach-tube. The spinal nerves with the central nervous system commonly escape. There is no temperature in the absence of complications. If death occurs, it is commonly eight or ten days after the poisoning, and is usually due to respiratory paralysis, or to some complication, such as pneumonia, or possibly asthenia from inanition.

THE SINECURE.

"WELL, my boy, and what are you going to do now?"

"Well, dad, I don't know. What I want is one of these fancy jobs where you do the least possible work for the very largest possible fee."

"Guess you are cut out for a corporation lawyer, my boy."

"No, dad. I was thinking of being a medical specialist." —*Cleveland Plain Dealer.*

Department of Physical Education.

WITH SPECIAL REGARD TO SYMMETRICAL DEVELOPMENT OF THE BODY

WAS PRESIDENT McKINLEY'S CASE BADLY MANAGED?

A CORRESPONDENT who does not care to have his name mentioned asks this question.

The editor of the GAZETTE fully appreciates the surprise and bitter disappointment that naturally followed the sudden and fatal termination of this phenomenal case after the hopeful announcements made by the eminent medical staff in attendance. In the very midst of services of praise and thanksgiving for the assurances of a sure and quick recovery came the blighting despatch that the President was dying!

We do not feel competent to criticize the treatment adopted by the eminent staff of medical and surgical advisers who gave such unremitting attention to the illustrious patient. If we were so disposed we have not the necessary data. "Beef tea" is not now considered of much value as food, and chicken soup is far from ideal, except among grandmas and domestic doctors. But the daily press may have substituted these names for other products of similar origin but of far more value. Reporters are marvelously wise, but they frequently perpetrate medical bulls that are decidedly funny when they are not too serious.

We do not, therefore, agree with those professional critics who assert that the President was starved to death.

We cannot understand how the medical men in attendance could commit themselves to such a hopeful prognosis in the face of the persistently high pulse-rate. The temperature, as reported, was never excessively high, but the pulse-rate remained most or all the time after the shooting above 120.

Such a pulse in a man of President McKinley's reputed vigor is ominous of great danger. It indicated severe vital depression. The attendant symptoms and the outcome prove that the physical condition of the patient was far from vigorous. The enormous and persistent strain imposed upon the head of a powerful nation, undergoing years of political stress, such as it has not known since the days of the Rebellion, is enough to try the best constitutions. When we add to this the terrible suspense and constant anxiety from the domestic trial through which President McKinley had just passed, and from which he could not have fully recovered, it is not to be wondered at that he could not recover from a gunshot wound that but a few years back would have been considered inevitably fatal.

To this may be added that he was an inveterate smoker, which certainly does not add to the chances of any invalid. One eminent critic of the treatment of the dead President expresses the opinion that his smoking had nothing to do with the fatal result; but we suspect that this commentator is himself a smoker. The heart-walls were described as very thin. It was undoubtedly to a certain degree a "smoker's heart," and for that reason certainly succumbed more easily.

We think the President died because his system was vitally degenerate and could not recoup from the shock of the assassin's bullet, as a more vigorous system, seconded by the rare surgical skill so promptly and efficiently invoked, would surely have done. Gangrene does not occur in tissues that are made scrupulously aseptic, as was surely done in this case, and that are normally nourished and vitally up to par.

SOME SUGGESTIONS REGARDING A DEPARTMENT OF SCHOOL HYGIENE.

In one of our Exchanges we find the following, by

LEIGH K. BAKER.

THOSE nations which have exercised a powerful and elevating influence have been those which have exercised a care for the health of their citizens. In a democracy, self-preservation demands an educated citizenship. An elemental condition of useful citizenship is a fair degree of physical health. It is both the interest and the duty of the State to insist that the physical basis in the educational structure be adequately and properly laid. It is strikingly true of the children of the cities that the desired improvement in health has not been attained. The dark, noisome alleys and tenements contain millions of the miserable offspring of ignorant foreigners, poorly born, poorly housed and fed, with crooked spines and misshapen skulls, with pathologic eyes or ears, and little in their environments to produce self-supporting, self-respecting citizens. The question resolves itself, Shall we put sufficient money into the school system to produce self-supporting citizens; or shall we later, on account of half-supporting them and paying insufficient attention to the health of the children, spend larger sums for the construction of hospitals, dispensaries, police stations, reform schools, etc.? Physicians, who of all classes of men are forced to carry this burden of indigency perhaps more than any other, should combine to place the right kind of men on school boards. The author outlines a systematic plan of organization with reference to the composition of the school board, the superintendent and teachers, and points out the dangers of allowing political influences to enter. The head of the department of school hygiene must be a medical man, who is at the same time a school sanitarian. Regular inspection of school children should be made, and plenty of assistance should be available to do it.

LETHAL EFFECT OF YEW.

THE sudden death of a patient, says the *Medical Press*, in Mullingar Asylum, from eating yew (taxus baccata) leaves arouses attention to the inadvisability of ornamenting the recreation grounds of asylums with plants and trees of well-known lethal properties. To both men and animals the yew is poisonous, as has been noted by classic writers including Cæsar, Virgil, and Livy. Bentley and Trimer state that the leaves and young branches in all circumstances act as a narcotic acrid poison. Numerous cases of poisoning are recorded in medical literature, as may be seen by reference to works on forensic medicine. That fatal results do not occur more often from the use of the leaves is greatly to be wondered at for the tree is common throughout the three kingdoms, and they are a favorite domestic remedy for worms, female irregularities, and less seldom as an hypnotic. At one time was recommended in the treatment of heart disease as a substitute for digitalis, over which it was said to possess the advantage of not being cumulative in its effects. In India the fruit and leaves were credited with antilithic properties, and some native physicians claimed litholytic properties for them. As a remedy for convulsions in children and for epilepsy in adults, the infusion of the leaves was once freely prescribed. Their active toxic action would imply that they possess properties that are well worth physiological examination, and they may possibly become a valuable addition to our therapeutic remedies. At present we practically know nothing more than that the tree yields a powerful poison for man and beast, and such knowledge is sufficient to warrant its exclusion from all places where the insane, children, or cattle may eat it.

We grow strong through assuming responsibilities—by bearing burdens and doing things, we acquire power.—*Elbert Hubbard.*

THE CRYING NEEDS OF MEDICAL JOURNALISM.

In a suggestive paper on this subject, in *American Medicine*, Dr. W. H. Burr, of Wilmington, Del., says:

In an experience of many years, during which I covered a large part of North America in the interests of a medical journal, I have had abundant opportunity to feel the professional pulse and ascertain the relation existing between medical journalism and the profession. Thinking that your readers may be interested in the subjoined notes, penned by the way, I submit them for review. I met thousands of physicians, in all sections of the country, including large metropolitan towns and the small cross roads, towns and post offices, and the question constantly propounded is, "What medical journal should I read?" The natural and inevitable reply is "The journal that I represent." But the intent of this paper is just, so personal consideration must be eliminated. It seems difficult to answer the query without somewhere giving offense. It has been intimated that of the 350 to 400 journals published in this country, two-thirds have no reasonable excuse for existence. In the effort to find a solution to the inquiry my experience has been unique. I have found it necessary not to classify the journals but the profession, location, habitat, etc. Startling results have followed this classification. For instance, in an experience of two years, covering most of the New England and Middle States (towns not under 5,000) less than twenty-five bona-fide subscribers were found for a journal which claims the largest circulation of any medical journal in the country. Indeed, I doubt that I found 100 bona-fide sub·scribers in the whole country. As a general proposition I would say that in towns of 5,000 and over, 85 per cent. of the profession took and read one or more of a list of seven weeklies and seven monthlies. This list refers to metropolitan journals and, with the exception of one national society organ which is included in the list, does not include the numerous local journals. In addition to this there are a few journals (monthlies) which claim to have, and do have, a national circulation, although it was a puzzle to locate the circulation until I had enlarged my sphere and canvassed smaller towns of 2,000 and less. Only recently in a town of 1,800, in the sunny South, I found four physicians and not one weekly in the town. In nine towns in the same section, containing fifty-six physicians, there were not more than ten who subscribed to a first-class journal, and it is my conviction (born through long experience) that all the arts of the most experienced solicitor would fail in converting these men, although many of them were graduates of standard colleges.

As an expression of sentiment regarding the manner in which the so-called first-class journal is held by some of these men, the following may prove of interest:

(1) "We want something to help us at the bedside. We care nothing for long articles on general or specialized subjects, about cases we shall never meet or matters with which we shall never deal. We want something practical." (2) "The trouble with Northern journals is that they discuss subjects that are of no interest here; climatic conditions are different, treatment is different. In pathology and surgery the journals are excellent, but we want treatment." (The assumption that Northern journals draw only from Northern contributors amuses one who reads journals.) (3) "Your journals are edited by college professors and contain little or nothing of interest to the general practitioner." (sic.) (College professors are supposed to have had no practical experience, and clinic cases drawn from the larger cities are invariably assumed to be of a different mould from material that meets the general practitioner. Then, too, the practice of the city is denominated theory by many country practitioners.) (4) "We want a journal edited by the people." (Who are the people?) (5) "We prefer to read text-books. The articles therein are more accurate and more care-

fully written, while journals are full of fantastic theories. The references in text-books are so handy." (It is evident they have not heard of a card index.) (6) "Journals were of some value when there were no text-books. They formerly represented the experiences of the men of the times. They are now outgrown and devoted to the vaporings of advertising doctors." (7) "The country doctor has not time to read journals."

This is the stock argument, and the last time it came from a man of the town before mentioned in which there were four physicians and no journals. I was in the town from 7 A.M. to 1 P.M. During that time, to my knowledge, there was one professional call, consuming perhaps one hour. The remaining portion of the time the men sat in their office and—waited. Generally these criticisms come from the towns of 2,000 and under class. I would not have it assumed that they represent the majority of country practitioners. On the contrary, some of the strongest and best equipped men I have met have been country practitioners, and if the original work done by some of these men, under great natural disadvantages, could find its way into some of the metropolitan magazines, it would enrich the literature of the country to an incalculable degree; but they will not write even though they read, and many of them have to contend with many side issues with which they are compelled to add to their income.

DELUSIVE STIMULATION.

Dr. T. Lauder Brunton, one of the most eminent authorities on the subject of nutrition, says: It is the child who pokes the fire from the top to break the coal and make it burn faster; the wise man pokes it from below so as to rake out the ashes and allow free access of oxygen. And so it is with the functions of life, only that, these being less understood, many a man acts in regard to them as a child does to the fire.

The man thinks that his brain is not acting because he has not supplied it with sufficient food. He takes meat three times a day, and beef tea, to supply its wants, as he thinks, and he puts in a poker to stir up, in the shape of a glass of sherry or a nip from the brandy bottle. And yet all the time what his brain is suffering from is not lack of fuel, but accumulation of ashes, and the more he continues to cram himself with food and to supply himself with stimulants, although they may help him for the moment, the worse does he ultimately become, just as the child's breaking the coal may cause a temporary blaze, but allows the fire all the more quickly to be smothered in ashes. It would seem that vital processes are much more readily arrested by the accumulation of waste products within the organs of the body than by the want of nutriment to the organs themselves.

DISINFECTION OF SICK-ROOM LINEN.

Sheets, pillow-slips, night-dresses, towels, etc., should be placed in a tub and over them poured a pint (one-half a bottle) of Platt's Chlorides and afterwards sufficient boiling water to completely cover the contents. The tub should then be closely covered for two hours, when the clothes may be removed, rinsed and washed in the usual way.

DISINFECTION OF DISCHARGES.

All excreta from the patient should be received in a porcelain vessel containing a mixture of one part Platt's Chlorides and four parts of water.

DISINFECTION OF UTENSILS.

Dishes, spoons and other utensils used by the sick person, should be placed in a metallic vessel holding not less than one gallon of water. The vessel should be placed outside of the door of the sick room, and twice in each twenty-four hours it should be removed to the kitchen range and its contents should be boiled for at least thirty minutes.

HOT AIR THERAPY.

THE fact that there are scores and scores of appliances for the therapeutic use of hot air is proof that this agent has come to be generally recognized as of great value.

It may be said that there is a large and constantly growing class of painful and heretofore reputedly incurable complaints. We refer to rheumatic joints and the numberless manifestations of rheumatic gout.

The cures of these that are being effected by means of the recently perfected apparatus now available are next to miraculous. One who has given the subject no study will be incredulous until demonstration convinces him. In this city the affable physician in charge of the Sprague Hospital, at 29 to 31 West 42d street, will at all reasonable hours give ample demonstration of the processes and apparatus employed. The most inveterate cases promptly succumb to a temperature of from 275° F. to 400° F. It is one of the modern miracles.

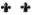

THE PROCESS OF HEALING IN FRACTURES.

BALDO ROSSI instituted a series of experiments on rabbits, in order to ascertain the effect of massage and early movement on the healing of fractures. One set of animals was treated by daily massage and movements, a second with immobilizing apparatus, and a third left to Nature. In the first set, the callus was found resistant on the third day (fifth day in the second set), and on the eighth day could be freed from all apparatus between the massage treatments, a result obtained on the twelfth to fourteenth day in the second set. Return of function came on the eighteenth day as against the thirtieth in the second set. As to the third set, the phenomena of recovery appeared a little later than in the animals treated by massage, and a little sooner than in those treated by immobilization. The results of microscopic researches bore out the clinical results.—*A'rchivio de Ortopedia,*

PREPARATION OF AN EASILY DIGESTED MILK FOR INFANT FEEDING.

S. STZEKELY (*Centralhalle*), has patented a process for the preparation of an easily digested milk food for the nutrition of infants, from the specifications of which we extract as follows: The milk, which must be fresh and "cow-warm" (*kuhwarme*), is brought in to a vessel capable of being hermetically closed against the atmosphere. Into this carbonic acid gas is introduced under a pressure of 20 atmospheres. If only cold milk can be got it should be artificially warmed to 100° F., by placing the vessel in warm water for a few minutes. When the pressure in the vessel reaches 20 atmospheres, the container is agitated for about three minutes, the gas allowed to escape, the milk removed and filtered off from the casein, which the treatment has precipitated to the extent of nearly one-half of the total contents.

The milk thus obtained, being robbed of so great a quantity of casein, becomes much nearer, in this respect, to human milk than any other substitute yet devised, containing not merely the proper quantity of casein, but the proper quality thereof. If it be desired to remove more casein, all that is necessary is to heat the milk to a higher temperature before treating with carbonic acid.

THE NUDITY CURE.

THERE is a village in Austria, near the Adriatic, where the nudity cure is practised. The debilitated, neurasthenics, the tired, etc., can go there and, in the costume of Adam, expose their individuals to the air, the sun's rays, or the rain. Thickets are carefully arranged so as to cut off all view of the patients; a hat and short trunks only are allowed; the sexes are separated. Baths, massage, gymnastics, and games are indulged in, and a strict vegetarian diet completes the treatment.—*Gaz. Hopitaux.*

"THE BLOOD OF THE NATION."

IN a paper under this title, in *Popular Science Monthly*, President Jordan, of Leland Stanford, Junior, University has the following: All great cities are destroyers of life. Scarcely one would hold its own in population or power were it not for the young men of the farms. In such destruction Paris has ever taken the lead. The concentration of the energies of France in the one great city of Paris is a potent agency in the impoverishment of the blood of the rural districts. To be a leader in a great city is an almost universal ideal. This ideal but few attain, and the lives of the rest are largely wasted. In Paris every night some few of these cast themselves into the Seine. Every morning they are brought to the Morgue behind the old church of Notre Dame. It is a long procession and a sad one from the provincial village to the strife and pitfalls of a great city, from hope and joy to absinthe and the Morgue. With all its pitiful aspects, the one which concerns us most is the steady drain on the life-blood of the nation, the steady lowering of the average of the parent stock of the future. In America the tendency to flock to great cities is becoming very great. And while the deterioration and waste in good stock are not so great with us as in some other parts of the world, effort should be made to divert a large proportion of this current of valuable human life and energy into healthier channels.

ANTIQUITY OF SOAP.

THE *Popular Science News* says that soap has been used for 3,000 years, and is twice mentioned in the Bible. A few years ago a soap-boiler's shop was discovered in Pompeii, having been buried beneath the terrible rain of ashes that fell upon that city 79 A. D. The soap found in the shop had not lost its efficacy although it had been buried 1800 years.

THEIR DESCENT TRACED FROM ADAM.

POPULAR interest in Albert Judson Fisher's unique love-story, "Daughter of Adam," in the *Ladies' Home Journal* for August, has been increased tenfold since it became known that the genealogical part of the story is not fiction, but fact. Not only is the marvelous line of descent, traced through 121 generations from Adam and Eve, absolutely genuine, but also the family names of the characters are the names of real people, for the line is actually that of Mr. and Mrs. John Smith Sargent, of Chicago, and Mrs. Sargent was formerly Miss Frances Moore, of Warren, Rhode Island. Even stranger still is the fact that, as shown in the story, Mr. and Mrs. Sargent had the same ancestor eight generations back.

THE TRUE AGE OF MAN.

A PROVERB there is with the popular seal
    (You hear it in various places),
That a man is as old as he happens to feel,
    A woman as old as her face is.
But Science, advancing with seven-league
    boots,
    Arousing the vulgar from coma,
The truth of the proverb most boldly disputes
    If one's arteries show atheroma.

    For we need to be told
    (So pathologists hold)
    That a man is as old
    As his arteries.

Robert Burns of the West, who first followed the plough,
    And later the trade of a poet,
In a popular song has been known to avow
    (Now most of the multitude know it)
That although in the case of a blue-blooded
    duke,
    The coat may be spicker and spanner,
For all that the coin in his pocket's a fluke
    And a man's still a man, in a manner.

But Rob ne'er was told
What pathologists hold,
That a man is as old
As his arteries.

So Shakespeare (or Bacon?) is totally
wrong
In talking of Man's Seven Ages.
And Burns is at sea in his topical song
On the fellow who sweats for his wages,
For when a poor beggar is nearing his end,
And with Death and the Devil he wrestles,
His looks or his feelings no succor can lend,
But only the state of his vessels.

So now you are told
What pathologists hold,
That a man is as old
As his arteries.

—Easton Weston, in *Edinburgh Dispatch*.

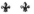

A PUBLIC PERIL.

Says the *New England Medical Monthly*: Most of those who have talked and written so convincingly against the Christian Science delusion have failed to emphasize the dangers to which the public is subjected through infection and the relations of the cult to state and local boards of health.

While for some reason not understood, the practice of this so-called cure is permitted in many of the states and it is therefore impossible to convict the guilty practitioner, no matter how flagrant the neglect, it is nevertheless within the power of the health authorities to make their lives a burden and we trust they will not fail to exercise their authority.

Within the past three weeks at least three instances have been reported in which individuals of this class, while suffering from diphtheria and smallpox, have disregarded all sanitary precautions and subjected many individuals to the dangers of infection. It is safe to assume that no case of infectious disease occurring among these people will ever be reported voluntarily to the various local boards. This being the case, the extent of the dangers which menace communities inoculated with these peculiar ideas is not difficult to appreciate.

Health boards fortunately have full police power in such cases and may not only institute an inspection of all dwellings containing suspicious cases, but may establish a most rigid quarantine and impose penalties for any breach of sanitary laws.

With the proper coöperation of its citizens, almost any community might easily rid itself of dangerous and otherwise undesirable people. Were the fatalities and misfortunes of the treatment sustained by its devotees only, no objection could be properly raised, but unfortunately there are thousands of children who, under present conditions, must suffer for the sins of their parents and guardians. While the profession is naturally unable to reach these cases, the health authorities may do good rescue work by simply exercising the prerogatives of their office.

A NEW CODE FOR DAILIES.

How the Philadelphia Times *Was Transformed in Two Hours Into a Sane Newspaper.*

From the Fourth Estate.

Newspaper men will be interested in the work that was done by the new proprietor who is the principal owner of the *New York Times,* when, within a period of two hours, on May 7, he transformed the *Philadelphia Times* from a discredited freak to a sane newspaper.

The actual transfer occurred at 4 o'clock in the afternoon. At 5 o'clock two tin signs announcing the new proprietorship were nailed on the fronts of the properties at Eighth and Chestnut streets, and 808 Sansom street.

At 7:30 the proprietor met the newspaper staff and made formal announcement of the changed ownership.

Then arose the problems as to the next day's issue. In reply to the inquiries of his editors and managers, the new proprietor gave directions, which may be codified as follows:

No red ink.
No pictures.
No double column heads.
No freak typography.
No free advertisements.
No free circulation.
No free notices to advertisers.
No reading matter advertisements without marks.
No medical advertisements.
No advertisements on first page.
No free passes from railroads.
No free theater tickets.
No collectors of advertising bills.
No Bryanism.
No coupon schemes.
No guessing contests.
No prize fighting details.
No advertisements that a self-respecting man would not read to his family.
. No concessions from the advertising rate card.
No personal journalism.
No pessimism.
No friends to favor.
No enemies to punish.
No drinking by employees.
No speculation by employees.
No private scandal.
No word contests.
No prize puzzles.
No advertisements
    Of immoral books.
    Of fortune tellers.
    Of secret diseases.
    Of guaranteed cures.
    Of clairvoyants.
    Of palmists.
    Of massage.
No advertisements.
    Of offers of large salaries.
    Of large guaranteed dividends.
    Of offers of something for nothing.

Following out the instructions given in this codification, a total of two and a half pages of objectionable advertising was thrown out in the first seven days of the new management.

Immediately after the transfer had been accomplished the reporters' force was increased and a large addition was made to the cable and domestic news service, and the large savings secured on the abandonment of freaks and foolishness were promptly applied to the improvement of the daily product.

PROPHYLAXIS in malaria Manson arranges under three heads:—Destruction of mosquitos, prevention of infection of mosquitos and prevention of mosquito bites, drainage, reclamation of swamps, and avoidance of unnecessary puddles where *Anopheles* can breed are required. "Painting" the water with petroleum frees it from mosquito larvæ, but the operation has to be frequently renewed. Prevention of mosquito infection might be attained by all-round drugging with quinine as Koch suggests, but this is perfectly impracticable. In this connection H. E. Durham points out that although quinine kills the asexual parasite it does not kill the sexual forms, at any rate rapidly. Protection of malarial patients from being bitten should be scrupulously observed, and deportation to a locality free from *Anopheles* has been advocated. W. N. Berkeley considers malaria should be notified, and inspection of infected houses made compulsory in order to ensure the destruction of mosquitos and the isolation of patients. Several observers, especially in tropical Africa, point to the native child as the great source of malarial infection. Christophers and Stephens find that *Anopheles* congregates wherever a clearing with native dwellings occurs. For Europeans settlement a mile from a native village would suffice. "To stamp out native malaria is at present chimerical." Malaria in the native child may present none of the characteristic signs of an attack of fever. Daniels emphasizes with equal force the danger of Europeans and natives living close together in a malarial country. He has also made postmortem investigations into the presence of malarial pigment in children and adults, and concludes that children acquire immunity probably by a previous attack.

Investigations made by the Liverpool Malaria Expedition at Nigeria show how prevalent is the parasite in native children, and how a European factory may be practically fever free if far enough removed from a native settlement, although situated in a brackish mangrove swamp swarming with *Anopheles*. The freedom from malaria afforded by protection from mosquito bites has been shown in the Campagna experiments. Sir William MacGregor points the moral of all the new teaching on malaria, and shows how administrators, school teachers, hospital authorities, nurses, and the general public must all reckon with this disease, and by administration, teaching, and organization seek to minimize the chances of infection and exposure. Leichman recommends a new method of applying Romanowsky's strain for the detection of the malarial parasite, which is approximately that of Maurer. The advantages claimed are that in all cases of tertian fever the infected red corpuscles show ruby red dots (Schuffner's dots), very young parasites and mixed infections are readily detected, and the method is simple. Thin cover-glass films of blood are fixed in absolute alcohol and ether, washed and dried. Weak watery solutions of eosin and of alkaline methylene blue are then poured simultaneously on the film. The nuclei of the leucocytes, the blood platelets, and in cases of tertian fever Schuffner's dots, are stained bright ruby red.

A MERITED REBUKE.

"Oh, you cruel boy, to take those eggs out of the nest! Think of the poor mother bird when she comes—"

"The mother bird's dead, miss."

"How do you know that?"

"I see it in your hat."—*London Punch.*

DRUGGISTS PREVENT FUNERALS.

"The laity has no idea," said a druggist, "of how many times a druggist keeps a doctor from causing a funeral. The doctors will deny this, but it is so. Somebody has said that every doctor sometime or other kills his man. Every doctor would kill two men if it wasn't for the druggist. We scan their prescriptions carefully, and if too large a quantity of some poisonous drug is given we have to limit the amount to as much as could be taken into the system without harm. Time and again if I had filled a prescription just as the doctor wrote it out there would have been a death instead of a cure in the case of the person the doctor was treating. My vigilance would save the patient, but the doctor would get the credit.

"One doctor whose prescriptions I filled was especially careless. More than that, he did not know any too much about medicine. I had corrected his prescriptions so many times that he got the idea that he could be as careless and as slovenly as he pleased in writing a prescription, as I would be sure to catch the mistake and correct the prescription. I got weary of this, and besides I was afraid that one of my new clerks who was disposed to take every piece of paper with a doctor's name to it as the law and gospel might some day fill one of these prescriptions and put in the full quantity of everything called for and then there would be a death that would involve me in trouble.

"One night a prescription came in that called for enough arsenic to kill a horse. I cut the amount down to the proper proportion. In an hour I called around at the doctor's office, and told him that his patient had come in, and, after having the prescription filled, had taken it and died in horrible agony a short time afterwards.

"'Well, well,' the doctor said, growing white, 'the prescription was all right. You put in too much arsenic.'

"I produced the prescription, showed him the amount of arsenic he had prescribed, and then demonstrated that it was about three times too much. 'Well, well,' he said, 'you should have known better.' 'But,' I said, 'you should have known better.'

"He was terribly frightened this time, and paced up and down the floor, and said: 'Why didn't you catch it?' Then he settled down in a chair, and when I thought he was going to faint he picked up the stub of his cigar, began to smoke, and said: 'Well, that fellow had to die some time or other, anyhow. Let this be a lesson to you to be more careful in filling prescriptions.'

"I had nothing more to say. The joke was on me. When the doctor heard next day that his patient had not reallly died he guyed me half to death, and was more careless than ever in writing prescriptions, and I had to institute a regular examining board, consisting of myself and two clerks, to pass on his prescriptions before we would fill them.

"But think of his wonderful nerve. 'Let this teach you to be more careful.' My, my, where would the doctors be if it wasn't for druggists?"—*N. E. Druggist.*

TO READ CHARACTER FROM THE FACE.

To read a person's character from his face is an accomplishment which few possess, but which many would like to have. The study is an absorbingly interesting one, and has not only an entertaining, but a practical side as well. An article on the subject will shortly be published in the *Ladies' Home Journal* giving careful details regarding the traits of character indicated by the different features of the face.

THE English way of making lemonade is as follows: To one quart of water, the juice of three lemons, using the rind of one, and two ounces of powdered sugar. Make the lemonade in a glass or earthen vessel of some kind, pouring the water over, when it is at the boiling point. Cover the vessel and set aside to cool before putting it in the icebox.

THE REPORT OF THE BRITISH MEDICAL ASSOCIATION'S COMMITTEE ON ANESTHETICS.

THE work of this committee has been carried on since 1891, the sub-committee consisting of Drs. Hutchinson, Childs, Buxton, Easter, Hewitt, and Rowell. Analyzing the cases studied, which were obtained partly from hospital, partly from private practice, they were subdivided into uncomplicated cases, complicated cases (the complications referable wholly or in part to the anesthetic), cases with minor complications, cases of anxiety, cases of danger, and cases of death, the symptoms mentioned in all these cases being due wholly or in part to the anesthetic.

There were forty-five various anesthetics or mixtures of anesthetics employed in all the 25,896 cases analyzed, in which chloroform was used 13,393 times, and ether 4,595, showing the great extent to which chloroform is used in Great Britain.

There were eighteen deaths under chloroform anesthesia, of which number three were considered to have been brought about entirely by the anesthetic, four to the anesthetic primarily, the patient's condition secondarily, and eleven where it was impossible to determine the relative *rôles* played by the anesthetic, the patient's condition, and the operation in the production of death.

Three deaths occurred under ether anesthesia, but of these not one seemed to be due entirely to the anesthetic.

Grouping all the fatal and dangerous cases together, this gives a danger-rate of .582 per cent. with chloroform anesthesia, and .065 per cent. with ether.

A LONDON physician declares that a person in robust health walks with his toes pointed to the front, while one with his health on the wane gradually turns his toes to the side and a bend is perceptible in the knees.

SOMETHING ABOUT BOILS.

Says the *American Druggist and Pharmaceutical Record:*

"Contrary to the common belief, boils are not indicative of blood disease. They are really indications of local poisoning by pus-bearing germs, and the boil is an abscess. Every pus prick, every scratch, every abrasion, every cut with a razor or pocketknife, every splinter that enters the skin may cause a boil. Nor need the wound be a serious one; it may be so minute as to be invisible to the unaided eye. Nor is the result always produced, for if it should be, every slight wound, every thorn prick, every scratch of a cat, every bite of a dog, every abrasion of the skin, would be followed by disastrous, if not fatal, consequences. The reason for this immunity is that there is a certain inherent power of the body to resist these noxious agents, and it is only when the powers of the body are weakened by disease that the morbific agents can thrive in the body and accomplish their evil work.

"In this sense, then, boils are diseases due to diseases of the blood, but it is not a disease in itself. High living also favors boils. Dr. Reid, speaking of pus, and incidentally of boils, says: 'Job was probably run down by a long period of debauchery. We read that the devil had him in tow some time before his boils broke out. If, now, he could have had the counsel of three good physicians, instead of as many tiresome theologains, he would have had his system toned up; his broken potsherd, with which "he scraped himself withal," thus spreading sympathy and infection, would have been taken from him, and he would have been taught a few lessons in sanitary science instead of theology.'

"The reason why a boil is always in the worst place is because that is the most exposed place. The back of the neck, where the collar rubs the microbes into the skin; the wrist, where the cuffs irritate and make the entrance of germs more easy; the top of the foot, where the shoe pinches; the razor-swept chin—are all favorite 'worst places.'"

TEN HYGIENIC TRUTHS.

THE late Dr. Frank H. Hamilton, of Bellevue Hospital, is said to have framed the following curious decalogue of health precepts:

"1. The best thing for the inside of a man is the outside of a horse.

"2. Blessed is he who invented sleep—but thrice blessed the man who will invent a cure for thinking.

"3. Light gives a bronzed or tan color to the skin; but where it uproots the lily it plants the rose.

"4. The lives of most men are in their own hands, and, as a rule, the just verdict after death would be—*felo de se.*

"5. Health must be earned—it can seldom be bought.

"6. A change of air is less valuable than a change of scene. The air is changed every time the wind is changed.

"7. Mould and decaying vegetables in a cellar weave shrouds for the upper chambers.

"8. Dirt, debauchery, disease, and death are successive links in the same chain.

"9. Calisthenics may be very genteel, and romping very ungenteel, but one is the shadow, the other the substance, of healthful exercise.

"10. Girls need health as much—nay, more than boys. They can only obtain it as boys do, by running, tumbling—by all sorts of innocent vagrancy. At least once a day girls should have their halters taken off, the bars let down, and be turned loose like young colts."

APHORISMS.

Every man stamps his value on himself. —*Schiller.*

Gratitude is the music of the heart.— *Robert Southey.*

Cheerfulness is the best promoter of health.—*Addison.*

We get out of Nature what we carry to her.—*Katherine Hager.*

WHAT A CARAT WEIGHS.

At a recent meeting of the Philadelphia College of Pharmacy an interesting note was furnished by W. E. Ridenour on the value of the carat as expressed in the metric system. He said that some time ago he was called upon to weigh a diamond and to state the weight in jeweler's terms, carats and fractions. It was necessary to find the equivalent in the metric system, as his weights were of the latter, and in looking the matter up found the following clipping from the *Mining and Scientific Press*, Oct. 27, 1900: "The weight by which diamonds and precious stones are calculated is 4 grains = 1 carat; 157¼ carats = 1 ounce, Troy. A fine diamond, perfectly white and pure, weighing 1 carat is worth $100; 2 carats, $400; 4 carats, $1,100; 5 carats, $1,750.

The diamond weighed .327 gramme, and, according to the above data, he reported its weight to be 1¼ carats. His report was made in the presence of the diamond salesman, who became indignant, as he had claimed the weight to be 1 carat ¼ — 1-16 and 1-32. The diamond was subsequently taken to several jewelers and the weight of 1 carat ¼ — 1-16 and 1-32 was verified in each case. Mr. Ridenour then weighed several 1 carat weights and found them all to weigh .205 gramme, being .055 gramme lighter than stated in the *Mining and Scientific Press*. This was subsequently confirmed by Henry Troemner, Philadelphia; so therefore 1 carat = .205 gramme = 3 2-13 grains.

THE SECRET.

Ella—Bella told me that you told her that secret I told you not to tell her.

Stella—She's a mean thing—I told her not to tell you I told her.

Ella—Well! I told her I wouldn't tell you she told me—so don't tell her I did.—*Brooklyn Life.*

WHY BATHING SOON AFTER A MEAL IS DANGEROUS.

M. Wertheimer, speaking before the Paris Academy of Science, developed some facts which will be well to bear in mind during any future bathing season. He showed that a sensation of cold on the skin acts on the circulation of the lower part of the trunk—that is to say, the veins, and also on the brain, in the same way as a mechanical or electrical stimulus of the sensitive nerves of the skin. This observation affords an explanation of the fact that a sudden immersion of the body in cold water after a meal, and while the process of digestion is going on, may be attended with danger. At this time the abdominal system is the seat of an intense physiological congestion, and the accumulation of blood in it is suddenly thrown back towards the nervous centers. The consequence may be a disorder resulting in death.

"Yes, I've been mistaken for all sorts and conditions during my wanderings," said Ernest Seton-Thompson. Hiding himself eyes deep in a garbage heap back of the Yellowstone Park Hotel, to watch the antics of some bears over their food, he had naturally put on the oldest clothes he could muster for the occasion. Digging away in that unsavory pile, he did not exactly convey the impression of opulence. "It really didn't occur to me, however, just how my actions might be interpreted," he said, "until some tourists hallooed to me from the edge of the wood:

"Say, my man," one of them called, "come out of that. Here's a plunk for you, and the cook'll give you something to eat up at the hotel."

Stendol says: "If the smoking habit continues for a century or two longer the intelligence of the world will end in its fumes, and the monkey will meet man as his equal."

THE HAIR IN TYPHOID FEVER.

H. M. LITTLE (*Montreal Med. Jour.,* May, 1901) has examined sixty-two cases some months after their typhoid, and noted the results as follows: Thirty-five had their hair cut in the hospital, and in only seven did the hair subsequently fall out. Of these seven, four were cut late. The ultimate result in all was a thicker growth of hair than ever before, and in two cases it was thought to be coarser. Twenty-seven did not have the hair cut, and in only three was there no falling out. Ten had to have the hair cut later to prevent baldness. In seven other cases not cut, four are very thin, two still falling, and one, before curly, is now thin and straight.

HARE (*American Journal of the Medical Sciences,* August, 1901) states that very few people even with grave cardiac and vascular disease die as the direct effect of an anesthetic. If statistics were looked into it would be found that a larger number of people die at stool or on going upstairs when suffering from disease of the heart than from anesthesia. He thinks that the majority of anesthesia accidents are the results of the shock of the operation and not of the anesthetic.

Dr. Ben. H. Brodnax asserts that a solution of Epsom salts, "1 to 16," applied to a scar, will remove the cicatricial tissue in a short time.

He also says that sponging the body twice a day with the same remedy, and a teaspoonful internally three times a day will reduce obesity rapidly.

In children a symmetrical pain about the shoulders should lead to a careful examination of the neck, for it is a frequent sign of beginning caries of the cervical vertebræ.

THOUGHTS ARE THINGS.

I HOLD it true that thoughts are things,
Endowed with being, breath and wings,
And that we send them forth to fill
The world with good results—or ill.

That which we call our secret thought
Speeds to the earth's remotest spot,
And leaves its blessings, or its woes,
Like tracks behind it as it goes.

It is God's law. Remember it
In your still chamber as you sit
With thoughts you would not dare have known,
And yet make comrades when alone.

These thoughts have life, and they will fly
And leave their impress by and by,
Like some marsh breeze whose poisoned breath
Breathes into homes its fevered death.

And after you have quite forgot,
Or all outgrown some vanished thought,
Back to your mind to make its home—
A dove or raven it will come.

Then let your secret thoughts be fair;
They have a vital part and share
In shaping worlds, and moulding fate—
God's system is so intricate.
—*Ella Wheeler Wilcox.*

If thou would'st be obeyed as a father, be obedient as a son.—*William Penn.*

Candor looks with equal fairness at both sides of a subject.—*Noah Webster.*

The non-observant man goes through the forest and sees no firewood.—*Johnson.*

Fools learn nothing from wise men, but wise men learn much from fools.—*Lavater.*

A lazy man is of no more use than a dead man, and he takes up more room.—*O. S. Marden.*

One of the best effects of thorough intellectual training is a knowledge of our own capacities.—*Bain.*

Brevity Club.

OVERTALK TO PATIENTS.

I HAVE waited a long time for some one more competent to say a sharp word or two on this subject, in the corner devoted to the pert and pithy comments, criticisms and suggestions of the Brevity Club. As no one has come to the rescue, I have pulled off my own coat and rolled up my sleeves. Let cowans and eavesdroppers beware the dog!

A great many otherwise very wise physicians tell their patients altogether too much. In the first place, they try to fully explain and describe their cases. This detracts from the mystery and seriousness of the sickness. Better say too little than too much. Patients are sure to want a definite name for every diseased manifestation and for every symptom of the same. Talk in riddles. Use learned words. A common cold is coryza, or specific influenza, or capillary congestion, or stenosis of the anterior nares. An obscure fever of which you are not quite sure of the type is an unidentified pyrexia, and so on throughout the list. Look as though you knew a great deal more than you do, and talk a great deal less than you think. Look a little mysterious when you are questioned about the symptoms. Every patient prefers to think that his is a remarkable and not at all a common case. And when it comes to the remedies make it an ironclad rule never to divulge the real name of any remedy. To the eager inquiry, "What are you giving me, doctor?" answer, "I am giving you one of the most recent and approved vasomotor sedatives," or "You are taking a cerebro-spinal tonic," or, an "intestinal antiseptic," or a "gastric corrective." It is a great mistake to mention any remedy by its common name. Your tonics will do ten times as much good if they are called "reconstructives," and your quinine will be more effective if called by a generic name, an antiperiodic, an antipyretic or, a plasmodial antagonist. Be-

sides, if you flatly show your hand by saying, "I am giving you hundredth grain doses of the arsenite of strychnia," or "fiftieth grain granules of atropia or nitroglycerine," your over-knowing patients will surely try to dose themselves next time they have similar symptoms. Look wise, talk little, and never tell a patient what he is taking.

WORK is for the worker! Did I say that once before? Very well, I think I'll print it twelve times a year. Work is for the worker. We become robust only through exercise, and every faculty of the mind and every attribute of the soul grows strong only as it is exercised. So you would better exercise only your highest and best, else you may give strength to habits or inclinations that may master you—to your great disadvantage. Work is for the worker and work is a blessing. There is a certain amount of work to do in the world, and the reason some folks have to work from daylight until dark is because many other folks never work at all. It was a Philistine who had to discover that, and voice it.

A certain amount of work is necessary to growth. Work is a blessing, not a curse, because through it we acquire strength—strength of mind and strength of body. To carry a responsibility gives a sense of power. Men who have borne responsibility know how to carry it, and with heads erect, and the burden well adjusted on their shoulders, they move steadily forward. Those who do not know better, drag their burdens behind them with a rope.

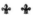

It has cost many a man life or fortune for not knowing what he thought he was sure of.—*J. S. White.*

The world is full of thoughts, and you will find them strewn everywhere in your path.—*Elihu Burritt.*

Notes and Queries.

Query 97. Broiled steak is universally admitted to be more digestible than fried steak; but will you please state some reasons why, and whether broiling is essentially preferable to roasting?

Again, I have never been free from an impression that roasted meats are dietetically preferable to boiled meats. Is this a mere prejudice?
C. L. H., Va.

Answer.—This question is taken up in one of the leading papers in this number of the GAZETTE. See that paper.

There are so many methods of broiling and so much difference in the processes of boiling that no set comparisons are possible. Broiling appliances have been and are still being greatly improved, and results depend largely on the particular methods employed. Various forms of heat are being utilized, varying from live coals to electricity. Done to perfection, broiling is the ideal method of cooking steaks, chops, etc., but, of course, it can not be applied to the cooking of large cuts and more or less bony parts used as roasts, etc. Roasting may be well or poorly done, and this will radically interfere with the results. When the juices of the meat are carefully retained and the oven heat is maintained evenly at the proper degree this process is also well-nigh ideal. If the surface be dried out or scorched, and the heart of it left raw and red it is anything but ideal.

Query 98. Is flesh the principal source of proteid food?
A. M. B., Cal.

Answer.—By no means. Eggs, milk, all the cereals, the legumes, beans, peas and lentils, nuts, fruits and most vegetable foods are sources of proteid elements. Some of them are much richer in this substance than flesh. It has been generally assumed that proteids derived from meats are more easily and quickly digested and assimilated than those derived from the vegetable world. This, no doubt, largely depends on their condition and mode of preparation.

Query 99. Is boiled milk constipating as is generally believed?
T. M., Mich.

Answer.—Not specially so. This universal belief is one of the current popular fallacies that seems to die hard. Boiling milk sterilizes it effectually and in addition it drives out its contained air and other gases. For this reason if for no other it is made less digestible. Its sterilization makes it a poor culture medium for any bacterial colonies that may be present in the alimentary canal, and thus it becomes a negative means of checking any form of bacterial diarrhœa that may be present. As certain species of bacteria are now being accredited with aiding the normal processes of digestion and maintaining the regular action of the bowels, boiled milk may to a certain extent interfere with this result. Hence the reputation it has acquired as a constipating agent.

Query 100. Are Belgian hares, now so extensively being raised in this country, a source of wholesome and nutritious food?
C. J. W., Cala.

Answer.—We have seen no analysis of the flesh of these animals, but it is very toothsome and dainty when properly and sufficiently cooked, and we have no doubt it is as nutritious as the average flesh-foods in use.

Note.

A number of questions lie over on account of the absence of the editor of this Department, who has been "doing vacation." Others have been received that are not quite in accord with our rules as to character.

We hope our readers will make more and more free use of this Department, and that those who do not wholly agree with replies made and ideas advanced will criticize them without hesitancy. And we repeat our request that all questions shall be of general interest.

WOERISHOFFER, one of the Wall street giants, who rose by his own efforts from poverty and became a millionaire, was downed by the tiny cigarette. He smoked constantly and boasted that he could quit when he liked, but the time came when he got so weak that he could not stand and he had to lie down to smoke. He then became alarmed when it was too late, for his millions could not save him, and he died a horrible death.

ONE day, in a town where he was to lecture, Henry Ward Beecher went into a barber shop to be shaved. The barber, not knowing him, asked him whether he was going to hear Beecher lecture.

"I guess so," was the reply.

"Well," continued the barber, "if you haven't got a ticket you can't get one. They're all sold, and you'll have to stand."

"That's just my luck," said Mr. Beecher. "I always did have to stand when I've heard that man talk."—*Ladies' Home Journal.*

ONE night when traveling through Virginia John Randolph stopped at an inn near the forks of two roads. The innkeeper was a fine old gentleman, and, knowing who his distinguished guest was, he endeavored during the evening to draw him into a conversation, but failed. But in the morning, when Mr. Randolph was ready to start, he called for his bill and paid it. The landlord, still anxious to have some conversation, tackled him again:

"Which way are you traveling, Mr. Randolph?"

"Sir!" said Mr. Randolph, with a look of displeasure.

"I asked," said the landlord, "which way you are traveling?"

"Have I paid you my bill?"

"Yes."

"Do I owe you anything more?"

"No."

"Well, I am going just where I please. Do you understand?"

"Yes."

The landlord had by this time got somewhat excited and Mr. Randolph drove off. But, to the landlord's surprise, in a few minutes he sent one of the servants to inquire which of the forks of the road he should take. Mr. Randolph still being within hearing distance, the landlord yelled at the top of his voice:

"Mr. Randolph, you don't owe me one cent; take whichever road you please."

BROKEN HEARTS.

WE often hear of broken hearts, and usually with a smile of incredulity, as though such a thing were not possible. Medical science has discovered that a literally broken heart is by no means as uncommon as one might fancy. A physician was recently called to a patient, a lady of middle age, who had experienced a severe shock. He found her dead, and as there was some discussion as to the cause of death, an autopsy was held, revealing the fact that the heart had burst at one side. Heart failure as a cause of death is about as satisfactory as to say "one dies for lack of breath," heart failure being merely a result of clearly defined conditions. Broken hearts can easily be brought about by a diet of sweetmeats, with a free use of fermented liquors. These weaken the tissues of the heart, and pave the way for a sudden dissolution. It has been supposed that fatty degeneration of the heart was an incurable disease, but this is another popular error, as such conditions are positively curable by a suitable diet, proper exercise and proper medical treatment.

THE actual application of the Klopfen treatment is as follows: The thorax is bared and greased. A silver paper knife of ordinary size is held with the wrist loose, and allowed to fall at rhythmic intervals on the surface of the chest, going systematically over the entire expanse, front and behind, but avoiding the mammæ, sternum clavicles and spine. Each sitting lasts about twelve minutes, and is repeated every day for about a month, when it is usual to omit the slapping for a week. The patients complain of a certain amount of smarting from the treatment, but find the afterglow agreeable. According to one observer, in thirty-nine out of forty-six patients with hemoptysis, hemorrhages did not recur after this treatment, but these somewhat favorable figures do not seem to be corroborated by other investigators.—*Medical Press.*

THE
DIETETIC AND HYGIENIC GAZETTE

A MONTHLY JOURNAL of PHYSIOLOGICAL MEDICINE

| Vol. XVII. | NEW YORK, NOVEMBER, 1901. | No. 11. |

WHAT THE CENTURY HAS TAUGHT US ABOUT LIVING.

By SAMUEL S. WALLIAN, A.M., M.D.

VIII.

HYGIENE BY ITEMS—SLEEP.

Sleep, that knits up the ravelled sleeve of care;
The death of each day's life; sore labor's bath;
Balm of hurt minds; great Nature's second
  course;
Chief nourisher in life's feast.

IT is the little foxes that gnaw the vines. Only an insignificant minority of human lives are ultimately wrecked by a single serious or overwhelming calamity. The countless majority succumb to a succession of comparatively insignificant and often unsuspected physiologic sins of omission or commission. It is this multiplication of little causes that finally saps the foundations and overthrows the structure. Phthisis, typhoid, rheumatism or renal failure may figure as the alleged and assigned causes, but they are all virtual results.

In the preceding section we have considered the more material but not more essential matters of the dwelling and its surroundings, the character and arrangement of the rooms, the furniture and hangings, and the equipment and conduct of the cookroom. Let us now pay our respects to some of the less obtrusive but not less vital items of everyday living.

Fashion, social customs and acquired habits have all combined to reverse the evident order of nature by turning the rational period for sleep into hours of waking. History does not tell us when the human race began to imitate the owl, which holds all its executive sessions during the night and turns daylight into a succession of siestas. It can hardly be questioned that in a state of nature human beings are inclined to rest and slumber as the day-god disappears behind the horizon. Darkness and slumber suggest each other, and are in a sense complementary. But darkness has been wellnigh extinguished by the inventive genius of the age; the brush of the dynamo has wiped the ink of midnight from the sky.

This may be labelled Art, but Art is as natural as any other evolutionary result. It is therefore a waste of words and breath to quarrel with Art.

Sleep is a normal condition of the body, involving partial or complete unconsciousness and occurring periodically. Its prime necessity is to enable the nervous system to recoup losses of energy that are constantly occurring during waking hours. During sleep the entire system rests, throws off waste matters and renews expended energies. All these functions and processes are essential to life. Rest is as necessary as food. Even the heart, which we usually accredit with unceasing work, regularly rests in the brief interval between pulsations. If it were not for this brief but constantly repeated interval of rest the heart would succumb to the strain, and "heart failure" would be the early and inevitable fate of every infant born into the world.

Darkness and silence are both inducive and conducive of sleep, but it is held by most physiologists that night sleep is more a matter of habit and tradition than of nature. The fact that darkness and stillness both invite to sleep is unanswerable as an argument against this theory. Habit, on the other hand, can easily adapt itself to new relations, and in time becomes a second nature. Hence the questionable conclusions of the physiologists.

Another definition of sleep is that it is a state of physiologic repose. It is both demanded and determined by the condition of the body.

The fact that many of the lower animals sleep in daytime and are active only in the night furnishes an argument for those who contend that the hours of sleep are a matter of habit. It would be quite as pertinent to assume that because certain animals spend several months at a time, including both day and night, in sleep, that man should be a hibernator.

The approach of sleep is accompanied by a series of sensations that somewhat resemble that of hunger, thirst, or the necessity for breathing. These sensations are usually referred to the head and neck, as that of hunger is referred to the stomach and thirst to the throat and mouth. When the feeling becomes intense the individual declares that he is "going asleep all over." There is, on the approach of sleep, more or less complete muscular relaxation. The eyelids droop, the head inclines forward or to one side and the lower jaw is inclined to drop. The power of equilibration is gradually relinquished, vagueness of thought ensues,

speech hesitates or is entirely lost, and the strong man becomes a helpless babe.

There are two degrees of sleep, profound, and partial or superficial. In the profound degree all psychic phenomena are abolished, —no dreams and no recollection of the state or of any accompanying experiences, on waking. Superficial sleep is accompanied by only partial obliteration of psychic phenomena. There are incoherent thoughts, illusions, dreams, and more or less distinct waking memories.

Kehlschütter devised a system of measuring the degree of intensity of sleep by the volume or intensity of sound required to awaken the sleeper. He found that during the first hour of sleep the required intensity rapidly increased. It continued to increase, sometimes rapidly and sometimes slowly, during the next two or three hours, and after that slowly till the hour of waking.

During calm sleep the breathing becomes slower and chiefly thoracic; the pulse slows down, the pupils are contracted, eyeballs rolled upward, and the eyes are not affected by light as in waking hours. All the secretions are reduced in quantity, and the peristaltic action of the alimentary tract is less active. While muscular relaxation is the rule certain sphincter muscles are more firmly contracted, especially the circular fibers of the iris, the action of which is to close the eyes.

In profound sleep the brain is comparatively bloodless and in a degree contracted. This condition favors the processes of repair and nutrition, hence sleep is especially necessary for those who do brain work and work that tires the nervous system. The circulation undergoes definite modifications during sleep. The lessened amount of blood in the brain is offset by an increase in the extremities and pelvic organs. Certain extraneous influences also affect the circulation during sleep, as for instance a loud noise or even a cold current of air. This sensitiveness to outside impressions may be likened to a vital alarm clock. Noise naturally suggests danger, and the system is thus kept semi-alert and ready to wake to full consciousness and repel intruders or any threatening influence. Dreams are frequently caused by impressions on the sensory nerves, impressions that disturb but do not possess a sufficient intensity to awaken the sleeper. These impressions frequently determine the direction and character of the half-roused faculties, the result being mental distortions and unaccountable vagaries of the fancy. If the sleeper be too lightly covered for warmth or comfort he is apt to dream of cold breezes, snow or ice. If too warmly covered, he may have a sensation of burning, etc., etc. In some cases there are consecutive thoughts so that speeches are made, discussions held with an imaginary opponent, or verses are written. Coleridge wrote or rather remembered the first stanzas of the most beautiful poem he had ever conceived as it occurred to him in a dream. He never ceased to mourn the loss of the body of the poem, all but the following having been lost, and a substitute written in his waking hours :

In Xanadu did Khubla Khan a stately pleasure
    dome decree,
Where Alph the Sacred River ran,
Through caverns measureless to man,
Down to a sunless sea.

Most dreams make too little impression on the mental faculties to cause their retention by the memory.

The dreamer lives in an ideal and fleeting world, a world that is not subject to the laws that govern matter and action in the real world. He has no cognizance of time or space. He flies at will, sails through the air without effort or wings, falls immense distances with impunity, and is sometimes transformed into some one else in the twinkling of an eye. He may be beset by bandits, shot through and through or pierced with daggers and yet is uninjured. Experiences and conversations that would require weeks of time to complete are matters of but a few moments in dreamland.

Somnambulism is one form of dream life. Certain subjects are addicted to it, and it seems to depend upon peculiar conditions that are possibly inherited.

The amount of sleep required varies with the age, sex, and habit of the individual. The very young sleep much more than half their time. There is an old adage that the child should sleep half its time, an adult one-third, while the gray-haired patriarch may be allowed to spend most of his time in sleeping and eating.

Habit is the controlling factor in determining the sleeping habit of the individual. Humbolt accustomed himself to as little as four or five hours and found it quite sufficient, living to a ripe old age and accomplishing wonders in the way of intellectual work. Many other philosophers and hard brain workers have similarly limited themselves in the matter of sleep. Napoleon slept but few hours although he belonged to the class of neurotics who are presumed to require much sleep. Nurses and mothers with ailing children get used to living with but brief snatches of sleep, and women seem to bear the loss of sleep better than men.

Speaking from the standpoint of the physiologist, the child requires much sleep for the reason that sleep favors the vegetative changes that are constantly taking place during the period of active growth. The adult needs less, seven or eight hours being ample for the average person.

Unnatural wakefulness or inability to sleep at proper times is called insomnia and becomes one of the most distressing as well as intractable of human ailments. It eventually undermines the health and renders its subjects incapable of efficient mental or physical labor. It may arise from innumerable causes, either of a physical or of a purely psychic nature. Intense grief, prolonged mental worry, or excessive study are prolific causes. Physical overwork and exhaustion from excesses of every kind may induce insomnia. Any cause that induces undue circulation in the brain results in sleeplessness. Finally, the reaction following the use of sleep-producing drugs causes insomnia of the most aggravated form.

POSTURE AS AN AID TO SLEEP.

The position of the body has considerable

to do with aiding or hindering sleep. Authorities differ very much in their advice on this point. A majority favor lying on one or the other side; a few insist upon the recumbent position as the best, while still others are recommending the prone position, or lying on the face. People who have no individual idiosyncrasies and who are in normal health may safely trust their own instincts in the matter, while those possessed of some inherited or acquired physical or mental whim, or some physical ailment, may find all rules irksome and inapplicable. The one thing to be guarded against is that position which will induce irregular heart action.

All the narcotics, alcohol, opium, cannabis indica, belladonna, tea, coffee, cocoa, etc., used continuously or to excess, result in more or less hyperesthesia of the brain and nerve centers and this condition causes insomnia.

Speaking from an esthetic and ideal point of view, the necessity for sleep is the one vital handicap of the human animal. For one-third of his existence man is compelled to become a helpless and unconscious lump of breathing clay. During this diurnally enforced condition he is powerless for his own self-defense, a prey to every prowling foe and a passive victim to accidents of flood or fire, cyclone or earthquake. He is dead to all that is good and beautiful and helpful—unresisting clay in the hands of any designing potter.

But these reflections are idle, the conditions involving a mortal entail, one of the few on which the incessant and universal law of evolution has yet made but nominal impression. Practically, we of the Twentieth require as much sleep as did our ancestors of the First century. For our efforts to abrogate the law the penalty is neurasthenia, the neurotic temperament, insomnia and premature decline.

Among the vitally practical questions in connection with the function of sleep is that of the materials from which we construct our couches. The question is more vitally important than is generally recognized or admitted. Works on physiology and hygiene scarcely advert to it. Medical schools barely mention it in connection with surgical procedures.

We spend one-third of our lives in bed— invalids all their weary hours—yet we passively continue the use of whatever material habit, tradition or inheritance has handed down to us, regardless of its sanitary or unsanitary qualities. Considering its importance and the progress of the age in other directions, it is both astonishing and unaccountable that this subject should have received so little attention, especially in an age that has made such strides in the study of personal hygiene and the origin of infections. How many modern forms of the commoner infectious diseases and complicated skin affections, which are the bête noir of medical practice everywhere, have their origin and source in the saturated, unsunned and unsanitary beds in which we spend so much of our time, in which we are born and in which we die, is a pathologic conundrum that no statistician has attempted to solve.

To begin with, we build our beds on all sorts of foundations, from the bunk of the pioneer with its brush bottom and the bamboo supports of the Oriental nations to the lacquered brass, woven wire springs and carved mahogany of the modern palace. With the taste and caprice expended in this direction the sanitarian has no quarrel, save perhaps as one or the other form involves more care or demonstrates its adaptability as a harbor of vermin. The student of hygiene is concerned with the materials of which the bedding is composed, and these vary all the way from feathers, hair, wool and cotton to chaff, straw, hay, corn husks, seagrass, various fibers, prepared sponge, spruce needles and balsam boughs.

Of all these materials, feathers, once considered the best, are in every sense not merely the poorest, but the worst. They are soft and warm—too soft and too warm, and without any other redeeming quality, since in spite of all possible cleansing precautions they are non-conductors and intrinsically reek of animal emanations. It would be hard to name any household item more hygienically abominable than the feather beds of our great-grandmothers, which in some communities and families are still in use. They are saturated with the dead emanations of half a dozen generations, charnel houses of all the uncremated ghosts since the landing of the Mayflower.

Among the well-to-do in most modern communities the use of feathers is now limited chiefly to pillows. The favored few can boast of "downy pillows," but the masses rest their weary heads on fluffy and odoriferous feather pillows. Social rank is measured by the size of these headrests. Ambitious housewives add bolsters, which indicate a further degree of social standing.

To sleep in a fashionable bed in the city, or the "spare bed" of the well-to-do country housewife, one must first make a bold advance on the formidable pile at the head of the bed, remove some artistically useless make-believes called "shams," and then either toss the pillows overboard or sit on end, propped up by pillows and bolster, like an asthmatic or an invalid.

High pillows of any material should never be tolerated. The habit of using them is purely habit and has no sanction in either anatomy, physiology or hygiene. Possibly the theory on which has arisen the Kirksville cult has a remote basis in fact. If so, the universal dislocations of the cervical vertebræ are to be accounted for by the use and abuse of pillows! In that case the "Osteopaths" have appeared none too soon. We must have our necks readjusted and take up the cudgel of life afresh.

Of all the other materials, except among the very poor, hair is much the most commonly used. There was a time, years agone, when a "curled hair" mattress meant the best foundation for a bed to be had in the market. That was before the effort to capture cheap trade had brought into use the filthy and ill-smelling scrapings of tanyards. Genuine curled hair, derived from the tails of neat cattle and the tails and manes of horses, when thoroughly cleansed and made aseptic, makes good mattresses and pillows that are immeasurably superior to feathers.

Cotton pillows are much cooler and more hygienic than either feathers or hair, and ordinary cotton mattresses are being used to some extent. They are makeshifts suitable to warm climates and summer weather, but made from ordinary or unprepared cotton are neither aseptic nor as elastic as those made from other material, nor do they retain their elasticity for any considerable length of time. When thoroughly freed from its natural oil, made aseptic, waterproof, germ, vermin and dust proof, by means of heat and peculiar chemic and mechanic processes that render it *permanently elastic*, cotton becomes ideally perfect as a material for mattresses and pillows.

Straw, hay, corn husks, moss, seagrass, excelsior and several foreign species of fiber are the other materials availed of for making bedding. Most of these are comparatively if not entirely wholesome, but none of them are extensively used except straw in the country and excelsior in cities. The straw pallet of literature is the synonym for poverty and asceticism. Like excelsior, it may or may not be sanitarily innocent, but at best neither is suggestive of solace or thrift.

For health, comfort and economy, by far the best material for mattresses is properly felted cotton—*Gossypium herbaceum*. It is easily cleansed and made aseptic, and it is susceptible of felting processes that make it delightfully and permanently elastic.

Patent Elastic Felt—is made from *Gossypium herbaceum*—a special cotton with unusually long tough fiber of great strength and resiliency, each minute fiber being a long tubular compound vegetable cell, one cell within another, the outer or enswathing sheet being a continuous skin-like cell of cellulose—and is a far more complicated structure than is generally supposed.

The raw material passes a most rigid inspection, and is carefully tested for elastic strength. It is loosely picked apart, thoroughly worked, beaten and lapped, forming loose, light, flaky, sheets that undergo a most vigorous mechanical treatment, opening up the fibers to remove all trace of natural vegetable oils, and permit the permeation of various solvents that expel all impurities. It is then subjected to the most intense heat, and certain chemical action, still further strengthening and toughening the fibers, and then so perfectly manipulated that it is rendered absolutely dry, free even from the water of hydration, and so entirely non-absorbent that it will float, possessing even more buoyancy than cork.

After all this treatment, which covers more work and exacting labor than you can imagine or than is easy to express, it is recarded, the fibers are straightened. and finally formed into light, airy, interlacing, silky, fibrous sheets of wonderful elasticity.

These sheets placed one over the other until the desired thickness is obtained, and enclosed within a tick will never spread, mat, pack, nor lose shape, and will remain in perfect condition for many years. It is free from any and all the objections that may be urged against feathers, hair, fiber or any other material thus far brought into use. Considering its durability, it is the most economical material proposed, and it is rapidly coming into popular favor. Too much can not be said in its praise, and the first trial of an elastic felted mattress is a revelation as well as a luxury. It is much more cushiony and inviting to the touch than hair, and is entirely devoid of the smothery and overheating sensations of feathers. It retains its elasticity indefinitely, never "packs," banishes bad dreams and woos the sufferer from insomnia. Blessings on the man who invented the felted mattress! Generations of his grandchildren and whole communities of invalids and former victims of "humpy" beds will rise up in their nightshirts and pajamas to call him blessed! His monument should be piled higher than Pompey's pillar, and his sepulcher should be lined with down-suggesting pillows!

And this brings us again to the subject of pillows. Any pillow that raises the head out of line with the body is anatomically unnatural and physiologically injurious. The thickness should never exceed one and a half or two inches, and some authorities urge that it is far better to entirely dispense with pillows.

Little need be said about bed coverings, for the material for these is usually determined by circumstances, and it is a waste of effort to preach to circumstances. Covering the mattress and materially protecting it it is well to use a quilted spread. This may be filled with down, wool or cotton, according to whim, purse and preference, cotton being much the most desirable. It can be removed daily for airing and sunning, when sunlight is at command. Linen and cotton are the time-honored materials used for sheets, woolen blankets being substituted by some hypersensitive people in cold weather.

Wool-filled blankets with cotton warp are about as warm and decidedly more economic to use, since they do not shrink and "full-up" so much.

For outer coverings down comforters are exquisitely light and pleasant to the touch, but they are too impervious, in a hygienic sense, and are too expensive for moderate purses. Light cotton puffs answer fairly well, but puffs filled with a layer of felted wool would be preferable in all cold climates. Even the counterpane or spread should by preference be of openwork or porous material. The close-woven goods are decidedly objectionable because they are so nearly air-tight.

Lastly, the most essential point is, that all bedding should be kept scrupulously clean and should be subjected to sunlight and fresh air daily, or as often as is practicable.

Dogs and some people sleep well on a full stomach. A large majority of the race find late or heavy suppers (dinners?) a mental, moral and physical incubus. The dog argument is inapt, because the conditions are all different. The dog partakes of a much simpler diet. sleeps on a hard floor or the ground and lies on his stomach. The human eats half a dozen courses, ending with indigestible lobster salad, and then curls up in a warm bed, with his overloaded stomach compressing his lungs, oppressing his heart and distressing every vital organ in his body.

Another item connected with sleep is too generally overlooked. It is that of segregation. Every human being, from the wailing infant to the tottering patriarch, man, woman and child, should have the exclusive use of a bed. No two persons should sleep in the same bed. This is especially true of those who are widely separated as to age.

It is unhygienic and one or the other of any and every two individuals who transgress this rule, inevitably suffers injury, in time. Husbands and wives, mothers and children should sleep apart.

SLEEP AND ITS RELATION TO HEALTH AND DISEASE.

By H. E. Peckham, A.B.

The old saying that an ounce of prevention is worth a pound of cure is just as true to-day as it was at the time the expression was first made. That we may prevent many forms of physical ailment which now afflict mankind by a proper attention to the phenomena of sleep and its relation to conditions of health and disease, perhaps has not occurred to many of the profession in all of its bearings and most important aspects.

It is my purpose in this short sketch, while recognizing that it is in many respects imperfect and in no way exhaustive, to state a few of the salient points in relation to this subject which should be of paramount interest to every practitioner, if in any way it may be understood by the people at large.

The subject may be divided for convenience into three principal heads.

First. Sleep and its relation and correlation to the phenomena of auto-intoxication.

Second. Sleep and its relation to diet.

Third. Sleep, modified for health or disease, by the position of the body during times of repose.

First.—The subject of auto-intoxication will be discussed from a scientific aspect, its chemistry, its physiological action and the theories which have been proposed for the causation of sleep. It is a well-known fact, especially among biologists and bacteriologists, that every living organism both animal and vegetable products in the course of its life history substances which are highly detrimental, if not fatal, to that organism, if it is compelled to live for a certain length of time in its own excretions. This is strikingly true of the lower forms of life, especially the unicellular forms. We have only to study the life of the common yeast plant to show how true this is. This organism will produce enough alcohol to kill itself if compelled to live in it for a certain length of time. The same is true of many of the disease germs as those of pneumonia, typhoid fever and many of those occurring in the intestines. The crises of pneumonia and typhoid mark the point when the germs have produced enough of their own poisons to kill them and the patient gets well because his cells are stronger than those of the organisms. It seems to be a universal law that the products of tissue metabolism, wherever found, are highly detrimental, if not fatal, to the organism which produces them. If we have a right to reason thus concerning the lower forms of life which represent only one cell, how much more have we the right to reason thus in regard to the more complex forms of higher life?

That normal tissues furnish us with some of the most complex problems in chemistry is apparent to every physiological investigator. That this subject might be considered at the present time only in its infancy is justified by the facts which have been revealed to us within the last fifteen or twenty years, especially since the discovery of bacteriology.

Confining our attention to the human organism and its especial metabolic phenomena, we have perhaps the most complex chemistry of all living organisms because, besides man's physical life and its varied movements and actions, he is also capable of the most intense and complex mental processes which are his especial distinction. Physiological chemistry has brought to light the fact that the products of tissue metabolism are among the most complex of all chemical substances. This is true of every tissue and every organ.

Man's bodily activities may be divided into two sets, those occurring during his waking hours and those that occur during periods of repose. Every one will concede that the most active of these occurs during his waking hours. Even though not engaged in muscular work his brain is always active, consequently, a man does not have to be actively engaged in muscular exertion in order to produce tissue waste. Perhaps his mental processes furnish more complex metabolic products than do his muscular activities. The nerve molecule is the most complex of all in the body and is the most influenced by slight metabolic changes; it is the hardest to build and the most easily broken down. So that those who are engaged in intellectual pursuits are more easily exhausted in the same length of time than are those engaged in hard physical labor. This is a matter of every-day observation; consequently those in the intellectual professions cannot and should not be expected to work the same length of time without intervening periods of rest, as those who are engaged in manual pursuits. The products of nerve metabolism are among the most complex in molecular structure because the nerve molecule is the most complex to begin with—in other words, because the anabolic process is so complex the katabolic product is equally complex. These metabolic products of nerve tissue form some of the least understood of all the products of tissue waste.

The human body is so constructed that it depends upon the healthy circulation of the blood for all of its anabolic and katabolic processes. Consequently, every cell is built according to the materials which are brought to it and according to the facility by which its excretions are carried away from it. Health, then, must resolve itself into a condition whereby there is a normal and constant exchange of proper nutritive substances to the cell and a proper disposition of the waste. I will not attempt to name the products of tissue metabolism in this article, for they can be found in any good work on physiological chemistry. I will only mention this fact, that in general the products of tissue metabolism are acid, especially those of the muscles. Perhaps the most prominent products of muscle metabolism are sarcolactic acid and carbon dioxid, while the most prominent products of nervous waste are lecithin, and the members of the xanthin series, especially those which, under favorable conditions, have a tendency to form the different leucomains. Now, it is known that healthy blood is always alkalin and never acid during life. An acid blood for any length of time seems certain death. The fact that the blood is alkalin has a significant bearing upon the question under discussion. During our waking hours, as said before, the body is in constant activity, whether muscular or mental; consequently the blood, being the medium by which the products of both muscular and nervous activity are removed from the body, is being constantly filled by these products. When the excretory glands, especially the liver and kidneys, and the lungs and intestines, are in proper working order, these acid substances are being constantly removed, during our times of greatest activity, so that the products of tissue metabolism, though in themselves highly poisonous, never cause any marked disturbance in the general physical economy, because they are not allowed to remain in the blood long enough—they are being constantly removed. By this means, then, the blood is kept to a certain degree in a uniform condition during our periods of exertion, but only to a certain point, when, the excretory apparatus becoming tired and worn out because its own functions are kept constantly at work, these organs fail to remove the excess of tissue waste. As I have said before, so long as the alkalinity of the blood is kept at a constant ratio in relation to the acid products poured into it, the general welfare of the tissues is kept constant; so that we might say that if the organs of excretion never became weakened through their normal functional and physiological activity, there never would be any reason for the rest of these organs or the recuperation of their own tissues. When, however, the deleterious products disturb the normal ratio above mentioned, to such an extent that what would be a normal alkalinity of the blood is reduced to an amount less than that which is proper for a healthy maintenance of tissue life, these deleterious substances are retained in the blood because of the failure on the part of the special excretory organs to remove them. It may be clearly seen, then, that the capacity of a person for work depends wholly upon the rapidity with which his excretory organs can remove these substances and the condition or natural resistance of his own cells against the products of their metabolism. This, in my mind, explains why many persons are capable of longer hours of hard labor, either mental or physical, than are others who apparently enjoy equally good health. It is merely a question of the condition of each individual's vegetative functions, the capacity for metabolism, the capacity for katabolism, and the condition of the excretory apparatus.

As I merely hinted before, the three principal organs which control this process of maintaining the blood in its proper degree of alkalinity are the liver, kidneys, and, to a larger extent than we are aware of, the lungs. As the kidney is largely an organ which r e m o v e s substances previously formed by other organs, and probably to a large extent by the liver, I shall consider it only as of secondary importance to the liver itself; in other words, I wish to show that in all probability it is the organ in which all these chemical processes take place, or possibly where certain complex substances given to the blood by the different cells of the body are worked over and put into such forms that they can be removed from the system or rendered inert. It may be that a great many of these complex substances are taken by the liver and made into the different constituents of the bile, and therefore made to serve the economical purposes which we notice in the intestine. It has been known for a long time that many poisons taken into the system, especially mineral poisons, are found actually incorporated into the liver cells. This is notably the case with such substances as iron, silver, mercury and others. It has been inferred from this that the liver stands on guard against all substances which might prove detrimental to the body if allowed to pass into the general circulation. When we come to study the physiology of this organ, great difficulties present themselves because even a small amount of experiment so alters the whole condition of the body as to render the results practically worthless. This only the more positively proves that the work of the liver is essential to life and health.

The relation which the hepatic circulation bears to the phenomena of sleep perhaps has never been fully understood, but it seems to me that we may explain this phenomenon largely by this means. Nearly every one has had the experience of becoming drowsy, apathetic and mentally dull after partaking of a heavy meal. In persons who have a weak digestion or slow peristalsis, this is no doubt due to the fact that the portal circulation is impeded and becomes sluggish, depending as it does upon the impetus given to its current by the blood being squeezed out of the capillaries during digestion, by the peristaltic contraction of the muscular walls of the alimentary tract. A sluggish liver is preceded by sluggish peristalsis. If the liver is to do its work it must have material to work upon, and this material is brought to it by the portal vein. In early life the portal circulation goes on unhindered, because all the digestive or nutritive functions in a healthy individual are very active; but if by injudicious feeding the liver is compelled to do an excessive amount of work, these substances which it should work over and pass out of the system are given back to the hepatic circulation and thus into the blood with a part of the excretions retained. So long as the general bodily tissues are in a normal condition these substances may be retained without any very deleterious effect, but if the injudicious manner of eating is continued day after day, possibly for years, the constant bathing of the different tissues by this vicious blood causes evidences of deterioration. The liver substance itself, depending as it does upon healthy blood, must necessarily be submitted to the same deleterious changes, consequently a vicious circle is established and the liver, giving over its products to the blood only partially worked over, is made less capable of normal processes by being obliged to feed upon this material. Possibly, too, the intestinal walls suffer from these changes, therefore destroying the normal contractility of their muscular walls, very materially interfering with, if not totally destroying, their power of propelling the blood through the intestinal veins. When this has been allowed to continue for any length of time there is bound to be, sooner or later, a condition of intestinal congestion, and in this way many of the forms of catarrhal enteritis are likely to occur. If, therefore, we wish to keep the blood in as pure a condition as possible, it seems to me the liver is the most important consideration, and every means should be used to facilitate a healthy portal circulation. Portal congestion obviously favors intestinal congestion; intestinal congestion, if not actually producing active forms of enteritis, will markedly interfere with the proper elimination of the poisons taken into the system through our various kinds of food by weakening the defensive character of the intestinal mucous membrane. Food, unless rendered strictly aseptic—which for many reasons is not advisable—contains many kinds of organisms, or if not the organisms themselves, at any rate some of their products. Bouchard in his work on auto-intoxication, a book every thinking physician should consult, has clearly pointed out that many forms of obscure disease may be directly traced to intestinal disorders. In my opinion, it is due to the fact that when the portal circulation is obstructed, either by lack of peristalsis in the intestines, by obstruction of the portal vein, by disease of the liver parenchyma, or heart troubles, the resorption of these poisonous substances into the circulation is bound to occur.

From the foregoing, then, it seems to me clear, in view of the fact that we are sufficiently aware of the marked deleterious effects of self-poisoning upon every cell of the body, and also of the fact that the liver plays such an important rôle in taking care of the poisons generated by the body, that if this organ is unable to perform its normal functions, these poisons will very materially affect every normal function of the entire organism. Bouchard, in his work, states that he has, by repeated experiment, shown that the toxicity of the urine produces two sets of phenomena; that the urine excreted during the day, or which represents certain products of tissue metabolism during hours of work, produces coma, while that excreted during sleep produces convulsions. These facts may directly explain the subject at hand. If the products of tissue metabolism caused by work will produce coma, there must be some relation between the amount of these metabolic products caused by mental and physical labor and the periods of rest and repose during which they are removed from the system. Bouchard merely hints at this possibility. While he has given us the results of an exhaustive research upon the toxicity of the renal and intestinal eliminations, he has, so far as I am aware, said very little about the toxicity of the pulmonary excretion. While I can give no experimental results to corroborate any views I may have in regard to this 'terra incognita of scientific research, theoretically, I am sure, judging from the rapid effects of bad air in producing coma, that diligent research in this field would yield an abundant harvest of very useful facts. It cannot be that carbon dioxid is responsible for all the poisonous effects of bad air. There must be some organic substances in expired air, either in gaseous or liquid form, which in very minute quantities produce very marked effects in depressing the vital functions. The pulmonary exhalations from patients suffering from renal or intestinal troubles, when in the last stages, show that the lungs are trying to eliminate the poisons of the entire system in their peculiar manner. The lungs for a time can take care of these poisons, but when the person dies it is not because the lungs are not able to transform the renal poisons into the pulmonary form of excretion (which I certainly believe they can do), but because the excretory cells of the lung give up the ghost from sheer exhaustion. They are poisoned by their own abnormally toxic excretions. I feel quite safe in assuming that many of the products of tissue metabolism which are instrumental in causing sleep are in the pulmonary excretion. A sluggish lung is just as bad for normal and refreshing sleep as a sluggish liver. Of course, the kidney is a very important organ and has an indispensable function in the bodily economy, but are not the poisons of the liver, lungs and intestine the most important from the standpoint of origin? Really, is the toxicity of the urine very great, if the other organs of emunction are in a vigorous, healthy condition? It is only when these fail that the kidney assumes a compensatory function, and, overcome by an extra amount of work, must increase its toxicity.

I wish now to mention the different theories which have been proposed for the causation of sleep. The first was that proposed by an Italian anatomist and histolo-gist, Cajal. His idea was based upon what is called the histological theory. This is, briefly stated, that certain nerve connections in the brain, evidently between those which are directly instrumental in forms of consciousness and the other forms of nervous activity, become broken—in other words, the dendrites of one neuron are withdrawn from the nerve-cell of the succeeding one, thereby destroying the possibility for nerve conduction.

The second is the so-called physiological theory which has as its basis the lowering of the blood pressure in the arteries of the brain, thereby causing anemia, and so a cessation of a part of its functions. The way this is brought about is through action on the vasomotor center in the medulla, thereby changing the degree of activity of the medullary functions, caused by lowered heart-action, and so a lessening of the blood-supply to the medulla itself. The lessened vasomotor activity allows the vasoconstrictors to act in some way so as to shut off the blood-supply to the brain and then anemia induces sleep. It is known that the brain is more anemic during sleep, but it is doubtful whether it suffers any greater degree of anemia than other parts of the body which have as great a vascular supply.

The third theory, the chemical theory, is that certain substances are produced in the body itself, which, acting upon the nerve-centers, cause changes in their function by depressing their normal action.

The first of these theories is now practically rejected, while the tendency is to give more weight to the last two, some endorsing one, some the other. It is my idea that the true explanation is to be found in the combination of both, and to show how this is so I wish to discuss the physiology of the two nervous systems, cerebro-spinal and sympathetic. Briefly stated, we may say that our conscious activities are relegated only to cerebro-spinal activity—by cerebro-spinal I mean the brain in its entirety and the peripheral nervous system, motor and sensory nerves. This part of the nervous system controls intellectual and physical life in all activities except those of anabolism and katabolism; in other words, it is our voluntary, objective life. The sympathetic, on the other hand, represented by the two chains of nerve ganglia situated within the pelvic, abdominal, thoracic and cervical portions of the body, while connected with the cerebro-spinal very intimately, still possesses a considerable degree of independence of action. It contains the power that builds every cell in the body and takes charge of the waste products. It represents all those activities concerned in nutrition, self-preservation and ultimately reproduction. Unlike the cerebro-spinal, it is wholly unconcerned with our involuntary actions. During our periods of work, both physical and intellectual, the cerebro-spinal is the one which is most active and consequently is producing very rapid tissue changes, the results of which are all the complex chemical substances just referred to. The sympathetic, too, is constantly at work preparing material for the nutrition of the cerebro-spinal nervous system and the muscular body which it controls. It is a constant and ceaseless worker and stands ever ready to keep the body in perfect repair in order that the cerebro-spinal functions, whether intellectual or physical, may be at their very best. Of course, these two processes go on side by side during our periods of activity, and so long as the sympathetic can remove the waste as fast as it is produced and also regenerate every cell by furnishing it with proper nutrition, the whole system is able to perform its normal functions. If, however, the cerebro-spinal system pushes its activities indefinitely, so that these products of tissue waste affect directly the organs of excretion, or, in other words, affect the domain of the sympathetic, the sympathetic becomes affected by these products of tissue waste as well as the rest of the body, and then these chemical substances which we have just seen are highly injurious if kept in the body, are not removed by the excretory apparatus,

because they have produced changes profound enough to interfere with their excretion. I believe (if it could only be absolutely proved) there is a direct relation between the phenomena of sleep and the alkalinity of the blood. There are some persons who require fewer hours of sleep than others and who do a tremendous amount of work while they are active. I believe this is due to the degree of the alkalinity of their blood. We know that Napoleon, than whom there was no one more active all his life, slept only five or six hours out of the twenty-four. And there are others who have been very active and seemed to maintain perfect health with such an amount of rest as to astonish us. In my opinion that is explained on no other basis than that they must have had a perfect excretory apparatus, enabling their blood to maintain a high degree of alkalinity. While we are active we are constantly filling the blood with such products as to reduce the normal ratio between alkalinity and acidity which is necessary for a healthy condition of the tissues. Now, when the blood becomes filled with this waste to such an extent that the sympathetic can not remove it and keep this ratio as it should be, these substances retained in the blood affect the cerebrospinal centers, especially the higher centers of the brain. It is known that some of these excretions are markedly depressant to the nervous system, that they cause a partial suspension of function. If this be true, we can see how, after a certain length of time, it is necessary for the cerebro-spinal activities to become suspended, or to entirely cease, so that these highly injurious products may be removed from the system. That is exactly what takes place. The sympathetic furnishes us with all the strength necessary, that we may carry on our conscious activities up to a certain point when, after the failure of the sympathetic to remove the waste as fast as formed, the sympathetic says to the cerebro-spinal: "You must stop and rest that I may remove the accumulation of dirt—it is time to clean house."

The depressant nature of the products of tissue metabolism, affecting as it does the higher cerebral centers, especially those of consciousness, acts, then, as a physiological anesthetic, and, whether we will or not, this state of anesthesia compels the cerebrospinal activities to cease. We then seek some place of repose, where it is quiet, so that all external sources of stimulation, in the nature both of light and sound, may be so excluded that the sympathetic may go to work and remove the harmful products from the blood. This is really the means by which the blood is restored to its normal alkalinity. When, after a certain number of hours of sleep, these depressant substances have been removed, or, we might say, the blood becomes sufficiently alkalin, we are more easily awakened. After the house has been sufficiently cleaned and everything put to rights by the sympathetic system, the cerebro-spinal is again ready to perform the functions of another day's labor.

Sleep, then, from the standpoint of autointoxication, is really a physiological anesthesia, and the process by which the blood is put into such a condition as to restore the proper activity of all bodily functions.

There can be no doubt that Americans are a race of dyspeptics, for two reasons: First, they eat too much and at any and all times; second, they use up energy almost as fast as it is generated. This applies both to the muscular and nervous systems. The first part of this subject has been treated in such a way that it must be apparent to every one that what we eat and the manner of our eating is of no small importance. If the poisons generated by the body can be so detrimental to its tissues, the food which these cells use determines largely their structure and the nature of the metabolic substances they produce. It is, therefore, all-important what the nature of our food is, and whether it is in such a form that the different digestive fluids of the body may so

transform it that all the needs of the body are supplied without giving to it those substances already of a poisonous metabolic nature, or whether these metabolic products are reduced to a minimum. I mean, we should not feed the body with foods which contain the products of tissue waste, thereby adding so much more to the already existing metabolic products, generated by the body itself. The question of diet, then, is a very important one, if we wish to keep the blood in as healthy a condition as possible. I believe that the vegetarian is right in many of his ideas, though, like every one who discovers a new principle and finds it works well, he no doubt pushes it to an absurd extreme. That some people can eat things which are poisonous to others is already a proverb. Each individual should study his or her physical wants and ascertain which foods will furnish the most strength for the body in general, a clear brain and refreshing sleep.

It is a fine art to fill exactly the needs of the body from the time we enter the world until the sunset of life, when old age requires only those physical things which will make age a blessing. What, then, are the proper foods? In general, the whole question hinges upon the condition of anabolism, katabolism and the excretory apparatus—in other words, the condition of the *vis a tergo*, the vital forces. No two people are constructed exactly alike; consequently, the needs and supply of each person should only be such as will keep the body of that person in perfect repair.

(To be concluded.)

DIETS FOR EVERY DAY USE.

By J. Warren Achorn, M.D.,

Boston.

OBESITY.

A state of obesity may be the physiological balance for some people, but with the majority it is due to overfeeding or an ill balanced diet, and for the remainder, race, heredity, laziness or a lazy liver, occupation and exercise, a small heart and lungs, mental peculiarities and temperament, small brains, age, sex and the frying pan, in addition, have to be considered. Obesity, then, is a many-sided problem, the solution of which rests in finding out what causes the fattening and then persuading the victim to practise abnegation or some other thing until he is rid of it.

The *frying pan* landed here in 1492, and from that day until very recent times it has ruled every kitchen and stomach in the land. The people of New England are still wedded to it, and in the South, where the standard of cooking is measured by the darkey mind, it reigns supreme. Fat people love fried food and fried food is indigestible. The frying pan has made more people miserable than alcohol; both congest the liver, but of the two, the first named is the greater sinner. Fat people are usually "cribgnawers"; they are always showing one how they eat something about the size of two half fingers, but the fact is, they are eating that something at all hours or are the victims of self-deception. Physicians would have no trouble with the plethoric variety if during the siege of Ladysmith their fat friends had all been there; they would have gotten their figures back. If

only one had an island in the sea, with a mermaid for a waitress, instructed to appear but once a day in an emerald green gown, bearing a silver tray with the right kind and amount of food on it, how easy the treatment of the majority of these cases would prove to be. Of course there should be a dog and a cow on the island and a hill, as aids to exercise, sweating and oxidation, with a starting point somewhere.

It is not wise to tell an obese patient that inheritance is in any way the cause of their disorder, as they will immediately surrender to the idea, lie down mentally and physically, and there is an end of it. They will make this their excuse ever after, and go on eating what they like rather than what they should have, until they burst. Inherited tendencies are a congenital defect, present in 50 per cent. of all cases. The treatment of obesity under these circumstances should be part of a child's bringing up.

Laying on fat late in life is due to the intake more often than to fault with the outgo, although we meet with cases that are under-fed, where the ration is lacking in tissue forming material and in consequence the patient is pale and flabby. The idea that avoirdupois is something in the world to be feared and admired, irrespective of how it looks or what it is made up of, is certainly a factor in the minds of some for preferring

NOTES.

Hot water as directed cannot usually be taken in quantity at first; one becomes quickly accustomed to it, however. Where so much water is taken between meals, there should be no thirst at meal time.

The condition of the kidneys and heart should always be known before an obesity diet is instituted.

The old rule—"two mouthfuls of meat to one of anything else," should not be followed in any case, plethoric or otherwise, even where the kidneys and heart are normal, unless hot water is faithfully taken, as a highly nitrogenous diet throws a great strain upon the kidneys.

Water in excess is indicated in plethora, whether associated or not with glycosuria, gout, lithemia or rheumatism, if the heart and kidneys admit of its use. If water in excess tends to keep the patient fat on account of slow circulation in the capillaries and deposition in consequence, salines should be used to drain the system.

In albuminuria, restricting the water is advantageous, as it is associated with cardo-vascular

disturbance. Restriction of fluids is also indicated in dilatation and heart weakness, arteriosclerosis, especially in anæmic cases where there is a tendency to dropsy.

Anæmic cases should be given iron; the blood corpuscles being crippled oxidation is retarded and obesity favored.

Restricting water with meals lessens the appetite; while water in quantity at meal time tends to fatten in some cases, by interfering with digestion, especially in dilatation of the stomach. When the use of water is restricted, the kidneys must be watched to see if the waste is still being eliminated. Two pints of water should be sufficient, no liquid being taken at meal time in case a dry diet is desired; or a cup of clear tea or coffee may be used night and morning, two glasses of wine and three of water in twenty-four hours, as a measure.

Red meat should be eaten but once a day on a dry diet.

All meat, fruit and fish should be free from skin or connective tissue. A reasonable amount of easily digested fat should be allowed in obesity, to remain corpulent; here is pride of person one way but none the other. A lawyer once said his ponderous abdomen cost him three thousand a year, but was worth ten thousand in his practice, because his clients could get behind it and feel protected. A generation hence public opinion will be so against undue corpulence that it will be looked upon as an evidence of ill breeding.

Some people can live on half as much as others and be fed; all such should have character enough to limit their food to their needs. The reaccumulation of fat after it has once been reduced, or inability to reduce it at all, is as often the result of lack of character as anything else.

Phillips Brooks has said that character is the greatest thing on earth. Patients without purpose, like logs in a stream, are simply "drifters"; they are looking for prescriptions and are always in need of them, but when it comes to acquiring a good habit, to replace a bad one, they are not up to it.

One can learn to like one or two at least of the foods suited to their use, in six weeks' time, if they will let the foods denied them religiously alone. It is simply learning over again to talk and walk in others and be fed; all such should have

accomplishment, because it has to be consciously dug out of the habits of a lifetime and often comes hard.

DIET IN OBESITY.

(Copyright.)

Drink one or two glasses of hot water on rising. The water may be flavored with lemon juice, weak tea or aromatic spirits of ammonia (a teaspoonful to a glass). Hot skimmed milk may be substituted for hot water, adding six grains of salt and six of soda to each glass.

BREAKFAST: *Cereals* — Cooked gluten (30 per cent.), other glutens with salt, meat or prune juice, or with a little butter or cream; rice with skimmed milk. Shredded wheat.

Meats ('red)—Round or rump steak, mutton chops, veal steak well done, scraped meat ball, served hot; pepper, salt, Chutney sauce, lemon juice, vinegar.

Fish (fresh only)—Cod, haddock, cunners, chicken halibut, smelts, flounder, the lean of shad or bluefish; perch, pickerel, trout, or other lake or brook fish. baked or roasted.

Eggs—Soft boiled or poached twice

---

especially when associated with nervous exhaustion.

More fat can be allowed those whose hearts are sound, as they can exercise vigorously. It has a greater satisfying power than any other form of food. This is why a raw egg will quickly allay hunger. Tea and coffee both satisfy hunger. Too great a variety of food tends to increase the appetite; so does the use of soup and condiments. A mild degree of starvation has to be maintained while the weight is being reduced for those whose lives are sedentary. The blood should be watched, as it is apt to thin along with the tissues.

When the urea and phosphates are below normal increase the exercise; when above normal, the amount of water and exercise being what they should, diminish the nitrogenous food, as there is renal insufficiency.

Hill climbing reduces fat. If practised to strengthen the heart's action, the patient should ston when palpitation comes on. but not sit down, and go on when it ceases.

Seaside living and bathing are good for obese patients. Cold baths cut down weight by heat

evaporation. Vapor baths facilitate oxidation; they may cause cardiac disturbance. In cases of fatty degeneration where exercise has to be restricted, sweating baths should be resorted to, but with caution.

A hot skimmed milk diet to commence with, two ounces every two hours, will cut down fat rapidly. Like a milk and egg diet it is only suited to patients in bed, beyond the first few days. The thing to keep at bay in the reduction of obesity is the carbo-hydrates; four to six ounces of starches and fat food together is the measure for the day. ordinarily. Two tablespoonfuls of sugar, repeated regularly will increase the body weight rapidly and sometimes outweighs anything one may be able to do within the limits of safety as an offset. Sugar is the most fattening of all foods. Whether one cuts down the starches or fats most is a matter of individual experience depending upon the case. In either event one is lessening the calories needed for daily burning and the fat stored up must be surrendered. It should be borne in mind that starches do not fatten; they simply offer themselves to protect the foods taken into the system, that do. Water starvation, sometimes.

a week. The whites may be eaten at any time.

Breads—Gluten bread, gluten and bran bread, bran bread, rye bread toasted and re-dried; unsweetened rusks, zwieback, hoe cakes, crusts. Butter in moderation. Orange marmalade.

Fruits—Raw, stewed or roasted, ripe sour apples, sour oranges, sour grapes, orange juice, pineapple juice, peaches, berries, cherries, grapefruit, white grapes, gooseberries, apricots, melons and unsweetened prunes.

Drinks—Black coffee with lemon juice, clear weak black tea, skimmed milk, water; one glass of either or none.

A. M. BETWEEN MEALS: Two glasses of hot water, hot skimmed milk, buttermilk, lemonade, cider; a gluten biscuit or a few almonds.

LUNCH: *Meats* (red)—Roast mutton, lamb or beef, sweetbreads.

Meats (white)—Stewed or roasted chicken, turkey, squab, capon. Any game bird except duck or goose. Mustard.

Any *fish* mentioned; shredded codfish, scrod.

Any *vegetable* mentioned; raw tomatoes with vinegar.

Any *bread* mentioned. French bread (dry), pilot bread, Bent's water crackers.

Any *fruit* mentioned.

Any *drink* mentioned.

Any *dessert* mentioned. Salted almonds, filberts, pecans with crackers or fruit.

P. M. BETWEEN MEALS: Weak tea with a rusk. Cider.

DINNER: *Soups*—(very little) St. Julien, plain consommé, oyster or clam broth, chicken, veal or lamb broth.

Any *fish* mentioned. Oysters raw, Little Neck clams, stewed clams.

Any *meat* mentioned.

Vegetables — Asparagus, spinach, water cresses, young onions, artichokes, oysterplant, m u s h r o o m s, Brussels sprouts, radishes, young peas, beans, lettuce, celery, tomatoes and white cabbage. One small baked potato, daily. Mustard.

Any *fruit* mentioned.

Any *drink* mentioned; claret, white wine, hock, still Moselle.

Desserts—Coffee jelly, calf's-foot jelly, strained cranberry, tamarind or rhubarb sauce; cottage, buttermilk or skimmed milk cheese; Parmesan, Dutch or Suffolk cheeses.

9 P. M.: Two glasses of hot water.

---

no matter what the patient eats, will certainly reduce weight.

Two ounces of bread and six of potato are about equal in carbo-hydrates; two ounces of bread and two of pea flour or rice are an offset.

Two ounces of bread equals one and a half of oatmeal, barley, maize, flour, corn flour, arrowroot, sago or tapioca.

Two ounces of bread equals ten or fifteen ounces of the sweeter fruits, or forty ounces of apple.

A quarter pound of bread a day should be sufficient.

A little Rochelle salts added to apple sauce makes it less tart and more palatable.

Nuts (except chestnuts) are particularly devoid of starch, and are therefore permissible when the digestion is good and fat is needed.

Sometimes the free use of vegetables, such as tomatoes, melons, cucumbers, etc., will maintain weight because they carry so much water; on the other hand, on account of the cellulose in them, they lessen hunger by giving the alimentary canal something to work on. Vegetables, generally speaking, are then indicated when a big appetite

has to be satisfied, and there are no contra-indications.

Patients with a tendency to gout, rheumatism, lithemia, headaches or neuralgia should let sugar and other sweets practically alone; they should not be allowed tea, coffee, viscera or red meat in excess, because they are uric acid yielders; or tomatoes, spinach, rhubarb, sorrel, asparagus and old onions, because they contain oxalate of lime.

Seven hours sleep should be sufficient, and no sleep should be taken during the day.

If the bowels are sluggish two teaspoonfuls of Carlsbad salts in hot water in the morning is useful if the stomach is not disturbed by it, especially in plethoric cases.

Medical gymnastics to reduce the size of the abdomen (or massage) and restore the figure, such as any one can practice for a few moments after the morning bath, or when convenient, are frequently essential to the successful operation of this diet.

This diet is intended for the *reduction* of obesity; it need not be so strictly adhered to after the weight and appetite are under control.

Department of Physiologic Chemistry.

WITH SPECIAL REFERENCE TO DIETETICS AND NUTRITION IN GENERAL.

INTESTINAL DISINFECTION.

PROFESSOR W. F. LOEBISCH, Director of the Laboratory for Applied Medical Chemistry at the Imperial and Royal University of Innsbruck, in a discourse held before the Medical Society of that city, published in the *Wiener Medicinische Presse*, Nos. 27 and 28, 1901, details at length the results of his experimental researches upon the influence of Urotropin upon intestinal decomposition. In spite of the demonstration of the inhibitory influence of the drug upon the development of the bacterium coli by Nicolaier, and of its destructive effect upon typhoid bacilli in the urine by Richardson, a direct influence of the Urotropin ingested upon intestinal fermentation itself was not thought of. Loebisch himself had his attention called to it quite accidentally. He was examining the urine of a man who was well nourished and upon a mixed diet, and who was taking Urotropin to the extent of 0.5 to 1 gram (7½ to 15 grains) daily for a posterior urethritis, and found that neither by Jaffé's or Obermayer's test could he get any reaction for indican. Now the presence of this substance in the urine is one of the most accessible and reliable indications of the occurrence of bacterial intestinal decomposition, and he was thus led to investigate the action of the drug upon these ordinary enteric changes.

Mr. Ernst Mayerhofer, assistant at his institute, made a series of personal experiments for the determination of the matter, during a period of twenty days. The diet was of the usual mixed variety. Only upon the last three days of the experimentation was it made uniform in quantity and quality.

As the tables presented by Loebisch clearly show, the indican in the urine examined decreased pari passu with the amount of Urotropin that was daily administered, until finally it disappeared altogether. The conclusion was inevitable that Urotropin, administered in daily doses of 2 grams (30 grains) to a healthy individual upon a mixed diet, inhibits ordinary bacterial intestinal putrefaction.

In view of the fact that the increased excretion of indican in the urine is an important symptom in various diseases, Loebisch next inquires whether this property of Urotropin to diminish or even abolish it in moderate daily doses of 2 grams (30 grains) cannot be utilized therapeutically.

Now both indol and skatol appear in the large intestine in consequence of a peculiar process of decomposition in which various aerobic and anaerobic bacteria are also concerned. Indol is not necessarily formed in ordinary albuminoid decomposition; apparently the aerobic indol-formers hinder this process. Under normal circumstances both the indols and the phenols are formed in the large intestine. Jaffé has shown that indican is increased in the urine in all cases in which the small intestine is occluded, as in incarceration from hernia or peritoneal adhesions; and H. Senator has found it augmented in chronic wasting processes, such as cancer of the stomach, etc., and even in simple coprostasis. Clinicians therefore look upon the increase of indican in the urine as an indication of a disturbance of the normal decomposition processes of the alimentary canal.

Disinfection of the intestinal canal is desirable in many cases in which agents like calomel, which cause diarrhea, are not appropriate. The contents must so far as possible be disinfected in situ; for which purpose the phenols, cresols, tribromphenol, thymol, and many other substances have been recommended. They have not obtained a very wide acceptance, however, perhaps for the reason that most of them are poisons, and the non-toxic medicinal dose may be readily overpassed.

Urotropin is a remedy that is very soluble in water, that by the above experiments has been proven to be inhibitory to intestinal decomposition, that has been found valuable in the treatment of various bladder diseases, and that has been proven to be harmless even when taken for weeks at a time in medicinal doses. Mayerhofer did not suffer from the least physical disturbance during the twenty days that he took the drug; I even had the impression that his complexion cleared, and that his physical energy was increased.

Loebisch then made a series of experiments as to the power of Urotropin to prevent the decomposition of non-sterile fibrin. They found that it had a hindering effect even when employed in very dilute ($1:10,000$) solution.

There is abundant evidence before us as to its power of inhibiting the development of the specific intestinal bacteria. Bacteriuria due to the bacterium coli (Nicolaier, Heubner) and the bacillus lactis aerogenes (Kruse) have been cured by its use. Loebisch has himself observed a case of recurrent bacteriuria which was always quickly relieved by a few doses of Urotropin. American, German, and English observers have testified to its beneficial influence upon typhoid bacilli in the urine. In view of these facts and of the foregoing experiments, there can be no doubt that Urotropin influences the bacteria of the intestinal canal in a similar manner. It is now the turn of the clinicians to experiment therapeutically with the drug in the many cases of abnormal intestinal decomposition.

⁂

IF you have something to do, do it now!

ON THE DIETETIC MANAGEMENT OF TYPHOID FEVER.*

DAVID INGLIS, M.D., OF DETROIT, MICH.,

AWAY back in the time when typhoid fever was first differentiated from the other continued fevers, some one originated the milk diet for this disease; and the medical profession, being subject to human frailties, has gone on accepting the milk diet as the proper treatment for typhoid fever, with a singular disregard of the facts, which pass under their observation, year after year. Theoretically, it would seem that physicians, in active practice, would reason out for themselves whether the milk diet were, really, what it is claimed to be or not; but it is a remarkable fact in all human history that men have accepted, for generations, not what they know to be true, but what they have assumed to be true, and so it has been with the medical profession and the milk diet in typhoid. It has been assumed that milk is a liquid and that it is readily assimilated and leaves little or nothing to pass through the bowels; and, upon this assumption, it has been further assumed that the nutritious qualities of the milk have served to keep up the patient's strength to the greatest possible degree, and that thus the two main indications in typhoid fever have been fulfilled; first, the avoidance of irritation of the ulcerated Peyer's patches, and therefore the prevention of hemorrhage, and, second, the maintenance of the general bodily nutrition. These assumptions have been quietly accepted by countless thousands of physicians, notwithstanding the fact that, at the termination of the fever, the patient has been found to be emaciated to an extreme degree, demonstrating visibly that the bodily nutrition has not been maintained to any high degree, but quite the contrary.

Let us take the first assumption, that milk is a liquid which is readily absorbed and leaves little or no detritus to pass through

* Read before the Detroit Academy of Medicine, and republished from *The Philadelphia Medical Journal*.

the intestines. The fact is that the serous portion of the milk is absorbed through the gastric mucous membrane, but this constitutes but a small part of the bulk of the milk. The casein of the milk is rapidly turned into a solid, which is not digested in the stomach but is passed on into the intestines. When a patient has a pretty steady diarrhea he usually succeeds in passing out the casein in small flocculent curds, and, as long as he succeeds in doing so, he remains tolerably safe from one of the dangers of this deceptive fluid. If, however, he does not have a sufficiently active diarrhea the casein is liable to form masses of scyballæ, not only in the large intestine but high up in the small intestine. Wilson, writing in the *Columbus Medical Journal*, says that, in a number of postmortems on typhoid fever cases, he had always found curds of undigested milk in the stomach and portions of these curds in the small bowel, where they were forming ideal foci for fermentation and breeding grounds for various microbes. Every physician who has had an extensive experience in typhoid fever is familiar with that exceedingly unpleasant complication which occurs, by no means unfrequently, toward the end of the fever, in cases in which the early diarrhea had stopped, or which occurs, even during the progress of the fever, in cases uncomplicated by milk diarrhea, the condition in which the rectum and colon become filled with impacted feces. The physician who has once scooped out from the rectum the dense, hard masses, so hard in many instances that, before attempting to break them up and remove them, it is necessary to soften them by injections of oil or soapsuds, every physician who has had this experience knows that this dense mass consists of nothing, practically, but milk. It is an entire mistake to regard milk as a liquid in diet. It is a liquid in the tumbler, but we ought always to think of it as solid food. It becomes a solid in the stomach, it enters the small intestine a solid, and it passes through a solid. If the original assumption be true, that it is wise to feed the patient so that there shall be as little as possible of

irritating detritus passing down over the ulcerated glands, then certainly milk does not fill the requirements.

Not only is the milk diet, in typhoid fever, logically unsound because of the large amount of solid substance which it sends down through the small intestine, where it is liable to act as an irritant, but it is a dangerous diet because it forms an admirable culture-medium for various bacteria. That it is an admirable medium for the spread of the specific bacillus of typhoid fever is undoubted. Whenever an epidemic breaks out and we attempt to trace the source of the intoxication, we search, first, for a defective water supply, and, if we do not find the source of contamination there, we immediately begin to follow the routes of the milkmen. A large number of epidemics have been traced accurately following a single milkman's route. If the milk can carry the poison into the patient in the first place, the large amount of undigested residue of solid milk, in the small intestines, would seem to form an admirable breeding-place for the further development of the specific germ of typhoid, but the question is a much wider one than simply the spreading of typhoid bacilli. At a recent meeting of the Detroit Academy of Medicine Dr. Dock read a paper on the treatment of typhoid fever. In the discussion I brought up the point just alluded to, and Dr. Dock's reply was to the effect that, after the first intoxication, in typhoid fever, the bacillus of Eberth was found, not so much in the intestinal canal or on the mucous membrane, but in the deeper structures of the intestinal wall, in the intestinal and mesenteric glands, as well as in more distant glandular structures. It was argued that, therefore, the attempt to produce intestinal asepsis was useless, as the specific bacilli were out of reach. Such an argument, while it may be technically correct, loses sight of a very essential series of facts. I suppose that no one would, for a moment, assert that all of the bacilli of Eberth left the intestine and were taken up in the glandular structures, for, were this so, there would not be the slightest danger of conveying the disease to others, by means of the dejecta of a typhoid fever patient. Now the fact is that, throughout the disease, the stools of the patient contain the specific germs in such quantities that we all thoroughly understand that it is from this source —practically from this source only—that the disease is propagated to others; it therefore is demonstrable that the specific bacilli of the disease remain in the intestinal canal, and there is every reason to believe that masses of undigested milk may very easily form a breeding ground for the bacilli, and so furnish a constant intoxication of the patient; but, even were there no typhoid bacilli left in the intestinal canal, there are other bacilli which will thrive with equal rapidity in milk, and there is every reason to believe that not only in typhoid fever but in many other diseases the real danger to the patient proceeds from the secondary intoxication. Stop, for a moment, to consider the phenomena of an ordinary case of consumption. The patient is infected with the tubercle bacillus. Under ordinary circumstances, as long as the infection is purely tuberculous, the patient's progress, from bad to worse, is but slow. He has, indeed, fever, cough, emaciation, and a small amount of expectoration, often almost none; so he may continue for a considerable time, slowly getting worse. Once let some portion of the lung substance become necrosed and a secondary streptococcus infection take place, notice what a rapid change occurs. He now develops hectic fever, night sweats, profuse expectoration, diarrhea. It might almost be said that the great danger of the tuberculous patient was that of a streptococcus infection. It is the secondary infection that starts him on the rapid downward course. Take, again, the phenomena of diphtheria. The primary infection is by the Löffler bacillus. The exudate in the throat is the result of the primary infection. While it is true that our efforts ought to be directed to overcoming the primary infection with all possible speed, does any physician feel justified in neglecting attention to the exudate?

Not at all. Indeed, he recognizes that the exudate forms a focus for a constant reinfection of the patient. Not only does the exudate form a focus of reinfection by the Löffler bacillus, but by the streptococcus as well. And again there is reason to believe that no small part of the danger of the diphtheritic patient arises from the secondary infection. We ought to keep precisely the same reasoning in mind in the management of typhoid fever. It does not seem a question of the primary infection of Eberth's bacillus alone, but anything which facilitates a constant reinfection by the Eberth bacillus or a secondary infection by streptococci or the colon bacilli adds enormously to the patient's dangers.

On these grounds, then, it seems to me that we have made a radical mistake in feeding milk to typhoid fever patients. Osborne, in an article in *The Philadelphia Medical Journal*, in December, 1899, has this to say:

"In typhoid fever, constipation keeps the partially digested milk or other nutriment long in the intestines, the mucus and ulcerative sloughs remain in situ, and thus beautiful culture grounds for all sorts of bacilli and cocci are formed, while in addition, the colon bacillus adds its toxims to the rest. Next, fermentation increases and gas is formed, and tympanites occurs with its discomfort and dangers of perforation and of hemorrhage from distention; meanwhile the action of the heart will be impaired as a consequence of abdominal distention. All of this increases the fever and the cerebral toxemia. If one has a doubt of what such bowel stoppage causes, he has but to recall instances in which a case of irregular chills, heavily coated tongue, profound headache, high and continued fever, concentrated urine, constipation, and tympanites has been proved, by absence of the malarial plasmodium from the blood and the negative Widal serum reaction, to be neither malarial nor typhoid; but a pure case of bowel infection."

Let us return now to the other assumption of the advantages of milk diet, to wit:

that milk keeps up the nutrition of the patient to the highest possible degree. Does it? Let any man who has carried his typhoid fever patient through, giving abundance of milk, and who sees his patient reduced to a skeleton, ask himself the question, "Does it?" The fact is it does not. The patient comes out at the end of the fever emaciated until he could hardly become emaciated any further. His pulse is weak; it could not become much weaker and the patient live. It would certainly seem that no other food could have brought the patient to a condition any worse, as far as his nutrition is concerned. I think the physician, looking at the emaciated typhoid skeleton, might even ask himself, "How much thinner would my patient have been if he had no food whatever?" It would seem, therefore, that the primary assumptions so commonly accepted on close examination are proven to be wrong one and all. Now there is another side. Before the patient calls the doctor, in typhoid fever, he usually has a period of from a week to ten days of general malaise during which he has a moderate degree of fever, a good deal of headache, and a moderate diarrhea, if any; he is sick, but he is not very sick. Finally the doctor is called. The patient is put to bed and measures are taken, one way or another, to moderate the fever. Theoretically he ought at once to begin to be somewhat better, or, at the very least, he ought not to grow rapidly worse, for now, lying in bed, he ought to save his strength and abate his fever, even if nothing were done for him. What happens? The officious doctor, eager to keep up his patient's strength, begins to insist on his taking considerable quantities of milk. The patient, led by nature's own indication, has been eating practically nothing. Now the fever begins to climb, step by step, day by day, until within three or four days it reaches its high point, and now the physician enters upon a long fight in which he endeavors to keep the fever within moderate bounds. It may be that the patient is put into the bath and the temperature is forced down, only to run rapidly up

in the next two or three hours, when another bath is given. So the temperature see-saws, inevitably rising as soon as the effect of the bath has passed off, and meantime the patient is being fed casein, although the doctor knows very well that the patient's digestive powers, as far as his stomach is concerned, have practically ceased, and the digestive power of his small intestine is even more precarious. Nevertheless, down goes the casein.

It has been my amusement to visit Mt. Clemens, the "Mecca" of rheumatic patients from all parts of the United States. I have seen patients who had scraped together, with great difficulty, enough money to come to Mt. Clemens, take a bath every morning, be rubbed, scrubbed, sweated, in a vigorous attempt to eliminate the rheumatic poison, and then, three times a day, sit down in the dining room, study over the bill of fare, in which the hotel keeper had provided an admirable menu consisting for the most part of meat and eggs, and then I have seen the patient eat more nitrogenous food at one meal than he could wash out of him by the bath the next morning. It seemed a most astonishing thing to see a man, three times a day, putting into himself, the very substances out of which is formed the poison which he is laboriously trying to get out of himself. Precisely analogous is the process of forcing food on our typhoid patients. The primary infection of the typhoid bacillus takes place by way of the sound mucous membrane. When the bacilli have begun to fill up the glandular structures connected with the intestine, the disease is established and must take its course, but without a fresh and continued infection it would seem reasonable to believe that the period of activity of the bacilli would come to an end within a reasonable time. If the intestines were emptied as far as possible of all substances which could form a culture ground for bacilli of any kind, the process of reinfection would, thereby, be reduced to a minimum. While the primary infection was pursuing its course, a certain waste of the tissues of the body would undoubtedly take place, but the probability is, that the febrile process would very soon become limited, by the absence of pabulum. In so far as the serous part of the milk is absorbed and, in so far as a portion of the casein is digested and absorbed, it is a question deserving of careful investigation, whether these foodstuffs do not simply serve to feed the fever. That the feeding of fevers in the so-called supporting treatment, is devoid of the striking advantages claimed for it, is shown by the statistics of the Massachusetts General Hospital. In these the mortality is shown to have been practically the same in the days when purging, bleeding, and low diet were employed, as it is when the feeding and supporting treatment are used. Now the old treatment of low diet included bleeding and purging. Our medical ancestors were as dangerous to their patients as we are to ours, only in a different way. If they had been content to let their patients have a low diet and lots of pure air and pure water they would, I think we will all agree, have had better results had they omitted the bleeding and used only so much purging as would keep the intestines fairly free from putrefying contents. They had a pretty good idea at the bottom of their purging process, but they overdid it. When the reaction came we went too far the other way, and, in a desperate attempt to support our patients, we also have sinned by overdoing.

A curious series of experiments on animals has been made, which has shown that feeding does not increase the vital resistance in fevers. Inoculated animals were found to survive any given infection, with little or no food better than those fed liberally. I know that it takes nerve to see a typhoid fever patient gradually wasting both strength and flesh as the fever goes on, and refrain from putting, what to a well man is nourishing food, into the patient. We do not see the dark red stomach, containing far more mucus than gastric juice; we cannot compel our imaginations to make real to us the swollen, cyanosed, almost or quite necrotic mucous membrane of the small intestine. If we could imagine these internal conditions so vividly that it was all as clear to us as the dusky face, the shrunken arms and legs, the hollow eyes, it would be easier for us to resist the impulse to put a lot of stuff down out of sight and hope for the best.

It has been my fortune to advocate the principles I now contend for, in consultation at the bedside. The doctor says: "Yes, doctor, I believe you are right in theory; I can see that the stomach is practically unable to digest food, that the intestinal mucous membrane not only has long since lost its normal function but is apt to be damaged by irritant substances and putrefying ones; you may be right that the fire of the fever would be less intense and would burn down sooner if we didn't keep piling on fuel, but just look at the patient! See how thin he is! How weak his pulse! Sometime I'd like to discuss your theory with you, but I guess this time I will go on feeding."

It takes nerve to take an infant suffering from cholera infantum, take it away from the mother's breast, cut off cow's milk, or food of any kind, and keep the baby on sterilized water and Epsom salts until the nearest approach possible to intestinal asepsis is secured, but, fortunately, the profession has learned that degree of courage.

I am well aware of the limitations of my own personal experience in typhoid fever. but at least I have seen this. I have seen patients whose fever kept springing up after the bath like a steel spring, patients whose brains were so poisoned that delirium was deepening into coma, come out into moderate fever and a clear head within 48 hours after the forced feeding was stopped and a water diet instituted.

We are oppressed by this fear of starvation. Starvation is a slow process. Dr. Tanner demonstrated that 40 days' starvation is endurable provided the patient drinks plenty of pure water.

The ideal diet for typhoid fever is pure water in abundance. This will keep the excretions by skin, lungs, kidneys, and liver up to their best, and our typhoid patients need to keep all means of elimination of poison in fullest activity, providing it be not a prostrating activity. The action of kidneys, liver, and skin induced by super-abundant water is never prostrating. This cannot be said of action induced by drugs. It is not enough to give the patient as much water as he may happen to crave, we must use our scientific imagination to picture the very large quantity of water which goes out by the lungs; notice how quickly the moistened tongue becomes parched; we must realize the evaporation from the skin; consider the diarrhea and the urinary needs; then put in water enough to keep all these in full activity.

People have imbibed enough of current medical opinion to make it difficult to stop our present dangerous overfeeding. Even were the attending physician convinced of the safety of the pure water diet, the friends will insist that the patient's strength must be kept up. In such cases any of the best advertised meat-juice foods (so-called) can be utilized. They contain little real food value, and are, fortunately, mostly absorbed in the stomach, and so leave little or no detritus to go through the bowels. There comes a time in the course of the fever when the patient's appetite returns. This is always a difficult period. Pressure by both the patient and the patient's friends is very great. It is hard to resist the cry for all kinds of food and lots of it, yet there is probably no man who reads this who has not had the bitter experience of seeing his patient quickly relapse after some newly tried indulgence in food. It seems to me that the best rule to follow is this: Give such foods as are most completely digested and absorbed in the stomach; keep steadily in mind that while the stomach may be acting but poorly, the intestinal condition is far worse. Still we should send down from the stomach as little detritus as possible. A tender lamb chop or a poached egg is safer than a tumbler of milk; safer now, safer all the way through.

One thing I wish to add in the matter of stimulation. Time has been when a conva-lescing typhoid patient drank alcohol in great quantities. The practice seems now largely gone by, and fortunately so, yet throughout these cases the physician knows the need and the value of an occasional stimulant. For a long time I have used, instead of alcohol, a small drink of good coffee. Those of us who know how a cup of coffee at—say from two to four in the afternoon, will keep us awake till two o'clock in the morning, know that the stim-ulant effect of coffee is not transient like that of alcohol, but lasts hour after hour—six, eight, ten hours. Now, what a typhoid convalescent needs is not a fillip which picks him up and drops him down again, he needs a good, steady, lasting lift, and coffee will give it to him. Don't have the friends give him watery coffee; a delicate after-dinner coffeecup full of good coffee with cream and sugar will taste good and do good, and keep on doing good.

One more practical point. I have urged that such foods as are given should be read-ily absorbed by the gastric mucous mem-brane; there is one food of which we are apt to think too little—sugar—we are apt to think of it as simply a means of sweet-ening foods; in reality it is highly nutri-tious—no other hydrocarbon is more promptly and easily absorbed—it leaves no detritus whatever. A man with muscles, tired from labor, can recuperate rapidly on sugar. A typhoid patient can take it up rapidly.

HOW NATURE BURNS UP THE FATS.

We find in *Good Health*, under the above caption, this terse and trimly, pertinent and incisive paper:

SUPPOSE you are suffering from obesity—what shall be done?—Burn up the fats. This cannot be done by the use of any kind of pill or any kind of medicine. But there is something that will prove effectual every time. When a man goes north to spend the winter, he must eat a quantity of fat-making material. When a bear is getting ready to hibernate, or to go into winter quarters, he eats nuts, honey, and all the fat-making things he can find, until he becomes fat enough to remain all winter in his hole.

For the same purpose the squirrels work all summer, eating, and hunting, and storing away all kinds of fat-making materials, especially nuts, to keep them warm during the long winter days and nights. During the winter this fat is burned up. What is it that burns up the fat? It is cold.

We have a hint as to one means of reducing fat in the effect of the application of cold water, as by the cold bath. The longer the bath is continued, if the patient is able to stand it, the more effectual it will be found in breaking down the fat. The notion that you can get rid of fat by sweating is a mistake. Sweating reduces the strength of the patient, but it does not reduce the fat; it makes no reduction except by the abstraction of water, and that leaves him so thirsty that he will soon make it up by drinking. You can also reduce flesh by starvation, but one will not then be healthy, because even if he falls sick and loses fat, when he gets well he will become fat again; so we must find a more physiological method. We have this physiological method in cold-water treatment—the cold shower, the cold douche, packing, and swimming in cold water.

Exercise is another means of burning up fat. But exercise is sometimes detrimental to the obese person, because he has such a heavy overcoat of fat. The writer has seen patients with overcoats of fat six inches thick in some places; one case of this kind weighed three hundred and fifty pounds. In these cases there is an enormous amount of fat to break down. When such a person is asked to take exercise, he is soon tired out. This patient's weight was so great that practically he had to carry one man on each shoulder, and of course it was a great task for him to take exercise.

Hot baths diminish and cold water increases the power to exercise. Cold water also gives capacity for exercise. It energizes the lungs, the muscles, and the heart. Some time ago we took one of the largest men in the house, and gave him a hot bath, and then tested his strength; he could lift only about half as much as before, and his total strength also was only a little more than half what it was before. Then we put him into a cold bath, and afterward tested his total strength, finding that he could lift a little more than he could before taking the hot bath.

Cold water will transform a weak man into a strong man. He may be so weak that he can hardly stand, but give him a cold bath, and in two minutes he will be stronger than before; there is energizing power in cold water. The obese man takes cold water, and that gives him strength and additional capacity for exercise, and exercise accumulates heat because the overcoat of fat retains heat; that is just what you would experience if in summer you should put on a thick overcoat, and take a bicycle ride or some other vigorous exercise. The obese man has a similar embarrassment as the result of an undue increase of heat. So, after exercising for a time, he has a fever, and then the exercise begins to tear down his muscles and nerves, and to break down his bodily structure—the structure which he depends upon to keep him strong and well. This effect we desire to avoid, so we begin by extracting heat from the obese patient by a cold bath, then making up that loss of heat by exercise; in this way some time will elapse before he is in danger of fever, because we have cured his fever before it begins.

The cold bath prepares a man for exercise. It is a good thing for the obese man to have a hot bath first to heat the skin to the point of perspiration—so that he may enjoy his cold bath. Heat, while it is seductive and enticing, is really unfriendly, for it decreases the power of resistance. But cold increases the power of resistance.

WHY DOES BREAD BECOME MOLDY?

In my early housekeeping days I, like most young housekeepers, accepted the traditional belief that bread when kept a few days—unless under the most favorable conditions—will become moldy and unfit for use, writes Mrs. Emma P. Ewing, in *Good Housekeeping* for October. I have, however, changed my belief. One evening some twenty years ago I discovered that a loaf of beautiful looking bread, baked four days previous, was moldy outside and "ropy" inside. This was a new experience, and I went to work to investigate the subject. After years of research, study and experiment I reached the conclusion that underdone bread is liable to become ropy as well as moldy in a short time, while bread thoroughly baked can be kept indefinitely. Thorough baking is a certain preventive of mold in bread. During the past fifteen years I have frequently kept bread two weeks and have never had a loaf of it go moldy. In September, 1898, I unintentionally left part of a French roll and part of a loaf of Vienna bread in a table drawer at Chautauqua. Upon my return there the following June I found both roll and loaf as free from mold as they were when baked, and they are still in the same condition—without a speck of mold on either.

There is a great deal of loose talk about yeast-raised bread becoming moldy, fermenting in the stomach, and giving people dyspepsia and other ailments, and Dr. Cyrus W. Edson some years ago wrote an article for a medical journal in which he pointed out the dangers that beset those who eat it. Now all the ills that afflict humanity may, and possibly do, lurk in the average loaf of bread which is improperly made and imperfectly baked, but yeast-raised bread properly made and thoroughly baked approaches nearly a perfect food and never molds, never ferments in the stomach and never gives the eater a dyspeptic pang.

Expert scientists tell us that exposure to a temperature of two hundred and seventy-five degrees will destroy yeast germs, spores of fungi, spores of bacilli and sporeless bacteria; and it is an established fact that bread cannot be properly baked at a lower temperature than three hundred and seventy-five degrees. Hence by subjecting bread, until thoroughly baked, to a temperature of three hundred and seventy-five degrees—a temperature that will brown flour in two or three minutes—it will be perfectly sterilized, its quality and flavor will be improved, and all danger of there being any living microorganisms in it will be overcome.

There is a vast difference in the flavor, digestibility and nutritive value of bread fresh from the oven, and bread three or four days old. It requires at least forty-eight hours for the rich, nutty flavor of good bread to become developed, and bread of the best quality seldom reaches its most perfect condition until the third day after it has been baked. People who persist in eating freshly baked bread—in most cases underdone—do not realize how enjoyable, digestible and satisfying a slice of bread is cut from a loaf that has been made scientifically, baked thoroughly and permitted to reach its best estate by ripening three or four days; but if they can be induced to give such bread a trial for a short period, they will never again be satisfied with the freshly baked, flavorless, indigestible, innutritious stuff that is now found upon the average table. Make your bread properly, bake it thoroughly, keep it in a well-ventilated box in a cool, dry place and you will never have a moldy loaf.

✤ ✤

ANTISEPTICS TESTED BACTERIOLOGICALLY.

There is much diversity of opinion respecting the value of the different antiseptics. Hence any contribution aiding in the establishment of the real facts is important. Dr. J. E. Weeks (*Archives of Opthalmology*), publishes a detailed account of numerous experiments bearing on this question. Taking as his pyogenic germ the Staphylococcus he has sought to ascertain the relative length of time required to kill it by antiseptics in solutions not strong enough to affect the tissues injuriously. The virulence of his fresh cultivations was tested by passing a little of the growth into the anterior chamber of a rabbit's eye. Destruction of the eye by panophthalmitis took place in every case.

Of bichloride of mercury solutions he found that 1:500 destroys the germs in ten seconds; 1:1,000 in forty-five seconds; 1:2,000 in one and one-third minutes; 1:4,000 in two and a half minutes; 1:5,000 in three minutes; 1:10,000 in five minutes; 1:20,000 twelve to fifteen minutes. Solutions of 1:4,000 rarely cause any irritation. Solutions 1:1,500 may be safely used on cut surfaces and abscess cavities.

Of nitrate of silver a solution of 1:10 destroys the germs in four seconds; 1:50 in eight seconds; 1:100 in twelve seconds; 1:500 in one and one-third minutes; 1:1,000 in four minutes. Thus it appears that nitrate of silver in weak solutions is a powerful germicide. Salicylic acid 1:600 destroys the germs in one minute; 1:1,000 in four minutes.

Absolute alcohol destroys the germs in four to twelve seconds. Ninety per cent. alcohol in twenty to thirty seconds.

Chlorine water in saturated solution is non-irritating to the conjunctiva and has about the same germicide power as the sublimate or nitrate of silver solutions.

Boric acid has no power to destroy the germs.

For the cleansing of instruments he commends sterilization by the use of hot water and the mechanical wiping with a clean linen towel.

We have not space to quote his conclusions respecting many other so-called antiseptics. Most of them are not available in work about the eye on account of irritating properties.

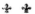

A PRIZE BREADMAKER TALKS.

I ALWAYS use distilled yeast. I have tried compressed yeast, and I have made my own yeast, but I have always had the best results from distillers' yeast. I use it immediately. I may keep it over night, but seldom longer than that. I set a sponge in the morning as soon as I get up. I don't like to set bread at night. There is no telling what may happen to it when you are asleep. The life may get chilled out of it, or it may get too warm and then sour, so it is best to start the job when you can watch it. I set a sponge at 6 o'clock in the morning, and at 10 it is out of the oven. Here are my measurements for a baking I do twice a week. They give me about three pounds of bread, one large loaf or two small ones. I use one cent's worth of yeast, a little more than a quarter of a cup. For wetting, I sometimes use half milk and half water, or all milk, generally the milk from which I have skimmed the cream for breakfast. If I happen to be out of milk, I use water, and the bread is almost as good. For a cent's worth of yeast I use one and a half cups of wetting, a level tablespoon of lard (why not butter? Editor GAZETTE), half a teaspoon of salt, a pinch of soda and one teaspoon of sugar. I don't scald the milk; simply have the wetting lukewarm. To this I add the yeast, then flour to make a thick batter. I set it in a warm place and generally in forty minutes it is light enough to make into dough. I turn it out on the bread board and knead it till it is as smooth as satin. One of the secrets of good bread is to knead in the least flour possible. Some women go on adding all the flour they can possibly work into dough, then they wonder why their loaves are tough and dry. After I have added all the flour that seems necessary, I use no more, except a pinch here and there where the dough sticks to the board. When it is smooth and elastic I return it to the bread pan and let it rise. The second time I put it on the board I give it the slightest kneading possible, simply enough to break every air bubble. An air bubble means a hole, and bread with a texture like a coarse sponge is pretty poor eating. I put my loaves in the pan and watch them. My rule is to let them rise to double their size, and I put enough dough in a pan to have a loaf that will round slightly over the top of the pan. When they rise higher than that they cut into slices that are not sightly. I don't consider a baking finished when the loaves are in the oven.

I plan to stay pretty near the stove during baking time. I turn every loaf after it has been in the oven five minutes. If one neglects this, the result is a loaf humped high on one side and low on the other. It may be good bread, but it is not sightly. I bake with a wood fire, which is hotter than coal, and generally thirty minutes after I set the loaves in the oven they are out again, cooling on a sieve. [Longer baking would greatly improve this bread. Editor GAZETTE.]—*Good Housekeeping* for October.

AN ERA OF LONGEVITY.

THAT the improved conditions of modern existence have added materially to the longevity of mankind is a matter that is being taken seriously in commercial circles. The Actuarial Society of America is to compile a new series of tables for the life insurance companies of the United States, which, the society maintains, will show a decreased mortality among the people of this country. This is expected to have the effect of decreasing the premium rates now charged, as the whole life insurance business is based on mortality tables. It cannot be doubted that, with sobriety and moderation in all things, the average man can live to an old age. The purification of foods, the marked advance in medicine and surgery, the wonders of modern science, are all assisting to prolong the existence of the man of the twentieth century. It remains for him to educate himself to enjoy that existence with contentment and success.—October *Success*.

THE INJURIOUS SUBSTANCES IN WHISKEY AND TOBACCO.

ACCORDING to the *Lancet*, it has been shown that, "comparatively speaking at any rate, fusel oil is not the injurious constituent of whiskey. It is rather the aldehydes, the partly oxidized alcohols in whiskey, which are mischievous, and the chief among them is furfurol. Old matured whiskey is free from furfurol, while freshly made or unmatured spirit contains a marked amount of this constituent, the source of the throbbing headache of the heavy drinker." It is very doubtful whether this piece of information adds anything to our knowledge. Ethyl alcohol, when taken in anything but quite small quantity, is injurious to mankind. This much is known for certain. The more alcohol the liquid contains, the more serious are the results of drinking it. The amount of aldehydes, fusel oil or ethers contained in the various drinks is of little moment, as compared with the percentage of ethyl alcohol. No physiologist has ever told us that "old matured whiskey" will not make a man drunk!

The *Lancet* also states that the amount of nicotine in Virginia tobacco does not often exceed one per cent., and that much of this is destroyed by the combustion. But new products are formed, consisting of tobacco tar oils, which are poisonous. "The composition of these oils indicates that they are very closely related to nicotine, and their chief constituent is pyridine, and it and its 'relatives' are responsible for the violent headache, trembling and giddiness following excessive smoking. The degree of toxicity of the smoke, however, probably depends largely upon the completeness of the combustion."

The *Lancet* eventually arrives at the conclusion that the cigarette is the least injurious form of smoking, that the pipe comes next, that the cigar is the most injurious of all.

THE HYGIENE OF FASTING.

ALMOST all the great founders of religions have deemed it salutary to prescribe a certain amount of fasting for their disciples. The reason for this, says a writer in the *Blätter für Volksgesundheitspflege*, as translated in the *Literary Digest*, is not only the knowledge that it is well for man to conquer his bodily desires, but also the experience that most persons eat too much. To overload the stomach with food is not less unhealthy than to deluge it with beverages; the more nutritious the food the more hazardous are the consequences when excess is habitual. Of all the sins of nutrition, the immoderate use of meat is certainly the most grievous. It gives to the body in a form that is favorable for easy assimilation the albumen that is absolutely necessary to life, and hence the earliest effect of its excessive use must be to surcharge the body with nutrients.

The chief point here is the critical examination of what is callēd hunger. Many persons believe that any and every sensation of hunger must be satisfied immediately, but this is a great mistake. An equally great, if not worse, mistake is the opinion that one must eat until a sense of satiety arises. These two mistakes combined lead to an unfavorable development of the human body, for the weight of the body grows to a degree that is detrimental to the activity of most of the chief and finer organs. For every stature an approximate weight may be stated that may be accepted as normal, and in accordance with this weight are adjusted the vital organs, particularly the heart. When a heart has volume sufficient only for a body of 150 pounds and is put to work to satisfy the demands of a body of 200 pounds, it soon shows that it is unequal to the task. It is just as if an engine that was built to pull only a prescribed weight were used to pull a large additional weight. The activity of the other organs, as well as of the heart, is hindered by the fat that is deposited about the latter. Excessive nutrition injures the mental capabilities also.

Of the particular consequences of excessive nutrition, such as hypochondria (the very name of which refers the reader to the region of the abdomen) and the gout, it is hardly necessary to speak.

MRS. SMITH'S BROWN BREAD.

MY Boston brown bread is different from any recipe I ever found in a cook book; it is one which has been made in our family for many years. I use two cups of sour milk, one well-beaten egg, half a cup of molasses—or less molasses and a tablespoonful of sugar when I wish bread that is not very dark and sweet. Then I add two level teaspoons of soda and three cups of graham flour. Nearly all recipes for brown bread mix rye, corn meal and Graham flour. I use the Graham flour alone; you have a nicer bread. Generally I steam brown bread in one-pound baking-powder cans. It makes neat slices, it keeps more moist than when a large loaf is cut, and it steams more quickly. Two and a half hours will be needed for brown bread when in small cans, three hours if it is steamed in a large pail. One secret of success with brown bread is keeping it covered as carefully as if it were a steamed pudding. I set a trivet in the bottom of an iron kettle, put in the bread and enough boiling water to come three-quarters of the way to the top. Then I put on the lid, set it over the fire and do not lift the lid again till the clock advises me it is ready. If water enough is put in at first it will not boil away, and it is not necessary to lift the lid to add more.—From *Good Housekeeping* for October.

The same journal says:
A baker who makes jam on a large scale says he never stirs it, but puts a large handful of marbles on the bottom of the kettle. These roll around when the jam boils and prevent it from burning.

POWDERING FOOD TO KEEP IT.

DESICCATED milk is one of the newer food products, and is prepared by causing a spray of ordinary fresh milk to enter a tank filled with hot air. The "atomized" fluid is carried upward, and its moisture being discharged in the form of vapor, the solid part of it is thrown down in another receptacle in the shape of a dry powder. Put up in suitable packages, this powder will keep fresh and good for a long time, and is readily made available for use by the addition of boiling water.

Eggs are now dried by a number of different processes, most of which in one way or another involve the use of a wheel that picks up the fluid eggstuff from a tank and carries it through a hot-air chamber, sometimes by the help of a belt, where it is finally scraped off automatically and discharged in a moisture-free condition into a box. One of the most notable inventors in this line is a woman.

Similar processes are applied in the manufacture of desiccated soups, of dried beef tea, and even of "pumpkin powder," which last furnishes an always-ready material for making pumpkin pies, no matter what the season may be.

On the same principle are constructed the latest machines for making what is called "continuous ice cream," the cream for which is taken up and frozen on the periphery of a rotating cylinder that contains ice or other refrigerating material.

The same "continuous" method is being utilized for making artificial ice, instead of the old process whereby the water was frozen in metal-lined tanks with the aid of ammonia pipes behind the iron plates. According to the new plan, the water is frozen on rotating cylinders, inside of which is the chilling agent, and is scraped off as fast as it is converted into ice. The ice particles are then pressed together, forming beautiful transparent cakes—*Saturday Evening Post.*

TEA AND COFFEE TWO HUNDRED YEARS AGO.

THE *Polyclinic* for May makes the following interesting excerpts from a Treatise on Foods, published in Paris in 1702 by M. Louis Lemery, "Regent-Doctor of the Faculty of Physick at Paris." Of tea M. Lemery says:

"Tea is very wholesome, since it produces many good effects and few bad ones. It may be preferred before coffee; for the immoderate use of coffee is sometimes very pernicious, but we see some who will drink ten or Twelve Dishes of Tea a Day without any hurt at all."

And again:

"It's good for the disorders of the Brain and Nerves. It refreshes the spirits, suppresses vapors, cures the Headache, prevents Drowsiness, helps digestion, purifies the blood; provokes urine and is good for phthisical and scorbutic persons. We do not find that Tea produces any ill effects; however it may if taken too liberally make the blood grow a little more subtil. It agrees at all times with any age and constitution."

The virtues of coffee are thus summed up by the author:

"It fortifies the stomach and Brain, promotes digestion, allays the headache, suppresses the Fumes caused by Wine or other liquors; promotes urine and Women's terms, opens some People's Bodies, makes the Memory and Fancy more quick and people that drink it brisk. It agrees when moderately taken especially in cold weather with Old People; with such as are phlegmatic and those who are fat and corpulent; but 'tis not so proper for bilious and melancholy persons. The use of Coffee to excess makes People lean, hinders them from Sleep, debilitates their Bodies, suppresses Venereal inclinations, and produces several other the like Inconveniences. Coffee drank to excess is at least as pernicious as the moderate use of it is wholesome to many persons. Many persons that have been used to drink too much coffee become infirm and paralytic as Willis and other physicians have observed."

[Thus the race was taught a habit that is quite as hard to abandon and well-nigh as disastrous as the use of spirituous liquors. Ed. GAZETTE.]

A NEW FOOD MADE FROM MILK.

PLASMON is a new creamery product, and is made both in Germany and in England from milk after the butter has been extracted. The name is taken from a Greek word, meaning "that which gives form." The fresh milk as it comes from the cow is put into a separator, all the cream being removed by this method. The separated milk is afterwards treated so as to coagulate all the proteids; and this coagulated mass is then kneaded and dried at a temperature of 70 degrees Centigrade under an atmosphere of carbon dioxid. When perfectly free from moisture, the plasmon is completely soluble in hot water.

Concerning the food value of this new product. it is claimed that one ounce of the powder is equal to three and a quarter pounds of the finest beefsteak! This means that it will take the place of between eleven and twelve pints of milk. The German government in using it in both the army and navy, and the department for the investigation of food for the troops has praised it highly as a portable and concentrated nutrient.

CEREALS AS FOODS.

FECULA and flours are often used as synonyms. Fecula are starches like that obtained from potatoes, corn, rice, etc. They are not digested in the stomach but in the intestines. and they are not converted into anything else but sugar. On the other hand, flour, from whatever cereal it may be derived, contains all the constituents of the

grain except cellulose, which is present in the husks. In addition to starch, therefore, it contains fat and mineral salts and proteids. Hence cereal flour resembles chemically the composition of eggs and contains all the elements of nutrition.—*Répertoire de Pharmacie.*

POTATO CHEESE.

POTATOES of good quality are chosen, usually large white ones, and these are boiled until they are "done." The skins are removed and the potatoes smoothly mashed, as though for making potatoes *à la maitre d' hôtel.* When quite cold, to every five parts of potatoes one part of unskimmed milk, freshly coagulated with rennet, is added, and the whole thoroughly incorporated, closely covered and set aside for five days. At the end of this time the mixture is again thoroughly tamped or mashed with a muller, and is placed in little wicker baskets and hung up to drain. When all superfluous moisture has drained off, the masses are removed from the baskets and placed on boards in a shady, cool place, to further dry out. They are then packed in layers in big jars or barrels, and kept for fifteen days. Finally each cheese is pressed into a tight terrine and hermetically sealed.

WHY AND WHEN WE FEEL HUNGRY: A GERMAN THEORY.

A GERMAN physician says we feel hungry when the blood-vessels of the stomach are comparatively empty. Many anemic patients have no appetite even when the stomach is empty; but the blood-vessels of the stomach are not empty in such cases, but rather congested. In healthy people lack of blood in the stomach acts upon a special nerve, and all the characteristic symptoms of hunger follow. Now this hunger nerve and the nerves of the mouth and tongue are branches of the same nerve-trunk. Hence, a stimulus applied to the tongue, by a spice for example, creates or increases appetite. On the other hand, when the nerves of the tongue are affected by a diseased condition of the mucous membrane of the mouth, the patient has no appetite, though his stomach may be empty, and he may be in actual need of food.

THE PHILOSOPHY OF EATING.

In a lecture before the Medical College of London, Gladstone laid great stress upon habits of eating as the secret of vitality and capacity for work at an advanced age. "Not only what you eat, but how you eat it, is important. You can train the taste so that hurtful dishes will become distasteful. Hold fast to plain food, good roast beef and mutton, bread, potatoes. Avoid highly spiced food, pastries, elaborate menus. Pure food is essential to a sound body, adulteration in the slightest degree is but poisoning the blood and shortening life. Chew every mouthful with systematic thoroughness. Experiments show remarkable and permanent ill effects from 'bolted' food. The kind of food is less responsible for a disordered stomach than the manner in which it is eaten. Food is our fuel. How long would a boiler do its work if fed with the haphazard recklessness we show in maintaining the human fire? There is a saying 'that with the French *chefs* came civilization.' Certainly the slow French dinner is a good example for dyspeptic Americans."

A CARNIVOROUS PARROT.

With one exception, all parrots are vegetarians. This exception is the strange New Zealand lory, the kea, which alone among its kind has developed the habit of eating flesh. From a psychological point of view the case is interesting, because it is the best recorded instance of the growth of a new and complex instinct under the eyes of human observers. The kea, before the arrival of the white man in New Zealand, was a mild-mannered, fruit-eating or honey-sucking bird. But as soon as sheep-stations were established, these degenerate parrots began to acquire a taste for raw mutton. At first they ate only the offal that was thrown out of the slaughter houses, picking the bones as clean of meat as a dog or a jackal. But in course of time, as the taste for blood grew, a new and debased idea entered their heads. If dead sheep are good food, are not living ones? The keas answered this question in the affirmative, and proceeding to act upon their conviction they invented a truly hideous mode of operation. A weak member of a flock of sheep is attacked, usually by a number of birds, and almost always after dark, the poor animal being worried to death by the combined efforts of the parrots, some of whom perch themselves upon its back and tear open the flesh, their efforts being to reach the kidneys which they devour at the earliest possible moment. As many as two hundred ewes are said to have been killed during one night upon a single sheep "station." Of course the New Zealand farmer resents the attacks of the keas, and as the result an attempt is being made to exterminate these carnivorous birds. The probability is that their existence will be limited to a few years.

WHY DO DOGS SWALLOW STONES, STICKS, ETC.?

It has recently been asserted that the presence of foreign substances like pebbles, glass and feathers in a dog's stomach show that the animal was affected with rabies. This is by no means correct. The dog is probably suffering from some stomach trouble, which may have given it convulsions and caused it to act in a manner which gave rise to the belief that it was rabid. When a dog is suffering from one or a complication of the disorders of the stomach or intestines, it will swallow bits of almost anything which comes to hand, hoping to find a counter-irritant and to get relief. A Baltimore physician, whose name I cannot remember, has expressed the opinion that the mere fact of finding foreign substances in a dog's stomach, although no proof of rabies, may indicate cerebro-spinal meningitis, which in its outward form resembles violent rabies, and is apt to make the dog behave somewhat in accordance with the popular conceptions of rabies. The fact that a dog swallows grass, and occasionally a small stone, does not indicate any serious disorder. The acids in the canine stomach are very strong and very plentiful. Sometimes the lining of the stomach becomes so charged with these acids, in excess of the quantity required to digest the food upon which the animal has been living, that the sufferer seeks an irritant which acts upon the walls of the stomach and causes an artificial flow of the acid. Grass is the counter-irritant provided by nature, and the one the dog prefers. It does not choose smooth grass, but that which has prickly edges and tickles the little vessels containing the acids. If grass is not around, most dogs will eat hair, which never does serious injury. When neither grass nor hair can be found, the poor animal will swallow other substances such as stones and wood. The latter is dangerous.

The moral is watch your dog and attend to any signs of sickness. Do not assume that he has rabies because he swallows foreign substances.—*Exchange.*

WOMEN AS SCIENTISTS.

THE problem whether women are fitted to succeed in scientific pursuits, says *The Philadelphia Medical Journal*, seems to have been solved satisfactorily by the late Eleanor Omerod. As a scientist Miss Omerod gained distinction in entomology, For years past she had been an authority in

that department, especially of entomology which relates to agriculture. She studied insects from the economic standpoint—that is, for their injurious effects upon agriculture, just as now we are beginning to study them more closely for their injurious effects upon human health. Hence Miss Omerod was a pioneer in a field which lies contiguous to that of human pathology. Her career was most interesting and instructive. From *Harper's Weekly* we learn that in early life she began to study insects on her father's country place in Gloucestershire. She studied their ravages in the fields and orchards, and the work became a life work. She contributed to the Royal Horticultural Society, and became entomologist to the Royal Agricultural Society. For twenty-four years she sent out an annual report of her work. Her fame spread abroad, and she was consulted by suffering agriculturists in all parts of the world. In recognition of her researches she received many medals, and last year she received (a rare thing in Britain) the degree of Doctor of Laws from the University of Edinburgh. Her work was untiring and unselfish, for it seems to have been done for the love of it and not for gain. At the age of seventy-three she died, having bequeathed to science the record of a great work, and to her sex the distinction of a fine career.

BARKER (*American Journal of the Medical Sciences*, October, 1901), writing of the recent outbreak of bubonic plague in San Francisco, points out that the Chinese in that city are, from a sanitary standpoint, much better off than their countrymen in cities of China, such as Hong Kong and Canton. They are on the whole well fed and clothed and he particularly emphasizes the fact that the Chinese in that city wear shoes, stockings and trousers, since it is believed by many that the bare legs and feet of the Chinese in Hong Kong and Canton had much to do with the frequency of infection with plague in those cities.

Department of Hygiene.

WITH SPECIAL REFERENCE TO STATE AND PREVENTIVE MEDICINE.

PUBLIC HYGIENE—STATE MEDICINE.*

By R. H. HARRISON, M.D., COLUMBUS, TEXAS.

THAT the foundations of sanitary science were laid early in the history of medicine, soon after the accumulation of sufficient data to furnish the elements of a special science—crude and irrational it is true, as is made manifest by the wearing of amulets for protection against evil influences—is almost a self-evident proposition. A little later the Hebrews adopted some systematic laws with respect to diet and cleanliness, evidently intended to protect the national health. But it was not until after the beginning of the Christian era that we find any distinct record of the control of sanitary measures by government. The provision of baths, even during the days of the Roman Empire, associated as they were with gymnasia for physical training, at governmental expense, was evidently for the protection of the public health, and the development of manly strength. Later, during the reign of Augustus, the public baths of the "Eternal City" were greatly enlarged, and placed under the control and direction of a physician. As time passed and civilization advanced, we find in various European nations record of the establishment, by their respective governments, of hospitals for the care of the sick and wounded. It was not until the beginning of the present century, however, that "State medicine" assumed definite proportions, and took the shape of an independent branch of science in that most enlightened and highly cultivated of all the nations of the earth—old England. The careful ob-

server of the facts of history will scarcely fail to perceive that the development of sanitary science has kept very even pace with the progress of our knowledge on other subjects. Respect for human life, and the effort to provide the means for its protection, affords significant evidence of the prevalent culture of the country in which it obtains. This fact finds apt illustration in the sanitary laws which have been adopted in the States in which wealth and high culture are congregated to the greatest extent. The old State of Massachusetts initiated the good work. New York, Pennsylvania and other States noted for wealth and intelligence followed suit, with results which testify, in unmistakable terms, to the incalculable value of good sanitary laws to the commonwealth. Yellow fever made its first appearance in Boston in 1693, but rarely since that date—her sanitary precautions having removed the conditions essential to its existence. Philadelphia had a similar experience with that fell disease in 1696; as did also, a few years later, the city of New York. Effective sanitary laws have long since rendered these cities immune to such death-dealing visitations.

The establishment of preventive medicine on a scientific basis probably dates no further back than to the first advent of cholera in Europe, some seventy or seventy-five years ago. Such legislation as had been had in both England and other European countries for the protection of the public health prior to that time was almost wholly confined to the provision of quarantine laws,

---

*Read before the Southern Texas Medical Association Republished from the *Texas Medical News.*

like those of our own State, against diseases of foreign origin, without any regard whatever to unsanitary conditions at home so often found fruitful of malignant disease, which should be prevented.

We are indebted to Mr. Edwin Chadwick, who was appointed secretary to the "Poor Law Board" of England about the year 1834, for the introduction of some sort of system into the administration of sanitary measures for the protection of the public health. Soon after entering upon the duties of his office, this gentleman surrounded himself by a corps of coadjutors, all of whom were imbued with the same statesmanlike and philanthropic impulses as himself, and under the title of "General Board of Health," the able body of men thus assembled addressed themselves with diligence to the investigation of the charge committed to their care. Their efforts resulted in a series of reports showing such a reckless waste of human life by reason of the unsanitary surroundings of the poor all over the nation that both the parliament and the public of England were startled into action; and while the resulting relief was intended for the most unfortunate and least important class of her citizens, its benefits were soon reflected to the entire body politic. The first decisive step in that direction was the creation, during the year 1843, of the "Royal Commission," consisting in part of laymen and partly of medical men, to inquire into the condition of the health of the larger towns and more populous districts of the country, and the best method of improving the public health in all classes of the community.

The beneficent work thus inaugurated was pursued with vigor and skill, and speedily culminated in the adoption, in the main, of the present elaborate system of laws for the protection of the public health which justly places England in the lead of all the nations of the earth in the care of the lives and property of her people from whatever source they may be menaced. This system of laws is there denominated "State Medicine."

The rapid reduction of the death-rate subsequent to the institution and practical application of these laws was so palpable that their propriety was at once placed beyond all doubt, and the general principles involved were promptly extended, until there was scarcely a county within the dominion left without their benefits. The establishment of county hospitals by the nobility and others of ample means followed, and in 1880 there were some three hundred and fifty institutions of that kind in operation within the kingdom—some counties with large manufacturing interests or other centers of population having three or four, while others less crowded had but one.

Sir John Simon, who so long held the position of chief officer of the Local Government Board (which was really the Central Board of Health) reported about this time more than fifteen hundred health organizations, each with its medical health officer, and all discharging their duties under the direction of and reporting to their common head. It is to be regretted that men of ample means in our own country—men who, having availed themselves of our liberal laws to accumulate large fortunes, have not imitated the example of our noble and wealthy English kinsman in the establishment of great charities of this character to a greater extent than they have done.

Sanitary science is subject to some natural and palpable divisions which we may, with propriety, consider. Sir John Simon, the great English author before referred to, says in a report now before me, "a recent American writer" (probably Dr. Bowditch, of Boston) announces as a principle of State medicine "it is the business of governments to do for the mass of individuals those things which cannot be so well done by individual action." This definition is sufficiently comprehensive but somewhat indefinite.

"State medicine" obviously comprises all laws which may be devised for the protection of the health of a State from the introduction of diseases of foreign origin; the protection of its people against the sale of impure foodstuffs and adulterated drugs; the provision of ample facilities for thorough medical education; the protection of the people against the impositions of ignorant pretenders to medical skill; the establishment of eleemosynary institutions for the care of the insane, the blind, deaf mutes and other unfortunates who are unable to care for themselves; the supervision of the sanitary condition of all public works, schools, prisons and private enterprises, which might become inimical to the public health; and, finally, the collection and preservation of the vital statistics of the State as a basis for the study of disease and the provision of means for its abatement. These duties are self-evident and need only to be indicated to secure recognition.

In a representative government like ours, each of its different divisions clearly has its peculiar duty. The national government should be charged with the duty of protecting its people from all diseases of foreign origin; and in default of the performance of that duty it should provide for the isolation and care of such cases whenever and wherever they find lodgment within our borders. The State should assume the duty of protecting her people against the introduction of diseases from one State into another; and in default thereof should provide for the isolation and care of all such cases as are permitted to gain access to the State through the insufficiency of law, or its defective administration. Counties and municipalities should be charged with the duty of maintaining good sanitary conditions within their respective limits, and the care of all such diseases as result from neglect of this duty should devolve upon such counties and municipalities. These duties of the different divisions of our government are so palpable that argument in their support seems to be unnecessary. They are in strict accord with the Constitution of our country; and a system of laws making the country boards the unit of organization, and requiring them to report to a State board; which in turn should be represented in, and required to report to, a national board of

health, would afford at once a more harmonious and practicable method of administering sanitary laws throughout the land than any other organization we can conceive of. A national board of health, so constituted, would afford the most practicable method of securing uniformity in the administration of sanitary laws, not only in the different States, but in the different counties of the several States; and obviate more effectually than any other, the necessity for the inefficient, impracticable and expensive quarantine regulations now so vainly depended upon.

The necessary limits of this paper forbid the consideration on the present occasion, of the application of medical science or its branches to the detection of crime, as a branch of State Medicine. That division of the subject must be reserved for another occasion.

[NOTE.—The facts which form the basis of this paper have been the common property of medical men of moderate reading so long, that credit of the sources from which they have been obtained is deemed unnecessary. Their pertinence to present conditions is so evident that public necessity justifies the work.]

HEBRA'S CONTINUOUS TEPID-WATER BATH.

We find the following very interesting description of this bath in the *Chicago Medical Journal and Examiner*:

THE continuous tepid-water bath occupies a prominent place among the elder Hebra's valuable contributions to general therapeutics. This bath consists of a large bath tub, in which an iron frame with transverse slats is suspended by chains, so that the patient may be withdrawn from and returned to the water by means of a crank. The iron frame is covered with a horsehair mattress, and furnished with comfortable pillows. The patient, perfectly nude—without any surgical dressing whatever—is placed in an easy position upon the mattress, and the bath tub is filled with water of 30-31° C. temperature. A sensation of chilliness is usually experienced at this period, which is immediately dispelled by the rapid elevation of the water's temperature to 38-40° C. The temperature of the bath is permanently maintained at this degree by the continuous renewal of the water. A sheet or other thin covering, may be thrown over the patient, and is useful by reason of its subjective effect.

The patient remains in the bath, day and night, except when withdrawn for the purpose of evacuation of the rectum or the bladder. There is no limit to the period of time which may be spent in the bath without detriment to the general health. Hebra has kept patients in the bath for periods of nine and ten months.

From this brief sketch it will be inferred that the pathological conditions which indicate the continuous tepid-water bath, are numerous and varied.

Burns, gangrenous wounds, bed-sores, and severe cases of pemphigus are notable examples of such conditions.

The best local treatment for burns—especially when a considerable extent of surface is involved—is to be found in the continuous bath. The terrible pain is relieved as by magic, psychic disturbance is quieted and the patient frequently falls into a refreshing sleep. The intense *thirst*—usually developed during the second stage—is slaked, without the imbibition of liquids, which are rejected as soon as swallowed. Of course, in severe burns this method of treatment is too frequently of a merely palliative character; the patient dies in the bath just as he does under other methods of treatment.

When, however, death does not immediately follow the burn, we have a method of local treatment, at once simple, painless, and effective. "The water protects the wound surfaces from contact with the atmospheric air, prevents the decomposition of the sphacelus, and favors its separation; it makes every dressing and change of dressing un-

necessary, limits the secretion of pus, and hastens cicatrization."—*Billroth.*

Gangrenous wounds—especially the "puerperal ulcers" of the vulva and vagina, during the *puerperium:* bed-sores, from all causes, but particularly from spinal injuries, are influenced in the most favorable way. The patient is spared the distress and fatigue of all change of dressing, the wounds receive absolute antiseptic attention, and the attendants are relieved of much tedious and unnecessary labor.

Dermatologists very generally admit that grave cases of pemphigus find the best local treatment in Hebra's continuous bath. The pain, itching and burning sensations of this distressing affection are relieved, and comparative ease and comfort gained. In these cases the action of simple water is both palliative and curative.

As at present informed, there is no hospital in America in which the continuous tepid-water bath of Hebra is an accepted institution. It is difficult to give a good reason for such wilful neglect of an invaluable therapeutic resource. The cost of construction and maintenance is relatively small, so that expense cannot be pleaded as an extenuating circumstance.

CREMATION IN ENGLAND.

AT Golders Green, among the open fields to the north of Hampstead Heath, the London Cremation Company, says the *London News,* has acquired twelve acres of land, which will be set apart for the cremation of the dead. A beautiful chapel is being built, the design of which, by Mr. Ernest Yeates, was exhibited at the Royal Academy this year, and the grounds, instead of being a wilderness of gravestones, will be laid out as a pleasantly wooded garden, surrounded by arched cloisters containing niches for the urns and caskets of the departed.

Up to the present all London cremations have had to be performed at Woking, the distance from London making the expense generally greater than that of a funeral. The actual charge for cremation itself is only £5, and as no grave is required and the coffin should be a mere light shell, the cost is not much greater than that of burial. At present, however, only one cremation a day is the average. If there were half a dozen or more the cost might be greatly reduced. The fuel for heating the furnace alone costs 14s., and the cost of labor and materials would not be more than twice as much for five or six cremations in one day. In Hull, where cremation is performed by the municipality, a charge of a guinea is made.

In all cases the remains are reduced to a pure white ash, the heat being so intense that no smoke or noxious gas is given off. The ashes of a full-sized adult person weigh about five pounds, and in bulk would just about fill an ordinary silk hat. After the cremation the ashes are placed in cinerary urns, caskets, or vases, many of which are of most graceful and artistic design. They are in earthenware, white and colored marble, bronze, or copper. Sometimes they are placed in tombs or sarcophagi, or in cloistered recesses with suitable inscriptions; sometimes the relatives prefer to take them home, or to have them buried at Woking or elsewhere, or even, for sentimental reasons, taken to sea and scattered to the waves. A husband and wife will occasionally leave directions that both are to be cremated after death and their ashes mingled in the same urn.

It was only in 1885, after the Cremation Society had existed for some years, that the use of the crematorium at Woking was first permitted, after strong official opposition. In that year three cremations took place, the body in one case being that of a Brahmin. But since then public prejudice against this form of disposal of the dead has greatly diminished, and last year 300 cremations took place. Probably the new Crematorium close to London will bring about a further increase.

The Roman Catholic Church still prohibits funeral rites over persons who are cremated, but many Catholics on sanitary grounds insist on this form of disposal of their remains. In the case of Jews the ashes are taken to the synagogue after cremation for the religious rites, while Church of England and Nonconformist clergymen and ministers generally hold a funeral service at the crematorium chapel.

One of the commonest popular objections to cremation is that it destroys the evidence of poison, and so facilitates crime. The reply to this is twofold. First, only a very limited number of cases of poisoning, those in which one or two metallic poisons have been used, could be detected for more than a short time after burial. Secondly, in every case of cremation a rigid system of certification both of the fact of death and of its cause is required. Thus any doubt is settled once for all, while under the present slipshod system of registration there is no guarantee that the cause of death has been accurately stated in the first instance. The doctor's certificate, being given to the family of the patient, often glosses over unfortunate facts, such, for instance, as ill-usage or death from alcohol. Proper certification, such as is required for cremation, would also prevent the dread possibility of the burial of the living.

On sanitary grounds the old system of burial has few defenders. The advocates of "earth to earth" burial point out that interring the body in a light wicker or other shell will cause it to be resolved into its elements much more quickly than if it were encased in a heavy coffin. But a quickening of the process of putrefaction does not diminish the total amount of contamination of earth and air and water.

To make burial a healthy and sanitary process is impossible where any large number of interments have to be provided for. Whether a body is to be consumed by fire or by slow underground decay the end is the same. By the agency of oxygen it has to be converted into its elements of mineral ash, gases and water. In an ideal burial a body should be placed in a light, porous soil, sufficiently deep above to render innocuous gases which escape to the air, and sufficiently deep below thoroughly to filter all escaping water before it reaches any underground channel. Then every shower of rain which saturates the soil will sink gradually down, carrying dissolved oxygen and drawing after it, as it drains away, new air from above. Oxidation will go on steadily and no harm will be done.

How different the conditions in the great cemeteries which encircle London, and around which populous suburbs are springing up! In the first place, most of these cemeteries are in clay soil. Nothing more utterly insanitary than a clay grave could well be devised. It is a watertight pit, dug in an impermeable soil, filled with broken and permeable material, and with a corpse at the bottom. Sometimes these pits are fourteen or fifteen feet deep, and contain as many as half-a-dozen superimposed coffins. The first fall of rain fills the bottom of the pit, the liquid has no escape, and as all dissolved oxygen is at once used up, anaerobic putrefaction of the most offensive type sets up in the body lying in the liquid. No fresh atmospheric oxygen can reach the coffins. When there is heavy rain the grave fills up, and the offensive liquid flows off on the surface to do unknown injury; while a hot, dry period gradually dries out the grave and causes a continual ascent of contaminating vapors into the air. If the grave is drained either at or near the bottom things are little better, for there is no porous soil to render harmless the escaping water, which flows into some channel from which it may do enormous harm.

This is true of a single clay grave, but what of the thousands of nameless dead herded together in the "common" graves of our London cemeteries, often with only a few inches of soil for decency's sake between coffin and coffin? Not a pretense of any protection by the soil can exist in such cases; the whole ground is saturated with corruption. London has now 100,000 burials per annum, enough to cover twelve acres of ground with graves without a footpath between. Practically all these interments take place in suburbs where the population is growing by leaps and bounds. Just as the old churchyards of the city have had to be cleared of their dead, so in a generation or so, unless cremation is soon adopted, we shall be faced with the tremendous problem of clearing Finchley and Highgate, Norwood, Tooting, and Nunhead.

THE FUTURE OF MEDICAL PRACTICE.

ACCORDING to the *New York Medical Journal:* A few years ago a young woman came to New York to pursue a course of study which would oblige her to stay here most of the time for rather a long period. Being a prudent person, she sought to insure her happiness as much as possible during her sojourn in a strange place. With this end in view, she asked her family physician for advice as to whom she should have recourse in case of illness. He gave her the names of a number of eminent specialists, but not that of a single general practitioner. Shortly after the girl arrived, when she had made a few acquaintances, she said to one of them: "My doctor has recommended a number of specialists to me, so that I know whom to go to if there's anything the matter with my eyes, with my skin, with my throat, with my nose, and so on, but the question I should like to have answered is, Whom shall I call in when I'm sick?"

This little tale represents rather accurately the perplexity into which the growth of specialism has cast many members of the community, but there is another side to the matter, that, namely, which involves the question of what is to become of the general practitioner. This problem has been discussed not a little, but by nobody so well, it strikes us, as by Dr. George E. Francis, of Worcester, in his recent annual discourse before the Massachusetts Medical Society, entitled "Medical Prospects." Dr. Francis is no pessimist, but while, like all the rest of us, he appreciates the work of the specialist in advancing medicine as a whole, he clearly recognizes the peril of the family doctor from the florid development of specialism—peril both from the educational point of view and from that of making a living. In the medical schools, he says, the division of the curriculum is constantly growing more and more minute; every endeavor is made by each instructor to render his own field so interesting in itself that, in the plenitude of attractive subjects of study, few of the students are likely to bear in mind that the main object of the study of medicine is not the microscopic investigation of some or all of the component parts, but that study of the separate departments is preliminary and subsidiary to that of medicine as a whole and to that of a man as a whole. "Medicine," he continues, "viewed as a science or as an art, is something far higher than a patchwork of its separate departments, precisely as man is far more than the joining together of a certain number of organs." It is, therefore, to be regretted that the increasing numerical preponderance in the teaching staff of specialists over men trained to view things broadly is making it every year more nearly impossible to so educate the student and so stock him with knowledge as to fit him for the general practice of medicine.

Dr. Francis takes a new view of the proposition that a student who intends to become a specialist ultimately should first spend some years in general practice; at least till he sheds a new light on it. He admits its excellence from the theoretical point of view, but he throws great doubt upon its general practicability. The point he makes is this: An absolute wall divides specialism from general practice. Over that wall nobody can climb gradually; if he is to pass it at all, he must vault over it. In other words, if a man in general practice attempts to glide slowly into a specialty, his fellow-practitioners will at once detect the effort, and, in self-defense, decline to send him patients as a specialist so long as he does any general practice, and specialists, as we all know, are largely dependent on

practice sent to them by the family doctors.

As to the effect of predominant specialism upon the general physician's means of making a livelihood, Dr. Francis entertains the common forebodings, and he even suggests that the time is not far away when the family doctor's advice will no longer be asked as to the choice of a specialist. This omission, he intimates, will first be made by the wealthy, and the example will soon be followed by the large class of those who are neither rich nor so very poor as to depend on the hospitals and dispensaries, but these latter will probably find exclusive dependence on specialists too expensive and return to the present order of things. However, there is a silver lining to the cloud depicted by Dr. Francis. "Very probably," he says, "the family doctor is about to be eclipsed for a time, perhaps to reappear later in a more glorified aspect."

FUTURE INCREASE OF OUR POPULATION.

THE remarkable increase of population predicted for the United States by Dr. H. S. Pritchett in a recent article in the *Popular Science Monthly* was noted not long ago in these columns. From a study of the past increase, the writer attempted to deduce the law governing it, and this law was then applied to estimate the future increase. This process, which is called by mathematicians "extrapolation," is acknowledged by them to be exceedingly risky, even in pure mathematics, and it is doubly so in application to matters where future conditions are imperfectly known. In a communication to the magazine in which Dr. Pritchett's article appeared, Charles E. Woodruff, an officer in the regular army, asserts that the writer has not even taken into account some very well-known conditions. He says:

"He does not seem to have taken into consideration the density of population and what we might call the saturation-point, or the maximum population which can be fed.

A population far below its saturation-point will increase rapidly, but when it saturates the land there is no increase, and as we approach our saturation-point our rate will rapidly diminish to zero.

"We do not know what our saturation-point is under the present conditions of food production; but we produce far more than is needed for our twenty people per square mile. Nor can we estimate our future saturation-point, for no one can presume to predict what science will enable us to do in the way of food production, other than what, by present methods, can be forced from the soil. We can only estimate our limit, basing it upon the known densities in countries which have always been populated to their limit.

"The saturation-point rises with civilization just as the saturation-point of air for water rises with the temperature. Cultivated land is said to produce 1,600 times as much food as an equal area of hunting land. Denmark, for instance, could support but 500 paleolithic people, and when their culture rose to the level of the present Patagonians, 1,000 could exist, and 1,500 of those on the level of the natives of Hudson's Bay. In the pastoral stage each family requires 2,000 acres, and France could not support 50,000 of such people. For centuries after the Norman conquest the whole of Europe could not support 100,000,000, or about 25 per square mile, while now there are 81."

The saturation-point may remain stationary in an arrested civilization, the writer notes. China, for instance, is said to have had 400,000,000 for many centuries. On the other hand, in lands where food can be bought from abroad and paid for by manufactured goods, the population can go beyond the saturation-point. Great Britain is said to import one-third of her food, and her 300 people per mile place her far beyond the point of saturation. When the countries from which she buys have no surplus for sale, her population must decrease to about 200 per mile, which is all that she can feed. Should her factories fail through foreign competition, so that she can not buy, she will also decrease in population, just as Ireland has done since the beginning of the last century. The writer goes on to say:

"America was saturated by savages in pre-Columbian times, and they were constantly at war for more room; but the land has always been far from saturation for civilized whites. Though we now export enough food for a large population, we can not produce very much more, for all the useful land is now taken up. Fully sixty per cent. of the desert lands west of the 100th degree of longitude will never have water on it, and that alone will forever prevent us being as densely populated as Europe. Perhaps we can now support fully 125,000,000, or 34 per mile, a point which Dr. Pritchett calculates we shall reach in 1925, at our present rate. By that time we shall have farms on ten or fifteen per cent. of the arid lands, the limit of possible irrigation, and perhaps then we can support 200,000,000, the calculated population for 1950; but it is difficult to see how we can feed 500,000,000, our calculated numbers a little over a century hence, for that would be a density of about 125 per mile—far greater than Europe.

"It is also difficult to see how science is to produce food indefinitely, for the real basis of food production is the soil and vegetation, such as the changing of cellulose into starches and sugars. The possible limit is the amount of the sun's energy we can capture through vegetation. The calculated population of a thousand years hence, 41,000,000,000, or 11,000 per mile, is not at present conceivable."

The law of population, the writer points out, is that its increase depends upon its density, irrespective of the birth-rate. At the saturation-point the death-rate and the birth-rate must be equal, as they are now in China, where there is at the same time a large birth-rate and also frightful destruction of life by pestilence, famine, and murder. He goes on to say:

"Our civilization will never tolerate such

mortality, nor can the surplus migrate, as it has been doing from Europe for four hundred years. Yet we need have no fear of future famines and pestilence due to overcrowding and so necessary in India and China, for the solution of the problem will come of its own accord in a natural limitation of the·size of families. . . . By the time we have reached our maximum growth it is quite likely that the number of children in American families will be less than three, or just enough to compensate for unavoidable deaths and still keep the population stationary. The deliberations of the Malthusian societies may appear very absurd, but they are merely discussing things which are sure to come about naturally and not artificially.

"Thus Dr. Pritchett's estimates of our future population of 11,000 per square mile being based upon the rates of increase in a country far below.its saturation-point, it seems that a better formula could have been obtained by taking the increases in European countries which probably have been saturated ever since the glacial times and supersaturated ever since they became maritime powers and could import food. Thus England had 5,500,000 in 1650, and only 6,500,000 in 1750, and less than 9,000,000 in 1800; since then, through food importations due to commerce, her rate of increase has been about thirteen per cent..per decade. Our rate, as above stated, was thirty-two per cent. in 1800, twenty-four per cent. in 1880, and the time it will be thirteen may be long before 1990, and it is quite likely to be zero with a century or two.

"Our country will never contain more people than it can feed, and the struggle for existence or the stress of life will not be a particle more severe than now. Since the first paleolithic man appeared on the scene, Europe has supported as many men as she could and has thus been at the saturation-point, ever on the verge of over-population, needing famines, wars of expansion, and other forms of death, so that there has always been the same struggle for existence we see now, and that struggle can never

be more severe than it has always been there. The course of civilization would even justify a prediction that life will be made easier, so that posterity may pity us as we pity our savage ancestors in their terrible struggle for existence."—*Literary Digest.*

HOW TO LIVE 100 YEARS.
By Bernard Morris, Centenarian.

Don't chew.
Don't smoke. .
Don't drink.
Eat only moderately.
Take plenty of rest and sleep.
Place implicit faith in God, who promises to care for all mankind.

"How do I feel on my one hundred and seventh birthday?" repeated Bernard Morris, the oldest employee in Greater New York, when a *World* reporter greeted him yesterday.

"Why, my lad, I feel as young and chipper as I did fifty years ago!"

And Barney—he is known by every one as Barney—looks as young to-day as he says he feels.

Born in County Cavan, Ireland, on June 10, 1792, Barney remained on a farm with his father until he was thirty-two years old. Then he came to America to try his fortune and settled in Brooklyn. He was a coach driver until eight years ago. Then he went to work for the city as a paper-picker in Prospect Park. Every day he can be seen around the picnic house mingling with the children, stopping a moment now and then to grasp the hands of old friends and to give advice to inquiring ones who stop to study the old man and listen with interest to his life story.

Barney is as sturdy as an oak. His hands and face are badly wrinkled, but his step is firm, his voice even, his eyesight much better than that of many men not half his age, and his hair only streaked with gray. He arises at 6 o'clock every morning, goes to work at 8, and labors steadily until 5 o'clock. Then he takes a car home, enjoys a hearty dinner with Mrs. Morris, reads the evening papers, and is in bed by 8 o'clock.

"I attribute my longevity to total abstinence from whiskey and tobacco," said Barney, "moderate eating, plenty of sleep and faith in God, who has promised to care for all.

"I never took but one drink of rum in my life. It was at a county fair in Ireland. I'll never forget the feeling I experienced, and I vowed never to take another drink. I read about people living to be one hundred years old who drink, smoke and chew. I tell you it is not necessary to do these things. I am a living example of a man who never touched them, and I am as well, strong and healthy as one could want to be.

"When I came to Brooklyn, in 1824, I was employed as a private coachman, after which I went into the hack business, driving carriages of my own. My first stand was at Fulton ferry, and my last at the Brooklyn City Hall. I was ninety-one years old when I quit the carriage business and went to work for the city.

"When I came to Brooklyn it was a small town. There were only eight churches here and not a brick building. Just beyond where the City Hall now stands was a wooden picnic ground called Post's Military Garden. In the summer people lived in tents in the woods around what is now Prospect Park.

"You may talk about your hold-ups in the West. Why, it was just as bad out around Jamaica when I first drove a cab there. I carried a pistol by my side and all the passengers had revolvers handy to repulse highwaymen."

Barney lives with his third wife, Mrs. Mary Morris, at No. 364 Warren street, Brooklyn. She has been his constant helpmeet and companion for thirty-nine years. He was sixty-eight and she only twenty-one years old when they were married.

"I don't know why I ever married my old man," said Mrs. Morris to a *World* reporter yesterday. "I was just a slip of a girl when I came to this country. One day I saw him with an eighteen-year-old girl, and I said to my mother, 'Mother, what does that young girl go with such an old man for; is he her father?'

"'Why, they are sparkin',' she replied.

"I didn't know what 'sparkin'' meant until mother explained that it was what we called 'courting' in the old country. In a few weeks I was introduced to the old man. I liked him from the start. I don't know why it was, but something just took hold of me, and I didn't care for any one else. So we were married, and he has made the best husband in the world. Not a cross word between us in all these years.

"Barney had to work to-day, but I haven't forgot his birthday. I have prepared a little surprise, and to-morrow all our friends will be here to celebrate the event."

WAS THE BOXER OUTBREAK AN ATTACK OF HYSTERIA?

EVERY abnormal phenomenon is treated nowadays from the standpoint of pathology; naughtiness in the child and drunkenness in the adult are alike regarded as, in a way, manifestations of disease. Now comes a French physician, Dr. J. Matignon, who asserts that the Boxers are nothing more than hysterical patients, and that this disease is one to which the Chinese, despite their proverbial calmness, are particularly prone. Dr. Matignon first calls our attention to the fact that most writers on Chinese subjects have contented themselves with very superficial observation. It is his opinion that hysteria is very widespread in China, notwithstanding the dictum of the average traveler that the race is patient, calm, and phlegmatic. The Chinese, he says, are children, from the Emperor down; they are marked especially by naiveté, credulity, and suggestibility, and also by impulsiveness, though one would not suspect this at first sight. Other characteristics are versatility of character, complete absence of precise ideas, and comparative insensibility to bodily pain. The author goes on to say:

"These mental and bodily phenomena have long made me suspect that hysteria was common in China. In the beginning of the spring of 1900 I undertook an investigation on the subject. . . . More than three hundred subjects were examined, and I proposed to extend my researches to three or four thousand cases. The serious events at Peking not only put a stop to my studies but caused my notes to disappear. The results that are at my disposal are therefore more in the nature of impressions and recollections than of precise statistical documents. My impression—which is shared by numbers of my fellow physicians who have practised in China—is that nervous disease is extremely common among the Celestials. . . . The fact that hysteria exists, and that we can easily find its chief symptoms throughout a great part of the population, seems to me to have a certain importance, and throws a new light on some phases of the moral history of the famous Boxers who have spread fire and sword over the north of China. Suggestion and hysteria have played the chief parts in the propagation of their doctrines and the recruiting of their adepts.

"It is far from my idea to show that the Boxer movement is only a manifestation of hysteria; nerve disease has been a secondary factor in it, although an important one. . . . The party chiefs, for the most part sincere, have found a rich soil in Chinese credulity and suggestibility. . . . In all their proclamations there is something of mystery, especially for simple minds. The Chinese believes the more as he understands less, and when he does not understand at all his faith becomes absolute.

"The natural suggestibility of the Chinese was raised to the paroxysmal point this last year. The whole Middle Kingdom was in a state of tense anxiety like that which the advent of the year 1000 must have produced in Europe. The year 1900 was to have an intercalary month; this was a grave omen, as had been proved by experience. . . . Suggestibility was exaggerated; every one felt its influence and in turn exerted it upon others."

The author goes on to recount the rapid increase of the Boxers, their rites, their initiations, etc., and sees in each the regular symptoms of hysteria, which would account also for their fanatical bravery. What is the remedy? Says M. Matignon:

"What suggestion has made it can unmake. When the court and the nobility show the Boxers no more favor, demonstrate that they believe no longer in their supernatural power, and proclaim that the foreigners are not doing injury to the country, the Celestial empire will be convinced. But I fear that the court, and especially the high officials, will not attempt to work thus by suggestion for a long time."—*The Literary Digest.*

SEASICKNESS.

In the many discussions which have taken place from time to time as to the cause of seasickness a strong tendency has manifested itself for the disputants to take onesided views. Some have maintained that the whole affection was an affair of vision, or of disturbance of equilibrium in the semicircular canals, or of derangement of the circulation in the brain, while not a few practically minded people, with their eyes fixed upon the final product as seen in the steward's basin, have held that bile is always at the bottom of the mischief. The truth is that no one of these explanations covers the entire field, while no one of them can be entirely neglected, and that seasickness is the summation of the effect of the motion of the ship upon a number of sensitive organs—in fact, upon the whole body. Some of these effects we cannot eliminate, some we can. By lying down we can to a certain extent lessen the effect upon the cerebral circulation, by shutting the eyes we can eliminate the effect on the visual center, and by carefully swaddling the abdomen in a long and wide flannel bandage one can to a considerable degree lessen the internal swashing of the intestinal contents. There is another point, however, to be considered, and that is the condition of the abdominal viscera at the time of starting. Dr. James Wortobet tells us that he has traveled more than 100,000 nautical miles, and has usually had under care several hundred passengers besides the crew. He therefore speaks from experience when he says that although there may be certain cases which are of cerebral origin, such cases are in the minority, and that in the majority of cases the symptoms start from the abdomen. People who are well inured to sea life and are usually quite free from sickness, may still suffer if they go to sea with loaded bowels, and he is quite sure that by the precautions often taken by experienced travelers they do, in fact, protect themselves from seasickness which would otherwise occur, such precautions being the taking of a saline purgative the day or so before traveling, adopting the recumbent posture, and avoiding oleaginous smells and the company of those who are seasick. He strongly advises those who suffer principally from gastric phenomena to provide themselves with a good flannel bandage, twelve feet long and six inches broad, and wind it around their trunk over the whole width of the abdominal region. This will afford great comfort by preventing the contents of the abdomen viscera from undue movements. He also says that for severe retching and persistent sickness nothing is so trustworthy as a hypodermic injection of morphine. [But it's dangerous! Ed. Gazette.]

There are about 2,500 hospitals and asylums in the United States. These give employment to 65,000 people and pay over $23,000,000 in salaries. These hospitals have 300,000 beds, are attended by 37,500 physicians, and treat over 1,000,000 patients during the year.

CHLORETONE INTERNALLY AND EXTERNALLY.

By P. H. Sumner, M.D.,

Camptown, Pa.

As an humble illustration of the general utility of chloretone in the usual course of routine practice I wish to cite the histories of two cases.

The first of these was a case of delirium tremens which had been under medical treatment, but, as I was informed, the patient had not slept for three weeks. I prescribed 20-grain doses of chloretone, to be given every three hours until eight doses in all had been taken. The result was the patient slept for ten hours and when he awoke the delirium had disappeared. Twenty grains of chloretone was given the succeeding night, which produced eleven hours' sleep. From that time on for about a week the treatment consisted of 1-30 grain of strychnine nitrate every four hours, when the case was dismissed.

The second case was that of a man whose hand had been caught in a grain binder. The packer had been forced through the center of the hand, tearing out between the middle and ring fingers. After the accident the man drove several miles from his farm to my office. Upon arrival his first statement was that the injury was so very painful that he wished I would apply something to relieve him while making preparation for the dressing.

I at once placed some absorbent cotton wet with a solution of chloretone upon each surface of the hand, and in a few minutes was asked by the patient what that was which I had used. "Why do you ask?" said I. "Because it has taken all the pain out of my hand," was the reply.

I then washed the wound with a bichloride solution, dusted it thoroughly with chloretone and covered the whole with absorbent cotton which was kept in place by means of a roller bandage. Three subsequent similar dressings at intervals of four days completed my treatment. The wound healed without pain or suppuration.

EPIDEMIC HYPNOTIC CRIMINAL SUGGESTION.

Says *American Medicine*: A child returned from a public execution to imitate after the manner of children, what he had seen, and killed himself by hanging. An epidemic of family murder by drowning helpless children is said to be prevalent in London. Several atrocious crimes of the Guldensuppe type followed, in New York, that terrible murder. In some part of the world there is almost every week chronicled these instances of epidemic crime incited by morbid suggestion derived from public or published initial examples. The newspapers give sinful accounts of the sins and thus encourage them. Pathologic suggestion and its dangers are facts the profession should urge upon legislators. Professor Gregory, of Iowa, says: "The excited reflection upon a shocking act by many thousands of persons, including numbers of low intelligence and morale, operates as a dangerous hypnotic suggestion to the crime." In the last five years there have been about 40,000 murders in the United period there have been but 597 legal executions. If capital punishment has the deterrent effect claimed for it, there should have been vastly more of them. We think they do not have that effect, but exactly the opposite one, and are certain it is so as to public executions.

INDIA'S DEATH BILL FROM NOXIOUS ANIMALS.

THE statistics of the Indian Empire, according to the *Medical Press* of March 20, 1901, bring home the responsibility of governing so vast a dependency. The last annual report of the government of India showed that no less than 2,966 persons died in the preceding year from the attacks of wild beasts, and 24,621 from snake bites. The increased number of deaths from the latter cause was partly attributed to the floods, which drove the snakes to the higher ground where the natives dwelt. Tigers killed 899 persons, wolves 238, bears 95, elephants 40, hyenas 27, jackals, crocodiles, and other wild animals 1,230. In addition, no fewer than 100,000 head of cattle were killed by predaceous animals, and 9,449 by snakes. On the other side of the balance 1,570 tigers, 4,538 leopards, 2,317 wolves, 776 hyenas, and 94,548 snakes were killed. Sir Joseph Fayrer, the great authority on Indian snakes, states that in the treatment of venomous snake-bite the only hope is to prevent the entry of the poison into the circulation by applying a tight bandage where possible and cutting out the bitten part. He appears not to have arrived at any satisfactory conclusion as to why nature should have endowed these creatures with so deadly a poison, which was not wanted for procuring food, since both innocent and poisonous snakes eat the same kind of food and swallow it in exactly the same kind of way. There can be little doubt that sooner or later progressive science will find a satisfactory antidote for the venom of snakes.

HOT AIR AS A THERAPEUTIC AGENT.

ORRIN S. WIGHTMAN, in the *New York Medical Journal*, says that:

Dry heat is a valuable pain-reliever without any of the depressant effects common to drugs.

In connection with constitutional and medicinal treatment, we have in it a positive curative agent.

It is a stimulant to rapid repair and absorption.

It is one of the most valuable eliminative agents we possess.

Where indicated, it possesses a sedative action on the nervous system obtained by no other means.

"TO REGENERATE THE HUMAN SPECIES."

According to a Paris Dispatch to *The New York Times,* a certain Count St. Ouen de Pierrecourt, who died recently, bequeathed to the city of Rouen his fortune of ten million francs—$2,000,000—on the novel condition that the city shall annually give a marriage present of 100,000 francs to a couple of giants, in order to regenerate the human species. The candidates are to be medically examined, and the healthiest couple must be chosen.

Unfortunately, gigantism and health very seldom go together. Had the French gentleman left his millions for the purpose of scientific education, much more might be accomplished, for even if a nation of persons of great size could be produced—which is improbable—they would present most of the characteristics of the giants of to-day, many of whom are monstrosities.

QUINSY.

Prof. Sajous, Philadelphia, says: Seen in the first twenty-four hours: Take every three hours one drachm of ammoniated tincture of guaiac to a teaspoonful of milk; gargle and swallow. After the third or fourth dose, the swelling of the tonsil subsides and the patient is much relieved; most likely he will have a diarrhea; this is the time to reduce the tincture to one-half drachm. When the case goes thirty-six hours without interference the treatment is different and difficult. Allow small pieces of ice in the mouth, while internally twenty grains of bromide of potassium combined with fifteen drops of wine of ergot, or six drops of tincture of belladonna every three hours, although the latter frequently causes headache; if the tonsil has a tendency to go to abscess, do not let it rupture spontaneously; find tender spot with finger; take curved bistoury and open, not cutting deeply; bind bistoury with cloth.

AN EXPLANATION OF THE FUNCTION OF THE PINEAL BODY.

The pineal body (sometimes called a gland), now named the epiphysis, was regarded by Descartes as the seat of the soul. Descartes, however, has been dead for about three hundred years, and our ideas concerning the soul have changed very considerably. The pineal body has recently been discovered to be a developmental remnant of a third eye, the elements of which have been distinctly traced in the New Zealand reptile, the sphenodon (or hatteria) by Mr. Baldwin Spencer. This pineal body occurs in all vertebrates, except the very lowest. In the hatteria it reaches the skin on the top of the head, and retains distinct traces of an eye-like formation—for instance, a complex retina. As the same vestigial hint of eye-structure has now been observed in several lizards, many naturalists are convinced that the pineal body in all animals is, in reality, the remnant of a parietal eye —an upward-looking sense-organ.—*Exchange.*

PASSIFLORA INCARNATA IN WHOOPING-COUGH.

Dr. Carties states that passiflora incarnata, a remedy little used in whooping-cough, serves well for sleeplessness, spasms, and certain nervous phenomena. Frequently when lying down at night the attacks are worse, and hyoscyamus, belladonna and conium will not serve as well as passiflora, five drops of the tincture at bedtime.

Another plan is to give two drops of the tincture immediately after each attack until the total quantity taken in the night is from six to twelve drops. The preparation of the tincture is important—it should be made from the wild plant and not the cultivated variety. To be sure that you obtain a reliable article, ask for Daniel's Conct. Passiflora Incarnata. There is the same difference between the aconite of the mountains and the garden variety.

SANITARY RULES TO GOVERN BARBER SHOPS.

THE HEALTH BOARD of San Francisco, Cal., recently sent the following rules to the supervisors to be adopted as an ordinance, and they will also be submitted to the State Barber Examiners for approval:

Mugs and shaving brushes shall be sterilized by immersion in boiling water after every separate use thereof.

Razors shall be wiped with alcohol both before and after they have been used.

Hair brushes known as "sanitary brushes" must be used after first being sterilized.

Razor strops must be kept clean and never wiped off with the hand or blown upon with the breath.

A separate clean towel shall be used for each person.

Barbers shall not blow away with breath any hairs after cutting, but use a towel or bulb or hairbrush.

Barbers shall keep their fingernails short-cut and clean; alum or other material used to stop the flow of blood shall be so used only in powder form and applied on a towel.

The use of powder-puffs, finger-bowls and sponges is prohibited.

No person shall be allowed to use any barber shop as a dormitory.

All barbers' instruments must be disinfected after using.

These rules shall be placed in a conspicuous place in the shops.—*American Medicine.*

A NEW THEORY OF LONGEVITY.

A NEW theory of longevity has lately made its appearance. "A man has a definite number of waking hours allotted to him," says the originator of the most recent idea, "and the fewer he uses up the longer will his life last. If, therefore, he is content to sleep for most of his days, there is no reason why he should not live for two hundred years." He adduces the case of the negroes as an illustration. The chances are that the only truth in this theory is the well-recognized fact that less than eight hours sleep is not sufficient for most mortals, and that those who habitually take less shorten their lives by so doing. But even if this novel elixir of life were what it claims to be, one may doubt whether the prescribed existence would be worth living. To our mind, the allotted three-score and ten years, without excessive sleep, would be preferable.—*Exchange.*

MILD CLIMATES AND CENTENARIANS.

IT is not surprising that more people live to be over 100 years old in warm climates than in the higher latitudes. The German Empire, with 55,000,000 population, has 778 centenarians. France, with 40,000,000, has 213. England has only 146; and Scotland, 46. Sweden has 10; Norway, 23; Belgium, 5; Denmark, 2; Spain, 401, and Switzerland none. Servia, with a population of 2,250,000, has 575 people over 100 years old. It is claimed that the oldest living person, one Bruno Cotrim, living in Rio de Janeiro, is 150 years old. He was born in Africa.

A BLIND PHYSICIAN.

DR. ROBERT H. BABCOCK, of Chicago, is one of the leading authorities in the West on tuberculosis and kindred pulmonary troubles. Yet since he was thirteen years old he has not seen a beam of sunlight. An accident led to blindness, and for thirty-six years he has acquired knowledge in darkness with almost as much readiness as would the ordinary man who sees. Dr. Babcock was born in Watertown, N. Y., forty-nine years ago. He obtained the degree of M.D. at the Chicago Medical College in 1878, following it with another degree of M.D. from the College of Physicians and Surgeons of New York in 1879. He was one of the ten honor men among 120 students in his class of '79. In 1880 he went to Germany and continued his medical studies for three years. After his return to Chicago he took up the practice of medicine and has won for himself a high reputation. Most of his present practice is in consultation with other physicians.—*Chicago Tribune.*

CATCHING COLD.

A REFORM is greatly needed in respect to "catching cold." Let the demon be exorcised first from the medical, and next from the popular mind! Let it be generally known and believed that few diseases are referable to the agency of cold, and that even the affection commonly called "a cold" is generally caused by other agencies; or, perhaps, by a special agent which may prove to be a microbe. Let the axiom, "a fever patient never catches cold," be reiterated until it becomes a household phrase! Let the restorative influence of cool, fresh, pure atmosphere be inculcated! Let it be understood that in therapeutics, as in hygiene, the single word *comfort* embodies the principles which should regulate coverings and clothing. Non-medicinal therapeutics will have gained much when this reform is accomplished. If most persons outside of the medical profession were to be asked what they considered as chiefly to be avoided in the management of sick people, the answer would probably be "catching cold." I suspect that this question would be answered in the same way by not a few physicians. Hence it is that sick-rooms are poorly ventilated, and patients are oppressed by a superabundance of garments and bedclothes. The air which patients are made to breathe, having been already breathed and rebreathed, is loaded with pulmonary exhalations. Cutaneous emanations are allowed to remain in contact with the body, as well as to pervade the atmosphere. Free exposure of the body is deemed hazardous, and still more so bathing or sponging, the entire surface of the body being exposed. Patients not confined to bed, especially those affected with pulmonary disease, are overloaded with clothing which becomes saturated with perspiration, and is seldom changed for fear of the dreaded "cold."—*Flint.*

CONCERNING THE HAND.

ONE of the most common signs of want of good breeding is a sort of uncomfortable consciousness of the hands, an obvious ignorance of what to do with them and a painful awkwardness in their adjustment. The hands of a gentleman seem perfectly at home without being occupied; they are habituated to elegant repose, or if they spontaneously move it is attractively. Some of Queen Elizabeth's courtiers made playing with their sword hilts an accomplishment, and the most efficient weapon of the Spanish coquette is her fan. Strength in the fingers is a sure token of mental aptitude. When Mutius burned his hand off before the eyes of his captors he gave the most indubitable proof we can imagine of fortitude, and it was natural that amid the ferocious bravery of feudal times a bloody hand in the center of an escutcheon should become the badge of a baronet of England.

AN interesting case of laboratory infection with bubonic plague was that which developed in a young man working in the laboratory of the University of Michigan. Dr. Novy (*American Journal of the Medical Sciences*, October, 1901) in reporting the case details the extreme violence and rapidity of the onset of his symptoms and relates the immediately good effect produced by large injections of Yersin's antipest serum. All told, the patient received within twenty-four hours 120 c.c. of serum, 1 dram injected intravenously. The case was plague of the pneumonic type. The patient recovered entirely, although extreme cardiac weakness existed for some time (more than two months) after the disease.

Department of Physical Education.

WITH SPECIAL REGARD TO SYMMETRICAL DEVELOPMENT OF THE BODY

MENTAL THERAPEUTICS.

FROM a long and valuable article contributed to the *Southern California Practitioner* by Dr. Norman Bridge upon this subject, we quote as follows:

A certain new few cardinal things are, I believe, necessary to be done in the care and culture of the people, and they are mental and moral mostly.

1. We must lessen the emotional attentions to infants. These wear out the brain energy and produce erethism that may last through life. Almost any infant can, in three months, be developed into an autocrat; and many of them have, before the end of the first year, true neurasthenia resulting from these influences.

2. As far as possible we ought to let the children alone, and stop the common incessant effort to entertain them. The effort continues the vicious effects of too much emotional attention in infancy. Let them entertain themselves; this will develop their minds and rest their emotions. We must observe them and talk about them in their presence less. Otherwise we are sure to provoke a series of most vicious emotions that grow into habits that influence them in a bad direction through life. Fairy tales and fairy talk are unwholesome. The average child already has too much imagination; it is a beautiful thing, but it is not necessary to increase it. There are difficulties with these rules for infants and children. Two motives actuate parents and children alike. The first is to make and have the children happy and pleasant now. The reflex effect on their elders is sweet; we like a happy child, and like to make a child happy. Thus we and the child conspire to the same end.

The second motive is to make sure that if possible the career of the child shall be long and successful. Both emotions are for the rising individual as we understand it, the one for the now, and the other for the future. Is it any wonder that we should generally sacrifice the future for the present? The child is incapable of foregoing a present pleasure for a future good, and the parents are too ready to agree not to count this day's indulgence when they know its ulterior effect is bad. The mother carries the child for hours to get it to sleep, not because it is necessary, but because it likes to be carried and refuses to sleep without it. She says the baby will not go to sleep otherwise, but if she thinks she knows this to be a tender-hearted fiction, her fault is lack of courage to break the habit. As the child gets older and begins to acquire habits that she fears may make him inelegant or impolite she has no hesitation in working for his future and she will drill him by the hour and worry by the day about his manners (that at fifteen he would spontaneously correct) and let him go on with nervous injuries that will last him through life. Parents think it a terrible thing if their boys smoke cigarettes, but they have allowed habits of the nervous system from babyhood up that are even worse for the future of a boy than smoking cigarettes in his teens. Parents who have perpetually entertained, coddled, and diverted their children, who have jumped to their call as to the command of a superior being, are by logic and nature estopped from objecting to cigarettes, coffee, wine or late hours, when they pass into youth and would still gratify their desires for all sorts of stimulating amusements. None of these sins against nature is so great as those that have been earlier fostered and encouraged. Indeed, had their earlier sins never been committed many of these later indulgences would not be sought. The exaltation due to the earlier mistakes cannot be ignored in later life.

Parents plead that their children ought to be obedient and self-denying as to indulgences that harm, because they, the parents, have been good to them in their infancy and childhood, have found amusements and pleasures for them, and denied them little or nothing of joy. This is the very gist of the sin they have committed. If the emotional propensities of the children had received as much tranquil rest as their muscles did, their brains would have grown up with more normal demands and with better resisting power.

3. We ought to stop making young ladies and gentlemen out of children. To push them into responsible social life, as early as is the rule in the best social stratum, is to develop emotions and cares, and subject them to tests and temptations that ought to be postponed for years. And the only justification we have for it is our and their unwholesome pleasure in all, and their hoped-for salvation from diffidence later. The truth is that the diffidence is an advantage and ought to be encouraged rather than otherwise.

4. We ought to minify the emotional struggles at school as far as possible. The strife for supremacy, the fear of failure, the envy and jealousy of others, constitute one of the most wearing tendencies on the brains of the young. Not all, by any means, but many of the school children suffer in this way. It is a duty to find out the ones most being harmed and worked for their lives.

5. An increase of the outdoor, athletic lives of the people as a whole would be one of the greatest gains of all. Indoor life keeps us below the par physiological, and to raise the standard of the system as a whole of course helps the brains.

To reduce and repress the unhappy emo-

tions that are engendered by the struggle to shine in society and in business, is one of the urgent needs, and hardest services to render. These emotions are envy, jealousy, fear of failure, sense of danger to our pride, all of which are wearing and depressing. This is the school experience carried into adult life; and with all its ramifications it does incalculable harm to the cerebral resisting power. To reduce the struggle itself as well as its bad emotions is quite as important. This ardor to do the duties that society and business seem to impose on us (and beyond the getting of bread) is not the whole cause of nervous overwork among men and women, but it is a very large influence in that direction.

When a woman gets neurasthenia from so-called nervous overwork, the chances are six in ten that the excess of work was a demand of some sort of social fiction, and was thus by the highest ethics unnecessary. With men the percentage is only a little less.

7. Less dress-parade in our lives is necessary. Reduce the everlasting dressing of our bodies, houses, tables and equipages. It all becomes a bugbear to the tired-out brain, and it tires the brain. It is what makes women say they feel like going crazy to think of packing their trunks for a trip to a fashionable resort, and it makes some of them really crazy. Such parade is a silly demand that our conceit and envy makes upon us, to the worry of the tired brains.

8. It is merely a truism to say that people who are carrying mind and body loads that are too heavy should have them lightened. If the load is apparently necessary and free from the vice of bad emotions, the rest is as truly necessary. Rest and change are demanded. These influences shift the bearings; take off the pressure from parts and powers that are tired, and put into exercise faculties that have been dormant, so that the man as a whole is brought up, his brain and body are refreshed, and mental wreck is fought off.

It is the influences that I have condemned, that make the apparently inevitable revolutions of the wheel of society. It is a spectacle that the old world has furnished, only in a lesser degree, again and again. Many resourceful American families eventually go to the wall in the greater world influences, while their places are taken by people who have come up from humbler beginnings. The rise to power of these is due to the fact that they have suffered less injury from the emotions that grind and wear out the nerve force. They have lived simpler lives nearer to nature, and have been moved by ambitions that are less carking and unwholsome.

This continual revolution of the wheel is self-acting and wholly conservative for the world. The race and company fit to command usually in the long run come up to power. The lessening of grasp due to the dissipations incident to the use of power—the miscalled rewards of power—causes its victims to drop out of the struggle and give place to those not belittled by such influences.

But must this debauchery of resources always go on? And is the revolution of the wheel inevitable?

BICYCLES FOR PHYSICIANS.

A DOCTOR said to me the other day, says Dr. E. C. Chamberlin in the *New York Herald*, "If I only dared to sell my horse and carriage I would do it and buy a wheel, but," said he, "if I do, then my patients will think that my practice is not as good as it was, and disastrous results might follow such a step;" so the poor man continues to ride on four wheels when he is anxious to ride on two.

The physician may have any attachment he choose put upon his wheel, in order to carry instruments or drugs. He is never troubled with coachman's hire, stable expenses, &c., and many other necessary outlays. Of course what I have said will only refer to a location where roads are good, as for instance, in a city practice.

On an avenue of asphalt, unless the distance be great, one need hardly consider time as a factor compared to the street cars, or cable, or even the "L." Provided the avenues be not crowded, a doctor can reach a point much quicker on his wheel than by any of the ways mentioned. This will be particularly applicable in a city not well favored by methods of rapid transit.

This point I have tested several times and find it true in every respect. A physician in a carriage riding from house to house gets fresh air, but his lungs are not being expanded in the least to receive it, whereas put the same man on a wheel and he combines healthful exercise and speed. Of course the physician must cater to the whims of his patients, and so, in some cases, perhaps, should he call on certain families with his wheel he might not be asked to call again. However, this notion of false pride is rapidly disappearing, for now the clergy are beginning to use the wheel, and why not the physician with equal dignity? The dress of a professional man need not consist of a long frock coat, gold headed cane, &c., but an ordinary sack coat, with long trousers, will appear quite as complete and genteel as you may desire. The novice might inquire what you do with your wheel when you make your calls.

If it be at an apartment house or hotel, leave it in the hall in charge of the hall boy; taking off your trousers guards you can go up stairs and no one need know but what your carriage stands at the door or that you came in the car. If it be at a private house, either chain it to the fence or place it in the area or leave in a corner drug store. For $2 a year you can insure against theft and for $4 against breakage. The only possible disadvantage in the wheel for a physician's use may be during a storm.

Of course, then the cars or a cab will carry you. The advantages of a wheel are numerous, not having mentioned the cheap little excursions that may be taken in the country; to enumerate, we have, first, physical exercise; second, cheapness; third, durability; fourth, speed; fifth, exhilaration; sixth, comfort, and not to mention various esthetic associations. The above list all combine to make the wheel a positive pleasure to many business men, as well as to physicians a decided necessity.

ATHLETICISM AND LONGEVITY.

THE point as to whether athletics, as carried on in colleges, is conducive to long life is a somewhat open question. Dr. James M. Whiton, a graduate of Yale in the class of 1853, tells the tale, in the *Boston Courier*, of the first Harvard-Yale rowing regatta, and presents some instructive figures bearing on the matter. He writes as follows: "It is noteworthy that, at the end of nearly forty-nine years, nearly one-half are still living—20 of 41, or 48.78 per cent. Of the 27 who rowed the race, 15 survive, or 55.55 per cent. But in the Yale Class of '53' though this included, as President Woolsey pertinently remarked, 'a great many boys,' only 50 now survive of 108, or 46.29 per cent.; of the Harvard Class of '53' but 40 of 90 survive, or 44.44 per cent." These facts would seem to show that the practice of athletics does not shorten life, but at the same time it must be borne in mind that in those days sport was not carried to excess. It was pursued more for the fun of the thing, and not, as nowadays, regarded as a very serious business, one almost of life or death. Training in colleges in America is at the present time abused, the result being in many cases a breakdown of the nervous and physical organization, not unfrequently ending in death.

EDUCATING THE LEFT HAND.

MODERN educators have, many of them, advised the training of the left hand, which in most persons is weaker and less capable than the right. Professor Arthur MacDonald in an article on the study of children, says on this subject, that to use the left hand more would increase symmetry and

uniformity in development. This theory seems very plausible, but recent investigation tends to show that right-handedness is natural, and that its superiority over the left hand increases with growth, also that the brightest pupils are, so to speak, more right-handed than the others. This suggests the modern tendency to become expert in one thing rather than be upon the surface of many things. The left hand does best when it supplements or helps the right hand. It is a general opinion that criminals have not only more left-handed people among them, but they are also more expert with both hands than people in general. Sometimes the finger muscles of the pickpocket are cut, so that he can apply either hand with greater dexterity.

HOUSEWORK AS EXERCISE.

TAKE the washtub first. Nothing can make that toil hygienic. One has to bend over the tub, using the arms with a steady, strenuous motion, and at every breath filling the lungs with hot steam. Washing may develop the muscles of the arms, but it cramps the back and contracts the chest. The only relief possible is to take a few minutes frequently for rest. I do not mean sitting down; that is not resting. Go to the door or window and take several long, deep breaths. Straighten up the body, throw back the shoulders and strike out with both arms. Exhale the breath and drop the arms. Repeat this exercise ten or twelve times during the morning's wash, and you will be astonished at how much less tired you are than usual. When sweeping, make both sides of the body do the work. Many a woman who would be classified by a dressmaker as a figure with one hip larger than the other, has cultivated this figure by constantly using the muscles of one side while sweeping or mopping. It is remarkable how a few years of doing certain work in a contracted, bad position will alter the poise of the body. I have heard it said that the student of physical development has a strange faculty, almost Sherlock Holmes-like, of telling by a glance at a man or woman what their calling is. Of course there are certain conditions—that they should have followed that calling a certain length of time and that it is a body physically untrained.

Bread kneading affords a better exercise than washing. The steam is not present and half an hour of steady motion such as given to well-made bread means good exercise for the forearm, provided the molding board is at a proper height and that one keeps the back and shoulders erect.—*Good Housekeeping* for October.

HARMONIZING TEMPER IN MARRIAGE.

FAR more difficult than the mere harmonizing of opinions in married life, is the harmonizing of tempers; since, while many people have no opinions worth mentioning on any subject, the humblest or most ignorant can set up a temper. Nothing can deal with tempers except conscience and time. I have known young married couples with whom it was unpleasant to be in the house during the first year of their marriage; and yet habit and sheer necessity made their society tolerable within two years, and positively agreeable in five. The presence of children is a help to this compatibleness, as being the one possession absolutely shared and necessarily accepted by each parent. Another great aid to the harmonizing of tempers—indeed something priceless, as a permanent rule—is to study mutually what may be called the equation of preferences—that is, to form a habit of considering, when husband and wife differ about any matter, which of the two has really the most reason to care about it. Thus it may sometimes make little difference to the wife whether breakfast is early or late, while a late breakfast may cost the husband his morning

train; or a carriage may be a very important matter to a wife with her skirts to take care of, while it may make no serious difference to the husband whether he walks or rides. It is surely better that one should make a little sacrifice, on any matter, than that the other should make a far greater one. Many a household jar which would have left prolonged stings behind it, if made a mere test of will and persistence, is settled easily when the equation of preferences is applied to it, and each is ready to make a little sacrifice to save the other from a greater one.—From "Success in Marriage," by Professor Thomas Wentworth Higginson, in October *Success.*

THE BEST WIFE FOR A DOCTOR.

WE find this spicy bit of advice in the *Alkaloidal Clinic:*

This is rather a delicate subject to discuss, for if the editor were to take very decided ground on the question, he would please a few readers and displease many more. So we will leave out all personalities, only hinting that if any one wants our private views on the absolutely perfect, ideal wife for a doctor, call around and we will gladly introduce him.

But whom should the doctor marry?

Max O'Rell says that authors should not marry at all; and saves himself by immediately adding—"for the sake of their wives." And that of course brings up the plaint of poor Jeanie Welsh Carlyle; that the world must have geniuses, but it was pretty hard on the woman who had to live with them. And one wonders what would have been the result to the world of letters, if Thomas Carlyle's doctor had known the significance of autotoxemia.

Don't marry the woman who thinks she has a career of her own. You will either clash or sink to the place of Mrs. ——'s husband.

Don't marry a woman devoted to society or fads. Inevitably she will look on you simply as a source of supplies, a ladder by which she can climb to eminence; and no matter how high she gets, she will blame you for not enabling her to get higher.

Don't marry a jealous woman. A doctor must deserve and have the entire confidence of his patrons, morally as well as professionally; and how can he expect this if his own wife, who presumedly knows him better than anyone else, considers him unfit to be trusted out of her sight?

Don't marry a woman mentally your superior.

Don't marry a fool, a sloven, a sensualist, a selfish, lazy or shrewish woman. Beware of the girl gifted with preternatural acuteness in picking flaws in others; or one who is always ready to attribute bad or unworthy motives to others.

If a woman was intended by nature to be a nun, don't interfere and coax her away into matrimony.

Look for a girl who has good health, who is brisk and tidy about the house and sings at her work, who is good and helpful to her mother, who is human enough to be unaffectedly happy that she has won a husband, and who is proud of him and of her wifehood, who has wit enough to make a delightful companion, and does not feel herself so superior that nothing her husband does is above criticism; who is old-fashioned enough to take pride in a clean house, a well-cooked meal, neatness of person and dress; one who can laugh, and who is on the lookout to meet her husband when he comes home from work.

"And the nights shall be filled with music,
  And the cares that infest the day
Shall fold their tents like the Arabs
  And as silently pass away."

The world is full of such women; pure, sweet and lovable; each one beyond all price to the man who wins her, loves her and treats her right. You can find them anywhere.

♣ ♣

THE ANTI-DRUG TENDENCY.

It cannot be denied that the average faith in drug-cures is steadily on the wane. Every reflective medical man begins to realize that most curable diseases disappear, if at all, spontaneously, and by natural processes, helped or hindered, as the case may be, by intelligent, mistaken or bungling art; that outside of Nature and a placebo we have little to rely on beyond a wise and persistent "expectancy"; which is either the result of an abiding faith that the *vis medicatrix naturæ* is all-sufficient, or a scientific and candid admission of helplessness and ignorance, and that the work of the enlightened physician is to bring into activity and carefully direct the forces of Nature —ine one word, *hygiene,* which is a comprehensive term, covering most of our honest efforts and giving us our most gratifying successes.

True, we cannot ignore the palpable duty of mitigating pain by temporizing anodynes and anesthetics, but we do not assume these to be other than palliators. To paralyze, temporarily, the sensory centers is not cure. And yet must we go on giving the placebo for its psychologic effect—the basis of "faith cure" and all medical credulity—and waiting for Nature to accomplish the readjustment we call curing.

By and by—it may be ages hence—we can judiciously withhold the placebo!

On the other hand, we cannot at once, nor perhaps ever, while human nature remains the same as now, dispense with all the apparent mystery and mythology of our art. No sane physician, physiologist or psychologist questions the fact that myth and mystery have their mission in the field of medicine. Without it we could not at all times enlist the faith and coöperation of our patients, whereas we all fully realize the potency and sometimes the all-importance of faith in the relief of human ailments.

It is by taking advantage of this weakness of human nature that the charlatan thrives; it is this that gives success to the unblushing vender of nostrums. No matter how cheap and nasty, or how inert and worthless his concoction, the fulsome laudations flaunted everywhere, and backed by scores of really "genuine certificates" wheedled from, and often even volunteered by, credulous dupes, who may not inaptly be styled pharmaco-maniacs, the sales of the vile trash reach fairly stupendous proportions, and the wily proprietors, who steal the livery of heaven in which to serve the devil, grow plethoric with gains wrenched from ignorant believers in medical mythology; while stupidly honest practitioners eke out a scanty existence by faithful plodding in overworked but underfed and underpaid fields of labor.

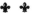

LET US ALL PROTEST.

THE *Philadelphia Medical Journal* thus protests against what it denominates a retrograde movement: The Post-office Department of our Government, like the United States Constitution, was made for the people, and not the people for it. It was not intended primarily as a money-making business. It is to serve the convenience of the public; to promote the interests, and, above all, to serve for the enlightenment of the populace. But there is great danger that some of these objects will be defeated if Third Assistant Postmaster General Madden is to have his way in ruling out of the privileges of second-class matter all periodicals that offer premiums to their subscribers. Mr. Madden seems to be worried because a certain concern sold tea-sets, claimed to be worth two dollars apiece, as premiums for a publication which was sold for one dollar a year. That certainly looks anything but a literary or educational enterprise, and may have been an imposition on the Department; but it does not follow that all the legitimate periodicals in the country that do an honest business by offering premiums (which, in most instances, are books) should be debarred from the privileges of going as second-class matter. Some discrimination should certainly be made; some judgment

and common sense should be displayed. We enter a protest here in the name of all legitimate journalism, and in the interest of the public which desires and must have its reading matter on reasonable terms. Let there be no tax on letters.

THE GEORGE JUNIOR REPUBLIC.

R. E. PHILLIPS, in *The World's Work.*

FROM all sources the number received since 1895 is 247. Of the whole number only one has been arrested after leaving the Republic. Another employed in a factory near Freeville was accused of stealing a wheel. A third has turned out to be a non-worker, and, while guilty of no offense, is not yet self-supporting. In all seven have been marked "unsatisfactory." That is, they either have no positions or have not filled them successfully. Of the rest four are working their way through college, five are in preparation and the others, without exception, hold good business positions. The naïve reply of a little girl who was asked, "What do you little citizens possess that we older persons do not?" who answered, "Self-control," shows the idea the Republic stands for. In short, the practical results that come from a clear appreciation of the broad, underlying principles of the Republic differentiate it from the "institution," and tend to give society a citizen rather than a criminal.

McKEESPORT IN STRIKE TIME.

IN *The World's Work* for October Mr. M. G. Cunniff writes of McKeesport in strike time, and draws a vivid comparison between the conditions there before the Steel Trust and the Amalgamated Association got their hold upon it and since. In a description of the founder of the W. Dewees Wood mill, he says:

"Every man in the works," said a striker

to me in McKeesport, "was 'Tom,' or 'Joe,' or 'Bill,' to him; every day he would walk about and joke with the workers at the furnaces and rolls; and, if a man looked ill, he would slap him on the back and tell him to take a few days off. He didn't take the vacation out of the man's time, either." When a man had been killed in the mill— and the list of cuts and burns and broken backs along the Monongahela is appalling —the widow and children regularly received the dead man's pay-envelope until they were able to take care of themselves. On his return from a journey he always made a round of the mills, shaking hands with every 'Tom' and 'Joe' and 'Bill' in the whole plant, like a man coming back to his family. Once, too, it is said, he was offered a chance to buy real estate to sell to his workmen— and the men working for him were of the kind that begin early to acquire homes—but his reported reply was, 'No. I will not take back from the men the money I have paid them in wages.' "

The growing city needed a library; the largest contributor was W. Dewees Wood. Nor did the men in the mill fail to respond. When, according to his habit, Mr. Wood advanced money to a man to tide him over a long illness—a man injured in the mill was supported outright —although the debt was never mentioned, every man gradually paid what he owed to the last dollar.

THEODORE ROOSEVELT — THE TYPICAL MAN OF THE TWENTIETH CENTURY.*

THEODORE ROOSEVELT as a type of what the representative American citizen should be, presents an extremely interesting study. Anthropologists agree that the man of this class should represent not merely one race in his ancestry, but several. In his veins should flow the blood of Ireland, Scotland, or Germany as well as England in order to determine if the descendant of a mixture of

* Day Allen Willey in *Modern Culture* for October.

these nations can be developed into the highest type of civilization. Many students of human nature have claimed that such a people cannot be depended upon to preserve the spirit of democratic institutions—to maintain such a republic as the United States. In the case of Theodore Roosevelt, however, pessimists encounter a serious obstacle. His ancestry represents not only Holland, as indicated by his name, but Scotland, Ireland, and France. Among them were the pioneer French Huguenots of the Southern States, the Dutch settlers of New Amsterdam, and Irish and Scotch refugees from Britain to New England. He has been a devotee of politics since he graduated from Harvard. His family moves in the most exclusive society and he is wealthy. Yet to-day he has reached a position through merely what he has accomplished for his city, his state, and the country at large, which places him among eminent Americans, though not yet past middle manhood.

Under any other but a Republican government, Mr. Roosevelt's ability would not have had such scope to be utilized for the common welfare, for he had only the opportunities afforded the average American, increased slightly by his family influence and means. But these factors would have amounted to nothing in his struggle against the political régime in the metropolis, for example, had he not been possessed of bravery and perseverance. As he said himself in the midst of that memorable contest: "We do not need genius in this fight, but courage, honesty and common sense. The rascals have the genius." Unfortunately, the latter assertion has proved to be true in many other instances. But the watchwords which led to the overthrow of the officials in power and in a brilliant victory for good government were those quoted— courage, honesty, and common sense.

His career illustrates forcibly what one man can accomplish single-handed in working for the common welfare. In fact this was and is his motto: "He who has not wealth owes his first duty to his family.

He who has wealth owes his first duty to his state. It is ignoble to heap money upon money. Such are the words as framed by his own lips. A century hence they may be classed among the world's wisest sayings.

J. PIERPONT MORGAN, THE WORLD'S GREAT MONEY MASTER.

COMPARATIVELY few people possess any very clear conception of what Mr. Morgan is or does in Wall Street. He is vaguely compared with Mr. Keene, who is a speculator; with Jay Gould, who was a wrecker; with Hill and Harriman, who are strictly railroad men; with the Astors, who are primarily real estate owners; with Mr. Carnegie, who was an ironmaster. But Mr. Morgan's business is purely that of a banker—a worker with money. He is not a practical railroad man, nor a steel manufacturer, nor a coal dealer, although he is interested in all these things, because he is constantly buying and selling railroad and steel and coal stocks. Sometimes for some specific purpose he buys so much of a railroad company's stock that he and his clients practically own the railroad, and he takes a strong position in directing its policy. Not long ago I heard an apparently intelligent speaker who conveyed the impression that Morgan bought a railroad out of his surplus cash as a farmer buys a cow. Nothing could be further from the truth. While Mr. Morgan must make use of his own large means it no doubt forms but a small part in his vast deals. The essence of successful banking is connections, otherwise friends. While coveting large earnings capital is proverbially shrinking and timid, fearing to strike out boldly for itself, and yet ever ready to trust itself with confidence to the leader whose skill, foresight, and cautious daring have been steadily fruitful of success. Such a money master is J. Pierpont Morgan.—Ray Stannard Baker, in *McClure's Magazine* for October.

SOME SAMPLE ADVERTISEMENTS OF YE OLDEN TIME.

IN the *Providence Gazette* of January 12, 1793, is an interesting item regarding a hog hunt.

Give ear all ye owners of swine that run at large in Providence Streets.—Such swine are by law forfeit to any person who will take them, and as they do mischief in gardens and meadows as well as are a nuisance in the streets, it is proposed to give chase to them on Monday next and afterwards to present them to the poor, so govern yourselves, hogs and pigs accordingly.

In the *Connecticut Gazette*, published at New London, in 1778, we find the following patriotic notice:

All gentlemen volunteers who are desirous of making their fortunes in six months' time are hereby informed that the noble privateer Brigantane Middletown, a prime sailer, mounting fourteen 6 and two 4-pounders, is now completely fitted and will be at New London by the first of December next, or sooner, and will sail from thence on a cruize of six months, against the enemies of the United States, and you may depend on good usage and accommodations.

NEGROES WERE SOLD THEN.

Going back to 1733, the *New York Gazette* advertises:

A likely negro girl, fit for town or country, has had the Small-Pox, she is about Fifteen years old; as also to be Sold sundry Drugs and Medicines by John Briggs over against the Meat Market in New York.

Coming up to 1777, New Yorkers one morning had this interesting item of information to read:

A Negro Wench. Run-Away. Supposed to Flatbush on Long Island where she was lately purchased of Cornelius Van Der Veer, Jun., is about twenty-two years old, called Betty, can speak both Dutch and English, is of a stubborn disposition especially when she drinks spirituous liquors, which she is sometimes too fond of; is a pretty stout wench but not tall, smooth fac'd and pretty black; 'tis probable she may be conceal'd in this city. Whoever harbors her will be prosecuted, but such as give information to William Tongue, her owner in Hanover Square, shall receive £5 reward with thanks. She usually wore a striped homespun pettycoat and gown.

STAYS IN THOSE DAYS.

That article of wearing apparel known in this day as corsets was known as stays by our great-great-grandmothers, and many of the advertisements regarding this subject were as cleverly put together as those of our own time on the more modern article. For instance, in 1735 we find in Bradford's *New York Gazette* the following interesting announcement:

James Munden, Partner with Thomas Butwell from London, Maketh Gentlewomen's Stays and Children's Coats in the Newest Fashion and so that Crooked Women and Children will appear strait. By whom Gentlewomen and Ladies in City and Country may be faithfully served.

In 1773, Richard Norris advertises his ability as a stay maker in Rivington's *New York Gazetter,* saying that he—

Takes this method to return his sincere thanks to his friends and customers for their past favors and to acquaint them that he now has the newest fashions from the Queen's Stay Maker in London, such as have not been made in these parts. He likewise makes all sorts of stays and jumps, plain and turned, for thick or thin ladies, at any distance, by sending their measure.

Of course in those good old days nobody who wanted to appear well before his friends or in society would think of allowing himself to be seen without a wig or a periwig, and advertisements regarding these obsolete articles of headdress are both numerous and amusing during the years preceding the Revolution. Alexander Miller advertises in Philadelphia, in 1746, that he has a fine supply of all sorts of wigs, done after the best and newest fashion, and he announces that he is ready to pay solid cash for the best live hair. Another interesting advertisement in the *Pennsylvania Gazette* for the same year is as follows:

Mary Catrel, from the city of Dublin, at Mr. Burk's, periwig maker, in Front street, Philadelphia, between Chestnut and Walnut streets, and almost facing Gray's alley, makes and sells all sorts of gentlemen's velvet caps, leather, &c.; also ladies' and children's caps, mantilets, pillareens, hoods, bonnets, long and short cloaks, mantles and scarfs, with black bags and roses for gentlemen's hair or wigs, all which she makes after the newest and neatest fashions and very cheap. N. B.—She also makes turbans for negroes.

Another advertisement in 1745, includes among articles which one tradesman has for sale, a seven-year-old negro boy, a plain gold watch and a lot of ground in New Brunswick, N. J.

In Zenger's *New York Journal* of August 26, 1734, forty shillings reward is offered for the following individual, who was so unruly as to run away from Johanna Kelsall:

A negro man, known by the name of Johnsey, here in town, but writes his name Jonathan Stow, about twenty-five years of age, of short stature, bandy legs, blubber lip, yellow complexion; his hair is neither negro nor Indian, but between both and pretty long. He had on when he went away a homespun jacket, a pair of trousers and a speckled shirt.

✦ ✦

PITHY PARAGRAPHS.

From the October *Ladies' Home Journal.*

BEING asked one day what one should do in order to become an efficient piano player Liszt replied laconically: "One must eat well and walk much."

The proper length of the forehead is one-third of the length of the face; the nose should also measure one-third, the mouth and chin together the other.

To make good tea and coffee the water should be taken at the first bubble. Remember, continued boiling causes the water to part with its gases and become flat. This is the cause of much bad tea and coffee.

A simple remedy for warts is a dram of salicylic acid with an ounce of collodion in a bottle which has a tiny brush run through the cork. Apply this mixture to the warts twice a day and in a few days they will dry up and fall off.

✦ ✦

Rudyard Kipling's latest animal story, "How the Leopard Got His Spots," has first place in the October *Ladies' Home Journal,* which is a truly notable number of this excellent magazine. "A Fifth Avenue Troubadour," the story of a bird in New York, by Ernest Seton-Thompson; "Some Things the President Does Not Do," and the last installment of "Miss Alcott's Letters to Her 'Laurie' " form a most interesting and varied trio. Miss Laura Spencer Portor's delightful love story, "A Gentleman of the Blue Grass," also begins in this number, and Josef Hofmann, the world-famed pianist, writes on "Playing the Piano Correctly." There is a crisp collection of anecdotes about Mr. Whistler, and a charming bit about "The Real 'Cranford,' " showing pictures of the places most mentioned in Mrs. Gaskell's great story. Mr. Bok's editorial is addressed "To a Young Man About to Marry." The remainder of the magazine is devoted to its enlarged editorial department, nine new editors, each with a special page, making their bows. Chief among these are Professor Griggs's talks on "The Education of a Child from Eleven to Eighteen," Professor S. C. Schmucker's "Seeing Things Outdoors," Miss Withey's "Speaking and Writing Correctly," "The Lady from Philadelphia," a new etiquette department, Doctor Walker's "Good Health for Girls" and Mrs. Sangster's answers to "Girls' Problems." The art features are most attractive. There is a double page of photographs of "Flowers that Bloom Above the Clouds," a page of remarkable photographs by Miss Watson, and a cover by Albert Herter. The Curtis Publishing Company, Philadelphia.

❧ ❧

A GOOD WOMAN.

ONE winter morning, the late Professor Swing was sauntering along the streets near his home. The pavements were coated with ice, and a woman who lived in the neighborhood was cautiously picking her way along. Suddenly her feet flew out and she came down hard upon the sidewalk. Professor Swing paused to satisfy himself that she was not seriously injured. Then he drily remarked: "Mrs. S——, in my opinion you are a very good woman." Piqued at his remark, and at the same time at her predicament, she retorted: "I don't know why you think so. What do you mean?" "Scripture has it," gravely replied Professor Swing, "that the wicked stand in slippery places. You seem to be sitting down."

PULEX IRRITANS M.D.

BY W. G. KEMPER, MANITOWOC, WIS.

A SURGEON I am known to be,
  With fame commensurate,
My talent is phlebotomy;
  My skill is simply great.

My name is Pulex Irritans;
  I treat the skin and hide;
I live and thrive in many land,
  And as a rule, I ride.

I'm free and very much at home
  In social gatherings;
I'm known in Paris and in Rome,
  And I consort with kings.

With noble ladies I have danced;
  My choice is aye the fair,
And maids that are by birth enhanced
  Are dainty ev'rywhere.

My courage is a wondrous trait;
  A lion I'll attack.
You see that tiger fierce and great?
  I'll leap upon his back.

A horse possesses not my strength,
  As I can prove with ease;
I leap a hundred times my length;
  Just watch me if you please.

You think as you this boaster hear,
  "A noted light is he,
Of men of birth and deeds a peer."
  O no—it is a flea!

NATURAL THERAPEUTICS.

THE great objects in the treatment of fever itself are to limit and reduce the pyrexia by direct and indirect means; to limit and repair destruction and degeneration of tissues and organs by alimentation; to provide matters for consumption in the abnormal production of heat, and thus to place the system in the most favorable condition for recuperation after the disease shall have run its course.

Book Reviews.

PROGRESSIVE MEDICINE, Vol. III., September, 1901. A Quarterly Digest of Advances, Discoveries and Improvements in the Medical and Surgical Sciences. Edited by Hobart Amory Hare, M.D., Professor of Therapeutics and Materia Medica in the Jefferson Medical College of Philadelphia. Octavo, handsomely bound in cloth, 428 pages, 16 illustrations. Per annum, in four cloth-bound volumes, $10.00. Lea Brothers & Co., Philadelphia and New York.

While not quite so bulky as preceding volumes, the present issue of this work is quite as valuable as any of its predecessors. The article on Pneumonia, Tuberculosis and other conditions of the Respiratory Tract is of especial importance, since it graphically sets forth the decided advances that have been made in the treatment of Pneumonia and Phthisis. Dr. Ewart also discusses the recently advocated methods of treating certain diseases of the Heart and Blood-vessels by medicated and other baths.

Dr. Spiller does ample justice to the subject of tumors and abscesses of the brain, and describes the commonest forms of some peculiar nervous diseases which so often baffle any but the expert neurologist.

Dr. Norris' paper on Obstetrics gives us the most recent views on the subjects of Symphysiotomy and Lumbar Anesthesia. There is not a dull section in the volume.

W.

PERU—HISTORY OF COCA. "The Divine Plant" of the Incas. With an introductory acount of the Incas, and of the Andrean Indians of to-day. By W. Golden Mortimer, M.D., Fellow of the New York Academy of Medicine; Member of the New York County Medical Society; Member of the New York Academy of Sciences; Member of the American Museum of Natural History; formerly Assistant Surgeon to the New York Throat and Nose Hospital, etc. With 178 illustrations; dedicated to Angelo Mariani, Paris, France, a recognized exponent of "The Divine Plant," and the first to render Coca available to the world. New York: J. H. Vail and Company, 1901. Price, $5.00.

Of six hundred and eight octavo pages, in the highest style of the printer's art, Dr. Mortimer's work is not only refreshing to the eye, but the feast spread therein is well fitted for the student of history, ethnography and geography, as well as physiology and the practice of medicine. The man of commerce desiring to study South America will find this work of great value. It should be in the library of every one of wide reading; those of the GAZETTE are specially interested in the physiological, dietetic and therapeutical researches. Dr. Mortimer has brushed away by his personal study, explorations and collective investigations, a mass of trashy ideas as to coca and gives its true scientific relations to man. The reviewer has for a number of years by virtue of his experience in practice, and by conversations with scientists who have adventured in South America, become convinced of the therapeutic value of coca specially as to the heart; that it "fed" nerve centers and promoted endurance when other means failed; these considerations alone are enough to warrant an investigation of the value of coca, but we find Dr. Mortimer has gone very thoroughly into the relations of coca to appetite, blood pressure, stimulation of circulation, digestive functions, heat of skin, mental and muscular stimulation, sedation and stimulation of nerves, improvement of nutrition, peripheral sensations, pupils and visions, secretions, sexual functions, sleep, etc. In therapeutics, the investigations and conclusions are as broad.

This book is heartily recommended, and when read, no one can again confound coca with cocoa.			J. A. C.

THE concluding paper on "The Therapeutic Value of Climate," will appear in the December GAZETTE.

Editor's Table.

Domestic Science Monthly for October is, as usual, full of good things. It would make a dead man hungry to read the assembled menus and appetizing recipes.

Good Housekeeping is another of our bright and interesting exchanges. It is a healthy sign of the times when we note the success of a long list of entertaining monthlies devoted to the science of Domestic Economy. While on this topic we will add the names of *What to Eat, The American Kitchen Magazine* and *Table Talk*. The housewife who cannot find among these all the practical help she needs must be hard to please—in fact, "pernickety."

From some of our brightest literary exchanges we have made liberal excerpts. We leave them to speak for themselves.

The World's Work is amply making good its original promises. There is nothing in the literary field that quite fills its place, and we are glad to note its rapidly increasing success. Notwithstanding the large editions provided each month the publishers almost invariably underestimate the demand and are compelled to return some late orders.

McClure's Magazine is better than ever, which is saying enough.

Lippincott's is not content with its long-enjoyed fame, but makes steady advances in the character of its literary matter. It is unique in the direction of completed stories and stories of unusual interest.

In its October issue, *Success* has published an industrial number that is interesting to all. The great progress of the nation, the stories of invention, and the problems of winning and developing the world's trade, are told by such notable men as Park Benjamin, Hudson Maxim, Charles R. Flint, and Sir Thomas Lipton. General Benjamin

F. Tracy, the eminent attorney, contributes a timely editorial in "Law as Part of a Business Education." Some interesting and inspiring information for middle-aged women will be found in an article by Margaret E. Sangster, and a subject that should appeal strongly to both sexes is Thomas Wentworth Higginson's "Success in Marriage," from which we have elsewhere quoted. The list of contributors contains some of the most noted names in the United States. *Success* is keeping up its reputation as a magazine of self-help and inspiration, and it has won fresh praise and power in its current effort to present the best interests of the United States.

"MODERN CULTURE" FOR OCTOBER.

Korea—"The Forbidden Kingdom."
(Illus.) F. W. Fitzpatrick.
The Missions of the Franciscans.
(Illus.) A Passage from Southwestern History. W. J. Spillman.
The Squire (concluded). (Illus.)
Florence E. Little.
King Alfred. Laurence M. Larson.
The Women of Ibsen's Plays.
Amalie K. Boguslawsky.
One of the Arradons—I.
Pauline Caro and Aimée Tourgée.
John S. Sargent. (Illus.)
N. Hudson Moore.
The Fishing Industry of the Great
Lakes. (Illus.) Walter E. Andrews.
A Glimpse of the Home Life of Governor Dole. (Illus.) Annabel Lee.
Theodore Roosevelt—The Typical
Man of the Twentieth Century.
Day Allen Willey.
Anarchism—A Study of Social Forces.
Henry Virstow.
A Humble Lorelei. Edward Bushnell.
Ignace Ian Paderewski—A Sketch.
Emma Henry Ferguson.
Rambles Out of Doors—Bush the
Black Squirrel. Orlando J. Stevenson.
Constancy. Anon.

Brevity Club.

WHAT SHALL WE DO FOR BREAD TO EAT?

By a Disgruntled Contributor.

Apropos of what has been said on the subject of bread in the columns of the Gazette, I want to say that the man who asserted that bread is the staff of life must either have lived in a far bygone age or else had very little regard for truth and veracity as those attributes are now defined.

Paraphrasing a recent criticism, the modern baker's loaf is an unpunished crime. It is a cross between semi-decomposed sponge and demoralized dextrine. How a sane baker can transform such thoroughly excellent flour as is everywhere available in our markets—in short, the best flour in the world—into such detestable, indigestible and innutritious bread is the culinary conundrum of the age. He should be indictable for systematized fraud, in that he deludes the unwary and ignorant consumer into the belief that he is sustaining his vital powers instead of insulting his digestive organs, when he devours the alum-toughened, ammonia-whitened and over-fermented loaf, and is told that it is bread. Much of the stuff is as tough as cotton batting, and some of it is fermented until it is as friable as a field pumpkin after it has braved the frosts of February.

A barrel of flour, such as our grandfathers never dreamed of as to quality, rich in all the essential elements that go to build and nourish the human frame, to make muscle and blood and brain, is doctored and diluted into three hundred loaves of ill-looking and ill-smelling stuff that sells for fifteen dollars and would be dear at half the price; or the high-toned baker-to-their-royal-highnesses, the upper ten (thousand), cuts down the yield to two hundred somewhat more sightly loaves, and sells them for twenty dollars. Sometimes he calls it "home-made" bread, and since the American housewife has about lost the art of

bread-making nobody knows enough to dispute him. The best of it is fourth rate, if compared with the real "home-made" bread our sainted mothers used to make, and samples of which can be met with at rare intervals even in these days of bread-famine.

Some of the self-styled "reformers" attribute the trouble to the quality of the flour of the day; but it is not the fault of the millers. The latter have made wonderful strides toward perfecting the product of their mills. They have learned the art of separating the starchy element in part and turning it over to the cracker and cake makers. The processes now in vogue, sometimes called patented, from the fact that certain forms of machinery used have been patented, afford flour of a quality of which our fathers did not even dream, and concerning which the "reformers" refuse to be enlightened, a quality that is the delight of the up-to-date physiologist. There is no possible excuse for the esthetic debasement and nutritive retrogradation of the loaves we are compelled to eat. In fact the more esthetic people are learning to avoid the stuff altogether. They turn to the prepared foods, shredded wheat, granose flakes, zwieback, whole-wheat crackers and the thousand and one breakfast cereals, all of which escape the devitalizing touch of the professional baker.

The remedy lies in ceasing to patronize the bakers and reverting to the wholesome, substantial and not essentially difficult art of bread-making at home. It isn't complicated nor mysterious. Every girl ten years old should learn to make good bread, and if more brides would master and practise the simple but essential art there would be fewer divorces and fewer suicides!

Abbott's Saline Laxative is highly esteemed by all my Clientèle. There is nothing more delightful, cooling and refrigerant. An elegant laxative.

Frank Gordon, M.D.
Morrellton, Ark.

Notes and Queries.

Query 101. *Editor* GAZETTE: I notice in a recent issue of your excellent journal some statements under the heading: "Erroneous Notions About the Toad."

Will you tell me if toads lay eggs, or do they all originate from tadpoles, and if they are from tadpoles, how do you account for them on dry land after a storm? Respectfully, W. R. MARTIN,

Editor *Roanoke Advocate.*

Answer.—Our esteemed confrère's question is a little mixed, and makes it necessary to supplement the brief paper published in the August GAZETTE.

First, the tadpole is not a primary form, but is the larval stage of the egg of the toad and frog family.

Certainly, all toads lay eggs, and a hatched egg is a tadpole. There are, however, two distinct species of toads, in regard to the egg business. The ordinary toad lays its eggs in the water in long rope-like tubes of transparent albumin, in which the eggs proper appear as black dots. Every schoolboy in the country is familiar with these soft, jelly-like coils of "toad's eggs."

The other species, no doubt, belonging to the batrachian Four Hundred, and looking with disdain on their plebeian neighbors, does not deposit its eggs in the water and then abandon them to their muddy fate. With this species the eggs are gallantly received by the waiting male toad and he deposits them on the back of the female, where they are encapsuled by folds of the skin. Here they hatch and the resulting tadpoles go through the required process of transformation—the shedding of tails and acquirement of legs—and emerge as perfected toads.

In case of the water-born tadpoles, they accomplish this metamorphosis in the water, and when they emerge as full-rigged toads, lose their hydropathic instincts and learn to breathe air, they make long pilgrimages on land, traveling during the night and hiding during the daytime. In case of a warm and sudden shower these little marauders emerge from their hiding places as if by magic. The idea that they rain down is a popular myth, the explanation being as above.

Toads, frogs and other reptiles never "rain down," except when—as rarely occurs—they are first drawn up from ponds or other places by a whirlwind or cyclone.

The toad and the frog belong to the same family. Both are technically batrachians, order *Bu*-

fonidæ, sub-order *Anura,* or tailless amphibians. Frogs differ from toads in having no teeth, in having only rudimentary or embryonic shoulder girdles, and in being more terrestrial in their habits.

There are ninety-two species that have been described, seventy-seven of which belong to the typical genus *Bufo.*

In this country we have about ten species of *Bufo.* The common eastern species is *Bufo lentiginosus.* In the middle States the variety is known as *Bufo Americanus.* The largest North American species is known as *Bufo boreas,* except that in tropical America there is a larger species called *Bufo maximus.* Specimens of this latter species measure eight inches in length and have voices to compete with the pedal bass of a pipe organ or the lower register of a mad bull.

Query 102. We thought we had settled the question of oatmeal cooking, but several correspondents have criticized our directions and asked various insinuating questions. We will not repeat all these questions since most of them are more insinuating than inquisitive. We will endeavor to "insinuate" a comprehensive embodiment of all the suggestions thus far received.

The use of oatmeal and oat flour should not be limited to breakfast porridge. It can be cooked in a hundred ways. The following methods will illustrate:

Ground oatmeal is made into various toothsome forms of bread, cakes and pie-crust. For the latter purpose it requires little or no shortening, as it is tender without.

Scotch Bannocks.—These are made from ground oatmeal, mixing the flour with cold water to the consistency of a not too thin batter or dough, adding a little salt. It is then rolled out rather thin, cut into squares or triangles and baked in a moderate oven.

Scotch Cakes are shortened with beef drippings and baking powder is added to make them light. The dough should be a little stiffer than for Bannocks.

For *Oatmeal Pie-crust.*—The ground oatmeal is scalded with boiling water, well mixed and kneaded, and rolled quite thin. It bakes quickly and is quite tender without shortening. The fruit selected should be of the tender, quick-cooking kind, or else it must be steamed or partly cooked in advance.

Oat Flour is very desirable as an addition to other flours, as buckwheat flour for pancakes, wheat flour used for pastry, cakes and bread, corn meal, etc.

Oatmeal Mush, sometimes called *porridge*—we do not approve of porridge. It is too thin. When people eat they should eat, not drink—was discussed pretty fully in this department in a recent number of the GAZETTE. We might have added many other recipes, and will now append a few:

First of all, *use the best oats*. The market is full of inferior qualities. Some brands sample well and soon deteriorate in quality. Find a reliable brand and insist upon that. Our preference is for the "Quaker" brand. It was good when first placed on the market and maintains its quality.

Cook in a double boiler at least half an hour. Two hours is better.

Get the knack of making it not too thick, but as thick as it can be readily stirred and cooked, so that it will be quite firm when it cools. In this form it will be much better masticated and insalivated; and this fact may be the prime factor in determining whether it will "agree" or not.

Oatmeal Mush with Fruit.—Punch the cores from tart apples, fill the holes with sugar, flavored with a little cinnamon. Bake the apples, place each one in an oatmeal dish and surround it with the mush. Serve with cream. Other kinds of fruit may be substituted for apples.

Oatmeal Gems.—Mix cold oatmeal mush with sweet milk, add a little salt and stir in wheat flour until a thick batter is formed. Sift into the wheat flour, before stirring it in, one or two teaspoonfuls of baking powder. Drop the batter from a spoon into heated iron gem pans and bake in a brisk oven until crisp and well done.

Quaker Rolls.—Make the mush in the usual way. To each cup of mush add one cup of Graham flour, two cups of wheat flour, a teaspoonful of salt and half a cake of compressed yeast. Mix well and set over night in a moderately warm place. In the morning roll out to about half an inch in thickness, cut with a large round cutter, fold in the center, wash over with milk, let rise again and bake to a nice brown in a hot oven.

Query 103. EDITOR NOTES AND QUERIES: Is the belief well founded that coffee drinking is the. or a, direct cause of so-called biliousness? (2) There is a fluid preparation on the market claiming to be coffee with the caffein extracted. Is such claim likely to be true? (3) For those who can not drink milk with comfort, and who dislike tea, the problem of what to drink with meals in a community that looks askance on a bottle of claret, is a difficult one. Have you a suggestion?
H. B. B., N. J.

Answer.—"Biliousness," as already set forth in these columns, is a very indefinite term. It oftener than otherwise means sluggish digestion, with more or less anto-infection or anto-intoxication. Coffee to a certain extent coöperates with other causes to bring about the sluggish condition, and therefore is to this extent a cause of "biliousness." It affects some persons, and especially sedentary people, much more than others. (2) We have never tested the fluid "coffee" from which the caffein is said to have been extracted. If the claim is true, it is perfectly safe to say that no coffee lover will accept it as a substitute for the real thing. It would be an insipid slop and no longer coffee. It would be trying to play "Hamlet" with the part of Hamlet omitted. (3) There are many substitutes for coffee, some of which imitate its color and flavor quite closely, and are at the same time entirely harmless and moderately nutritious.

Of these substitutes the writer has personally tested all that have came to his immediate notice. Several are fairly good. The one finally adopted and used for the past three or four years with satisfaction is the *Postum Cereal,* prepared by the company of that name at Battle Creek, Mich.

Don't be tempted by the claret!

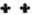

ALL ROADS LEAD TO NEW YORK.

ST. LOUIS has for many years been almost preëminent as the rallying ground of large manufacturers of pharmaceutical preparations.

As long as their various products found their market exclusively on this continent there was no essential drawback to the location; but when their customers in Europe and other foreign countries begin to be numbered by thousands the question of location assumes quite a different aspect.

These companies are gradually realizing this fact and are acting accordingly. The Rio Chemical Company has just removed its plant to this city, and established headquarters at 56 Thomas street. We heartily welcome this company to the center of the world and wish for it a long life and prosperity.

To discover truth is the best happiness of an individual; to communicate it, the greatest blessing he can bestow upon society.—*Townsend.*

THE
DIETETIC AND HYGIENIC GAZETTE
A MONTHLY JOURNAL OF PHYSIOLOGICAL MEDICINE

| Vol. XVII. | NEW YORK, DECEMBER, 1901. | No. 12. |

SLEEP AND ITS RELATIONS TO HEALTH AND DISEASE.

By H. E. PECKHAM, A.B.

(Concluded from page 653.)

THERE are five forms of food necessary for the body, proteids, carbohydrates, fats, salts and water. The most perfect food for the growing infant is milk. This, taken directly from the breast of a healthy woman, contains no organisms of any kind, consequently, Nature intended this to be the greatest means by which infant life is saved from disease. Therefore, the very best diet for a child, up to the age of a year at least, is its mother's milk. During childhood and until puberty has become well established, the dietary should be studied more carefully than at any other period of life. This should be adapted to suit the strength of the digestive system, the amount of exercise taken, and especially the amount of oxidation taking place in the tissues. Children should we weaned from an exclusive milk diet gradually, and then the most easily digested foods should be given first. A small amount of thoroughly boiled rice is probably the best to start with. Nature does not like sudden changes, and she makes a fuss here as in everything else. After a child has enough teeth to make mastication easy and complete, a generous diet from those foods of vegetable origin containing all the food principles needed in the body is most desirable. These are found in such foods as good whole-wheat bread, well baked, and boiled or baked potatoes, which furnish a large amount of carbo-hydrate, and peas or beans, which contain a large per cent. of proteids. Milk in moderate amounts is also good, providing there have been no digestive disturbances during infancy. As for meat, I would not exclude a moderate amount of it after the age of three or four years, providing it is thoroughly cooked, either boiled or roasted. This should be restricted to turkey, chicken, mutton and good beef. Thick, greasy gravies, veal, pork, and many forms of game are abominations, and can be digested only by mature and healthy stomachs. The best form of fat, in case the child requires it, is butter, since it is a product of milk which is a natural food. The salts, which are necessary for the system, other than the common salt used in seasoning, are contained chiefly in the vegetable diet.

Fruits that are perfectly ripe and fresh should have a large place in a child's dietary, but here, also, certain kinds should be proscribed. Those containing a large per cent. of raw starch, like bananas, should be given sparingly and in small amounts. Oranges, pears, peaches and apples, when fully ripe, are probably the very best fruits to eat raw. I think the apple stands king among all fruits for continual use. Seedy fruits (unless the seeds are removed) should be taken only in small quantities by either old or young, and best during a regular meal. The small sharp seeds of strawberries, cranberries and huckleberries especially, when eaten in large quantities, are directly responsive for scybala in the large intestine, which are a great source of irritation, resulting in inflammation, mucous colitis and chronic ulcers, on the one hand, or chronic constipation and intestinal paresis, on the other. The old idea that figs are beneficial because the seeds irritate the colic mucous membrane, in the light of present scientific knowledge, should be consigned to a dark and barbarous past. Figs or strawberries, if taken in medicinal quantities, can have nothing but disastrous sequelæ in reducing the normal and healthy tonic condition of the whole large intestine, especially the rectum. As in a furnace clogged with ashes, the fires of life will not burn unless there be a regular and copious evacuation from the intestine. A physician told me of a case from whom, after a high flushing, he removed eleven pounds of hard scybala, containing the seeds of a fruit eaten two years previous. The patient knew it was so because no fruit of that kind had been eaten since that time. The disastrous results of a sluggish intestine may be appreciated when it is estimated that one normal evacuation from the intestine contains enough poison to kill the individual, should it be absorbed back into the system. The selection of a fruit, then, depends, as in other articles of food, upon the condition of the excretory apparatus; in this instance more particularly, the intestine. Seedy fruits cannot by any logical argument be given in any but small quantities to persons who suffer with weak intestinal peristalsis. Even those possessing a strong and vigorous intestine should take care of it in this regard, and consider the possibilities of any indiscretion. I am sure any one who will examine the plicate arrangement of the colic mucous membrane, can understand the relation of scybala of the colon to sluggish peristalsis, and thence to auto-intoxication, abnormal drowsiness and sleep. The early habit of evacuating the rectum at least once a day, preferably just before retiring, will bless any one with good sleep, a useful life and a happy old age.

I think few realize the importance of water as a food. We forget that the body itself is about two-thirds water; therefore, every tissue is constantly bathed by a circulation of fluids of different kinds which are from eight- to nine-tenths water. Water is one of the finest means for keeping the system free from metabolic poisons. A great many of the tissue poisons, if not soluble in water, are suspendid in it, reducing their toxicity and enhancing their elimination through the kidneys and lungs. Water is necessary particularly in the renal and pulmonary excretions. Carbon dioxid is carried to the lungs as soluble carbonates of potassium and sodium, hence a proper amount of water is necessary for this excretion, besides other deadly organic poisons which find their exit through the lungs. As a general rule, people drink too little—I mean pure water. When they do drink, it is usually in the form of tea, coffee, beer or some kind of alcoholic liquor containing substances which Nature tries to get out of the system. The soda fountain and ice-cream table have spoiled many a vigorous digestion.

The waters of different localities vary so much in character, that I am sure enough has not been said about the influence which they exert upon the inhabitants of these places. Surface water in many localities contains the carbonate of lime held in solution more or less by the amount of free carbonic acid present, making it more difficult of absorption than the organic phosphate of lime. Hard water is not the best for protracted use and is certainly detrimental to the health of those who have weak absorptive powers. Surface water containing any great quantity of sulphates is not a good one. Dentists have told me that they can almost tell where a person is born by the hardness of his teeth. Those who drink surface water full of sulphates are more likely to have brittle teeth than are those who have been fortunate enough to have used the water from springs or wells of hilly or mountainous districts.

I mention these things to show how we can reduce the nature of the poisons generated by the tissues of the body to a minimum that the different organs, especially those of digestion, can have healthy material with which to build the different tissues and not be continually clogged and worn out by taking care of an abnormal amount of waste. It may be seen, then, that foods which represent a large amount of excretory matter, such as meat extracts and blood extracts, must contain a large amount of these excretory products; also that such organs as the liver, kidney and blood, whose function it is to take care of the waste products of the body, must contain in greater or less degree these very same poisons. Therefore, if we wish to select an animal food which will contain the least possible amount of excretory matter, we should study the food upon which this animal lives, as well as its habits and environment.

Those forms of life which live upon decayed or dead animal matter, such as certain forms of shellfish, the oyster, the lobster, the mussel, certain kinds of fish, and some land animals, cannot be recommended as articles of diet for any except those who are blessed with a strong and vigorous excretory system. I do not wish to be understood as saying that no one should indulge in these articles of food, I only wish to point out that when they do so they are adding substances to the body which can certainly be of no practical benefit and only increase the amount of work which the defensive forces of the body must do to render them inert. Those creatures which live upon decayed material, referred to above, will be found to have enormous livers, or like anatomical arrangements, which remove these poisons from their systems. Such an arrangement is absolutely necessary for the life of these creatures. This is why the oyster, lobster, and many of the creatures of the sea which are known to live upon dead matter exclusively, have such large livers, and, strange to say, this is the very part of these so-called delicacies of diet which seems so desirable.

Knowing as we do that the poisons of animal tissues are carried away by the blood, and that they are highly injurious to the system, it seems to me that when we talk about the food value of pure blood extracts, which do not represent the fibrin of the meat in some predigested form, we do not take into consideration that these excretory products are reduced to a highly concentrated state, and, therefore, the poisonous effects of meat and blood extracts, as they are put upon the market, represent a greater degree of toxicity than would an equal amount of fresh meat. The same might be said of soups, the principal part of which is the extract of some meat—they contain merely the products of tissue metabolism. While they are no doubt stimulating because they increase the activity of the excretory organs to remove them, it is doubtful whether the small amount of nutritive value they possess is a full compensation for the amount of poisonous substances taken in with them. There cannot be a shadow of a doubt that many people have been starved to death by beef tea, so carefully prepared by loving friends and relatives, whereas they should have had the fibrin of the meat in a predigested form, which is in reality the only nutritious part of an animal diet. So that, while we cannot disregard the place which meat should have in our diet, it behooves us to study the nature of that meat.

The evil results of irregular eating are too well known to require a detailed account here. The pernicious effects of retiring to bed with a stomach filled with the abominable stuff which constitutes the usual midnight lunch or banquet will receive due attention in the third part of this article.

The relation of sleep to diet, then, can be readily understood by associating this part of my subject with the first part. If the products of tissue metabolism are active in causing sleep; if we wish to keep from sleeping three-fourths of the time we are supposed to be awake, we should not take into the system those substances which directly depress the nervous centers, clog the brain, and destroy our acutest mental and physical activities. I cannot recommend anything but the closest study of this subject.

There can be no doubt that the position of the body during sleep is responsible for a great many troubles, the cause of which has been attributed to other conditions, or entirely overlooked. This part of my subject is perhaps more important than that on the relation of sleep to auto-intoxication.

In the beginning, I wish to state that man is practically the only animal that is handicapped by the upright position of his body. The fact that the entire weight of all his internal viscera is supported by the spine and the tonic condition of the abdominal and thoracic muscles, makes it exceedingly important that these visceral attachments be kept in a perfectly healthy condition; that is, that they receive perfect nutrition and perfect innervation through the circulation of blood and lymph. When we consider that one-third of a person's life is spent in bed, we may easily see how the position of the body during that time may affect the nutrition of the spinal centers and the innervation of the abdominal supports for the viscera. Few associate the position during sleep with the functions of the parts of the body just referred to. It may be further stated that man is practically the only animal that sleeps upon its back. This has a direct effect upon every visceral function. The spinal cord, situated as it is in a bony canal, is so placed that it may not receive external injury, and, also, that it may not suffer any great degree of circulatory disturbance. It is quite as necessary, as in case of the brain, that the spinal cord and its centers receive an equable amount of blood and also that there be no venous congestion interfering with the return of the blood. If it is important then, that the functions of the spinal cord should not be interfered with, every precaution should be used to avoid the possibility of circulatory disturbances or stasis. The thoracic viscera, situated as they are in a bony cage, perhaps suffer the least disturbance in this respect directly; however,

they do suffer indirectly, as I shall point out later. The abdominal viscera, on the other hand, are not favored to this extent. The liver, which weighs five or six pounds, is the largest viscus in the abdominal cavity and is dependent for its normal position upon its peritoneal attachments to the diaphragm, the ribs of the right side and by the lesser omentum to the stomach. The intestines, also, with their contents constitute no small part of the weight of the body, and the stomach when full weighs at least three pounds. We can, therefore, see that if a person lies upon the back it sets up several phenomena: the spinal column comes in contact with the surface upon which the body rests, and the heat generated because of this contact is apt to produce a relaxation of the spinal vessels favoring spinal congestion, and, therefore, an over activity of all the spinal centers. Another condition resulting from such a position is the effect upon the sympathetic nervous system. The principal plexuses which govern the abdominal viscera are the solar, the hypogastric and the pelvic. The sympathetic system directly controls by means of its vaso-motor nerves the blood supply to every tissue of the body. When we fully understand the delicate mechanism which the vaso-motor system represents, we will readily see how any derangement of its functions, either by stimulation or inhibition, will produce the localized congestion seen in different parts of the body, and resulting therefrom in different forms of disease. If the contents of the abdominal cavity rest with their full weight upon these plexuses, it must be clear that they will directly disturb the vascular supply to every part of the body. When one lies upon the back the liver has a tendency to fall forward and downward. This puts the falciform ligament upon a stretch, pulling upon the diaphragm and interfering with its normal relaxation and contraction. This will disturb respiration, which, I tried to point out in discussing auto-intoxication, is exceedingly important. This position of the liver would also constrict the inferior vena cava, retarding the return of the venous blood to the heart, causing functional derangement in the cardiac cycle above the diaphragm and congestion of the liver and all the abdominal viscera drained by the portal vein below. A person retiring with a full stomach, if he sleep upon his back, will suffer from different forms of mental activity, such as dreams and nightmare, because the stomach rests directly upon the solar plexus. The solar plexus being disturbed will also derange the innervation to the heart through the cervical ganglia of the sympathetic, accelerating its action, thereby causing more blood to enter the brain, stimulating especially the subconscious centers. The power of associating ideas being removed by the cessation of consciousness, the nerve cells, which have received certain perceptive stimuli, run riot without any logical connection, causing dreams and nightmare. This, in my mind, is the direct connection between digestion and dreams. The same rise of blood pressure favors different forms of spinal congestion, thereby disturbing the cord reflexes by a hyperemic condition. This spinal hyperemia causes greater activity, and if the general vasomotor action of the entire body is disturbed by pressure upon the sympathetic centers, to such an extent that the poisonous products of the blood are deposited in the peripheral parts of the body, there will occur certain muscular twitchings from which many suffer during sleep, because the poisons of the blood stimulate the terminal sense organs of the skin, directly causing abnormal reflexes through the reflex arc. I think that it should be clear that going to bed with a full stomach and sleeping upon the back is very detrimental, not only to good sleep, but for a healthy condition of the body in general. The effect of late suppers for those persons who are not exceedingly strong is no small item for consideration.

Byrom Robinson, in a recent and very instructive article* has shown that dilation of the stomach and the first half of the duo-

* The Cincinnati Lancet Clinic, Dec. 8, 1900.

denum is caused by the pressure of the superior mesenteric artery, vein and nerve upon the transverse duodenum, and says, "It might appear strange that the mechanical arrangements of animal structure should tend to destroy its own existence." This is not so strange, if we consider lying upon the back unnatural—that Nature, in constructing the "mechanical arrangements" of man, never intended that he should assume such a position, either awake or asleep, as would tend to destroy his own existence. When sleeping upon the back a full stomach cannot help exerting pressure upon every structure lying behind it. It deranges the solar plexus, the great vasomotor center of distribution for the entire abdominal vascular supply, resulting in all kinds of venous and arterial ischemia and hyperemia. The reason Nature is good to most of us, is because we are endowed with a sympathetic nerve so strong that the involuntary muscular structures innervated by it, will force anything through the alimentary canal, even though there be considerable resistance. Such conditions as Robinson describes are no doubt either acquired by lying upon the back both while awake and asleep, or congenital when a child is born with an abnormally long mesentery (for the longer the mesentery the greater the pressure exerted upon the superior mesenteric structures), or both congenital and acquired, when a child is born with a long messentery, a weak sympathetic nervous system, and is allowed to stay too much upon the back during infancy. One can readily understand that those animals which walk upon all four limbs are less subject to circulatory and nervous disturbances than is man, for no other reason than that the horizontal position of the spinal column will constrict or obstruct none of the vital forces. The same position is taken both awake and asleep—the spinal cord is above the abdominal viscera instead of below them. I think the profession should seriously consider the propriety of allowing sick persons to lie too much upon the back—that is, without frequent changes. I cannot logically see how such a position does not prolong disease by interfering with the source of all health, the sympathetic nervous system. Man, because of his upright position, suffers greater sympathetic derangement than do other members of the animal kingdom, whose viscera fall away from the spinal column, leaving the great sympathetic centers free and unobstructed. The mere fact that man's vital forces have to change their action to accommodate the circulation every time he arises from the horizontal to the upright position, puts him at a disadvantage when compared with other animals that never change in any marked degree the vascular supply to the different parts of the body, whether awake or asleep. There is always a regular supply of blood because the spinal column is always horizontal. This change of position so often from the horizontal to the vertical and vice versa, necessitates a very finely adjusted vaso-motor apparatus, which should not and cannot be deranged without very serious results. The most fruitful source of vaso-motor derangement is spending too much time upon the back.

In a similar manner the intestines disturb sympathetic rhythm by pressure upon the hypogastric plexus and indirectly the pelvic plexus. The pelvic plexus, because of its intimate connection with the pelvic viscera should be freest from too great a disturbance, either through the solar plexus itself or directly by the condition of the pelvic contents. Here, again, sleeping upon the back causes many troubles, especially among women. Women who suffer with lax abdominal walls which favor enteroptosis, should be exceedingly careful about assuming this position, whether awake or asleep. In some cases of this nature there can be no doubt that through the disturbance of the solar and hypogastric plexuses the vaso-motor control of all the pelvic vessels is greatly disturbed, favoring the retention of poisons, thus weakening the pelvic tissues. Every gynecologist knows the results of pelvic displacements and their effects upon the vegetative functions. The

whole sympathetic system is disturbed from the pelvis to the top of the head. A most fruitful source of irritation here in the pelvis is sleeping upon the back when the bladder is full. A full bladder practically fills the whole of the true pelvis; consequently, both the hypogastric and pelvic plexuses are very easily pressed upon when this viscus is full and helped by the pressure of gravity. Consequently, persons who drink a great deal should never resist the calls of Nature in this regard, especially at night.

If, as I mentioned in the first part of this article, the sympathetic while we are asleep is instrumental in removing the toxic products generated during hours of work, I think I have logically pointed out the direct effects of disturbance in this most important part of the nervous system by sleeping upon the back. It is certainly abnormal, unnatural and very disastrous in all its results. I would not recommend it even for those who are well and strong; it certainly does not increase their physical or mental capacity and only throws more work upon the sympathetic system, which is the life or death of every individual.

It might be asked, then, What is the best position during sleep? Of course, it can be seen that from an anatomical and physiological standpoint the best position is upon the abdomen, or some position which will favor the minimum amount of spinal pressure or congestion. Very few ever train themselves to assume this position for the simple reason that it is not taught to them during infancy and childhood.

Parenthetically, I might say that I think parents make a great mistake in allowing their infants to sleep as much as they do upon the back. Pardoning the digression, I will state that in a new-born child the liver is out of all proportion in size to the other organs in the abdomen, weighing anywhere from one and a half to two pounds. The pressure of this gland upon the abdominal contents, favoring a disturbance of the function of the diaphragm, should be avoided at that time of life as well as during maturity. The liver in a child is the most active organ it possesses, and I think I sufficiently proved the disastrous results of interference with the portal circulation in the discussion of auto-intoxication. When the child lies upon its back the greater part of the time, the weight of the liver can not help exerting some pressure upon the portal vein, interfering with a healthy hepatic circulation. The metabolism of the child, being very rapid, calls for feeding at short intervals, keeping the stomach full, thus exerting pressure upon the solar plexus with the results noted above. No doubt children would fare just as well if placed for a part of the time upon the side, preferably the right side, as this will release the weight and pressure of the large liver, favor the passage of the gastric contents into the intestine, and release the action of the heart.

Returning to the point of digression, if our parents have not trained us to assume the right position in our earlier years we can do much in the right direction ourselves. After the habit has once been acquired of sleeping upon the abdomen, it is not so very difficult to keep this position, although it means considerable of a struggle, extending over some time. However, if this position is impossible to some, the next best is upon the right side. Probably the best way is to lie upon the right side for the first part of the night, or until there is need of evacuating the bladder, and then assuming a position upon the left side for the rest of the night, when the stomach has become empty.

The fact that a person lies upon the side, however, does not remove the possibility for other serious troubles than those mentioned. Few of this generation, living as we do amidst great nervous excitement, realize the great importance of complete physical and mental relaxation for conserving the vital forces. Frequently after retiring, the lawyer thinks and worries about some client he must exonerate from blame and help out of trouble; the physician is kept awake in the acutest mental activity, planning how he can save a patient hovering between life

and death; the merchant worries for fear some irresponsible person may set fire to his store and cause his financial ruin; the broker, dealing in stocks, fears the least fluctuation in money values, and lies awake wondering whether with the coming morn he will be a millionaire or a pauper. And so it is in nearly all walks of life. More persons than we are aware of never sleep in a condition of perfect physical and mental relaxation. To obtain the greatest value from sleep we must be able to induce by every means possible a perfect cessation of all cerebrospinal activities. To pass into unconsciousness with every muscle tightly drawn, because of too great cerebral activity, can not have the desired result, perfect rest. Unconsciousness does not always mean rest. A person may work a great deal harder during sleep and awake a great deal more exhausted and tired than when he went to bed.

We should also lie in such a position as not to disturb a free circulation to every tissue in the body. Therefore, the body should lie in as straight a position as possible, that the blood may reach all parts equally. The lower limbs should not be flexed to too great a degree, either the thighs upon the pelvis or the lower legs upon the thighs, for shutting off the normal blood supply to the lower extremities will have a tendency to cause abdominal congestion, and possibly cerebral congestion. The arms should not be left above the head, nor in such a position as to shut off the terminal circulation. The habit of going to bed with cold feet, when the vaso-constrictors have shut down tightly upon the terminal circulation, is a bad one, especially for children, because they will flex the lower limbs upon the body in the endeavor to get them warm. If flexion of the limbs interferes with the circulation the child's object in assuming such a position is defeated and its feet are never warm.

In concluding this article I wish to make a few final suggestions:

First: Take care of the liver, the kidneys, the lungs, and the intestines. Never allow any condition to exist which interferes with a healthy and vigorous portal circulation.

Second: Sleep is a physiological anesthesia induced by the metabolic poisons of the body itself.

Third: Keep the body healthy by a well cooked vegetable diet with a small amount of perfectly healthy and easily digested animal food, together with plenty of good water, all of which will reduce to a minimum the work of the excretory apparatus and increase the capacity for intellectual or physical labor.

Fourth: Assume such a position during sleep as to relieve pressure of every kind upon the sympathetic nervous system.

Fifth: Assume such a position during sleep that the circulation to every tissue of the body is normal and regular.

Sixth: THE GREATEST AMOUNT OF GOOD CAN BE DONE IN RELATION TO THIS SUBJECT BY PUTTING THESE SUGGESTIONS INTO PRACTICE DURING INFANCY AND CHILDHOOD. AN OUNCE OF PREVENTION IS WORTH A POUND OF CURE.

OCCUPATIONS WHICH HASTEN DEATH.

MORTALITY OF NON-WORKERS GREATEST OF ALL.

IT has long been recognized by life insurance companies, says a writer in the *New York Times*, that there are certain occupations which are almost certain to bring life to a premature end. So important is the settlement of the question of the effects of various occupations upon the duration of life regarded by insurance concerns that, at the present time, the actuaries of America are engaged in an effort of magnitudinous proportions to collect exact statistics on the subject. * * *

The actuary deals essentially with averages. He takes the experience of many insurance companies and sees what effect certain causes have upon men of every age and occupation. The tables which estimate the effect of occupation upon the duration of life are made up of the experience of companies with regard to all men regularly engaged in a specific occupation. All occupations with which the companies have had experience are included. Men with no occupations are placed in a class by themselves and an exclusive average thus obtained. It is found that so many men out of every thousand with a regular occupation die every year. The average occupied man is then said to die with this average rapidity. Specific occupations are then grouped, and the average death rate in each of them is computed. The experience of American companies has not been as completely set forth as those of English concerns. so insurance in the United States must be based in so far as occupation is concerned largely upon the result of English experience, which must be slightly different from what it is here, though not enough to make more than a fractional difference in the average percentages.

A well-known New York actuary said a few days ago that the latest compilations which have been made show that the cutlery manufacturing trade is one of the most dangerous of all occupations. In every factory where cutlery is made the air is laden with invisible metal dust caused by the grinding of the steel, and this being carried into the lungs, produces asthma, and eventually consumption. The grinders bending over their work inhale such enormous quantities of the dust that they rarely live above the age of forty, while a needle polisher who begins to work at his trade at seventeen may feel that he is unusually fortunate if he is alive at thirty-seven.

All metal trades, in fact, says this actuary, are very hazardous. Phthisis, or tubercular affections, and respiratory diseases are the principal penalties of these pursuits. Records show that filemakers are dying more rapidly year by year. Files are now being manufactured in much greater abundance than formerly, and the mixture of metals from which they are made is more injurious to the human system when inhaled than was formerly the case. Filemakers are beginning to suffer from chronic lead poisoning, a disease with which in former years they were not troubled at all. The lowest mortality for metal workers is among blacksmiths.

Experience of recent years shows that the mortality among those connected with the supply of liquors is enormous. Brewers, for example, die about 50 per cent. faster than the average man who works at a regular calling. Brewers, contrary to the general impression, die extensively from alcoholism, while gout is an enemy which makes itself sorely felt in this occupation. Brewers are also more than ordinarily subject to diabetes, liver diseases, and Bright's disease. The general mortality among saloon keepers is just twice as high as the average, and saloon keepers die from alcoholism just seven times as fast as do the average of men of other occupations, six and one-half times as fast from diseases of the liver, six times as fast from gout, and more than double as fast from diseases of the urinary system, from rheumatic fever, from diabetes, and from suicide.

One of the most terrible diseases is that which attacks wool sorters and all who handle untanned skins, for not only do they breathe the poisonous fumes which arise from the skins before they have been preserved, and which invariably cause consumption or diphtheria, but they are also subject to anthrax. At the time of being killed, the animal may not have been in a healthy state, and therefore poison lurks in the skin. Then, if the worker chances to have a cut on his hand, some of the moisture touches the wound, and anthrax follows inevitably. The worker sickens, goes into delirium, and after suffering the most terrible agony for several days dies.

Among butchers, the mortality is usually very high. Strange to relate, the butcher's trade seems to be one which leads him particularly to alcoholism. The latest statistics, too, show that there were twice as many deaths among butchers from alcoholism as was the case in the reports of a decade ago. The effects of the butcher's trade proper seem to be most manifest in the diseases of gout, rheumatic fever, diabetes, and cancer.

Bakers, too, are more than normally subject to premature death. In the first place, there is great danger from accident in the striking of a match or taking a light into a room in which flour dust is floating. In case this is done, there follows an explosion which is likely to be very dangerous. Then in the flour itself there is a very small microbe which eventually has its effect upon the teeth, causing them to break away at the roots. This little microbe also attacks the drums of the ears and causes deafness, to say nothing of fanning the spark of consumption. Bakers, unlike butchers, do not die much from alcoholism, but they are peculiarly subject to diseases of the liver, rheumatic fever, diabetes, and urinary troubles.

All the building trades are very dangerous. The plumber, the painter, and the glazier, according to the actuary interviewed on this subject, show a very high mortality. With the development of these trades of recent years, too, the mortality does not seem to decrease. These workers suffer very severely from lead poisoning, this being the principal cause of their excessive death rate. The painter is paralyzed through mixing paints owing to the large quantities of arsenic and white lead which they contain. The occupation of the plumber is also subject to an undue mortality from phthisis, cancer, and rheumatic fever.

The glass blower, no matter how strong his constitution, cannot long escape the certain death of his trade. Life insurance companies are now extremely reluctant to take risks in this occupation at all. These workers are assailed by a multitude of troubles. In all glass factories millions of jagged fragments of glass are constantly floating in the air. These, being inhaled, wound the lungs, causing hemorrhage, and premature death. Glass workers are also apt to grow dumb through a peculiar complaint induced by handling the glass, and which attacks the jaws and ends in paralysis. In mirror factories, in addition to the dangers already mentioned, there is that of mercurial poisoning. This deadens the sight, crumbles away the jaws, and ultimately kills long before death is due. The average mortality among those who have worked in glass for more than twenty years is, according to recent actuarial tables, more than 60 per cent. Glass workers, in addition to the dangers of their work proper, are apt to be led into alcoholic troubles and nervous diseases. They suffer from these twice as much as do persons following ordinary occupations.

The occupation of the miner is dangerous both from its liability to accident and from his inevitable susceptibility to certain dread diseases. No other class of men suffer so heavily from consumption, and the life underground is apt to produce blindness and ague. Paralysis follows if work is persisted in after these ailments first manifest themselves. Sometimes the loss of reason is the next step. In lead, copper, and quicksilver mines the results are even more disastrous. Mineral poison becomes injected into the system, and besides originating blindness and paralysis causes the teeth to fall out, while a "copper canker," as it is called, eats into the flesh in precisely the same way as does leprosy. Coal miners are the healthiest of all miners. They are unusually free from phthisis, and they suffer inappreciably from alcoholism. In recent years, too, the liability among coal miners to accident has decreased very considerably.

The actuary said that one of the most curious problems life insurance companies had been called upon to consider in recent years was the matter of insuring the lives of divers. Divers do not live long, and those who dive to great depths are of extremely short lives. The diver generally dies from accident. The first warning the deep-sea diver has of the effect that the high pressure he has undergone is about to end his life is copious bleeding of the nose, accompanied by occasional fits of giddiness. From this, in case he escapes alive, two results may accrue: either total collapse of the nervous system or a disease known as diver's palsy. Both of these result in the victim becoming a permanent invalid.

The man who works on high places seems to suffer from troubles very similar to those of the diver. The man who works in cellars and basements, on the other hand, is liable at any time to be struck down by a malignant fever. If he recovers from this he is left weak and decrepit for the remainder of his life. The mortality among ordinary laborers exceeds that among the average of men by about 25 per cent.

The layman might suppose that sailors, living as they do in air where there is always so much ozone, would be of an unusually healthy class. As a matter of fact, however, sailors are subject to scurvy, a most malignant disease, which either brings its victims to an early grave or leaves them weak and helpless during all the rest of their lives. Moreover, the lack of shade during the hot weather at sea and the brilliance of the sun upon the water impair the eyesight, and in later years the sailor may, without the slightest warning, go suddenly blind.

Chemists and druggists seem to be peculiarly addicted to suicide. From rheumatism those engaged in these occupations die twice as fast as the average, while they are four and one-half times as susceptible to gout. Among tobacco dealers the mortality from diabetes is double as high as is the case among the average of men. Dairymen are peculiarly subject to gout, while a large number of them commit suicide. Among grocers and keepers of fruit stands, diabetes seems to be a very prevalent cause of death. Drapers die faster than the average from phthisis, influenza, and rheumatic fever. The jeweler is liable to suffer from the most violent of all solid poisons, diamond dust. Cataracts and loss of sight are common ailments among those who set jewels.

The worker in match factories suffers from a peculiar complaint known as "phossy jaw." This was at one time the most deadly of all trade maladies, but matchmakers studied the problem and they now use a newly invented kind of phosphorus which reduces the number of fatal cases to a minimum. Nevertheless, a large number of workers in these factories succumb to this trouble every year, and insurance companies are extremely loath to insure the life of any man in a match factory. The symptoms of "phossy jaw" are a crumbling away of the jawbone, this ending ultimately in total paralysis and death.

Dyers, bleachers, and all who labor in factories where chemicals are largely used seldom reach their fortieth year. The chlorine, used so extensively by dyers and chemists in general, attacks the lungs and burns them away gradually but surely. Those occupied in making chlorine gas are well aware that if they continue in that employment they cannot expect to live more than ten years. Hatters, shoemakers, and tailors show very high mortality from phthisis.

Physicians die just a little faster than their patients, upon an average. Only three causes of death in this occupation show a lower proportion than is the case in the average occupation: phthisis, diseases of the respiratory system, and accident. On the other hand, mortality from diseases of the liver, of the circulatory and urinary systems, as well as from suicide, appears to be greatly in excess. From gout and diabetes, physicians suffer about three times as heavily as do the average men of occupations. Among doctors and members of the legal and clerical professions diseases of the heart are the most frequent of all causes of death.

Lawyers are most generally subject to influenza, cancer, nervous diseases, diseases of the liver, Bright's disease, and diabetes. Diabetes is the principal disease in this occupation. The profession suffers less severely than the average of occupied males from phthisis, heart disease, lung disease, and their mortality from accident is much below the average.

Among commercial travelers the mortality is very high. This is due to the nature of their employment and the large proportion of time they must spend in the open air in all kinds of weather. Not so many of them die from accident as might be supposed. Diseases of the liver, alcoholism, diabetes, cancer, and Bright's disease are particularly prevalent as the causes of death in this occupation, which, however, suffers less than the average male population from phthisis and diseases of the respiratory organs. The railway employe does not die nearly so rapidly as might be supposed, his mortality being below that of the sailor and the miner.

The profession in which there is the lowest mortality is the clergy. Insurance men say that many people consider that there is a Providential provision in this. The mortality in this class from phthisis and respiratory diseases is represented by figures which are, respectively, only 36 and 31 per cent. of the average of all classes. On the other hand, the clergy experience more than double the average mortality from diabetes and one and a half times the average from rheumatic fever. They suffer slightly more than the average from influenza, and also from diseases of the digestive organs other than the liver. Among local diseases, affections of the circulatory system are collectively the most frequent cause of death among the clergy.

Among the causes of death of occupied men in general, phthisis and diseases of the respiratory organs most generally cause death. Alcoholism, gout, cancer, and suicide are more common in city life, while in rural and industrial districts diseases of the nervous and respiratory systems are more than ordinarily frequent. Phthisis and alcoholism are far below the average among agricultural workers. Records of recent years show that cancer is increasing slightly, while phthisis and all other tubercular diseases are decreasing.

What is perhaps the most peculiar of all mortality facts is that insurance companies had rather take a risk on a man with an occupation than upon a "gentleman of leisure." The latest compilation of experience in both the United States and England is to the effect that the mortality of unoccupied men exceeds that of the average of occupied men by 132 per cent.

THE NEED FOR MORE EFFICIENT SANITATION.

"THE problem above all others which awaits solution is not how to invent the most deadly weapon of offense or defense, nor to evolve the best means of living cheaply, nor to discover a specific for each and every disease; nor is it in the sphere of high politics; but the problem is" (*Med. Record*) "to devise the most effective methods of improving the sanitary conditions of cities and teaching and enabling the poorer classes throughout the world to lead a healthy life—in short, to endeavor to banish disease by rational preventive measures. It would be superfluous here to do more than point to the curtailment of disease already brought about by various modes of thorough sanitation intelligently carried out. Suffice it to say that the results have been so illuminating that they have shed a bright light upon the possibilities of the future, and have acted as a beacon for the guidance of social reformers. The question of sanitation, however, is such a wide one that within the limits of an article it will be possible to deal with only a few of its more salient features.

"At the Pan-American Congress just held in Havana, Dr. Walter Wyman, Surgeon-General M. H. S., gave an able address on the subject, and especially urged that municipalities should more fully recognize their responsibility and their duty to the community by insisting that the cities and towns under their control should be kept clean and wholesome throughout; and he rightly drew attention to the fact that in order to bring about this state of affairs it will be necessary to cultivate among the people a demand for municipal sanitary excellence, and as great an abhorrence of municipal filth and neglect of sanitary engineering as there is of uncleanly dwellings and of uncleanliness of person. A good water supply, perfect sewerage, and proper disposal of garbage, good street paving and street cleaning, should be the first boast of every municipality. But these are no new truths; and although it is perfectly right that they should be constantly ventilated, and that, if possible, the mass of the people should be educated to appreciate their full significance, and while at the same time thinking persons of all grades of society have come or are coming to a belief in the virtues of proper municipal sanitation, and take a pride in the beauty of the town in which they live, yet the difficulty is that the real root of the evil is not grappled with, and that the localities in which disease is nourished and the sources from which it is spread far and wide are too often untouched. As Dr. Wyman pertinently remarks: 'There is no reason whatever for the existence of slums in any city. Relatively speaking, too much attention is paid to public parks and handsome municipal buildings. The city's improvements should be in the alleys, around the docks, in the tenement-house quarters; and great as may be the appreciation of public art as manifested by statues and public gardens, and of the parks and boulevards, let these wait upon the less showy but more important features of municipal life. The old saying, "What the eye does not see the heart does not grieve for," applies with equal force to cities as to individuals.

" 'The faults that do not obtrude themselves upon the observation are by the majority of people passed by heedlessly. The plague spots of large centres of population are invariably in out-of-the-way places. Therefore the sewerage, paving, light and ventilation of these, the worst sections, should receive the first and most constant attention. Unfortunately, it is notorious that this is not the case, and the energies of the municipal authorities are for the most part concentrated upon the effort to keep the principal thoroughfares in a satisfactory sanitary condition to the neglect of the disease-breeding purlieus. The wealthy and presumably better-educated portion of the community display in this connection a lamentable lack of foresight, and their apathy with regard to the unsanitary conditions of the districts inhabited by the poor classes in many instances may be termed almost suicidal." Dr. Wyman puts the situation plainly when he says: "It is an interesting matter for conjecture—What would be the effect upon the prevalence of contagious disease if there could be a complete wiping out of all slums and low tenement-house districts in all our cities? It matters not that an epidemic once started may prevail as violently or more violently in the better portions of a city, and that cleanliness and sanitation may then have but little effect upon its progress. The fact remains that for the perpetuation of these diseases among the people filth and bad environment are essential; and when we reflect how easy and natural is the upward gradation of infection, how readily through successive grades it may ascend the social scale from the lowest to the highest, the direct and personal interest of the wealthy and more intelligent classes of a community in the condition of the poor and ignorant becomes manifest." The fact is that well-to-do citizens are both directly and indirectly concerned with the physical and moral welfare of their poorer brethren, and that a failure to realize their true position in the matter will inevitably recoil disastrously upon their own heads. The men of almost unlimited wealth, "rich beyond the dreams of avarice," who are more numerous in this country than in any other, and who, to their credit be it said, are as a class by no means backward in furthering charitable schemes, seem not as yet to have become impressed either with the need of or with the good to be done by assisting with their money the cause of efficient sanitation.

"In Europe and in Great Britain especially, many philanthropists of ample means have expended large sums in improving the dwellings of the poor, with on the whole most satisfactory results. The writer of the address to which reference has been made, comments upon the immense amount—$61,-000,000—which has been contributed during the past year to educational, religious, and charitable objects and institutions in the United States, and makes the just reflection that while such lavish benevolence is a magnificent manifestation of prosperity and philanthropy combined, yet in the list of benefactions there is no mention of purely sanitary gifts or endowments. He is of the opinion that more practical and beneficial results would have been obtained if this $61,000,000, instead of being expended upon educational, religious, and charitable institutions, had been devoted to reclaiming the slums, and in the purchase and destruction of rookeries, with the erection in their stead of modern sanitary tenement houses; and that, too, even though the money had not been expended outright as a gift, but as a safe though moderately paying investment. The tendency of up-to-date treatment of disease is rather to prevent than to cure. The policy is assuredly a wise one. But so long as districts reeking with filth, overcrowded, lacking light, air, and ventilation are allowed to exist, the hope of stamping out or even checking disease to any great extent must be dismissed as Utopian. Sanitation carried out thoroughly and rigorously is the only panacea."

⁂

AMERICANS ARE GROWING LONGER LIVED.

THE recent publication by the chief statistician of the United States census for 1900, of the vital statistics of the country, gives an opportunity, says the *Med. Times*, for some interesting comparisons and deductions. In the registration areas so far made public there has been a decrease in the death-rate for the country in the past ten years of 1.8 per one thousand of population, or a decrease of nearly 10 per cent.

When it comes to the study of great centers of population some interesting facts are shown. Curiously enough, among the large cities, Chicago shows the smallest death-rate per one thousand of the population, *viz.*: 16.2 for 1900, as against 19.1 for 1890; St. Louis, its old-time rival, stands a good second, with 17.9 against 17.4 in 1890, a slight increase in rate during the ten years. Boston comes third, with a distinctly higher rate, that of 20.1, although it is reduced from 23.4 in 1890. New York City comes a close fourth, with 20.4 as against 25.3, showing a great decrease in the ten years, probably due to the efforts of such practical reformers as Riis. Baltimore comes fifth, with 21. as against 22.9, while Philadelphia comes next, with 21.2 as against 21.3 in 1890. Philadelphia is a remarkably healthy city outside of its death-rate from typhoid fever, due to its water supply, a defect which will be removed within the coming year through the introduction of an elaborate system of filtration.

The smaller cities show a distinctly better death-rate, beginning with Buffalo, the exposition city, with a death-rate of 14.8 as against 18.4 a decade ago. Milwaukee stands second, with 15.9 as against 18.8; Detroit comes third, with 17.1 as against 18.7, but it is tied with Cleveland's, whose 1890 rate was 20.2. Cincinnati comes next, with 19.1 as against 21, and San Francisco last among the cities of the second class, with 20.5 as against 22.5.

Some cities show a decided increase in the death-rate, notably New Orleans, which has the enormous rate of 28.9, while it was in 1890, 26.3. All the Southern cities for 1900 show high rates of mortality: Mobile 25.9, San Antonio 23.6, Atlanta 26.6, while Savannah shows the rate of 34.3, and Charleston the terrific mortality of 37.5, or more than twice other cities of the same size.

These figures show definitely that more care is shown in sanitation, in the science of living, the introduction of new methods of life, of advances in surgery, etc.

There is one thought in regard to the Western cities with low mortalities compared to Eastern towns with higher which may cause some of these figures to be misleading. There has been a great rush for twenty years of younger people to the West; this has a double effect; it tends to raise the average mortality among the older people left at home, while it lowers that of the regions into which they move.

Still, the figures are encouraging and are a definite refutation to the croakers who feel that the American is growing shorter-lived.

✤ ✤

SOMETHING ABOUT FROGS.

Apropos of what was said in the November issue of the GAZETTE, we republish the following, by Mary Rogers Miller, in the November *Country Life in America:* The author tells, in graphic language, the "Life-story of the Frog," with pictorial illustrations from photographs, of his growth from the wriggling tadpole to the large, jumping, croaking frog.

"A frog's egg," says Mrs. Miller, "looks like a small black bead. Great numbers of these are found together, surrounded by a quantity of the jelly. As the sun warms the water the eggs feel its quickening force and development begins. In the course of a week or two the tiny tadpoles squirm free and swim away into the pond. If taken from the water they would die as quickly as one of us would if forced to exchange places with them. Lungs for air-breathing are fast replacing the gills which did duty in the tad-pole stage. The young frog frequently pokes his nose out of the water as his lungs grow more lung-like, to try them. The mouth, too, must widen and the eyes grow larger and more bulging. When all is complete, the tail will no longer stand in the way.

"The little tadpole, or polliwog, has no family ties. He wots nothing of brothers and sisters. He goes to no school save that of daily experience. To-day a fish may teach him how to dodge, or his own grandfather give him a lesson in deep diving, but in both cases it is to escape making a meal for his teachers that he dodges or dives. The main business of the day is eating—or being eaten. If he escapes the latter for six weeks or two months the common frog finds himself possessed of two hind legs—later of two front ones. Then his tadpole days are over and he enters into the state of froghood.

"Of frogs there are many kinds, including the giant hoarse-voiced bull-frog, which is said to attain a length of twenty-two inches, the leopard frog, the green frog and the wood-frog. All these are found in the ponds in spring, whither they go, if not there already, to deposit their eggs or 'spawn.' With the efficient help of true toads and tree-toads they make up the nocturnal orchestra of the ponds and marshes. Whether the nights are thus made hideous or melodious depends entirely upon the audience. The orchestra is in tune with nature. What if a few strong voices sometimes drown out the fainter ones? One must needs sit down on a log and become a part of the landscape. Then will the music begin, perhaps with a bass solo. A few trial notes, then, gathering volume, it will soon wake the echoes, *Zoom, zoom, zoom!* Resonant, booming, manful,—it is worth going miles to hear."

LIGHT AS A THERAPEUTIC AGENT.

LIGHT has always been looked upon as a beneficent agent, and darkness held to be a subject of dread and evil. Through the sensitive surface of the retina light instantaneously produces very profound effects upon the entire nervous system. Light, however, is found to be not simple but compound—each of the seven primary colors has its distinct influence and produces its characteristic impression. There have been various efforts to determine which of these rays is most potent as a healing agent. There was the blue-glass craze, purple-glass fads, etc. The photographer finds it necessary to perform most of his chemical manipulations behind ruby glass. Formerly he used only the yellow rays.

Further investigation has demonstrated that light as a whole without reference to single rays is divisible into three groups, *viz.:* heat rays, light rays, and chemic rays.

Each of these groups of rays has its distinct activities. Neither the chemic nor the heat rays are perceptible to the eye, but they are not less wonderful in their influence over the animal economy. It is the chemic rays that cause delicate colors to fade, that produce certain bleaching effects, and that change the composition of certain compounds when exposed to strong sunlight.

The heat rays produce the usual effects of heat and need not be discussed at this time. No doubt future experiments will demonstrate that direct sun-heat—for all heat is indirectly sun-heat—can be made far more effective than any so-called artificial form of heat.

Just now it is the chemic rays that are attracting attention. Prof. Finsen, of Copenhagen, has been a pioneer in this investigation. This eminent experimenter has apparently demonstrated that the particular forms of bacteria which are causative of the severer forms of skin diseases can be destroyed by a thorough and prolonged application of the chemic rays of light. Lupus vulgaris or tuberculosis of the skin has heretofore proved a *bête noire* to both physician and surgeon. By means of the chemic rays this destructive lesion can be successfully removed, and as far as yet tested the cure promises to be permanent. This is a great triumph of science.

Whether the deep-seated forms of tuberculosis will eventually be reached by this potent agency, remains to be demonstrated.

TAKING COLD.

TAKING cold is nothing but a *vulgarity,* says a prominent writer. If this be true, and undoubtedly it is in the great majority of instances, what a world of sickness and deaths can be prevented.

Apropos of this subject we find the following in *The Hospital:*

Some remarks recently made by Professor Clifford Allbutt in regard to the influence of chill as a cause of disease serve to illustrate how quickly the pendulum of medical fashion swings as new ideas gain currency in the minds of medical practitioners. Time was when all sorts of ailments were with the utmost confidence attributed to "chill," and when physicians in gravely putting down the origin of colds, pneumonias, and fevers of all kinds to this cause, did so without the slightest suspicion that they were talking nonsense. Then came the time when with one accord the profession bent the knee before the microbe. In proportion as we accepted the theory that febrile and even other maladies were due to germs and micro-organisms, it seemed absurd to talk of chill as provocative of such ailments. We laughed at the ignorance of our fathers, and if here and there a few of us, being skeptical, still talked of chill as an efficient cause of illness, we spoke with bated breath, for the microbe held the field. Then came the turn of the tide. It soon became evident that these wonderful germs were present in all sorts of unexpected places, and that if they really possessed the powers which some had attributed to them we ought all of us long ago to have been dead men. So we looked around for "predisposing" or contributory causes, influences by aid of which the microbes were enabled to take root, and among these we soon found our old friend "chill." As Professor Allbutt says, clinical physicians in their respect for bacteriology had of late rarely ventured to invoke chill and the like as causes of pneumonia, pleurisy, dysentery, and so forth; but, as things were now, he would urge that, so far from being remote, these might often be the immediate causes —so-called exciting causes; in other words, that of a score of persons carrying morbific bacteria about them only the few subjected

to the immediate cause of chill might become affected with disease. So our grandmothers were right after all!

PROGRESS IN THE STUDY OF CANCER.

THE one disease, aside from leprosy, of which we know but little, is carcinoma. Now and then some excited or unscrupulous investigator announces its germ, or a cure for it. But the germ turns out to be an optical illusion and the cures all prove cruel delusions.

Some progress, however, is being made in this important study.

In the London *Lancet*, Dr. Webb advances several rather novel but very reasonable ideas. He seems to have demonstrated that, while it is autoinfective, it is not communicable, or, in other words, contagious.

He says in substance that, "Cholesterine in the economy is in solution, and is kept in this condition by its natural aqueous solvent—soap. It is the loss of this soap that permits cholesterine to separate from the living cell, and cell-cancer to start. The uncholesterine cell is the uncontrolled cell. Cholesterine is at fault in this disease as the bad odor shows. As treatment, the writer uses injections of soap. A bit is dissolved in boiling distilled water and strained. Never more than a teaspoonful should be administered at a time. When thyroid is not contraindicated, it is given per os. This treatment has met with excellent success. When the soap injection is given even alone, pain and odor have been avoided in most trying cases, such as cancer of the tongue. The writer defines malignancy as the crystallization of cholesterine from the living cell."

Department of Physiologic Chemistry.

WITH SPECIAL REFERENCE TO DIETETICS AND NUTRITION IN GENERAL.

MORE ADVICE TO THE CORPULENT.

WE have published numerous admonitions and systems of advice to those who are too much inclined to embonpoint, of late, but the subject will not down. Every month we have further inquiries, suggestions and criticisms. Practically it is found that in a certain number of cases all the diet systems and all the drugs prescribed fail of their object. For all ordinary cases perhaps enough has been said. Those who will not benefit by advice and who will not restrict themselves enough to even approximately carry out any system can not expect relief and do not deserve it. For the minority, those who have faithfully tried Bantingism, Oertelism and all the other isms recommended for the purpose of reducing flesh something more is needed.

What is the fundamental cause of this malady, for it is as much a disease as tabes or typhoid. Happily, there is no longer any room for discussion on this point. *It is essentially a want of adequate oxidation;* tissue metamorphosis too slowly and too imperfectly performed. While this condition persists, the diet may be ideal, and yet the accumulation will go on.

For these unfortunates, what is the rational remedy? Certainly not any one precaution, however desirable as an aid, not any one restriction, however effective it may be in the majority of cases. Unquestionably, the remedy must consist essentially of more oxygen and less CO_2, more exercise, and more perfect elimination. This is simple to say, and has been said and resaid over and over again until it has become an old story. How to secure and utilize the requisite oxygen and exercise, and escape the CO_2, without investing in a chemical laboratory and a gymnasium, is the problem we have to face.

To begin with, every vouchsafed chapter of advice must take into account the association of weak, fat-smothered hearts that sooner or later become prominent and often serious symptoms in all cases of obesity. Any system or regimen that ignores this complication is liable to do more harm than good, and even to endanger the lives of the unfortunates who attempt to profit by it.

First, *teach patients to breathe.* They think they know all about breathing, but they don't. They are continually handicapped by habit and restricted by clothing. Loosen up and lighten the clothes, so that no organ is in the least inpeded in its work. Make them breathe clear down, and thus enlist the diaphragm and abdominal muscles. It is these that churn the food so that digestion, assimilation and elimination can be perfectly performed.

Second, say to them: *teach the skin to breathe;* a function it was surely designed to perform quite as naturally as it attends to the perspiratory act. To do this, expose the entire body to the open, or at least fresh air as often and as long as you can find the time to do it, every day or twice a day. Invigorate it by the regular daily use of the cold bath and vigorous friction. This advice you have heard until it has become a very ancient and worm-eaten chestnut; and you generally pass it by with a little shudder and a promise of "by and by." The shudder is silly, for within a week or two you can make the ordeal a privilege and pleasure rather than a dreaded duty. If hypersensitive, as many people are, especially you who are addicted to too much flesh, take a very hot bath, for five minutes, *à la* the Japanese, and follow this with a sudden and fearless cold plunge or vigorous shower. You will soon grow to delight in the tonic and inspiriting effects that will follow, and will lose all dread of the cold bath. Bear in mind that *it is cold not heat* that stimulates increased oxidation, and it is increased oxidation that you are after. Follow this with a flesh brush, a rough hair mitten, thirty-nine lashes with a cat-o-nine tails made of hard rope, and all the kneading, punching, slapping and massage you have breath and muscle to give yourself or can bribe some one else to do for you. But do not depend on an attendant. *Work yourself.* Half the benefit comes from the exercise. You will voluntarily want the plunge or shower to be made cooler and cooler as you become accustomed and inured to it.

Of course, a sensible diet is essential, but you do not need to starve yourself and brave collapse and heart weakness from insufficient nutrition, although in most cases there is very little danger of this. Find out the exact needs of the body and supply them, without adding a single crumb for waste, as a vital storage battery, or for a rainy day. A little experience ought to settle this point; but bear in mind that you are quite inclined to deceive yourself, pettifog with your sensations and become self-indulgent. You crave sweets and you nibble, without even noticing it yourself; and then you deny it. It has been dinned into your ears day and night that you must religiously let sweets, fats and pastries alone, but you don't do it. You can not resist candy, and have no idea how much you dispose of, all the while flattering yourself that you are abstemious and self-denying.

Lean meats, little starch, plenty of fruits of the acid and subacid varieties, watery vegetables that give much bulk and little nutrition—these are the standard saws that are the stock in trade of all your advisers. All these and numerous others that are equally familiar are important, and it isn't safe to ignore them; but none of them are as important as the point regarding increased oxidation and more perfect metamorphosis.

Ventilate the house from cellar to garret. Never sit, live or sleep in a close room, winter or summer. Especially make it a point to sleep with a window wide open, and forever banish the "taking cold" bugaboo. Practise a system of forced respiratory exercises, not spasmodically, but regularly and punctiliously, and the oftener the better, even if it be a hundred times a day. No apparatus is necessary, and no time need be lost in the process. Simply fill the lungs with perfectly fresh, cool air—the coolest that is available—retain it as long as convenient and expire it slowly. Take, every day, without fail, just as much general exercise as the state of your muscles and heart will warrant, and let it be exercise that calls into play all the principal sets of muscles, not merely a few of the less important ones. Increased oxidation can not be effectively stimulated without the assistance of the muscles. But don't delude yourself into believing that carriage riding is exercise. Stride a horse or a wheel, or each alternately. Climb hills every time you can get a chance. Learn to ride the wheel upgrade; but get at all these vigorous exercises gradually and with reasonable circumspection, and then stick to them. Too many who set out with the best of intentions are too easily discouraged and succumb to shiftlessness. Only the Spartans win.

Rope-climbing has been recommended in these columns. It is one of the very best of all exercises for those who have omental accumulations—large abdomens. Fifteen minutes night and morning at this sailor practice will do wonders for those whose principal deformity hides their toes. At first you can not climb very high—perhaps not a foot from the floor; but in a short time, if you persist and are in earnest, you will make progress and will finally be able to reach the ceiling. As you acquire facility and rise on the rope your confidence in results will rise. You will rapidly or, at least, steadily lose weight and gain lung power, which is the thing you most lack. If you add a spirometer to your accessories and use it daily and often as a lung developer, it will prove a valuable auxiliary. Those who are inclined to embonpoint almost without exception have small lungs.

When you have faithfully practised these various methods and can readily climb to the highest ceiling, half a dozen times at each séance, the scales will probably show that your ambition and your avoirdupois are on speaking terms and ready to arbitrate their differences; while with every pound you lose your general health will improve, your muscles will grow firm, complexion clear, and spirits exuberant.

If this prescription had cost you a thousand dollars you would no doubt have great respect for it and would move heaven and earth, and jeopardize the peace of mind of all your friends in order to carry it out. Don't be such an idiot! Get in earnest, once in your life. *Go to work for yourself.* There's nothing on earth to hinder you from making yourself over from an over-indulgent and over-sensitive physical coward and degenerate to a live, **aggressive and contented human being.**

And then they can undertake to teach their dumpy and out-of-breath next neighbors how to accomplish this same process of physical emancipation and regeneration.

FOOD PRESERVATIVES AND THEIR EFFECTS.*

By H. E. BARNARD, CHEMIST, NEW HAMPSHIRE LABORATORY OF HYGIENE.

WITHIN the last quarter of a century numerous new methods for the preservation of foods have been introduced, some of which have been wonderfully beneficial; others are of questionable nature and value, while still others are open to the most weighty objections.

The refrigerator has become a household article, the ice machine has been invented and perfected, and cold storage introduced in packing house, market, and transporta-

*Sanitary Bulletin State Board of Health.

tion cars; the antiseptic and toxic properties of chemicals have been studied, and the preparation and sale of chemical preservatives have become a distinct industry.

It is now a common thing for druggists, grocers, and dealers in dairy supplies to advertise as a recent discovery some article of "wonderful preservative properties, but entirely wholesome."

On account of the perishable nature of many foods, it is obvious that a substance having the properties claimed for the various food preservatives would be of incalculable value. At the same time it is of the utmost importance that nothing should be added to foods which is toxic in itself, or which interferes even to the slightest extent with the process of digestion.

This last point is especially important in its relation to invalids and children. Food treated with antiseptic drugs may, perhaps, be eaten with impunity by adults who are in good health, and yet turn the scale against an infant or invalid whose life is in the balance; and indeed we cannot say, that the continued use of small amounts even of those antiseptic chemicals which seem to interfere least with the normal functions of the body will not exert a deleterious influence in time.

Again we must remember that the absence of food preservatives is often an indication of wholesome food, at least so far as cleanly methods and appliances, complete sterilization, and careful, efficient management can make it wholesome.

On the other hand, the presence of preservatives may often be taken as an indication that food products have been prepared by shiftless, slovenly, uncleanly and generally inefficient methods.

In using preservatives of unknown composition, reliable and well-meaning food manufacturers may unknowingly commit two wrongs. First, they may add to their products a compound of markedly toxic properties; second, they may violate the law. Dependence cannot be placed on the claims of dealers. Representations of wholesomeness are worthless, because they accompany every food preservative. The statement that a given preservative may be used according to directions without violating the provisions of any pure food law is always false.

Among the various chemicals used as preservatives are borax and boric acid, benzoic acid, salicylic acid, or its sodium salt, and formaldehyde. Both borax and boric acid are extensively employed for the preservation of meat, fish and dairy products.

While boric acid and borax are not as objectionable as some other preservatives they are toxic compounds and their use is to be condemned.

Salicylic acid has been used in enormous quantities to preserve fruit, meat and vegetables, but the mass of evidence resulting from physiological studies with salicylic acid tends to condemn the addition of this substance to foods under all circumstances.

It is possible that the majority of persons in sound health may suffer no evident injury from small amounts of salicylic acid, but its use by aged and infirm persons is attended with great danger.

We have recently examined a sample of "Preservit," prepared by Preservit Co., Newburgh, N. Y., and advertised by them as a household necessity for preserving fruit, milk, butter, eggs, etc. The preparation is in the form of tablets and the directions for use call for the addition of one tablet to each pint of fruit or one quart of milk.

An examination of this preparation shows it to consist of salicylate of soda, salt, and flour compounded as follows:

Salicylate of soda 32.46
Sodium chloride 30.01
Flour 37.53

This preparation retails at one dollar ($1.00) per package, yet the cost of manufacture is probably less than ten cents ($.10).

Formaldehyde has been used as a disinfectant and germicide for a number of years, but its use as a preservative was not advocated until 1895. It is now very extensively employed for the preservation of milk, and has been reported in other articles of food.

The addition of formaldehyde to foods is undoubtedly objectionable, and its use is prohibited by law in nearly all States and countries. Not only does it interfere with digestion to a marked extent but it has been definitely proved that a compound is formed with the caseine of milk which causes the latter, when treated with dilute acid, such as exists in the gastric juice, to separate in hard lumps that are attacked only with difficulty by digestive ferments.

Preservatives have been and are used in this State, especially by unscrupulous milk dealers and market men, and many preparations are on the market for private use in canning fruit, etc.

It is the intention of the State Board of Health, through the recently established Laboratory of Hygiene, to investigate thoroughly the use of food and milk preservatives, and in coöperation with local health officers and the people at large to see that our excellent laws ensuring us pure foods are enforced. In New Hampshire the sale of articles of food to which preservatives have been added is strictly prohibited by Chapter 269 of the Public Statutes, as follows:

SECTION 3. If any food or substance to be eaten or used in the manner of food or drink contains a less quantity of any valuable constituent than is contained in the genuine article weight for weight, *or contains any substance foreign to the well-known article under whose name it is sold,* or is colored, coated, polished, or powdered, whereby damage is concealed, or contains any added poisonous ingredient, or consists wholly or partly of any decomposed, putrid, or deceased substance, or has become offensive or injured from age or improper care it shall be deemed to be adulterated within the meaning of this chapter.

THE persons who make the most fuss about hay-fever are those who live in clover.
—September *"New" Lippincott.*

THE FLORA OF THE HUMAN BODY AND THE EVILS OF THE LARGE INTESTINE.

E. METCHNIKOFF, according to the *Journal of the American Medical Association*, in a lecture delivered at Manchester, states that the human body shelters from sixty to seventy different kinds of microbes. There are less on the skin than elsewhere; about thirty are found in the mouth, where their secretions attract the leucocytes, and are thus beneficial; about thirty in the stomach; fourteen in the small intestine; and forty-five in the rest of the intestines. The microbes in the gastrointestinal canal do not seem to influence digestion, but certain species evidently prevent the development of others. The cholera vibrio, for instance, kills a nursing rabbit, while it is completely harmless for the adult rabbit, after its intestines are tenanted by microbes. Most of the products secreted by the microbes inhabiting the large intestine are poisonous for the human organism, and the auto-intoxication may assume all forms. Even a chronic inflammation of the large arteries has been noticed in calves as the result of intestinal auto-intoxication. During our entire existence we have to submit to noxious action of the poisons secreted by our intestinal flora.

Attempts to sterilize the intestines have proved futile. The best means of getting rid of the microbian flora in the intestines would be to follow the example of the birds, and evacuate the contents of the intestines the moment that digestion is finished. Recent experiences have shown that persons can survive in good health after the removal of a considerable portion of the alimentary canal—four individuals are now alive whose stomachs have been removed. Ciechomski, of Warsaw, has reported the case of a woman of fifty who had carried a spontaneous abdominal fistula for more than three years without its interfering with her occupations or child-bearing. The entire large intestine was found completely atrophied.

Comparative anatomy shows that the vertebrates with the smallest amount of large intestine are the longest lived. Parrots and ravens live from sixty to one hundred years, while the horse, with its exceptionally developed large intestine, lives but twenty. Ostriches and cassowaries live only twenty-three to thirty-five years, and these are the only large birds with a large intestine. Man is not immunized against his microbial flora, and natural selection has failed to liberate him from his large intestine, which is an absolutely harmful and dangerous organ, not merely from the poisonous products of its microbian tenants, but also because it is the seat of many fatal lesions. Most of the poisons which intoxicate, which gradually enfeeble us, and which render us old before our time, originate in the large intestine.

If it is still impossible to attack the evil at its root by having the surgeon remove the large intestine, there is yet a possibility of relief by means of microbicidal and antitoxic serums, and by reinforcing the noble elements of our organs. The cytotoxins which Metchnikoff and his pupils have produced, which in large doses destroy red corpuscles, spermatozoids, kidney and liver cells, etc., injected in small doses, have an opposite effect, stimulating instead of destroying the functions of the elements in question.

⁕ ⁕

APPETITE AND APPETITES.

LIFE as we see it, says the *Pacific Health Journal*, is dependent upon appetite. Every cell, every animal from the least to the greatest lives because it has an appetite. There is something that calls for nourishment, and causes the organism to seek it. This is the instinct of self-preservation. As a rule, the gratification of the appetite is the means of preserving the individual and the species. But many of these appetites have become perverted, so that their gratification tends to decay rather than life. In some lower forms of life the gratification of the sexual function, while it preserves the species, causes the death of the organisms concerned. In the higher forms of life the use of this function is attended by the expenditure of a great amount of vital force; and where, through perverted appetite, it is unduly used, or abused, it leads to early decay, physical, mental and moral. Nothing will so surely wreck a person's prospects in life as will over indulgence in this line. As we look over the world we see hosts of incompetent, unreliable persons, never making a success of anything, wondering, perhaps, why they are in the world, having no aim in life outside of a mere comfortable existence; or, if they have a higher aim, despondent because they see the hopelessness of reaching what they desire We see nervous wrecks, self-centered and miserable, making their friends miserable. We see those who in their teens gave every promise of success, suddenly lose their hold on life and drop into a speedy decline. We see, everywhere, painters, carpenters, seamstresses, bookkeepers, physicians—men and women in all professions and trades, who are not masters of their occupation, but who simply "pass in the crowd." Part of this is due to hereditary influence, part to wrong education, but very largely to the misuse of that function which should be to us most sacred. In these cases, an unhealthy appetite leads its votaries on to destruction.

The appetite for food, implanted by the Creator to serve as a conservator of life, becomes often the tyrant which drives to perdition. As has been said of fire, appetite is a faithful servant but a hard master. To parley with it is to fall. Hesitation is fatal; one must say no, and mean it, to every temptation to wrong indulgence, for every time one yields it is the harder next time to resist. On the other hand, "Each victory will help us some other to win."

Healthy appetites mean healthy lives. Unhealthy appetites, yielded to, become stronger; resisted, become weaker. It is possible for every individual, with divine help, to crush every unhealthy, abnormal appetite, and cultivate such appetites as will make the most healthful life the most natural life.

Sometimes one, while not indulging in an appetite physically, does so mentally; a course, which, if persisted in, will eventually result in the physical indulgence. Those who have given up the use of meat sometimes express themselves as longing for a tender steak or a piece of chicken. The admission of such longings to the mind makes it more clamorous for recognition, and increases the difficulty of overcoming the appetite.

Mental unchastity is about as evil in its effects as physical unchastity. In fact, one usually results in the other sooner or later. The time to deal with a wrong thought or emotion is at its inception. By watching, one can know when a wrong thought is entering the mind, and nip it in the bud, not by keeping the mind fixed on the evil thought, but by filling the mind with good thoughts.

✤ ✤

WHY GERMANY BARS AMERICAN PORK.

THERE has been a good deal of international acrimony indulged over the action of German authorities in relation to the admission of American products, especially with reference to alleged "measly pork."

German health authorities have charged an increasing prevalence of trichinosis to the eating of pork imported from this country. We have ridiculed the idea, but *American Medicine* puts a phase on the question that probably has not occurred to the respective disputants. It ought to prove an international peacemaker: That uncooked meat should be eaten by civilized people, and to such an extent as to make it a matter of the highest national and economic concern between two of the most progressive of nations, would, at first sight, seem absurd, and yet the habit of the German people of eating raw pork brings about tariff disputes and economic wars with America. Thousands of microscopists are employed in Germany to prevent trichinosis. A tithe of the expense and trouble expended in preventing foolish people from eating raw meat would accomplish the result much more perfectly. And this under a government both grandmotherly and great-grandmotherly! Dr. Stiles finds that in 274 cases of trichinosis in America, 208 were in Germans. The fact is of significance also as an illustration of the slowness of the acceptance of science by the people, and of how indifferent we may become in the matter. Among the most scientific people, and with a most perfectly organized profession, the simple and effective method of preventing the disease in question is ignored and interest devoted to silly tariff and ineffective protective devices. Science has in many things outrun practical realization. There is needed a more determined effort on the part of the profession and of government to bring home to the people the knowledge as yet entirely too theoretic.

FRUIT FOR THIRST.

SOMEWHAT late in the year the *Lancet* has discovered that fruit is the best thirst quencher. But though late the *Lancet's* conclusions are good. "The question, what to drink, might," it says, "on sound physiological reasoning, be answered, eat sound, ripe, juicy fruit. It is noticeable that as fruit enters into the diet the indulgence in alcoholic drinks is diminished. Moreover, the juice of fresh-cut fruit is perfectly free from microbes, is as sterile as freshly clean-drawn milk, and the fruit acids tend to inhibit the power of those disease-producing bacteria which flourish in neutral or alkaline media. The marked anti-scorbutic properties of fresh fruit, due to the vegetable acids and their salts in the juice, are of great importance. For the most part these acids are combined with potash, and hence a free diet of fruit preserves a healthy alkaline condition of the blood, and there is consequently a reduced tendency to the depositing of acids in the tissues. It is a common experience that the more a person drinks to satisfy the demands of thirst, in hot weather, the worse he feels. The temptation is to gulp down huge quantities of fluid, with the result that excessive perspiration sets in, and a very uncomfortable and unrelieved feeling follows. On the other hand, a judicious amount of sound, ripe, juicy fruit, whilst containing all the water necessary to assuage thirst, would lead to no such distress, and would exercise other healthy effects on the bodily functions.

THE EFFECT OF DIET ON CHARACTER.

A FRENCH medical journal attributes the following to an "eminent English physician":

An exclusively pork diet tends infallibly to pessimism.

Beef, if persevered in for months, makes a man strong, energetic and audacious.

A mutton diet, continued for any length of time, tends to melancholia, while veal-eaters gradually lose energy and gaiety.

The free use of eggs and milk tend to make women healthy and vivacious.

Butter used in excess renders its users phlegmatic and lazy.

Apples are excellent for brain workers, and everybody who has much intellectual work to do should eat them freely. Potatoes, on the contrary, render one dull, invidious and lazy, when eaten constantly and in excess.

To preserve the memory, even to an advanced age, nothing is better than mustard.

[This last item may be taken with a grain of—salt.—Ed. GAZETTE.]

VEGETARIANISM.

By J. D. Craig, of Chicago.

As the Gazette invites views from all sides on the diet question, the advocates of a vegetarian diet should not allow their side to go by default. If it were true, as stated by the *Medical Age*, that there are not so many advocates of vegetarianism now as formerly, we should hear less of it, whereas it is doubtful if there ever has been a time when it has been more generally discussed than now. And, furthermore, there never has been a time when as many persons, and particularly physicians, have abandoned the use of flesh meat as there is at this time. Vegetarianism is growing rapidly.

The attention of the medical profession has been directed to the subject very largely by the writings of Dr. Haig, and if the advocates of a flesh, or mixed diet will search for facts instead of publishing mere opinions, they will find that the foundation for their faith is anything but a firm one.

In both articles on vegetarianism in the Gazette for September there are statements made that are not true. No one who has any knowledge of the donkey and Shetland pony will deny that they are capable of carrying, for days together, from twice to four times their weight, and it is doubtful if the writer can find a vegetarian man or woman in Europe or America, between twenty and fifty years of age, that cannot do nearly as well.

This and Rosenheim's statement are fully answered, I think, in an article of mine published in the *Pacific Health Journal* for June, which I reproduce here.

In the table appended to this paper it will be seen that the vegetable kingdom supplies all of the proteids needed for any purpose, whatever, and, although neither milk, butter, cheese nor eggs are necessary to nourish the human body, the one who uses these articles in his dietary is no less a vegetarian than one who does not. Vegetarianism means simply the abstinence from the flesh of animals as food, and that is all it does now or ever did mean.

A NEW SOURCE OF FOOD.

The common horse-chestnut, *Æsculus hippocastanum*, generally considered poisonous by the average rustic who makes no use of the nut except to shy one at every stray canine that comes within range. Contrary to this popular belief, the nut is really full of nutrition and is harmless. It, however, contains a bitter, resinous principle and a fat oil that is unpleasant to the taste. It is, no doubt, owing to these two principles that the flesh of this nut has acquired some therapeutic repute.

Dried and pulverized, it has been used as a catarrh snuff, and is not without curative properties in proper cases.

Hitherto, the tree, which is a rapid grower and prolific bearer of fruit, has been considered merely ornamental and the nuts a waste product. Chemists have long known that the nut is rich in starch and albumen, and therefore highly nutritious, but until recently no effort has been made to utilize it as a food product. Scientific interest has culminated in the perfection of a process by which the bitter resin and oil are extracted and the remaining substance made palatable and appetizing. The process consists in moderate roasting to facilitate the removal of the outer shell. The "meat" is then pulverized and placed in a closed percolator containing ethyl alcohol. The mixture is maintained at a moderate temperature for a week, during which time the resin has been dissolved. The resulting tincture is then drawn off, the alcohol evaporated, recovered by condensation and returned to the powder and the maceration continued for another week, in order to remove all trace of the resinoid.

In fact, the process is repeated by an automatic arrangement of the apparatus until the chestnut meat is wholly free from the bitter taste. The alcohol is finally all driven off by distillation and the dried meat becomes a pleasant and very nutritious food.

The tree flourishes in the temperate climate in almost any soil, is a vigorous grower and the crop of nuts annually yielded ought to make it a profitable investment, provided the new process proves all that is claimed for it and not too expensive for commercial purposes.

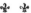

"COME AND EAT."

By Clara Marshall.

"Do you know, sir," asked a supercilious waiter of a ragged Confederate soldier who had strayed into a Richmond restaurant, "that you have seated yourself at the table with General Magruder?"

"Oh, I don't care who I eat with, jest so the vittals is clean," was the nonchalant reply.

This spirit of meal-time indifference to anything and everything except what is set before one in the way of eatables is more excusable in starving soldiers than in many other animals possessed of the gift of speech. "It is true, I never had a day's sickness all the time I was with Stonewall Jackson," observed a reminiscent rebel; "but, then," he went on plaintively, "what is the use of being in high health when a fellow is hungry all the time?"

A man like this, fresh from hardtack fare, is not expected to be good company at table—at any rate, not for the first twenty minutes or so—but the case is different among civilians; and so it is to be desired, for hygienic as well as less practical reasons, that the invitation, "Come and eat," so often heard in rural districts, shall not be responded to so literally. All good people have at their tongue's ends the Solomonic saying: "Better is a dinner of herbs where love is than a stalled ox and contention therewith"; but it does not seem to occur to them all that love should not be mute at mealtimes.

"We had little wit at our feast," observes the Vicar of Wakefield, "but there was much laughter, and that did quite as well."

All doctors agree that the best served meal is better for a sauce of cheerful talk, wise or otherwise, the latter quality perhaps being preferable. That mute and *mauvais quatre d'un heure* prevailing in too many family dining rooms at feeding time provides work for the doctor, and possibly the conscienceless practitioner may enjoy "listening to his table-fellows saying nothing," while plying their knives and forks. But we are sure that the court physician of China, whose salary is stopped when any member of the Royal Family is ill, would insist that this family shall keep time with their chopsticks to the music of cheerful chatter.

"Talk nonsense rather than sit mum," said a man of the world to his young sisters.

They followed this advice, in the dining room as well as the parlor, and this, no doubt, was one of the reasons why the young physician who attended to the health of that part of the country never had occasion to pay them any *professional* visits. In that family dining room it was not, "Come and eat," but, "Come and make merry."

The scientist may indeed trace our origin to languageless animals, but after all these eons of evolution it is only reasonable to protest in the name of health as well as of civilization against men and women being as conversationless at meal times as are those quadrupeds that feed with their forefeet in the trough.

HOW TO SERVE APPLES.

THE apple is an important, most wholesome and most delicious article of diet. One good way to prepare it is to thinly slice a ripe, mellow sweeting and pour over it a modicum of sweet cream.

Again, grate or scrape a well-flavored apple into a small dessert glass of whipped cream, slightly sweetened, and you have a delicate tid-bit to close any meal, in place of richer dessert.

An enjoyable supper is the following: Take large Greenings or Baldwins, wash, core, but not peel, fill the apertures with sugar, and, if you like, a couple of raisins and a bit of cinnamon; place in a granite baking dish, deep and large, pour over a half cup of boiling water and set in a quick oven. When the skins are burst and the flesh thoroughly done, take out all except one and carefully place in the serving dish. Take the skin from the one reserved, sweeten a little more if need be, add a pinch of salt to the ripe juice, which should measure a large cup full, give a dash of nutmeg, and pour the juice thickened with the mashed apple over those heaped in the dish. Set aside to cool, and when served, say truly if you have ever tasted anything more delectable. Accompany it with thin slices of whole wheat bread and butter, and a cup of cocoa, and you have all the ingredients for a most enjoyable supper.—*Golden Age.*

WE can beat the above "out of sight." Thus:

Pare, slice and eat out of hand, without any extraneous addition of salt, cinnamon, nutmeg, saltpetre or what not, any variety of good, ripe, moderately tart apples, such as Greenings, Spitz, Baldwins, Bellefleurs, Newtown Pippins, Northern Spies, Winesaps, Kings or Seek-no-furthers.

Make this your dessert after each and every meal, leaving puddings and salads to the dyspeptics.—ED. GAZETTE.

✤ ✤

NEW JERSEY'S new food law went into effect on Friday of last week. The new law makes a local board of health its own inspector, with power to act under State authority—an innovation that is considered a move in the right direction for several reasons. In the first place, it will insure a more complete inspection of foods and drugs than was possible under the previous arrangements; again, the work can be done at much smaller expense to the State, while the possibility of friction between the State inspectors and inspectors from the local health board will be obviated.

THE DOSIMETRIC SYSTEM.

A CORRESPONDENT asks us to explain the essential principles on which this system of medication is founded.

It was originated by a Dr. Burggraeve, formerly a professor in one of the German Universities. He conceived the idea that ordinary pharmaceutic preparations vary so much in alkaloidal strength, on which their virtues depend, that no medical practice based on their use can be accurate. Thus the crude herbs, such as aconite, belladonna, digitalis and the like, are found to yield very uncertain percentages of the alkaloids, aconitin, atropin and digitalin, and that tinctures and fluid extracts of these very active and powerful agents may possess all the way from one to twenty per cent. of therapeutic potency. No physician and few pharmacists can accurately test a given sample of any of these products, without much delay and considerable expense, and hence is helplessly at sea as to the probable effects of a stated dose.

Other plants yield several distinct alkaloids, as for example hyoscyamin and hyoscin from hyoscyamus. When the tinctures, decoctions or fluid·extracts of such plants are prescribed the prescriber ought to know that he is giving both alkaloids, and must expect mixed results.

Again, Burggraeve's experiments showed that the physiologic action of any drug can only be determined in any individual case by test. What would be a maximum and possibly toxic dose in one case might be moderate and entirely safe in another individual. Hence he adopted the principle of first separating or isolating the active principle of each plant or drug and using this in minute but definite dosage. This insures accuracy.

Then he went further and determined to his satisfaction a minimal dose of each drug in use, making this so small that it would be entirely safe to administer in any case, no matter how sensitive to drug action or what peculiar idiosyncrasy the patient might prove to have. This dosage, in any emergency, to be repeated at very short intervals until the physiologic action of the drug is manifest and then to be given less frequently to maintain such action. He thus proposed, as a result of his experiments, extending over years of practice among the large European hospitals, to provide the practitioner with what has been styled "arms of precision" in his battle with disease.

In carrying out this system all the powerful alkaloids are first isolated and purified, and are then mixed with any negative excipient that may be required to preserve it from chemical change or the action of the atmosphere and subdivided into minute doses to correspond with his theory. Thus the initial, model or minimal dose of strychnine is gm. .0004 or gr. $1\text{-}134$. The dose of hyoscyamin is gm. .00026 or gr. $1\text{-}250$; of hyoscin gm. .000065 or gr. $1\text{-}1000$.

It will be seen that these doses are by no means homœpathic, and yet the size of the little granules except in color representing them much resemble the infinitesimal doses of the "little pill" doctors.

They are active and accurate subdivisions of the drug in every case, and the doctor who prescribes them never needs to worry lest he has given an overdose to some particularly susceptible patient.

This minimal dosage may be repeated in all cases of emergency and suffering, as often as every ten minutes until the symptoms abate or the physiologic action of the drug is apparent.

There are other characteristics of the practice which might be mentioned, but our correspondent had better study them at first hands through some of the numerous volumes treating of the subject. For a time it made little headway with American physicians, partly on account of the cost of procuring the accredited preparations, which were made only in Paris. But within a few years a Chicago firm* has made it quite unnecessary to send abroad for reliable preparations.

Castro's work on the Dosemetric system is published by the Appletons.

* The Abbott Alkaloidal Co.

THE CARE OF EPILEPTICS.

THE happiness and well-being of a confirmed epileptic depends largely, says the Nursery Section of *The Hospital*, upon the social and professional qualities of the attendants. Necessarily the companionship is close and constant, since such a patient cannot safely be left much alone. As a rule, epileptics are not easy persons to manage; the temperament is apt to be unstable, the temper fractious, and the entire disposition variable and *difficile*. Epileptic fits are commonly preceded by periods of irritability and "nerve storm." Usually the patient tends towards mental depression and melancholia. It is an absolute necessity to find bright interests and occupations for epileptics cut off by the nature of their disease from the ordinary social amusements of daily life. The apathy—which so often accompanies epilepsy—makes it a difficult task to provide congenial hobbies and occupations for patients on whose hands time is apt to hang specially dull and heavy.

GLASSES AND GAMES.

Failing, or deficient eyesight, is a common accompaniment of the disease, and this in itself interferes with many pursuits and interests otherwise possible. In some severe cases, the doctor may not think it desirable for glasses to be used constantly, owing to the danger of injury if a patient fall in a fit whilst wearing them. Even when no definite eye trouble exists, any over strain or over use of the sight is apt to give rise to a seizure. So that in finding employment for "idle hands to do," the nurse must bear in mind the necessity for occupation without eye-strain. All open-air games and interests are good, so long as they are not pushed to a fatiguing point. Croquet is an admirable game for epileptics, though I have met with some cases in which the game had to be limited to one hour daily. Many patients complain that croquet causes considerable strain to the eyes and brings on headache. Thus, over-use of the croquet lawn has been found to aggravate and induce fits in some confirmed cases. An important point which needs emphasis is the fact that the midday heat and sun glare of summer is an immediate cause of fits in the epileptic. Epileptic seizures are much more common in summer than in winter. A very great authority on this disease invariably warns his patients to remain indoors between twelve and four P.M. during the hot summer months.

SYMPATHETIC CO-OPERATION WANTED.

People who have suffered from epilepsy since their childhood are usually neglected from an educational point of view. Commonly they are neither taught to play the piano, to paint, or to draw. In too many cases they have been allowed to drift into listless, uninterested ways, sitting for hours in a state of apathy. And a deficiency in the powers of observation is very noticeable in some epileptics. To draw these patients into the common interests of life calls for the most sympathetic co-operation on the part of a nurse. The mental outlook of so many epileptics is cheerless in the extreme. Girl and women patients suffering from this disease are apt to fall into careless customs as to dress and appearance. Cut off as they are from all but a very restricted social circle, they easily acquire a habit of thinking "it doesn't matter how they look." It is a great point to the good to rouse a wholesome vanity and care for personal appearance in patients who tend to drift into this hopeless mental attitude.

CLOTHING AND HABITS.

A very important point in the personal hygiene of epileptics is that they should not wear tight cl―― ― A "pulled-in" corset is c; ―sponsible for a seizure or a series of seizures; female epileptics aggravate the tendency to fits by putting their hair at night into very tight crimping and curling pins. There are no such things as trifles where epilepsy is concerned. In many cases where the tendency is strong, a very small stimulus will cause a fit. Personal and domestic hygiene is an all-important

factor in their care. Healthy regular habits, plenty of fresh air and outdoor exercise, careful dieting, and bright, unexciting interests do much to ward off the recurrence of attacks and to make otherwise dull, dreary lives comparatively cheerful and happy.

DIET.

Cases of epilepsy differ materially. Some patients have their fits in "crops." That is to say, they have a succession of attacks —three, four, or more perhaps within twenty-four hours—after which they may be quite free from fits two or three weeks. In other cases the attacks come singly and very frequently. Some patients tend to have their seizures in the daytime, while in others the attacks are confined almost exclusively to the night. When three to four fits have taken place during the night the patient will usually be considerably exhausted in the morning. The "nerve storm" has been violent, and a reaction of depression almost surely sets in. Fits are sometimes followed by extreme nausea, going on to violent vomiting. This is more especially true of the type of patients whose fits come in "crops." In these cases the dietary must be simple and light. Broths and weak beef teas [Bovinine is better.—ED. GAZETTE], small quantities of Valentine's meat juice given in aerated water, peptonized cocoa and milk, are all suited to the nausea and vomiting of an epileptic.

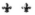

SENATOR VEST'S TRIBUTE TO THE DOG.

ONE of the most eloquent tributes ever paid to the dog was delivered by Senator Vest, of Missouri, some years ago. He was attending court in a country town, and while waiting for the trial of a case in which he was interested was urged by the attorneys in a dog case to help them. Voluminous evidence was introduced to show that *the defendant had shot the dog in malice*, while other evidence went to show that the dog had attacked defendant. Vest took no part in the trial and was not disposed to speak. The attorneys, however, urged him to speak. Being thus urged he arose, scanned the face of each juryman for a monment, and said:

"Gentlemen of the Jury: The best friend a man has in the world may turn against him and become his enemy. His son or daughter that he has reared with loving care may prove ungrateful. Those who are nearest and dearest to us, those whom we trust with our happiness and our good name, may become traitors to their faith. The money that a man has he may lose. It flies away from him, perhaps when he needs it most. A man's reputation may be sacrificed in a moment of ill-considered action. The people who are prone to fall on their knees to do us honor when success is with us may be the first to throw the stone of malice when failure settles its cloud upon our heads. The one absolutely unselfish friend that man can have in this selfish world, the one that never deserts him, the one that never proves ungrateful or treacherous, is his dog. A man's dog stands by him in prosperity and in poverty, in health and in sickness. He will sleep on the cold ground, where the wintry winds blow and the snow drives fiercely, if only he may be near his master's side. He will kiss the hand that has no food to offer; he will lick the wounds and sores that come in encounter with the roughness of the world. He guards the sleep of his pauper master as if he were a prince. When all other friends desert he remains. When riches take wings and reputation falls to pieces he is as constant in his love as the sun in its journeys through the heavens. If fortune drives the master forth an outcast in the world, friendless and homeless, the faithful dog asks no higher privilege than that of accompanying him, to guard against danger, to fight against his enemies. And when the last scene of all comes, and death takes the master in its embrace, and his body is laid away in the cold ground, no matter if all other friends pursue their way, there by the graveside will the noble dog be found,

his head between his paws, his eyes sad, but open in alert watchfulness, faithful and true even in death."

Then Vest sat down. He had spoken in a low voice, without a gesture. He made no reference to the evidence or the merits of the case. When he finished judge and jury were wiping their eyes. The jury filed out but soon entered with a verdict of $500 for the plaintiff, whose dog was shot; and it was said that some of the jurors wanted to hang the defendant.—*Nashville American.*

EXPRESSIONS OF THE EYE.

WOMAN'S weapon is her eye, and the latest importation is a code for the manipulation of that organ. Within a certain range the female of our species has an instinctive perception of the manner in which her optical apparatus should be employed upon her complementary creature in pantaloons; but science has reduced the subject to exact terms. Charts have been prepared—Washington girls are studying them—showing that the eye has 729 distinctive expressions, conveying as many different shades of meaning.

The proper thing to do is to procure one of these charts, and reproduce with your own eyes the 729 expressions before a mirror. When you have mastered them all try them on other people and see how they work. It is popularly imagined that the eyeball itself is an expressive thing, but as a matter of fact the ball of the eye has scarce any expression at all. That all depends upon the lids and brows. The upper lid does the intellectual; its position is regulated by the sort of thinking you are doing. The lower lid expresses, by its draw, rosy or otherwise, the senses. The eyebrows are emotional, and so on.

All this, however, is only the beginning. Certain it would appear that young ladies of the future, trained to make eyes on exact principles, will be much more seductive creatures than hitherto. But you must not be surprised if you find a Washington girl winking at you; it is ten to one that she is practising the novel science of ocular expression.

✤ ✤

EUTRAPELIA AND EUTRAPELOUS.

THE question of the day, or, to be accurate, the question of next week, is, "Have you eutrapelia?" The word comes from La Crosse. Wis., through the American Ecclesiastical Review, to which it is sent by the Rev. Anselm Kroll. It is what Mr. Kipling calls clean mirth, and the learned sponsor of the word quotes many authorities to define and distinguish it, and shows that it is characteristic of the true Christian, and is jest without jeer, laughter without scorn, wit without malice, joke without offense to one's neighbor. It "gives a pleasant taste of happiness in all diversions." It has nothing in common with that fondness for sport that weakens the religious sentiment, but blends piety and natural joy. This seems to indicate that booby-traps, football scrimmages, Chimmie Fadden stories, Mr. Peter Newell's pictures of hydrocephalous boys, Mr. Croker's remarks about Mr. Moss, the compliments passing between Mr. Osborne and Mr. Weeks, Mr. Krüger's definition of Queen Victoria, and Mr. Joseph Smith's praises of the British lion are not eutrapelous. Neither are explosive bullets, attempts to confer freedom with a bayonet point, or happiness by the destruction of commerce; but the writings of Miss Jewett, Mr. Birrell, Mr. Kenneth Grahame, E. Nesbit, F. Anstey; the drawings of Mr. Herford and Mr. Reed; Mr. Seton-Thompson's bears and Mr. Hopkinson Smith's cap'ns; Mr. Kipling's fishermen; Mr. Joel Chandler Harris's darkies, children, and menagerie; "Santa Claus's Partner," and Miss Repplier's criticism and cat are eutrapelous. What a lovely world it will be when its clever folk cease to strive to be satirical or sarcastic, and resolve to be eutrapelous. Everybody must hope to see his neighbor begin.—*The New York Times Saturday Review.*

PASTEUR.

PASTEUR, the great French scientist, often appeared very irascible in public owing to his uncompromising hatred of error and falsehood, which made him a most severe critic of the work of his pupils and assistants, as well as his own. It is related that upon one occasion his ridicule of some operations performed by the veteran surgeon, Jules Guérin, so exasperated that gentleman that he sent a challenge to Pasteur. The secretaries of the Académie de Médecine were, however, successful in settling the quarrel, and prevented the absurdity of bloodshed over a dispute as to the means of saving life. But apart from such controversies, Pasteur seems to have been one of the gentlest and kindest of men, a tender and devoted son, husband and father, and entirely happy in his close and numerous friendships. "The Life of Pasteur," which McClure, Phillips & Co. have recently published, has as its motto the words of Dr. Roux, a noted pupil of Pasteur, to whom the world is indebted for the antitoxin treatment of diphtheria, who declares that "it is necessary to have lived in intimacy with the man to know all the goodness of his heart." R. Vallery-Rabot, the author of the biography, has had that privilege. He is Pasteur's son-in-law, and his life-story of the famous scientist is filled with interesting incidents which reveal his admirable qualities.

✤ ✤

SUCCESSFUL PRACTITIONERS.

THE large personal estate, some $1,875,-000, left by the late Sir Willam Jenner, of London, makes it interesting to recall the big fortunes left by other fashionable and successful medicos of recent times in England.

The next largest personalty to that of Sir W. Jenner's was that of Sir William Gull. He died in 1890, leaving $1,720,110 behind him. This, of course, was the result of professional fees, a large portion of which for a long series of years had been excellently invested.

Then comes the late Sir Andrew Clark, though there is a large falling off in the amount, $1,034,465. Sir Andrew sank a good round sum in real estate. Another big fortune was Sir Oscar Clayton's, about $735,000, and yet another of quite recent date, Sir Richard Quain's, about $585,000. Dr. Thomas Armitage left over $1,000,-000, but the bulk of this was certainly not professional earnings. Dr. Paul, of Camberwell, amassed over $500,000, but he owned one, if not two, lucrative private lunatic asylums.

Sir William Bowman, the oculist, Sir Prescott Hewett, Sir George Paget and Sir Risdon Bennett left substantial fortunes, but all were well under the $500,000 mark. There has been speculation as to what incomes some of these successful doctors earned; $15,000 or $20,000 a year is a big income for a professional man, but at one time Sir William Gull's professional fees most certainly averaged $1,000 a week, if not more, while Sir Andrew Clark's takings at the zenith of his career must have amounted to an average of over $1,500 for every six working days. There are prizes in the medical profession, without a doubt.

MYSTERIOUS MUSIC.

A STRIKING example of the magical effects capable of being produced by any one conversant with the laws of sound was shown by the late Professor Tyndall in one of his lectures. He placed on the floor of the room an ordinary guitar. No one was near, and yet some unseen hand drew music from it, so that all could hear. The guitar was replaced by a harp, with the same result. A wooden tray was then substituted, and even from that issued mysterious harmonies. The marvelous effect was simply due to the sound-conducting quality of wood. In a room beneath, and separated by two floors,

was a piano; and connecting the rooms was a tin tube containing a deal rod, the end of which emerged from the floor. The rod was clasped by rubber bands so as to close the tube, and the lower end of the rod then rested on the sound-board of the piano. As the guitar rested upon the upper end of the rod, the sounds were reproduced from the piano; and when the sound-board of the harp was placed on the rod it seemed as though the actual notes of the harp were heard.

WHY MONARCHS WERE INSANE.

PATHOLOGISTS have often pointed out the fact that physical and mental enervation are apt to go hand in hand, and the intellectual degeneracy of etiquette monarchs may have a good deal to do with the Sybaritism of their palace life.

The plebeian functions which mediæval sovereigns were obliged to perform by proxy included the adjustment of their gala gloves. They had flunkies to remove their cravats and warm their nightshirts, unplait their pigtails, and tuck up their bedclothes around their shoulders. In the morning courtiers competed for the honor of holding their wash-basin; peers of the realm waited on bended knees to buckle their shoes. If the inheritor of a legitimate throne lifted a spoon to break an egg, lynx-eyed lackeys anticipated his needs with the agility of trained conjurers. If he intimated a desire to break the Seventh Commandment, calligraphic secretaries wrote his love letters. Like his food, his information on current topics was served ready dressed and cooked, till he turned into a masticating machine and repeater of conventional twaddle.—*From Lippincott's.*

ONLY a few years ago the business most despised in New York was perhaps that of the sandwich board man. Now it has achieved the dignity of a union whose members are as rigid in the enforcement of their rights as the men in any other trade.

BILLBOARDS are responsible for the sore eyes, the hunger, the indigestion, and the liver troubles, as well as a multitude of other ills with which the people of Chicago are afflicted, according to evidence introduced this morning before Master in Chancery Rush. Dr. Sara C. Buckley, who was a witness in a suit for an injunction to restrain the city from interfering with advertising signs, declared she had known persons who, when they saw the advertisement or the sign of an eye specialist, became immediately afflicted with eye trouble and came to her for treatment.

"The same thing is true of advertisements for all kinds of medicine," she insisted. "People become convinced that they are afflicted with a disease when they see its remedy advertised. The process of suggestion is responsible for this, and the bill boards are the cause of it."

WHAT REALLY EDUCATES A CHILD.

THE child who runs for a day over an ocean ship has laid in a store of observations worth more than much teaching of mechanical invention and means of transportation. A few weeks spent in making a little garden, planting seeds, caring for the tender growths, gathering and utilizing such produce as may come, will bring the child nearer to the great Nature-mother than much school work and even many excursions for Nature-study. It is play, work, love that educate; spontaneous self-expression, action compelled by inner or outer forces. relations to other individuals.—Edward Howard Griggs, in the *Ladies' Home Journal.*

SAYS the *American Grocer:* "We agree with the position assumed by Dr. Wiley, Chief Chemist of the Department of Agriculture, that 'Unless a preservative is known to be injurious to health, in the quantities used, the sale of foods containing it should be permitted, if the character of the preservative and the amount employed be plainly marked upon the label.'

"This entire question of food adulteration is easily settled if all legislation is based on the proposition that the sale of foods known to be unwholesome should be absolutely prohibited. Many foods are cheapened by mixture with other substances of a wholesome character, but that is not sufficient to prohibit their sale. Let such foods be sold for what they are, and under such legal supervision as will secure honest labeling. The prejudice of consumers will quickly disappear when experience has demonstrated that an article labeled as containing some preservative, coloring matter, glucose or sweetener other than sugar, is found to be wholesome."

Dr. W. M. Wilson, who startled the national convention of weather forecasters at Milwaukee, by declaring that there is no appreciable difference in air, the world over, and that mountain health resorts are a fad, evidently aspires to be the Triggs of his profession.

Let Dr. Wilson spend three months in the Rocky Mountains, or climbing the Cuyamacas in Southern California, and he will be ready to repent his rashness and retract his words. Those who have tried "mountain air" do not need to be told this. No, Doctor. There is no comparison between the air of Milwaukee and that of Middle Park or Manitou.

Department of Hygiene.

WITH SPECIAL REFERENCE TO STATE AND PREVENTIVE MEDICINE.

THE THERAPEUTIC VALUE OF CLIMATE.

Sixth Paper.

SPECIAL FEATURES AND LOCALITIES OF SOUTHERN CALIFORNIA.

MORE than a century and a quarter ago, headed by that impersonation of both intrepid courage and fanatical zeal, Father Junipero Serra, barefooted Franciscan friars tore their feet and tortured their hands on the savage cacti that everywhere in Southern California dispute the presence and aggressions of the human family. They bravely and patiently faced the multiple dangers from savage tribes and savage beasts, from scorching sands and blazing sun, from treeless plains and trackless deserts.

Don Cabrillo was no saint, but even the devil could play escort to saints, if he had a purpose behind his apparent condescension.

The Puritans would have execrated him as a pirate, and no doubt the same religious zealots would have ascribed to even Fra Junipero an overweening ambition for pious conquest, propagandism and personal dominion over ignorant and pliable subjects. Whether his piety prevented him from dreaming of prospective discoveries of hidden treasures and golden sands may never be known. However, there is no question but that suffering and sacrifice were the foundation stones on which all the early missions were built. It is an unwarranted libel to assume that the fever of conquest, the lust of gain and of power was the prime motive that prompted the adventurous spirits who founded missions, made the desert to blossom as the rose, and gave

their lives for the sake of ameliorating the spiritual condition of the barbaric tribes that once made this region their favorite rendezvous, their summer and winter stamping ground for special fêtes and festivals, for fetichism and athletic games. It is easy for modern carpers to say that the friars were mercenary hypocrites and cared more for enslaving bodies than for saving souls; but the palpable and admitted results of these early missionary efforts give the lie to the libel. Even if their motives were tainted with selfishness, superstition and loyalty to an ecclesiastic oligarchy whose history is smirched with crimes without number and cruelties unparalleled, then these zealots or pretenders builded better than they knew. They opened up a new world, and they discovered a climatic realm that still remains without a peer on the face of the globe. As evidence of their worldly selfishness it is quoted that they were in no hurry to make known the possibilities of the Paradise into which they had blundered; but we must give them credit for the full measure of what they did accomplish, for it is what men do and not what they talk that tells. They brought to the new Land of Promise the olive, the orange and the vine; they planted in that virgin soil that had never before known the man with the hoe; they built primitive viaducts that brought water from the mountain streams to feed the thirsty earth and make to grow blooming and luxuriant gardens where before was only dry sands and desolation.

And thus they transformed a sun-scorched desert into a

Realm of the golden fruit, realm of the
    bleeding vine,
Where the soil says to the husbandman,
    "Give me my meed of water and I will give
    you wine!"

True, they impressed the superstitious aborigines, as fast as they could bring them under control, to carry their burdens and perform all their manual tasks, and in order to accomplish this end they no doubt resorted to pious fraud and the power that strong and unscrupulous minds have over the weak and untutored. They instituted a religious despotism and practised many forms of cruelty toward their fear-haunted wards that would not now be tolerated. No doubt they interpreted the Seventh Commandment with a spirit of charity, and appropriated many red-skinned Ramonas who would have otherwise blushed unseen and wasted their fragrance on the commonplace lover-braves of their own tribes.

But in spite of all their shortcomings—for human nature is weak and has been the same since time began—these devotees of a decaying system had their mission in the history of the New World in its developmental stage, and all these crumbling missions are their monuments. But for their zeal, patience and obstinate perseverance, in the face of difficulties that would have appalled less determined or less infatuated natures, possibly California would to-day remain a part of old Mexico, and the friars of old, in their successors, would still be dreaming away their lives in the shade of palm and olive planted by themselves, and warming their veins with the blood of the vines they brought from Spanish vineyards.

At all events it was they who demonstrated the soil possibilities of a region whose climatic felicities would have otherwise remained practically unknown save to the savage who did not care to invite the outside world to share his privileges. They proved these possibilities; they developed systems of irrigation; they built dams and aqueducts that are still in existence to attest their ingenuity and perseverance. Under their inspiration the palm and the olive supplanted the chapparal, and vineyards and fig trees took the place of cacti and sagebrush.

The monastery bells they hung, and by the solemn music of which they conquered and awed the crude but plastic natures of the red men of the west, are dumb and dismantled, and the altars before which they led their coerced converts have crumbled into dishonored dust, in the presence of the advancing spirit of civilization. The outcome of their century of strenuous effort and iron rule, of victorious conquest over arid soil and barbaric men, is—California!

It is a land of which much has been written and sung and painted by paragrapher, poet and photographer, but of which the last word has not yet been said and mayhap never will be said. It is a land of promise and possibilities that no poet, philosopher or political economist can weigh or estimate, because it has never had a counterpart by which to be measured. As yet its day of recompense and realization has not come, for it is still in the throes of development and reclamation. Its anxious and oftentimes discouraged people are slowly solving the two basic problems of water-supply and motive power. These solutions will finally be made easy, and then will follow an era of which the present is but a vague hint and prophecy.

This much in a general and discursive way. And now to turn to the more practical topics pertaining to the subject.

All that is climatically desirable in Southern California is either seacoast or mid-mountain country. There are no plains or broad plateaus in this section of the west. The coast country extends unevenly and in widely varying degrees of desirability, for two-hundred and fifty miles southeasterly, from Point Conception to the Mexican line. It varies in width from five to twenty-five or thirty miles. Its area is stated at nearly

45,000 square miles, but it may be safely asserted that two-thirds of this surface is either undesirable or unavailable except to hawks and the hunted coyote. Viewed from the top of any centrally located mountain peak, one sees an apparently unbroken panorama of rocky summits, a wilderness of waste, mere clefts among ragged rocks that seem to monopolize the landscape, obliterate the valleys and crowd out every vestige of green save here and there a skirting of stunted trees. The appearance is that of a countless series of extinct volcanoes and rocky remnants of geologic upheavals that might have occurred but yesterday. Everywhere a monotony of lava-like rocks, serrated and seamed and forbidding.

At a distance it gives one a sense of arid and unrelieved desolation, almost as appalling as the desert proper, almost as dire as Death Valley itself.

On descending one is surprised to find quite extensive valleys, refreshingly fertile, with groves of live oak, sycamores and evergreens. Here and there cool springs gush from green hillsides and rush together to form running streams that lose themselves in the sands below. As one nears the ocean, that basks in almost perpetual sunshine and is never sullen, there are broad reaches of arable land on which the white man has been exploiting his miracles of cultivation,—in the newer sections only for a few months, and in the older ones for a quarter of a century. The rich, deep green of the orange and lemon orchards forms an artistic contrast that merges into blending with the gray-green tint of the olive, and this again with the prune and apricot, the walnut, almond and pecan, and other deciduous fruits. One never tires of the pictures. As orchard after orchard and grove after grove is revealed surprise deepens into astonishment and delight.

There is everywhere climate enough and to spare, but, no matter what the land agents may assert, the really delectable spots are mere patches, oases in a Sahara of bare, burnt rocks, scoria and sagebrush. Santa Barbara at the extreme north-

western limit is the center of the first of these oases.

For a distance of nearly seventy miles from Point Conception the trend of the coast line is nearly due east. Hence Santa Barbara county faces a southern sea. This Point is an abrupt salient that thrusts its blunt angle into the Pacific in such a way as to divert and break the force of its Monster Current. The result is a bit of meteorologic legerdemain. The passenger coming down the coast from San Francisco— a delightful trip at any season of the year— notes the sudden and wonderful transition as the steamer rounds this Point and glides into the calmer and warmer waters that lave the divergent shore line in front of Santa Barbara. And, too, the alert and busy mariner smiles a smile of relief and relaxes his vigilance when the time arrives to port his helm and drift into the quiet waters of the unruffled sea that greets him as he rounds Conception.

Northward from this Point the climate resembles that of San Francisco, with cold currents and frequent fogs that harass and depress the sensitive invalid. Below the Point soft breezes greet him and prevail all the way to San Diego. Such is the contrast that at Lompoc on the west coast of Santa Barbara county above the Point, apples grow to perfection, while on the south coast, at Montecito, prize medal lemons are the boast of the horticulturist.

To the northward of Santa Barbara rises the Santa Ynez range of mountains, forming a near-by wall three thousand feet high that acts as an effectual barrier against the cool north winds that follow down the coast from Oakland and San Francisco. To complete the exceptional conditions that prevail at Santa Barbara, Nature interposed a system of rock-anchored jetties, in a cordon of islands that twenty-five miles from the coast rise abruptly and form a breakwater that cannot be undermined and that will never depend upon the vigilance of man or the government for repairs. Thus, the surf is always a moderate one and there is no undertow to endanger the lives of bathers. With a mountain barrier protecting her on the north, with protecting islands that stem the fiercer onslaughts of old ocean and a placid beach in front of it, Santa Barbara becomes at once a Paradise Regained!

This tells the whole story without the usual appeal to either lying or incoherent statistics, which can be made to bolster the most uncomfortable climate in the world. A summary of the "average" temperatures, rainfall, humidity, clear and cloudy days, wind-movement, etc., will be adverted to in a general way when other localities are considered.

HOT AIR TREATMENT.

THE application of hot air in the treatment of a number of painful, intractable and incorrigible diseases is not at all new, having been in vogue almost since the advent of the Christian era. The "Thermae" of ancient Greece and Rome and the "Hammam" of the Turks are duplicated all over the country under the name of Turkish and Russian baths and bath cabinets. These have their thousands of regular or spasmodic patrons and purchasers, and accomplish a world of good in their limited way. We use the word "limited" intentionally, for the reason that these baths do not reach the masses, or rather the masses do not reach the baths. Of our 76,000,000 people not the half of one per cent. have ever reached "the sublime consciousness of being clean," as Edwin Forrest used to put it, by personally experiencing the luxury of a thorough Turkish bath. All these baths aim chiefly at cleanliness. Incidentally, no doubt the effects of heat are realized to a certain extent; but it is in most cases moist heat, and moist heat cannot be carried to any high degree. It is simply unendurable, when the temperature exceeds a definite and not very elevated range. It would be instant death to expose a human being to a moist heat at anywhere near the boiling point of water, whereas dry heat can be endured up to 400° or even 500° F. without harm to the tissues thus exposed.

The discovery of this fact dates back some years, and occurred in this way: A gentleman, in an emergency, had occasion to enter a compartment used as a desiccating room in which the temperature was regularly maintained at about 300° F. He remained in this immense oven for some minutes and escaped unharmed, save that wherever the metal frame of his spectacles touched the skin he was severely blistered.

This dry heat of high degree is now being utilized for therapeutic purposes, and some of its results are fairly astonishing. For example, enlarged and anchylosed joints are reduced to natural size and made movable; deep-seated inflammations, as arthritis, synovitis and the like, are readily overcome, and exudations resulting from chronic joint inflammation are promptly resolved and dispersed. Rheumatic joints are relieved of all pain and made supple again. Even the lancinating pains of gout are quickly ameliorated, and with the aid of proper constitutional and dietetic auxiliaries, its unfortunate victims are made almost as good as new. As these are the cases that baffle physicians and systems of treatment everywhere any treatment that will relieve and cure them assumes a degree of importance that ordinary language fails to express.

As it is easy to surmise, some ingenuity is required to make the treatment by dry heat available in that large class of painful cases to which it is applicable and for which it promises most relief.

Expensive and rather elaborate apparatus is required to generate the heat and to make it applicable at such portions of the body as suffer from these painful, deforming diseases. A novice can hardly imagine or foresee the many difficulties to be overcome. In the first place, the extreme degree of heat required for the best results causes both perspiration and evaporation, which at once transforms dry into moist heat and thus defeats its chief object. Much ingenuity has been expended in the effort to perfect appliances by which the high degree of heat required can be readily engendered and maintained for a considerable time without causing the exposed surfaces to exude rapidly, whether perspiration, or blood serum and the watery portion of internal tissues, if not of the blood itself. This would prevent the full action of the heat by converting it into moist heat and would thus negative results. The acknowledged efficiency of the principle has elicited apparatus of every variety, most of it, however, having no higher ambition than to cause the patient or victim to perspire freely, whereby eliminative results of wonderful scope are proposed and promised. Thus "Turkish Bath Cabinets" are advertised in all the magazines and are offered at all prices from $3 up. But from a scientific and therapeutic point of view these cheap contrivances are even cheaper in their effects, and at the same time have a restricted range. One may "sweat out" a common cold or "open the pores" by means of one of these simple and inexpensive affairs. But they have no claim when it comes to the scientific application of high degrees of dry heat. This result can not be accomplished without more elaborate appointments.

At last a thoroughly efficient apparatus has been invented and is now on the market. We do not know the inventor, but the apparatus, as commercially exploited, is named the Sprague Hot Air Apparatus. It costs something, as all good things do, but it is a marvel of efficiency. Not every general practitioner will find it feasible to possess or use this invention in his practice; but those who have proper office room and appurtenances, as well as hospitals, sanitariums and the like, will find a hot air plant not only desirable but essential. There is nothing that can possibly take its place, speaking from the standpoint of the orthopedists and specialists in the treatment of chronic joint affections.

This apparatus, as has already been stated, has been brought to a high state of perfection and efficiency, and such of our readers as will make it in their way to investigate it thoroughly will thank us for having called their attention to it.

Apropos of this subject we reproduce from *The Alkaloidal Clinic*, the following paper, entitled:

SOME THERAPEUTIC VALUES OF HEAT.*

By C. Stuart Hutchison, M.Sc., M.D.

Many misconceptions have been gathered around the subject of heat as a therapeutic agent.

In the summer of 1898 my attention was called to the experiments that were being carried on in the Cook County Hospital, Chicago, showing the fact that the human body could tolerate an excessive amount of dry heat.

The fact that the entire body can comfortably be placed in a temperature of 300 degrees F. for an hour, and a limb in a temperature of 500 degrees F. is worthy of consideration. Heat has always been known, by both the profession and the laity, to relieve pain. Who of you has not been called to see a suffering patient and found a hot iron to her back or a hot dinner-plate over the stomach? Heat can relieve pain and subdue local inflammation, or awaken tissues from the slow death of atrophy. Heat may be applied locally to a part, to the entire body, or inhaled with benefit in many disorders to which the human body is subject. White heat is a cautery and antiseptic. Hot air locally stimulates the skin and muscles. When applied to the entire body it acts as a diaphoretic, stimulating the peripheral nerves and dilating the capillary blood-vessels. The pulse is increased, the heart-action strengthened and body-temperature rises, respiration is increased, deepened and quickened.

To the nervous system prolonged heat is a sedative, producing relaxation of the muscles followed by drowsiness. Heat promotes absorption and hastens elimination, by stimulating circulation and respiration.

The treatment of any disease or disorder must be governed by the symptoms and

*Read before the Central District Medical Association, of Iowa.

conditions of each individual case. Therefore to ascertain the cases suitable for the treatment of dry hot air, we can only state facts in a general way.

First of all the rheumatics, both muscular and articular. We will not discuss the etiology at this time, but suffice to say that uric acid plays a very important part in both rheumatism and gout.

It has been the experience of the writer when an acute articular rheumatic member is placed in a dry air-chamber at the temperature of 400 degrees F. for an hour, the pain is relieved, swelling diminished and comparatively free motion can be had after a thorough massage.

The stiffness, pain and disagreeable symptoms of muscular rheumatism are relieved after a few hot baths of the entire body (except the head), at a temperature of 225 degrees F. Thus we may say acute articular rheumatism, muscular rheumatism, lumbago, torticollis, pleurodynia, sciatic and other rheumatic affections, with acute and chronic gout, may be relieved if not entirely cured. In dry, scaly skin troubles, where stimulation is required, diaphoresis can be produced and relief often follows.

In sprains of ankles, wrists, knees or elbows, nothing can compare with the relief obtained from a treatment of dry hot air at the temperature of 450 to 500 degrees F. It relieves pain, diminishes swelling and permits free massage. In spasmodic affections involving the muscles a local appliance of heat relieves much of the distress.

Dysmenorrhea due to the neuralgic or rheumatic diathesis, inflammation within the pelvis and parenchymatous nephritis, may be relieved by increasing the elimination through the skin and bowels. Repeated baths cause functional hypertrophy of the sweat-glands and eventually enable them to do more work. In colds the congestion of the nasal mucous membrane can be relieved by one treatment. Syphilitics obtain the same result as from the Hot Springs.

Chronic ulcers are stimulated by heat, and with cleanliness granulation will be produced and often permanent cures established. Recent literature shows that a reduction of the obese can be accomplished with heat more rapidly than with drugs. However, care must be taken with those suffering from fatty degeneration or marked valvular lesion of the heart, on account of the stimulating effect on the circulation.

In no case do I rely entirely on the heat alone, but employ such measures, either medical or surgical, as the case requires; enforcing hygienic rules and correcting dietetic errors.

Hot air has been pushed forward by Dr. Palmer, who invented a system of applying dry heat to the cavities. Dr. Woodward applied it more extensively and used it in the treatment of disease of the nose, throat and lungs.

The operation is simple. The machine is lighted and let run a few minutes to eliminate all odors. The patient removes all clothing, puts on a Turkish bath-robe and mounts to a table covered by a Turkish sheet; the feet are placed in Turkish stockings and hands in mittens, and then wrapped in toweling; the Turkish sheet is then drawn over the entire outfit and fastened by means of a small hook, so as to make a complete sack with the head only exposed. This permits the patient to turn from side to side at ease, without any danger of loosening a towel, and a part becoming exposed to the direct heat. The table is then placed in the hot cylinder and the front closed by heavy canvas, leaving the head only exposed. In twenty minutes the heat can be brought to a temperature of 250 degrees without discomfort to the patient. The body temperature rises to 100 or 102, pulse to 100 or 120, respiration is deepened and becomes quicker, sometimes to thirty-five per minute. The head is kept cool by cold applications and iced drinks given freely. At the end of the bath the lights are turned down and small slides opened on top; a few minutes later the table is withdrawn, one part of the body exposed at a time and thoroughly massaged. After massage the skin is gently rubbed with alcohol, and the patient wrapped in blankets and allowed to rest in a comfortable position. They generally sleep, and in an hour are rested and ready to go home.

Ames, Ia.

The editor of *The Alkaloidal Clinic* adds: "Dr. Hutchison is not the only one who has become justly enthusiastic over the results of hot air treatment. I cannot comprehend how a progressive, up-to-date physician can permit his competitors to monopolize this useful invention."

NASAL CATARRH.

THIS universal scourge is thus discussed in London *Health:*

Under the name of nasal catarrh, or chronic coryza, we refer to an affection ill-understood, ill-defined, characterized by a hypertrophy of the nasal mucous membrane, with or without secretion. The patient passes through alternating periods of easy and difficult respiration. The passages of the nose insensibly become closed, especially towards three or four o'clock in the morning. Thus are explained those obstructions of breathing which suddenly wake patients, chiefly children. Breathing through the nose was natural while they were asleep. Gradually the nose becomes obstructed by swelling of the mucous membrane; the secretions from this effectually complete the blocking of the passage. It is the same as when you apply a tracheotomy tube to an anæsthetized dog. Close the canula gradually, and the animal will make the greatest efforts at respiration; at any given moment he would wake, absolutely suffocated, struggling for air with might and main. Open the canula, and all becomes natural and peaceful. We know a traveler who suddenly wakes up at night, a prey to the greatest anguish, unable to breathe. He rushes to the window, and the paroxysm is over!

If the nasal passages close insensibly and gradually, they generally become clear quite suddenly; most frequently without any appreciable cause, or under the influence of emotion, cold, heat, certain powders (boracic acid, cocaine, menthol, tobacco). Most snuff-takers have chronic coryza, and take it to clear the nostrils. The patient is conscious of the sensation when they become clear. He hears a slight liquid noise, and the passage is open. If he lies on one side, this side becomes stuffed up, while the other clears.

CHRONIC CORYZA

is present wherever there exist nasal polypi, deviations of the septum, vegetations on the septum, adenoid growths, enlarged tonsils. It is thus very important to examine the nose thoroughly in all cases of nasal catarrh, so as to arrive at a definite conclusion as to its cause. A mother whose child breathes with the mouth open is guilty of negligence if she does not consult a physician, but allays her conscience with the popular prejudice, so dangerous, that the child "will grow out of it."

In the treatment of nasal catarrh, the first thing is to keep the nose thoroughly clean. To remove the secretions, dust, etc., we utilize a nasal syphon, and wash out the nostrils night and morning with a powder composed of bicarbonate of soda, chloride of sodium, and borax, of each seven grains. This is to dissolved in a half-tumbler of warm water, and passed into the nostrils by means of a tube. This nasal douche is not so much a medicament as a measure for keeping the nostrils absolutely clean. They can then be made accessible to any curative or alleviative medication which may be suitable in the eyes of the surgeon. If there are growths, etc., these may be removed by electrolysis, cauterization, scarification of the mucous membrane, section of the septum, etc. All these operations may be performed without pain, without interfering with the occupation or treatment in other directions. The important thing is, that they should be done by a skilled hand. To cauterize, to cut a membrane is not difficult, especially when the patient has no control over the affair, but to do it well is another matter:

and the patient knows it as he waits, perhaps for hours, ill-affording, though not begrudging, the time that he may attend the man of skill and repute.

✤ ✤

THE HYGIENE OF THE NOSE.

LITTLE is said about the care of this organ, and yet it is a statistical fact that nine out of ten persons find it a troublesome member, and the trade in handkerchiefs—not the dainty bits of ornamental lace that cost as much as a suit of clothes or a fine horse, but the regular business article, that is as

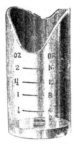

necessary as the coat one wears or food one eats—is something enormous.

Nose specialists, it is true, have devised douches, best nasal syringes and all that, but the nasal douche, as ordinarily used, is a dangerous procedure, and the post-nasal syringe should never be used by any but an expert, lest it do harm. The douche as ordinarily used is made to cleanse the postnasal surfaces by a stream of liquid of some kind thrown into the parts with more or less force, and frequently results in damage to the Eustachian tubes and through these to the hearing apparatus.

Even the passive douches, by means of tubes of various design, are most of them either awkward or inefficient. The latest device,* which is herewith illustrated, is designed to overcome all, or nearly all, the objections to its predecessors. A glance at the

* McKesson & Robbins, N. Y.

cut shows that it consists of a graduated glass cup so shaped as to be applicable to the nasal organ and to permit the hygiene of the nose, too generally neglected or imperfectly performed, to be easily, pleasantly and effectively accomplished by any one without discomfort or injury of any kind.

In use, the proper solution having been accurately made, the higher lip or curve of the cup is adjusted to upper lip and base of the nose and the cup tilted until it is easy to sniff the contents slowly and gently into one or both nostrils.

The process is that of practically "drinking through the nose," except that the solution is not swallowed. It readily passes back into the nasopharynx and cleanses all the parts with which it is brought in contact. When extreme thoroughness is aimed at, the fluid may be drawn entirely through the passages and expelled by the mouth.

Altogether this simple device seems destined to fill an important want, and will be found desirable by very many people who do not complain of nasal catarrh. It is a valuable aid to every one, as contributing to a more perfect personal hygiene.

✤ ✤

THE BEST ALKALIN WASH.

BY W. HARPUR SLOAN, M.D.,

Chief Ear Dept., Medico-Chirurgical College, Philadelphia, Pa.

THERE are many alkalin preparations on the market that are used daily with varied results in conditions where such a preparation is indicated. I have tried most of them in all conditions, and after an impartial trial I am compelled to say that the preparation known as "Glyco-Thymoline," made by the Kress & Owen Co., stands at the head of the list. Its formula is one that commends its use, the ingredients being of an antiseptic and non-irritating nature.

Having formed this opinion of "Glyco Thymoline," I have concluded to report a few clinical cases in which it has given me good results.

Case No. 1.—M. L., 23 years, came under my care suffering with a distressing case of ozena. The turbinated bones on both sides of her nose presented a condition of marked atrophy; there was a complete loss of smell and taste, and a formation of crusts in the nasal chamber; the stench of same was foul. She complained of continual headache, and other symptoms of a depleted and run-down system. I placed her on a tonic of iron, arsenic and strychnia, internally; locally, the use of "Glyco Thymoline," diluted, in a Bermingham douche, three times a day. After one month's treatment the crusts had ceased to form; there was a complete restoration of taste and a slight return of smell; general health improved; patient well satisfied with results.

Case No. 2.—C. A., age 8 years, came to me suffering with a severe otorrhœa, following scarlet fever. There was a mucopurulent discharge from both ears, child completely deaf; the auditory canal was excoriated and sore, and the general health below par. I used cod liver oil internally and syringed the ears three times a day with "Glyco Thymoline." At the end of one month the discharge of pus had stopped; hearing much improved and the child's general health very much better.

Case No. 3.—J. W., age 25 years, came under my care suffering with an aggravated case of cystitis, which had been treated by several of our best physicians without much improvement. He had great pain in the region of the bladder and loins, worse on urination; a heavy deposit of mucus and some blood in the urine; temperature 100°, which would rise a degree during the periods of pain. I used the usual treatment for such cases without positive results, when I thought of irrigating the bladder with "Glyco-Thymoline" (dilute). This I did once in twenty-four hours, at the same time giving the remedy internally, in teaspoonful doses, every three hours. For the first two days not much improvement; third day no blood and less mucus in the urine. Treatment continued two weeks, when I discharged him cured.

Case No. 4.—J. H., age 35 years, consulted me for pruritus ani, which had troubled him for several years; his business compelled him to sit the best part of the day. He had used various ointments, prescriptions, etc., for this troublesome affection, with only temporary relief. At his first visit I ordered him to bathe the rectum twice daily with castile soap and warm water, then to apply "Glyco Thymoline," half strength, to the parts. After persisting for a time the swelling and severe itching was lessened, and then left him altogether.

RUBEOLA AND RUBELLA.

IF one consults the medical dictionaries he finds that the word rubeola receives two definitions. The first makes it a synonym for rubella, or that which is more commonly known in this country as German measles, and the second gives the word as a synonym for measles. There is, therefore, some confusion as to the proper significance of the terms rubella and rubeola. Jürgensen (Nothnagel's Special Pathology and Therapeutics, Vol. V, Part II.) shows that rubella is a nosological entity, and that it has nothing to do with either measles or scarlet fever. Furthermore, the majority of recent writers describe the two diseases separately. The following, as is well known, are the chief differences between measles and rubella:

In measles the period of incubation is from 5 to 14 days, or an average of about 12 days, while in rubella, or German measles, this period is from 7 to 21 days. In measles the onset is gradual with anorexia, fever, and marked catarrhal symptoms, while in rubella the onset is usually without symptoms until just before the rash appears. Enlargement of the cervical, axillary, and inguinal glands is very common in the latter. In measles the febrile stage is rather more pronounced than in rubella, and in the former disease the eruption does not appear until the fourth day, whereas in rubella it

appears on the second day. This eruption
in measles is coarse, papular, dark red, and
much more pronounced than in rubella.
Finally, there are many more complications
or sequelæ in measles than in rubella.
Among these complications are the following: Purulent conjunctivitis, stomatitis,
bronchitis, catarrhal pneumonia, otitis media, and intestinal derangements. One way
out of the difficulty caused by this unfortunate misuse of terms would be to always
use the word rubella to signify rötheln, or
German measles, but a still better way
would be to drop the term rubeola altogether
and refer to the two diseases as measles and
rubella. We doubt, however, whether any
of these Latin terms, namely roseola, rubella
and rubeola will ever become popular with
the profession. Even now many of the
best-read men will hesitate a moment if
they are asked for a prompt definition of
these individual terms. On the other hand,
the terms measles and rötheln, or German
measles, are perfectly well understood, and
are not liable to be mistaken.

THERMOMETRIC SCALES.

It is now more than eight years since the
centigrade (also called the Celsius) thermometer was legalized in Prussia, and, we
believe, in the rest of the German Empire;
yet, as late as June 4 of this year, the ministry at Würtemberg issued a circular calling the attention of officials to the fact that
"in all official communications, reports and
publications, the centigrade thermometric
scale must be used." The circular also
stated that in order to completely and immediately set aside forever the Réaumur instrument in the government offices and
buildings, centigrade instruments would be
furnished by the ministry, and, further, that
all instruments bearing the double scale
(centigrade and Réaumur's), must be done
away with in their offices by January 1,
1906, at the latest.

"It is hard," says the proverb, "to teach an

old dog new tricks," and it is true; but what
is harder, is to make him forget his old
tricks. As with dogs, so with men, and we
can conceive of no more difficult task than
that of the reformer who undertakes to eliminate from the life of a people an institution
or system, or a custom of any description, to
which they were born and bred.

Here is the Réaumur scale, for instance,
based originally upon an error, both in
theory and in practice, inconvenient
and antiquated, yet it still hangs
on, in spite of official proclamations,
even among the "bureaucrats" themselves. It has been claimed that the
continued popularity of this system in Germany was due entirely to the celebrated
meteorologist, Dove, who, while recognizing
the great advantages of the centigrade scale,
said to his pupils, "Do what you please
after I am dead and gone, but while I linger
please do not force me to change my customs—I am too old." We doubt it—it
would have been the same then had the meteorologist never uttered his pathetic plea.

It is the same with the Fahrenheit scale in
England and her colonies, and the United
States, and, in spite of all the great advantages offered by the centigrade system—the
fact that it is based upon two constants of
nature, its great simplicity, etc., generations
will pass away before it supplants the
Fahrenheit scale among English-speaking
people.

One could better understand this trait did
national pride enter into the matter, but, as
has been observed by M. Brenan, in his
"History of the Thermometer," the English-
speaking peoples use the system of a Dane
(Fahrenheit), the French that of a Swede
(Celsius), and the Germans that of a
Frenchman (Réaumur). To complete the
paradox, we may add that Hanau, a German, made definite the system of Fahrenheit,
and Cristin, a Frenchman, that of Celsius.

In none of the systems now in use is the
scale graduated as originally designed. In
Réaumur's early scales the boiling point of
water was placed at 100, and sometimes
even higher. Fahrenheit's system was at

first based on nothing definite. While he was experimenting there occurred a very severe spell of cold, and the point reached by the mercury on that occasion he assumed as his zero. In like manner he assumed 24 as representing the greatest heat of summer. Later on he divided his degrees into four parts. In 1737 Hanau wrote, "According to the most accurate thermometer that M. Romer, of Dantzig, has been able to procure (construct?) for M. Fahrenheit, water boils at 212°, and freezes at 32°.

Celsius, five years later, or in 1742, published his method of grading his thermometers. At that period he marked the temperature of boiling water as zero (0°) and that of melting ice, or freezing water at 100°. Subsequently, he reversed this scale. About this time Cristin, member of the Académie des Beaux Arts, Lyons, published a series of "Notes on the Graduation of Mercurial Thermometers." December 11, 1743, he wrote: "If the public will adopt the new division of 100° between the freezing and boiling points of water, I think it will do wisely; but if it doesn't, I will not worry about it (*je n'en serais pas faché*). I shall always have the satisfaction of having done my best." As Cristin left the thermometer of Celsius, we have it to-day. It has been claimed that Celsius reversed his scale of his own notion, and independently of Cristin. It may be that he did so, but Cristin's publication appeared about a year after the paper of Celsius, above referred to, in which boiling water was the zero.

Réaumur established his scale as follows: Having established by experiment that a certain quantity of hydrated alcohol, occupying a space, at the temperature of freezing water (0°, or zero) which he assumed as 1,000, on being placed in boiling water increased its volume to 1.080, he took as his basis of division the amount of heat necessary to dilate the alcohol one thousandth (0.001) part of its volume. He thought in this manner to divide the interval between the boiling and the freezing points of water into 80 equal parts. Both his theory and his process were faulty, however, and

the result was that he divided a space, approximating very closely to 80° of Celsius's, or of the centigrade thermometer, into 80 parts, so that if his practical *method* were followed, instead of his *directions*, or *theory*, his thermometers, by a singular chance, would now have degrees almost exactly those of the centigrade instrument.

"Thus," says *La Nature*, "the physicists of Germany, by linking a faulty process to a faulty theory, have an established system which they have found it very difficult to eradicate."

A CORRECTOR OF IODISM.

By W. H. MORSE,

American Member of Bureau of Materia Medica, Westfield, N. J.

H. W. LeFevre, a leading dentist of Denver, Colorado, writes me, under date of January 31st, concerning the use of Iodia for asthma. After making narration of a case in which he is greatly interested, he inquires as to the composition of Iodia, and says: "From the name, I suppose it to be made up largely of iodide of potassium." Then he adds: "She has taken [referring to the patient] a great deal of the iodide, and it invariably causes trouble with her stomach, and she declares she will never take another drop of it; and she can detect it at once. Consequently, if Iodia is made up largely of it, there will be no use for me to try to get her to take it."

I quote this letter, as the same matter of question has come to other physicians from time to time, and the circumstances are not always such that a lucid answer can be given, even where the clinical experience with Iodia has been large, and the success attending its use has been beyond question. Iodia is not "made up largely of iodide of potassium," although its five grains of that salt to three of ferric phosphate, with the other components, go to give it the governing quality. But these same components are there not only to fortify the iodide, but as well to correct it in its incidental effects and defects. These, of course, are comprised under the term "iodism." Iodia never disposes to cause iodism in any of its three forms, and, in fact, insures the system against it in two, and more than measurably in the third. To understand this we have to consider that there are three forms of the affection—the first as a true cachexia, comprising a number of disturbances of the general nutrition and its conditions. The second develops as nervous disturbances and anomalies of secretion, together with affections of the skin. The third is due to the irritation produced by the agent in the gastro-intestinal tract.

HUMAN AND BOVINE TUBERCULOSIS.

ON this subject evidence and argument are in order. We give the following from a well-known advocate of pure milk and healthy kine. Dr. E. R. Brush, of Mount Vernon, N. J., says: "One simple fact that strengthens my belief that human bacillary tuberculosis is all derived from the bovine species is that where this animal does not exist pulmonary consumption is unknown. The Kirghiz on the Steppes of Russia who have no cows have domesticated the horse, using his meat, milk, and skin, and a case of pulmonary tuberculosis has never been known to exist among the tribe. The Esquimau has no cows, neither has he pulmonary consumption; and I think it can be laid down as a fact that where dairy cows are unknown consumption is unknown. He further says that the reason that tuberculosis is not more frequently transmitted from cattle to man is accounted for in the difference of temperature. A germ cultivated in the cow is a tropical growth, because her average temperature is between 101° and 103°. The human race, by this mode of illustration, represents the temperate zone. The bacillus introduced from the cow into the healthy man finds a difference of temperature of four or five degrees, and although it may live, and in a lessened degree increase, it does not become virulent until, from some other cause, the temperature of the man is increased, when it rapidly multiplies, and thereafter creates its own proper temperature, such as we find in most cases of tuberculosis.—*Sanitarian.*

THE LATEST POPULATION STATISTICS.

THE Census Bureau issued a bulletin October 11th showing the population of the United States by sex, general nativity and color, for 1900. Of the total population of the United States, there were 39,059,242 males and 37,244,145 females. The native element numbered 65,843,302, and the foreign born 10,460,085. Of the colored population there was a total of 9,319,585, divided as follows: Colored, 8,840,789; Chinese, 119,050; Japanese, 85,986, and Indians, taxed, 137,242; untaxed, 129,519. There has been practically no change in the proportions of the sexes since 1890. The foreign-born element has increased since 1890 only 12.4 per cent. of its former number, as against 22.5 per cent. in the native-born gain. There has been a slight decrease during the past ten years of persons of colored descent, the proportion now being 11 6 per cent. In 1890 it was 11.9 per cent. The Chinese show a loss, and the Indians have decreased 2.5 per cent. In the United States proper, the largest proportion of foreign-born is found in North Dakota, where this element comprises 35.4 per cent. of the total population; the next largest percentages of foreign-born being found in Rhode Island, with 31.4 per cent.; Massachusetts with 28.9, and Minnesota, Montana, Connecticut and New York, with about 26 per cent. each. The native Indians of Alaska number 29,536, a gain of 16.5 per cent. since 1890.

ANOTHER NEW CURE FOR CONSUMPTION.

DR. WILFRED G. FRALICK, visiting surgeon to the Metropolitan Hospital and consulting surgeon to the Brooklyn Memorial Hospital, is at work perfecting a remedy which he believes will cure tuberculosis and other bacterial processes. Until he has satisfied himself that his fluid is perfect, Dr. Fralick does not intend to publish its composition. The solution is injected intravenously, and has already caused great improvement in a number of cases. Though he has only employed this formula for six weeks, he is simply overwhelmed by phthisical patients from all over the world. While all bacteria are destroyed by this means, Dr. Fralick states that the solution will not build up tissues which are already destroyed. He intends to study its limitations, dosage, and exact effect, believing that premature publication of a remedy does more harm than good.

MADE IT PLAIN.

He was a German, and couldn't understand the intricacies of the law. He was trying to mortgage his share of the old homestead. The lawyer couldn't quite see what he was driving at, and at last the German in desperation cried:

"Vell, at the expiration of my mother's death dot property is to be divided yet!"

This is almost as good as the way the German got off that familiar but vulgar expression, "He has no more show than a bull with his tail cut short in fly time." He said: "He has not more show den a bull mit his tail cut short off when de time flies."

THE BIRTH-RATE OF GREATER NEW YORK.

The Health Department returns show that in the last quarter reported by the Board, there were 144 births of children of Bohemian parentage, of whom 143 were born in New York County and only one in Brooklyn. In the same period there were 187 births of children of Swedish parents, and of these 103 were in Brooklyn and only 84

in New York County. There were 1,465 children born of Austrian parents in New York—Hungarians, Poles or Germans—and of these 1,352 were born in New York County and only 112 in Brooklyn. The same disparity in favor of New York County is to be seen in the case of the children of Irish, Italian and Russian parentage. But the number of children born of Scotch parentage, as well as of Swiss, Danish, Norwegian and Finn parentage, is as large in Brooklyn as in New York County, and the children of Canadian parentage nearly as large. Brooklyn retains as a borough its distinction of having the largest number of births of children of American parentage. It is the most truly American of the five boroughs which constitute the present city of New York. Manhattan is the most cosmopolitan.

THE TREATMENT OF DYSMENOR-RHEA.

Prof. Schwarze (*Therapeutische Mo natshefte*) writes upon the treatment of the forms of dysmenorrhea associated with pathological anteflexion, retroflexion in the virgin uterus, and the different forms of congenital deformity of the uterus. This class includes stenosis of the external and internal os and all forms of dysmenorrhea in which no anatomical changes can be demonstrated. He believes the coal-tar analgesics are of use, as well as the preparations of iron, and sodium salicylate. In many cases it is necessary to administer codeine in small doses and the tablet of "Antikamnia and Codeine" would seem to have been specially prepared in its proportions, for just these indications. Begin by taking one tablet every three hours on the day previous to expected period and continue until relieved. The introduction of a sound into the uterus just before the menstrual period, removing the pathological anteflexion and dilating the canal, is often followed by relief of symptoms. Rapid dilatation of the cervical canal, a day before the period, is the better method.

THE KLOPFEN TREATMENT OF TUBERCULOSIS.

THE method of treatment of pulmonary tuberculosis known as the "Klopfen" plan consists in slapping with a silver paper-cutter the surface of the chest in front, behind, and at the sides. A scientific examination into the advantages said to result from this process appears to justify the conclusion that this practice is really a powerful means of mechanically stimulating the pulmonary apparatus and of dissipating the tendency to congestion, and in this manner promotes spontaneous healing of tuberculous lesions.

MR. BOK'S ADVICE ON MARRIAGE.

A YOUNG man recently wrote to the editor of *The Ladies' Home Journal* asking: "What have you to say, squarely and fairly, to a young man of twenty-nine who is about to marry?" In the October *Journal* Mr. Bok uses a page for his answer. Its salient points are these: that a man should make the woman of his choice his chum, as well as his wife; that he should show her the highest consideration as well as love her; that he should remember that he owes his wife to her mother, and treat his mother-in-law with respect, at least; that he should keep his wife informed as to his income; that he should give her a regular allowance and that he should have his life insured in her favor. And above all, that when a young man marries he must remember that he leaves a world of self and enters into a world of another and self.

TORPEDOES, when first employed by the Americans against the English in the revolutionary war, were called American turtles, and their use was pronounced infamous and worthy only of savages.

Book Reviews.

A SYSTEM OF PHYSIOLOGIC THERAPEUTICS. A Practical Exposition of the Methods, other than Drug-Giving, Useful in the Prevention of Disease and in the Treatment of the Sick. Edited by Solomon Solis Cohen, A.M., M.D., Professor of Medicine and Therapeutics in the Philadelphia Polyclinic; Lecturer on Clinical Medicine at Jefferson Medical College; Physician to the Philadelphia Hospital, etc. Volume III., Climatology, Health Resorts, Mineral Springs. By F. Parkes Weber, M.A., M.D., F.R.C.P. (Lond.), Physician to the German Hospital, Dalston; Assistant Physician North London Hospital for Consumption, etc. With the Collaboration for America of Guy Hinsdale, A.M., M.D., Secretary of the American Climatological Association, etc. In two books. Book I.—Principles of Climatotherapy, Ocean Voyages, Mediterranean, European and British Health Resorts. Book II.—Mineral Springs, Therapeutics, etc. Illustrated with maps. Price for the complete set, $22.00 net.

These are the third and fourth volumes of Cohen's "System of Physiologic Therapeutics," whose timeliness has already been commented upon. The first part treats of the factors of climate, with their effect on physiologic functions and pathological conditions, and describes the fundamental principles that underlie the application of climates, health resorts and mineral springs in the prevention of disease, and to promote the comfort and recovery of the sick.

The second part describes health resorts, and the third part discusses in detail the special climatic treatment of various diseases and different classes of patients. Book II. also describes the health resorts in Africa, Asia, Australasia and America.

In Book I. ocean voyages are first treated of with considerable detail, and their advantages and disadvantages, indications and counter-indications as a therapeutic measure, are pointed out. As very little exact information on this important subject exists in an available form, this chapter should be of great use to physicians. The subject of altitude is treated in a similarly full and definite manner, and not only are we told what classes of patients and disorders are benefited by Alpine and Rocky Mountain climates, but also what classes are unsuitable for such treatment. The difference between summer and winter climates in Switzerland, and the therapeutic indications for the different seasons are discussed at length. In addition, the sea-coast and inland health resorts of the Mediterranean countries, those of Continental Europe and those oi the British Islands, including mountain stations of various elevations, plains, and mineral water spas, are described, with no waste of words, but with a fulness of detail unusual in medical books. Not only geographic and climatic features are pointed out, but also social and other characteristics so important in selecting a resort that shall be suitable to the tastes and means of the individual patient, as well as beneficial in his disease. Throughout this section allusion is made to the special medical uses of the various resorts described, and to the particular form of treatment for which any one is famous.

The existence of sanatoriums for special diseases, as those at seaside resorts for scrofulous and weakly children, and in various regions for consumption, nervous affections, diseases of women, and the like, are specified; and the mere lists of such places, as found in the index, are likely to prove invaluable for reference. We know none other so complete. A mere glance at the closely printed pages of the index will show how unusually full is the treatment of special resorts and their particular qualities. Like the preceding volumes these are thoroughly scientific and eminently practical, a combination that reflects credit alike on authors and editor.

NEW METHODS IN EDUCATION. By J. Liberty Todd. The Orange Judd Company, Springfield, New York and Chicago. Students' Abridged Edition, pp. 352.

This abridgement of Mr. Todd's complete work, of which an addition *de luxe* was issued two years ago, has been issued in response to an imperative demand for a smaller and more compact work for the use of teachers and students.

The original work, scarcely two years old, has exerted a profound influence throughout the educational world, the most competent authorities pronouncing the highest encomiums in its praise.

In his preface the author very aptly says: "Largely as a result of imperfect training or wrong methods of education in youth, beauty and high quality of product are too commonly lacking in mechanical industries and in the world of literature and the fine arts. Our people excel in quantity of product, but not in quality." How true this is in literature, and especially in medical literature. Adapting Carlyle's sweeping criticism, "the (medical) world is afloat on a sea of words." This work is an earnest effort to improve the quality of what we produce, whether the product of muscle, mind or fancy. It suggests new methods of education, but only those that have stood the test of many years' searching investigation and practical experience.

THE WOMAN BEAUTIFUL, a practical Treatise on the Development and Preservation of Woman's Health and Beauty, and the Principles of Taste in Dress. By Ella Adelia Fletcher. New York: Brentano's, 1901.

This handsome volume is dedicated to "The Lovely Women Sixty Years Young, whose noble womanhood wins beauty from the passing years."

If we were to criticize this work it would be on account of its size. It comprises 535 pages of a rather unusual size—6x9½. This may not be objectionable to many readers who will prize the work as a book of reference on the topics treated. For a larger class, who are so busy and so impatient that they seldom read except as they run, a severe ordeal of condensation would have proved valuable. But when an author is so genuinely in earnest, as evidently was the author of this book, the would-be critic's pen is blunted and the acid in his ink is all neutralized.

Miss Fletcher advocates high ideals, and her "practical" suggestions are generally practical, which is saying a good deal.

The directions for muscular and respiratory exercises are very full, and with few exceptions invulnerable to criticism. The recipes, which are lavishly inserted, are of the approved pattern, without being at all novel. Women who value health and appreciate beauty can not fail to find in this volume material aid in their quest for either or both.

THE PHYSICIAN'S VISITING LIST FOR 1902. Philadelphia: P. Blakiston's Son & Co.

This List has become one of the institutions of this country, professionally speaking. This being the fifty-first year of its appearance, the rank and file of the profession do not need to have their attention called to this standard publication. Only the younger members—recent graduates—need to be reminded of its special features, which have been constantly advanced as the needs of the busy practitioner have suggested changes, until it is now at about high-water mark of perfection.

Very few publications live half a century. Its stability is its best certificate of character.

McClure's Magazine for November is fully up to its traditional high standard. The illustrations are exceptionally fine. The forthcoming holiday number will be a souvenir worth preserving.

Success for November excels any of its previous issues. Its name was a prophecy, which its progress amply fulfils.

THE new *Lippincott's Magazine* for December—its annual Christmas number—is full of good things. Here is the list:

Ralph Tarrant, Louis Evan Shipman.

King Edward's Coronation, Mrs. Belloc-Lowndes.

Sister Theresa, Meribah Reed.

The Captain of H. B. M. Ship Diamond Rock, Rev. Cyrus Townsend Brady.

Bethlehem, Zitella Cocke.

The Oppression of Gifts, Agnes Repplier.

The Storm, Charles Elmer Jenney.

The Best Books, Edmund Gosse, LL.D.

Life's Answer, Mary E. Stickney.

Morning and Night Pieces, I. Zangwill.

The Visiting of Mother Danbury, Paul Laurence Dunbar.

The Little Gate of Fairyland, E. Ayrton.

Christmas Stories of the Saints, Abbie Farwell Brown.

The Ballad of the Scullion-Maid, Theodosia Garrison.

The Unfinished Elegy, Karl Edwin Harriman.

✢ ✢

BOOKS AND PAMPHLETS RECEIVED.

HISTORY OF MEDICINE. By Alexander Wilder, M.D., New Salem, Me. The New England Eclectic Publishing Co., 1901.

SYPHILIS, ITS DIAGNOSIS AND TREATMENT. By William S. Gottheil, M.D. Chicago: G. P. Engelhard & Co., 1901.

FOOD VALUE OF MEAT. By W. R. C. Latson, M.D. New York: The Health Culture Co.

REPORT OF SANITARY INVESTIGATIONS. Delaware State Board of Health. Springfield: Phillips Bros., 1901.

THE COST OF FOOD. By Ellen H. Richards.

HANDBOOK OF SANITATION. By George M. Price, M.D. New York: John Wiley & Sons, 1901.

THE RELATION OF THE MEDICAL EDITOR TO ORIGINAL COMMUNICATIONS. By Harold N. Moyer, M.D. Reprint from Annals of Gynecology and Pediatrics.

SEXUAL HYGIENE. By the Editorial Staff of the Alkaloidal Clinic. Chicago: The Clinic Publishing Co., 1901.

HOME ECONOMICS. By Maria Parloa, New York. The Century Company.

THE CENTURY COOKBOOK. By Mary Ronald, New York. The Century Company.

Department of Physical Education.

WITH SPECIAL REGARD TO SYMMETRICAL DEVELOPMENT OF THE BODY

NOTES ON NEURITIS AND ITS RADICAL TREATMENT.

By G. H. Patchen, M.D.,

Medical Director of the Zander Improved Movement Cure Institute.

THIS not uncommon disorder is dreaded by both physician and patient; by the physician because of its intractableness to ordinary methods of treatment, and by the patient both on account of the suffering it occasions, and the serious impairment of the usefulness of the affected member which sometimes follows.

Neuritis is an inflammation of a nerve or its covering, and, according to all accepted authorities, is a disease of many varieties and causes. Several varieties have received names which are intended to explain the nature or cause of the inflammation. But, whatever the cause, form or name may be, there is one basic condition, common to all, which controls the pathological situation and which must be removed before a cure, by any therapeutic method, can be accomplished. This is the inflammation itself, considered entirely apart from the causes which have produced it. For, although inflammation is an effect which may be due to a variety of causes, its essential factors are few and always the same.

A recent writer of prominence and authority defines inflammation as the "manifestations of the attempt at repair of actual or referred injury to a part." He further says that the "inciting cause of inflammation is irritation and its object is to remove irritation." Again, he says that "it may occur in any tissue of the body, but in whatever tissue or organ it occurs, the pathological process is essentially the same."

Practically, therefore, we never have to deal with but one kind of inflammation.

That it bears different names according to the nature or location of the region of the body involved, is of no therapeutic significance. Curative measures, really worthy of the name, are equally effective in the treatment of any of the so-called forms.

Neuritis, like all other inflammations, is brought about by the coöperation of two distinct kinds of causes, (1) the exciting, as injury, cold, dampness, or nervous strain, occasioned by emotional excitement, as grief, anxiety, suspense and other forms of distress and misfortune, and (2) the predisposing, as a deficient supply of healthy blood from lack of proper food and air, the presence of certain autogenetic impurities in the blood or of poisons introduced from without, deprivation of healthy nerve influence, old age, etc.

From a therapeutic point of view the predisposing causes are the most important and are the ones to which remedial effort, for the most part, should be directed, as they are in constant operation. The exciting causes are usually too transient in their action either to admit of or require treatment. Exceptionally, they are continuously active, as when they form an unfavorable part of the patient's environment. In these instances their influence is as pernicious as are the predisposing causes, and their prompt and radical removal is as imperative.

Of the predisposing causes there are but two which are dominant and seriously interfere with recovery. These are, (1) the presence of autogenetic impurities or extraneous poisons in the blood, and (2) some hindrance, defect or irregularity of the blood supply, resulting in congestion and stagnation of the blood currents in the venous or arterial capillaries.

As congestion is a necessary factor of inflammation, it is evident that, if perfect freedom of the circulation existed in every part of the body—if the outflow through the veins were momentarily equal to the inflow through the arteries—inflammation could not occur because it would be deprived of one of the chief elements of its production. On the other hand, were the blood pure and free from all foreign elements, inflammation could not exist because the exciting cause of irritation would be lacking.

The symptoms of neuritis are too well known to require mentioning. On account, however, of the similarity of many of them to those of rheumatism, it is often mistaken for, and treated as, the latter disease. Although such an error is more negatively than positively harmful, it is, nevertheless, a very serious one. The treatment usually prescribed is necessarily as erroneous as the diagnosis, and, therefore, not as specifically relevant as it should be. The consequence is not only a loss of valuable time in getting control of the disease, but a corresponding prolongation of suffering on the part of the anxious and confiding patient.

The prognosis is usually favorable, except in those cases in which the parenchyma of the nerves is severely affected. This condition, according to an eminent authority, "is more properly a neural degeneration, and produces the same alterations which we have learned to be the result of nerve section."

TREATMENT.

In regard to the treatment of neuritis, it should not be forgotten that, as in all other abnormal conditions, the manifestations we are pleased to call the disease are really processes of cure—the methods employed by Nature to remove the local irritation and repair the damage its presence has caused.

Since all curative power resides in and consists of vital action, it is not the part of therapeutic wisdom to interfere with it. It is better to do nothing at all than to do anything which is opposed or contrary to the remedial plans and processes which Nature has ordained, and which she always follows.

But, although Nature is always the real physician, the medical attendant, nominally in charge, need not think there is nothing for him to do but to enact the rôle of a silent and inactive observer. The position he assumes as Nature's chief assistant is one involving both work and responsibility, and there is much he can do to assist her recuperative efforts.

In the first place, he can ferret out and remove, as far as possible, all exciting causes and make such changes in the patient's environment that he will no longer be subjected to their baneful influence. In the second place, he can minimize, if he cannot entirely control, the activity and force of the predisposing causes by the use of such hygienic measures as will establish a more perfect degree of activity of the vital functions of respiration, circulation, digestion, assimilation and elimination, thereby securing for his patient more abundant nutrition and vitality. Parenthetically, it may be stated that the more perfectly these desirable results can be accomplished, the less there will be to do in a more directly curative way, for, unless there is some impairment of one or more of the vital functions just mentioned, it is impossible for disease of any kind to exist. In the third place, he can see that only such distinctly curative measures shall be employed as are known to be in harmony with the efforts Nature is making in the same direction.

The remedies for neuritis are of two kinds: those which are merely palliative, and those which are radically curative. Palliative measures which inhibit or interfere with the orderly processes of nutrition should not be employed. Although the patient may desire them on account of their power to mitigate temporary suffering, they neither add to his vitality nor aid or accelerate the vital processes by whose action alone a cure is made possible. On the contrary, by preventing the free and rapid elimination of waste matter, already too abundant, palliative measures, of the kind referred to, actually prolong the disease, and often become the unsuspected cause of serious complications.

Happily, in these latter days so many both efficient and harmless palliatives are available that no excuse, but ignorance, can be offered for depending upon the more ancient and pernicious kinds. Besides, every remedy which is radically curative is, at the same time, palliative in the highest degree.

Among the remedies classified as curative are water, heat, cold, electricity, acupuncture and a long list of drugs. They are all of more or less service, some being used to combat symptoms which appear at one stage of the disease, others to overcome conditions which are manifested at an earlier or later period, but none is sufficiently reliable and effective to entitle it to be called a specific.

There is a remedy, however. which, simply on its merits, clearly deserves this distinction. It is adapted to and meets all the remedial requirements of every variety and stage of the disease, whether it be acute or chronic, mild or severe, and as well, also, whether the victim is otherwise strong or feeble, old or young.

Like electricity, this remedy is not new except in its completed form and more perfected methods of administration. It may be said to have been discovered in sections, because of the long intervals of time which have existed between the discovery and use of its different parts.

As the whole is greater than any of its parts, so this remedy, in its entirety, possesses much more curative virtue, both in range and intensity, than any of the factors which compose it, however valuable they may have proved to be. Physicians, therefore, and others, who have formed an opinion of its merits from the effects produced by any of its integral parts, can have no adequate conception of its remedial powers as a whole.

The name of this invaluable therapeutic agent is MOTION. One form of it, under the name of friction or rubbing, was, without question, used in an empirical way by our earliest ancestors. This variety of motion was undoubtedly the precursor of manual massage, which is now justly recognized as a superior remedy for many serious diseases, and whose methods and processes are administered, by those properly qualified, in a most scientific manner. Swedish movements comprise another remedial form of motion. These were classified and arranged upon a scientific basis by Ling in 1805 to 1812. They, also, have won recognition and favor, and have a limited but definite field of usefulness. Later, the remedial scope and power of motion has been largely augmented by the most ingenious mechanical inventions for giving massage and vibrations at rates both slower and much more rapid than those possible to the hand. Other devices, equally ingenious and effective, have also been perfected by means of which both active and passive movements may be applied, with accuracy and precision, to any desired part of the trunk or limbs.

These mechanical appliances have proved, practically, to be medical resources of great value. They not only materially lessen the labor of the masseur and medical gymnast, but produce therapeutic results impossible to be attained in any other known way.

To give those without experience a general idea of the power and relevancy of motion as a remedy, it will only be necessary to call their attention to three physiological facts. First, that vital action proceeds in the same regular and established order both in illness and in health, and from this order there can be no variation except in degree. Second, that health and even life itself depends upon the forms and kinds of motion which are exhibited by, and are a part of, the various bodily functions; and, third, that all remedies, of whatever nature, are of value only as they are able either to modify or promote these motions.

To explain what are the effects of the different forms of motion and what, according to the teachings of a large and extended clinical experience, is the best manner of using them to overcome the disease in question, will require so much space and time that it must be left for another occasion.

RESPIRATORY GYMNASTICS.

WHILE we are all agreed, says an editorial in the *Southern California Practitioner,* that the placing of the patient in the proper climate is an essential factor in the relief of certain diseases, especially tuberculosis, there is a question as to whether or not we are sufficiently impressed with the importance of instructing our patients how to properly use air so that it may be of the greatest value to them. Usually, the amount of air that is taken into the lungs is largely regulated by the amount of exercise that the subject takes. There are many patients to whom exercise, especially of an active kind, is practically forbidden, and it is particularly to this class of patients that systematic respiratory practice may be of great value. I was particularly impressed with this by an article in the International Clinics, Volume III., 1900, by Dr. Fernand La Grange, of France, from whom I take the liberty of quoting freely.

If it be true that practically three times the amount of air is taken into the lungs during an active walk that is taken into the lungs when in a recumbent position, we can readily understand how much good can be accomplished by a little instruction along this line of respiratory gymnastics. Air is practically a food to the blood. The increasing of this food, with the majority of the patients, can prove only beneficial, for, unlike forced feeding of the stomach, which may bring about disturbances of digestion, forced feeding of oxygen to the blood is invariably beneficial. It is not irrational to believe, also, that many patients, who, through a want of sufficient exercise, through want of a proper knowledge of the right way of breathing, have much dormant space in the respiratory apparatus. By proper methods

this dormant space may be utilized, and with it will come increased capacity for the reception of oxygen by the blood in the portion of lung that has been accustomed to do poor work.

Not only is the lung tissue affected by having less than the normal amount of oxygen supplied, but the general nutrition of the body is also interfered with. The increased amount of oxygen taken in by improved respiration acts, by supplying the blood with more oxygen, as a general tonic and invigorator. The anemic condition of the blood that usually accompanies tuberculosis tends to be overcome by this increased supply of oxygen, and a general invigoration of the system results.

There are many ways by which patients may be taught to amplify their respiratory movements, as, for instance, systematic breathing exercises, the use of the spirometer, singing, playing upon wind instruments, and reading aloud. The extra amount of air required for reading and speaking amounts to considerable. This is well shown by the fact that since the introduction of the phonetic method of education for deaf mutes, tuberculosis is said to have materially diminished among that class of unfortunates. As La Grange, in the article above referred to, well says, "before the phonetic method was introduced, tuberculosis among deaf mutes was particularly noticeable. It is not difficult to understand how this should become lessened when they are taught the power of vocalization, for articular speech requires much respiratory activity. The lungs must alternately fill and empty themselves with energy to produce the current of air that causes the glottis, tongue and lips to vibrate at each spoken word. In children who do not speak, this form of pulmonary exercise is totally lacking, and they fall into the habit of respiratory inertia (the lungs using only the number of cells required for breathing), so that in learning to produce articular sounds such children have the greatest difficulty in making respiratory efforts sufficiently energetic to cause the organs of phonation to vibrate. That this idiosyncrasy accounts for the predisposition of these children to tuberculosis is shown by the beneficent results derived from teaching them to speak like other people. The phonetic method enables them to make the sounds of speech which they cannot hear, but which they may read on the lips of those around them. This method not only permits these unfortunates to mingle in society, but since its introduction tuberculosis has markedly decreased among them.

Oertel's method of exercising, of course, greatly increases the respiratory power. But unfortunately many patients who have fully developed tuberculosis are practically forbidden violent exercise, because of the fatigue and possible danger of hemorrhage, in some cases, that would ensue. However, I believe there are no patients, at least among those who have a reasonable chance of recovery, who are not able to undertake systematic breathing exercises.

The simplest form of respiratory gymnastics would be to take a number of the amplest and deepest inspirations that the capacity of one's lungs will allow, and to follow each inspiration with a forced expiration to empty the lungs as completely as possible. This is, in fact, an excellent way of increasing respiratory activity, and is really the foundation of the Swedish method. All the latter does in addition is to add a certain number of movements which amplify the results to which the respiratory efforts would be restricted if the subject remained motionless while making them. There are certain movements and attitudes that facilitate breathing to which patients instinctively resort when troubled with difficulty in breathing. These are utilized by the Swedish method to give more efficacy to systematized respiratory efforts and exercise. While the patient fills his chest with air to the utmost limit, the arms are raised vertically, separated and carried backward; then during expiration they are lowered and brought forward. This is the fundamental process of which all the Swedish breathing movements are but variations; for these are based on the fact that the action of raising the arms and carrying them outward when not hindered, and especially when assisted by a simultaneous, voluntary effort of inspiration, raises the ribs upward and outward by means of the muscles which connect the thorax with the arms and shoulders. The bringing into play of these muscles, combined with the voluntary inspiratory effort, increases the expansion of the chest to its maximum. The patient who follows this method derives, in a state of complete calm, all the benefit that a patient in a crisis of dyspnea would obtain from forced breathing. In this there is a two-fold advantage: an immediate one, in that the quantity of air taken into the chest is increased, and a secondary one, in that the muscles of complemetary breathing are exercised, and thereby become better developed and more efficient.

The habit of deeper breathing has a beneficial influence, even upon the structure of the lungs, by obliging parts that are customarily inactive to take part mechanically in the act of respiration. Air cells collapsed from disuse become distended by the air which is drawn in by the vigorous inspiratory act, and regain their normal dimensions. By thus resuming active participation in the pulmonary function, the volume of the lungs diminished by disuse is increased, often with the most astonishing rapidity.

As a consequence of this modification in the volume of its contents, the chest changes in form. The ribs no longer yielding to atmospheric pressure, the chest measure increases without thickening of the walls of the thorax. This increase in the perimeter of the chest is a measure of the lung expansion.

While it is not intended to convey the idea that respiratory gymnastics will cure tuberculous patients, it nevertheless may become an adjunct of other lines of treatment, and we, as physicians, living in a climate to which many invalids wend their way, should be ever mindful of the good in this direction that can be achieved. It should be considered in the same catagory with instruction as to diet, proper clothing, exercise, and the general mode of living. The patient who leaves a cold climate and comes to California and shuts himself up in a north room, economizes in every way possible, takes little or no exercise, clothes his body with insufficient clothing, under the impression that he is in a warm climate, breathes as little air as possible, without attention of any kind directed to the benefits to be derived from systematic breathing, certainly cannot hope to show great improvement. Our advice should be concerning these things, as well as concerning the medicines that he is to use to aid in eradicating his malady.

BICYCLING: ITS INDICATIONS AND CONTRAINDICATIONS.

By means of a gasometer attached to a bicycle the air expired by the rider has been collected for analysis, and the amount of energy liberated in the course of metabolism by this form of physiological exercise has thus been estimated. L. Zuntz (*Fortschritte d. Med.*, Sept. 22, 1901) shows that a rider who covers 15 kilometers in an hour liberates ten per cent. more energy than does a pedestrian who walks 6 kilometers in the same period; if the wheelman rides 21 kilometers the energy requirement is almost twice as great as that of the 6-kilometer pedestrian. Inasmuch as bicycling involves so extraordinary a consumption of energy and is accompanied by relatively slight sensations of fatigue, its place in the treatment of obesity would seem to be theoretically established. Like all active muscular exercise bicycling diminishes the quantity of sugar in the urine in diabetes. In slight degrees of anemia bicycling is of advantage as a stimulus to metabolism; in severe cases this form of exercise makes such demands upon the

heart that it is contra-indicated. The use of the bicycle favors assimilation in chronic obstipation. Earlier literature contained frequent references to cases of inflammation of the knee-joint, said to be due to bicycling. Recently such cases have ceased to be reported, and it is probable that those originally cited related to individuals predisposed to arthritis. Faulty posture while riding no doubt leads to spinal deformity, and the danger of this result is especially to be guarded against in youthful riders. F. A. Schmidt goes so far as to advise that riding be forbidden to all children under twelve years of age. Many writers have recorded happy results from the adoption of wheeling by neurasthenics.

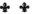

A MASSACHUSETTS IDEA WORTH COPYING.

Six years ago, when a woman who had served the town in many useful capacities died in Deerfield, Mass., her friends decided to erect a fitting memorial. And in place of a tablet or fountain or other token of small use, they conceived the idea of a Village Club Room. In *The Ladies' Home Journal* for October Mary E. Allen tells of this appropriate and novel tribute and the way it is conducted. It consists of a large room with an open fireplace, cozy window seats and low bookcases, a coat-room, a small kitchen and closets. The book shelves contain a free library of about four hundred books. A piano has been loaned and some other furniture given. A number of folding chairs and tables were bought. By means of these an audience may be seated or a supper served. The Martha Goulding Pratt Memorial is owned by a regularly incorporated body, controlled by seven trustees. A committee of twelve women is appointed to see that things are kept in order.

THE
Dietetic and Hygienic
Gazette

A Monthly Journal of Physiological Medicine

VOLUME XVII

1901

THE GAZETTE PUBLISHING COMPANY

NEW YORK

THE
DIETETIC AND HYGIENIC
GAZETTE

INDEX TO VOLUME XVII

A

Absinthe and its Effects.................... 25
Acoustic Exercises for Deaf-Mutes. Dr. V.
  Urbantsclistch 53
Acquired Tendencies, Inheritance of........ 272
Adrenalin, Clinical Experience with. Emil
  Mayer, M. D............................. 502
Advertisements, Some Sample of Ye Olden
  Time 697
Alcohol—Infection Increased by Use........ 40
Alcoholism, Treatment of Acute. Dr. J. K.
  Bauduy 56
Alcoholism; A Crime or a Disease? Dr. F.
  E. Fronczac.............................. 174
Alcoholism, Dangers of 560
Alcohol Nutrition and Inebriety............ 603
American Pork, Why Germany Bars........ 726
Americans are Growing Longer Lived....... 717
American Medicine.—ED.................... 304
American Medical Editors, The Ass'n of.... 461
American Woman's Physique. Dr. C. A. L.
  Reed 440
Amusements, The Beneficial Effects of...... 183
Among Our Exchanges.—ED................. 377
Animals, Physiological Experimentation of.
  Sir Edward Foster........................ 39
Anesthetics, Report of British Medical Asso-
  ciation's Committee on................... 634
Anopheles, Anent the. Newman W. Fynn... 419
Antiphlogistic Action of Cold, Concerning
  the. Dr. Emmert......................... 591
Antiseptics, Ozoniferous Essences as........ 235
Antisepsis, Intestinal. Dr. Chas. F. Hope... 477
Antiseptics Tested Bacteriologically......... 665
Appendicitis, Relations of Influenza and..... 227
Aphorisms, Some Medical.................. 442
Appetite and Appetites.................... 725
Apples, How to Serve...................... 729
Army Ration in the Tropics, The. Surg. J.
  R. Kean, U. S. V........................ 20

Artemus Ward, Reminiscences of.—ED...... 507
Athletics and Practical Physiology in Med-
  ical Schools. Dr. Bayard Holmes........ 50
Augean Stable, An.—ED.................... 486

B

Baboon, The Chackma...................... 64
Baking Alive 104
Baby's Diet, The.......................... 213
Banana, Food Value and Digestibility of.... 542
Bathing, Recreation After. Dr. Baruch..... 288
Barber Shops, Sanitary Rules to Govern.... 687
Beverages, Non-Alcoholic. Dr. E. M. Cos-
  grave.................................... 28
Beautiful, How to Grow, With the Years.
  Jeanette Thorpe 357
Bicycles for Physicians 691
Blood of the Martyrs, The. Brevity Club.... 253
Blind Physician, A. R. H. Babcock.......... 687
Boxer Outbreak—Was it an Attack of Hys-
  teria?.. 682
Body Coverings, The Physiology of.—ED.... 81
Body, A Plea for the Education of the. C. E.
  Ehinger, M.D... 244
Boils, Something About.................... 635
Bright's Disease, The Question of Diet in.. 85
Breathing, Deep. Dr. J. H. Pryor......... 179
Breathing, the Lost Art of. S. S. Wallian,
  A.M., M.D............................... 513
Breathe, How to 405
Brain, Do We Think with One-Half of Our? 204
Bread, A New Kind of..................... 212
Bread, White vs. Brown.................... 338
Bread, A Beauty........................... 341
Bread Supply, Population and.............. 597
Bread, Why Does It Become Mouldy?...... 665
Bread Maker, A Prize, Talks............... 666
Bronchial Diseases, Treatment of by Posture. 183
Brown Bread, Mrs. Smith's................. 668

PAGE

Butter Without Salt or Other Chemicals.... 157
Business Outlook in Med. Practice........ 312
Business Hints, Timely, for Professional Men.
　H. W. Perkins, M.D...................... 433

C

Carbolic Acid, The Revival of.............. 39
Catfish "Salmon"........................... 64
Causative or Executive.—Brevity Club....... 253
Caterer Cornered, A....................... 284
Cır Sanitation. Dr. S. H. Woodbridge..... 286
Causes, Getting at the.—Ed................. 329
Carbuncles, Some Points in their Treatment 366
Catarrh of Nose, The Treatment of Simple
　Chronic.. 367
Catarrh, Nasal............................ 743
Cancer, Progress in the Study of.......... 720
Carat, What It Weighs. W. E. Ridenour.... 636
Carbohydrates, The Dynamic Value of...... 479
Children, Aphorisms for................... 59
Cheese—Is It Wholesome?—Ed............. 209
Christian Science Miracle, The Recent...... 282
Chlorosis.. 455
Children, American 473
Character, The Effect of Diet on........... 727
Civilization, Bathing and 549
Climate, Therapeutic Value of. 1st paper. Ed. 289
　"　　　"　　　"　"　2d　"　"　353
　"　　　"　　　"　"　3d　"　"　423
　"　　　"　　　"　"　4th　"　"　481
　"　　　"　　　"　"　5th　"　"　609
　"　　　"　　　"　"　6th　"　"　737
Clergy, The, and the Doctors 602
Cleanliness Without Soap.................. 619
Clubs, A Word About.—Brevity Club....... 571
Colds 601
Cold-Catching. Prof. Flint................. 688
Consumption, Treatment of, in England.... 286
Consumptives, Directions to 106
Consumptives, State Sanatoria for. Dr. H.
　L. Taylor............................... 295
Cocaine, The Habit of..................... 236
Cocaine Debauchery 348
Cold, Effects of, Upon the Mind........... 108
Colds, How to Avoid 185
Colds.—Editorial.......................... 594
"Come and Eat".......................... 729
Coughing as a Fine Art. Dr. G. A. Young.. 365
Cook and the Doctor, The. C. Champeaux.. 55
Cookery, Ruskin's Views on................ 159
Cooking, Old Housekeeper on.............. 596
Constipation.. 84
Corns, Cure of, on Sole of Foot............ 107
Cocoa, Its Proper Preparation............. 151
Color Nut for Psychics to Crack.......... 158
Colors and the Mind....................... 223
Complexion, Methods of Improving the..... 238
Colorado Desert, Redeeming the........... 467

PAGE

Cooling the Air, Devices for................ 560
Cousins, Should They Marry?.............. 595
Consumption, Another New Cure for. Dr.
　W. G. Fralick 748
Corpulent, More Advice to the.—Ed 721
Cremation and Crime...................... 621
Cremation in England...................... 676
Cremation.. 350
Crematorium, First Municipal, in Great
　Britain 234
Curvature, Spinal, from Wrong Sitting Posi-
　tions.. 312
Cyclist, Hygiene of the 184

D

Dailies, A New Code for................... 631
Daily Exercise, Some Reasons for.......... 182
Death, Hour of. Dr. Pilgrim.............. 287
Death, Occupations which Hasten 712
Death Rate in the State of New York...... 238
Dental Caries as a Factor of Disease....... 158
Development, Symmetrical 177
Die Rich, Die Disgraced. Andrew Carnegie.. 58
Diet, Some Current Absurdities in.......... 276
Diet, A Harvard Student's................. 59
Diet, Vegetable........................... 95
Diet, Medical Press on.—Ed................ 147
Diets for Every-Day Use. J. Warren
　Achorn, M.D.
　　Diet in Constipation 13
　"　"　Dyspepsia 77
　"　"　Biliousness 141
　"　"　Bright's Disease 206
　"　"　Heart Disease 269
　"　"　Bronchitis 333
　"　"　Eczema 457
　"　"　Rheumatism 521
　"　"　Obesity 653
Dieting to Reduce Flesh................... 410
Dietary. Dr. Thomas...................... 489
Dietetic Dunce, The.—Ed.................. 401
Dietetics, Scientific. Dr. J. J. Black......... 29
　"　　Purpose of...................... 86
Disease, Flies as Disseminators of.......... 463
Disease, The Origin of..................... 41
Diversion, Ethics and the Doctor.—Ed....... 417
Disorders, Nervous 469
Digestive Ferments, Digestion and the. C.
　W. Canan, M.D........................... 478
Dish Washing............................. 489
Disinfection, Intestinal. Prof. Loebisch..... 657
Diabetes Mellitus, The Dietetic and Medicinal
　Treatment of. R. B. Glass, M.D......... 44
Diabetes Mellitus, Its Etiology and Treat-
　ment. A. B. Williams, M.D............. 165
Diabetes, Dietetic Treatment of. Dr. N. P.
　Davis, Jr................................ 80
Diacetic Acid Diet and Diabetes. Chas. Platt,
　M.D.................................... 257

PAGE

Doctors, Proportion Among Men of Genius 408
Dog, Senator Vest's Tribute to the.......... 732
Domestic Medicine—Doctors, Druggists, and.
  —ED.................................... 97
Dosimetric System 730
Dreams, What Are? 552
Drinking Water—Examination of, in Ill.... 37
Dysmenorrhea, The Treatment of.......... 749

E

Eating, The Philosophy of. Gladstone...... 671
Early School Life, Some Considerations Re-
  garding the Hygiene of................... 491
Editors, Doctors, and..................... 120
Eggs, The Chemistry and Dietetic Value of.
  Dr. E. V. Parrott....................... 392
Eggs, The Uses of........................ 413
Electricity, Nerve Force and.............. 437
Elementary Gases of Our Atmosphere, The
  Newly Discovered. Theodore W. Schaefer,
  M.D...................................... 65
Emotions, The Value of Healthy.......... 437
Energy, Intelligent Direction of.......... 346
Enzyms, The 538
Eutrapelia and Eutrapellous 734
Epileptics, The Care of................... 731
Euformol, The Germicidal and Deodorant
  Properties of. Thomas Maben, F. C. S.... 103
Evil, The Problem of...................... 336
Exertion 180
Exercise, Dr. Germain See on............. 311
Exaggeration, Value of 615
Eve, Expressions of the................... 733

F

Family Doctor, Must the, Go?............. 297
Fats, How Nature Burns Up the........... 663
Fasting, the Hygiene of 668
Feeding the Sick, Practical Points On. Dr.
  E. A. Irwin.............................. 67
Feeding, Infant. Joseph E. Winters, M.D... 430
Feeding, Infant 540
Feeding According to Climate. Dr. L. L.
  Seaman 504
Fermentation by Yeast 220
Fire, That Kindles Power, the............. 54
Filter, A Cheap Home Made................ 495
Flora of the Human Body, The, and the Evils
  of the Large Intestine. E. Metchnikoff.... 725
Food of Mixed Diet, The Availability of the
  Different Classes of Nutrients in. U. S. Ex.
  Station Reports 82
Foods, Notes on 149
Food Preservatives 154
  " Before Sleep. Dr. Cathell........... 155
Foods, Nutritive Value of Certain........ 155
Food Economy, Are the Teachings of Science
  Regarding, Practical? A. P. Bryant....... 198

PAGE

Food, Clean.. 280
  " Adulteration 405
Foods, The Evolution of.—ED.............. 414
Food as a Factor in the Causation of Disease.
  Dr. Elmer Lee........................... 420
Food Before Sleep 466
  " Alum in 535
  " Powdering to Keep It................. 669
Food, A New Source of.—ED.............. 728
  " Preservatives and Their Effects. H. E.
  Barnard 723
Formaldehyd in Milk....................... 22
Forestry and Its Relation to Health........ 496
Fruits, Medical Uses of................... 92
  " Food Value of........................ 94
  " Medical Uses of 340
Fruit Breakfasts.. 425
Frozen Meats, How They Deteriorate....... 221
Fractures, Process of Healing in. Baldo
  Rossi 629
Frogs, Something About.................... 718
Funerals, Druggists Prevent................ 633

G

Gastric Affections, Olive Oil. Dr. Cohnheim. 17
Gastric Ulcer, The Prophylaxis of........ 108
Gastralgia, Nature and Treatment of. Mos-
  turo Jones, M.D.......................... 237
Glands, The Digestive 152
Gould, Dr. and the Phila. Med. Journal.—ED. 189
Gout and Rheumatism, Nature's Alkaline
  Treatment of. Dr. C. H. Brandt.......... 229
Gout, Strawberries and.................... 280
Gowns, Ella Wheeler Wilcox's............. 313
Gold Coin Supplanting Paper............... 426
Grape Cure, The 240
Grippe, Statistics of in N. Y. State.......... 366
Greater New York, The Birth Rate of....... 749
Gymnastic Training, Purpose of New Rational
  Educational System.. 306
Gymnastic Training in New Jersey State Nor-
  mal College. H. B. Boice, M.D........... 497
Gymnastics, Respiratory 756

H

Half Truths and Humdrum in the Field of
  Hygiene.—ED.... 34
Hands, Disinfection by Means of Essences... 48
Ham, Sir Henry Thompson's Method of
  Cooking 471
Happiness.. 93
  " The Problem of 585
Hair, Heads Without.—ED................. 145
Handkerchief, Hygiene of the.............. 163
Hand, Concerning the..................... 688
Health and Longevity, The Essentials of. W.
  G. Kemper, M.D........................... 1
Health, A Birth-right and How to Maintain
  It. Alexander Wilder, M.D............... 76

PAGE

Health, Economics of. Alexander Wilder, M.D......... 259
Health and Repose........................... 346
Health Hints. Brevity Club................... 506
Health Resorts and Country Houses, The Sanitation of 556
Headache, Causes of 281
Heat, Employment of, as a Therapeutic and Diagnostic Measure.. 435
Heat, Some Therapeutic Values of. C. S. Hutchison, M.Sc., M.D.................. 741
High Altitudes, The Hygiene of............ 208
Hints, Useful.. 623
Hot Air as a Therapeutic Agent. O. S. Wightman................................ 685
Hot Air Treatment.—ED................... 740
Hot Air Cure............................... 470
Hot Water, The Therapeutical Drinking of— Its Use and Origin. Ephraim Cutter, M.D., LL.D................................ 69
Hotel and Restaurant Cooking, Dreary Monotony of 544
House Work as Exercise................... 692
House-cleaning, Spring. Dr. H. Bashore.... 139
How Nature Cures.......................... 110
Honey, Medicinal Value of................. 112
Human Eye, The, and How to Care for It. Dr. Reik 54
Human System, Foreign Bodies in the...... 618
Human Species, To Regenerate the......... 686
Hygiene, Public—State Medicine. R. H. Harrison, M.D............................. 673
Hygiene, Personal, in Diseases of the Nose and Throat 299
Hygienic and Physical Condition of Slums, to Improve the 622
Hypnotic Criminal Suggestion, Epidemic.... 685
Hysteria, The Old Way or the New of Treating It? D. L. Stocking, M.D.............. 438
Hyperemia, Artificially Produced, as a Therapeutic Measure. Prof. Bier............. 398
Hydrogen Dioxid as a Local Anæsthetic. Dr. H. E. Kendall.......................... 48
Hydrogen Dioxid, On the Proper Use of. Dr. R. S. Morris............................. 617

Idleness, Organized 376
Imagination, Choked by.................... 121
Immunes, A Race of....................... 156
Immunity 175
Insomnia, Tea and Coffee as Causes of...... 156
Inebriety, The Curability of by Med. Treatment. Dr. T. D. Crothers................ 56
Infant Feeding, Whey Cream, Modifications in.. 212
Infants, Feeding of in Health and Disease... 214
Individual Resistance in Disease............ 43
Iodism, A Corrector of... 747

K

Karnice, The 438

L

PAGE

Left Hand, Educating the. Prof. MacDonald 692
Light as a Therapeutic Agent.—ED.......... 719
Littleness of Soul vs. Littleness of Fortune.. 620
Longevity, A New Era of.................. 667
"   Athleticism and 692

M

"Malaria." Brevity Club.................... 378
"   Stamping Out in Italy. Prof. Grassi................................. 47
Man, Masquerading as a.................... 475
"   The Future. Prof. McGee.......... 559
"   Parthenogenerated, The ....
Mania, The Hygiene of. Dr. Antoimie...... 46
"   Nostrum 374
Marriage, Talk of.......................... 372
"   Harmonizing Temper in......... 693
Married Life and Long Life................ 372
Marcus Aurelius Antoninus, Wisdom of..... 315
Massage, General. Haldor Sneve, M.D..... 308
Massage, Brush. F. B. Fry................ 371
"   In Japan. Dr. X. C. Wood......... 51
"   A Scientific Therapeutic Measure... 180
Medicine, Mathematics in.................. 474
"   Preventive.... 119
Medication, Non-Alcoholic. M. S. Whetstone, M.D............................... 4
Medical Profession, Why is it Traduced?— ED...................................... 225
Medical Practice, The Future of............ 678
Medical Journalism, Crying Needs of....... 627
Mere Mention.............................. 436
Methods to Increase Birth-rate, French..... 490
Meat, Value of, in the Prevention and Treatment of Pulmonary Tuberculosis. F. Parks Weaver 96
Milk Secretion, The Influence of Food Upon. Dr. Temesvary 19
Milk, Modification of .....·.............. 156
Milk, Clean.. 493
Milk, Preparation of for Infant Feeding. S. Stzekely.................................. 629
Milk, A New Food Made from.............. 670
Milk, Noiseless.. 95
Mind, Physical Basis of. B. F. Beebe, M.D.. 9
Miles and Meals.—ED...................... 400
Microbes, Among the...................... 171
Mixed Diet, The Advantages of. Dr. Cosgrave.................................... 24
Mosquitoes, The Predatory................. 60
Mosquito Bites, Sulphur as a Preventive of.. 120
Mosquitoes, The Fight Against............. 589
Mouth, Breathing and its Relation to Diseases of the Throat, Nose. etc. Dr. Mayo Collier 52
Mouth, Acidity of the, During Sleep........ 95
Modern Education, Effect of on Children. U. M. D'A. Cahart, M.D.................. 52

PAGE

Morgan, J. Pierpont......................... 697
Monarchs. Why They Were Insane.......... 735
Mushrooms as Food. Dr. Andrew Wilson... 216
Muscular Exertion, Effects of Sudden and
　Prolonged in Young Adolescents......... 369
Music, Mysterious. Prof. Tyndall.......... 735

N

Nausea, To Cure............................ 75
Nature, Aiding. A. D. McComachie, M.D... 135
　"　As a Doctor...................... 406
Nation, The Blood of the................... 630
Napoleon's Tomb at Paris................... 622
Neurasthenia and Melancholia, The Toxic
　Origin of. Dr. M. A. Starr............... 524
Neuritis and its Radical Treatment, Notes on.
　G. H. Patchen, M.D...................... 753
Next!—Ed.................................. 273
Nitrous Acid in Water, Demonstration of by
　Erdmann's Method. Dr. H. Mennicke.... 233
Nineteenth Century, The Surgeon of the. F.
　Treves, F.R.C.S.......................... 394
Nose, Hygiene of.—Ed...................... 744
Normal Body Temperature, How Maintained
　in Cold Weather 73

O

Oatmeal, Cooking.—Ed..................... 534
Obesity, Therapeutics and Hygiene of....... 187
Obesity, Treatment of by Massage.......... 305
Obesity, "Hypurgie" of.—Ed................ 427
Octogenarian. A Well Preserved........... 406
Old Age, The Dread of.................... 113
One Hundred and Five Years Old........... 605
One Hundred Years, How to Live. Bernard
　Morris.................................. 681
Opium Narcosis. 590
Opportunity, A Waiting.—Ed............... 529
Organs, Regeneration of 156
Ounce of Prevention, The.—Ed............ 33
Over-fat, Some Advice for the. Dr. Strebel.. 479
Over-fat, A Word to the.—Ed.............. 593
Oxalic Acid in Urine, The Source of. Dr.
　Lommel................................ 18
Oxygen, Value of in Cardiac Lesions. B. C.. 124
Oysters and Disease.................. 27, 169

P

Pan-American, On the.—Ed................ 614
Patients. Over-talk to. B. C................ 638
Parrot, A Carnivorous....................... 671
Pasteur 734
Paris Cook, Art of the 91
Parthenogenesis........................... 338
Perfumes, Artificial 204

PAGE

People, Dangerous Class of................ 235
Perspiration, Does it Increase Elimination?
　G. H. Patchen, M.D..................... 577
Peril, A Public 631
Physiology, Huxley on.................... 592
Physicians, The Mortality and Morbidity of.. 111
Physicians' Strikes 415
Physician Who Advertises, The........... 459
Physical Training—The Fundamental Part of
　Universal Education. W. W. Hastings.... 49
Phthisical Patients, The Sweat of.......... 111
Physical Culture 114
Physical Education, The Elements of Pleas-
　ure in 173
Physical Education, The Hope of the Nation. 242
Physical Education, Ideals in.............. 562
Physical Development. Dr. A. H. Kinnicutt.. 370
Philosophy, Anti-malarial 303
Physiologic, Chemic Literature, Gleanings
　from Recent.—Ed....................... 465
Phthisis, Is Wetness of Soil a Cause of?.... 227
Pine Needle Oil.......................... 476
Pithy Paragraphs 698
Posture, Sleeping. Mrs. E. L. Sessions...... 50
Position of the Head in Sleep, The......... 205
Poisoning, Sausage 624
Population, Future Increase of Our......... 679
Population Statistics, The Latest........... 748
Polypharmacy With a Vengeance. G. T.
　Welch, M.D............................. 518
Progress in Med. and Surg., A Century's. S.
　S. Wallian, A.M., M.D.................. 129
Profession and the People, Want of Touch
　Between.—Ed.......................... 293
Prospects, Medical. Dr. G. E. Francis...... 527
President McKinley's Case, Was it Badly
　Managed?—Ed.......................... 625
Protest, Let Us All....................... 695
Prophylaxis in Malaria. Dr. Manson....... 632
Promotion, A Well-earned.—Ed............ 462
Pulex Irritans, M.D. A. G. Kemper....... 699
Pure Butter Law, Cannot Enforce. State
　Board of Health........................ 48

Q

Question, A Cold 347
Quinine 460

R

Raw Milk, A Plea for. Dr. Louis Fischer.... 211
　"　"　Feeding. The Disadvantages of.
　Louis Fischer, M.D..................... 18
Rabies, Pasteur Treatment of.............. 472
Readers, A Word With Our.—Ed........... 241
Remedies, What Are?—Ed................. 545
Republic, The George Junior.............. 695

PAGE

Remittent Malarial and Yellow Fever, A Few
   Remarks on the Diagnosis of. I. P. Agos-
   tini, A. A. Surg., U. S. A................ 99
Rheumatism, Concerning the Treatment of.
   Dr. W. T. Parker........................ 363
Rheumatism—What It Really Is...:........ 409
Rheumatism, The Microbes of............. 412
Rhus................................... 373
Right of Way. Physicians Have the........ 488
Roosevelt, Theodore 696
Rubeola and Rubella 745

                        S

Saint Bernard, The Genuine................ 403
Saleratus and Cream of Tartar............. 402
Sanitary Science, Hygiene and............. 495
Sanitation and the Motorists.............. 105
Sanitation, The Effect of More Efficient...... 716
Sciatica, Diet in Treatment of. Dr. A. P.
   Williamson.............................. 80
Schools, Vacation. E. C. Putnam, A.B., M.D. 116
School Rooms, Unhealthy 185
School Children, Med. Supervision of....... 395
School Children, The Preservation of the
   Teeth of 558
School Hygiene, Suggestions Regarding a
   Dept. of. L. K. Baker................... 626
Science Between the Acts................... 364
Scientists, The Recreations of............. 604
Scientific Work, Concentration in.......... 621
Scientists, Women as 672
Scales, Thermometric 746
Sea Sickness............................. 683
   "   "   "Eucalyptus Rostrata" in....... 236
Sea Sickness, Some Suggestions on. D. R.
   Brower, M.D., LL.D...................... 455
Services, Doctor May Refuse 375
Sensibility to Pain, Measure of............ 500
Sight, The Training of the. M. Brudenell
   Carter................................. 53
Skin, General Care of..................... 123
   "   "   "   " ......:......... 360
Sleep, Artificial—A Special Process for Pro-
   ducing 428
Sleep, Healthy 469
   " Positions that Affect. Dr. Granville... 239
   " Why Do We?......................... 552
   " and Its Relations to Health and Dis-
      ease. H. E. Peckham, A.B........... 647
Sleep and its Relations to Health and Dis-
   ease, concluded. H. E. Peckham, A.B..... 647
Smallpox in the U. S...................... 303
Smallpox, Diagnosis of the................ 362
   "   A Preventable Disease........... 430
Snake-bite. Dr. McFarland................. 352
Solidified Air 403
Sound, Transmission of 592
Specific Gravity, Corporeal 618
Splints, Home-made. Dr. Thompson Baird.. 374

PAGE

Spending, The Science of.................. 376
Spinsters, A Paradise of. C. D. Wright..... 431
Spleen—The Rôle in the Pancreatic Digestion
   of Proteids. Dr. H. F. Bellamy.......... 20
Span of Life—Is It True that It Is Lengthen-
   ing? 55
Spitting Nuisance, The—In Public Convey-
   ances.—ED.............................. 161
Sprains, Massage in 179
Spitting Nuisance, The Public 235
Sterilizing and Pasteurizing Milk, Advantages
   and Limitations of. Dr. Blackader........ 37
Sterilized Milk, Advantages of. Dr. A. D.
   Blackader.............................. 153
Stomach, Some Plain Talk About the. C. F.
   Ulrich, A.M., M.D...................... 195
Stomach, Massage of the. Gustaf Nortrom.. 242
Staple Foods, Carelessness in the Interdiction
   of 537
Standards, Advancing the. Prof. G. D.
   Somers................................. 561
Stones, Sticks, Etc., Why Do Dogs Swallow? 671
Stimulation, Delusive. Dr. T. L. Brunton... 628
Stammering 232
Summer Diarrhœa of Infants, The Hygienic
   Treatment of. H. C. Hazen, M.D........ 501
Summer Diarrhœa of Infants and Children—
   After Treatment of..................... 550
Summer, What to Eat in................... 541
Suggestive Infection, Case of.............. 407
Sunlight or Sleep for Children?............ 426
Sunlight, Tesla's New 349
Sucramine, A New Sweetening Agent. M. J.
   Bellier................................ 543
Summer Clothing, Selection of............. 556
Sugar and the Doctor 339
   " Dietetic Value of.................... 344
Sword, Song of the....................... 371

                        T

Table Talk. F. S. Rook................... 278
Table Drinking........................... 599
Taking Cold 719
Tea, The Influence of, on Digestion. Dr. J.
   W. Fraser.............................. 94
Tea, Rubbish 343
Tea and Coffee Two Hundred Years Ago... 669
Teeth of School Children, The Preservation
   of 110
Teeth of the Nation, The................. 123
   "   Bleaching 144
   " Care of. Dr. Richter................ 159
Tears, The Chemistry of................... 220
Tendency, Anti Drug...................... 694
Therapeutics, Mental 689
Thirst, Fruit for 727
Thought, Education and Liberal............ 404
Thought, Money Cannot Organize.......... 404
Thoughts Are Things. Ella Wheeler Wilcox. 637
Toad—Erroneous Notions About............ 462
Tobacco—The Use of on Active Service.... 38

PAGE

Tobacco Heart, The........................ 279
Tongue, The, in Health and Disease. Dr.
  J. Muller................................. 140
Topics of the Times. Dr. Wyman.......... 226
Tropics, Meat Ration in the. Dr. Egan, Surg.,
  U. S. A.................................. 274
Truths, Ten Hygienic. Dr. F. H. Hamilton... 635
Tuberculosis. Food in. Mitchell Bruce...... 19
  "   British Congress on 173
Tuberculosis, The Nature. Treatment of..... 176
Tuberculous Joints, Sun Baths in Treatment
  of.. 281
Tuberculosis, Fresh Air and................. 298
Tuberculosis, Progress in the Sanatorium
  Treatment of............................. 328
Tuberculosis, Home Treatment of. Dr. L. F.
  Flick..................................... 365
Tuberculosis, Human and Bovine............ 748
Tuberculosis, Concerning Bovine. Dr. G. M.
  Edwards.................................. 548
Tuberculosis, The Klopfen Treatment of..... 750
Tub Bath, The Sacrosanct.................... 463
Typhoid Fever, Feeding in. F. L. Keays.... 17
  "   "   "   Dr. G. W. More-
  house..................................... 43
Typhoid Fever, Exclusive Soup Diet and Rec-
  tal Irrigations in. Dr. A. Siebert.......... 57
Typhoid Fever, Some Practical Methods of
  Bathing in. Dr. S. Baruch............... 239
Typhoid Fever, Dietetic Management of.... 658
Twentieth Century, The Physician in the. Dr.
  A. H. Smith.............................. 100

U

Ugliness that Costs Money.................. 494
Unborn, Hospital for the................... 283
Unfermented Grape Juice, Preparation of.... 21
Unsterilized Cows' Milk, Feeding the Infants'
  of the Poor with.......................... 222

V

Vegetarianism and Insanity.—ED....... 210, 536
  "   Tesla on.. 604
  "   J. D. Craig 728
  "   Views on 539
Vegetables as Medicine 343
Vital Force, Nature of..................... 594
Voices, Judged by Their................... 375

W

Wash, The Best 744
Waste in the Kitchen...................... 543
Water Purification, Extemporaneous Methods
  of 48
Water. Dr. C. S. Dremsen................. 71
  "   Drinking 88
  "   Brevity Club.................... 190
Water Bath, Tepid, Hebra's Continuous.... 675
Water Purified 172
What Really Educates a Child.............. 736

PAGE

Whey Cream Modifications in Infant Feed-
  ing.. 212
Whiskey and Tobacco, Injurious Substance
  in 667
Wheel, The Hygiene of the................ 567
Why Don't I Get Well? Dr. S. F. Meacham. 217
Wife, The Best for a Doctor.............. 693
Window, The Open........................ 557
Work. Elbert Hubbard 638

Y

Yeast, What Is? 23
Yellow Fever, The Etiology of. Surgeons
  Reed and Agramonte, U. S. A............ 492
Yew, Lethal Effect of 626
Youth and Years.—ED..................... 337

On the Editor's Table......... 445, 510, 574, 701

Notes and Queries: 61, 62, 63, 127, 191, 255,
  ....318, 384, 447, 511, 575, 639, 703

Editorials:
  "American Medicine" 304
  Artemus Ward, A Reminiscence of........ 507
  Augean Stable, An....................... 486
  Awards at the Pan-American ....
  Body Coverings, The Physiology of....... 81
  Causes, Getting at the................... 329
  Cheese, Is It Wholesome?................ 209
  Climate, Therapeutic Value of—1st paper.. 289
    "   "   "   " —2nd " .. 353
    "   "   "   " —3rd " .. 423
    "   "   "   " —4th " .. 481
    "   "   "   " —5th " .. 609
    "   "   "   " —6th " .. 737
  Colds 594
  Corpulent, More Advice to the........... 721
  Dietetic Dunce, The...................... 401
  Diet, Med. Press on..................... 147
  Diversion, Ethics and the Doctor......... 417
  Doctors, Druggists and Domestic Med..... 97
  Food, A New Source of................. 728
  Foods, the Evolution of.................. 414
  Gould, Dr., and The Phil. Med. Jour..... 189
  Hair, Heads Without..................... 145
  Half Truths and Humdrum in the Field
    of Hygiene 34
  Hot Air Treatment....................... 740
  Light as a Therapeutic Agent............. 719
  Legislature, The N. Y. and the Pseudo-
    paths 241
  Med. Profession, Why Is It Traduced?.... 225
  Miles and Meals 400
  Next ! 273
  Nose, Hygiene of 744
  Oatmeal, Cooking 534
  Opportunity, A Waiting.................. 529

PAGE

Ounce of Prevention, The................ 33
Over Fat, A Word to the................ 593
Pan-American, Lesson of the............ 614
Physiologic-Chemic Literature, Gleanings
  from Recent 465
Profession and the People, Want of Touch
  Between 293
Profession, A Smirched ....
Promotion, A Well Earned............... 462
President McKinley's Case—Was It Badly
  Managed? 625
Readers, A Word With Our............. 241
Remedies, What Are? 545
Spitting Nuisance in Public Conveyances,
  The 161
Vegetarianism and Insanity.............. 210
Youth and Years 337

Book Reviews:

Cook for the Sick and Invalids, How to.
  Helena V. Sachse 508
Cocoa, Peru, History of. W. G. Mortimer,
  M.D....... 700
Education, New Methods in. J. L. Todd.. 751
Food and the Principles of Dietetics. Rob-
  ert Hutchison, M.D................... 444
Hypnotism 316
Infant Feeding in Health and Disease.
  Louis Fischer, M.D.................... 382
Medicine and Surgery, American Year
  Book of for 1901..................... 252
Physiologic Therapeutics, A System of,
  Vol. I. S. S. Cohen, A.M., M.D........ 750
Physiologic Therapeutics, A System of,
  Vol. II. S. S. Cohen, A.M., M.D....... 508
Physicians' Visiting List, 1902. P. Blakis-
  ton Sons & Co........................ 752

PAGE

Pocket Formulary, Medical News. E. I.
  Thornton, M.D......................... 383
Progressive Medicine, Vol. I, 1901. H. H.
  Hare, M.D............................. 316
Progressive Medicine, Vol. II, June, 1901.
  H. H. Hare, M.D...................... 509
Progressive Medicine, Vol. III., 1901. H.
  H. Hare, M.D......................... 700
Progressive Medicine, Vol. IV., December,
  1900. H. H. Hare, M.D................ 126
Practical Medicine, Analytical Encyclo-
  pedia of. C. de M. Sajous, M.D........ 574
Respiratory Organs, Diseases of the, Acute
  and Chronic. William F. Waugh, A.M.,
  M.D....... 508
Twenty-first Annual Report of the State
  Board of Health in the State of Rhode
  Island 382
Woman, Beautiful, The. Ella A. Fletcher.
  Brentano's, 1901...................... 751

Brevity Club:

Blood of the Martyrs, The.............. 253
Bread to Eat, What Shall We Do for?..... 702
Causative or Executive? 253
Clubs, A Word About................... 571
Fight for Life, The 506
Health Hints 506
History of the Club and Proceedings of,
  First Meeting 124
In Re the Brevity Club................. 317
"In Re," Another 378
Maiden Effort, A New Member's......... 442
Malaria 378
Overtalk to Patients 638
Oxygen, Value of in Cardiac Lesions.... 124
Water 190

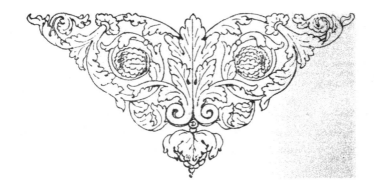

Lightning Source UK Ltd.
Milton Keynes UK
UKHW02n1239130218
317658UK00004B/211/P